The Mind's Machine
Foundations of Brain and Behavior
FOURTH EDITION

The Mind's Machine
Foundations of Brain and Behavior

FOURTH EDITION

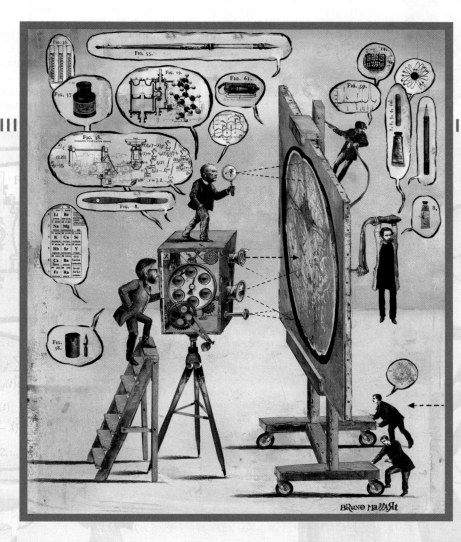

Neil V. Watson • S. Marc Breedlove

Simon Fraser University   *Michigan State University*

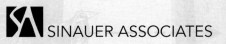 SINAUER ASSOCIATES

NEW YORK   OXFORD
OXFORD UNIVERSITY PRESS

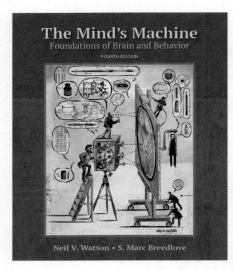

About the Cover and Chapter Opener Images

Bruno Mallart is one of the most talented European artists, his work having appeared in some of the world's premier publications: The New York Times, The Wall Street Journal, and the New Scientist, to name a few. A freelance illustrator since 1986, Mallart first worked for several children's book publishers and advertising agencies, using a classical realistic watercolor and ink style. Some years later he began working in a more imaginative way, inventing a mix of drawing, painting, and collage. His work speaks of a surrealistic and absurd world and engages the viewer's imagination and sense of fun. Despite the recurring use of the brain in his art, Mallart's background is not scientific—though his parents were both neurobiologists. He uses the brain as a symbol for abstract concepts such as intelligence, thinking, feeling, ideas, and knowledge. Attracted to all that is mechanical, Mallart's art frequently includes machine parts such as gears and wheels that imply movement and rhythm. These features together, in their abstract representation, beautifully illustrate the topics discussed in The Mind's Machine, Fourth Edition, and even include a glimpse of Neil and Marc at work. To see more of Bruno Mallart's art, please go to his website: www.brunomallart.com.

Eye icon © donets/123RF

Oxford University Press is a department of the University of Oxford. It furthers the University's objective of excellence in research, scholarship, and education by publishing worldwide. Oxford is a registered trade mark of Oxford University Press in the UK and certain other countries.

Published in the United States of America by Oxford University Press
198 Madison Avenue, New York, NY 10016, United States of America

Address editorial correspondence to:

Sinauer Associates
23 Plumtree Road
Sunderland, MA 01375 U.S.A.

Address orders, sales, license, permissions, and translation inquiries to:

Oxford University Press U.S.A.
2001 Evans Road
Cary, NC 27513 U.S.A.
Orders: 1-800-445-9714

ACCESSIBLE CONTENT   Every opportunity has been taken to ensure that the content herein is fully accessible to those who have difficulty perceiving color. However, some of these Figures and activities will be less accessible to some readers due to the intrinsic nature of the colors and activities.

Library of Congress Cataloging-in-Publication Data

Names: Watson, Neil V. (Neil Verne), 1962- author. | Breedlove, S. Marc, author.

Title: The mind's machine : foundations of brain and behavior / Neil V. Watson, Simon Fraser University, S. Marc Breedlove, Michigan State University.

Description: Fourth edition. | New York, NY : Sinauer Associates/Oxford University Press, 2021. | Includes bibliographical references and index. | Summary: "The Mind's Machine, introduced in 2012, was written to present the interdisciplinary topics of introductory behavioral neuroscience to students from non-science majors, to psychology, life sciences, and neuroscience. This engaging and user-friendly text brings in relevance to students of all backgrounds through coverage of contemporary research, clinical cases and experimental studies, as well as through the use of clear learning objectives and concept checks, and Acrobatiq courseware for adaptive learning integrated with interactive learning tools"-- Provided by publisher.

Identifiers: LCCN 2020030747 (print) | LCCN 2020030748 (ebook) | ISBN 9781605359731 (paperback) | ISBN 9780197542248 (epub)

Subjects: LCSH: Brain--Textbooks. | Brain--Physiology--Textbooks. | Human behavior--Physiological aspects--Textbooks. | Psychobiology--Textbooks. | Neurophysiology--Textbooks. | Neuropsychology--Textbooks.

Classification: LCC QP376 .W26 2021 (print) | LCC QP376 (ebook) | DDC 612.8/2--dc23

LC record available at https://lccn.loc.gov/2020030747

LC ebook record available at https://lccn.loc.gov/2020030748

9 8 7 6 5 4 3 2 1
Printed in the United States of America

For Kathaleen Emerson and Sydney Carroll,
with affection and appreciation for their sharp eyes, calm nerves, and warm friendship.
Their fingerprints—and red pencil marks—are all over our books.

N. V. W.   S. M. B.

Brief Contents

Table of Contents

2 Neurophysiology The Generation, Transmission, and Integration of Neural Signals 54

3 The Chemistry of Behavior Neurotransmitters and Neuropharmacology 82

4 Development of the Brain   120

5 The Sensorimotor System   142

6   Hearing, Balance, Taste, and Smell   176

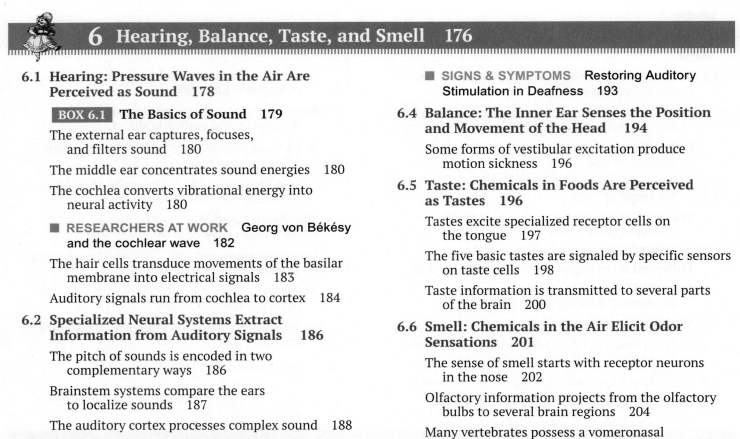

7   Vision   From Eye to Brain   210

8 Hormones and Sex 244

9 Homeostasis Active Regulation of the Internal Environment   290

10 Biological Rhythms and Sleep   316

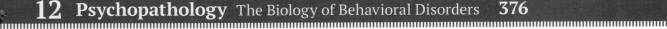

Preface

Who has not pondered their own consciousness, marveled at their many sensory experiences, or wondered how a small and lumpy organ can process so much information? Neuroscience boils down to the mind studying its own machine, an intrinsically fascinating topic that seems to fill every media channel nowadays. But another reason neuroscience is in the news so frequently is simply that it has become one of the most active branches of science. The pace of discoveries about brain and behavior has increased at an exponential rate over the last few decades, and continues to accelerate.

Every new edition of one of our books requires substantial updating because so much is happening all the time. (It's exciting, but wow, do we read a lot of reports and articles!) In fact, by far the hardest part of our job as authors lies in deciding which discoveries to include and which to (reluctantly) leave out: As the Red Queen remarked to Alice in Wonderland, "it takes all the running you can do, to keep in the same place." Our neuroscience news website (oup.com/he/watson-breedlove4e/news) boasts a collection of more than 25,000 news stories, drawn from the mainstream media, relating to the topics of this book. You can follow updates on the website, via email, or Facebook (www.facebook.com/BehavioralNeuroscience).

While we are sampling from this almost boundless scientific smorgasbord, we have to watch our weight. Our goal for *The Mind's Machine*, Fourth Edition is to introduce you to the basics of behavioral neuroscience in a way that focuses on the foundational topics in the field—with a generous sprinkling of the newest and most fascinating discoveries—and leaves you with an appetite for more. Whether you are beginning a program of study centered on the brain and behavior, or are just adding some breadth to your education, you will find that behavioral neuroscience now permeates all aspects of modern psychology, along with related life sciences like physiology, biology, and the health sciences. But that's not all. The tools and techniques of behavioral neuroscience also create new ways of looking at questions in many other areas, such as economics, the performing arts, anthropology, sociology, computer science, and engineering. Researchers are beginning to probe mental processes that seemed impenetrable only a decade or two ago: the neural bases of decision making, love and attachment, memory and learning, consciousness, and much of what we call the mind. Our aim in *The Mind's Machine*, Fourth Edition is to provide a foundation that places these and other important topics in a unified scientific context, delivered in clear, inclusive, and gender-neutral language.

We've found that students enrolled in our courses have diverse academic backgrounds and personal interests. In this book, we've tried to avoid making too many assumptions about our readers, and have focused on providing both behavioral and biological perspectives on major topics. If you've had some high-school level biology you should have no trouble with most of the material in the book.

For those readers who have more experience in science—or who want more detail—we have peppered the chapters with embedded links to more advanced material located in Oxford Learning Link. These links, called *A Step Further*, are just one of several novel features we have included to aid your learning. Throughout the book you will find web links that will connect you to animated versions of many figures, video clips, and more.

Each chapter also features at least one segment called *Researchers at Work*, which illustrates the nuts and bolts of experimentation through real-world examples, and a segment called *Signs & Symptoms* that relates a real-world clinical issue relevant to the chapter topic. To help you gauge your progress, each chapter is divided into several major topics bracketed by features called *The Road Ahead*, specifying your learning objectives for the material that follows, and *How's It Going?*, providing self-test conceptual questions. Every chapter also ends with a Visual Summary, an innovative combination of the main points and figures from the chapter, which you can also view in an interactive format in Oxford Learning Link. We encourage you to explore Oxford Learning Link (oup.com/he/watson-breedlove4e), which contains a comprehensive set of study questions. This tool is a powerful companion to the textbook that enhances the learning experience with a variety of multimedia resources.

The chapter lineup in this edition of *The Mind's Machine* encompasses several major themes. In the opening chapters, we trace the origins of behavioral neuroscience and introduce you to the structure of the brain, both as seen by the naked eye and as revealed through the microscope. We discuss how the cells of the brain use electrical signals to process information, and how they transmit that information to other cells within larger circuits. Along the way we'll look at the ways in which drugs affect nerve cells in order to change behavior, as well as some of the remarkable technology that lets us study the activity of the conscious brain as it perceives and thinks. New for this edition, Chapter 4 delves into developmental neuroscience: the continual remodeling of the nervous system and behavior as we grow up and grow old.

In the middle part of the book we look at the neural systems that underlie fundamental capabilities like feeling, moving, seeing, smelling, and hearing. We'll also consider biological and behavioral aspects of "mission-critical" functions such as feeding, sleeping, and sexual behavior. And we'll look at how the endocrine system acts as an interface between the brain and the rest of the body, as well as the reverse—ways in which the environment and behavior alter hormones and thus alter brain activity.

In the latter part of the book we turn to high-level emotional and cognitive processes that color our lives and define us as individuals. We'll survey the systems that allow us to learn and remember information and skills, and the brain systems dedicated to language and spatial cognition. Research on processes of attention has made great progress in recent years, and we'll also consider consciousness and decision-making from a neuroscientific perspective. Finally, we'll review some of the consequences of brain dysfunction, ranging from psychopathology to behavioral manifestations of brain damage, and some of the innovative strategies being developed to counter these problems.

As you make your way through the book, you'll learn that one of the outstanding features of the brain is its ability to remodel. Every new experience, every piece of information that you learn, every skill that you master, causes changes in the brain that can alter your future behavior. The changes may involve physical alterations in the connections between cells, or in the chemicals they use to communicate, or even the addition of whole new cells and circuits. It's a property that we neuroscientists refer to as "plasticity." And it's something that we aim to exploit—if we've done our job properly, *The Mind's Machine*, Fourth Edition should cause lots of changes in your brain. We hope you enjoy the process.

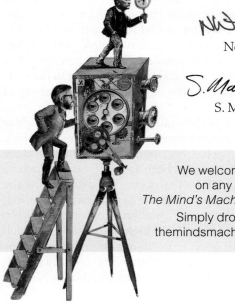

Neil V. Watson

S. Marc Breedlove

We welcome feedback
on any aspect of
The Mind's Machine, Fourth Edition.
Simply drop us a line at
themindsmachine@gmail.com.

Acknowledgments

This book bears the strong imprint of our late colleagues and coauthors Arnold L. Leiman (1932–2000) and Mark R. Rosenzweig (1922–2009). Arnie and Mark prepared the earliest editions of our more advanced text, *Behavioral Neuroscience*, and many illustrations and concepts in *this* book originated in their minds' machines.

In writing this book we benefited from the help of many highly skilled people. These include members of the staff of the Sinauer Associates branch of Oxford University Press: Jess Fiorillo, Editor; Alison Hornbeck and Kathaleen Emerson, Production Editors; Joan Gemme, Production Manager and Book Designer; Richard Neilsen and Meg Britton Clark, Production Specialists; Jason Dirks, Digital Resource Development Manager; and Peter Lacey, Digital Resource Development Editor. Copy Editor Lou Doucette skillfully edited the text, and Photo Researchers Mark Siddall and David McIntyre sourced many of the photographs. For over 25 years now we've been working with Mike Demaray, Craig Durant, and colleagues at Dragonfly Media Group, who so skillfully transform our rough sketches and wish lists into the handsome and dynamic art program you'll enjoy throughout the book.

Our greatest source of inspiration (and critical feedback) has undoubtedly been the thousands of students to whom we have had the privilege of introducing the mysteries and delights of behavioral neuroscience, over the past decade (or two or three or <ahem> four). We have benefited from wisdom generously contributed by a legion of academic colleagues, whose advice and critical reviews have enormously improved our books. In particular we are grateful to: Brian Adams, John Agnew, Duane Albrecht, David L. Allen, Dionisio A. Amodeo, A. Michael Anch, Anne E. Powell Anderson, Michael Antle, Benoit Bacon, Francis R. Bambico, Scott Baron, Alo C. Basu, Jeffrey S. Bedwell, Mark S. Blumberg, William Boggan, Beth Bowin, Sunny K. Boyd, Eliot A. Brenowitz, Chris Brill, Susanne Brummelte, Peter C. Brunjes, Rebecca D. Burwell, Aryn Bush, Joshua M. Carlson, Vanessa Cerda, Evangelia Chrysikou, Suzanne Clerkin, Kenneth J. Colodner, Catherine P. Cramer, Jennifer A. Cummings, Gregory L. Dam, Derek Daniels, Katherine M. Daniels, Heidi Day, Betty Deckard, Brian Derrick, Karen De Valois, Russell De Valois, Rachel A. Diana, Tiffany Donaldson, Gary L. Dunbar, Rena Durr, Steven I. Dworkin, Lena Ficco, Thomas Fischer, Julia Fisher, Loretta M. Flanagan-Cato, Francis W. Flynn, Lauren A. Fowler, Michael Foy, Joyce A. Furfaro, Philip A. Gable, Kara Gabriel, John D. E. Gabrieli, Jack Gallant, Eric W. Gobel, Kimberley P. Good, Christopher Goode, Diane C. Gooding, Janet M. Gray, Gary Greenberg, James Gross, Ervin Hafter, Ian A. Harrington, Mary E. Harrington, Ron Harris, Laura M. Harrison, Christian Hart, Chris Hayashi, Steven J. Hayduk, Wendy Heller, Brian J. Hock, Mark Hollins, Dave Holtzman, Rick Howe, Karin Hu, Richard Ivry, Lucia Jacobs, Karen Jennings, Tephillah Jeyaraj-Powell, Janice Juraska, Jessica M. Karanian, Erin Keen-Rinehart, Dacher Keltner, Raymond E. Kesner, Mike Kisley, Keith R. Kluender, Leah A.

Krubitzer, Joseph E. LeDoux, Diane Lee, Robert Lennartz, Michael A. Leon, Simon LeVay, Jeannie Loeb, Stephen G. Lomber, Jeffrey Love, Christopher M. Lowry, Donna Maney, Stephen A. Maren, Joe L. Martinez, Jr., Melissa Masicampo, John J. McDonald, Robert J. McDonald, James L. McGaugh, Robert L. Meisel, Paul Merritt, Julia E. Meyers-Manor, Ralph E. Mistlberger, Jeffrey S. Mogil, Daniel Montoya, Randy J. Nelson, Chris Newland, Miguel Nicolelis, Michelle Niculescu, Antonio A. Nunez, Lee Osterhout, Kathleen Page, John Pellitteri, Linda Perrotti, James Pfaus, John D. Pierce, Jr., Eleni Pinnow, Helene S. Porte, Joseph Porter, George V. Rebec, Thomas Ritz, Scott R. Robinson, David A. Rosenbaum, Jennifer K. Roth, Lawrence Ryan, Stephen Sammut, Martin F. Sarter, Jeffrey D. Schall, Stan Schein, Frederick Seil, Andrea J. Sell, Dale R. Sengelaub, Victor Shamas, Matthew Shapiro, Arthur Shimamura, Kezia C. Shirkey, Rachel Shoup, Rae Silver, Cheryl L. Sisk, Laura Smale, Ken Sobel, D. J. Spear, Robert L. Spencer, Scott F. Stoltenberg, Jeffrey Stowell, Steve St. John, Patrick Steffen, Steven K. Sutton, Bruce Svare, Harald K. Taukulis, Earl Thomas, Jessica Thompson, Jennifer L. Thomson, Oscar V. Torres, Sandra Trafalis, Brian Trainor, Lucy J. Troup, Meg Upchurch, Franco J. Vaccarino, David R. Vago, Thomas E. Van Cantfort, Cyma Van Petten, Charles J. Vierck, Beth Wee, Carmen Westerberg, Robert Wickesberg, Christoph Wiedenmayer, Eric P. Wiertelak, Walter Wilczynski, Christina L. Williams, S. Mark Williams, Adrienne Williamson, Guangying Wu, Richard D. Wright, Melana Yanos, Heather J. Yu, Mark C. Zrull, and Irving Zucker.

The following external reviewers read and critiqued chapters of the Third Edition of *The Mind's Machine*; their contributions and corrections really helped us to hone this, the Fourth Edition. Any errors that remain are thus entirely our fault.

Katelyn Black, *Tulane University*
Renee A. Countryman, *Austin College*
Sarah E. Holstein, *Lycoming College*
Paul Meyer, *University of Buffalo*
Daniel Montoya, *Fayetteville State University*
John Moore, *Olivet College*
Mark Schmidt, *Columbus State University*
Rachel J. Smith, *Texas A&M University*
Steven St. John, *Rollins University*
Alicia A. Walf, *Rensselaer Polytechnic Institute*
Eric P. Wiertelak, *Macalester College*

Finally, we would like to thank all our colleagues whose ideas and discoveries make behavioral neuroscience so much fun.

Digital Resources

to accompany **The Mind's Machine:**
Foundations of Brain and Behavior, Fourth Edition

Oxford Learning Link
(oup.com/he/watson-breedlove4e)

For the Student

The Mind's Machine, Fourth Edition Oxford Learning Link contains a wide range of study and review resources to help students master the material presented in the text and to help engage them in the subject with fascinating examples. Tightly integrated with the text, these online resources greatly enhance the learning experience. Oxford Learning Link includes:

- *The Mind's Machine*, Fourth Edition e-book, with all the print book's contents in a digital format.

- *Animations* and *Videos* that illustrate dynamic processes and show examples of interesting phenomena.

- *Activities* that help the student learn and understand complex concepts and anatomical (and other) terms.

- *"A Step Further"* readings that offer additional coverage of selected topics.

- Online, interactive versions of the *Visual Summaries*, with links to key chapter figures, animations and videos, and activities.

- *Flashcards*, to help the student master the hundreds of new terms introduced in the textbook.

- *Biological Psychology NewsLink* (www.biopsychology.com/news), an invaluable online resource, has thousands of news stories updated 3-4 times a week to help students make connections between the science of biological psychology and their daily lives.

Optimize Student Learning with Oxford Insight

The Mind's Machine, Fourth Edition is available powered by Oxford Insight. Oxford Insight delivers the trusted and student-focused content of *The Mind's Machine* within powerful, data-driven courseware designed to optimize student success. Developed with a foundation in learning science, Insight enables instructors to deliver a personalized and engaging learning experience that empowers students by actively engaging them with assigned reading. This adaptivity, paired with real-time actionable data about student performance, helps instructors ensure that each student is best supported along their unique learning path.

For more information on how *The Mind's Machine*, Fourth Edition powered by Oxford Insight can enrich the teaching and learning experience in your course, please visit **oxfordinsight.oup.com** or contact your Oxford University Press representative.

For the Instructor

Oxford Learning Link provides instructors using *The Mind's Machine*, Fourth Edition with a wealth of resources for use in course planning, lecture development, and assessment. Content includes:

- *Textbook Figures and Tables*: All the figures and tables from the textbook are provided in a PowerPoint presentation.

- *PowerPoint Lecture presentations* that include text covering the entire chapter, with selected figures.

- *Videos* that illustrate interesting concepts and phenomena.

- *Instructor's Manual* that provides instructors with a variety of resources to aid in planning their course and developing their lectures. For each chapter, the manual includes:

  - Chapter overview
  - Chapter outline
  - Detailed key concepts
  - References for lecture development, including books, journal articles, and online resources
  - Detailed media references for animations and videos
  - Key terms

- *Test Bank*: The Test Bank consists of a broad range of questions covering all the key facts and concepts in each chapter. Each chapter includes multiple choice, short answer, and essay questions.

- *Computerized Test Bank*: The entire test bank is provided in TestGen software. This software makes it easy to assemble quizzes and exams from any combination of publisher-provided questions and instructor-created questions.

- *Test Bank Only cartridge*: The entire test bank is offered in an interoperable cartridge that is compatible with all major learning management systems.

Value Options

eBook

(ISBN 978-0-19754-224-8)

The Mind's Machine is available as an eBook, in several different formats, including RedShelf, VitalSource, and Chegg. All major mobile devices are supported.

The Mind's Machine, Fourth Edition
Oxford Learning Link animations, videos, and activities:

Animations & Videos

1.1	Inside the Brain	8.3	Chemical Communication Systems
1.2	Brain Explorer	8.4	Mechanisms of Hormone Action
1.3	Brain Development	8.5	The Hypothalamus and Endocrine Function
1.4	Visualizing the Living Human Brain	8.6	Organizational Effects of Testosterone
2.1	Electrical Stimulation of the Brain	9.1	Regaining the Weight
2.2	Brain Explorer	9.2	Brain Explorer
2.3	The Resting Membrane Potential	9.3	Negative Feedback
2.4	The Action Potential	9.4	Thermoregulation in Humans
2.5	Action Potential Propagation	9.5	Anorexia
2.6	Spatial Summation	10.1	Narcolepsy
2.7	Synaptic Transmission	10.2	Brain Explorer
3.1	Synaptic Transmission	10.3	Biological Rhythms
3.2	Brain Explorer	10.4	A Molecular Clock
3.3	Neurotransmitter Pathways	10.5	Animal Sleep Activity
3.4	Agonists and Antagonists	10.6	Narcoleptic Dogs
4.1	Blindness and the Brain	10.7	REM Behavior Disorder
4.2	Brain Explorer	11.1	The Case of S.M.
4.3	Stages of Neuronal Development	11.2	Brain Explorer
4.4	Migration of a Neuron along a Radial Glial Cell	11.3	Stress
5.1	Sensory Systems	12.1	Lobotomy
5.2	Brain Explorer	12.2	Brain Explorer
5.3	Somatosensory Receptive Fields	12.3	Tardive Dyskinesia
5.4	The Stretch Reflex Circuit	13.1	Memory
6.1	Inside the Ear	13.2	Brain Explorer
6.2	Brain Explorer	13.3	AMPA and NMDA Receptors
6.3	Sound Transduction	13.4	Morris Water Maze
6.4	Mapping Auditory Frequencies	14.1	Attention and Perception
6.5	The Vestibular System	14.2	Brain Explorer
6.6	The Human Olfactory System	14.3	Inattentional Blindness
7.1	Object Recognition	14.4	From Input to Output
7.2	Brain Explorer	14.5	Reconstructing Brain Activity
7.3	Visual Pathways in the Human Brain	15.1	Global Aphasia
7.4	Receptive Fields in the Retina	15.2	Brain Explorer
7.5	Spatial Frequencies	15.3	Split-Brain Research
8.1	Gender	15.4	Face Blindness
8.2	Brain Explorer	A.1	Gel Electrophoresis

Activities

The Mind's Machine
Foundations of Brain and Behavior
FOURTH EDITION

Introduction:
Building the Mind's Machine

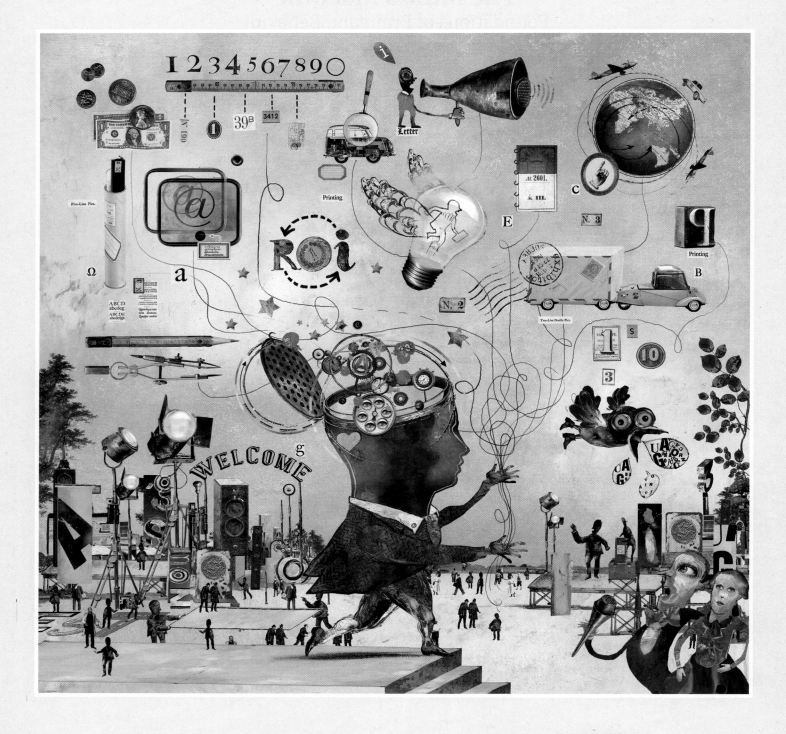

We humans have a long history of using contemporary technology as a metaphor for the mysterious workings of the brain, so today it is commonplace to see the brain described as a computer, complete with "hardware" and "software." Perhaps tomorrow's neuroscientists will describe the brain in terms of quantum devices, wormholes, or a technology that has yet to be imagined. But while modern research aims to describe the complicated machine within each of our heads, we also want to know how the operation of the brain produces the *mind*—the perceptions, emotions, thoughts, self-awareness, and other cognitive processes that inform our behavior.

During the twentieth century, a lot of ink was spilled over the "nature–nurture" controversy, with scholars arguing passionately about the extent to which mental characteristics and abilities are the result of learning experiences versus "innate, hardwired" genetic programs. The two perspectives have often been presented as mutually incompatible alternatives, but thanks to more-powerful techniques, we have come to realize that there is nothing controversial about nature versus nurture: they are two sides of the same coin. Consider the case of rat pups who have inattentive mothers. As adults, the formerly neglected pups show elevated stress hormone responses to stressors that have little effect on rats that were not neglected as pups (O'Donnell and Meaney, 2020). How does this lasting reactivity develop—through experience or as a result of inborn biological factors? Both, it turns out. As we'll see later in this Introduction, and throughout the book, the mind and its machine are shaped by a precise combination of genes and experience, inextricably tied together.

There are now nearly 8 billion of us, and while we can debate whether to fear or celebrate that number, there is no doubt that each of those billions of human brains will at times contemplate its own existence and meaning. How does the operation of a three-pound organ generate our sense of self, express our unique personalities, record information, and guide our actions? Evolution has shaped our bodies and brains so that we closely resemble one another, yet our brains remain malleable throughout life, continually remolded by our environments, experiences, and interactions with other people. So, through a remarkable intersection of genetic heritage and environmental influences, billions of unique individuals have been formed, and we literally change each other's minds on a daily basis.

See Video Intro.1:
Nature and Nurture

Intro.1 Behavioral Neuroscience Spans Past, Present, and Future

THE ROAD AHEAD

We open the book by situating behavioral neuroscience in its historical context, considering its relationship to different branches of brain science, and reviewing some of the important developments that will propel brain research into the future. Reading this section should prepare you to:

Intro.1.1 Define *behavioral neuroscience*, identify its synonyms, describe the scope of the field, and situate it relative to other branches of brain science.

Intro.1.2 Trace the history of our understanding of the role of the brain, as articulated by scholars across the millennia.

Intro.1.3 Name and briefly describe some of the most influential concepts, emerging topics, and future goals for brain research.

The general field of **neuroscience**—the scientific study of the nervous system—is divided into many subdisciplines because the topic is so vast. The first scholars to study the relationships between brain and behavior called themselves philosophers, because it was philosophy that established the *scientific method* as our best tool for finding new knowledge. Philosophers had long been concerned with the sources of human behavior, so **behavioral neuroscience**, the field that relates behavior to bodily processes, naturally evolved from those beginnings. The names *biological psychology, brain and behavior,* and *physiological psychology* are all synonyms for *behavioral neuroscience,* but whichever name is used, the main goal of this field is to understand the brain structures and functions that respond to experiences and generate behavior.

Researchers with dramatically varied backgrounds—psychologists, biologists, physiologists, engineers, neurologists, psychiatrists, and many others—together make up the field of behavioral neuroscience. It is a field that spans both academia and industry, with focus that ranges from pure research on basic processes to entirely applied work directly translating findings into goods and services (Hitt, 2007). The diverse branches of science that overlap with behavioral neuroscience are mapped in **FIGURE Intro.1**.

An early textbook famously opened with the observation that, as a science, "psychology has a long past but only a short history" (Ebbinghaus, 1908). That's certainly an apt description of behavioral neuroscience. The modern era of behavioral neuroscience—characterized by objective experimentation and use of the scientific method to test hypotheses—has a formal history of only 100 years or so. But curiosity about the genesis of behavior reaches much further into the past, shaped by religious ideas, folk knowledge, and ancient observations about the biology of humans and nonhuman animals.

What is this?

In each chapter of the book, you will find several of these small features, entitled **THE ROAD AHEAD.** They are intended to provide you with a road map for the reading you are about to do, giving you a sense of where the following section is going and what we hope you will get from it (i.e., your learning objectives).

View Animation Intro.2: Brain Explorer

neuroscience   The scientific study of the nervous system.

behavioral neuroscience   Also called *biological psychology, brain and behavior,* and *physiological psychology.* The study of the biological bases of psychological processes and behavior.

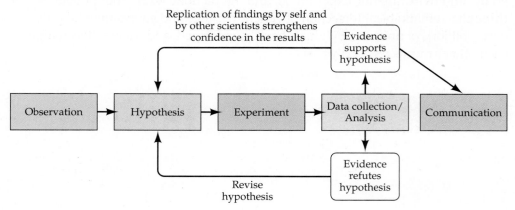

The Scientific Method   Scientists use a formal system of hypothesis testing and refinement to gradually develop understanding of neural processes.

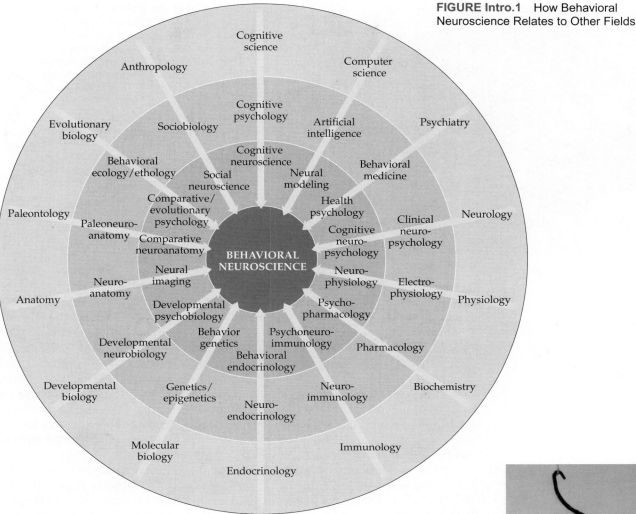

FIGURE Intro.1   How Behavioral
Neuroscience Relates to Other Fields

An understanding of the brain's role in behavior has developed over centuries

The elaborate preparation of tombs and careful mummification of important people in ancient Egypt (especially about 1500–1000 BCE) reflected the belief that the dead would enter an afterlife that entailed both struggle and—for the adequately equipped individual—great reward. So, in addition to embalming the body with special salts and oils, the usual practice was to preserve four important organs in alabaster jars in the tomb: liver, lungs, stomach, and intestines. The heart, being especially esteemed, was preserved in its place within the body. The brain, however, was picked out though the nostrils and thrown away; apparently, it was considered to be of little value in the afterlife.

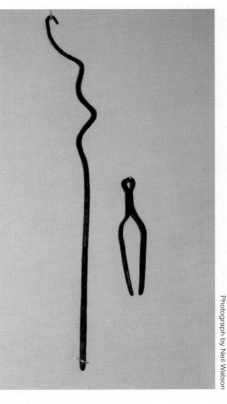

Brain Extraction Kit   It seems the ancient Egyptians had little regard for the brain. During the mummification process, embalmers used specialized tools, like these examples in the British Museum, to first break up the small bones behind the nose and then extract the brain through the opening. Unlike other major organs, the brain was discarded, and the cranium was stuffed with linen or straw.

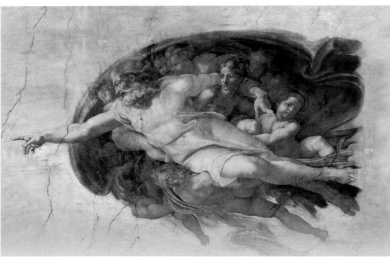

A Brain on the Ceiling of the Sistine Chapel?
Between 1508 and 1512, Michelangelo painted the Sistine Chapel in the Vatican. In one panel of Michelangelo's masterpiece, God is depicted reaching out to bestow the gift of life upon humanity, through Adam. But neuroscientists have noted that the oddly shaped drapery behind God, and the arrangement of his attendants, closely resembles the human brain (Meshberger, 1990); compare it with the midsagittal view in Figure 1.16A. A keen student of anatomy, Michelangelo probably knew perfectly well what a dissected human brain looks like. So, was Michelangelo having some fun, making a subtle commentary about the origins of human behavior? We probably will never know, but modern research tools are helping us to understand how our distinctive human qualities—language, reason, emotion, and the rest—are products of the brain.

There is little or no mention of the brain in the Quran, and it is likewise never mentioned in either the Old Testament or New Testament of the Bible, but the heart is mentioned hundreds of times, along with several references each to the liver, the stomach, and the bowels as the seats of passion, courage, and pity, respectively. Aristotle (about 350 BCE), the most prominent scientist of ancient Greece, likewise considered mental capacities to be properties of the heart. When we call people kindhearted, openhearted, fainthearted, hardhearted, or heartless, and when we speak of learning by heart, we are using language echoing this ancient notion. Aristotle thought the brain was little more than a cooling system for hot blood from the heart. But Aristotle's near contemporary, the great Greek physician Hippocrates (about 400 BCE), already suspected that Aristotle's view was—ahem—wrongheaded, and he instead ascribed emotion, perception, and thought to the functioning of the brain.

By the second century CE, this brain-centered view of mental processes had become more accepted, appearing in the writings of the Greco-Roman physician Galen (the "Father of Medicine"). Galen's experiences in treating head injuries of gladiators led him to propose that behavior results from the movement of "animal spirits" from the brain through nerves to the body, but his understanding of the relevant anatomy was poor because the dissection of humans was outlawed in Rome at that time. Not until much later were techniques developed for making highly detailed anatomical studies of the fine structure of the brain.

Skillfully applying newly developed innovations in drawing technique, Renaissance painter and scientist Leonardo da Vinci (1452–1519) produced exquisite neuroanatomical illustrations of nerves and brain structures (**FIGURE Intro.2**). Religious dogma dominated Renaissance science—just ask Galileo—with the result that scientific writing from that era often presents the brain as a mysterious and intricate gift from God. But perhaps some thinkers of the day secretly held a more secular view of neuroscience; for example, it

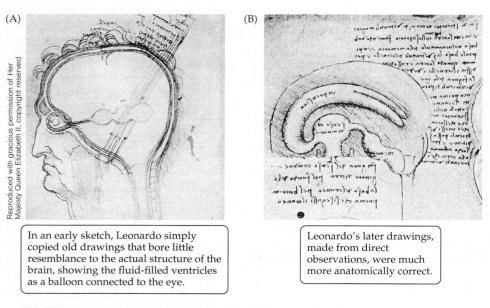

(A)

In an early sketch, Leonardo simply copied old drawings that bore little resemblance to the actual structure of the brain, showing the fluid-filled ventricles as a balloon connected to the eye.

(B)

Leonardo's later drawings, made from direct observations, were much more anatomically correct.

FIGURE Intro.2 Leonardo da Vinci's Changing View of the Brain has been observed that certain depictions of God on the ceiling of the Sistine Chapel, painted by Michelangelo (1475–1564), bear a striking resemblance to the human brain (Meshberger, 1990; Suk and Tamargo, 2010). It is believed that Michelangelo was conducting dissections of cadavers at about the time that the painting was created.

In any event, weighing religious notions of the soul against increasingly mechanistic views of the brain became a major preoccupation for later scholars. Among his many contributions to math and science, René Descartes (1596–1650) tried to explain how the control of behavior might resemble the workings of a machine, proposing the concept of spinal reflexes and a neural pathway for them (FIGURE Intro.3). But Descartes also argued (perhaps in order to deflect criticism) that free will and moral choice could not arise from a mere machine. So Descartes asserted that humans, at least, had a nonmaterial soul as well as a material body and that the soul governed behavior through a point of contact (possibly the pineal gland) in the brain. This notion of **dualism** spread widely and left other thinkers with the task of trying to explain *how* a nonmaterial soul could exert influence over a material body and brain. Today, almost all neuroscientists have discarded dualism in favor of the much simpler view that the workings of the mind can be understood as purely physical processes taking place in the material brain.

Thanks in large part to systematic studies of the relation between various disorders and damage to regions of the human brain that were conducted by the English physician Thomas Willis (1621–1675), the notion that the brain coordinates and controls behavior eventually became widely accepted (Zimmer, 2004). A pseudoscientific fad of the early 1800s called **phrenology** (FIGURE Intro.4A) capitalized on the emerging idea that specific behaviors, feelings, and personality traits were controlled by corresponding specific regions of the brain. Although phrenology was plainly wrong in several fundamental

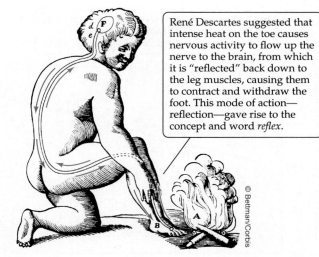

René Descartes suggested that intense heat on the toe causes nervous activity to flow up the nerve to the brain, from which it is "reflected" back down to the leg muscles, causing them to contract and withdraw the foot. This mode of action—reflection—gave rise to the concept and word *reflex*.

FIGURE Intro.3   An Early Account of Reflexes

dualism   The notion, promoted by René Descartes, that the mind has an immaterial aspect that is distinct from the material body and brain.

phrenology   The belief that bumps on the skull reflect enlargements of brain regions responsible for certain behavioral faculties.

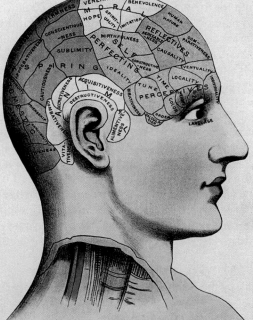

In the nineteenth century phrenologists associated arbitrary "faculties" with bumps on the skull, using maps like this to infer an individual's talents, personality, and temperament.

(A)

FIGURE Intro.4   Mapping Behavior: Then and Now (B after M. J. Nichols and W. T. Newsome, 1999. *Nature* 402: C35.)

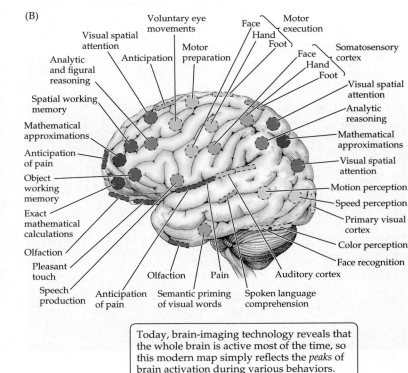

(B)

Voluntary eye movements
Visual spatial attention
Analytic and figural reasoning
Spatial working memory
Mathematical approximations
Anticipation of pain
Object working memory
Exact mathematical calculations
Olfaction
Pleasant touch
Speech production
Anticipation
Motor preparation
Face Hand Foot
Motor execution
Face Hand Foot
Somatosensory cortex
Visual spatial attention
Analytic reasoning
Mathematical approximations
Visual spatial attention
Motion perception
Speed perception
Primary visual cortex
Color perception
Face recognition
Auditory cortex
Olfaction
Pain
Semantic priming of visual words
Spoken language comprehension
Anticipation of pain

Today, brain-imaging technology reveals that the whole brain is active most of the time, so this modern map simply reflects the *peaks* of brain activation during various behaviors.

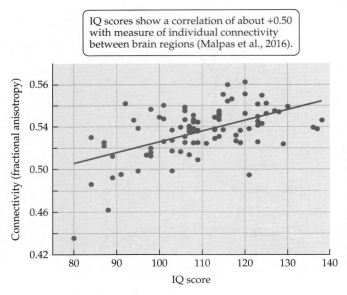

IQ scores show a correlation of about +0.50 with measure of individual connectivity between brain regions (Malpas et al., 2016).

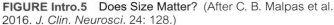

FIGURE Intro.5   Does Size Matter? (After C. B. Malpas et al. 2016. *J. Clin. Neurosci.* 24: 128.)

localization of function   The concept that different brain regions specialize in specific behaviors.

ways—for example, phrenologists believed they could "read" a person's character by feeling the bumps on that person's head—the field helped establish the concept of **localization of function**, which asserts that different brain regions specialize in specific behaviors.

Later researchers found that damage to specific regions of the brain causes predictable impairments in people; for example, Paul Broca (1824–1880) noted that damage to a particular region of the left side of the brain reliably causes problems with speech production (see Chapter 15). Neuroscientists today accept that the localization of function within the brain is more or less true. Although the whole brain is active most of the time, when we are performing particular tasks, certain brain regions become even more activated, and different tasks activate different networks of brain regions. So modern functional maps of the human brain track the locations where these peaks of activation occur (**FIGURE Intro.4B**). A parallel concern that harks back to the phrenologists has been the importance of brain size to intellectual function. After a couple of centuries of study, the evidence indicates that while the overall size of your brain matters, it matters a lot less than you might expect. Initial evidence suggests that IQ measures may instead show a stronger relationship to individual differences in connectivity than to brain size (**FIGURE Intro.5**; Malpas et al., 2016).

In 1890, William James's book *Principles of Psychology* signaled the beginnings of a modern approach to behavioral neuroscience. In James's work, psychological ideas such as consciousness and other aspects of human experience came to be seen as properties of the nervous system. A true behavioral neuroscience began to emerge from this approach. By the beginning of the twentieth century, researchers were applying newly developed tools to study mental processes that had previously seemed unknowable. Rapid progress was made in developing techniques for measuring learning and memory in humans and animals, and Russian physiologist Ivan P. Pavlov (1849–1936) made his landmark discoveries of classical conditioning in animals— Nobel Prize–winning work that influences scientists to this day.

This rapid progress prompted a parallel interest in understanding the neural basis of learning, marked by one of the first true behavioral neuroscience research programs: the "search for the engram" by Karl Lashley (1890–1958). Although he would not accomplish his goal of linking a specific brain region to the formation of a specific long-term memory (an "engram"), Lashley gave us the idea (now well established) that memory is not localized to only one region of the brain. Behavioral neuroscience also bears the strong imprint of Canadian psychologist Donald O. Hebb (1904–1985), who showed that cognitive processing could be accomplished by networks of active neurons, molded by repeated activation patterns into functional circuits. His hypothesis about how neurons strengthen their connections as a consequence of experiences led to the idea of the *Hebbian synapse*, a type of plastic (changeable) connection between neurons that remains a hot topic in contemporary neuroscience research, as discussed in Chapter 13.

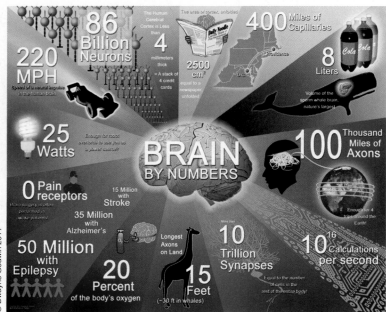

Your Brain, by the Numbers

Research objectives reflect specific theoretical orientations

In designing their research programs, present-day behavioral neuroscientists seek answers to well-defined, specific questions that build on the discoveries of scientists who have gone before. In developing the questions that they wish to study, researchers draw on multiple different research perspectives. Here are some of the major ones:

1. *Systematic description of behavior*   Until we describe what we want to study, we cannot accomplish much. Depending on our goals, we may describe behavior in terms of detailed acts or processes, or in terms of results or functions. To be useful for scientific study, a description must be precise, using accurately defined terms and units.

2. *The evolution of brain and behavior*   Charles Darwin's theory of evolution through natural selection is central to all modern biology and psychology. Behavioral neuroscientists employ evolutionary theory in two ways: by evaluating similarities among species that reflect shared ancestry, and by looking for species-specific differences in behavior and biology that have evolved as adaptations to different environments. We will discuss many examples of both perspectives in this book.

3. *Life span development of the brain and behavior*   **Ontogeny** is the process by which an individual changes in the course of its lifetime—that is, grows up and grows old. Observing the way a particular behavior changes during ontogeny may give us clues to its functions and mechanisms. For example, we know that learning and memory abilities in monkeys increase over the first years of life. Therefore, we can speculate that prolonged maturation of brain circuits is required for complex learning tasks.

4. *The biological mechanisms of behavior*   To understand the underlying mechanisms of behavior, we must regard the organism (with all due respect) as a "machine." Accordingly, behavior is the collaborative project of nerve cells, or **neurons**: about 86 billion of them in the case of the human brain (Herculano-Houzel, 2012). In a sense, the mechanistic questions are the "how" questions of behavioral neuroscience, in contrast to the "why" questions that derive from the evolutionary and developmental perspectives. So in the case of learning and memory, for example, we might try to understand how a sequence of electrical and biochemical processes allows us to store information in our brains, and how a different process retrieves it.

5. *Applications of behavioral neuroscience discoveries*   The practical application of fundamental discoveries in behavioral neuroscience can improve our lives, and as in so many other branches of science, basic and applied research inform each other in a reciprocal manner. We'll see numerous examples of this reciprocity in the book, ranging from genome-based treatment of brain diseases to technological approaches for understanding brain mechanisms of learning, memory, and consciousness.

The future of behavioral neuroscience is in interdisciplinary discovery and knowledge translation

New discoveries from behavioral neuroscience labs are leading to greater understanding of brain disorders and, with time, will result in the development of effective treatments. This is an urgent problem of much greater scale than many people realize: even excluding addiction and developmental disorders, one in five U.S. residents lived with a mental illness in 2016 (SAMHSA, 2017), and for many disorders the prevalence appears to be on the rise (Hidaka, 2012; Duffy et al., 2019). Neurological and psychiatric disorders vary tremendously both in their severity—from illnesses that can be managed with suitable treatments, to devastating conditions that completely disable—and

ontogeny   The process by which an individual changes in the course of its lifetime.

neuron   Also called *nerve cell*. The basic unit of the nervous system.

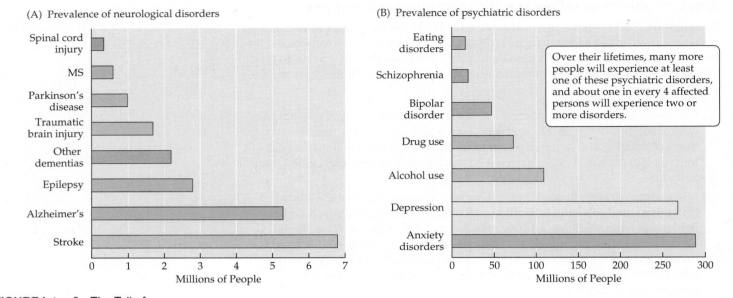

(A) Prevalence of neurological disorders

(B) Prevalence of psychiatric disorders

Over their lifetimes, many more people will experience at least one of these psychiatric disorders, and about one in every 4 affected persons will experience two or more disorders.

FIGURE Intro.6   The Toll of **Brain Disorders** (Data for A from C. L. Gooch et al. 2017. *Annu. Neurol.* 81: 479-484. B after H. Ritchie and M. Roser. 2019. "Mental Health." Published online at OurWorldInData. org. Retrieved from: https://ourworld-indata.org/mental-health. Underlying data available from http://ghdx. healthdata.org/gbd-results-tool.)

neuroplasticity   Also called *plasticity*. The ability of the nervous system to change in response to experience or the environment.

in their incidence (**FIGURE Intro.6**). The economic toll of so much illness is staggering: the cost for treatment of dementia (severely disordered thinking) alone exceeds the costs of treating cancer and heart disease combined.

As the quest to understand and relieve these diseases gathers speed, some of the historical distinction between clinical and laboratory approaches has begun to fade away. For example, when clinicians encounter a pair of twins, one of whom has schizophrenia while the other seems healthy, the discovery of structural differences in their brains (**FIGURE Intro.7**) immediately raises questions for laboratory scientists: Did the structural differences arise before the symptoms of schizophrenia, or the other way around? Were the brain differences present at birth, or did they arise during puberty? Does medication that reduces symptoms affect brain structure? (We'll consider schizophrenia again in Chapter 12.)

The twenty-first century has brought an explosion of new research areas and perspectives to behavioral neuroscience. In addition to the rapid progress in the more established topic areas of behavioral neuroscience, which we survey in this book, some emerging research areas are attracting intense interest. In the paragraphs that follow, we'll take a brief look at a handful of these.

NEUROPLASTICITY   When you think about it, the only explanation for our ability to learn skills and form memories is that the brain physically changes in some way to encode and store that information. In this book we'll see many examples of how behavior and experiences alter the physical brain—a phenomenon called **neuroplasticity** (or just *plasticity*; from the Greek plassein, "to mold or form")—but much remains to be discovered about mechanisms of neuroplasticity.

We know that experiences can alter the size of brain regions and interconnections between neurons, and cellular changes have been discovered that could be mechanisms for storing memories. We also know that certain

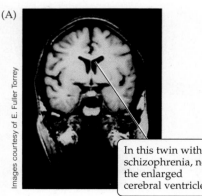

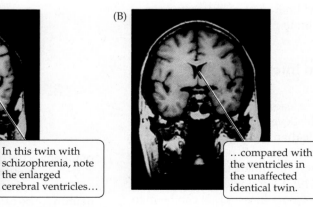

(A)

(B)

In this twin with schizophrenia, note the enlarged cerebral ventricles…

…compared with the ventricles in the unaffected identical twin.

Images courtesy of E. Fuller Torrey

FIGURE Intro.7   Identical Twins but Nonidentical Brains and Behavior experiences and physiological states can modify the rate at which new neurons are born in the adult brain, but again, the functional significance of this **adult neurogenesis** (see Chapter 13) remains to be explored. Perhaps nothing distinguishes behavioral neuroscience from other neurosciences more clearly than a fascination with neuroplasticity and the role of experience.

SOCIAL NEUROSCIENCE   Because of neuroplasticity, even simple interactions with other people can remodel our brains. Indeed, the whole point of coming to a lecture hall is to have the instructor use words and figures to alter your brain so that you can retrieve that information in the future (in other words, they are teaching you something). Most aspects of our social behavior are learned—from the language we speak to the clothes we wear and the kinds of foods we eat, as well as our identity in belonging to larger groups (clubs, teams, schools, nationalities, and so on).

Social neuroscience is an emerging discipline that uses the tools of neuroscience to discover how biological and social factors continually interact and affect each other as behavior unfolds. For example, the amount of testosterone in a male's circulation affects his dominance behavior and aggression, expressed in social settings ranging from friendly games to overt physical aggression (see Chapter 11). But the outcome of those contests can cause changes in relative testosterone levels—winners show more testosterone, and losers have less—so testosterone concentration in the blood at any particular moment is determined (in part) by the male's recent history of dominant/submissive social experience. The modified testosterone level, in turn, helps determine the male's dominance and aggression in the future. So it goes.

EVOLUTIONARY PSYCHOLOGY   Zoologists have long viewed animal behaviors as adaptations that evolved to solve specific ecological pressures, such as the need to find food and avoid predators. More recently, speculations about how natural selection might have shaped our own behavior, including specific cognitive abilities, have given rise to a lively and controversial field called **evolutionary psychology** (Buss, 2013). For example, it has been argued that sexual selection was crucial for evolution of the human brain. If early ancestors of modern humans came to favor mates who sang, made jokes, or produced artistic works, an "arms race" might have ensued as the ever more discriminating brains of one sex demanded ever more impressive performances from the brains of the other sex. Did humor, song, and art originate from the drive to be sexy? And does sexual selection account for the large size of the human brain?

Although evolutionary psychology excels at generating intriguing hypothetical accounts of the evolution of behaviors, the challenge for the future is to come up with ways to test and potentially disprove these hypotheses.

EPIGENETICS   Nearly all of the cells in your body have a complete copy of your genome (i.e., a copy of all your genes), but each cell uses only a small subset of those genes at any one time. **Epigenetics** is a young field focusing on factors that have a lasting effect on patterns of **gene expression**—the turning on or off of specific genes—without changing the structure of the genes themselves. In some cases, the acquired alteration in gene expression is passed down through generations, from parent to child, despite the absence of genetic modifications.

Earlier, we described rats that will show heightened stress reactivity throughout their lives if neglected by their mothers while they are pups, and we asked whether this phenomenon was more attributable to "nature" or to "nurture." The answer is: neither. Or perhaps both. It is an epigenetic phenomenon, in which the maternal neglect causes lasting inactivation of a gene—a process called *methylation* (see Chapter 13)—that causes the pup to be hyperresponsive to stress for the rest of its life. So, early experience produces a permanent change in the way in which genes are expressed in the brain of the neglected rat, thus altering its behavior in adulthood—nurture and nature.

adult neurogenesis   The creation of new neurons in the brain of an adult.

social neuroscience   A field of study that uses the tools of neuroscience to discover both the biological bases of social behavior and the effects of social circumstances on brain activity.

evolutionary psychology   A field of study devoted to asking how natural selection has shaped behavior in humans and other animals.

epigenetics   The study of factors that affect gene expression without making any changes in the nucleotide sequence of the genes themselves.

gene expression   The turning on or off of specific genes.

neuroeconomics The study of brain mechanisms at work during decision making.

consciousness The state of awareness of one's own existence, thoughts, emotions, and experiences.

This same gene is also more likely to be methylated in the postmortem brains of humans who have committed suicide, but only if the victim was subjected to childhood abuse (McGowan et al., 2009). So, methylation of the gene in abused children may make them more susceptible to stress as adults and put them at risk for suicide—a powerful demonstration of epigenetic influences on behavior. Epigenetic modifications are increasingly understood to have a major role in the development of individual differences in mental health disorders such as depression and stress pathology (Gray et al., 2017; Manoli and Tollkuhn, 2018). (For additional examples of social influences on the structure of the brain, see **A STEP FURTHER Intro.1**, on the website.)

NEUROECONOMICS A growing number of neuroscience labs focus on the neural bases of decision making. Involving perspectives ranging from philosophy to social psychology to cognitive psychology, neuroscience, and economics, **neuroeconomics** aims to identify brain regions that are especially active when decisions are being made: while playing games, managing resources, making strategic choices, and so on. Naturally, this research has some shorter-term benefits relating to product marketing—what makes us want to buy something—but researchers mostly hope that, over the longer term, we will develop a more complete understanding of both the massive brain networks that are active while we choose among various alternatives and decide what to do next, and the ways in which we perceive and express our free will (as well as if, indeed, we actually *have* free will!).

Early indications are that we possess brain mechanisms dedicated to neuroeconomic evaluations, assessing the relative value of each choice available and then sifting through the evaluated choices in order to make a conscious decision (Kable and Glimcher, 2009; Ojala et al., 2018), along with mechanisms to inhibit impulsive decision making (Muhlert and Lawrence, 2015; Heilbronner and Hayden, 2016). There is good reason to expect exciting new discoveries about how these neural systems interact with other cognitive systems to produce our conscious feeling of self.

THE TRULY FINAL FRONTIER: CONSCIOUSNESS Ultimately, many of the traditional and emerging topics in behavioral neuroscience converge on the problem of **consciousness**: the personal, private awareness of our emotions, intentions, thoughts, and movements and of the sensations that impinge upon us. How is it possible that you are aware of the words on this page, the room you're occupying, the goals you have in life? Scientists have laid some of the groundwork for conceptualizing consciousness as a property of the brain and for establishing it as an area of scientific inquiry (Zeman, 2002), but the devil is in the details. Later in the book we will consider experiments that demonstrate properties of consciousness, including the role of arousal systems of the brain, and evidence that synchronized activity within large cortical networks gives rise to conscious introspection (Raichle, 2015). And some of these experiments lead us to interesting—possibly disturbing—conclusions that our consciousness may track the operation of our brains much less accurately than we perceive (as discussed in Chapter 14).

However it is brought about, any satisfying account of consciousness should be able to explain, for example, why a certain pattern of activity in your brain causes you to experience the sensation of blue when looking at the sky. And a really good theory should tell us how we could cause you to experience the sky as yellow, just by changing your brain activity for you (not, of course, by simply fitting you with colored goggles, but rather through a change in the deeper conscious experience of the world around you). However, we are nowhere near understanding consciousness this clearly. We generally have no idea what the actual inner experience of a human or animal is—only what an individual's behavior tells us about it. So even if you tell me that the sky is blue to you, I can't tell whether blue feels the same in your mind as it does in mine. Until we can get a more complete grasp of these complex issues of brain and behavior, we are in no position to know whether complicated machines like computers are, or

"How Beautifully Blue the Sky"
We would all agree that this sky is the color we call "blue." But in Chapter 14 we'll ask whether everyone who sees that sky has the same experience of the color.

The goal of massive projects in both the USA and Europe is to have a digital re-creation of the neurons and connections found in a human brain. As this projection from the European project (bluebrain.epfl.ch) shows, this would require an "exascale" computer capable of a mind-bending quintillion (one billion billion) operations per second, and a truly staggering amount of computer memory.

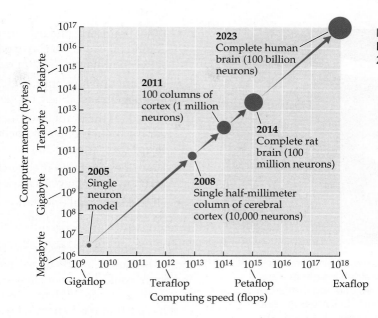

FIGURE Intro.8 The Human Brain Project (After M. M. Waldrop. 2012. *Nature* 482: 456.)

might one day be, conscious. Several large research projects are currently engaged in the Herculean task of mapping the neural networks within an entire human brain (Waldrop, 2012), which will require computer systems with almost unimaginable processing power and memory (**FIGURE Intro.8**).

HOW'S IT GOING ❓

1. Define *behavioral neuroscience*. Name some fields that are closely allied to behavioral neuroscience.
2. What do we mean when we say that behavioral neuroscience has a long past but only a short history? Review the prehistory of behavioral neuroscience and the gradual process of elimination that linked the brain and behavior.
3. Discuss the concept of localization of function.
4. Comment on the prevalence of psychiatric and neurological disorders in contemporary society, and discuss their economic and emotional impact.
5. Describe the five major theoretical perspectives employed by modern behavioral neuroscientists that we discussed in the chapter: behavioral description, evolution, development, biological mechanisms, and applications.
6. Where is behavioral neuroscience headed? Discuss some of the probable hot topics for future behavioral neuroscientists.

Looking forward: A glimpse inside *The Mind's Machine*

Our mission in this book is to acquaint you with the broad topic of behavioral neuroscience, from historical underpinnings to cutting-edge investigations of the most complex aspects of our intellect. Along the way, we are going to touch on hundreds of the most interesting questions in modern neuroscience; here are just a few examples:

• How does the brain grow, maintain, and repair itself over the life span, and how are these capacities related to the growth and development of the mind and behavior from the womb to the tomb? (See Chapter 4.)

• How does the nervous system capture, process, and represent information about the environment? (See Chapter 5, Chapter 6, and Chapter 7.) For example, sometimes brain damage causes a person to lose the ability to identify other people's faces; what does that tell us about how the brain works during face recognition? (See Chapter 14.)

What is this?

Sprinkled throughout every chapter, sections entitled **HOW'S IT GOING?** provide conceptual questions that will help you check your learning and ensure you are meeting the objectives set out in **THE ROAD AHEAD.**

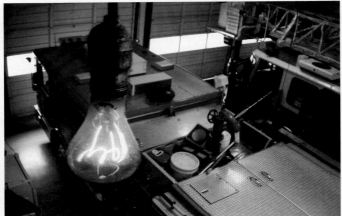

A Bright Idea The symbolic lightbulb coming on over someone's head, representing a sudden insight or idea, is an especially apt metaphor for the functioning of the brain, given the lightbulb's rapid action and ability to penetrate the gloom (both literal and metaphorical). This particular lightbulb, in a fire station in Livermore, California, is the world's longest-burning bulb (you can check in on it, live, at www.centennialbulb.org/cam.htm). It has been continually lit for more than 1 million hours (about 117 years)—since the dawn of the scientific discipline of behavioral neuroscience.

- What brain sites and activities underlie feelings and emotional expression? Are particular parts of the brain active in romantic love, for example? (See Chapter 11.)
- Why are different brain regions active during different language tasks? (See Chapter 15.)
- How does the brain track the passage of time, and trigger the regular bouts of unconsciousness that we call sleep? (See Chapter 10.)
- How does the brain manage to change during learning, and how are memories retrieved? (See Chapter 13.)
- How does sexual orientation develop? How can gender be defined? (See Chapter 8.)

The relationship between the brain and behavior is very mysterious because it is difficult to understand how a physical device, the brain, could be responsible for our subjective experiences of fear, love, and awe. Perhaps it is the "everyday miracle" aspect of the topic that has generated so much folk wisdom—and unfounded mythology—about the brain (Pasquinelli, 2012). For example, the oft-repeated claim that we normally use only 10% of the brain is commonplace—a survey of teachers found that nearly half of them agreed with this cockamamie notion (Howard-Jones, 2014). In fact, brain scans show that the entire brain is active most of the time while we go about normal daily activities. There are lots of other examples of commonplace beliefs about the brain (Macdonald et al., 2017). We've compiled a few of these in **A STEP FURTHER Intro.2** on the website. (Throughout the book you'll find similar opportunities for you to explore selected topics in more detail by going **A STEP FURTHER Intro.3**).

Of course, it wasn't that long ago that the idea of making light from electricity seemed far-fetched. With each passing year, technological developments and the progress of thousands of neuroscientists in labs around the world provide a clearer view of what is happening when a lightbulb goes on in the mind and someone has a clever idea. Our hope for this book is that it will turn on a few lightbulbs for you too.

Recommended Reading

Cacioppo, S., and Cacioppo, J. T. (2020). *Introduction to Social Neuroscience.* Princeton, NJ: Princeton University Press.

Dehaene, S. (2014). *Consciousness and the Brain: Deciphering How the Brain Codes Our Thoughts.* New York, NY: Penguin Books.

Finger, S. (2001). *Origins of Neuroscience.* New York, NY: Oxford University Press.

Godfrey-Smith, P. (2017). *Other Minds: The Octopus, the Sea, and the Deep Origins of Consciousness.* New York, NY: Farrar, Straus and Giroux.

Kaku, M. (2015). *The Future of the Mind: The Scientific Quest to Understand, Enhance, and Empower the Mind.* New York, NY: Random House.

Koch, C. (2012). *Consciousness: Confessions of a Romantic Reductionist.* Cambridge, MA: MIT Press.

Wickens, A. P. (2014). *A History of the Brain: From Stone Age Surgery to Modern Neuroscience.* New York, NY: Psychology Press.

© Caters News/Zuma Press

You should be able to relate each summary to the adjacent illustration, including structures and processes. The online version of this **Visual Summary** includes links to figures, animations, and activities that will help you consolidate the material.

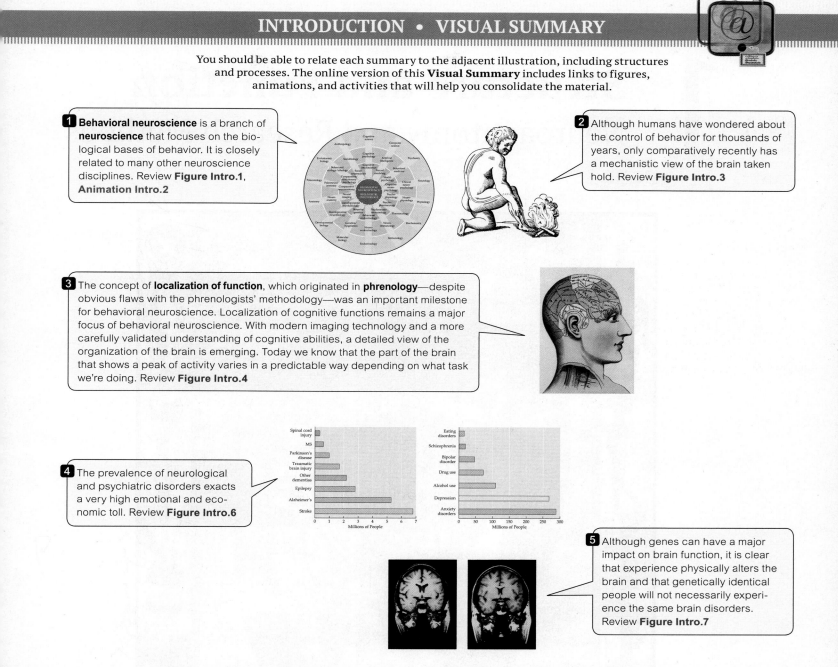

1 **Behavioral neuroscience** is a branch of **neuroscience** that focuses on the biological bases of behavior. It is closely related to many other neuroscience disciplines. Review **Figure Intro.1**, **Animation Intro.2**

2 Although humans have wondered about the control of behavior for thousands of years, only comparatively recently has a mechanistic view of the brain taken hold. Review **Figure Intro.3**

3 The concept of **localization of function**, which originated in **phrenology**—despite obvious flaws with the phrenologists' methodology—was an important milestone for behavioral neuroscience. Localization of cognitive functions remains a major focus of behavioral neuroscience. With modern imaging technology and a more carefully validated understanding of cognitive abilities, a detailed view of the organization of the brain is emerging. Today we know that the part of the brain that shows a peak of activity varies in a predictable way depending on what task we're doing. Review **Figure Intro.4**

4 The prevalence of neurological and psychiatric disorders exacts a very high emotional and economic toll. Review **Figure Intro.6**

5 Although genes can have a major impact on brain function, it is clear that experience physically alters the brain and that genetically identical people will not necessarily experience the same brain disorders. Review **Figure Intro.7**

The Mind's Machine digital resources include additional videos, flashcards, and other study tools.

1

Structure and Function
Neuroanatomy and Research Methods

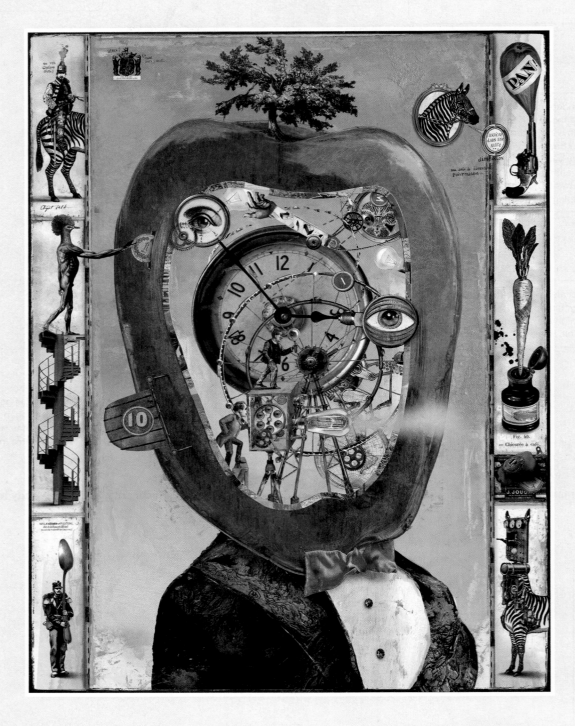

Electrical Storm

Sam had been feeling a bit odd all day; he thought perhaps he was coming down with a bug. But when he collapsed unconscious to the floor of the lunchroom at work and began twitching and jerking, it was clear that he had a much bigger problem than the flu. Sam was having a *seizure*, a type of uncontrollable convulsion that he'd never had before. By the time Sam arrived at the hospital, the seizure had stopped, and although he was confused and slow to respond to commands, he didn't seem to be in distress. But when Sam smiled at Dr. Cheng, the attending neurologist, and offered to shake her hand, Dr. Cheng ordered immediate brain scans: Sam could offer only half a smile, because only the left side of his face was working, and he was unable to grip Dr. Cheng's hand at all.

How can an understanding of the pathways between brain and body provide clues about Sam's problem? We now know quite a bit about the neural organization of basic functions, but the control of complex cognition remains a tantalizing mystery. However, the advent of sophisticated brain-imaging technology has invigorated the search for answers to fundamental questions about brain organization: Does each brain region control a specific behavior, or is the pattern of connections within the brain more important? Do some regions of the brain act as general purpose information processors? Is everybody's brain organized in the same way?

Almost everything about us—our thoughts, feelings, and behavior, however serious or silly—is the product of a knobbly three-pound organ that, despite its unremarkable appearance, is the most complicated object in the known universe. In this chapter we'll have a look at the structure of the brain, first at the cellular level and then zooming out to survey the brain's larger-scale anatomical landscape. We'll also take a brief look at the elements of research design that all neuroscientists must consider when designing their studies, and some of the amazing technologies that allow researchers to probe the mysteries of the cells and structures that make up the mind's machine.

See Video 1.1:
Inside the Brain

1.1 The Nervous System Is Made of Specialized Cells

 THE ROAD AHEAD

The first part of the chapter is concerned with the cells of the nervous system. By the end of the section, you should be able to:

1.1.1 Name and describe the general functions of the four main parts of a neuron.

1.1.2 Classify neurons according to both structure and function.

1.1.3 Outline the key components of a synapse and the major steps in neurotransmission.

1.1.4 Describe the four principal types of glial cells and their basic functions.

**View Animation 1.2:
Brain Explorer**

neuron Also called *nerve cell*. The basic unit of the nervous system, each composed of receptive extensions called *dendrites*, an integrating cell body, a conducting axon, and a transmitting axon terminal.

glial cells Also called *glia*. Nonneuronal brain cells that provide structural, nutritional, and other types of support to the brain.

synapse The cellular location at which information is transmitted from a neuron to another cell.

All of your organs and muscles are in communication with the nervous system, which, like all other living tissue, is made up of highly specialized cells. The most important of these are the **neurons** (or *nerve cells*), arranged into the circuits that underlie all forms of behavior, from simple reflexes to complex cognition. Each neuron receives inputs from many other cells, integrates those inputs, and then distributes the processed information to other neurons. Your brain contains 80–90 billion of these tiny cellular computers (Herculano-Houzel, 2012), working together to process vast amounts of information with apparent ease. An even larger number of **glial cells** (sometimes called just *glia*) are found in the human brain, mostly providing a variety of support functions but also participating in information processing. Because neurons are larger and produce readily measured electrical signals, we know much more about them than about glial cells.

An important early controversy in neuroscience concerned the functional independence of individual neurons: Was each neuron a discrete component? Or were the cells of the nervous system fused together into larger functional units, like continuous circuits? Through painstaking study of the fine details of individual neurons, the celebrated Spanish anatomist Santiago Ramón y Cajal (1852–1934) was able to show that although neurons come very close together, they are not quite *continuous* with one another. Ramón y Cajal and his contemporaries established what came to be known as the *neuron doctrine*: (1) neurons and other cells of the brain are structurally, metabolically, and functionally independent, and (2) information is transmitted from neuron to neuron across tiny gaps, later named **synapses**.

It's impossible to measure exactly how many synapses there are in the brain, but scientists think there may be as many as 10^{15} (a *quadrillion*) synapses. That's a number too huge for most of us to comprehend: if you gathered a quadrillion grains of sand, each a millimeter in diameter, they would fill a cube that is longer on each side than an American football field—well over a million cubic yards, or 750,000 cubic meters (in more familiar units that's about 260 million gallons of sand, or 750 million liters)! These vast networks of connections are responsible for all of our achievements.

The neuron has four principal divisions

Although neurons come in hundreds of different shapes and sizes, they all share certain features. Like other cells of the body, a neuron contains genes encoded in DNA inside a cell nucleus, as well as a wide assortment of organelles performing basic functions like producing energy (the mitochondria) to power cellular operations, or translating genetic instructions (the ribosomes) into the specialized proteins essential for the structure and functioning of the neuron (consult the Appendix if you need a refresher on cell biology). But neurons also share a set of unique, highly

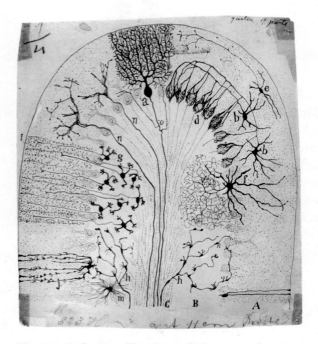

Nineteenth-Century Drawings of Neurons Santiago Ramón y Cajal created detailed drawings of the many types of neurons found in the brain (labeled here by Cajal with lowercase letters). Based on his studies of neurons, Cajal and his collaborators proposed that neurons are discrete cells that communicate via tiny contacts, which were later named *synapses*.

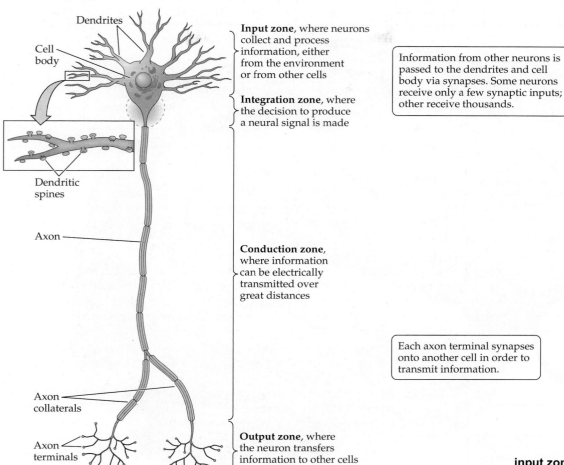

Input zone, where neurons collect and process information, either from the environment or from other cells

Information from other neurons is passed to the dendrites and cell body via synapses. Some neurons receive only a few synaptic inputs; other receive thousands.

Integration zone, where the decision to produce a neural signal is made

Conduction zone, where information can be electrically transmitted over great distances

Each axon terminal synapses onto another cell in order to transmit information.

Output zone, where the neuron transfers information to other cells

Dendrites

Cell body

Dendritic spines

Axon

Axon collaterals

Axon terminals

FIGURE 1.1   The Major Parts of the Neuron

specialized components that allow them to collect input signals from multiple sources, process and combine this information, and distribute the results of this processing to other cells. These information-processing features, illustrated in **FIGURE 1.1**, can be viewed as belonging to four functional zones:

1. **Input zone**   At cellular extensions called **dendrites** (from the Greek *dendron*, "tree"), neurons receive information via synapses from other neurons. Some neurons have dendrites that are elaborately branched, providing room for many synapses. Dendrites may be covered in *dendritic spines*, small projections from the surface of the dendrite that add additional space for synapses.

2. **Integration zone**   In addition to receiving additional synaptic inputs, the neuron's **cell body** (or *soma*, plural *somata*) integrates (combines) the information that has been received to determine whether or not to send a signal of its own.

3. **Conduction zone**   A single extension, the **axon** (or *nerve fiber*), carries the neuron's own electrical signals away from the cell body. Toward its end, the axon may split into multiple branches called **axon collaterals**.

4. **Output zone**   Specialized swellings at the ends of the axon, called **axon terminals** (or *synaptic boutons*), transmit the neuron's signals across synapses to other cells.

input zone   The part of a neuron that receives information from other neurons or from specialized sensory structures.

dendrite   An extension of the cell body that receives information from other neurons.

integration zone   The part of a neuron that initiates neural electrical activity.

cell body   Also called *soma*. The region of a neuron that is defined by the presence of the cell nucleus.

conduction zone   The part of a neuron—typically the axon—over which the action potential is actively propagated.

axon   Also called *nerve fiber*. A single extension from the nerve cell that carries action potentials from the cell body toward the axon terminals.

axon collateral   A branch of an axon.

output zone   The part of a neuron at which the cell sends information to another cell.

axon terminal   Also called *synaptic bouton*. The end of an axon or axon collateral, which forms a synapse onto a neuron or other target cell and thus serves as the output zone.

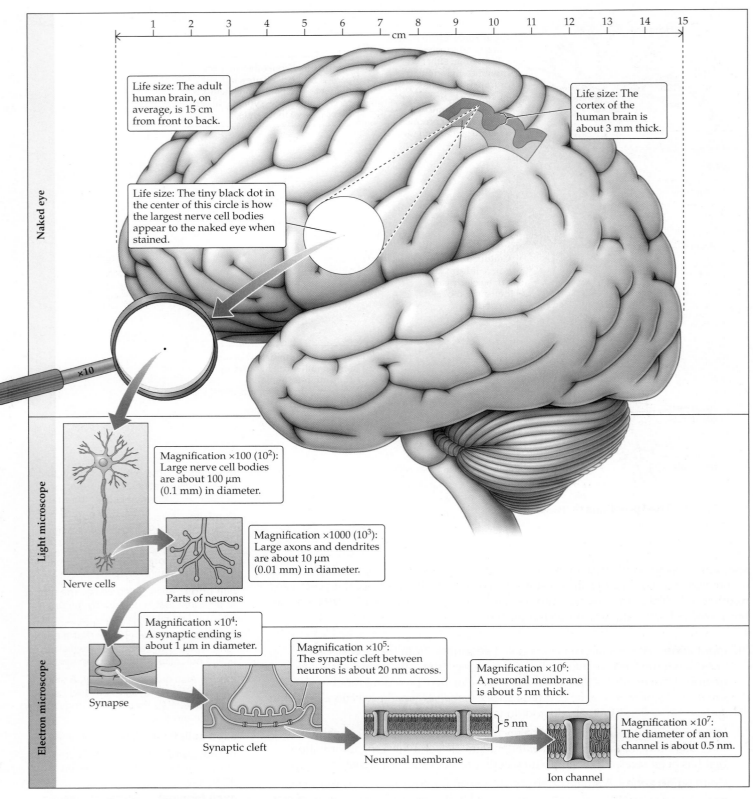

cm

Life size: The adult human brain, on average, is 15 cm from front to back.

Life size: The cortex of the human brain is about 3 mm thick.

Life size: The tiny black dot in the center of this circle is how the largest nerve cell bodies appear to the naked eye when stained.

×10

Naked eye

Magnification ×100 (10^2): Large nerve cell bodies are about 100 μm (0.1 mm) in diameter.

Magnification ×1000 (10^3): Large axons and dendrites are about 10 μm (0.01 mm) in diameter.

Nerve cells

Parts of neurons

Light microscope

Magnification ×10^4: A synaptic ending is about 1 μm in diameter.

Magnification ×10^5: The synaptic cleft between neurons is about 20 nm across.

Magnification ×10^6: A neuronal membrane is about 5 nm thick.

Magnification ×10^7: The diameter of an ion channel is about 0.5 nm.

Synapse

Synaptic cleft

5 nm

Neuronal membrane

Ion channel

Electron microscope

FIGURE 1.2 Sizes of Some Neural Structures and the Units of Measure and Magnification Used in Studying Them

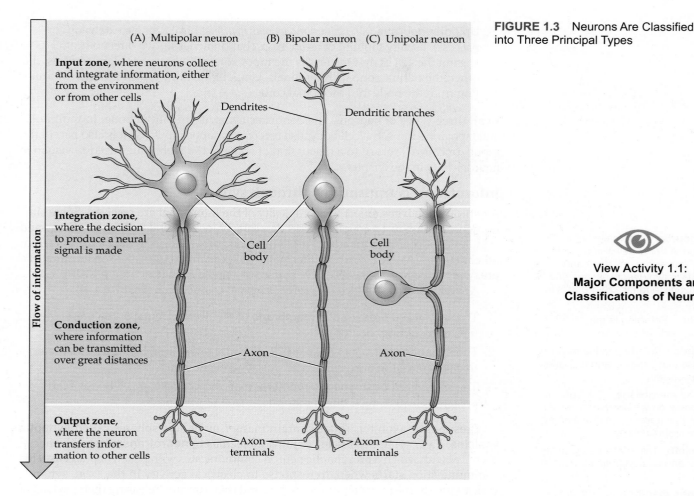

FIGURE 1.3 Neurons Are Classified into Three Principal Types

View Activity 1.1:
Major Components and Classifications of Neurons

The tremendous diversity of sizes, and shapes, and functions of neurons reflects their differing processing functions. For example, **motor neurons** (also called *motoneurons*) are large with long axons reaching out to synapse on muscles, causing muscular contractions. As their name implies, **sensory neurons** are specialized to gather sensory information, and they take many different shapes depending on whether they detect light or sound or touch and so on. Most of the neurons in the brain are **interneurons**, which analyze information gathered from one set of neurons and communicate with others. The axons of interneurons may measure only a few micrometers (μm; a micrometer is a millionth of a meter), while motor neurons and sensory neurons may have axons a meter or more in length, conveying information to and from the most distant parts of the body. In general, larger neurons tend to have more-complex inputs and outputs, cover greater distances, and/or convey information more rapidly than smaller neurons. The relative sizes of neural structures that we will be discussing throughout the book are illustrated in **FIGURE 1.2**.

In addition to size, neuroscientists classify neurons into three general categories of shape, each specialized for a particular kind of information processing (**FIGURE 1.3**):

1. **Multipolar neurons** have many dendrites and a single axon. They are the most common type of neuron.

2. **Bipolar neurons** have a single dendrite at one end of the cell and a single axon at the other end. Bipolar neurons are especially common in sensory systems, such as vision.

motor neuron   Also called *motoneuron*. A neuron that transmits neural messages to muscles (or glands).

sensory neuron   A nerve cell that is directly affected by changes in the environment, such as light, odor, or touch.

interneuron   A nerve cell that is neither a sensory neuron nor a motor neuron. Interneurons receive input from and send output to other neurons.

multipolar neuron   A nerve cell that has many dendrites and a single axon.

bipolar neuron   A nerve cell that has a single dendrite at one end and a single axon at the other end.

3. **Unipolar neurons** (also called *monopolar neurons*) have a single extension (or process), usually thought of as an axon, that branches in two directions after leaving the cell body. One end is the input zone with branches like dendrites; the other, the output zone with terminals. Unipolar neurons transmit touch information from the body into the spinal cord.

In all three types of neurons, the dendrites comprise the input zone. In multipolar and bipolar neurons, the cell body also receives synaptic inputs, so it is also part of the input zone. We'll return to a discussion of some of the techniques used to visualize neurons later in the chapter.

Information is transmitted through synapses

A neuron's dendrites reflect the complexity of the inputs that are received. Some simple neurons have just a couple of short dendritic branches, while others have huge and complex dendritic trees (or *arbors*) receiving many thousands of synaptic contacts from other neurons. At each synapse, information is transmitted from an axon terminal of a **presynaptic** neuron to the receptive surface of a **postsynaptic** neuron (**FIGURE 1.4A**).

A synapse can be divided into three principal components (**FIGURE 1.4B**):

1. The specialized **presynaptic membrane** of the axon terminal of the presynaptic (i.e., transmitting) neuron
2. The **synaptic cleft**, a gap of about 20–40 nanometers (nm; billionths of a meter) that separates the presynaptic and postsynaptic neurons
3. The specialized **postsynaptic membrane** on the dendrite or cell body of the postsynaptic (i.e., receiving) neuron

Presynaptic axon terminals contain many tiny hollow spheres called **synaptic vesicles**. Each synaptic vesicle contains molecules of **neurotransmitter**, the special chemical with which a presynaptic neuron communicates with postsynaptic cells. This communication starts when, in response to electrical activity in the axon, synaptic vesicles fuse to the presynaptic membrane and then rupture, releasing their payload of neurotransmitter molecules into the synaptic cleft (see Figure 1.4B). After crossing the cleft, the released neurotransmitter molecules interact with matching **neurotransmitter receptors** that stud the postsynaptic membrane. The receptors capture and react to molecules of the neurotransmitter, altering the level of excitation of the postsynaptic neuron. This action affects the likelihood that the postsynaptic neuron will in turn release its own neurotransmitter from its axon terminals. Molecules of neurotransmitter generally do not enter the postsynaptic neuron; they simply bind to the outside of the receptors momentarily to induce a response, and then detach and diffuse away.

The configuration of synapses on a neuron's dendrites and cell body is constantly changing—synapses come and go, dendrites change their shapes, dendritic spines wax and wane—in response to new patterns of synaptic activity and the formation of new neural circuits. We use the general term **neuroplasticity** to refer to this capacity for continual remodeling of the connections between neurons. We will take a much more detailed look at neurotransmission in Chapter 2 and Chapter 3.

The axon integrates and then transmits information

Most neurons feature a distinctive cone-shaped enlargement on the cell body called an **axon hillock** ("little hill"), from which the neuron's axon extends. The axon hillock has unique properties that allow it to gather and integrate the information arriving from the synapses on the dendrites and cell body. As we will discuss in more detail later, this process of integration determines when the neuron will produce neural signals of its own. The neuron's output information, encoded in a stream of electrical impulses, then races down the axon toward the targets that the neuron is said to **innervate**.

unipolar neuron Also called *monopolar neuron*. A nerve cell with a single branch that leaves the cell body and then extends in two directions; one end is the input zone, and the other end is the output zone.

presynaptic Referring to the "transmitting" side of a synapse.

postsynaptic Referring to the region of a synapse that receives and responds to neurotransmitter.

presynaptic membrane The specialized membrane on the axon terminal of a nerve cell that transmits information by releasing neurotransmitter.

synaptic cleft The space between the presynaptic and postsynaptic neurons at a synapse.

postsynaptic membrane The specialized membrane on the surface of a neuron that receives information by responding to neurotransmitter from a presynaptic neuron.

synaptic vesicle A small, spherical structure that contains molecules of neurotransmitter.

neurotransmitter Also called *synaptic transmitter*, *chemical transmitter*, or simply *transmitter*. The chemical released from the presynaptic axon terminal that serves as the basis of communication between neurons.

neurotransmitter receptor Also called simply *receptor*. A specialized protein that selectively senses and reacts to molecules of a corresponding neurotransmitter or hormone.

neuroplasticity Also called *neural plasticity*. The ability of the nervous system to change in response to experience or the environment.

axon hillock The cone-shaped area on the cell body from which the axon originates.

innervate To provide neural input to.

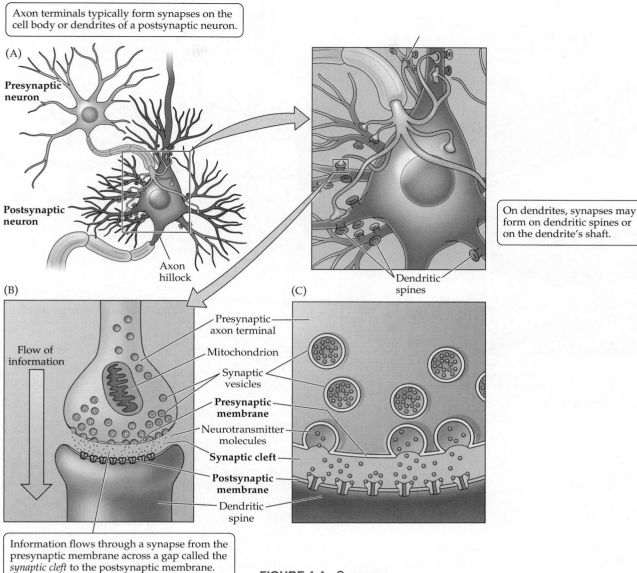

Axon terminals typically form synapses on the cell body or dendrites of a postsynaptic neuron.

(A)

Presynaptic neuron

Postsynaptic neuron

Axon hillock

On dendrites, synapses may form on dendritic spines or on the dendrite's shaft.

Dendritic spines

(B)

Flow of information

Presynaptic axon terminal

Mitochondrion

Synaptic vesicles

Presynaptic membrane

Neurotransmitter molecules

Synaptic cleft

Postsynaptic membrane

Dendritic spine

(C)

Information flows through a synapse from the presynaptic membrane across a gap called the *synaptic cleft* to the postsynaptic membrane.

FIGURE 1.4   Synapses

The axon is a hollow tube, and various important substances, such as enzymes and structural proteins, are conveyed through the interior of the axon from the cell body, where they are produced, to the axon terminals, where they are used. This **axonal transport** works in both directions: *anterograde transport* moves materials toward the axon terminals, and *retrograde transport* moves used materials back to the cell body for recycling. So, it's important to understand that the axon has two quite different functions: the rapid transmission of electrical signals along the outer membrane (like a wire), and the much slower transportation of substances within the axon, to and from the axon terminals (like a pipe).

axonal transport   The transportation of materials from the neuronal cell body toward the axon terminals, and from the axon terminals back toward the cell body.

Glial cells protect and assist neurons

Early neuroscientists had little regard for glial cells, viewing them as a mere filler holding the neurons together (in Greek *glia* means "glue"). But we now know that glial cells are much more important than that. Glial cells directly affect neuronal processes by providing neurons with raw materials, chemical signals, and specialized structural components.

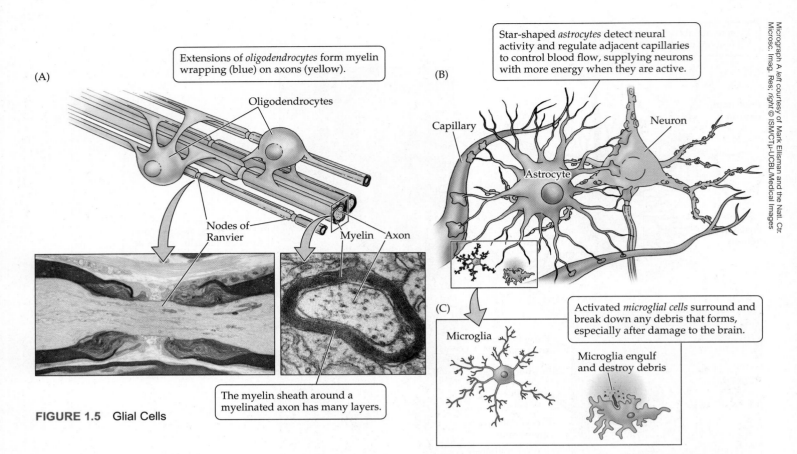

(A)

Extensions of *oligodendrocytes* form myelin wrapping (blue) on axons (yellow).

Oligodendrocytes

Nodes of Ranvier

Myelin   Axon

The myelin sheath around a myelinated axon has many layers.

FIGURE 1.5 Glial Cells

(B)

Star-shaped *astrocytes* detect neural activity and regulate adjacent capillaries to control blood flow, supplying neurons with more energy when they are active.

Capillary

Neuron

Astrocyte

(C)

Microglia

Activated *microglial cells* surround and break down any debris that forms, especially after damage to the brain.

Microglia engulf and destroy debris

oligodendrocyte A type of glial cell that forms myelin in the central nervous system.

Schwann cell A type of glial cell that forms myelin in the peripheral nervous system.

myelin The fatty insulation around an axon, formed by glial cells. This sheath boosts the speed at which nerve impulses are conducted.

node of Ranvier A gap between successive segments of the myelin sheath where the axon membrane is exposed.

astrocyte A star-shaped glial cell with numerous processes (extensions) that run in all directions.

microglial cells Also called *microglia*. Extremely small motile glial cells that remove cellular debris from injured or dead cells.

There are more glial cells than neurons in the brain (Herculano-Houzel, 2014), but in contrast to the hundreds of types of neurons that have been identified, there are just four main kinds of glial cells (**FIGURE 1.5**). Two of these four types of glia—**oligodendrocytes** and **Schwann cells**—wrap around successive segments of axons to insulate them with a fatty substance called **myelin**. These myelin sheaths give an axon the appearance of a string of elongated slender beads. Between adjacent beads, small uninsulated patches of axonal membrane, called **nodes of Ranvier**, remain exposed (**FIGURE 1.5A**). Within the brain and spinal cord, myelination is provided by the oligodendrocytes, each cell typically supplying myelin beads to several nearby axons (also illustrated in Figure 1.5A). In the rest of the body, it is Schwann cells that do the ensheathing, with each Schwann cell wrapping itself around a segment of one axon to provide a single bead of myelin. But whether it is provided by oligodendrocytes or by Schwann cells, myelination has the same result: a large increase in the speed with which electrical signals pass down the axon, jumping from one node of Ranvier to the next. (In Chapter 2 we discuss the diverse abnormalities that arise when the myelin insulation is compromised in the disease multiple sclerosis [MS].)

The other two types of glial cells—astrocytes and microglial cells—perform more diverse functions in the brain. **Astrocytes** (from the Greek *astron*, "star," for their usual shape) weave around and between neurons with tentacle-like extensions (**FIGURE 1.5B**). Some astrocytes stretch between neurons and fine blood vessels, controlling local blood flow to increase the amount of blood reaching more-active brain regions (Schummers et al., 2008). Astrocytes help to form the tough outer membranes that swaddle the brain, and they also secrete chemical signals that affect synaptic transmission and the formation of synapses (Perea et al., 2009; Eroglu and Barres, 2010). In contrast, **microglial cells** (or *microglia*) are tiny and mobile (**FIGURE 1.5C**). Their primary job appears to be to contain and clean up sites of injury (S. A. Wolf et al., 2017). However, astrocytes and microglia may also worsen some problems, such as harmful swelling (*edema*) following brain injury, and degenerative processes like Alzheimer's disease (Chapter 4) and Parkinson's disease (Chapter 11) (W. S. Chung et al., 2015; Liddelow et al., 2017).

Supported and influenced by glial cells, and sharing information through synapses, neurons form the vast ensembles of information-processing circuits that give the brain its visible form. Powerful anatomical and genetic initiatives, such as the Allen Institute brain-mapping project (www.brain-map.org), are creating detailed maps of the cellular composition of the major divisions of the nervous system. These major divisions are our next topic.

HOW'S IT GOING ?

1. What are the four "zones" common to all neurons, and what are their functions?
2. Compare and contrast axonal signal transmission and axonal transport.
3. Describe the three main components of the synapse. What are some of the specialized structures found on each side of the synapse?
4. What are the names and general functions of the four types of glial cells?
5. What special properties does myelin have?

1.2 The Nervous System Extends throughout the Body

THE ROAD AHEAD

The second part of the chapter surveys the major components of the nervous system. By the end of the section, you should be able to:

1.2.1 Explain what a nerve is, and distinguish between somatic and autonomic nerves.

1.2.2 Identify the cranial and spinal nerves by name and function.

1.2.3 Describe the general functions of the two divisions of the autonomic nervous system.

1.2.4 Name the main anatomical structures that make up the two cerebral hemispheres.

1.2.5 Summarize the anatomical conventions used to describe locations and projections within the nervous system, and distinguish between gray matter and white matter structures.

1.2.6 Describe the fetal development of the brain, and catalog the major adult brain divisions that arise from each fetal region.

Neuronal cell bodies, dendrites, axons, and glial cells mass together to form the tissues that define the **gross neuroanatomy** of the nervous system—the neural structures that are visible to the unaided eye (in this context *gross* means "large," not "yucky," but you may feel otherwise). The gross view of the entire human nervous system presented in **FIGURE 1.6** reveals the basic division between the **central nervous system** (**CNS**; consisting of the brain and spinal cord) and the **peripheral nervous system** (everything else). Let's take a closer look at the anatomical organization of these systems.

The peripheral nervous system has two divisions

The peripheral nervous system consists of **nerves**—collections of axons bundled together—that extend throughout the body. Some nerves, called **motor nerves**,

gross neuroanatomy   Anatomical features of the nervous system that are apparent to the naked eye.

central nervous system (CNS)   The portion of the nervous system that includes the brain and the spinal cord.

peripheral nervous system   The portion of the nervous system that includes all the nerves and neurons outside the brain and spinal cord.

nerve   A collection of axons bundled together outside the central nervous system.

motor nerve   A nerve that transmits information from the central nervous system to the muscles and glands.

(A)

Here, a modern view of the central nervous system (CNS) is superimposed on the peripheral nervous system as drawn by Andreas Vesalius (1514–1564). The peripheral nervous system connects the body to the CNS.

Central nervous system

Peripheral nervous system

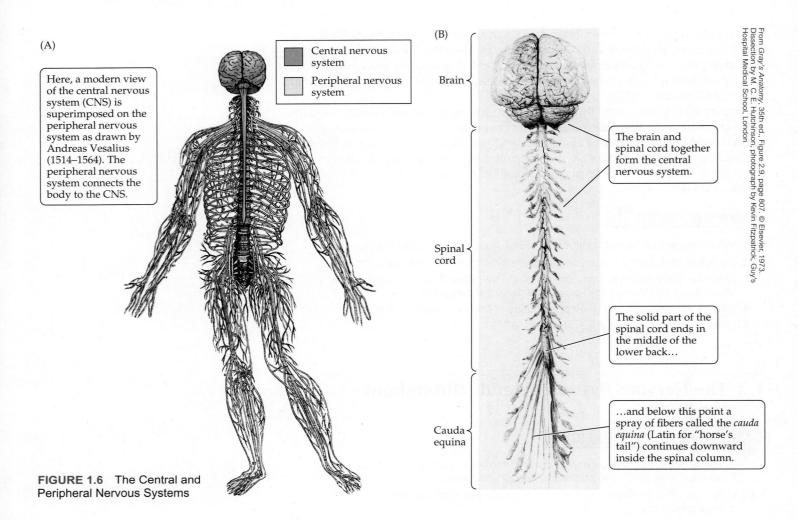

FIGURE 1.6 The Central and Peripheral Nervous Systems

(B)

Brain

The brain and spinal cord together form the central nervous system.

Spinal cord

The solid part of the spinal cord ends in the middle of the lower back…

Cauda equina

…and below this point a spray of fibers called the *cauda equina* (Latin for "horse's tail") continues downward inside the spinal column.

From *Gray's Anatomy*, 35th ed., Figure 2.9, page 807. © Elsevier, 1973. Dissection by M. C. E. Hutchinson, photograph by Kevin Fitzpatrick, Guy's Hospital Medical School, London.

transmit information from the spinal cord and brain to muscles and glands; others, called **sensory nerves**, convey information from the body to the CNS. The various nerves of the body are divided into two distinct systems:

1. The **somatic nervous system**, which consists of nerves that interconnect the brain and the major muscles and sensory systems of the body

2. The **autonomic nervous system**, which consists of nerves that connect primarily to the viscera (internal organs)

THE SOMATIC NERVOUS SYSTEM Taking its name from the Latin word for "body"—*soma*—the somatic nervous system is the main pathway through which the brain controls movement and receives sensory information from the body and from the sensory organs of the head. The nerves that make up the somatic nervous system form two anatomical groups: the cranial nerves and the spinal nerves.

We each have 12 pairs (left and right) of **cranial nerves** that arise from the brain and innervate the head, neck, and visceral organs directly, without ever joining the spinal cord. As you can see in **FIGURE 1.7**, some of these nerves are exclusively sensory: the olfactory (I) nerves transmit information about smell, the optic (II) nerves carry visual information from the eyes, and the vestibulocochlear (VIII) nerves convey information about hearing and balance. Five pairs of cranial nerves are exclusively motor pathways from the brain: the oculomotor (III), trochlear (IV), and abducens (VI) nerves innervate muscles to move the eyes; the spinal accessory (XI) nerves control

sensory nerve A nerve that conveys information from the body to the central nervous system.

somatic nervous system A part of the peripheral nervous system that supplies neural connections mostly to the skeletal muscles and sensory systems of the body. It consists of cranial nerves and spinal nerves.

autonomic nervous system A part of the peripheral nervous system that provides the main neural connections to the internal organs.

cranial nerve A nerve that is connected directly to the brain.

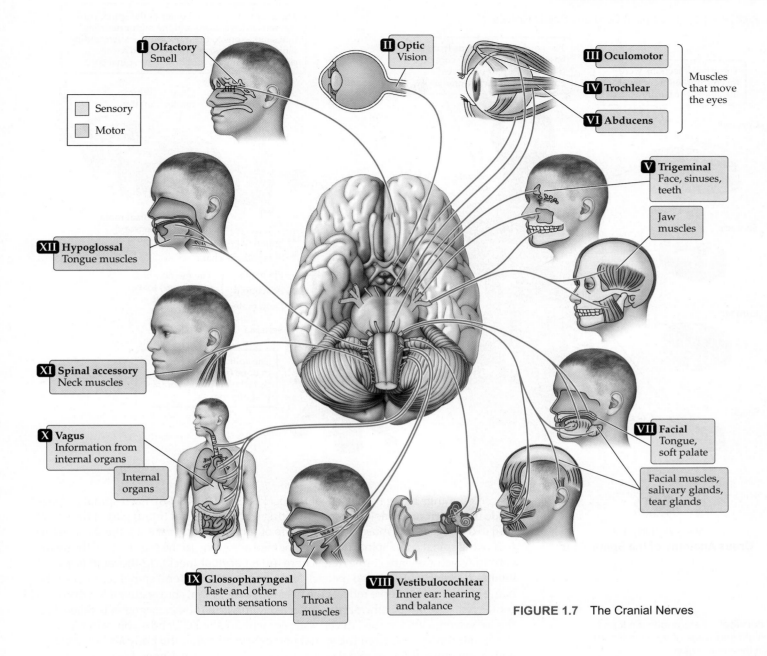

FIGURE 1.7 The Cranial Nerves

neck muscles; and the hypoglossal (XII) nerves control the tongue. The remaining cranial nerves have both sensory and motor functions. The trigeminal (V) nerves, for example, transmit facial sensation through some axons but control the chewing muscles through other axons. The facial (VII) nerves control facial muscles and receive some taste sensation, and the glossopharyngeal (IX) nerves receive additional taste sensations and sensations from the throat and also control the muscles there. The vagus (X) nerve extends far from the head, running to the heart, liver, and intestines, and other organs. Its long, convoluted route is the reason for its name, which is Latin for "wandering." The vagus is the primary route by which the brain both controls and receives information from many visceral organs, and it participates in such varied functions as sweating, digestion, and heart rate (Shaffer et al., 2014).

Along the length of the spinal cord, an additional 31 pairs of **spinal nerves**—again, one member of each pair serves each side of the body—emerge through regularly

**View Activity 1.2:
The Cranial Nerves**

spinal nerve A nerve that emerges from the spinal cord.

FIGURE 1.8 The Spinal Cord and Spinal Nerves

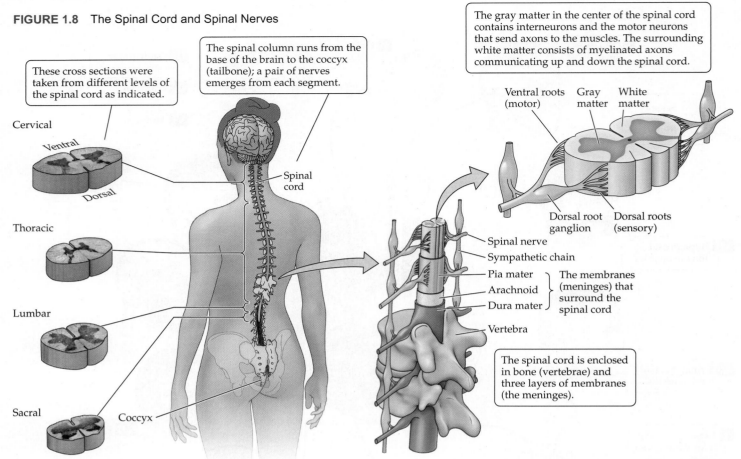

These cross sections were taken from different levels of the spinal cord as indicated.

The spinal column runs from the base of the brain to the coccyx (tailbone); a pair of nerves emerges from each segment.

The gray matter in the center of the spinal cord contains interneurons and the motor neurons that send axons to the muscles. The surrounding white matter consists of myelinated axons communicating up and down the spinal cord.

Cervical
Ventral
Dorsal

Thoracic

Lumbar

Sacral
Coccyx

Spinal cord

Ventral roots (motor)
Gray matter
White matter

Dorsal root ganglion
Dorsal roots (sensory)

Spinal nerve
Sympathetic chain
Pia mater
Arachnoid
Dura mater
} The membranes (meninges) that surround the spinal cord

Vertebra

The spinal cord is enclosed in bone (vertebrae) and three layers of membranes (the meninges).

View Activity 1.3:
Gross Anatomy of the Spinal Cord

cervical   Referring to the topmost eight segments of the spinal cord, in the neck region.

thoracic   Referring to the 12 spinal segments below the cervical (neck) portion of the spinal cord, in the torso.

lumbar   Referring to the five spinal segments in the upper part of the lower back.

sacral   Referring to the five spinal segments in the lower part of the lower back.

coccygeal   Referring to the lowest spinal vertebra (the coccyx, or "tailbone").

sympathetic nervous system   The part of the autonomic nervous system that generally prepares the body for action.

parasympathetic nervous system   The part of the autonomic nervous system that generally prepares the body to relax and recuperate.

spaced openings along both sides of the backbone (**FIGURE 1.8**). Each spinal nerve is made up of a group of motor fibers, projecting from the ventral (front) part of the spinal cord to the organs and muscles, and a group of sensory fibers that enter the dorsal (rear) part of the spinal cord. Spinal nerves are named according to the segments of the spinal cord to which they are connected. There are 8 **cervical** (neck), 12 **thoracic** (torso), 5 **lumbar** (lower back), 5 **sacral** (pelvic), and 1 **coccygeal** (bottom) spinal segments. The name of each spinal nerve reflects the position of the spinal cord segment to which it is connected; for example, the nerve connected to the 12th thoracic segment is called *T12*, the nerve connected to the 7th cervical segment is called *C7*, and so on. After leaving the spinal cord, axons from the spinal nerves spread out in the body and may merge with axons from different spinal nerves to form the various peripheral nerves.

THE AUTONOMIC NERVOUS SYSTEM   Although it is "autonomous" in the sense that we have little conscious, voluntary control over its actions, the autonomic nervous system is the brain's main system for controlling the organs of the body. The activity of our organs is determined by a balance between the two major divisions of the autonomic nervous system—called the *sympathetic* and *parasympathetic nervous systems*—that act more or less in opposition to each other (**FIGURE 1.9**).

Axons of the **sympathetic nervous system** exit from the middle parts of the spinal cord, travel a short distance, and then innervate the *sympathetic ganglia* (small clusters of neurons found outside the CNS), which run in two chains along the spinal column, one on each side (see Figure 1.9 *left*). Axons from the sympathetic ganglia then spread throughout the body, innervating all the major organ systems. In general, sympathetic innervation prepares the body for immediate action: blood pressure increases, the pupils of the eyes widen, the heart quickens, and so on. This set of reactions is sometimes called the *fight-or-flight response*.

FIGURE 1.9   The Autonomic Nervous System

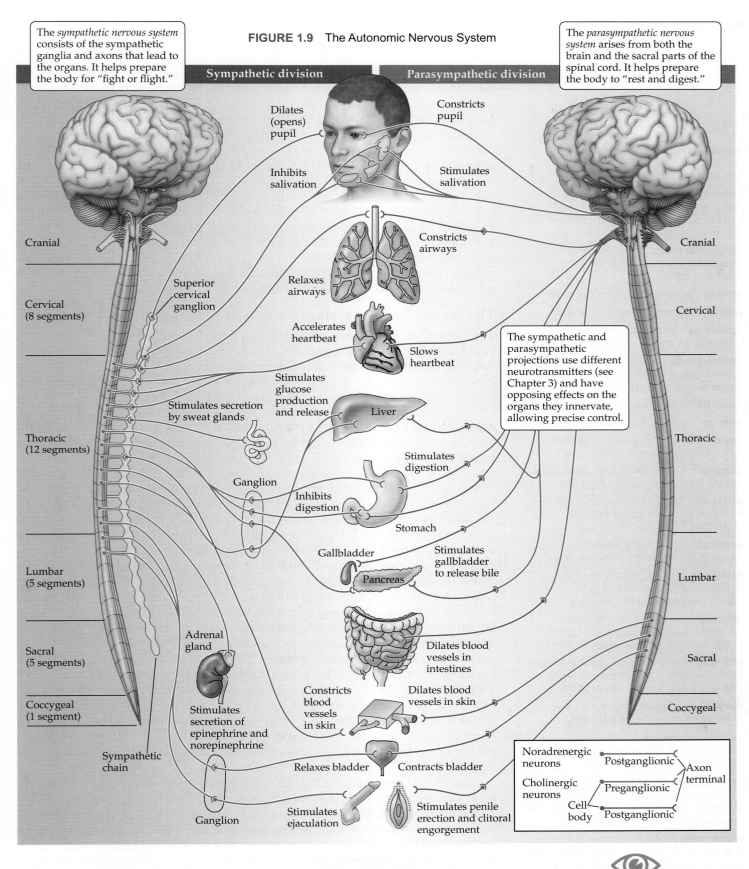

Sympathetic division

Parasympathetic division

The *sympathetic nervous system* consists of the sympathetic ganglia and axons that lead to the organs. It helps prepare the body for "fight or flight."

The *parasympathetic nervous system* arises from both the brain and the sacral parts of the spinal cord. It helps prepare the body to "rest and digest."

Dilates (opens) pupil

Constricts pupil

Inhibits salivation

Stimulates salivation

Cranial

Cervical (8 segments)

Superior cervical ganglion

Constricts airways

Relaxes airways

Cranial

Cervical

The sympathetic and parasympathetic projections use different neurotransmitters (see Chapter 3) and have opposing effects on the organs they innervate, allowing precise control.

Accelerates heartbeat

Slows heartbeat

Stimulates glucose production and release

Stimulates secretion by sweat glands

Liver

Thoracic (12 segments)

Ganglion

Stimulates digestion

Inhibits digestion

Stomach

Thoracic

Gallbladder

Pancreas

Stimulates gallbladder to release bile

Lumbar (5 segments)

Lumbar

Sacral (5 segments)

Adrenal gland

Dilates blood vessels in intestines

Sacral

Coccygeal (1 segment)

Stimulates secretion of epinephrine and norepinephrine

Constricts blood vessels in skin

Dilates blood vessels in skin

Coccygeal

Sympathetic chain

Relaxes bladder

Contracts bladder

Noradrenergic neurons

Cholinergic neurons

Postganglionic

Axon terminal

Preganglionic

Cell body

Postganglionic

Ganglion

Stimulates ejaculation

Stimulates penile erection and clitoral engorgement

In contrast to the effects of sympathetic activity, the **parasympathetic nervous system** generally helps the body to relax, recuperate, and prepare for future action— sometimes called the *rest-and-digest response*. Anatomically, nerves of the parasympathetic system originate in the brainstem (above the sympathetic nerves) and in the

**View Activity 1.4:
Concept Matching:
Sympathetic vs. Parasympathetic**

sagittal plane The plane that divides the body or brain into right and left portions.

coronal plane Also called *frontal plane* or *transverse plane*. The plane that divides the body or brain into front and back parts.

horizontal plane The plane that divides the body or brain into upper and lower parts.

medial In anatomy, toward the middle..

lateral In anatomy, toward one side.

ipsilateral In anatomy, pertaining to a location on the same side of the body.

contralateral In anatomy, pertaining to a location on the opposite side of the body.

superior In anatomy, above.

inferior In anatomy, below.

basal "Toward the base" or "toward the bottom" of a structure.

anterior Also called *rostral*. In anatomy, toward the head end of an organism.

posterior Also called *caudal*. In anatomy, toward the tail end of an organism.

proximal In anatomy, near the trunk or center of an organism. Compare *distal*.

distal In anatomy, toward the periphery of an organism or toward the end of a limb.

afferent Carrying action potentials toward the brain, or toward one region of interest from another region of interest.

efferent Carrying action potentials away from the brain, or away from one region of interest toward another region of interest.

dorsal In anatomy, toward the back of the body or the top of the brain.

ventral In anatomy, toward the belly or front of the body, or the bottom of the brain.

gray matter Areas of the brain that are dominated by cell bodies and are devoid of myelin. Gray matter mostly receives and processes information.

white matter A light-colored layer of tissue, consisting mostly of myelin-sheathed axons, that lies underneath the gray matter of the cortex. White matter mostly transmits information.

cerebral hemisphere One of the two halves—right or left—of the forebrain.

sacral spinal cord (below the sympathetic nerves), which explains the name: the Greek *para* means "around" (see Figure 1.9 *right*). Compared with sympathetic nerves, parasympathetic nerves travel a longer distance before terminating in parasympathetic ganglia, clusters of neurons that are usually located close to the organs they serve.

The sympathetic and parasympathetic systems have very different effects on individual organs because the organs receive different neurotransmitters from the two opposing systems (*norepinephrine* from sympathetic nerves and *acetylcholine* from parasympathetic nerves; see Chapter 2 and Figure 11.19). The balance between the two systems determines the state of the internal organs at any given moment. So, for example, when parasympathetic activity predominates, heart rate slows, blood pressure drops, and digestive processes are activated. As the brain causes the balance of autonomic activity to become predominantly sympathetic, opposite effects are seen: increased heart rate and blood pressure, inhibited digestion, and so on. This tension between parasympathetic and sympathetic activity ensures that the individual is appropriately prepared for current circumstances.

The central nervous system consists of the brain and spinal cord

The spinal cord funnels sensory information from the body up to the brain and conveys the brain's motor commands out to the body. The spinal cord also contains circuits that perform local processing and control simple units of behavior, such as reflexes. We will discuss other aspects of the spinal cord in later chapters, so for now let's focus on the anatomy of the executive portion of the CNS: the brain.

ANATOMICAL CONVENTIONS FOR DESCRIBING THE ANATOMY OF THE BRAIN
Because the nervous system is a three-dimensional structure, two-dimensional illustrations and diagrams cannot represent it completely. Anatomists use standard terminology to help identify structures, locations, and directions in the brain. It's a bit of a chore, but learning the anatomical lingo now will make later discussions of brain organization much easier to follow. As illustrated in **FIGURE 1.10**, the brain is usually visualized in one of three main planes to obtain a two-dimensional section from this three-dimensional object. The plane that divides the brain into right and left portions is called the **sagittal plane**. The plane that divides front (anterior) from back (posterior) is called the **coronal plane** (also known as the *frontal plane*), and the **horizontal plane** divides between upper and lower parts.

In addition to the three planes of dissection, locations in the nervous system are described using directional terms. **Medial** means "toward the middle," whereas **lateral** means "toward the side." **Ipsilateral** means "on the same side," as opposed to **contralateral**, which means "on the opposite side." These terms are all relative, as are the terms **superior** ("above"), **inferior** ("below"), and **basal** ("toward the bottom"). Locations toward the front of the brain are **anterior** or *rostral*, locations toward the rear are **posterior** or *caudal* (from the Latin *cauda*, "tail"). **Proximal** means "near" and **distal** means "far" or "toward the end of a limb." And a nerve or pathway is **afferent** if it carries information into a region that we're interested in, and it's **efferent** if it carries information away from the region of interest (a handy way to remember this is that *e*fferents *e*xit but *a*fferents *a*rrive, relative to the region of interest). Lastly (phew!), **dorsal** means "toward the back," and **ventral** means "toward the belly."

Most people have heard brain tissue referred to as **gray matter**. When you cut into a brain, you see that the outer layers of the cortex have a darker grayish shade (see Figure 1.10). This is because they contain a preponderance of neuronal cell bodies and dendrites. In contrast, the underlying **white matter** gets its snowy appearance from the whitish fatty myelin that insulates many axons. So, a simple view is that gray matter mostly receives and processes information, while white matter mostly transmits information.

THE OUTER SURFACE OF THE BRAIN
On average, the human brain weighs only 1,400 grams (about 3 pounds), accounting for just 2% of the average body weight. Put your two fists together and you get a sense of the size of the two **cerebral hemispheres**—

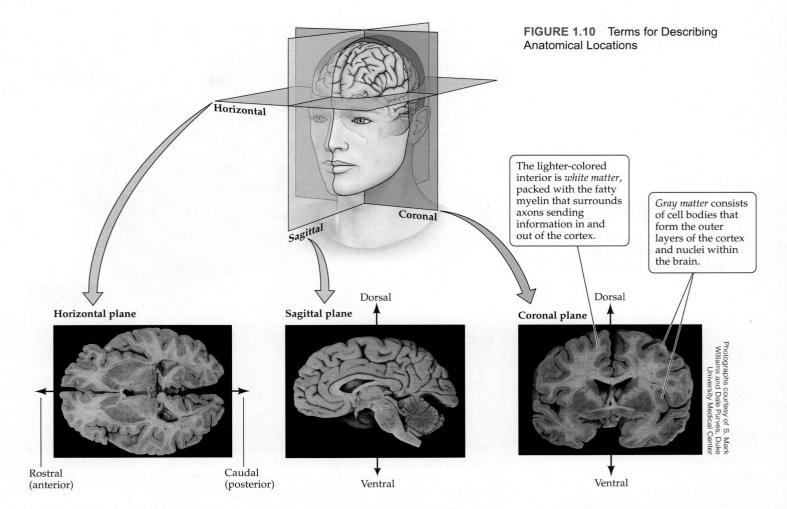

FIGURE 1.10 Terms for Describing Anatomical Locations

Horizontal

Sagittal

Coronal

The lighter-colored interior is *white matter*, packed with the fatty myelin that surrounds axons sending information in and out of the cortex.

Gray matter consists of cell bodies that form the outer layers of the cortex and nuclei within the brain.

Horizontal plane

Sagittal plane

Dorsal

Coronal plane

Dorsal

Rostral (anterior)

Caudal (posterior)

Ventral

Ventral

Photographs courtesy of S. Mark Williams and Dale Purves, Duke University Medical Center

smaller than most people expect. But what the brain lacks in size and weight it makes up for in intricacy. One obvious complication of the brain is its lumpy, convoluted surface—the result of elaborate folding of a thick sheet of tissue, mostly the dendrites, cell bodies, and axonal projections of neurons, called the **cerebral cortex** (or sometimes just *cortex*). The resultant ridges of tissue, called **gyri** (singular *gyrus*), are separated from each other by crevices called **sulci** (singular *sulcus*). Folding up the tissue in this way greatly increases the amount of cortex that can be crammed into the confines of the skull, and about two-thirds of the cerebral cortex is hidden in the depths of these folds. The pattern of folding is not random; in fact, it is similar enough between brains that we can name the various gyri and sulci and group them together into *lobes*.

Using a combination of landmarks and anatomical conventions, neuroscientists distinguish four major cortical regions of each cerebral hemisphere: the **frontal**, **parietal**, **temporal**, and **occipital lobes** (**FIGURE 1.11**). In some cases, the boundaries between adjacent lobes are very clear; for example, the **Sylvian fissure** (or *lateral sulcus*) divides the temporal lobe from other regions of the hemisphere. The **central sulcus** provides a distinct landmark dividing the frontal and parietal lobes. The physical boundaries between the occipital lobe and the temporal and parietal lobes are less obvious, but the lobes are quite different with regard to the functions they perform.

The cortex is the seat of complex cognition. Depending on the specific regions affected, cortical damage can cause symptoms ranging from impairments of movement or body sensation; through speech errors, memory problems, and personality changes; to many kinds of visual impairments. In people with undamaged brains, the four lobes of the cortex are continually communicating and collaborating in order to produce the seamless control of complex behavior that distinguishes us as individuals.

cerebral cortex Also called simply *cortex*. The outer covering of the cerebral hemispheres, which consists largely of nerve cell bodies and their branches.

gyrus A ridged or raised portion of the cortical surface.

sulcus A crevice or valley of the cortical surface.

frontal lobe The most anterior portion of the cerebral cortex.

parietal lobe The large region of cortex lying between the frontal and occipital lobes in each cerebral hemisphere.

temporal lobe The large lateral region of cortex in each cerebral hemisphere. It is continuous with the parietal lobe posteriorly and separated from the frontal lobe by the Sylvian fissure.

occipital lobe A large region of cortex that covers much of the posterior part of each cerebral hemisphere.

Sylvian fissure Also called *lateral sulcus*. A deep fissure that demarcates the temporal lobe.

central sulcus A fissure that divides the frontal lobe from the parietal lobe.

FIGURE 1.11 The Human Brain Has Four Distinct Lobes

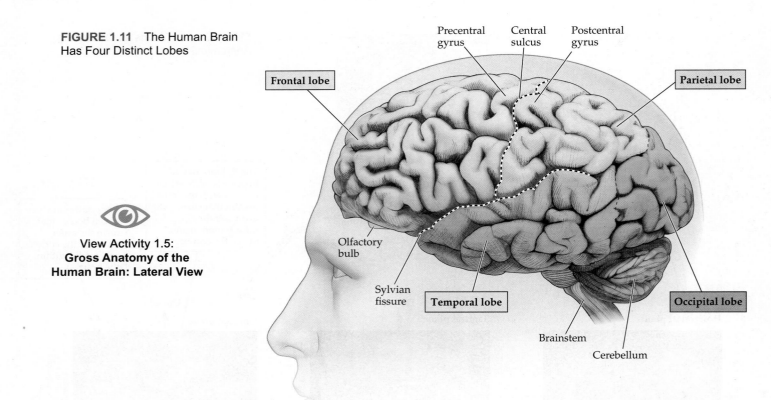

View Activity 1.5:
Gross Anatomy of the Human Brain: Lateral View

corpus callosum The main band of axons that connects the two cerebral hemispheres.

postcentral gyrus The strip of parietal cortex, just posterior to (behind) the central sulcus, that receives somatosensory information from the entire body.

precentral gyrus The strip of frontal cortex, just anterior to (in front of) the central sulcus, that is crucial for motor control.

neural tube An embryonic structure with subdivisions that correspond to the future forebrain, midbrain, and hindbrain.

forebrain The frontal division the neural tube, containing the cerebral hemispheres, the thalamus, and the hypothalamus.

midbrain The middle division of the brain.

hindbrain The rear division of the brain, which in the mature vertebrate contains the cerebellum, pons, and medulla.

telencephalon The anterior part of the fetal forebrain, which will become the cerebral hemispheres in the adult brain.

diencephalon The posterior part of the fetal forebrain, which will become the thalamus and hypothalamus in the adult brain.

brainstem The region of the brain that consists of the midbrain, the pons, and the medulla.

Furthermore, hundreds of millions of axons connect the left and right hemispheres via the **corpus callosum**, allowing the brain to act as a single entity during complex processing. Some life-sustaining functions—heart rate and respiration, reflexes, balance, and the like—are governed by lower, subcortical brain regions.

The sense of touch is mediated by a strip of parietal cortex just behind the central sulcus called the **postcentral gyrus** (see Figure 1.11), so it is often referred to as the *primary somatosensory cortex*. In front of the central sulcus, the **precentral gyrus**—*primary motor cortex*—of the frontal lobe is crucial for motor control. As we will see in later chapters, both gyri exhibit *somatotopic organization*, which means that they precisely map the various parts of the contralateral side of the body (Penfield and Rasmussen, 1950). The occipital lobes are crucial for vision, and the temporal lobes receive auditory inputs and help in memory formation. But each lobe of the brain also performs a wide variety of other high-level functions. These will be major topics in later chapters.

DEVELOPMENT OF SUBDIVISIONS WITHIN THE BRAIN It can be difficult to understand the origin of some of the regional names applied to the adult human brain. For example, part of the brain closest to the back of the head is anatomically identified as part of the forebrain. Why? The key to understanding this confusing terminology is to consider how the gross anatomy of the brain develops early in life.

In a very young embryo of any vertebrate, the CNS looks like a tube (Chapter 4). The walls of this **neural tube** are made of cells, and the interior is filled with fluid. A few weeks after conception, the human neural tube begins to show three separate swellings at the head end (**FIGURE 1.12A**): the **forebrain**, the **midbrain**, and the **hindbrain**; the remainder of the neural tube eventually forms the spinal cord. By about 50 days, the fetal forebrain features two clear subdivisions. At the very front is the **telencephalon** (from the Greek *encephalon*, "brain"), which will become the cerebral hemispheres (consisting of cortex plus some deeper structures). The other part of the forebrain is the **diencephalon**, which will go on to become the thalamus and the hypothalamus, two of the many subcortical structures of the forebrain.

Similarly, the hindbrain further develops into several large structures: the cerebellum, pons, and medulla. The term **brainstem** usually refers to the midbrain, pons, and medulla combined (some scientists include the diencephalon too). **FIGURES 1.12B** and **C** show the positions of these structures and their relative sizes in the adult human brain. Even when the brain achieves its adult form, it is still a fluid-filled tube, but a tube of very complicated shape.

The main sections of the brain can be subdivided in turn. We can work our way from the largest, most general divisions of the nervous system on the left of the schematic in Figure 1.12B to more-specific ones on the right.

Within and between the major brain regions are collections of neurons called **nuclei** (singular *nucleus*) and bundles of axons called **tracts**. Recall that outside the CNS, collections of neurons are called *ganglia*, and bundles of axons are called *nerves*. Unfortunately, the word *nucleus* can mean either "a collection of neurons in the CNS" or "the spherical DNA-containing organelle within a single cell." You must rely on the context to understand which meaning is intended. Because brain tracts and nuclei are the same in different individuals, and often the same in different species, they have names too (many, many names).

You are probably more interested in the functions of all these parts of the brain than in their names, but as we noted earlier, each region serves more than one function, and

nucleus   Here, a collection of neuronal cell bodies within the central nervous system (e.g., the caudate nucleus).

tract   A bundle of axons found within the central nervous system.

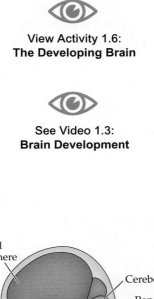

View Activity 1.6:
The Developing Brain

See Video 1.3:
Brain Development

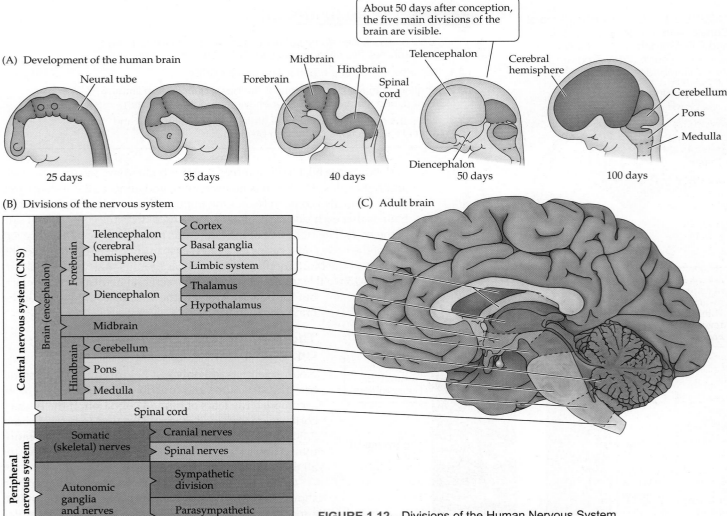

(A) Development of the human brain

About 50 days after conception, the five main divisions of the brain are visible.

Neural tube

Forebrain   Midbrain   Hindbrain   Spinal cord   Telencephalon   Cerebral hemisphere   Cerebellum   Pons   Medulla   Diencephalon

25 days   35 days   40 days   50 days   100 days

(B) Divisions of the nervous system

(C) Adult brain

FIGURE 1.12   Divisions of the Human Nervous System in the Embryo and the Adult

our knowledge of the functional organization of the brain is continually being updated with new research findings. So, with that caution in mind, we'll briefly survey the functions of specific brain structures next, leaving the detailed discussion for later chapters.

View Activity 1.7: The Basal Ganglia and Activity 1.8: The Limbic System

HOW'S IT GOING ❓

1. Name and briefly describe the major divisions of the peripheral nervous system. What general function does each part perform?
2. Briefly sketch and describe the anatomical organization of the cranial nerves. How many nerves are there? Now do the same for the spinal nerves.
3. Give some examples of how each division of the autonomic nervous system affects organs of the body.
4. Why does the cortex look so lumpy on the outside?
5. What is special about the pre- and postcentral gyri?
6. Review the fetal development of the brain, and the major divisions of the brain that arise from the earlier fetal form of the nervous system.

1.3 The Brain Shows Regional Specialization of Functions

THE ROAD AHEAD

Functional neuroanatomy connects behaviors to brain regions. By the end of this section, you should be able to:

1.3.1 Describe the cellular organization of the cortex.

1.3.2 Identify the major components of the basal ganglia and limbic system, and state some of the behavioral functions of each.

1.3.3 Name the major divisions of the brainstem and midbrain, and identify key functions performed by each.

Vertebrates are bilaterally symmetrical: our bodies have mirror-image left and right sides. The brain is no exception, and almost all the structures of the brain also come in twos. One important principle of the vertebrate brain is that each side of the brain generally controls the contralateral side of the body. The right side of the brain thus controls movement of the left side of the body and receives left-sided sensory information. Likewise, the left side of the brain monitors and controls the right side of the body. In Chapter 15 we'll learn about how the two cerebral hemispheres interact, but for now let's review the various components of the brain and their functions.

The cerebral cortex performs complex cognitive processing

Neuroscientists are only just beginning to understand how the structures and functions of the cerebral cortex accomplish the feats of human cognition. If the human cortex were unfolded, it would occupy an area of about 2,000 square centimeters (315 square inches)—more than 3 times the area of this book's front cover. How are all those millions of cells arranged?

Cortical neurons make up six distinct layers, as shown in **FIGURE 1.13**. Each cortical layer has a unique appearance because it consists of either a band of similar neurons, or a particular pattern of dendrites or axons.

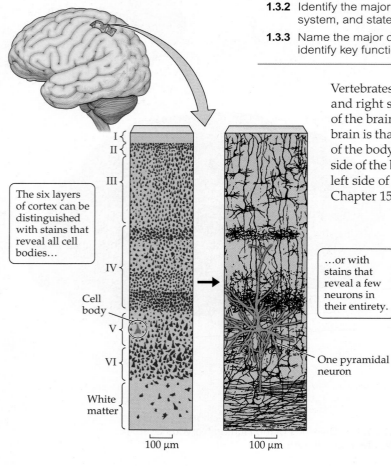

FIGURE 1.13 Layers of the Cerebral Cortex (After P. Rakic, in F. O. Schmitt and F. G. Worden, 1979. *The Neurosciences: Fourth Study Program.* MIT Press: Cambridge, MA.)

The six layers of cortex can be distinguished with stains that reveal all cell bodies…

…or with stains that reveal a few neurons in their entirety.

Cell body

One pyramidal neuron

White matter

100 μm   100 μm

I
II
III
IV
V
VI

For example, the outermost layer, layer I, is distinct because it has few cell bodies, while layers V and VI stand out because of their many neurons with large cell bodies. The most prominent kind of neuron in the cerebral cortex—the **pyramidal cell**—usually has its pyramid-shaped cell body in layer III or V.

In some regions of the cerebral cortex, neurons are organized into regular columns, perpendicular to the layers, that seem to serve as information-processing units (Horton and Adams, 2005). These **cortical columns** extend through the entire thickness of the cortex, from the white matter to the surface. Within each column, most of the synaptic interconnections of neurons are vertical, although there are some horizontal connections as well (Mountcastle, 1979; Sakmann, 2017).

Important nuclei are hidden beneath the cerebral cortex

Buried within the cerebral hemispheres are several large gray matter structures, richly connected to each other and to other brain regions and contributing to a wide variety of behaviors. One prominent cluster—the **basal ganglia**, consisting primarily of the *caudate nucleus*, the *putamen*, and the *globus pallidus* (**FIGURE 1.14A**)—plays a critical role in the control of movement (see Chapter 5).

Curving through each hemisphere, alongside the basal ganglia, lies a loose network of structures called the **limbic system** (identified in **FIGURE 1.14B**) that is involved in emotion and learning. The **amygdala** is a limbic structure involved in emotional regulation (see Chapter 11) and the perception of odor (see Chapter 6). The **hippocampus** and **fornix** are important for learning and memory (see Chapter 13). A strip of cortex atop the corpus callosum in each hemisphere, called the **cingulate gyrus**, is implicated in many cognitive functions, including the direction of attention (see Chapter 14), and the **olfactory bulb** processes the sense of smell. Other limbic structures near the base of the brain, especially the hypothalamus, help to govern motivated behaviors, like sex and aggression, and to regulate the hormonal systems of the body.

Toward the medial (middle) and basal (bottom) aspects of the forebrain are found the **thalamus** and the **hypothalamus** (the latter means simply "under thalamus"). You can see both the hypothalamus and thalamus in Figure 1.14B and Figure 1.15A. The thalamus is the brain's traffic cop, directing virtually all incoming sensory information

pyramidal cell   A type of large nerve cell that has a roughly pyramid-shaped cell body and is found in the cerebral cortex.

cortical column   One of the vertical columns that constitute the basic organization of the cerebral cortex.

basal ganglia   A group of forebrain nuclei, including the caudate nucleus, globus pallidus, and putamen, found deep within the cerebral hemispheres.

limbic system   A loosely defined, widespread group of brain nuclei that innervate each other and form a network.

amygdala   A group of nuclei in the medial anterior part of the temporal lobe.

hippocampus   A medial temporal lobe structure that is important for learning and memory.

fornix   A fiber tract that extends from the hippocampus to the mammillary body.

cingulate gyrus   A strip of cortex, found in the frontal and parietal midline, that is part of the limbic system and is implicated in many cognitive functions.

olfactory bulb   An anterior projection of the brain that terminates in the upper nasal passages and provides the primary inputs for the sense of smell.

thalamus   Paired structures to either side of the third ventricle that direct the flow of sensory information to and from the cortex.

hypothalamus   Part of the diencephalon, lying ventral to the thalamus.

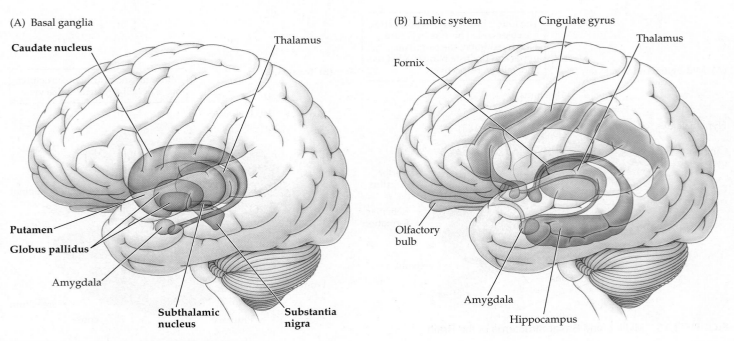

(A) Basal ganglia

Caudate nucleus
Thalamus
Putamen
Globus pallidus
Amygdala
Subthalamic nucleus
Substantia nigra

(B) Limbic system

Cingulate gyrus
Thalamus
Fornix
Olfactory bulb
Amygdala
Hippocampus

FIGURE 1.14   Two Important Brain Systems

tectum   The dorsal portion of the midbrain, consisting of the inferior and superior colliculi.

superior colliculi   Paired gray matter structures of the dorsal midbrain that process visual information.

inferior colliculi   Paired gray matter structures of the dorsal midbrain that process auditory information.

tegmentum   The main body of the midbrain, containing the substantia nigra, periaqueductal gray, part of the reticular formation, and multiple fiber tracts.

substantia nigra   A brainstem structure that innervates the basal ganglia and is a major source of dopaminergic projections.

periaqueductal gray   A midbrain region involved in pain perception.

reticular formation   An extensive region of the brainstem, extending from the medulla through the thalamus, that is involved in sleep and arousal.

cerebellum   A structure located at the back of the brain, dorsal to the pons, that is involved in the central regulation of movement and in some forms of learning.

View Activity 1.9:
Gross Anatomy of the Human Brain: Midsagittal View
and Activity 1.10:
Gross Anatomy of the Human Brain: Basal View

to the appropriate regions of the cortex for further processing, and receiving instructions back from the cortex about which sensory information is to be transmitted. The small but mighty hypothalamus has a much different role: it is packed with discrete nuclei involved in many vital functions, such as hunger, thirst, temperature regulation, sex, and many more. Furthermore, because the hypothalamus also controls the pituitary gland, it serves as the brain's main interface with the hormonal systems of the body. We'll encounter the hypothalamus again in several later chapters.

The midbrain has sensory and motor components

Compared with the forebrain and hindbrain, the midbrain doesn't encompass a lot of tissue, but that doesn't mean its components are unimportant. The top part of the midbrain, called the **tectum** (from the Latin for "roof," because it's atop the midbrain), features two pairs of bumps—one pair in each hemisphere—with specific roles in sensory processing. The more rostral bumps are called the **superior colliculi** (singular *colliculus*), and they have specific roles in visual processing. The more caudal bumps, called the **inferior colliculi** (see Figure 1.15A), process information about sound.

The main body of the midbrain is called the **tegmentum**, and it also contains several important structures. The **substantia nigra** is in many ways a part of the basal ganglia, and loss of its neurons (which normally release the neurotransmitter dopamine within the forebrain) leads to Parkinson's disease, discussed in Chapter 5. The **periaqueductal gray** is a midbrain structure implicated in the perception of pain (see Chapter 3). The **reticular formation** (*reticular* means "netlike") is a loose collection of neurons that are important in a variety of behaviors, including sleep and arousal (see Chapter 10). Multiple large tracts of nerve fibers run in, out, and through the midbrain to connect the brain to the spinal cord.

The brainstem controls vital body functions

The midsagittal and basal views of the brain in **FIGURE 1.15** show the hemispheres of the **cerebellum**, which is tucked up under the posterior cortex and attached to the dorsal brainstem. Like the cerebral cortex, the cerebellum is highly convoluted, but it is made up of a simpler three-layered tissue instead of the six layers found in the cerebral cortex. The cerebellum has long been known to be crucial for motor coordination and

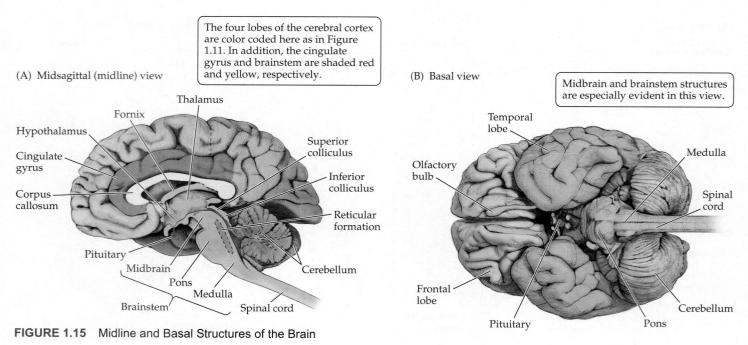

(A) Midsagittal (midline) view

The four lobes of the cerebral cortex are color coded here as in Figure 1.11. In addition, the cingulate gyrus and brainstem are shaded red and yellow, respectively.

Thalamus
Fornix
Hypothalamus
Cingulate gyrus
Corpus callosum
Pituitary
Midbrain
Pons
Medulla
Brainstem
Spinal cord
Superior colliculus
Inferior colliculus
Reticular formation
Cerebellum

(B) Basal view

Midbrain and brainstem structures are especially evident in this view.

Temporal lobe
Olfactory bulb
Medulla
Spinal cord
Frontal lobe
Pituitary
Pons
Cerebellum

FIGURE 1.15   Midline and Basal Structures of the Brain

control, but we now know that it also participates in certain aspects of cognition, including learning. The adjacent **pons** (from the Latin word for "bridge") contains many nerve fibers and important motor control and sensory nuclei; it is the point of origin for several cranial nerves. The reticular formation, which we first saw in the midbrain, stretches down through the pons and ends in the medulla.

The **medulla** marks the transition from the brain to the spinal cord. In addition to conveying all of the major motor and sensory fibers to and from the body, the medulla contains nuclei that drive such essential processes as respiration and heart rate, so brainstem injuries are often lethal. And like other parts of the brainstem, the medulla gives rise to several cranial nerves.

pons The portion of the brainstem that connects the midbrain to the medulla.

medulla The posterior part of the hindbrain, continuous with the spinal cord.

Behaviors and cognitive processes depend on networks of brain regions

In order to understand the neural origins of our most complex behaviors and experiences—thought, language, music—it will be necessary to understand how different brain regions with distinct functions collaborate in larger-scale networks. This applies to functional units as small as the individual cortical columns we mentioned earlier and to much larger assemblages of millions of cells making up substantial parts of cortical lobes.

Cortical regions communicate with one another via tracts of axons looping through the underlying white matter. Some of these connections are short pathways to nearby cortical regions; others travel longer distances through and between the two cerebral hemispheres and subcortical structures like the basal ganglia. Progress in describing the *"connectome"* of the human brain (Glasser, Coalson et al., 2016)—the network map that completely describes the functional connections within and between brain regions, based on huge volumes of human and nonhuman animal neuroanatomical data (van Essen and Glasser, 2018; Suárez et al., 2020)—is rapidly transforming the field of behavioral neuroscience.

HOW'S IT GOING ?

1. How are the cells of the cerebral cortex organized?
2. Name the major components of the basal ganglia and the limbic system. What behaviors especially rely on these systems?
3. What functions are served by the thalamus and hypothalamus?
4. Name and describe the general functions of the major components of the midbrain and hindbrain.
5. Why are injuries to the medulla often fatal?
6. Define the connectome, and discuss its significance for understanding the functioning of the brain.

1.4 Specialized Support Systems Protect and Nourish the Brain

THE ROAD AHEAD

Next, we consider the specialized structures and fluids that support the operations of the brain. By the end of this section, you should be able to:

1.4.1 Name and describe the meninges, ventricular system, and glymphatic system, and review their clinical significance.

1.4.2 Give an outline of the vascular supply of the brain, and note the signs and symptoms of stroke.

meninges　The three protective membranes—dura mater, pia mater, and arachnoid—that surround the brain and spinal cord.

dura mater　The outermost of the three meninges that surround the brain and spinal cord.

pia mater　The innermost of the three meninges that surround the brain and spinal cord.

arachnoid　The thin covering (one of the three meninges) of the brain that lies between the dura mater and the pia mater.

cerebrospinal fluid (CSF)　The fluid that fills the cerebral ventricles.

meningitis　An acute inflammation of the meninges, usually caused by a viral or bacterial infection.

meningioma　A noninvasive tumor of the meninges.

ventricular system　A system of fluid-filled cavities inside the brain.

lateral ventricle　A complex C-shaped lateral portion of the ventricular system within each hemisphere of the brain.

choroid plexus　A specialized membrane lining the ventricles that produces cerebrospinal fluid by filtering blood.

third ventricle　The midline ventricle that conducts cerebrospinal fluid from the lateral ventricles to the fourth ventricle.

fourth ventricle　The passageway within the pons that receives cerebrospinal fluid from the third ventricle and releases it to surround the brain and spinal cord.

The brain is relatively soft and easily damaged. It also needs a steady and substantial supply of fuel to maintain normal functioning, and thus keep us alive. Fortunately, the brain is equipped with systems to protect and cushion it and to provide a continual source of energy, nutrients, and important chemicals.

The brain floats within layers of membranes

Within the bony skull and vertebrae, the brain and spinal cord are swaddled by three protective membranes called **meninges** (see Figure 1.8). Between a tough outer sheet called the **dura mater** (in Latin, literally "tough mother") and the delicate **pia mater** ("tender mother") that adheres tightly to the surface of the brain, a webby substance called the **arachnoid** ("spiderweb-like") creates a reservoir called the *subarachnoid space* that suspends the brain in a bath of a watery liquid called **cerebrospinal fluid** (**CSF**). The meninges can become inflamed by infections, termed **meningitis**, or distorted by a hemorrhage; either situation is a medical emergency because the brain is squeezed and impaired. Tumors called **meningiomas** can form in the meninges and are technically benign, because they don't spread, but any mass that takes up space in the enclosed cranium is far from harmless.

The brain relies on two fluids for survival

The brain essentially floats in cerebrospinal fluid within the subarachnoid space, cushioning it from minor blows to the head. But CSF has additional important roles, passing into the substance of the brain, conveying nutrients and signaling chemicals, and picking up waste matter for later clearance. Inside the brain is a series of chambers called the *cerebral ventricles*, which are filled with CSF (**FIGURE 1.16**). These chambers comprise the **ventricular system**. Each hemisphere of the brain contains a **lateral ventricle** extending into all four lobes of the hemisphere. The lateral ventricles are lined with a specialized membrane called the **choroid plexus**, which produces CSF by filtering blood. The CSF flows from the lateral ventricles into a midline **third ventricle** (so named because it follows the two lateral ventricles) and continues down a narrow passage (the *cerebral aqueduct*) to the **fourth ventricle**, which lies between the cerebellum and the pons. Just below the cerebellum, three small openings allow CSF to exit the ventricular system and circulate over the outer surface of the brain and spinal cord. The CSF is absorbed back into the circulatory system through large veins

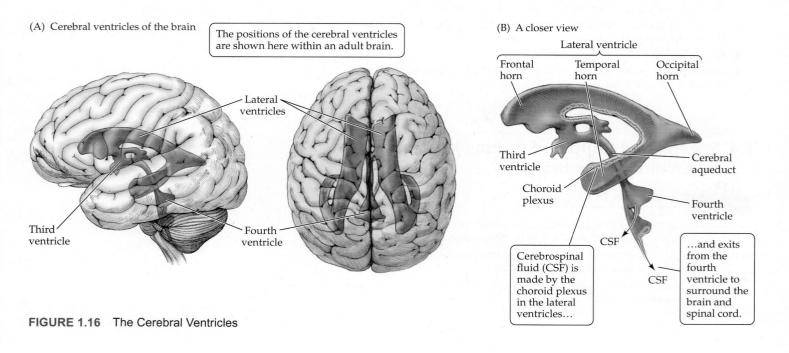

(A) Cerebral ventricles of the brain

The positions of the cerebral ventricles are shown here within an adult brain.

Lateral ventricles

Third ventricle

Fourth ventricle

(B) A closer view

Lateral ventricle

Frontal horn

Temporal horn

Occipital horn

Third ventricle

Choroid plexus

Cerebral aqueduct

Fourth ventricle

CSF

CSF

Cerebrospinal fluid (CSF) is made by the choroid plexus in the lateral ventricles…

…and exits from the fourth ventricle to surround the brain and spinal cord.

FIGURE 1.16　The Cerebral Ventricles

beneath the top of the skull. A problem that blocks the flow of CSF through the ventricular system may result in **hydrocephalus**, a ballooning of the ventricles as they accumulate fluid, resulting in greatly varying symptoms.

Although the brain had long been thought to lack the lymphatic system found in other tissues, the recently discovered **glymphatic system** (**FIGURE 1.17**; the name reflects the involvement of glial cells) provides for drainage of waste-bearing CSF-derived fluids from the brain as well as the distribution of various nutrients, immune system components, and signaling substances (Jessen et al., 2015; Mestre et al., 2020). Curiously, glymphatic clearance occurs primarily while we sleep, and

hydrocephalus A ballooning of the ventricles, at the expense of the surrounding brain, which may occur when the circulation of CSF is blocked.

glymphatic system A lymphatic system in the brain that participates in removal of wastes and the movement of nutrients and signaling compounds.

**View Activity 1.11:
The Cerebral Ventricles**

Glymphatic drainage, which occurs primarily during sleep, helps clear debris and wastes from the brain, including proteins that have been implicated in Alzheimer's disease.

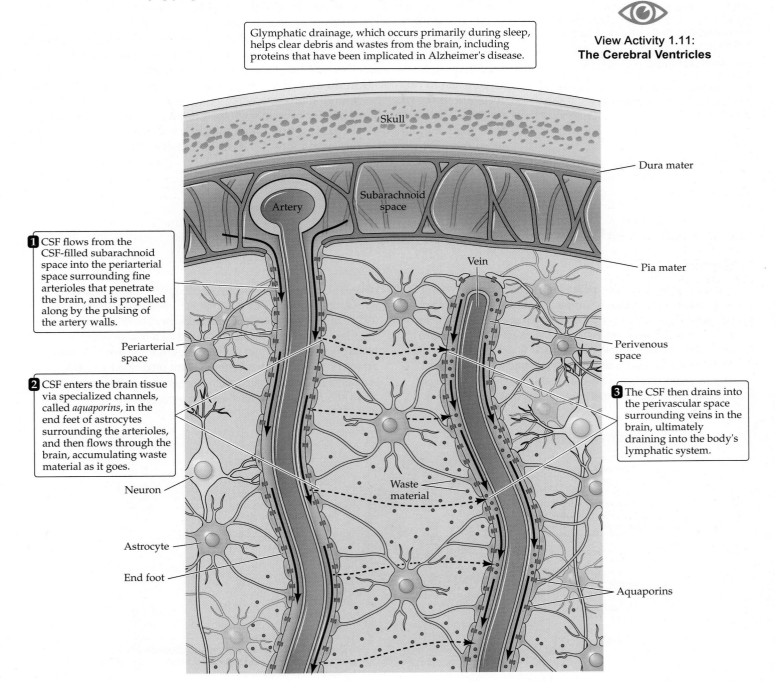

1 CSF flows from the CSF-filled subarachnoid space into the periarterial space surrounding fine arterioles that penetrate the brain, and is propelled along by the pulsing of the artery walls.

2 CSF enters the brain tissue via specialized channels, called *aquaporins*, in the end feet of astrocytes surrounding the arterioles, and then flows through the brain, accumulating waste material as it goes.

3 The CSF then drains into the perivascular space surrounding veins in the brain, ultimately draining into the body's lymphatic system.

Skull

Dura mater

Subarachnoid space

Artery

Vein

Pia mater

Periarterial space

Perivenous space

Neuron

Waste material

Astrocyte

End foot

Aquaporins

FIGURE 1.17 **The Glymphatic System** (After M. Nedergaard and S. A. Goldman. 2016. *Sci. Am.* 314: 44–49.)

cerebral arteries   The three pairs of large arteries within the skull that supply blood to the cerebral cortex.

blood-brain barrier   The mechanisms that make the movement of substances from blood vessels into cells more difficult in the brain than in other body organs, thus affording the brain greater protection from exposure to some substances found in the blood.

stroke   Damage to a region of brain tissue that results from the blockage or rupture of vessels that supply blood to that region.

transient ischemic attack (TIA) A temporary blood restriction to part of the brain that causes stroke-like symptoms that quickly resolve, serving as a warning of elevated stroke risk.

researchers are working to understand how this system may protect against neurological problems such as Alzheimer's disease, stroke, and multiple sclerosis (M. K. Rasmussen et al., 2018).

The second crucial fluid for the brain is, of course, blood. Without a lavish supply of oxygen- and nutrient-rich blood, the tissue of the brain would swiftly die. That's because brain tissue is unusually needy: it accounts for only 2% of the average human body but consumes more than 20% of the body's energy at rest. So the brain is critically dependent on a set of large blood vessels. Blood arrives in the brain via two pairs of arteries: the *carotid arteries* in the neck, and the *vertebral arteries* that ascend within each side of the vertebrae of the neck, fusing to form the *basilar artery* inside the skull. These arteries give rise to a set of three pairs of **cerebral arteries** that supply the cortex, plus a number of smaller vessels that penetrate and supply other regions of the brain. Fine vessels and capillaries branching off from the arteries deliver nutrients and other substances to brain cells and remove waste products. In contrast to capillaries in the rest of the body, capillaries in the brain are highly resistant to the passage of large molecules across their walls and into neighboring neurons. This **blood-brain barrier** probably evolved to help protect the brain from infections and blood-borne toxins, but it also makes the delivery of drugs to the brain more difficult. You can learn more about the brain's elaborate vascular system in **A STEP FURTHER 1.1**, on the website.

SIGNS & SYMPTOMS

Stroke

The general term **stroke** applies to a situation in which a clot, a narrowing, or a rupture interrupts the supply of blood to a particular brain region, causing the affected region to stop functioning or die (**FIGURE 1.18**). Although the exact effects of stroke depend on the region of the brain that is affected, the five most common warning signs are sudden numbness or weakness, altered vision, dizziness, severe headache, and confusion or difficulty speaking. Effective treatments are available to help

restore blood flow and minimize the long-term damage of a stroke, but only if the victim is treated immediately (Albers et al., 2018). Some people experience temporary stroke-like symptoms lasting for a few minutes. Caused by a brief interruption of blood supply to some part of the brain, this **transient ischemic attack** (from the Greek *ischemia*, "interrupted blood"), or **TIA**, is a serious warning sign that a major stroke may be imminent, and it should be treated as a medical emergency.

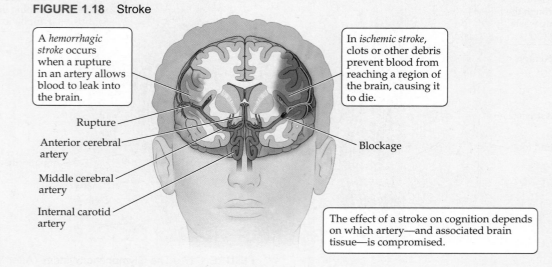

FIGURE 1.18   Stroke

A *hemorrhagic stroke* occurs when a rupture in an artery allows blood to leak into the brain.

In *ischemic stroke*, clots or other debris prevent blood from reaching a region of the brain, causing it to die.

Rupture

Anterior cerebral artery

Middle cerebral artery

Internal carotid artery

Blockage

The effect of a stroke on cognition depends on which artery—and associated brain tissue—is compromised.

1. Name the three meninges, and describe how they're organized. Identify one special characteristic of each.
2. What is CSF? What function does it serve, where does it come from, and where does it go?
3. Describe the ventricular system of the brain.
4. What is the blood-brain barrier?
5. What are the two types of stroke, and what are some common symptoms of a stroke?

1.5 Scientists Have Devised Clever Techniques for Studying the Structure and Function of the Nervous System

THE ROAD AHEAD

Our focus now turns to experimental approaches researchers use to probe the nervous system. By the end of this section, you should be able to:

1.5.1 Distinguish between invasive and noninvasive experimental techniques.

1.5.2 Review the techniques for studying the detailed, cellular structure and function of the brain, and review their application in various types of studies.

1.5.3 Summarize the major brain-imaging technologies used to study living human brains, highlighting their differing uses and limitations.

Because it is both fantastically complex and somewhat inaccessible, the brain poses special challenges when it comes to formulating research questions and designing experiments to answer those questions. Researchers have long sought methods that would allow them to study the detailed structure and function of the nervous system, from mapping the molecular components of the various cells that make up the brain to tracking the moment-by-moment activity of large neural networks during the execution of complex behaviors. These techniques vary in terms of their *invasiveness*: to study the brain at the cellular level, we generally need to work with postmortem tissue samples or biopsies, whereas the larger-scale activity of the brain can be studied using less-invasive functional-imaging technologies.

Histological techniques let us view the cells of the nervous system in varying ways

Over the last 150 years or so, technical advances in **histology**—the study of the composition of body tissues—have made it possible to selectively stain different parts of neurons and glia. Nowadays, scientists use specialized staining procedures to study the numbers, shapes, distribution, and interconnections of neurons within targeted regions of the brain. We can group these techniques based on the types of experiments they enable.

REGIONAL CELL COUNTS   Using **Nissl stains**, scientists can visualize all of the cell bodies in a tissue section, making it possible to measure the size and number of cell bodies in particular regions (**FIGURE 1.19A**).

INDIVIDUAL CELL SHAPES   Mysteriously, and in contrast to Nissl stains, **Golgi stains** label only a small minority of neurons in a sample, but the affected cells are stained very completely, revealing fine details of cell structure such as the branches of

histology   The study of tissue structure.

Nissl stain   A tissue stain that outlines all cell bodies because the dyes are attracted to RNA, which encircles the nucleus.

Golgi stain   A tissue stain that completely fills a small proportion of neurons with a dark, silver-based precipitate.

FIGURE 1.19 Histological Methods for Studying Neurons

A **Nissl stains** label all cell bodies in a region.

B **Golgi stains** reveal fine details of individual neurons.

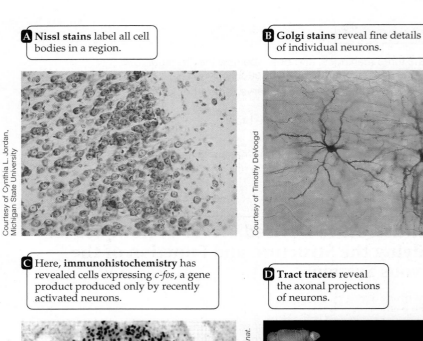

Courtesy of Cynthia L. Jordan, Michigan State University

Courtesy of Timothy DeVoogd

C Here, **immunohistochemistry** has revealed cells expressing *c-fos*, a gene product produced only by recently activated neurons.

D **Tract tracers** reveal the axonal projections of neurons.

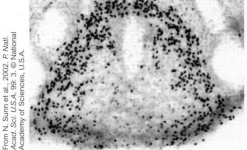

From N. Sunn et al., 2002. *P. Natl. Acad. Sci. U.S.A.* 99: 3. © National Academy of Sciences, U.S.A.

From J. Yuan et al. 2015. *Front. Neuroanat.* 9: 70, courtesy of Dr. Qingming Luo

E The **Brainbow** technique vividly illustrates the interconnections of many neurons simultaneously.

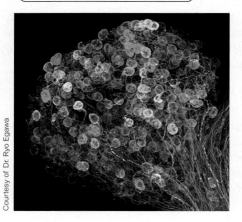

Courtesy of Dr. Ryo Egawa

autoradiography A staining technique that shows the distribution of radioactive chemicals in tissues. See Box 8.1.

dendrites and axons. Neurons stained with the Golgi method (and similar techniques, such as filling cells with fluorescent dye) stand out in sharp contrast to their unstained neighbors, so Golgi staining is useful for identifying the types and precise shapes of neurons in a region. (**FIGURE 1.19B**)

EXPRESSION OF CELLULAR PRODUCTS   Often, neuroscientists would like to know the distribution of neurons that exhibit a specific property. In **autoradiography**, for example, animals are treated with radioactive versions of experimental drugs, and then thin slices of the brain are placed alongside photographic film. Radioactivity emitted by the labeled compound in the tissue "exposes" the emulsion—like light striking film—so the brain essentially takes a picture of itself, highlighting the specific brain regions where the drug has become selectively concentrated. An alternative way to visualize cells that have an attribute in common—termed **immunohistochemistry (IHC)** (**FIGURE 1.19C**)—involves creating antibodies against a protein of interest (we can create antibodies to almost any protein). Equipped with colorful labels, these antibodies can selectively seek out and attach themselves to their target proteins within neurons in a brain slice, revealing the distribution of only those neurons that make the target protein. A related procedure called **in situ hybridization** goes a step further and, using radioactively labeled lengths of nucleic acid (RNA or DNA, see the Appendix), labels only those neurons in which a gene of interest has been turned on.

INTERCONNECTIONS BETWEEN NEURONS   Many research questions are more concerned with the pattern of connections between neurons than with their cellular structure (**FIGURE 1.19D**). To accomplish this goal, scientists have developed many sorts of **tract tracers**, substances that are taken up by neurons and transported over the routes of their axons. Some tract tracers can even jump across synapses, or work their way backward through the length of the neural pathway, leaving visible molecules of label all along the way. In "Brainbow" experiments, inserted genes cause neurons to express fluorescent proteins in hundreds of different hues (**FIGURE 1.19E**), powerfully aiding the study of interconnections of neurons (Lichtman et al., 2008; Weissman and Pan, 2015).

Brain-imaging techniques reveal the structure and function of the living brain

How can we study intact and functioning brains? Unlike older, more invasive techniques, modern brain-imaging technology permits study of the brains of living participants, revealing both structure and patterns of activity in the brain.

COMPUTERIZED AXIAL TOMOGRAPHY   In **computerized axial tomography** (**CAT or CT scans**), X-ray energy is used to generate images by moving an X-ray source in steps around the head. At each point, detectors on the opposite side of the head measure the amount of X-ray radiation that is absorbed; this value is proportional to the density of the tissue the X-rays passed through. When this process is repeated from many angles, the results are mathematically combined into a computer-generated anatomical image of the brain based on density (**FIGURE 1.20A**). CT scans are medium-resolution images, useful for visualizing problems such as strokes, tumors, or cortical shrinkage.

Sam, whom we met at the beginning of the chapter, had developed a meningioma that was pressing on and deforming the motor cortex on the left side of his brain. The tumor impaired the functioning of regions of the motor cortex responsible for voluntary control of the muscles of Sam's right arm and the right side of his face, producing his alarming symptoms. Fortunately, his emergency CT scan pinpointed the meningioma, and following surgical removal of the tumor, Sam experienced immediate improvement; he has been healthy ever since.

MAGNETIC RESONANCE IMAGING   Using magnetic fields and radio waves instead of X-rays, **magnetic resonance imaging** (**MRI**) provides higher-resolution images than CT, with fewer damaging effects. For an MRI image of the brain, the person's head is first placed in an extremely powerful magnet that causes all the protons in the brain to line up in parallel, instead of in their usual random orientations (protons are found in the nuclei of atoms; in body tissues, most protons are found within water molecules). Next, the protons are knocked over by a powerful pulse of radio waves. When this pulse is turned off, the protons relax back to their original configuration, emitting radio waves as they go. Detectors surrounding the head measure those radio waves, which differ for tissues of varying densities. This density-based information is

immunohistochemistry (IHC)
A histological technique in which labeled antibodies are used to visualize specific proteins within tissues.

in situ hybridization   A method for detecting particular RNA transcripts in tissue sections by providing a nucleotide probe that is complementary to, and will therefore hybridize with, the transcript of interest. See Box 8.1; Appendix Figure A.4.

tract tracer   A substance used to visualize the axonal connections of neurons.

computerized axial tomography (CAT or CT scans)   A noninvasive technique for examining brain structure through computer analysis of X-ray absorption at several positions around the head.

magnetic resonance imaging (MRI)
A noninvasive brain-imaging technology that uses magnetism and radio-frequency energy to create images of the gross structure of the living brain.

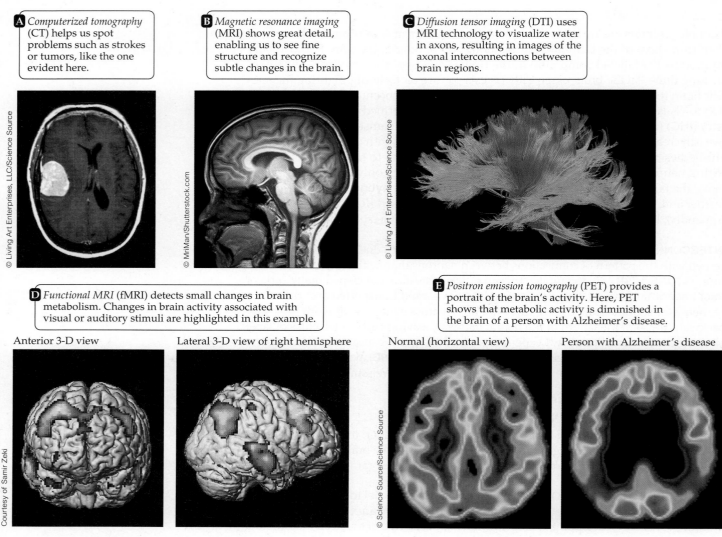

A *Computerized tomography* (CT) helps us spot problems such as strokes or tumors, like the one evident here.

B *Magnetic resonance imaging* (MRI) shows great detail, enabling us to see fine structure and recognize subtle changes in the brain.

C *Diffusion tensor imaging* (DTI) uses MRI technology to visualize water in axons, resulting in images of the axonal interconnections between brain regions.

D *Functional MRI* (fMRI) detects small changes in brain metabolism. Changes in brain activity associated with visual or auditory stimuli are highlighted in this example.

Anterior 3-D view   Lateral 3-D view of right hemisphere

E *Positron emission tomography* (PET) provides a portrait of the brain's activity. Here, PET shows that metabolic activity is diminished in the brain of a person with Alzheimer's disease.

Normal (horizontal view)   Person with Alzheimer's disease

FIGURE 1.20 Visualizing the Living Human Brain

then used by a computer to create a detailed cross-sectional view of the brain (**FIGURE 1.20B**) that scientists use to evaluate the size and shape of distinct brain regions. MRI images can also reveal subtle changes in the brain, such as the local loss of myelin that is characteristic of multiple sclerosis. A variant of MRI, called **diffusion tensor imaging** (**DTI**), exploits a signal associated with the diffusion of water within axons in order to visualize axonal fiber tracts within the brain. This kind of research, generally known as *tractography*, is helping us to learn how networks of brain structures work together in various forms of complex cognition and consciousness.

FUNCTIONAL BRAIN IMAGING   With its ability to image localized changes in the brain's activity, rather than details of its structure, **functional MRI (fMRI)** has revolutionized cognitive neuroscience. Offering both reasonable speed (temporal resolution) and sharpness (spatial resolution) at the gross anatomical level, fMRI uses rapidly oscillating magnetic fields to detect regional changes in brain metabolism, particularly patterns of oxygen use and blood flow in the most active regions of the brain. Scientists can use fMRI data to create "difference images" of the specific activity of different parts of the brain while people engage in various experimental tasks. Although fMRI cannot resolve the fine cellular structure of the brain and is too slow to track rapid, moment-by-moment changes in the activity of networks of neurons, fMRI combined with conventional anatomical MRI has revealed many important clues about how networks of brain structures collaborate on complex cognitive processes (**FIGURES 1.20C** and **D**). An additional consideration is

diffusion tensor imaging (DTI)
A modified form of MRI in which the diffusion of water in a confined space is exploited to produce images of axonal fiber tracts.

functional MRI (fMRI)   Magnetic resonance imaging that detects changes in blood flow and therefore identifies regions of the brain that are particularly active during a given task.

that, as in other imaging techniques, fMRI imagery is not photographic: it is created by a computer, based on mathematical models. There is concern among researchers that the computer algorithms used in this process may sometimes be misleading (Eklund et al., 2016; Poldrack et al., 2017).

Like fMRI, **positron emission tomography** (**PET**) depicts the brain's activity during behavioral tasks. Short-lived radioactive chemicals are injected into the bloodstream, and radiation detectors encircling the head map the destination of these chemicals in the brain. A particularly effective strategy is to inject radioactively labeled glucose ("blood sugar") while the person is engaged in a cognitive task of interest to the researcher. Because the radioactive glucose is selectively taken up and used by the most active parts of the brain, a moment-to-moment color-coded portrait of brain activity can be created (**FIGURE 1.20E**) (P. E. Roland, 1993; Chiaravalloti et al., 2019). Although PET can't match the detailed resolution of fMRI, it tends to be faster and thus better able to track quick changes in brain activity.

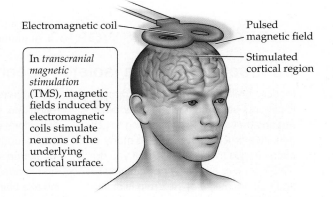

In *transcranial magnetic stimulation* (TMS), magnetic fields induced by electromagnetic coils stimulate neurons of the underlying cortical surface.

FIGURE 1.21   Transcranial Magnetic Stimulation

MAGNETIC STIMULATION AND MAPPING   It is a simple matter to pass magnetic fields into the brain. However, it is technically more challenging to project magnetic fields in a highly focused and precise manner. In **transcranial magnetic stimulation** (**TMS**) (**FIGURE 1.21**), focal magnetic currents are used to briefly stimulate the cortex of alert people directly, without any lasting physical alterations or surgery. Using TMS allows experimenters to map cortical surfaces by activating discrete areas of the brain while simultaneously tracking any resulting changes in behavior, and it can be powerfully combined with functional brain-imaging techniques like PET (Tremblay et al., 2020).

Not only can magnets stimulate neurons, but neurons also act as tiny electromagnets themselves! In **magnetoencephalography** (**MEG**), a large array of ultrasensitive detectors measures the minuscule magnetic fields produced by the electrical activity of cortical neurons. This information is used to construct real-time maps of brain activity during ongoing cognitive processing (**FIGURE 1.22**). Because MEG can track quick, moment-by-moment changes in brain activity, it is excellent for studying the rapidly shifting patterns of brain activity in cortical circuits that fMRI is too slow to track (Baillet, 2017; Gross, 2019).

Now let's look a little more closely at a process scientists use to distinguish the brain activity underlying a specific behavior from the background activity of the busy conscious brain.

positron emission tomography (PET)
A brain-imaging technology that tracks the metabolism of injected radioactive substances in the brain, in order to map brain activity.

transcranial magnetic stimulation (TMS)   A noninvasive technique for examining brain function that applies strong magnetic fields to stimulate cortical neurons in order to identify discrete areas of the brain that are particularly active during specific behaviors.

magnetoencephalography (MEG)
A noninvasive brain-imaging technology that creates maps of brain activity during cognitive tasks by measuring tiny magnetic fields produced by active neurons.

(A) Face

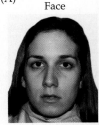

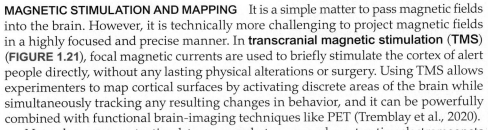

Magnetoencephalography (MEG) measures the minuscule magnetic fields given off by ensembles of cortical cells during specific behavioral functions. Here, MEG maps brain activity associated with viewing faces…

(B) Object

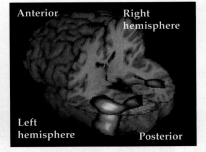

…versus viewing nonface objects.

View Animation 1.4:
Visualizing the Living Human Brain

FIGURE 1.22   Animal Magnetism

RESEARCHERS AT WORK |||||||||||||||||||||||||||||||||||||||||||||||||||||||||||||||||||||||||||||||||||||||||||||||||||||

Subtractive analysis isolates specific brain activity

Modern brain imaging provides dramatic pictures showing the particular brain regions that are activated during specific cognitive processes; there are many such images in this book. But if you do a PET scan of a healthy person, you find that almost all of the brain is active at any given moment (showing that the old notion that "we use only 10% of our brain" is nonsense). How do researchers obtain these highly specific images of brain activity?

In order to associate specific brain regions with particular cognitive operations, researchers developed a sort of algebraic technique, in which activity during one behavioral condition is subtracted from activity during a different condition. So, for example, the data from a control PET scan made while a person was gazing at a blank wall might be subtracted from the data from a PET scan collected while that person studied a complex visual stimulus. Averaged over enough trials, the specific regions that are almost always active during the processing task become apparent, even though, on casual inspection, a single experimental scan might not look much different from a single control scan (**FIGURE 1.23**). It is important to keep in mind that although functional brain images seem unambiguous and easy to label, they are computer-generated composites—not actual brain images—and thus only as accurate as the assumptions and algorithms with which they are created (Racine et al., 2005; Poldrack et al., 2017).

FIGURE 1.23 Isolating Specific Brain Activity

■ **Hypothesis**

Brain regions engaged in a specific behavior can be isolated by algebraic means, subtracting resting scans from scans during activity.

■ **Test**

Participants are scanned twice—once while looking at a blank screen, and once while looking at test stimuli. The control scan is then subtracted from the test scan.

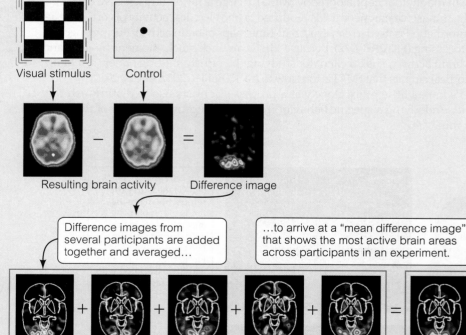

Visual stimulus   Control

Resulting brain activity   Difference image

■ **Result**

By repeating the process and averaging the results across multiple participants, a stable "difference image" showing activation of just a few brain regions is formed. Averaging such difference images from several people increases confidence that this brain region is indeed involved in that activity.

Difference images from several participants are added together and averaged…

…to arrive at a "mean difference image" that shows the most active brain areas across participants in an experiment.

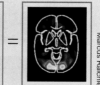

Mean difference image

Courtesy of Marcus Raichle

■ **Conclusion**

The activated brain regions in the difference image—in this case, in the occipital cortex—are selectively involved in the particular cognitive processing required by the stimulus.

1. Compare and contrast the main methods for producing still images of the structure of the brain. What do you think are some of the advantages and disadvantages of each method?

2. Compare and contrast the main functional-imaging technologies used for visualizing the activity of brain regions. What do you think are some of the advantages and disadvantages of each method?

3. Describe the process that neuroscientists can use to isolate brain activity associated with a specific behavior, as visualized by functional-imaging techniques.

1.6 Careful Research Design Is Essential for Progress in Behavioral Neuroscience

THE ROAD AHEAD

In the final section of the chapter, we turn our attention to factors that neuroscientists consider in designing research: both the formal layout of experiments and the theoretical considerations on which research questions are based. Studying this section should prepare you to:

1.6.1 Describe and distinguish between correlational studies and experimental studies—in which either the body is altered and behavior is measured, or behavior is manipulated and bodily changes are measured—and explain how scientists rely on all three types of studies to develop research programs.

1.6.2 Discuss the major theoretical perspectives that inform research in behavioral neuroscience.

1.6.3 Discuss important issues that modern behavioral neuroscience must contend with, such as the use of animals in research, and the replication crisis in behavioral research.

1.6.4 Explain the different levels of analysis that may be focused on by behavioral neuroscientists, and describe how they may relate to one another.

The complexity of human behavior, and the organ by which it is produced, necessitate the use of indirect means to manipulate behavior and the activity of the brain. This complexity also contributes to an emerging crisis in behavioral neuroscience: difficulty in replicating numerous influential earlier findings (De Boeck and Jeon, 2018). These complications underscore the importance of careful research design based on detailed observation, precise control of experimental variables, and selection of appropriate research participants, and they are the impetus driving rapid evolution of research methodology across the behavioral sciences.

Three types of study designs probe brain-behavior relationships

Behavioral neuroscientists use three general types of studies for research. In an experiment employing **somatic intervention** (**FIGURE 1.24A**), we alter a structure or function of the brain or body to see how this alteration changes behavior. In this sort of experiment, the physical alteration is an **independent variable** (a general term used to describe the manipulated aspect of any experiment), and the behavioral effect is the **dependent variable** (a general term used to describe the measured consequence of an experimental manipulation). Some examples of somatic intervention experiments include (1) administering a hormone to some animals, but not others, and comparing their sexual behavior; (2) electrically stimulating a specific brain region and measuring alterations in movement; and (3) destroying a specific region in the brain and observing subsequent changes in sleep patterns. In each case, the behavioral measurements

somatic intervention   An approach to finding relations between body variables and behavioral variables that involves manipulating body structure or function and looking for resultant changes in behavior. See Figure 1.24. Compare *behavioral intervention*.

independent variable   The factor that is manipulated by an experimenter.

dependent variable   The factor that an experimenter measures to monitor a change in response to manipulations of an independent variable.

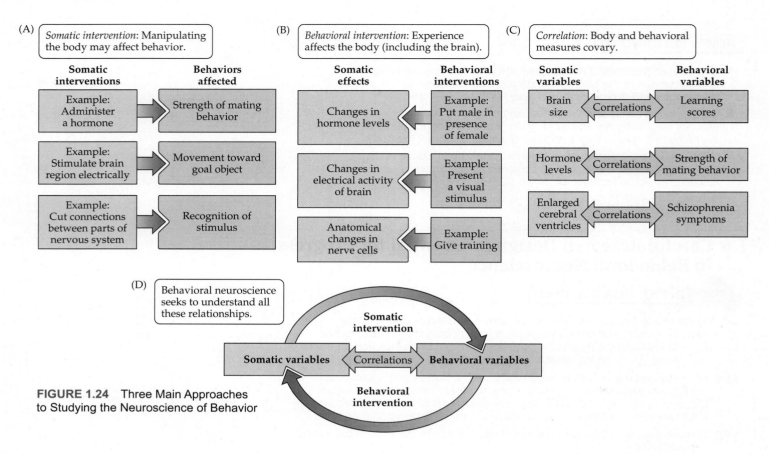

FIGURE 1.24 Three Main Approaches to Studying the Neuroscience of Behavior

follow the bodily intervention; furthermore, in each case the behavioral measurements are compared with those of a **control group**. In a **within-participants experiment**, the control group is simply the same individuals, tested before the somatic intervention occurs. In a **between-participants experiment**, the experimental group of individuals is compared with a different group of individuals who are treated identically in every way except that they don't receive the somatic intervention.

The approach opposite to somatic intervention is **behavioral intervention** (**FIGURE 1.24B**). In this approach the scientist alters or controls the behavior of an organism and looks for resulting changes in body structure or function. Here, behavior is the independent variable, and change in the body is the dependent variable. A few examples include (1) allowing adults of each sex to interact and then measuring their hormone levels, (2) having a person perform a cognitive task while in a brain scanner and then measuring changes in activity in specific regions of the brain, and (3) training an animal to fear a previously neutral stimulus and then observing electrical changes in the brain that may encode the newly learned association. As with somatic intervention, these experimental approaches may employ either within-group or between-groups designs.

The third type of study is **correlation** (**FIGURE 1.24C**), which measures how closely changes in one variable are associated with changes in another variable. Two examples of correlational studies include (1) observing the extent to which memory ability is associated with the size of a certain brain structure, and (2) noting that increases in a certain hormone are accompanied by increases in aggressive behavior. Note that while this type of study tells us if the measured variables are associated in some way, it can't tell us which causes the other. We can't tell, for example, whether the hormones cause the aggression or aggression increases the hormones. But even though it can't establish **causality**, correlational research can help researchers identify which things are linked, directly or indirectly, and thus it helps us to develop hypotheses that can be tested experimentally using behavioral and somatic interventions.

Combining these three approaches yields the circle diagram of **FIGURE 1.24D**, showing how the three types of studies complement each other. It also underscores that the effects of brain and behavior are reciprocal: each affects the other in an ongoing cycle.

Animal research is an essential part of life sciences research, including behavioral neuroscience

Human beings' involvement and concern with other species predates recorded history; early humans had to study animal behavior and physiology in order to escape some species and hunt others. To study the biological bases of behavior inevitably requires research on animals of other species, as well as on human beings. Psychology students usually underestimate the contributions of animal research to psychology because the most widely used introductory psychology textbooks often present major findings from animal research as if they were obtained with human participants (Domjan and Purdy, 1995).

A vocal minority of people believe that research with animals, even if it does lead to lasting benefits, is unethical. Others argue that animal research is acceptable only when it produces immediate and measurable benefits. The potential cost in taking this perspective lies in the fact that we have no way of predicting which experiments will lead to a breakthrough. The whole point of studying the unknown is that it is unknown; there is a long history of chance observation, based on the steady accumulation of basic knowledge, leading to unexpected benefits.

There's no denying that animal research can cause stress and discomfort, and researchers have a strong ethical obligation to hold pain and stress to the absolute minimum levels possible. Animal research has itself provided us with the drugs and techniques that make most research painless for lab animals, while also leading to improved veterinary care for our animal companions (Sunstein and Nussbaum, 2004), and researchers are ethically bound to continually refine lab practices, with animal well-being a primary concern. Researchers are also bound by animal protection legislation and are subject to continual administrative oversight to ensure adherence to nationally mandated animal care policies that emphasize the use of as few animals as possible without jeopardizing research integrity, as well as the use of the simplest species that can answer the questions under study.

As human beings with the full range of emotions and empathetic feelings toward animals, we all wish there were an alternative to the use of animals in research. But if we want to understand how the nervous system works, we have to actually study it, in detail. The life sciences would slow to a crawl without the basic knowledge that we derive from studying animals.

How do similarities and differences among people and animals fit into behavioral neuroscience? Each person is in some ways like all other people, in some ways like some other people, and in some ways like no other person. As shown in **FIGURE 1.25**, we can extend this observation to the much broader range of animal life. The electrical messages used by nerve cells (see Chapter 2) are essentially the same in a jellyfish, a cockroach, and a human being, and many species employ identical hormones. These characteristics are said to be **conserved**, meaning that they first arose in a shared ancestor. But mere similarity of a feature between species does not guarantee that the feature came from a common ancestral species. Our eyes resemble those of octopuses, but certain key differences reveal that their eyes and our eyes evolved separately.

With respect to each biological property, researchers must determine how animals are identical and how they are different. When we seek animal models for studying human behavior or biological processes, we must ask the following question: Does the proposed animal model *really* have some things in common with the process at work in humans? In later chapters we will see many cases in which it does, but even within the same species, individuals differ from one another: cat from cat, blue jay from blue jay, and person from person. Behavioral neuroscience seeks to understand individual differences as well as similarities.

correlation The tendency of two measures to vary in concert, such that a change in one measure is matched by a change in the other.

causality The relation of cause and effect, such that we can conclude that an experimental manipulation has specifically caused an observed result.

conserved In the context of evolution, referring to a trait that is passed on from a common ancestor to two or more descendant species.

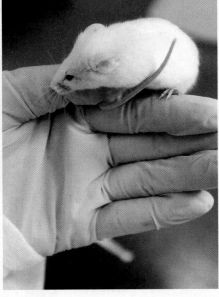

Animal Research is Crucial In studying something as complicated as the mammalian brain, there is often no option but to study the brains of lab animals, the vast majority of which are rats and mice. Much of the research you will read about in this book has relied on studies of animals. Very high standards of care are provided to research animals, as a result of extensive legislative requirements, the need to protect the integrity of research, and the researchers' ethical and empathetic concern for their research subjects.

Each person has some characteristics shared by...

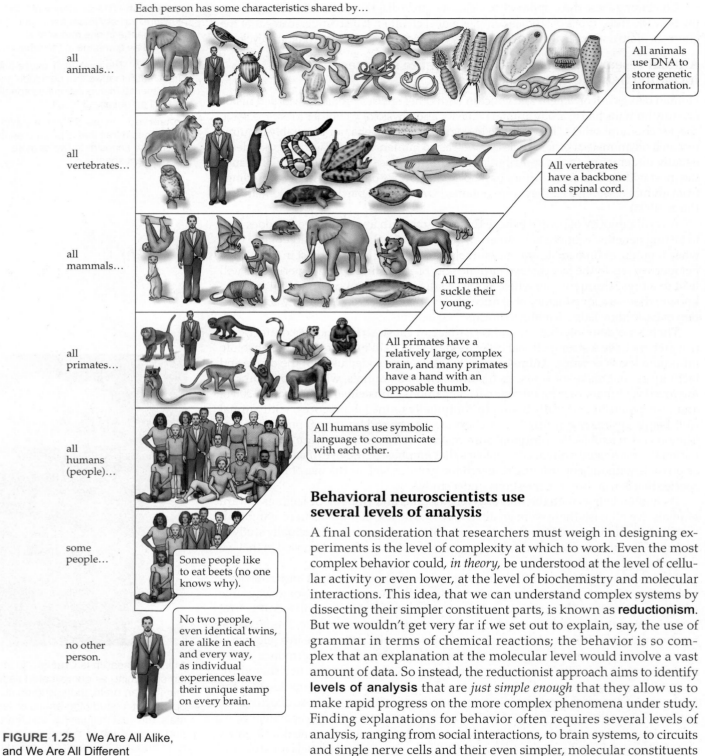

all animals...

All animals use DNA to store genetic information.

all vertebrates...

All vertebrates have a backbone and spinal cord.

all mammals...

All mammals suckle their young.

all primates...

All primates have a relatively large, complex brain, and many primates have a hand with an opposable thumb.

all humans (people)...

All humans use symbolic language to communicate with each other.

some people...

Some people like to eat beets (no one knows why).

no other person.

No two people, even identical twins, are alike in each and every way, as individual experiences leave their unique stamp on every brain.

FIGURE 1.25 We Are All Alike, and We Are All Different

reductionism The scientific strategy of breaking a system down into increasingly smaller parts in order to understand it.

Behavioral neuroscientists use several levels of analysis

A final consideration that researchers must weigh in designing experiments is the level of complexity at which to work. Even the most complex behavior could, *in theory*, be understood at the level of cellular activity or even lower, at the level of biochemistry and molecular interactions. This idea, that we can understand complex systems by dissecting their simpler constituent parts, is known as **reductionism**. But we wouldn't get very far if we set out to explain, say, the use of grammar in terms of chemical reactions; the behavior is so complex that an explanation at the molecular level would involve a vast amount of data. So instead, the reductionist approach aims to identify **levels of analysis** that are *just simple enough* that they allow us to make rapid progress on the more complex phenomena under study. Finding explanations for behavior often requires several levels of analysis, ranging from social interactions, to brain systems, to circuits and single nerve cells and their even simpler, molecular constituents (**FIGURE 1.26**).

Naturally, different problems are carried to different levels of analysis, and fruitful work is often being done simultaneously by different workers at several levels. For example, in their research on visual perception, some cognitive psychologists carefully analyze behavior. They try to determine how the eyes move while looking at a visual pattern, or how the contrast among parts of the pattern determines its visibility.

Meanwhile, other behavioral neuroscientists study the differences in visual abilities among species and try to determine the adaptive significance of these differences. For example, how is the presence (or absence) of color vision related to the lifestyle of a species? At the same time, other investigators trace out brain structures and networks involved in different visual tasks. Still other scientists try to understand the electrical and chemical events that occur in the brain during vision.

Some people doubt whether our "merely human" brains will ever be able to understand something as complicated as the human brain, to a level where we can fully explain mysterious properties like consciousness, identity, or the perception of free will. Nevertheless, the gains we are making in understanding how the brain works—the subject of this book—bring us closer to that goal every day.

level of analysis The scope of an experimental approach. A scientist may try to understand behavior by monitoring molecules, nerve cells, brain regions, or social environments or using some combination of these levels of analysis.

HOW'S IT GOING ?

1. What are the three general forms of research studies in behavioral neuroscience? What is the issue of "causality"? How do the three research perspectives inform and shape one another?

2. Define *independent variable*, *dependent variable*, *control group*, *within-participants experiment*, and *between-participants experiment*.

3. Consider both sides of the debate over animal research, weighing the pros and cons of the "for" and "against" positions. How do you think animal use should be regulated?

4. What is the general principle behind reductionism? How does this influence the level of analysis at which a researcher works? For that matter, what is meant by "level of analysis"?

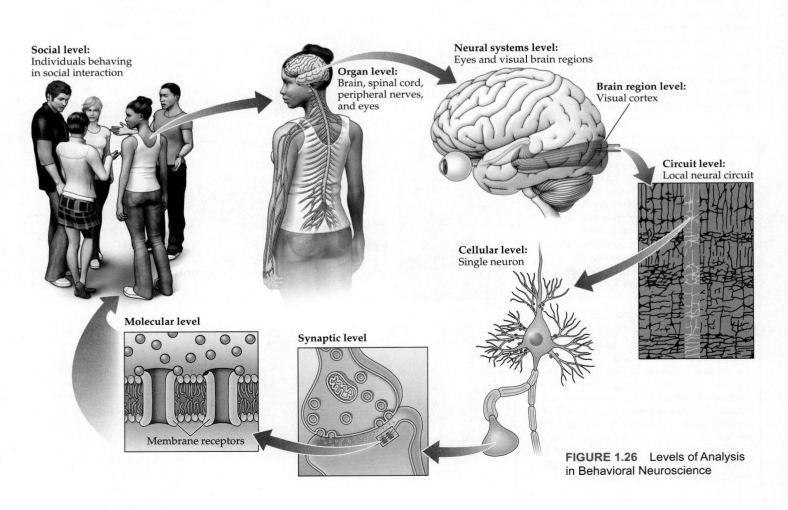

Social level:
Individuals behaving in social interaction

Organ level:
Brain, spinal cord, peripheral nerves, and eyes

Neural systems level:
Eyes and visual brain regions

Brain region level:
Visual cortex

Circuit level:
Local neural circuit

Cellular level:
Single neuron

Molecular level

Membrane receptors

Synaptic level

FIGURE 1.26 Levels of Analysis in Behavioral Neuroscience

Recommended Reading

Bausell, R. B. (2015). *The Design and Conduct of Meaningful Experiments Involving Human Participants: 25 Scientific Principles*. New York, NY: Oxford University Press.

Blumenfeld, H. (2021). *Neuroanatomy through Clinical Cases* (3rd ed.). Sunderland, MA: Oxford University Press/Sinauer.

Huettel, S. A., Song, A. W., and McCarthy, G. (2014). *Functional Magnetic Resonance Imaging* (3rd ed.). Sunderland, MA: Oxford University Press/Sinauer.

Papanicolau, A. C. (Ed.). (2017). *The Oxford Handbook of Functional Brain Imaging in Neuropsychology and Cognitive Neurosciences*. Oxford, UK: Oxford University Press.

Schoonover, C. (2010). *Portraits of the Mind: Visualizing the Brain from Antiquity to the 21st Century*. New York, NY: Abrams.

Swanson, L. W., Newman, E., Araque, A., and Dubinsky, J. M. (2017). *The Beautiful Brain: The Drawings of Santiago Ramón y Cajal*. New York, NY: Abrams.

Vanderah, T., and Gould, D. J. (2020). *Nolte's The Human Brain: An Introduction to Its Functional Anatomy* (8th ed.). New York, NY: Elsevier.

1 • VISUAL SUMMARY

You should be able to relate each summary to the adjacent illustration, including structures and processes. The online version of this **Visual Summary** includes links to figures, animations, and activities that will help you consolidate the material.

1 **Neurons** (nerve cells) are the basic units of the nervous system. The typical neuron has four main parts: (1) **dendrites** receive information; (2) the **cell body** (soma) integrates the information; (3) an **axon** carries impulses from the neuron; and (4) **axon terminals** transmit the neuron's signals to other cells. Neurons almost universally feature an **input zone**, an **integration zone**, a **conduction zone**, and an **output zone**. Review **Figure 1.1, Animation 1.2**

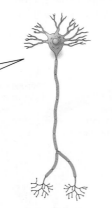

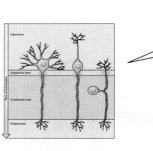

2 Neurons take numerous forms and may be **multipolar**, **bipolar**, or **unipolar**. The exact shape of a neuron is determined by the type of information it gathers, the processing it performs, and the destination to which it transmits the processed information. Thus each neuron gathers, analyzes, and transmits information. Review **Figure 1.3, Activity 1.1**

3 Neurons make functional contacts with other cells at specialized junctions called **synapses**. By changing their shape or function in response to experiences, synapses exhibit **neuroplasticity**. At most synapses a chemical **neurotransmitter** released from the **presynaptic membrane** diffuses across the **synaptic cleft** and binds to special **neurotransmitter receptor** molecules in the **postsynaptic membrane**. Review **Figure 1.4**

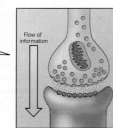

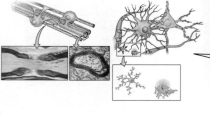

4 **Glial cells** provide support to neurons, form **myelin**, maintain the brain, and contribute to neural activity. Review **Figure 1.5**

5 To the naked eye, the nervous system of vertebrates is divided into the **central nervous system** (**CNS**—the brain and spinal cord) and the **peripheral nervous system**. The peripheral nervous system, in turn, consists of two parts: the **somatic nervous system** and the **autonomic nervous system**. Twelve pairs of **cranial nerves**, which make up one part of the somatic nervous system, arise from the brain to directly take in information or send out commands to the body, mostly the head and neck. Review **Figures 1.6** and **1.7, Activity 1.2**

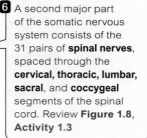

6 A second major part of the somatic nervous system consists of the 31 pairs of **spinal nerves**, spaced through the **cervical, thoracic, lumbar, sacral**, and **coccygeal** segments of the spinal cord. Review **Figure 1.8, Activity 1.3**

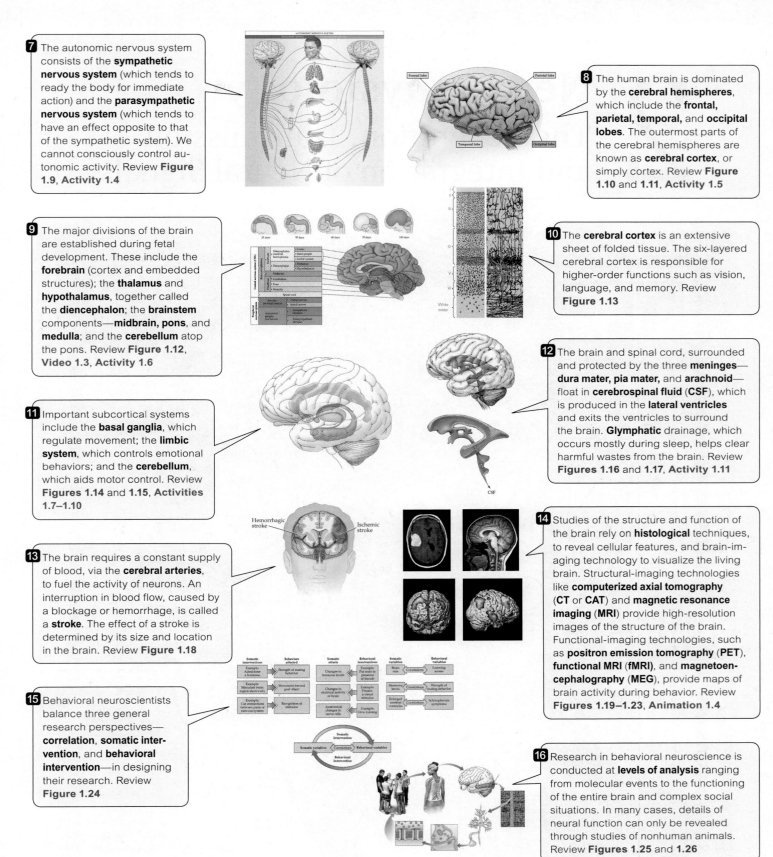

7 The autonomic nervous system consists of the **sympathetic nervous system** (which tends to ready the body for immediate action) and the **parasympathetic nervous system** (which tends to have an effect opposite to that of the sympathetic system). We cannot consciously control autonomic activity. Review **Figure 1.9**, **Activity 1.4**

8 The human brain is dominated by the **cerebral hemispheres**, which include the **frontal, parietal, temporal,** and **occipital lobes**. The outermost parts of the cerebral hemispheres are known as **cerebral cortex**, or simply cortex. Review **Figure 1.10** and **1.11**, **Activity 1.5**

9 The major divisions of the brain are established during fetal development. These include the **forebrain** (cortex and embedded structures); the **thalamus** and **hypothalamus**, together called the **diencephalon**; the **brainstem** components—**midbrain, pons**, and **medulla**; and the **cerebellum** atop the pons. Review **Figure 1.12**, **Video 1.3**, **Activity 1.6**

10 The **cerebral cortex** is an extensive sheet of folded tissue. The six-layered cerebral cortex is responsible for higher-order functions such as vision, language, and memory. Review **Figure 1.13**

11 Important subcortical systems include the **basal ganglia**, which regulate movement; the **limbic system**, which controls emotional behaviors; and the **cerebellum**, which aids motor control. Review **Figures 1.14** and **1.15**, **Activities 1.7–1.10**

12 The brain and spinal cord, surrounded and protected by the three **meninges**—**dura mater, pia mater,** and **arachnoid**—float in **cerebrospinal fluid** (**CSF**), which is produced in the **lateral ventricles** and exits the ventricles to surround the brain. **Glymphatic** drainage, which occurs mostly during sleep, helps clear harmful wastes from the brain. Review **Figures 1.16** and **1.17**, **Activity 1.11**

13 The brain requires a constant supply of blood, via the **cerebral arteries**, to fuel the activity of neurons. An interruption in blood flow, caused by a blockage or hemorrhage, is called a **stroke**. The effect of a stroke is determined by its size and location in the brain. Review **Figure 1.18**

14 Studies of the structure and function of the brain rely on **histological** techniques, to reveal cellular features, and brain-imaging technology to visualize the living brain. Structural-imaging technologies like **computerized axial tomography** (**CT** or **CAT**) and **magnetic resonance imaging** (**MRI**) provide high-resolution images of the structure of the brain. Functional-imaging technologies, such as **positron emission tomography** (**PET**), **functional MRI** (**fMRI**), and **magnetoencephalography** (**MEG**), provide maps of brain activity during behavior. Review **Figures 1.19–1.23**, **Animation 1.4**

15 Behavioral neuroscientists balance three general research perspectives—**correlation, somatic intervention**, and **behavioral intervention**—in designing their research. Review **Figure 1.24**

16 Research in behavioral neuroscience is conducted at **levels of analysis** ranging from molecular events to the functioning of the entire brain and complex social situations. In many cases, details of neural function can only be revealed through studies of nonhuman animals. Review **Figures 1.25** and **1.26**

The Mind's Machine digital resources include additional videos, flashcards, and other study tools.

2 Neurophysiology

The Generation, Transmission, and Integration of Neural Signals

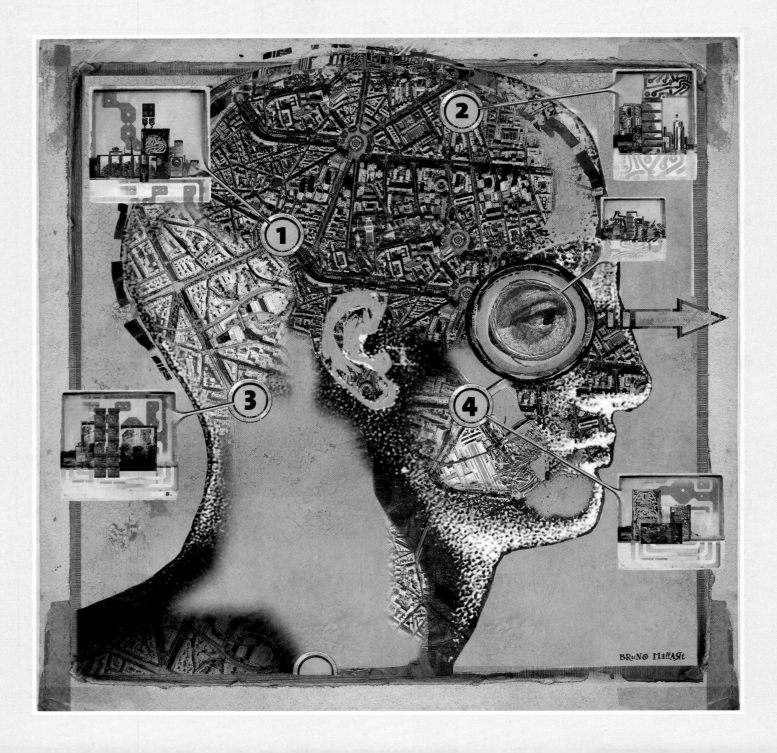

BRuNO MallARt

Grab the Bull by the Brains

Perhaps the most dramatic neuroscience demonstration in history occurred in 1964 when Yale professor José Delgado strolled into an arena in Spain to face an enraged bull trained to attack humans. Armed only with a remote control, Delgado watched the massive bull paw the earth, lower its head, and charge right at him. Just before the bull reached him, Delgado pressed a button on the remote control that caused a wire, called an *electrode*, in the bull's brain to deliver a tiny trickle of electricity. The bull stopped cold. When Delgado electrically stimulated another part of the bull's brain, the animal turned to the right and calmly trotted away. Repeated stimulations rendered the bull docile for several minutes (Marzullo, 2017). Other bulls responded differently to brain stimulation, depending on the brain region targeted. One animal produced a single "moo" for every button press—a hundred times in a row.

Delgado also electrically stimulated electrodes in the brains of people, in an attempt to pinpoint the cause of a neurological disorder. Depending on which part of the brain was stimulated, patients might suddenly become anxious or angry (Delgado, 1969). In this #MeToo era, probably the creepiest response elicited by one brain stimulation site was in women who suddenly became romantically interested in the man interviewing them. Yet as soon as the electrical stimulation of their brains stopped, the women returned to their usual reserved behavior.

Why does a tiny bit of electrical stimulation in the brain produce such profound changes in mood and behavior? The reason is that neurons normally use electrical signals to sum up vast amounts of information. When Delgado electrically stimulated the brain, he was triggering those normal electrical signals in a very abnormal way, with sometimes startling results. To understand how even a tiny electrical charge to the brain can so dramatically affect the mind, we need to understand how electrical signaling works in the brain.

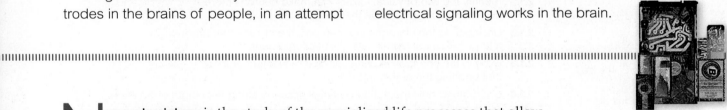

See Video 2.1:
Electrical Stimulation of the Brain

Neurophysiology is the study of the specialized life processes that allow neurons to use chemical and electrical signals to process and transmit information. In this chapter we'll study the electrical processes at work within a neuron; in Chapter 3 we'll look at the chemical signals that pass between neurons. We'll see that brain function is an alternating series of electrical signals within neurons and of chemical signals between neurons.

For example, a doctor may use a small rubber mallet to strike just below your knee and watch your leg kick upward in what is known as the *knee-jerk reflex*. Simple as it appears, a lot happens during this test. First, sensory neurons in the muscle detect the hammer tap and send a rapid electrical signal along their axons to your spinal cord. That rapid electrical signal along the axons from knee to spinal cord is called an *action potential,* which is a major topic in this chapter. When the action potential reaches the axon terminals, they release a chemical, called a *neurotransmitter,* to stimulate spinal motor neurons.

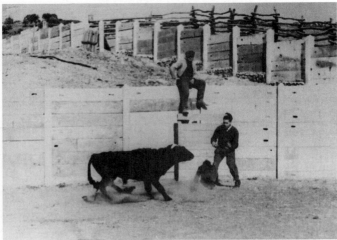

Courtesy of the Delgado estate and José Carlos Delgado

Hold It Right There! Dr. José Delgado stops a bull in the middle of a charge, using the remote control in his hand.

In response to the neurotransmitter, the motor neurons send action potentials down their own axons to release yet another neurotransmitter onto muscles. In response to that neurotransmitter, the muscles contract, kicking your foot into the air. Problems in electrical or chemical signaling in this circuit might cause the kick to be stronger or weaker, faster or slower, than it should be.

So this "simple" behavior involves several rounds of signaling: first electrical (along sensory neuron axons), then chemical (sensory neurons to motor neurons), then electrical again (along motor neuron axons), and finally chemical again (motor neurons to muscle). This is the classic pattern of neural function: information flows *within* a neuron via electrical signals (action potentials) and passes *between* neurons through chemical signals (neurotransmitters). This sequence also reflects the organization of this chapter. First we explain how neurons produce action potentials and send them along their axons. Then we describe how the action potential causes axon terminals to release neurotransmitter into the synapse. Next we discuss how the neurotransmitter affects the electrical state of the neuron on the other side of the synapse. And we conclude the chapter by discussing how electrical probing of the brain revealed that the brain's surface reflects a map of the body. All this will prepare us for Chapter 3, where we will learn more details about the chemical signals between neurons.

View Animation 2.2: Brain Explorer

2.1 Electrical Signals Are the Vocabulary of the Nervous System

THE ROAD AHEAD

The first section of this chapter explains how neurons use electrical forces to process information. Reading this material should enable you to:

2.1.1 Identify the two physical forces that make neurons more negatively charged inside than outside.

2.1.2 Understand the changes in a neuron's membrane that produce a large electrical signal called an *action potential*.

2.1.3 Explain the changes in channels and movement of ions that underlie the action potential.

2.1.4 Understand how the action potential spreads along the length of an axon.

2.1.5 Understand how each neuron uses these electrical signals to integrate information from other neurons.

neurophysiology The study of the life processes of neurons.

ion An atom or molecule that has acquired an electrical charge by gaining or losing one or more electrons.

anion A negatively charged ion, such as a protein or a chloride ion.

cation A positively charged ion, such as a potassium or sodium ion.

intracellular fluid Also called *cytoplasm*. The watery solution found within cells.

extracellular fluid Also called *interstitial fluid*. The fluid in the spaces between cells.

cell membrane The lipid bilayer that encloses a cell.

microelectrode An especially small electrode used to record electrical potentials inside living cells.

Like all living cells, neurons are more negative on the inside than on the outside, so we say they are *polarized*, meaning there is a difference in electrical charge between the inside and outside of the cell. Let's consider a neuron at rest, neither perturbed by other neurons nor producing its own signals. Of the many **ions** (electrically charged molecules) that a neuron contains, a majority are **anions** ("ANN-eye-ons"; negatively charged ions), especially large protein anions that cannot exit the cell. The rest are **cations** ("CAT-eye-ons"; positively charged ions). (It may help you to remember that the letter *t*, which occurs in the word *cation*, is shaped a bit like a plus sign, +.) All of these ions are dissolved in the **intracellular fluid** inside the cell and the **extracellular fluid** outside the **cell membrane**.

If we insert a fine **microelectrode** into the interior of a neuron and place another electrode in the extracellular fluid and take a reading (as in **FIGURE 2.1**), we find that the inside of the neuron is more negative than the fluid around it. Specifically, a

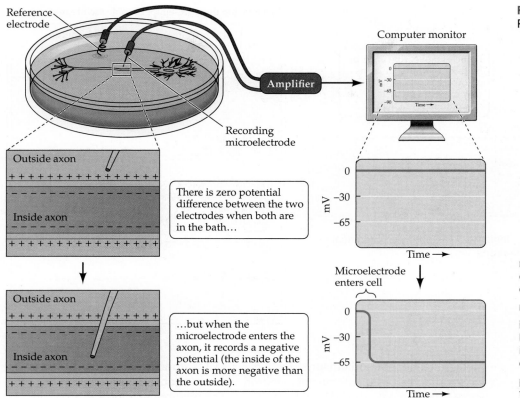

FIGURE 2.1 Measuring the Resting Potential

Reference electrode

Recording microelectrode

Amplifier

Computer monitor

Outside axon

Inside axon

There is zero potential difference between the two electrodes when both are in the bath…

Outside axon

Inside axon

…but when the microelectrode enters the axon, it records a negative potential (the inside of the axon is more negative than the outside).

Microelectrode enters cell

Time →

Time →

View Activity 2.1: Distribution of Ions

resting potential   The difference in electrical potential across the membrane of a nerve cell at rest.

millivolt (mV)   A thousandth of a volt.

ion channel   A pore in the cell membrane that permits the passage of certain ions through the membrane when the channel is open.

potassium ion (K⁺)   A potassium atom that carries a positive charge.

neuron at rest exhibits a characteristic **resting potential** (an electrical difference across the membrane) of about −50 to −80 thousandths of a volt, or **millivolts** (**mV**) (the negative sign indicates that the cell's interior is more negative than the outside). To understand how this negative membrane potential comes about, we have to consider some special properties of the cell membrane, as well as two forces that drive ions across it.

The cell membrane is a double layer of fatty molecules studded with many sorts of specialized proteins. One important type of membrane-spanning protein is the **ion channel**, a tube-like pore that allows ions of a specific type to pass through the membrane (**FIGURE 2.2**). As we'll see later, some types of ion channels are gated: they can open and close rapidly in response to various influences. But some ion channels stay open all the time, and the cell membrane of a neuron contains many such channels that selectively allow **potassium ions (K⁺)** to cross the

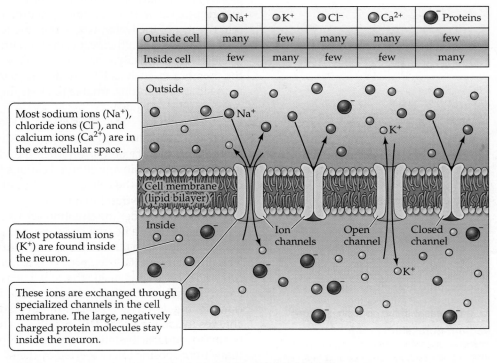

	Na^+	K^+	Cl^-	Ca^{2+}	Proteins
Outside cell	many	few	many	many	few
Inside cell	few	many	few	few	many

Outside

Most sodium ions (Na^+), chloride ions (Cl^-), and calcium ions (Ca^{2+}) are in the extracellular space.

Cell membrane (lipid bilayer)

Inside

Most potassium ions (K^+) are found inside the neuron.

Ion channels

Open channel

Closed channel

These ions are exchanged through specialized channels in the cell membrane. The large, negatively charged protein molecules stay inside the neuron.

FIGURE 2.2   The Distribution of Ions Inside and Outside a Neuron

(A) Diffusion

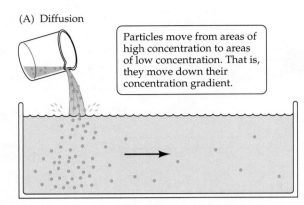

Particles move from areas of high concentration to areas of low concentration. That is, they move down their concentration gradient.

(B) Diffusion through semipermeable membranes

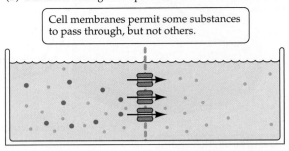

Cell membranes permit some substances to pass through, but not others.

(C) Electrostatic forces

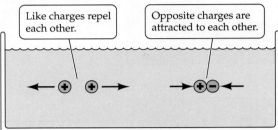

Like charges repel each other.

Opposite charges are attracted to each other.

FIGURE 2.3 Ionic Forces Underlying Electrical Signaling in Neurons

sodium ion (Na⁺) A sodium atom that carries a positive charge.

selective permeability The property of a membrane that allows some substances to pass through, but not others.

diffusion The spontaneous spread of molecules from an area of high concentration to an area of low concentration.

electrostatic pressure The propensity of charged molecules or ions to move toward areas with the opposite charge.

sodium-potassium pump The energetically expensive mechanism that pushes sodium ions out of a cell, and potassium ions in.

membrane, but not **sodium ions (Na⁺)**. Because it is studded with these K⁺ channels, we say that the cell membrane of a neuron exhibits **selective permeability**, allowing some things to pass through, but not others. The membrane allows K⁺ ions, but not Na⁺ ions, to enter or exit the cell fairly freely.

The resting potential of the neuron reflects a balancing act between two opposing processes that drive K⁺ ions in and out of the neuron. The first of these is **diffusion** (**FIGURE 2.3A**), which is the tendency for molecules of a substance to spread from regions of high concentration to regions of low concentration. For example, when placed in a glass of water, the molecules in a drop of ink will tend to spread from the drop out into the rest of the water, where they are less concentrated. So we say that molecules tend to "move down their concentration gradient" until they are evenly distributed. If a selectively permeable membrane divides the fluid, particles that can pass through the membrane, such as K⁺, will diffuse across until they are equally concentrated on both sides. Other ions, unable to cross the membrane, will remain concentrated on one side (**FIGURE 2.3B**).

The second force at work is **electrostatic pressure**, which arises from the distribution of electrical charges rather than the distribution of molecules. Charged particles exert electrical force on one another: like charges repel, and opposite charges attract (**FIGURE 2.3C**). Positively charged cations like K⁺ are thus attracted to the negatively charged interior of the cell; conversely, anions are repelled by the cell interior and so tend to exit to the extracellular fluid.

Now let's consider the situation across a neuron's cell membrane. Much of the energy consumed by a neuron goes into operating specialized membrane proteins called **sodium-potassium pumps** that pump three Na⁺ ions out of the cell for every two K⁺ ions pumped in (**FIGURE 2.4A**). This action results in a buildup of K⁺ ions inside the cell (and reduces Na⁺ inside the cell), but as we explained earlier, the membrane is selectively permeable to K⁺ ions (but not Na⁺ ions). Therefore, K⁺ ions can leave the interior, moving down their concentration gradient and causing a net buildup of negative charges inside the cell (**FIGURE 2.4B**). As negative charge builds up inside the cell, it begins to exert electrostatic pressure to pull positively charged K⁺ ions back inside. Eventually the opposing forces exerted by the K⁺ concentration gradient and by electrostatic pressure reach the **equilibrium potential**, the electrical charge that exactly balances the

(A) The sodium-potassium pump

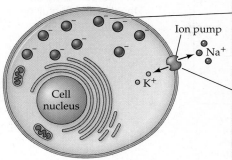

Ion pump

Na+

K+

Cell nucleus

Cells contain many large, negatively charged molecules, such as proteins, that do not cross the membrane.

The sodium-potassium (Na+-K+) pump continually pushes Na+ ions out and pulls K+ ions in. This ion pump requires considerable energy.

FIGURE 2.4 The Ionic Basis of the Resting Potential

(B) Membrane permeability to ions

K+ channel

K+

K+

K+

K+

Na+

The membrane is permeable to K+ ions, which pass back out again through channels down their concentration gradient. The departure of K+ ions leaves the inside of the cell more negative than the outside. Na+ ions cannot pass back inside.

(C) Equilibrium potential

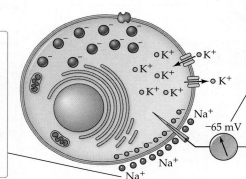

Cations like Na+ push against the membrane's exterior, attracted to the negative interior. Likewise, anions coat the interior of the cell membrane, attracted to cations on the other side. Most of the cell's potential difference is due to these charges immediately surrounding the membrane.

K+

K+

K+

K+

K+

Na+

Na+

Na+

−65 mV

When enough K+ ions have departed to bring the membrane potential to −65 mV or so, the electrical attraction pulling K+ in is exactly balanced by the concentration gradient pushing K+ out. This is the K+ equilibrium potential, approximately the cell's resting potential.

concentration gradient: any further movement of K+ ions into the cell (drawn by electrostatic attraction) is matched by the flow of K+ ions out of the cell (moving down their concentration gradient). This point approximates the cell's resting potential of about −65 mV (values may range between −50 and −80 mV), as **FIGURE 2.4C** depicts.

The resting potential of a neuron provides a baseline level of polarization found in all cells. But unlike most other cells, neurons routinely undergo a brief but radical change in polarization, sending an electrical signal from one end of the neuron to the other, as we'll discuss next.

A threshold amount of depolarization triggers an action potential

Action potentials are very brief but large changes in neuronal polarization that arise in the initial segment of the axon, just after the **axon hillock** (the cone-shaped region where the axon emerges from the cell body; see Figure 1.4A), and then move rapidly down the axon. The information that a neuron sends to other cells is encoded in patterns of these action potentials, so we need to understand their properties—where they come from, how they race down the axon, and how they send information across synapses to other cells. Let's turn first to the creation of the action potential.

Two concepts are central to understanding how action potentials are triggered. **Hyperpolarization** is an increase in membrane potential (i.e., the neuron becomes *even more negative* on the inside, relative to the outside). So if the neuron already has a resting potential of, say, −65 mV, hyperpolarization makes it even *farther from zero*, maybe −70 mV. **Depolarization** is the reverse, referring to a decrease in membrane potential. The depolarization of a neuron from a resting potential of −65 mV to, say, −50 mV makes the inside of the neuron more like the outside. In other words, depolarization of a neuron brings its membrane potential *closer to zero*.

Let's use an apparatus to apply hyperpolarizing and depolarizing stimuli to a neuron, via electrodes. (Later we'll talk about how synapses produce similar hyperpolarizations and depolarizations.) Applying a *hyperpolarizing* stimulus to the membrane

View Animation 2.3:
The Resting Membrane Potential

equilibrium potential The point at which the movement of ions across the cell membrane is balanced, as the electrostatic pressure pulling ions in one direction is offset by the diffusion force pushing them in the opposite direction.

axon hillock The cone-shaped area on the cell body from which the axon originates.

hyperpolarization An increase in membrane potential (the interior of the neuron becomes even more negative).

depolarization A decrease in membrane potential (the interior of the neuron becomes less negative).

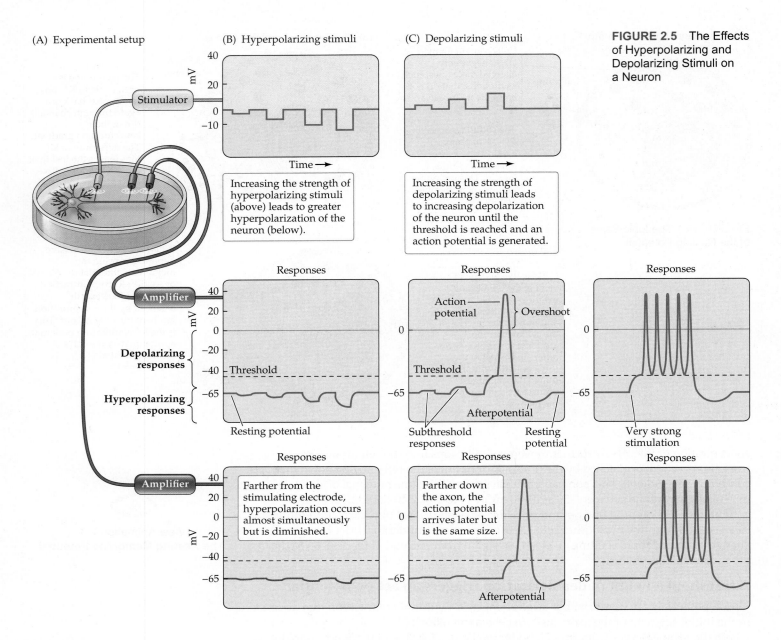

(A) Experimental setup

(B) Hyperpolarizing stimuli

Increasing the strength of hyperpolarizing stimuli (above) leads to greater hyperpolarization of the neuron (below).

(C) Depolarizing stimuli

Increasing the strength of depolarizing stimuli leads to increasing depolarization of the neuron until the threshold is reached and an action potential is generated.

FIGURE 2.5 The Effects of Hyperpolarizing and Depolarizing Stimuli on a Neuron

Responses — Threshold — Depolarizing responses — Hyperpolarizing responses — Resting potential

Responses — Action potential — Overshoot — Threshold — Subthreshold responses — Afterpotential — Resting potential

Responses — Very strong stimulation

Farther from the stimulating electrode, hyperpolarization occurs almost simultaneously but is diminished.

Farther down the axon, the action potential arrives later but is the same size.

Afterpotential

local potential An electrical potential that is initiated by stimulation at a specific site, is a graded response that spreads passively across the cell membrane, and decreases in strength with time and distance.

threshold The stimulus intensity that is just adequate to trigger an action potential in an axon.

action potential Also called *spike*. A rapid reversal of the membrane potential that momentarily makes the inside of a neuron positive with respect to the outside.

produces an immediate response that passively mirrors the stimulus pulse (**FIGURES 2.5A** and **B**). The greater the stimulus, the greater the response, so these changes in the neuron's potential are *graded responses*.

If we measured the membrane response at locations farther and farther away from the stimulus location, we would see another way in which the membrane response seems passive. Like the ripples spreading from a pebble dropped in a pond, these graded **local potentials** across the membrane get smaller as they spread away from the point of stimulation (see Figure 2.5B *bottom*).

Up to a point, the application of *depolarizing* pulses to the membrane follows the same pattern as for hyperpolarizing stimuli, producing local, graded responses. However, the situation changes suddenly if the stimulus depolarizes the axon to −40 mV or so (the exact value varies slightly among neurons). At this point, known as the **threshold**, a sudden and brief (0.5- to 2.0-millisecond) response—the **action potential**, sometimes referred to as a *spike* because of its shape—is provoked (**FIGURE 2.5C**). An action potential is a rapid reversal of the membrane potential that momentarily makes the inside of the neuron *positive* with respect to the outside. Unlike the passive graded potentials that we have been discussing, the action potential is actively reproduced (or *propagated*) down the axon, through mechanisms that we'll discuss shortly.

Applying strong stimuli to produce depolarizations that far exceed the neuron's threshold reveals another important property of action potentials: larger depolarizations do not produce larger action potentials. In other words, the size (or *amplitude*) of the action potential is independent of stimulus size. This characteristic is referred to as the **all-or-none property** of the action potential: either it fires at its full amplitude, or it doesn't fire at all. It turns out that neurons encode information by changes in the *number* of action potentials rather than in their amplitude. With stronger stimuli, *more* action potentials are produced, but the size of each action potential remains the same.

A closer look at the form of the action potential shows that the return to baseline membrane potential is not simple. Many axons exhibit small potential changes immediately following the spike; these changes are called **afterpotentials** (see Figure 2.5C), and they are also related to the movement of ions in and out of the cell, which we take up next.

Ionic mechanisms underlie the action potential

What events explain the action potential? The action potential is created by the sudden movement of Na^+ ions into the axon (Hodgkin and Katz, 1949). At its peak, the action potential reaches about +40 mV, approaching the equilibrium potential for Na^+, when the concentration gradient pushing Na^+ ions *into* the cell would be exactly balanced by the positive charge pushing them *out*. The action potential thus involves a rapid shift in membrane properties, switching suddenly from the potassium-dependent resting state to a primarily sodium-dependent active state and then swiftly returning to the resting state. This shift is accomplished through the actions of a very special kind of ion channel: the **voltage-gated Na^+ channel**. Like other ion channels, this channel is a tubular, membrane-spanning protein, but its central Na^+-selective pore is *gated*. The gate is ordinarily closed. But if we electrically stimulate the neuron, or if synapses affect the neuron in ways we'll describe later, then the axon may be depolarized. If the axon is depolarized enough to reach threshold levels, the channel's shape changes, opening the "gate" to allow Na^+ ions through for a short while.

This tiny protein molecule, the voltage-gated Na^+ channel, is really a quite complicated machine. It monitors the axon's membrane potential, and at threshold the channel changes its shape to open the pore, shutting down again just a millisecond later. The channel then "remembers" that it was recently open and refuses to open again for a short time. These properties of the voltage-gated Na^+ channel are responsible for the characteristics of the action potential.

You might wonder whether the repeated inrush of Na^+ ions would allow them to build up, affecting the cell's resting potential. In fact, relatively few Na^+ ions need to enter to change the membrane potential, and the K^+ ions quickly restore the resting potential. In the long run, the sodium-potassium pump enforces the concentrations of ions that maintain the resting potential.

Consider what happens when a patch of axonal membrane depolarizes. As long as the depolarization is below threshold, Na^+ channels remain closed. But when the depolarization reaches threshold, a few Na^+ channels open at first, allowing a few ions to start entering the neuron. The positive charges of those ions depolarize the membrane even further, opening still more Na^+ channels. Thus, the process accelerates until the barriers are removed and Na^+ ions rush in (**FIGURE 2.6**).

The voltage-gated Na^+ channels stay open for a little less than a millisecond, and then they automatically close again. By this time, the membrane potential has shot up to about +40 mV. Positive charges inside the nerve cell start to push K^+ ions out, aided by the opening of additional voltage-gated K^+ channels that let lots of K^+ ions rush out quickly, restoring the resting potential.

View Animation 2.4:
The Action Potential

all-or-none property   The condition that the size (amplitude) of the action potential is independent of the size of the stimulus.

afterpotential   The positive or negative change in membrane potential that may follow an action potential.

voltage-gated Na^+ channel
A Na^+-selective channel that opens or closes in response to changes in the voltage of the local membrane potential. It mediates the action potential.

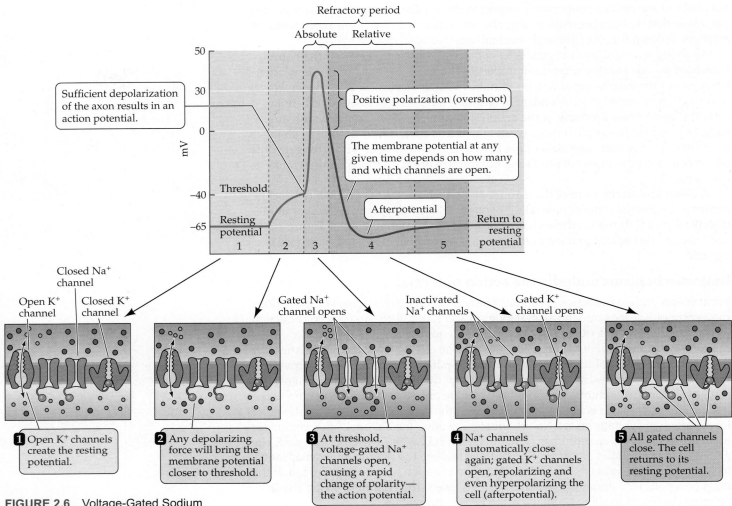

Refractory period

Absolute | Relative

Sufficient depolarization of the axon results in an action potential.

Positive polarization (overshoot)

The membrane potential at any given time depends on how many and which channels are open.

Threshold

Afterpotential

Resting potential

Return to resting potential

Closed Na⁺ channel

Open K⁺ channel | Closed K⁺ channel

Gated Na⁺ channel opens

Inactivated Na⁺ channels

Gated K⁺ channel opens

1 Open K⁺ channels create the resting potential.

2 Any depolarizing force will bring the membrane potential closer to threshold.

3 At threshold, voltage-gated Na⁺ channels open, causing a rapid change of polarity—the action potential.

4 Na⁺ channels automatically close again; gated K⁺ channels open, repolarizing and even hyperpolarizing the cell (afterpotential).

5 All gated channels close. The cell returns to its resting potential.

FIGURE 2.6 Voltage-Gated Sodium Channels Produce the Action Potential

refractory Temporarily unresponsive or inactivated.

absolute refractory phase A brief period of complete insensitivity to stimuli.

relative refractory phase A period of reduced sensitivity during which only strong stimulation produces an action potential.

Applying very strong stimuli reveals another important property of axonal membranes. As we bombard the axon with ever-stronger stimuli, an upper limit to the frequency of action potentials becomes apparent at about 1,200 spikes per second. (Many neurons have even slower maximum rates of response.) Similarly, applying pairs of stimuli that are spaced closer and closer together reveals a related phenomenon: beyond a certain point, only the first stimulus is able to elicit an action potential. The axonal membrane is said to be **refractory** (unresponsive) to the second stimulus.

Refractoriness has two phases: During the **absolute refractory phase**, a brief period immediately following the production of an action potential, no amount of stimulation can induce another action potential, because the voltage-gated Na⁺ channels can't respond (in Figure 2.6, see the brackets above the graph, as well as step 4). The absolute phase is followed by a period of reduced sensitivity, the **relative refractory phase**, during which only strong stimulation can depolarize the axon to threshold to produce another action potential. The neuron is *relatively* refractory because K⁺ ions are still flowing out, so the cell is temporarily hyperpolarized after firing an action potential (see Figure 2.6, step 4). The overall duration of the refractory phase is what determines a neuron's maximal rate of firing.

In general, the transmission of action potentials is limited to axons. Cell bodies and dendrites usually have few voltage-gated Na⁺ channels, so they do not conduct action potentials. The ion channels on the cell body and dendrites are stimulated chemically at synapses, as we'll discuss later in this chapter. Because the axon has many such channels, an action potential that occurs at the origin of the axon regenerates itself down the length of the axon, as we discuss next.

HOW'S IT GOING

1. What does it mean if a neuron is depolarized or hyperpolarized, and which action brings the cell closer to threshold?
2. Describe how the polarity of a neuron changes during the phases of an action potential.
3. How does the flow of ions account for that sequence of changes in electrical potential?
4. What mechanisms underlie the two phases of the refractory period?

Action potentials are actively propagated along the axon

Now that we've explored how voltage-gated channels underlie action potentials, we can turn to the question of how action potentials spread down the axon—another function for which voltage-gated channels are crucial. Consider an experimental setup like the one pictured in **FIGURE 2.7**: recording electrodes are positioned along the length of the axon, allowing us to record an action potential at various points on the axon. Recordings like this show that an action potential begun at the axon hillock spreads in a sort of chain reaction down the length of the axon.

How does the action potential travel? It is important to understand that the action potential is regenerated along the length of the axon. Remember, the action potential is a spike of depolarizing electrical activity (with a peak of about +40 mV), so it strongly

**View Animation 2.5:
Action Potential Propagation**

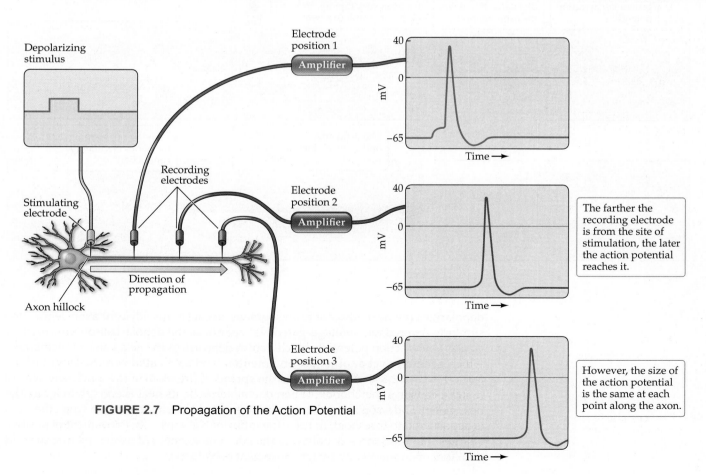

FIGURE 2.7 Propagation of the Action Potential

FIGURE 2.8 Conduction along Unmyelinated versus Myelinated Axons

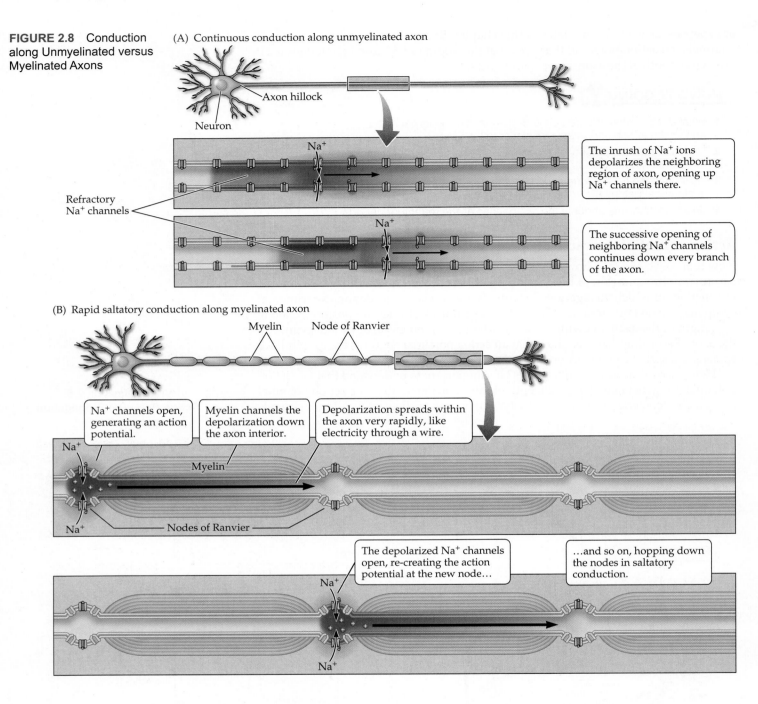

(A) Continuous conduction along unmyelinated axon

Axon hillock

Neuron

Na⁺

Refractory Na⁺ channels

The inrush of Na⁺ ions depolarizes the neighboring region of axon, opening up Na⁺ channels there.

Na⁺

The successive opening of neighboring Na⁺ channels continues down every branch of the axon.

(B) Rapid saltatory conduction along myelinated axon

Myelin   Node of Ranvier

Na⁺ channels open, generating an action potential.

Myelin channels the depolarization down the axon interior.

Depolarization spreads within the axon very rapidly, like electricity through a wire.

Na⁺

Myelin

Na⁺

Nodes of Ranvier

The depolarized Na⁺ channels open, re-creating the action potential at the new node…

…and so on, hopping down the nodes in saltatory conduction.

Na⁺

Na⁺

depolarizes the next adjacent axon segment. Because this adjacent axon segment is similarly covered with voltage-gated Na⁺ channels, the depolarization immediately creates a new action potential, which in turn depolarizes the next patch of membrane, which generates yet another action potential, and so on all down the length of the axon (**FIGURE 2.8A**). An analogy is the spread of fire along a row of closely spaced match heads in a matchbook. When one match is lit, its heat is enough to ignite the next match, and so on along the row. Voltage-gated Na⁺ channels open when the axon is depolarized to threshold. In turn, the influx of Na⁺ ions—the movement of positive charges into the axon—depolarizes the adjacent segment of axonal membrane and therefore opens new gates for the movement of Na⁺ ions.

BOX 2.1 How Is an Axon Like a Toilet?

It might help you to remember basic facts about action potentials if you consider how much they resemble a flushing toilet. For example, if you gently push the lever on a toilet, nothing much happens. As you gradually increase the force you apply to the lever, you will eventually find the threshold—the amount of force that is just enough to trigger a flush (step 1 of the figure). Likewise, the neuron has a *threshold*—the amount of depolarization that is just enough to trigger an action potential at the start of an axon. Once you're past the threshold, it doesn't matter how hard you pushed the (traditional style) toilet lever; the flush will always be the same. Similarly, once the neuron is pushed past threshold, the action potential will be the same. This is the *all-or-none* property of action potentials (step 2).

After a toilet has flushed, it takes a while (about a minute) before it can flush again (step 3). Likewise, after a neuron fires, it takes a while (about a millisecond) before it can fire again. This is the neuron's *refractory period*. Why do neurons have a refractory period for action potentials? As you may remember, the voltage-gated sodium channels always slam shut for a while after they've opened, no matter what the membrane potential is. Until that time is up, the sodium channels won't open again. If the situation is urgent, we can flush our toilet about 60 times per hour or fire our neurons about 1,000 times per second. (If things are *really* urgent, we might do both.)

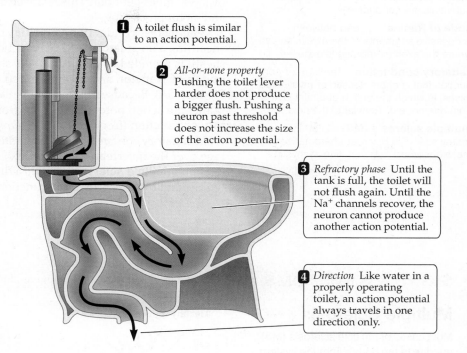

1 A toilet flush is similar to an action potential.

2 *All-or-none property* Pushing the toilet lever harder does not produce a bigger flush. Pushing a neuron past threshold does not increase the size of the action potential.

3 *Refractory phase* Until the tank is full, the toilet will not flush again. Until the Na$^+$ channels recover, the neuron cannot produce another action potential.

4 *Direction* Like water in a properly operating toilet, an action potential always travels in one direction only.

Also notice that when a properly working toilet flushes, the water always goes in the same direction (no one wants a toilet that sometimes flushes backward!) (step 4). Likewise, the neuron's action potential goes in only one direction down the axon, from the end attached to the cell body to the axon terminals.

Of course, neurons are different from toilets in many ways. The outflow of a toilet goes only to the single sewer line leaving a house, but an action potential may flow down many axon branches, to communicate with hundreds of other neurons. Voltage-gated sodium channels on the axon branches ensure that the action potential is just as large in each branch, so it's not diminished by spreading out among branches. A toilet has only one lever, but each neuron has hundreds or thousands of synapses, and by producing different sorts of local, graded potentials, some synapses make the neuron more likely to reach threshold, while others make it less likely.

The axon normally conducts action potentials in only one direction—from the axon hillock toward the axon terminals—because, as it progresses along the axon, the action potential leaves in its wake a stretch of refractory membrane (see Figure 2.8A). The action potential does not spread back over the axon hillock and the cell body and dendrites, because the membranes there have too few voltage-gated Na$^+$ channels to be able to produce an action potential.

Many of the characteristics of action potentials have been whimsically likened to the action of a toilet, as **BOX 2.1** explores.

If we record the speed of action potentials along axons that differ in diameter, we see that **conduction velocity** varies with the diameter of the axon. Larger axons allow the depolarization to spread faster through the interior. In mammals, the conduction velocity in large fibers may be as fast as 150 meters per second. (We will discuss axon

conduction velocity The speed at which an action potential is propagated along the length of an axon.

myelin   The fatty insulation around an axon, formed by glial cells. The myelin sheath boosts the speed at which action potentials are conducted.

node of Ranvier   A gap between successive segments of the myelin sheath where the axon membrane is exposed.

saltatory conduction   The form of conduction that is characteristic of myelinated axons, in which the action potential jumps from one node of Ranvier to the next.

multiple sclerosis (MS)   Literally "many scars." A disorder characterized by the widespread degeneration of myelin.

diameter and conduction velocity again in Chapter 5.) Although not as fast as the speed of light (as was once believed), neural conduction can nevertheless be very fast: over 300 miles per hour. This relatively high rate of conduction ensures rapid sensory and motor processing.

The fastest conduction velocities require more than just large axons. **Myelin** sheathing also greatly speeds conduction. As we described in Chapter 1, the myelin sheath is provided by glial cells. This sheath surrounding the axon is interrupted by **nodes of Ranvier**, small gaps spaced about every millimeter along the axon (see Figure 1.5A). Because the myelin insulation resists the flow of ions across the membrane, the action potential "jumps" from node to node. This process is called **saltatory conduction** (from the Latin *saltare*, "to jump") (**FIGURE 2.8B**). The evolution of rapid saltatory conduction in vertebrates has given them a major behavioral advantage over the invertebrates, whose axons are unmyelinated and thus slower in conduction. **Multiple sclerosis (MS)** is a disease in which myelin is compromised, with highly variable effects on brain function, as described in Signs & Symptoms next.

SIGNS & SYMPTOMS ||||||||||||||||||||||||||||||||||||||||||||||||||||||||||||||||||||||||||||||||||||||||||||||

Multiple Sclerosis

Most cases of multiple sclerosis (MS) are due to the body's immune system generating antibodies that attack one or more molecules in myelin. If the myelin is damaged enough, then saltatory conduction of axon potentials is disrupted, throwing off the brain's timing in coordinating behavior and interpreting sensory input (**FIGURE 2.9**). MS can present with a bewildering variety of motor and/or sensory symptoms, depending on where, exactly, myelin damage occurs. For many people, the first symptoms they notice are blurred vision or poor color perception. For others, the first symptoms are unexpected tingling sensations, or a difficulty coordinating their walking, with the feeling of stiff legs. Eventually, almost all MS patients experience fatigue. The various symptoms wax and wane for reasons no one understands. While MS symptoms generally worsen over time, the rate of change varies a great deal across patients, making it impossible to predict how the disease might progress.

There is currently no cure for MS, but there are medicines to manage the

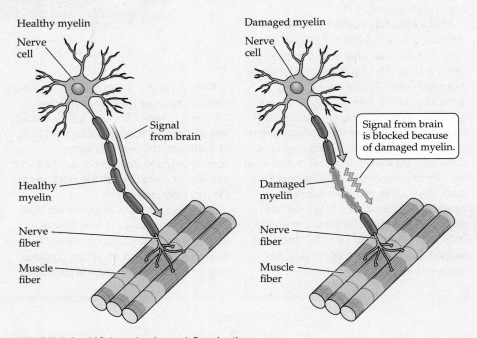

FIGURE 2.9   MS Impairs Axonal Conduction

symptoms, mostly by interfering with the immune system to curtail myelin damage. It's also important to get physical therapy to learn how to maintain normal activity despite the symptoms. Smoking increases the risk of MS. It is also more common in women than in men. Symptoms tend

to be reduced during pregnancy when estrogen levels are high (Voskuhl and Momtazee, 2017), so there is growing interest in whether hormones might offer an effective treatment.

HOW'S IT GOING ❓

1. How is the action potential propagated along the axon?
2. What factor causes saltatory conduction, and why does it speed propagation of the action potential?
3. Why do action potentials move only away from the cell body?
4. What is the underlying cause of multiple sclerosis, and what are some symptoms of the disease?

Synapses cause local changes in the postsynaptic membrane potential

At the beginning of the chapter, we told you that when the action potential reaches the end of an axon, it causes the axon to release a chemical, called a **neurotransmitter** (or *transmitter*), into the synapse. We will discuss the many different types of transmitters in detail in Chapter 4. For now, what you need to know is that when an axon releases neurotransmitter molecules into a synapse, they briefly alter the membrane potential of the other cell. Because information is moving from the axon to the target cell on the other side of the synapse, we say the axon is from the **presynaptic** cell, and the target neuron on the other side of the synapse is the **postsynaptic** cell.

The brief changes in the membrane potential of the postsynaptic cell in response to neurotransmitter are called, naturally enough, **postsynaptic potentials**. A given neuron, receiving synapses from many other cells, is subject to hundreds or thousands of postsynaptic potentials. When added together, this massive array of local potentials determines whether the axon hillock's membrane potential will reach threshold and therefore trigger an action potential. The nervous system employs electrical synapses too (see **A STEP FURTHER 2.1**, on the website), but the vast majority of synapses use neurotransmitters to produce postsynaptic potentials.

We can study postsynaptic potentials with a setup like that shown in **FIGURE 2.10**. This setup allows us to compare the effects of activity of excitatory versus inhibitory

neurotransmitter   Also called simply *transmitter*, *synaptic transmitter*, or *chemical transmitter*. The chemical released from the presynaptic axon terminal that serves as the basis of communication between neurons.

presynaptic   Located on the "transmitting" side of a synapse.

postsynaptic   Referring to the region of a synapse that receives and responds to neurotransmitter.

postsynaptic potential   A local potential that is initiated by stimulation at a synapse, can vary in amplitude, and spreads passively across the cell membrane, decreasing in strength with time and distance.

FIGURE 2.10   Recording Postsynaptic Potentials

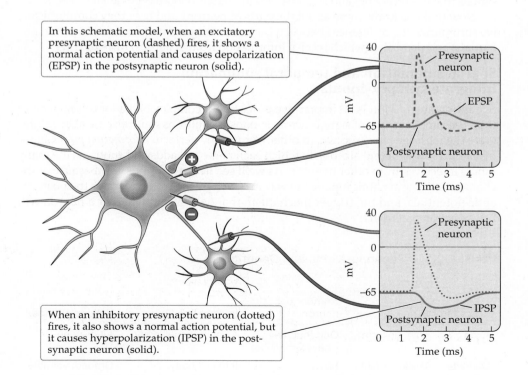

In this schematic model, when an excitatory presynaptic neuron (dashed) fires, it shows a normal action potential and causes depolarization (EPSP) in the postsynaptic neuron (solid).

When an inhibitory presynaptic neuron (dotted) fires, it also shows a normal action potential, but it causes hyperpolarization (IPSP) in the postsynaptic neuron (solid).

excitatory postsynaptic potential (EPSP) A depolarizing potential in a neuron that is normally caused by synaptic excitation. EPSPs increase the probability that the postsynaptic neuron will fire an action potential.

inhibitory postsynaptic potential (IPSP) A hyperpolarizing potential in a neuron. IPSPs decrease the probability that the postsynaptic neuron will fire an action potential.

chloride ion (Cl⁻) A chlorine atom that carries a negative charge.

View Animation 2.6: Spatial Summation

synapses on the local membrane potential of a postsynaptic cell. The responses of the presynaptic and postsynaptic cells are shown on similar graphs in Figure 2.10 for easy comparison of their timing. It is important to remember that excitatory and inhibitory neurons get their names from their *actions on postsynaptic neurons*, not from their effects on behavior.

Stimulation of the excitatory presynaptic neuron (red in Figure 2.10) causes it to produce an all-or-none action potential that spreads to the end of the axon, releasing transmitter. After a brief delay, the postsynaptic cell (yellow) displays a small local depolarization, as Na^+ channels open to let the positive ions in. This postsynaptic membrane depolarization is known as an **excitatory postsynaptic potential** (**EPSP**) because it pushes the postsynaptic cell a little closer to the threshold for an action potential.

The action potential of the inhibitory presynaptic neuron (blue in Figure 2.10) looks exactly like that of the excitatory presynaptic neuron; all neurons use the same kind of action potential. But the effect on the postsynaptic side is quite different. When the inhibitory presynaptic neuron is activated, the postsynaptic membrane potential becomes even more negative, or hyperpolarized. This hyperpolarization moves the cell membrane potential away from threshold—it decreases the probability that the neuron will fire an action potential—so it is called an **inhibitory postsynaptic potential** (**IPSP**).

Usually IPSPs result from the opening of channels that permit **chloride ions** (**Cl⁻**) to enter the cell. Because Cl⁻ ions are much more concentrated outside the cell than inside (see Figure 2.2), they rush into the cell, making its membrane potential more negative. What determines whether a synapse excites or inhibits the postsynaptic cell? One factor is the particular neurotransmitter released by the presynaptic cell. Some transmitters typically generate an EPSP in the postsynaptic cells; others typically generate an IPSP. Sometimes the same neurotransmitter can be excitatory at one synapse and inhibitory at another, depending on what sort of receptor the postsynaptic cell possesses. So in the end, whether a neuron fires an action potential at any given moment is decided by the balance between the number of excitatory and the number of inhibitory signals that it is receiving, and it receives many signals of both types at all times.

Now that you know more about the parts of neurons and how they communicate, we summarize the differences between axons (which send information via action potentials) and dendrites (which receive information from synapses) in **TABLE 2.1**.

Spatial summation and temporal summation integrate synaptic inputs

Synaptic transmission is an impressive process, but complex behavior requires more than the simple arrival of signals across synapses. Neurons must also be able to integrate the messages they receive. In other words, they perform *information processing*—by using a sort of neural algebra, in which each nerve cell adds and subtracts the many inputs it receives from other neurons. As we'll see next, this is possible because of the characteristics of synaptic inputs, the way in which the neuron integrates the postsynaptic potentials, and the trigger mechanism that determines whether a neuron will fire an action potential.

TABLE 2.1 Comparing Axons and Dendrites

	Property			
	Size	Number per neuron	Information flow	Voltage changes
Axon	Thin, uniform	One (but may have branches)	Away from cell body	All-or-none
Dendrite	Thick, variable	Many	Into cell body	Graded, variable

We've seen that postsynaptic potentials are caused by transmitter chemicals that can be either depolarizing (excitatory) or hyperpolarizing (inhibitory). From their points of origin on the dendrites and cell body, these graded EPSPs and IPSPs spread passively over the postsynaptic neuron, decreasing in strength over time and distance. Whether the postsynaptic neuron will fire depends on whether a depolarization exceeding threshold reaches the axon hillock, triggering an action potential. If many EPSPs are received, the axon may reach threshold and fire. But if both EPSPs and IPSPs arrive at the axon hillock, they partially cancel each other. Thus, the net effect is the *difference* between the two: the neuron subtracts the IPSPs from the EPSPs. Simple arithmetic, right?

Well, yes, summed EPSPs and IPSPs do tend to cancel each other out. But because postsynaptic potentials spread passively and dissipate as they cross the cell membrane, the resulting sum is also influenced by *distance.* For example, EPSPs from synapses close to the axon hillock will produce a larger effect there than will EPSPs from farther away. The summation of potentials originating from different physical locations across the cell body is called **spatial summation**. Only if the overall sum of *all* the potentials—both EPSPs and IPSPs—is sufficient to depolarize the cell to threshold at the axon hillock is an action potential triggered (**FIGURE 2.11A**). Usually it takes excitatory messages from many presynaptic neurons to cause a postsynaptic neuron to fire an action potential.

Postsynaptic effects that are not absolutely simultaneous can also be summed, because the postsynaptic potentials last a few milliseconds before fading away. The closer they are in time, the greater is the overlap and the more complete is the summation, which in this case is called **temporal summation**. Temporal summation is easily understood if you imagine a neuron with only one input. If EPSPs arrive one right after the other, they sum, and the postsynaptic cell eventually reaches threshold and produces an action potential (**FIGURE 2.11B**). But these graded potentials fade quickly, so if too much time passes between successive EPSPs, they will never sum and no action potentials will be triggered.

spatial summation   The summation of postsynaptic potentials that reach the axon hillock from different locations across the cell body. If this summation reaches threshold, an action potential is triggered.

temporal summation   The summation of postsynaptic potentials that reach the axon hillock at different times. The closer in time the potentials occur, the greater the summation.

FIGURE 2.11   Spatial versus Temporal Summation

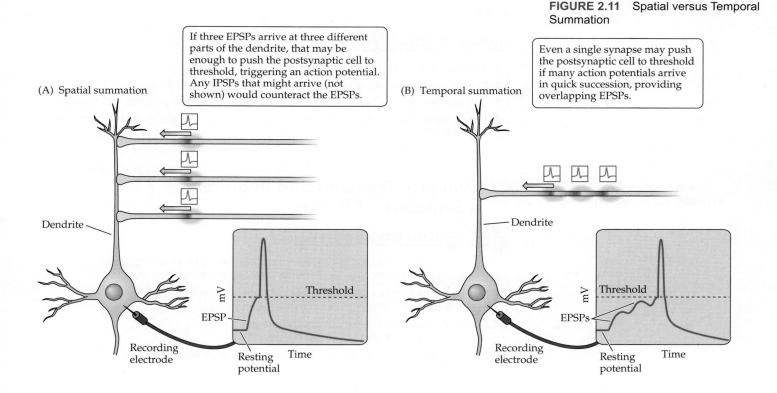

(A) Spatial summation

If three EPSPs arrive at three different parts of the dendrite, that may be enough to push the postsynaptic cell to threshold, triggering an action potential. Any IPSPs that might arrive (not shown) would counteract the EPSPs.

Dendrite

Recording electrode

mV

Threshold

EPSP

Resting potential

Time

(B) Temporal summation

Even a single synapse may push the postsynaptic cell to threshold if many action potentials arrive in quick succession, providing overlapping EPSPs.

Dendrite

Recording electrode

mV

Threshold

EPSPs

Resting potential

Time

TABLE 2.2 Characteristics of Electrical Signals of Nerve Cells

Type of signal	Signaling role	Typical duration (ms)	Amplitude	Character	Mode of propagation	Ion channel opening	Channel sensitive to:
Action potential	Conduction along an axon	1–2	Overshooting, 100 mV	All-or-none, digital	Actively propagated, regenerative	First Na⁺, then K⁺, in different channels	Voltage (depolarization)
Excitatory postsynaptic potential (EPSP)	Transmission between neurons	10–100	Depolarizing, from less than 1 to more than 20 mV	Graded, analog	Local, passive spread	Na⁺, K⁺	Chemical (neurotransmitter)
Inhibitory postsynaptic potential (IPSP)	Transmission between neurons	10–100	Hyperpolarizing, from less than 1 to about 15 mV	Graded, analog	Local, passive spread	Cl⁻, K⁺	Chemical (neurotransmitter)

TABLE 2.2 summarizes the many properties of action potentials, EPSPs, and IPSPs, noting the similarities and differences among the three kinds of neural potentials.

It should now be clear that although action potentials are all-or-none phenomena, the postsynaptic effect they produce is graded in size and determined by the processing of many inputs occurring close together in time. The membrane potential at the axon hillock thus reflects the moment-to-moment integration of all the neuron's inputs, which the axon hillock encodes into action potentials.

Dendrites add to the story of neuronal integration. A vast number of synaptic inputs, arrayed across the dendrites and cell body, can induce postsynaptic potentials. So dendrites expand the receptive surface of the neuron and increase the amount of input the neuron can handle. All other things being equal, the farther out on a dendrite a potential occurs, the less effect it should have at the axon, because the potential decreases in size as it passively spreads. When the potential arises at a dendritic spine (see Figure 1.4), its effect is even smaller because it has to spread down the shaft of the spine. Thus, information arriving at various parts of the neuron is weighted, in terms of the distance to the axon hillock and the path resistance along the way.

HOW'S IT GOING ?

1. What are EPSPs and IPSPs?
2. Compare and contrast spatial summation versus temporal summation.
3. Discuss the electrical properties of a neuron that allow it to process information.
4. Where does information enter a neuron, and how does a neuron send information to other cells?

View Animation 2.7: Synaptic Transmission

2.2 Synaptic Transmission Requires a Sequence of Events

THE ROAD AHEAD

This portion of the chapter explains how neurons release chemicals to signal one another. After reading this material, you should be able to:

2.2.1 Identify the sequence of steps that take place when one neuron releases a chemical signal to affect another.

2.2.2 Understand how a variety of chemical signals enables a diversity of neuronal responses to other neurons.

2.2.3 Identify the interactions between neurons and muscles that underlie a simple reflex.

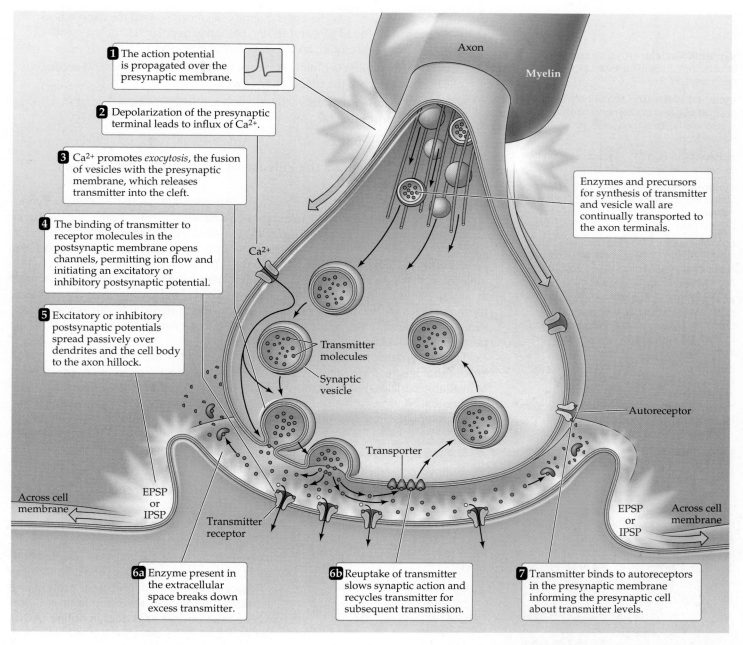

1 The action potential is propagated over the presynaptic membrane.

2 Depolarization of the presynaptic terminal leads to influx of Ca^{2+}.

3 Ca^{2+} promotes *exocytosis*, the fusion of vesicles with the presynaptic membrane, which releases transmitter into the cleft.

4 The binding of transmitter to receptor molecules in the postsynaptic membrane opens channels, permitting ion flow and initiating an excitatory or inhibitory postsynaptic potential.

5 Excitatory or inhibitory postsynaptic potentials spread passively over dendrites and the cell body to the axon hillock.

Axon

Myelin

Enzymes and precursors for synthesis of transmitter and vesicle wall are continually transported to the axon terminals.

Ca^{2+}

Transmitter molecules

Synaptic vesicle

Autoreceptor

Transporter

Across cell membrane

EPSP or IPSP

Transmitter receptor

EPSP or IPSP

Across cell membrane

6a Enzyme present in the extracellular space breaks down excess transmitter.

6b Reuptake of transmitter slows synaptic action and recycles transmitter for subsequent transmission.

7 Transmitter binds to autoreceptors in the presynaptic membrane informing the presynaptic cell about transmitter levels.

FIGURE 2.12 Steps in Transmission at a Chemical Synapse

The steps that take place during chemical synaptic transmission are summarized in **FIGURE 2.12**:

1. The action potential arrives at the presynaptic axon terminal.

2. Voltage-gated calcium channels in the membrane of the axon terminal open, allowing calcium ions (Ca^{2+}) to enter.

3. Ca^{2+} causes synaptic vesicles filled with neurotransmitter to fuse with the presynaptic membrane and rupture, releasing the transmitter molecules into the synaptic cleft.

4. Transmitter molecules bind to special receptor molecules in the postsynaptic membrane, leading—directly or indirectly—to the opening of ion channels in the postsynaptic membrane. The resulting flow of ions creates a local EPSP or IPSP in the postsynaptic neuron.

synaptic vesicle A small, spherical structure that contains molecules of neurotransmitter.

synaptic cleft The space between the presynaptic and postsynaptic cells at a synapse. This gap measures about 20–40 nanometers.

calcium ion (Ca^{2+}) A calcium atom that carries a double positive charge.

synaptic delay The brief delay between the arrival of an action potential at the axon terminal and the creation of a postsynaptic potential.

ligand A substance that binds to receptor molecules, such as a neurotransmitter or drug that binds to postsynaptic receptors.

acetylcholine (ACh) A neurotransmitter that is produced and released by parasympathetic postganglionic neurons, by motor neurons, and by many neurons in the brain.

neurotransmitter receptor Also called simply *receptor*. A specialized protein, embedded in the cell membrane, that selectively senses and reacts to molecules of a corresponding neurotransmitter.

5. The IPSPs and EPSPs in the postsynaptic cell spread toward the axon hillock. (If the sum of all the EPSPs and IPSPs ultimately depolarizes the axon hillock enough to reach threshold, an action potential will arise.)

6. Synaptic transmission is rapidly stopped, so the message is brief and accurately reflects the activity of the presynaptic cell.

7. Synaptic transmitter may also activate presynaptic receptors, resulting in a decrease in transmitter release.

Let's look at these seven steps in a little more detail.

Action potentials cause the release of transmitter molecules into the synaptic cleft

When an action potential reaches a presynaptic terminal, it causes hundreds of **synaptic vesicles** near the presynaptic membrane to fuse with the membrane and discharge their contents—molecules of neurotransmitter—into the **synaptic cleft** (the space between the presynaptic and postsynaptic membranes). The key event in this process is an influx of **calcium ions (Ca^{2+})**, rather than K^+ or Na^+, into the axon terminal. These ions enter through voltage-gated Ca^{2+} channels opening in response to the arrival of an action potential. **Synaptic delay** is the time needed for Ca^{2+} to enter the terminal, for the vesicles to fuse with the membrane, for the transmitter to diffuse across the synaptic cleft, and for transmitter molecules to interact with their receptors before the postsynaptic cell responds.

The presynaptic terminal normally produces and stores enough transmitter to ensure that it is ready for activity. Intense activity of the neuron reduces the number of available vesicles, but soon more vesicles are produced to replace those that were discharged. Neurons differ in their ability to keep pace with a rapid rate of incoming action potentials. Furthermore, the rate of making the transmitter is regulated by enzymes that are manufactured in the neuronal cell body and transported down the axons to the terminals.

Receptor molecules recognize transmitters

The action of a key in a lock is a good analogy for the action of a transmitter on a receptor protein. Just as a particular key can open a door, a molecule of the correct shape, called a **ligand** (see Chapter 3), can fit into a receptor protein and activate or block it. So, for example, at synapses where the transmitter is **acetylcholine (ACh)**, the ACh fits into areas called *ligand-binding sites* in **neurotransmitter receptor** molecules located in the postsynaptic membrane (**FIGURE 2.13**).

The nature of the postsynaptic receptors at a synapse determines the action of the transmitter (see Chapter 3). For example, ACh can function as either an inhibitory or an excitatory neurotransmitter, at different synapses. At excitatory synapses, binding of ACh to one type of receptor opens channels for Na^+ and K^+ ions. At inhibitory synapses, ACh may act on another type of receptor to open channels that allow Cl^- ions to enter, thereby hyperpolarizing the membrane (i.e., making it more negative and so less likely to create an action potential).

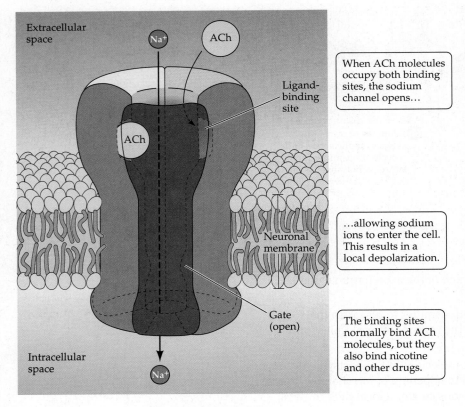

When ACh molecules occupy both binding sites, the sodium channel opens…

…allowing sodium ions to enter the cell. This results in a local depolarization.

The binding sites normally bind ACh molecules, but they also bind nicotine and other drugs.

FIGURE 2.13 A Nicotinic Acetylcholine Receptor

The lock-and-key analogy is strengthened by the observation that various chemicals can fit onto receptor proteins and block the entrance of the key. Some of the preparations used in this research sound like the ingredients for a witches' brew. As an example, consider some potent poisons that block ACh receptors: curare and bungarotoxin. **Curare** is an arrowhead poison used by native South Americans. Extracted from a plant, it greatly increases the efficiency of hunting: if the hunter hits any part of the prey, the arrow's poison soon blocks ACh receptors on muscles, paralyzing the animal. **Bungarotoxin**, another blocker of ACh receptors, is found in the venom of the many-banded krait (*Bungarus multicinctus*), a snake native to China and Southeast Asia.

The chemical nicotine, found in tobacco products, mimics the action of ACh at some synapses, increasing alertness and heart rate. Molecules such as nicotine that act like transmitters at a receptor are called **agonists** (from the Greek *agon*, "contest" or "struggle") of that transmitter. Conversely, molecules that interfere with or prevent the action of a transmitter, like curare, are called **antagonists**.

Just as there are master keys that fit many different locks, there are submaster keys that fit a certain group of locks, as well as keys that each fit only a single lock. Similarly, each chemical transmitter binds to several different receptor molecules. ACh acts on at least four subtypes of **cholinergic** receptors. Nicotinic cholinergic receptors—yes, the subtype on which nicotine exerts its effects—are found at synapses on muscles and in autonomic ganglia; it is the blockade of these receptors that causes paralysis brought on by curare and bungarotoxin. Most nicotinic sites are excitatory, but there are also inhibitory nicotinic synapses. The many "flavors" of receptors for each transmitter have evolved to enable a variety of actions in the nervous system.

The nicotinic ACh receptor resembles a lopsided dumbbell with a tube running down its central axis (see Figure 2.13). The handle of the dumbbell spans the cell membrane, with two sites on the outside that fit ACh molecules (Karlin, 2002). For the channel to open, both of the ACh-binding sites must be occupied. Receptors for some of the synaptic transmitter molecules that we will consider in later chapters, such as gamma-aminobutyric acid (GABA), glycine, and glutamate, are similar. In Chapter 3, we'll learn about another common type of neurotransmitter receptor that alters the internal chemistry of the postsynaptic cell to either open separate ion channels or trigger longer-lasting changes (see Figure 3.2).

The coordination of different transmitter systems of the brain is incredibly complex. Each subtype of neurotransmitter receptor has a unique pattern of distribution within the brain. Different receptor systems become active at different times in fetal life. The number of any given type of receptor remains plastic in adulthood: not only are there seasonal variations, but many kinds of receptors show a regular daily variation of 50% or more in number, affecting the sensitivity of cells to that particular transmitter. Similarly, the numbers of some receptors have been found to vary with the use of drugs. We'll learn more about these properties of neurotransmitter receptors in Chapter 3.

The action of synaptic transmitters is stopped rapidly

When a chemical transmitter such as ACh is released into the synaptic cleft, its postsynaptic action is not only prompt but usually very brief as well. It is important that each activation of the synapse be brief in order to maximize how much information can be transmitted. Think of it this way: the worst doorbell in the world is one that, when the button is pushed, rings forever. Such a doorbell would be able to transmit only one piece of information, and only once. But a doorbell that could ring as fast as a thousand times per minute would be able to send a lot of information—Morse code maybe. Likewise, a synapse can signal over a thousand times per *second*, potentially sending a lot of information (but not by Morse code).

Two processes bring transmitter effects to a prompt halt:

1. *Degradation* Transmitter molecules can be rapidly broken down and thus inactivated by special enzymes—a process known as **degradation** (step 6a in Figure 2.12).

curare   A neurotoxin that causes paralysis by blocking acetylcholine receptors in muscle.

bungarotoxin   A neurotoxin, isolated from the venom of the many-banded krait, that selectively blocks acetylcholine receptors.

agonist   A substance that mimics or boosts the actions of a transmitter or other signaling molecule.

antagonist   A substance that blocks or reduces the actions of a transmitter or other signaling molecule.

cholinergic   Referring to cells that use acetylcholine as their synaptic transmitter.

degradation   The chemical breakdown of a neurotransmitter into inactive metabolites.

acetylcholinesterase (AChE)
An enzyme that inactivates the transmitter acetylcholine.

reuptake The process by which released synaptic transmitter molecules are taken up and reused by the presynaptic neuron, thus stopping synaptic activity.

transporter A specialized membrane component that returns transmitter molecules to the presynaptic neuron for reuse.

axo-dendritic synapse A synapse at which a presynaptic axon terminal synapses onto a dendrite of the postsynaptic neuron, either via a dendritic spine or directly onto the dendrite itself.

axo-somatic synapse A synapse at which a presynaptic axon terminal synapses onto the cell body (soma) of the postsynaptic neuron.

axo-axonic synapse A synapse at which a presynaptic axon terminal synapses onto the axon terminal of another neuron.

dendro-dendritic synapse A synapse at which a synaptic connection forms between the dendrites of two neurons.

knee-jerk reflex A variant of the stretch reflex in which stretching of the tendon beneath the knee leads to an upward kick of the leg.

For example, the enzyme that inactivates ACh is **acetylcholinesterase (AChE)**. AChE breaks down ACh very rapidly into products that are recycled (at least in part) to make more ACh in the axon terminal.

2. *Reuptake* Alternatively, transmitter molecules may be swiftly cleared from the synaptic cleft by being absorbed back into the axon terminal that released them—a process known as **reuptake** (step 6b in Figure 2.12). Norepinephrine, dopamine, and serotonin are examples of transmitters whose activity is terminated mainly by reuptake. In these cases, special receptors for the transmitter, called **transporters**, are located on the presynaptic axon terminal and bring the transmitter back inside. Once taken up into the presynaptic terminal, transmitter molecules may be repackaged into newly formed synaptic vesicles to await release, conserving the resources that would be needed to make new transmitter molecules. Malfunction of reuptake mechanisms is suspected as the cause of some kinds of mental illness, such as depression (see Chapter 12).

Neural circuits underlie reflexes

For simplicity, so far we have focused on the classic **axo-dendritic synapses** (from axon to dendrite) and **axo-somatic synapses** (from axon to cell body, or soma). But many nonclassic forms of chemical synapses exist in the nervous system. As the name implies, **axo-axonic synapses** form on axons, often near the axon terminal, allowing the presynaptic neuron to strongly facilitate or inhibit the activity of the postsynaptic axon terminal. Similarly, neurons may form **dendro-dendritic synapses**, allowing coordination of their activities (**FIGURE 2.14**).

Now that we know more about the electrical signaling that takes place within each neuron and the neurotransmitter signaling that goes on between neurons, we can revisit the **knee-jerk reflex** that we discussed at the start of the chapter (**FIGURE 2.15**). Note that this reflex is extremely fast: only about 40 milliseconds elapse between the hammer tap and the start of the kick. Several factors account for this speed: (1) both the sensory and

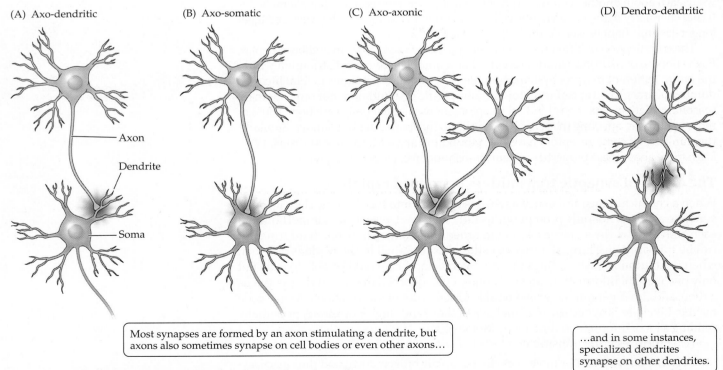

(A) Axo-dendritic   (B) Axo-somatic   (C) Axo-axonic   (D) Dendro-dendritic

Axon

Dendrite

Soma

Most synapses are formed by an axon stimulating a dendrite, but axons also sometimes synapse on cell bodies or even other axons…

…and in some instances, specialized dendrites synapse on other dendrites.

FIGURE 2.14 **Different Types of Synaptic Connections** In reality, neurons typically summate input from hundreds or even thousands of synapses.

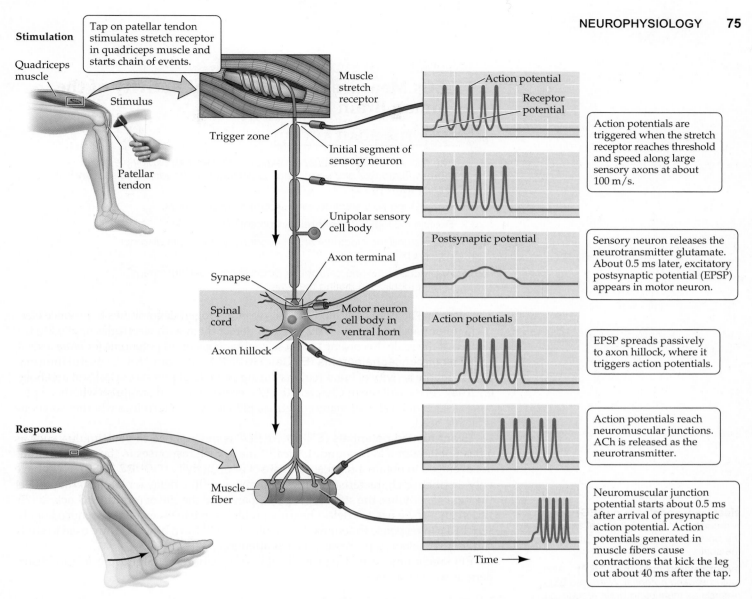

Stimulation

Quadriceps muscle

Tap on patellar tendon stimulates stretch receptor in quadriceps muscle and starts chain of events.

Stimulus

Patellar tendon

Muscle stretch receptor

Trigger zone

Initial segment of sensory neuron

Unipolar sensory cell body

Axon terminal

Synapse

Spinal cord

Motor neuron cell body in ventral horn

Axon hillock

Response

Muscle fiber

Action potential

Receptor potential

Action potentials are triggered when the stretch receptor reaches threshold and speed along large sensory axons at about 100 m/s.

Postsynaptic potential

Sensory neuron releases the neurotransmitter glutamate. About 0.5 ms later, excitatory postsynaptic potential (EPSP) appears in motor neuron.

Action potentials

EPSP spreads passively to axon hillock, where it triggers action potentials.

Action potentials reach neuromuscular junctions. ACh is released as the neurotransmitter.

Neuromuscular junction potential starts about 0.5 ms after arrival of presynaptic action potential. Action potentials generated in muscle fibers cause contractions that kick the leg out about 40 ms after the tap.

Time ⟶

FIGURE 2.15 The Knee-Jerk Reflex

the motor axons involved are myelinated and of large diameter, so they conduct action potentials rapidly; (2) the sensory cells synapse directly on the motor neurons; and (3) both the central synapse and the neuromuscular junction are fast synapses. We discuss other aspects of neural circuits in **A STEP FURTHER 2.2**, on the website.

We offered this reflex at the start of the chapter as an example of neural processing—electrical signaling *within* each neuron alternating with chemical signaling between neurons. Chapter 3 will explain how drugs can interfere with the chemical signaling *between* neurons. For the final part of this chapter, let's see how scientists exploit the electrical signaling within neurons to learn more about brain function.

HOW'S IT GOING ?

1. Recount the seven steps in synaptic transmission, including processes that end the signal.
2. What ion must enter the axon terminal to trigger neurotransmitter release?
3. What are agonists and antagonists?
4. Describe how information is processed within neurons by electrical signals yet communicated to other neurons by chemical signals.

2.3 EEGs Measure Gross Electrical Activity of the Human Brain

> **THE ROAD AHEAD**
>
> *The final section of the chapter explains how we can exploit electrical signals to monitor and understand brain function. Reading this section should allow you to:*
>
> **2.3.1** Understand how electroencephalograms (EEGs) work.
>
> **2.3.2** Explain the logic of event-related potentials.
>
> **2.3.3** Understand the electrical activity underlying the brain disorder called epilepsy.
>
> **2.3.4** Appreciate how neurosurgeons discovered important "maps" by electrically stimulating the brain.

The electrical activity of millions of cells working together combines to produce electrical potentials large enough that we can detect them with electrodes applied to the surface of the scalp. Recordings of these spontaneous brain potentials (or *brain waves*), called **electroencephalograms** (**EEGs**) (**FIGURE 2.16A**), can provide useful information about the activity of brain regions during behavioral processes (Jackson and Bolger, 2014). As we will see in Chapter 10, EEG recordings can distinguish whether a person is asleep or awake. In many countries, EEG activity determines whether someone is legally dead.

Event-related potentials (**ERPs**) are EEG responses to a single stimulus, such as a flash of light or a loud sound. Typically, many ERP responses to the same stimulus are averaged to obtain a reliable estimate of brain activity (**FIGURE 2.16B**). ERPs have very distinctive characteristics of wave shape and time delay (or latency) that reflect the type of stimulus, the state of the participant, and the site of recording (Luck, 2005). ERPs can also be used to detect hearing problems in babies, evident as reduced or absent ERPs in response to sounds. In Chapter 14 we'll learn how ERPs are used to study subtler psychological processes, such as attention.

EEG recordings can also provide vital information for diagnosing seizure disorders, as we discuss next.

Electrical storms in the brain can cause seizures

Since the dawn of civilization, people have pondered the causes of **epilepsy**, a disorder in which **seizures** lasting for a few seconds or minutes may produce dramatic behavioral changes such as alterations or loss of consciousness and rhythmic convulsions of the body. Worldwide, about 30 million people suffer from epilepsy, which we now know to be a disorder of electrical potentials in the brain.

In the normal, active brain, electrical activity tends to be desynchronized; that is, different brain regions carry on their functions more or less independently. In contrast, during a seizure there is widespread synchronization of electrical activity: broad stretches of the brain start firing in simultaneous waves, which are evident in the EEGs as an abnormal "spike-and-wave" pattern of brain activity. Many factors, such as trauma, injury, or metabolic problems, can predispose brain tissue to produce such synchronized activity, which, once begun, may readily spread from one brain region to others.

There are several major categories of seizure disorders. The most severe, with loss of consciousness and rhythmic convulsions, are called **tonic-clonic seizures** (formerly known as *grand mal seizures*) and are accompanied by abnormal EEG activity all over the brain (**FIGURE 2.17A**). In the more subtle **simple partial seizures** (or *absence attacks*, formerly known as *petit mal seizures*), the characteristic spike-and-wave EEG activity is evident for 5–15 seconds at a time (**FIGURE 2.17B**), sometimes occurring

electroencephalogram (EEG) A recording of gross electrical activity of the brain via large electrodes placed on the scalp.

event-related potential (ERP) Also called *evoked potential*. Averaged EEG recordings measuring brain responses to repeated presentations of a stimulus. Components of the ERP tend to be reliable because the background noise of the cortex has been averaged out.

epilepsy A brain disorder marked by major, sudden changes in the electrophysiological state of the brain that are referred to as *seizures*.

seizure A wave of abnormally synchronous electrical activity in the brain.

tonic-clonic seizure Also called *grand mal seizure*. A type of generalized epileptic seizure in which nerve cells fire in high-frequency bursts, usually accompanied by involuntary rhythmic contractions of the body.

simple partial seizure Also called *absence attack*. A seizure that is characterized by a spike-and-wave EEG and often involves a loss of awareness and inability to recall events surrounding the seizure.

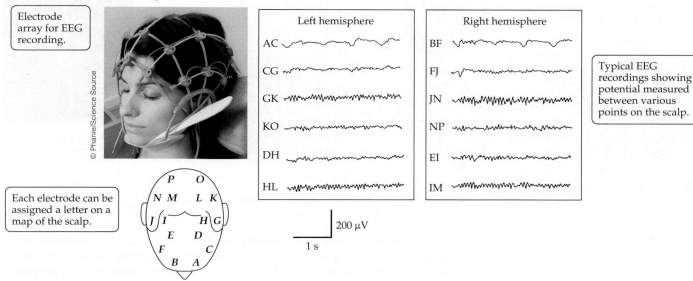

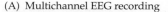

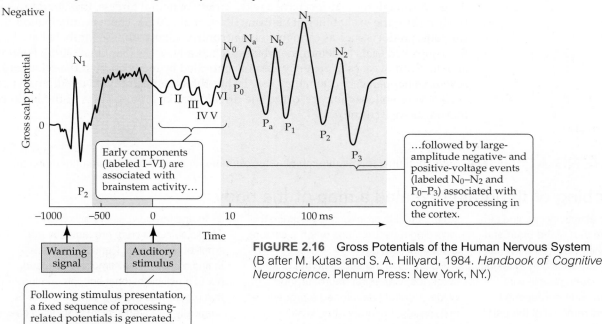

FIGURE 2.16 Gross Potentials of the Human Nervous System (B after M. Kutas and S. A. Hillyard, 1984. *Handbook of Cognitive Neuroscience*. Plenum Press: New York, NY.)

many times per day. The person is unaware of the environment during these periods and later cannot recall events that occurred during the episodes. Behaviorally, people experiencing simple partial seizures show no unusual muscle activity; they just stop what they're doing and seem to stare into space.

Complex partial seizures do not involve the entire brain and thus can produce a wide variety of symptoms, often preceded by an unusual sensation, or **aura**. In one example, a woman felt an unusual sensation in the abdomen, a sense of foreboding, and tingling in both hands before the seizure spread. At the height of the episode, she was unresponsive and rocked her body back and forth while speaking nonsensically, twisting her left arm, and looking toward the right. Of course, her seemingly random

complex partial seizure A type of seizure that doesn't involve the entire brain and therefore can cause a wide variety of symptoms.

aura In epilepsy, the unusual sensations or premonition that may precede the beginning of a seizure.

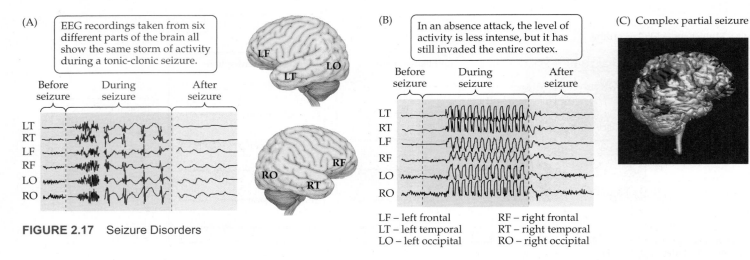

(A)

EEG recordings taken from six different parts of the brain all show the same storm of activity during a tonic-clonic seizure.

| Before seizure | During seizure | After seizure |

LF
LT
LO

LT
RT
LF
RF
LO
RO

FIGURE 2.17   Seizure Disorders

(B)

In an absence attack, the level of activity is less intense, but it has still invaded the entire cortex.

| Before seizure | During seizure | After seizure |

LT
RT
LF
RF
LO
RO

RF
RO
RT

LF – left frontal   RF – right frontal
LT – left temporal   RT – right temporal
LO – left occipital   RO – right occipital

(C) Complex partial seizure

set of behavioral symptoms actually reflected the functions of the particular brain regions activated by the seizure (**FIGURE 2.17C**); others experiencing seizures would produce a completely different set of behaviors. In some individuals, complex partial seizures may be provoked by stimuli like loud noises or flashing lights.

Many seizure disorders can be effectively controlled with the aid of antiepileptic drugs. Although these drugs have a wide variety of neural targets, they tend to selectively reduce the excitability of neurons (Park et al., 2019). There is anticipation that cannabis products such as cannabidiol may control seizures, but so far there have been few controlled trials to determine whether it actually works (Samanta, 2019). For now, about a third of cases of epilepsy are not controlled by medication. If the seizures are severe, or happen very often, they may be life-threatening. Individuals suffering from such severe epilepsy may resort to the drastic step of having parts of the brain removed, as we'll see next.

RESEARCHERS AT WORK ||||||||||||||||||||||||||||||||||||||||||||||||||||||||||||||||||||||||||||||||||||||||

Surgical probing of the brain revealed a map of the body

Usually the electrical activity causing seizures begins in one part of the brain and then spreads to others. So in the twentieth century, neurosurgeons began taking drastic measures to help people with severe epilepsy that did not respond to medication: surgical removal of the part of the brain where the seizures begin. The trick, of course, is to remove the part of the brain where the seizures begin, and *only* that part. Otherwise the patient might take the risks of surgery and still suffer from seizures, or might suffer impairment of a vital function, such as verbal or memory skills, if healthy tissue is removed. One way to locate the origin of the seizures is to compare EEG readings from different places on the skull (see Figure 2.17). But this approach gives only a rough idea of where the seizures

begin, and it is problematic because the recording must be made when a seizure is actually starting.

To improve the success rate of such surgeries, Canadian neurosurgeon Wilder Penfield developed a procedure that, nearly a century later, is still compelling (Foerster and Penfield, 1930). Using only local anesthesia to deaden the pain of cutting the scalp and opening up the skull, Penfield had patients remain awake and alert as he exposed the brain. Then he used electrodes to provide a tiny electrical stimulation to the surface of the cortex, asking the patient to report the results. One strategy for people whose epileptic seizures were preceded by an aura was to try to find the point where stimulation recreated the aura.

In one famous case of a woman whose seizures were preceded by the smell of burnt toast, Penfield was able to find a spot where stimulation caused her to smell burnt toast and, presuming that region was the origin of the seizures, surgically removed it. (The brain itself has no pain receptors, so cutting the cortex didn't hurt.) Using this refined technique, Penfield was able to cure about half of his patients, and seizures were reduced in another 25%. Later, José Delgado also stimulated patients' brains to seek the origin of seizures, as we discussed at the start of the chapter. Delgado altered the technique by implanting several electrodes temporarily, so the patient could walk around while doctors electrically stimulated different brain regions and observed the results. In Chapter 5 and

Chapter 12 we'll learn that today electrodes are sometimes implanted in the brain as a treatment for other disorders.

In his pioneering work, Penfield did more than help his patients. He also made major discoveries about the organization of the human cortex (**FIGURE 2.18**). By carefully recording the effects of stimulating different regions of the brain, he found that stimulation of occipital cortex often caused the patient to "see" flashes of light. Stimulating another region might cause the person's thumb to tingle, while stimulation elsewhere might cause the patient's leg to move. Through these studies, Penfield confirmed that each side of the cortex receives information from, and sends commands to, the opposite side of the body. He found that stimulating the postcentral gyrus of the parietal cortex caused patients to experience sensations on various parts of the body in a way that was consistent from one person

to another (see Figure 5.9). Just across the central sulcus from each site, in the precentral gyrus, stimulations caused that same part of the body to move (see Figure 5.22). These "maps" of how the various parts of the body are laid out on the cortex (Jasper and Penfield, 1954) have been reproduced in countless textbooks, providing the basis of what is called the *homunculus*, the "little man" drawn on the surface of the cortex to depict Penfield's maps, as we will discuss further in Chapter 5.

These groundbreaking observations taught us that brain function is organized in a map that reproduces body parts. We also learned that the map is distorted, in the sense that parts of the body that are especially sensitive to touch, such as the lips or fingers, are monitored by a relatively large area of cortex compared with, say, the backs of the legs.

Penfield's studies also stimulated a rich store of speculation about the

relationship between the workings of the brain and the mind. In a small minority of patients, electrical stimulation in some sites would sometimes elicit a memory of, for example, sitting on the porch step and hearing a relative's voice, or hearing a snatch of music. As we saw at the start of this chapter, other researchers would find that electrical stimulation of the brain could make people think they loved their examiner or could make an angry, murderous bull peaceful and calm. In another case, electrical stimulation of one part of her brain caused a young woman to find whatever was happening around her to be humorous (Fried et al., 1998).

These startling observations—showing that electrical stimulation of the brain triggers mental processes—remain a cornerstone of neuroscience, and a tantalizing demonstration that our mind is a result of physical processes at work in the machine we call the brain.

■ Hypothesis

Sensory information from the body arrives in an organized fashion in the cortex.

■ Experiment

Electrically stimulate the surface of the cortex in alert patients, carefully recording the patient's experience with stimulation at each site. Compare these maps in various patients.

■ Result

Each side of the brain receives sensory information from the opposite side of the body, organized along the postcentral gyrus of the parietal lobe. Across the central sulcus, in the precentral gyrus, cortical regions control movement of that same part of the body so that sensory and motor regions are aligned.

■ Conclusion

The maps of sensory cortex and motor cortex are remarkably consistent from one person to another.

FIGURE 2.18 Mapping the Human Brain

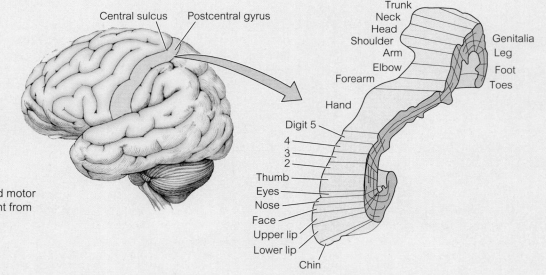

Central sulcus   Postcentral gyrus

Trunk
Neck
Head
Shoulder
Arm
Elbow
Forearm
Hand

Genitalia
Leg
Foot
Toes

Digit 5
4
3
2
Thumb
Eyes
Nose
Face
Upper lip
Lower lip
Chin

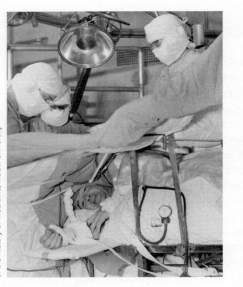

Brain Stimulation   Surgeon Wilder Penfield electrically stimulating the surface of the exposed brain in an awake patient.

1. What are EEGs and ERPs? How have these techniques been useful?
2. What are the three main categories of epileptic seizures, and what are the main characteristics of each type?
3. Describe Penfield's surgical procedure and what it revealed about organization of the brain.

Recommended Reading

Kandel, E. R., Schwartz, J. H., Jessell, T. M., Siegelbaum, S. A., et al. (2013). *Principles of Neural Science* (5th ed.). New York, NY: McGraw-Hill.

Nicholls, J. G., Martin, A. R., Fuchs, P. A., Brown, D. A., et al. (2021). *From Neuron to Brain* (6th ed.). Sunderland, MA: Oxford University Press/Sinauer.

Purves, D., Augustine, G. J., Fitzpatrick, D., Hall, W. C., et al. (2017). *Neuroscience* (6th ed.). Sunderland, MA: Oxford University Press/Sinauer.

Sapolsky, R. M. (2018). *Behave: The Biology of Humans at Our Best and Worst*. New York, NY: Penguin Books.

Valenstein, E. S. (2005). *The War of the Soups and the Sparks: The Discovery of Neurotransmitters and the Dispute over How Neurons Communicate*. New York, NY: Columbia University Press.

You should be able to relate each summary to the adjacent illustration, including structures and processes. The online version of this **Visual Summary** includes links to figures, animations, and activities that will help you consolidate the material.

1 Chemical signals transmit information between neurons; electrical signals transmit information within a neuron. The **resting potential** is a small electrical potential across the neuron's membrane. Review **Figure 2.1, Animation 2.2**

2 Different concentrations of ions inside and outside the neuron—especially **potassium ions (K^+),** to which the resting membrane is **selectively permeable**—account for the resting potential. At the K^+ **equilibrium potential**, the **electrostatic pressure** pulling K^+ ions into the neuron is balanced by the **diffusion** pushing them out. Review **Figures 2.2–2.4**, **Activity 2.1**, **Animation 2.3**

3 **Depolarizing** the axon (reducing its resting potential) until it reaches a **threshold** value opens **voltage-gated Na^+ channels**, making the membrane permeable to Na^+. The **sodium ions (Na^+)** rush in, and the axon becomes briefly more positive inside than outside. This event is called an **action potential**. Review **Figure 2.5, Animation 2.4**

4 Following the action potential, the resting potential is quickly restored by the influx of K^+ ions. **Sodium-potassium pumps** maintain the resting potential in the long run, counteracting the influx of Na^+ ions during action potentials. Review **Figure 2.6**

5 The action potential strongly depolarizes the adjacent patch of axonal membrane, causing it to generate its own action potential, propagating down the axon. **Saltatory conduction** of the action potential along the **nodes of Ranvier** between **myelin** sheaths speeds propagation along the axon. Review **Figures 2.7–2.9, Animation 2.5**

6 Like all other **local potentials, postsynaptic potentials** spread very rapidly but are not regenerated, so they diminish as they spread passively along dendrites and the cell body. **Excitatory postsynaptic potentials** (**EPSPs**) are depolarizing (they decrease the resting potential) and increase the likelihood that the neuron will fire an action potential. **Inhibitory postsynaptic potentials** (**IPSPs**) result in **hyperpolarization**, decreasing the likelihood that the neuron will fire. Review **Figure 2.10**

7 Neurons process information by integrating the postsynaptic potentials through both **spatial summation** (summing potentials from different locations) and **temporal summation** (summing potentials across time). Review **Figure 2.11, Animation 2.6**

8 Action potentials are initiated near the **axon hillock** when the excess of EPSPs over IPSPs reaches threshold. During the action potential, the neuron cannot be excited by a second stimulus; it is **absolutely refractory**. For a few milliseconds afterward, the neuron is **relatively refractory**, requiring a stronger stimulation than usual in order to fire. Review **Figure 2.6**

9 Synaptic transmission occurs when a chemical neurotransmitter diffuses across the **synaptic cleft** and binds to **neurotransmitter receptors** in the postsynaptic membrane. Review **Figures 2.12** and **2.13, Box 2.1, Animation 2.7**

10 Summing electrical activity over millions of nerve cells as detected by electrodes on the scalp, **electroencephalograms** (**EEGs**) can reveal rapid changes in brain function—for example, in response to a brief, controlled stimulus that evokes an **event-related potential** (**ERP**). They can also reveal a **seizure** in someone with **epilepsy**. Review **Figures 2.16–2.18**

The Mind's Machine digital resources include additional videos, flashcards, and other study tools.

3 The Chemistry of Behavior
Neurotransmitters and Neuropharmacology

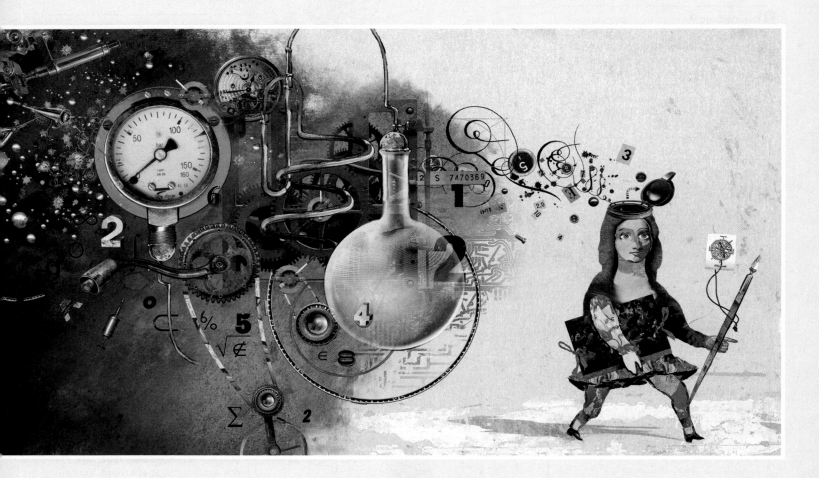

Living the Dream

As the twentieth century began, scientists knew that neurons were important for brain function, but controversy swirled about how neurons communicated. What happened at those newly discovered synapses between one neuron and another? Did sparks of electricity pass from cell to cell? Or was some unknown chemical substance involved? Some scientists, nicknamed "sparks," favored the idea that electrical signals crossed synapses; other scientists, the "soups," thought neurons released a chemical that flowed across synapses. No one knew how to figure out which account was correct.

Otto Loewi was so consumed with the question of neural communication that he even dreamed about it. One night he suddenly awoke, having dreamed of an experiment that could finally answer whether the "soups" or the "sparks" were right. He made a few notes and went back to sleep, only to discover the next day that he couldn't make any sense of his scribblings from the night before. So when he had the same dream again the following night, he got up and went straight to the lab to do the experiment while it was still fresh in his mind. The result was a discovery that would revolutionize the study of the brain.

Throughout the ages, people have experimented with **exogenous** substances (substances from outside the body) to try to change the functioning of their bodies and brains. Our ancestors sipped, swallowed, and smoked their way to euphoria, calmness, pain relief, and hallucination. They discovered deadly poisons in frogs, miraculous antibiotics in mold, powerful painkillers in poppies, and all the rest of a vast catalog of helpful and harmful substances. By studying the physiological actions of these substances, modern scientists have been able to unlock many mysteries of brain function.

The preceding chapters showed us that the brain is an electrochemical system. Today we know that, in general, each neuron *electrically* processes information received through many synapses and then releases a *chemical* to pass the result of that information processing to the next cell. Specifically, a presynaptic neuron releases an **endogenous** substance (a substance from inside the body), a chemical called a *neurotransmitter*. The neurotransmitter then communicates with the postsynaptic cell. As you might have guessed, most drugs that affect behavior do so by meddling with this chemical communication process at millions, or even billions, of synapses. So, we open our discussion with a detailed look at the sequence of electrochemical events in synaptic transmission.

**See Video 3.1:
Synaptic Transmission**

exogenous Arising from outside the body.

endogenous Produced inside the body.

View Animation 3.2:
Brain Explorer

3.1 Synaptic Transmission Is a Complex Electrochemical Process

THE ROAD AHEAD

We open with a detailed look at the sequence of electrochemical events in synaptic transmission. After reading this section, you should be able to:

3.1.1 Review the neuronal processes leading to the release of neurotransmitter into a synapse.

3.1.2 Explain how receptors capture, recognize, and respond to molecules of neurotransmitter.

3.1.3 Give a general overview of the concept of receptor subtypes and how their existence adds complexity to neural signaling.

FIGURE 3.1 A Review of Synaptic Activity EPSP, excitatory postsynaptic potential; IPSP, inhibitory postsynaptic potential.

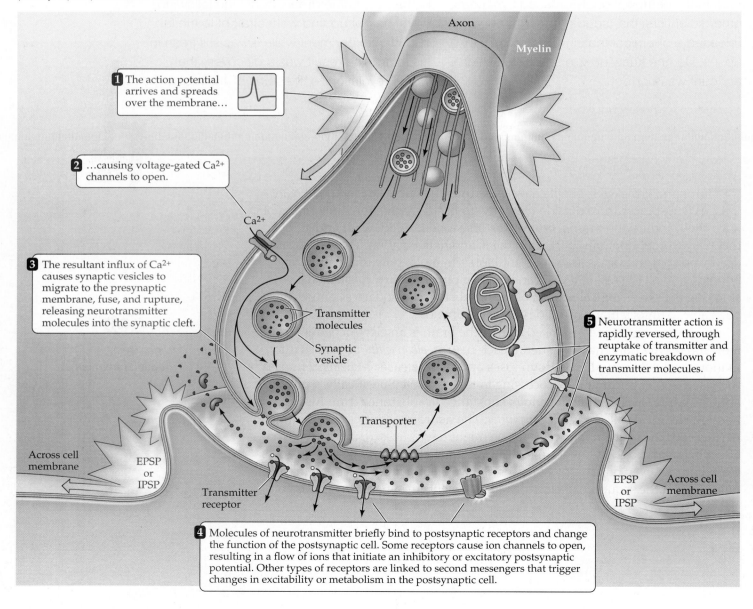

As we learned in Chapter 2, the typical neuron integrates a variety of inputs and, if sufficiently excited (i.e., *depolarized*), fires a distinctive, brief electrical signal called an *action potential* that rapidly sweeps down the axon toward the *axon terminals*, each of which forms the **presynaptic** side of a **synapse**. **FIGURE 3.1** recaps the events that follow the arrival of the action potential. First, because the arrival of the action potential strongly depolarizes the axon terminal, voltage-gated calcium (Ca^{2+}) channels in the terminal membrane are induced to open. The resulting inflow of Ca^{2+} ions drives the migration of synaptic vesicles to the nearby presynaptic membrane, where specialized proteins on the walls of the vesicles and corresponding proteins on the synaptic membrane interact and cause the vesicles to release their cargo of molecules of **neurotransmitter** (or just *transmitter*) into the synaptic cleft (a process called *exocytosis*). In Chapter 2 we also saw that following their diffusion across the cleft, neurotransmitter molecules briefly bind to their corresponding **neurotransmitter receptors**—protein molecules embedded in the **postsynaptic** membrane that recognize a specific transmitter—which then mediate a response on the postsynaptic side. Eventually the neurotransmitter molecules are either (1) broken down by enzymes into simpler chemicals or (2) brought back into the presynaptic terminal in a process called **reuptake** (see Figure 3.1). Reuptake of transmitters relies on specialized proteins, called **transporters**, that bind molecules of neurotransmitter and conduct them back inside the presynaptic terminal. Once inside, the neurotransmitter molecules can be recycled.

Neurotransmitter receptors are very selective about the substances that they will respond to: as we saw in Chapter 2, the action of transmitters on receptors is often likened to a key opening a lock. Nevertheless, the various neurotransmitter receptors can all be categorized as belonging to one of two general kinds: ionotropic receptors or metabotropic receptors. An **ionotropic receptor** is really just a fancy ion channel; when bound by a neurotransmitter molecule, an ionotropic receptor quickly changes shape, opening (or closing) its integral ion channel (**FIGURE 3.2**). The opening

presynaptic   Located on the "transmitting" side of a synapse.

synapse   The cellular location at which information is transmitted from a neuron to another cell.

neurotransmitter   Also called simply *transmitter*. A signaling chemical, released by a presynaptic neuron, that diffuses across the synaptic cleft to alter the functioning of the postsynaptic neuron.

neurotransmitter receptor   Also called simply *receptor*. A specialized protein that is embedded in the cell membrane, allowing it to selectively sense and react to molecules of the corresponding neurotransmitter.

postsynaptic   Located on the "receiving" side of a synapse.

reuptake   The reabsorption of molecules of neurotransmitter by the neurons that released them, thereby ending the signaling activity of the transmitter molecules.

transporter   A specialized membrane component that returns transmitter molecules to the presynaptic neuron for reuse.

ionotropic receptor   Also called *ligand-gated ion channel*. A receptor protein containing an ion channel that opens when the receptor is bound by an agonist.

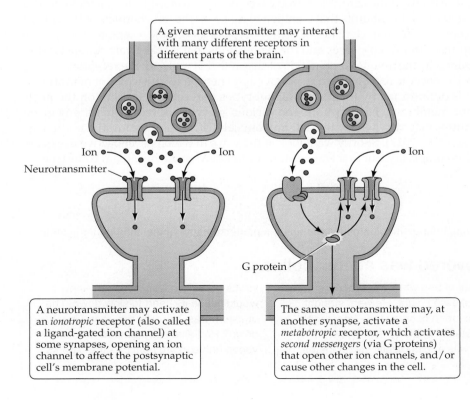

A given neurotransmitter may interact with many different receptors in different parts of the brain.

Ion

Neurotransmitter

Ion

Ion

G protein

A neurotransmitter may activate an *ionotropic* receptor (also called a ligand-gated ion channel) at some synapses, opening an ion channel to affect the postsynaptic cell's membrane potential.

The same neurotransmitter may, at another synapse, activate a *metabotropic* receptor, which activates *second messengers* (via G proteins) that open other ion channels, and/or cause other changes in the cell.

FIGURE 3.2   The Versatility of Neurotransmitters

(or closing) of channels in the postsynaptic membrane allows more (or fewer) of the channels' favored ions to flow into or out of the postsynaptic neuron, thus changing the local membrane potential. If the change in the postsynaptic membrane potential is a depolarization, bringing the cell closer to its threshold for producing an action potential, we call it an **excitatory synapse**. Conversely, if the result is a local hyperpolarization of the postsynaptic cell, making it less likely that the cell will produce an action potential, we call it an **inhibitory synapse**.

But not all receptors contain an ion channel. Receptors belonging to the other major category—the **metabotropic receptors**—don't pass ions or other substances through the cell membrane. Instead, they provide a link across the cell membrane to complicated chemical machinery—called *G proteins*—inside the postsynaptic neuron (see Figure 3.2). When activated, metabotropic receptors alter the inner workings of the postsynaptic cell, using internal chemical signals called *second messengers* that are activated by the G proteins. This two-step signaling process can cause changes in excitability of the postsynaptic cell, or it can cause other, slower but larger-scale responses. For example, the metabotropic receptor may kick off a chain of chemical reactions that will affect gene expression (the use of genes to produce proteins; see the Appendix). Changes in gene expression can have many lasting effects, such as changing the excitability of the postsynaptic neuron, remodeling its connections to other cells, or stimulating the production of more receptors and signaling chemicals.

Together, the two major families of transmitter receptors allow not only rapid responses where timing is crucial, but also more complex, integrative, slower behaviors such as emotional responses, social behavior, and so on. Receptors add an important layer of complexity in neural signaling, because any given transmitter may affect various kinds of receptors that differ from one another in structure. This diversity of **receptor subtypes** is true for both metabotropic receptors and ionotropic receptors. In mammals and almost all other organisms, a gene "superfamily" encodes hundreds of different kinds of **G protein–coupled receptors** (GPCRs), including the many and various types of metabotropic neurotransmitter receptors that we'll be seeing again later in the book. In the case of ionotropic receptors, a diverse group of genes encodes the various protein subunits that combine to make up the ion channels at the core of the receptors. The characteristics of each subtype of ionotropic receptor—the specific neurotransmitter it recognizes and the type of ions that it selectively conducts—are determined by the unique combination of subunits that make up the receptor.

So, the specific response of any postsynaptic neuron to molecules of neurotransmitter is determined by the particular subtypes of receptors present on the postsynaptic membrane. Furthermore, the various subtypes of receptors for any given transmitter may vary widely in their anatomical distribution within the brain (e.g., Beliveau et al., 2017). Shortly we'll look at the ways in which psychoactive drugs exploit this complexity, but first let's see how Otto Loewi made his dream come true.

excitatory synapse   A type of synapse that, when active, causes a local depolarization that increases the likelihood the neuron will fire an action potential.

inhibitory synapse   A type of synapse that, when active, causes a local hyperpolarization that decreases the likelihood the neuron will fire an action potential.

metabotropic receptor   A receptor protein that does not contain ion channels but may, when activated, use a second-messenger system to open nearby ion channels or to produce other cellular effects.

receptor subtype   Any type of receptor having functional characteristics that distinguish it from other types of receptors for the same neurotransmitter.

G protein–coupled receptor (GPCR) A type of receptor that, when activated extracellularly, initiates a G protein signaling mechanism inside the cell.

RESEARCHERS AT WORK

The first transmitter to be discovered was acetylcholine

Our chapter began with the classic story of Otto Loewi's dream of an experiment that would reveal the first neurotransmitter. After forgetting the details of the dream the first night, Loewi was quick to get out of bed when the dream returned the following night. He went straight to the lab to conduct the experiment depicted in **FIGURE 3.3**. Loewi's first step was to electrically stimulate the vagus nerve in a frog, which he knew would cause its heart to slow down. The question was, Why did the heart slow down? Had electricity jumped from the vagus nerve to the heart, as the "sparks"

RESEARCHERS AT WORK *(continued)* ||||||||||||||||||||||||||||||||||||||||||||||||||||||

believed? Or were the "soups" right? Had the nerve released a chemical to slow the heart?

Loewi's critical, dream-inspired experiment was to collect the fluid that surrounded the slowing heart. Then he applied that fluid to the heart of another frog. If the first heart had been slowed by electrical signals from the vagus, then the fluid should have no effect on the second heart. But if activation of the vagus caused it to release a chemical that slowed the beating of the heart, then the fluid from the first heart should alter the beating of the second. In fact, the transferred fluid caused the second heart to slow its rate, providing Loewi with conclusive evidence of chemical neurotransmission (and a nice shiny Nobel Prize, in 1936). The neurotransmitter was later chemically identified as **acetylcholine** (**ACh** for short). The "soups" were vindicated.

■ Question

Do neurons release a chemical to communicate with other cells, or is the communication based on electrical signals?

■ Experiment

Step I: Stimulate the vagus nerve to slow the heart.

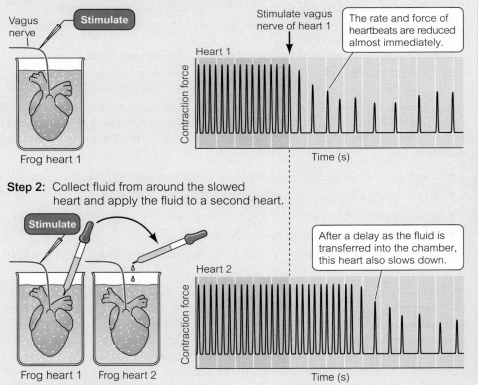

Step 2: Collect fluid from around the slowed heart and apply the fluid to a second heart.

■ Result

The second heart also slowed.

■ Conclusion

The vagus nerve uses a chemical neurotransmitter, not a direct electrical connection, to communicate to cells of the heart and cause it to slow down.

FIGURE 3.3 "Soups" versus "Sparks": The First Neurotransmitter

acetylcholine (ACh) A neurotransmitter that is produced and released by the autonomic nervous system, by motor neurons, and by neurons throughout the brain.

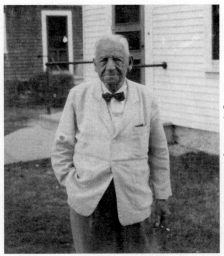

Photograph courtesy of Dr. Edward D. Rockstein

Otto Loewi Following the Nazi annexation of Austria in 1938, Loewi, then a professor at the University of Graz, was forced to flee to the United States, where he remained for the rest of his life. He was photographed in the summer of 1955 by his associate, Dr. Morris Rockstein, at the Woods Hole Marine Biological Laboratory.

HOW'S IT GOING ?

1. Distinguish between endogenous and exogenous substances, and give a few examples of each.
2. Review the sequence of events that occurs when an action potential arrives at the axon terminal and causes a release of neurotransmitter. Use the following terms in your answer: *exocytosis, receptors, ionotropic, metabotropic, reuptake*.
3. Describe how the first neurotransmitter was discovered. Why do you think we selected this discovery for this chapter's "Researchers at Work" feature?

3.2 Neurotransmitter Substances Differ in Their Chemical Structure and in Their Distribution within the Brain

THE ROAD AHEAD

Next we survey the major families of neurotransmitters and their distribution in the brain. After reading this section, you should be able to:

3.2.1 Identify general properties shared by most neurotransmitters, summarizing the criteria for establishing that a substance acts as a neurotransmitter.

3.2.2 Name the major neurotransmitters, and briefly describe the chemical families of transmitters to which they belong.

3.2.3 Trace the anatomical distribution of the major transmitters in the brain.

3.2.4 Briefly discuss some of the major functional roles of the classical transmitters.

In the years since Loewi's discovery, neuroscientists have agreed on some basic principles for deciding whether a brain chemical qualifies as a classical neurotransmitter. We can conclude that a candidate substance is a transmitter if it meets the following qualifications:

- It can be synthesized by presynaptic neurons and stored in axon terminals.
- It is released when action potentials reach the terminals.
- It is recognized by specific receptors located on the postsynaptic membrane.
- It causes changes in the postsynaptic cell.
- Blocking its release interferes with the ability of the presynaptic cell to affect the postsynaptic cell.

The brain contains many different chemicals that meet these criteria and are therefore considered classic neurotransmitters. Considering the rate at which these substances are being discovered, it would not be surprising if there turned out to be several hundred different neurotransmitters at work in synapses throughout the central nervous system. But for now, let's content ourselves with a look at a few of the best-known neurotransmitter systems in the brain.

TABLE 3.1 summarizes the major neurotransmitters and the chemical families to which they belong. **Amino acid neurotransmitters** and **peptide neurotransmitters** (or *neuropeptides*), as their names suggest, are based on single amino acid molecules or on short chains of amino acids (called *peptides*), respectively. A different family—the **amine neurotransmitters**—includes some of the best-known classical transmitters, such as acetylcholine, dopamine, and serotonin. Each year the list of probable neurotransmitters grows, and the search for new transmitters has occasionally yielded surprises like the **gas neurotransmitters**, soluble gases that diffuse between neurons to alter ongoing processes (and defy several of the criteria for transmitters that we just listed!).

amino acid neurotransmitter
A neurotransmitter that is itself an amino acid. Examples include GABA, glycine, and glutamate.

peptide neurotransmitter   Also called *neuropeptide*. A neurotransmitter consisting of a short chain of amino acids.

amine neurotransmitter   A neurotransmitter based on modifications of a single amino acid nucleus. Examples include acetylcholine, serotonin, and dopamine.

gas neurotransmitter   A neurotransmitter that is a soluble gas. Examples include nitric oxide and carbon monoxide.

TABLE 3.1 Some Synaptic Transmitters and Families of Transmitters

Family and subfamily	Transmitter(s)
AMINO ACIDS	Gamma-aminobutyric acid (GABA), glutamate, glycine, histamine
AMINES	
Quaternary amines	Acetylcholine (ACh)
Monoamines	*Catecholamines*: Norepinephrine (NE), epinephrine (adrenaline), dopamine (DA)
	Indoleamines: Serotonin (5-hydroxytryptamine [5-HT]), melatonin
NEUROPEPTIDES	
Opioid peptides	*Enkephalins*: Met-enkephalin, leu-enkephalin
	Endorphins: Beta-endorphin
	Dynorphins: Dynorphin A
Other neuropeptides	Oxytocin, substance P, cholecystokinin (CCK), vasopressin, neuropeptide Y (NPY), hypothalamic releasing hormones
GASES	Nitric oxide, carbon monoxide

The most abundant neurotransmitters are amino acids

A majority of synapses in the brain rely on amino acid transmitters for communication. Of this group, the two best studied are **glutamate**, the most widespread excitatory transmitter in the brain, and **gamma-aminobutyric acid** (**GABA**), the most widespread inhibitory transmitter. Both have wide-ranging effects at synapses throughout the central nervous system, and from an evolutionary perspective they are among the most ancient transmitters.

GLUTAMATE Glutamate interacts with several subtypes of receptors, which are named after drugs that selectively activate them. Activation of the ionotropic AMPA receptors, the most plentiful receptors in the brain, has rapid excitatory effects. NMDA receptors are another subtype of ionotropic glutamate receptors, with unique characteristics that suggest they play a central role in memory formation (discussed in Chapter 13 and on the website in **A STEP FURTHER 3.1**). There are also several metabotropic glutamate receptors (mGluRs), which act more slowly because they work through second messengers.

GABA Among the subtypes of receptors for GABA, the $GABA_A$ receptors have received decades of special scrutiny because of their relationship to anxiety relief. $GABA_A$ receptors are ionotropic; when activated, they allow more Cl^- ions to flow into the postsynaptic cell, resulting in a rapid-onset local hyperpolarization that inhibits the cell's activity. Compounds that mimic this action of $GABA_A$ tend to be effective calming agents because they produce a widespread decrease in neural activity. In fact, drugs belonging to the family of *benzodiazepines*—examples include Xanax (alprazolam) and Ativan (lorazepam)—potently activate $GABA_A$ receptors and are widely used to treat anxiety and panic attacks, as well as to aid muscle relaxation, sleep induction, and the like. $GABA_B$ receptors, in contrast, are metabotropic receptors with slower postsynaptic effects (Gassman and Bettler, 2012); $GABA_B$-selective drugs may be helpful for treating diverse chronic problems such as pain and mood disorders (Pin and Bettler, 2016).

Four classical neurotransmitters modulate brain activity

It is possible to stain brain tissue in such a way that only the neurons that make a particular neurotransmitter end up being labeled (see Box 1.1). Studies of brain sections stained in this way have shown that transmitters are found in complex

glutamate An amino acid transmitter, the most common excitatory transmitter.

gamma-aminobutyric acid (GABA) A widely distributed amino acid transmitter, the main inhibitory transmitter in the mammalian nervous system.

FIGURE 3.4 Neurotransmitter Pathways in the Brain

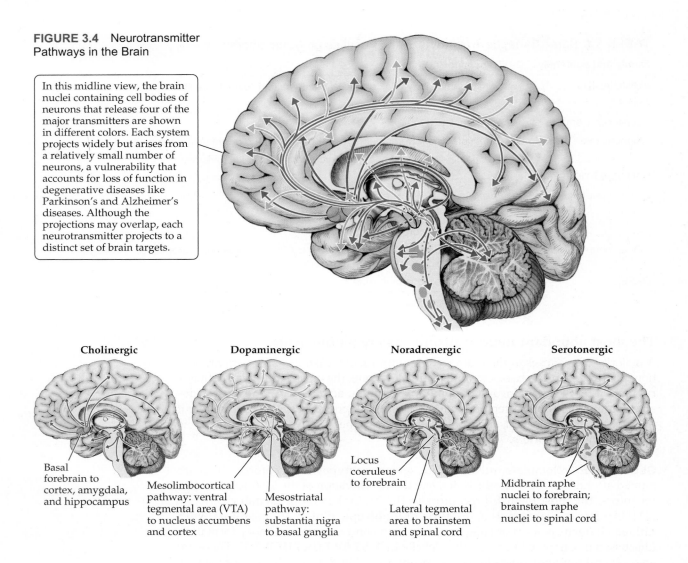

In this midline view, the brain nuclei containing cell bodies of neurons that release four of the major transmitters are shown in different colors. Each system projects widely but arises from a relatively small number of neurons, a vulnerability that accounts for loss of function in degenerative diseases like Parkinson's and Alzheimer's diseases. Although the projections may overlap, each neurotransmitter projects to a distinct set of brain targets.

Cholinergic

Basal forebrain to cortex, amygdala, and hippocampus

Dopaminergic

Mesolimbocortical pathway: ventral tegmental area (VTA) to nucleus accumbens and cortex

Mesostriatal pathway: substantia nigra to basal ganglia

Noradrenergic

Locus coeruleus to forebrain

Lateral tegmental area to brainstem and spinal cord

Serotonergic

Midbrain raphe nuclei to forebrain; brainstem raphe nuclei to spinal cord

View Animation 3.3: Neurotransmitter Pathways

co-localization The synthesis and release of more than one type of neurotransmitter by a given presynaptic neuron.

networks of neurons that extend throughout the brain. In **FIGURE 3.4**, this complicated anatomy is depicted for acetylcholine plus just three of the most famous classical amine transmitters: dopamine, serotonin, and norepinephrine (amines are nitrogen-containing compounds related to ammonia, often derived from an amino acid). Acetylcholine and the amine transmitters have been implicated in many categories of behavior and pathology, so these transmitter systems are major targets for drug development. We'll encounter them in many locations throughout the book. (To learn more about how neurons synthesize neurotransmitters, see **A STEP FURTHER 3.2**, on the website.) A key point to remember is that each of these classical neurotransmitters is carried by a different set of axons, and those axons project to different brain regions. Each type of neurotransmitter is thus talking to a distinct set of brain targets, and there may be overlap as two different transmitters arrive at the same target. How those targets respond depends on which neurotransmitter is being released and which kind of receptors the target neurons possess (**TABLE 3.2**). And despite its gnarly appearance, Figure 3.4 is actually a simplification; there are many more transmitters at work than the four we have shown here, and they are arranged in much more complicated networks. Furthermore, we now know that some neurons make and release more than one type of transmitter—a phenomenon known as neurotransmitter **co-localization**.

TABLE 3.2 The Bewildering Multiplicity of Transmitter Receptor Subtypes

Transmitter	Known receptor subtypes	Function
Glutamate	AMPA, kainate, and NMDA receptors (ionotropic); mGluRs (**m**etabotropic **glu**tamate **r**eceptors)	Glutamate is the most abundant of all neurotransmitters and the most important excitatory transmitter. Glutamate receptors are crucial for excitatory signals, and NMDA receptors are especially implicated in learning and memory.
Gamma-aminobutyric acid (GABA)	GABA$_A$ (ionotropic)	GABA receptors mediate most of the brain's inhibitory activity, balancing the excitatory actions of glutamate. GABA$_A$ receptors are inhibitory in many brain regions, reducing excitability and preventing seizure activity.
	GABA$_B$ (metabotropic)	GABA$_B$ receptors are also inhibitory, by a different mechanism.
Acetylcholine (ACh)	Muscarinic receptors (metabotropic)	Both types of receptors are involved in cholinergic transmission in the cortex.
	Nicotinic receptors (ionotropic)	Nicotinic receptors are crucial for muscle contraction.
Dopamine (DA)	D$_1$ through D$_5$ receptors (all metabotropic)	DA receptors are found throughout the forebrain. DA receptors are involved in complex behaviors, including motor function, reward, and higher cognition.
Norepinephrine (NE)	α_1, α_2, β_1, β_2, and β_3 receptors (all metabotropic)	NE has multiple effects in visceral organs, important in sympathetic nervous system and fight-or-flight responses. In the brain, NE transmission provides an alerting and arousing function.
Serotonin	5-HT$_1$ receptor family (5 members)	Different subtypes differ in their distribution in the brain.
	5-HT$_2$ receptor family (3 members)	5-HT$_2$ receptors may be involved in mood, sleep, and higher cognition.
	5-HT$_3$ through 5-HT$_7$ receptors (All but one subtype [5-HT$_3$] metabotropic)	5-HT$_3$ receptors are particularly involved in nausea.
Miscellaneous peptides	Many specific receptors for peptides such as opiates (delta, kappa, and mu receptors), cholecystokinin (CCK), neurotensin, neuropeptide Y (NPY), and dozens more (all metabotropic)	Peptide transmitters have many different functions, depending on their anatomical localization. Some important examples include the control of feeding, sexual behaviors, and social functions.

ACETYLCHOLINE We now know that acetylcholine (ACh) plays a major role in neurotransmission in the forebrain. Many **cholinergic** (ACh-containing) neurons are found in nuclei within the **basal forebrain**. These cholinergic cells project widely in the brain, to sites such as the cerebral cortex, amygdala, and hippocampus (see Figure 3.4). Widespread loss of cholinergic neurons is associated with Alzheimer's disease, and experimental disruption of cholinergic pathways in rats interferes with learning and memory.

DOPAMINE Out of more than 80 billion neurons in the human brain, only about a million synthesize **dopamine** (**DA**), but they are critically important for many aspects of behavior. Figure 3.4 shows the paths of the major **dopaminergic** projections. One of these projections is called the *mesostriatal pathway* because it originates in the midbrain (mesencephalon) around the **substantia nigra** and projects axons to regions of the basal ganglia (aka the *striatum*). There aren't all that many neurons in the system—hundreds of thousands—but keep in mind that a single axon can divide to supply thousands of synapses. Those synapses play a crucial role in motor control. When people lose a significant number of mesostriatal dopaminergic neurons, from either exposure to toxins or just old age, they develop the

cholinergic Referring to cells that use acetylcholine as their synaptic transmitter.

basal forebrain A region, ventral to the basal ganglia, that is the major source of cholinergic projections in the brain.

dopamine (DA) A monoamine transmitter found in the midbrain—especially the substantia nigra—and in the basal forebrain.

dopaminergic Referring to cells that use dopamine as their synaptic transmitter.

substantia nigra A brainstem structure that innervates the basal ganglia and is a major source of dopaminergic projections.

profound movement problems of Parkinson's disease (described in Chapter 5), including tremors.

Another dopaminergic projection, called the *mesolimbocortical pathway*, also originates in the midbrain, in a region called the **ventral tegmental area** (**VTA**) (see Figure 3.4). From there, the pathway projects to various locations in the limbic system (see Chapter 2) and cortex. The mesolimbocortical system appears to be especially important for the processing of reward; it's probably where feelings of pleasure arise. Thus, it makes sense that the mesolimbocortical dopamine system is important for learning that is shaped by positive reinforcement (which usually involves a reward; see Chapter 13), especially via the D_2 dopamine receptor subtype. Abnormalities in the mesolimbocortical pathway are associated with some of the symptoms of schizophrenia, as we discuss in Chapter 12. At the end of this chapter we'll look at the role of this pathway in addictive behaviors.

SEROTONIN   Dopaminergic neurons may be scarce, but there are even fewer **serotonergic** neurons in the human brain—just 200,000 or so. Nevertheless, wide expanses of the brain are innervated by serotonergic fibers, originating from neurons sprinkled along the midline of the midbrain and brainstem in the **raphe nuclei** (*raphe* is pronounced "rafay" and is Latin for "seam") (see Figure 3.4).

Serotonin (**5-HT**, short for its chemical name, 5-hydroxytryptamine) participates in the control of all sorts of behaviors: mood, vision, sexual behavior, anxiety, sleep, and many other functions. As we'll see a little later, drugs that increase serotonergic activity are often prescribed for depression and anxiety. The precise behavioral actions of serotonergic drugs depend on which of the many 5-HT receptor subtypes are affected (see Table 3.2) (Gorzalka et al., 1990; Carr and Lucki, 2011).

NOREPINEPHRINE   As Figure 3.4 shows, many of the brain's **noradrenergic** neurons—given this name because **norepinephrine** (**NE**) is also known as *noradrenaline*—have their cell bodies in two regions of the brainstem and midbrain: the **locus coeruleus** ("blue spot") and the **lateral tegmental area**. Noradrenergic axons from these regions project broadly throughout the cerebrum, including the cerebral cortex, limbic system, and thalamic nuclei. They participate in the control of behaviors ranging from alertness to mood to sexual behavior (and many more).

Many peptides function as neurotransmitters

Peptides are very important signaling chemicals both in the brain and in the other organs of the body. Here are just a few examples of peptides that act as neurotransmitters:

- The **opioid peptides**, a group of endogenous substances with actions that resemble those of opiate drugs like morphine: some key opioids are met-enkephalin, leu-enkephalin, beta-endorphin, and dynorphin. As with morphine, these peptides act as analgesics (painkillers) and have rewarding properties.

- A diverse group of peptides originally discovered in the periphery—especially in the organs of the gut (which explains some of their names)—that are also made by neurons in the spinal cord and brain. These peptides may act as synaptic transmitters, and they are often co-localized with classical transmitters. Examples include vasoactive intestinal polypeptide (VIP), substance P, cholecystokinin (CCK), neurotensin, and neuropeptide Y (NPY).

- Various peptide hormones, such as oxytocin and vasopressin, that are produced by the hypothalamus and pituitary. These two peptides are involved in an astonishing variety of functions, ranging from basic housekeeping like urine production through to higher-level functions like memory, pair-bonding (see Chapter 8), and social processes.

---

ventral tegmental area (VTA)
A portion of the midbrain that projects dopaminergic fibers to the nucleus accumbens.

serotonergic   Referring to cells that use serotonin as their synaptic transmitter.

raphe nuclei   A string of nuclei in the midline of the midbrain and brainstem that contain most of the serotonergic neurons of the brain.

serotonin (5-HT)   A synaptic transmitter that is produced in the raphe nuclei and is active in structures throughout the cerebral hemispheres.

noradrenergic   Referring to cells using norepinephrine (noradrenaline) as a transmitter.

norepinephrine (NE)   Also called *noradrenaline*. A neurotransmitter produced and released by sympathetic postganglionic neurons to accelerate organ activity.

locus coeruleus   A small nucleus in the brainstem whose neurons produce norepinephrine and modulate large areas of the forebrain.

lateral tegmental area   A brainstem region that provides some of the norepinephrine-containing projections of the brain.

opioid peptide   A type of endogenous peptide that mimics the effects of morphine in binding to opioid receptors and producing marked analgesia and reward.

Some neurotransmitters are gases

Neurons sometimes use certain gas molecules to communicate information; the best studied of these is nitric oxide (not to be confused with "laughing gas," which is nitr*ous* oxide). Carbon monoxide also serves as a transmitter in some cells. Although we call them *gas neurotransmitters*, these substances are different from traditional neurotransmitters in at least three important ways:

1. Gas transmitters are produced in cellular locations other than the axon terminals, especially in the dendrites, and are not held in vesicles; the substance simply diffuses out of the neuron as it is produced.

2. No receptors in the membrane of the target cell are involved. Instead, the gas transmitter diffuses into the target cell to trigger second messengers inside.

3. Most important, these gases can function as **retrograde transmitters**: by diffusing from the postsynaptic neuron back to the presynaptic neuron, a gas transmitter conveys information that is used to physically change the synapse. This process may be crucial for memory formation (see Chapter 13), but gas transmitters also have been implicated in functions as diverse as hair growth and penile erections (Meldrum et al., 2014).

Now that we've surveyed the major neurotransmission mechanisms of the brain, let's turn our attention to chemicals from outside the body that affect the function of the brain: drugs and toxins.

retrograde transmitter   A neurotransmitter that diffuses from the postsynaptic neuron back to the presynaptic neuron.

View Activity 3.1:
Families of Transmitters

HOW'S IT GOING ❓

1. Identify the criteria that are used to establish whether a substance in the brain can be considered a neurotransmitter. Briefly discuss why each one is important.
2. Name and briefly describe each of the major categories of neurotransmitters.
3. What are the main excitatory and inhibitory amino acid transmitters of the brain, and what importance do they have?
4. Name and describe the anatomical organization of the four major "classical" amine neurotransmitters. What are some of the functions in which each transmitter has been implicated?
5. What is a peptide? Where do peptides come from—give a few examples—and what are some functions they perform?
6. Discuss the ways in which the gas transmitters resemble and differ from traditional amine transmitters.

3.3 Drugs Fit Like Keys into Molecular Locks

THE ROAD AHEAD

The effects of drugs depend on the types of receptors they interact with. After reading this section, you should be able to:

3.3.1 Distinguish between agonist, antagonist, and partial agonist drug actions.

3.3.2 Explain the concepts of binding affinity and efficacy, and discuss the general relationship between a drug's dose and its effects.

3.3.3 Summarize the routes of administration of drugs and the ways in which the brain and body adapt to the presence of drugs over time.

In everyday English, we use the term *drug* in different ways. One common meaning is "a medicine used in the treatment of a disease" (as in *prescription drug* or *over-the-counter drug*). Many *psychoactive drugs*—compounds that alter the function of the brain and

ligand   A substance that binds to receptor molecules, such as a neurotransmitter or drug that binds postsynaptic receptors.

agonist   A substance that mimics or potentiates the actions of a transmitter or other signaling molecule.

antagonist   A substance that blocks or attenuates the actions of a transmitter or other signaling molecule.

partial agonist   A drug that, when bound to a receptor, has less effect than the endogenous ligand would.

View Animation 3.4:
Agonists and Antagonists

FIGURE 3.5 Examples of Agonistic and Antagonistic Actions of Drugs on Receptors

thereby affect conscious experiences—fall into this category, and they may be useful in psychiatric settings. Some psychoactive drugs are used recreationally, with varying degrees of risk to the user; these are sometimes referred to as *drugs of abuse*, although such substances may also have therapeutic value. Some psychoactive drugs affect the brain by altering enzyme action or modifying other internal cellular processes, but as you may have guessed, most of the drugs that are of interest in neuroscience act via receptors.

Recall from Chapter 2 that any substance that binds to a receptor is termed a **ligand**. The natural ligands for receptors are molecules of neurotransmitters, of course. But as you may have guessed, many (but not all) drugs that affect the brain are also receptor ligands. The actions of drugs on ionotropic and metabotropic receptors are illustrated in **FIGURE 3.5**. Drugs that mimic or potentiate the actions of a transmitter are called **agonists**. A substance that mimics the normal action of a neurotransmitter on its receptors by binding to the receptors and activating them is thus a *receptor agonist*. Similarly, drugs that reduce the normal actions of a neurotransmitter system are called **antagonists**. Drugs classified as *receptor antagonists* bind to receptors but do *not* activate them—instead, they block the receptors from being activated by their normal neurotransmitter. For that reason, drugs with this action are sometimes called receptor *blockers*. Some important drugs, called **partial agonists**, are useful because they produce only a middling response. And still other drugs have agonistic or antagonistic effects that are not receptor mediated, such as drugs that alter the synthesis or release of transmitter by presynaptic neurons.

Many drugs—caffeine, opium, nicotine, and cocaine are just a few examples—originally evolved in plants, often as a defense against being eaten. Other modern

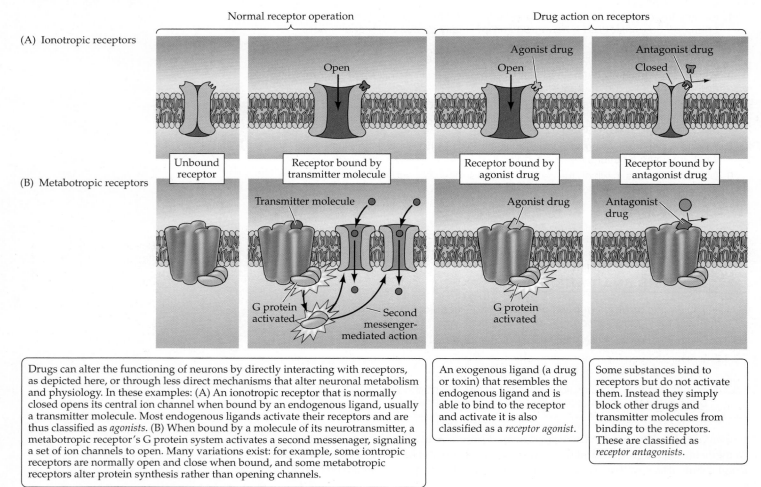

| Normal receptor operation | | Drug action on receptors | |

(A) Ionotropic receptors

Open — Receptor bound by transmitter molecule

Unbound receptor

Agonist drug — Open — Receptor bound by agonist drug

Antagonist drug — Closed — Receptor bound by antagonist drug

(B) Metabotropic receptors

Transmitter molecule
G protein activated
Second messenger-mediated action

Agonist drug
G protein activated

Antagonist drug

Drugs can alter the functioning of neurons by directly interacting with receptors, as depicted here, or through less direct mechanisms that alter neuronal metabolism and physiology. In these examples: (A) An ionotropic receptor that is normally closed opens its central ion channel when bound by an endogenous ligand, usually a transmitter molecule. Most endogenous ligands activate their receptors and are thus classified as *agonists*. (B) When bound by a molecule of its neurotransmitter, a metabotropic receptor's G protein system activates a second messenager, signaling a set of ion channels to open. Many variations exist: for example, some iontropic receptors are normally open and close when bound, and some metabotropic receptors alter protein synthesis rather than opening channels.

An exogenous ligand (a drug or toxin) that resembles the endogenous ligand and is able to bind to the receptor and activate it is also classified as a *receptor agonist*.

Some substances bind to receptors but do not activate them. Instead they simply block other drugs and transmitter molecules from binding to the receptors. These are classified as *receptor antagonists*.

drugs are synthetic (human-made) and tuned to target specific transmitter systems. For example, benzodiazepine antianxiety drugs like lorazepam (trade name Ativan) enhance GABA neurotransmission; classic antipsychotics like haloperidol (trade name Haldol) block dopamine receptors; selective serotonin reuptake inhibitors like fluoxetine (Prozac) are antidepressants. So to understand how drugs work, we must perform analyses at many levels—from molecules to anatomical systems to behavioral effects and experiences.

Earlier we said that a given neurotransmitter interacts with a variety of different *subtypes* of receptors. To get a sense of just how diverse the transmitter receptor subtypes can be, take another look at Table 3.2. For example, there are more than a dozen different subtypes of serotonin receptors. Some are inhibitory, some excitatory, some ionotropic, some metabotropic; in fact, the only thing they all really share is that they are normally stimulated by serotonin. They even differ in their anatomical distribution within the brain. This division of transmitter receptors into multiple subtypes presents us with an opportunity because, although the natural transmitter will act on *all* its receptor subtypes, we humans can craftily design drugs that fit into only one or a few receptor subtypes. Selectively activating or blocking specific subtypes of receptors can produce diverse effects, some of which are beneficial. For example, treating someone with large doses of the neurotransmitter serotonin would necessarily activate *all* of the different subtypes of serotonin receptors in their brain, producing a confusing welter of different effects. But drugs that selectively block $5\text{-}HT_3$ receptors while ignoring other subtypes of serotonin receptors produce a powerful and specific anti-nausea effect that brings relief to people undergoing cancer chemotherapy.

Drugs are administered and eliminated in many different ways

Drug molecules aren't magic bullets; they don't somehow know where to go to find particular receptor molecules. Instead, drug molecules just spread widely throughout the body, binding to their selective receptors when they happen to encounter them. This binding triggers a chain of cellular events, but it is usually temporary, and when the drug (or transmitter) breaks away from the receptor, the receptor resumes its unbound shape and functioning.

The amount of a drug that gets to the brain, and how fast it gets there, depends in part on the drug's route of administration. Some routes, such as smoking or intravenous injection, rapidly ramp up the amount of drug that is **bioavailable**: free to act on the target tissue, and thus not in use elsewhere or in the process of being eliminated. With other routes, such as ingestion (swallowing), the concentration of drug builds up more slowly over longer periods of time. The duration of a drug effect also depends on how the drug is metabolized and excreted from the body—via the kidneys, liver, lungs, or other routes. In some cases, the metabolites of drugs are themselves active; this **biotransformation** of drugs can produce substances with beneficial or harmful actions. The factors that affect the movement of a drug into, through, and out of the body are collectively referred to as **pharmacokinetics**.

The effects of a drug depend on its dose

The tuning of drug molecules to receptor subtypes is not absolutely specific. In reality, a particular drug will generally bind strongly to one kind of receptor, more weakly to a few other types, and not at all to many others. This chemical attraction is known as **binding affinity** (or simply *affinity*). At low doses, when relatively few drug molecules are in circulation, drugs will preferentially bind to their highest-affinity receptors. At higher doses, enough molecules of the drug are available to bind both the highest-affinity receptors and some of the lower-affinity receptors. It's interesting to note that neurotransmitter molecules are low-affinity ligands: they bind only comparatively weakly to their receptors, so they can rapidly detach a moment later, allowing the synapse to reset in preparation for the next presynaptic signal.

Once it is bound to a receptor, the extent to which a drug molecule *activates* the receptor is termed its **efficacy** (or *intrinsic activity*). As you might guess, agonists have

bioavailable Referring to a substance, usually a drug, that is present in the body in a form that is able to interact with physiological mechanisms.

biotransformation The process in which enzymes convert a drug into a metabolite that is itself active, possibly in ways that are substantially different from the actions of the original substance.

pharmacokinetics Collective name for all the factors that affect the movement of a drug into, through, and out of the body.

binding affinity Also called simply *affinity*. The propensity of molecules of a drug (or other ligand) to bind to receptors.

efficacy Also called *intrinsic activity*. The extent to which a drug activates a response when it binds to a receptor.

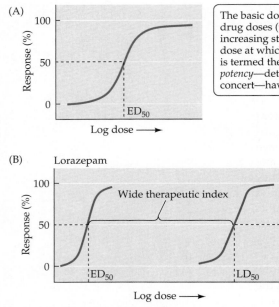

(A)

The basic dose-response curve (DRC) plots increasing drug doses (usually on a logarithmic scale) against increasing strength of the response being studied. The dose at which the drug shows half of its maximal effect is termed the *effective dose 50%* (ED_{50}). Drugs with high *potency*—determined by affinity and efficacy in concert—have a lower ED_{50}.

(B)

The *therapeutic index* refers to the separation between useful doses of the drug and dangerous doses. This is determined by comparing the ED_{50} dose of the drug with the dose at which 50% of the animals either show symptoms of toxicity (*toxic dose 50%*; TD_{50}) or outright die (*lethal dose 50%*; LD_{50}). In this example, a greater difference between ED_{50} and LD_{50} is observed for the anti-anxiety drug lorazepam (Ativan) than for the older anti-anxiety drug pheno-barbital, indicating that lorazepam is the safer drug. Many deaths—accidental and not—have resulted from phenobarbital overdose.

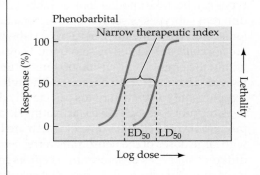

FIGURE 3.6 The Dose-Response Curve

high efficacy: they tend to activate the receptors they bind to. Conversely, antagonists have low or no efficacy (see Figure 3.5). Partial agonists, unsurprisingly, have appreciable but submaximal efficacy. So it is a combination of affinity and efficacy—where it binds and what it does—that determines the overall action of a drug. For example, the classic antipsychotic drugs tend to have high affinity and low efficacy at the D_2 subtype of dopamine receptors; in other words, they are D_2 blockers. It's a topic we'll revisit in Chapter 12.

Giving larger doses of a drug ultimately increases the proportion of receptors that are bound and affected by the drug. Within certain limits, this increase in receptor binding also increases the response to the drug; in other words, greater doses tend to produce greater effects. When plotted as a graph, the relationship between drug doses and observed effects is called a **dose-response curve** (**DRC**), typically taking the sigmoidal shape shown in **FIGURE 3.6A**. Careful analysis of DRCs reveals many aspects of a drug's activity, such as useful and safe dose ranges (**FIGURE 3.6B**), and it is one of the main tools for understanding the functional relationships between drugs and their targets.

Humans have devised a variety of ingenious techniques for introducing substances into the body; these are summarized in **TABLE 3.3**. In Chapter 1 we described how tight junctions between the cells of the walls of blood vessels create a **blood-brain barrier** that inhibits the movement of larger molecules out of the bloodstream and into the brain. This barrier poses a major challenge for neuropharmacology because many drugs that might be useful are too large to cross the blood-brain barrier into the brain. To a limited extent this problem can be circumvented by administering the drugs directly into the brain, but that is a drastic step. Alternatively, some drugs can take advantage of active transport systems that normally move nutrients out of the bloodstream and into the brain.

Repeated treatments may reduce the effectiveness of drugs

Our bodies are well equipped to maintain a constant internal environment, optimized for cellular activities, and to counteract physiological challenges. In the case of drugs, the body's ability to adapt to challenges may result in the development of **drug tolerance**,

dose-response curve (DRC) A formal graph of a drug's effects (on the *y*-axis) versus the dose given (on the *x*-axis).

blood-brain barrier The protective property of cerebral blood vessels that impedes the movement of some harmful substances from the bloodstream into the brain.

drug tolerance Also called simply *tolerance*. A condition in which, with repeated exposure to a drug, an individual becomes less responsive to a constant dose.

TABLE 3.3 The Relationship between Routes of Administration and Effects of Drugs

Route of administration	Examples and mechanisms	Typical speed of effects

INGESTION
  Tablets and capsules
  Syrups
  Infusions and teas
  Suppositories
	Many sorts of drugs and remedies: ingestion depends on absorption by the gut, which is somewhat slower than most other routes and affected by digestive factors such as acidity of the stomach and the presence of food.	Slow to moderate

INHALATION
  Smoking
  Nasal absorption (snorting)
  Inhaled gases, powders, and
  sprays
	Nicotine, cocaine, organic solvents such as airplane glue and gasoline, other drugs of abuse, and a variety of prescription drugs and hormone treatments: inhalation methods take advantage of the rich vascularization of the nose and lungs to convey drugs directly into the bloodstream.	Moderate to fast

PERIPHERAL INJECTION
  Subcutaneous
  Intramuscular
  Intraperitoneal (abdominal)
  Intravenous
	Many drugs: subcutaneous (under the skin) injections tend to have the slowest effects because they must diffuse into nearby tissue in order to reach the bloodstream; intravenous injections have very rapid effects because the drug is placed directly into circulation.	Moderate to fast

CENTRAL INJECTION
  Intracerebroventricular (into
  ventricular system)
  Intrathecal (into the cerebrospinal
  fluid of the spine)
  Epidural (under the dura mater)
  Intracerebral (directly into a brain
  region)
	Central methods involve injection directly into the central nervous system and are used in order to circumvent the blood-brain barrier, to rule out peripheral effects, or to directly affect a discrete brain location.	Fast to very fast

where a drug's effectiveness diminishes with repeated treatments. Consequently, successively larger and larger doses of a drug are needed to produce the same effect.

Drug tolerance can develop in several different ways. Some drugs provoke **metabolic tolerance**, in which the body (especially metabolic organs, such as the liver with its specialized enzymes) becomes more effective at eliminating the drug from the bloodstream before it can have an effect. Alternatively, the target tissue may change its sensitivity to the drug—a phenomenon called **functional tolerance**. One important way in which a cell develops functional tolerance is by changing how many receptors it has on its surface. So, for example, after repeated doses of an *agonist* drug, neurons may **down-regulate** their receptors (decrease the number of receptors available to the drug), thereby becoming less sensitive and countering the drug effect. If the drug is an *antagonist*, target neurons may instead **up-regulate** (increase) the number of receptors, to become more sensitive and thus counteract the drug effect. Indeed, continual modification of receptor densities is a key feature of synapses and is crucial for neurotransmission and plasticity (Choquet and Triller, 2013).

Tolerance to a particular drug often generalizes to other drugs of the same chemical class; this effect is termed **cross-tolerance**. For example, people who have developed tolerance to heroin tend to exhibit a degree of tolerance to all the other drugs in the opiate category, including codeine, morphine, and methadone. This phenomenon occurs because all those drugs act on the same family of receptors.

metabolic tolerance   The form of drug tolerance that arises when repeated exposure to the drug causes the metabolic machinery of the body to become more efficient at clearing the drug.

functional tolerance   The form of drug tolerance that arises when repeated exposure to the drug causes receptors to be up-regulated or down-regulated.

down-regulation   A compensatory decrease in receptor availability at the synapses of a neuron.

up-regulation   A compensatory increase in receptor availability at the synapses of a neuron.

cross-tolerance   A condition in which the development of tolerance for one drug causes an individual to develop tolerance for another drug.

HOW'S IT GOING ❓

1. Briefly explain agonist and antagonist actions of a ligand, with respect to effects on receptors.
2. What are receptor subtypes? What is their significance for drug development?
3. Briefly explain how dose-response curves are calculated and why they are useful to pharmacologists. Distinguish between a drug's binding affinity and its efficacy.

4. Provide a review of the different ways in which drugs can be administered, in particular noting some considerations that are taken into account when deciding on a route of administration.

5. How does repeated exposure to a drug alter its effects? (*Hint*: Use the words *tolerance* and *regulate* in your answer.)

3.4 Drugs Affect Each Stage of Neural Conduction and Synaptic Transmission

THE ROAD AHEAD

Drugs affect many stages of synaptic transmission. After reading this section, you should be able to:

3.4.1 Summarize the ways in which drugs alter presynaptic processes, with examples.

3.4.2 Summarize drug effects on postsynaptic processes, with examples.

3.4.3 Define autoreceptors and explain their function, using caffeine as an example.

3.4.4 Review the processes that terminate transmitter action at synapses.

As the saying goes, it takes two to tango. Synaptic transmission involves a complicated choreography of the two participating neurons, and drugs that affect the brain and behavior may act on either side of the synapse. Let's consider these two sites of action in turn.

Some drugs alter presynaptic processes

One of the ways that a drug may change synaptic transmission is by affecting the presynaptic neuron, changing the system that converts an electrical signal (an action potential) into a chemical signal (secretion of neurotransmitter). As **FIGURE 3.7** illustrates, the most common presynaptic drug effects can be grouped into three main categories: effects on transmitter *production*, effects on transmitter *release*, and effects on transmitter *clearance*.

TRANSMITTER PRODUCTION   In order for the presynaptic neuron to produce neurotransmitter, a steady supply of raw materials and enzymes must arrive at the axon terminals and carry out the needed reactions. Drugs are available that alter this process in various ways (**FIGURE 3.7A**). For example, a drug may inhibit an enzyme that neurons need in order to synthesize a particular neurotransmitter, resulting in depletion of that transmitter. Alternatively, drugs that block axonal transport prevent raw materials from reaching the axon terminals in the first place, which could also cause the presynaptic terminals to run out of neurotransmitter. In both cases, affected presynaptic neurons are prevented from having their usual effects on postsynaptic neurons, with sometimes profound effects on behavior. A third class of drug (e.g., reserpine) doesn't prevent the *production* of transmitter but instead interferes with the cell's ability to *store* the transmitter in synaptic vesicles for later release. The effect on behavior may be complicated, depending on how much transmitter can still reach the postsynaptic cell.

TRANSMITTER RELEASE   As we saw in Chapter 3, transmitter is released when action potentials arrive at the axon terminal and trigger an inflow of calcium ions. But a number of drugs and toxins can block those action potentials from ever arriving. For example, compounds that block sodium channels (like the toxin that makes puffer fish a dangerous delicacy, called *tetrodotoxin*) prevent axons from firing action potentials, shutting down synaptic transmission with deadly results. And drugs called *calcium channel blockers* do exactly as their name suggests, blocking the calcium influx

A Effects on Transmitter Production

1 Inhibition of transmitter synthesis
Example: *Para*-chlorophenylalanine inhibits tryptophan hydroxylase, preventing synthesis of serotonin from its metabolic precursor.

2 Blockade of axonal transport
Example: Colchicine impairs maintenance of microtubules and blocks axonal transport.

3 Interference with the storage of transmitters
Example: Reserpine blocks the packaging of transmitter molecules within vesicles, thereby allowing the transmitter to be broken down by enzymes.

B Effects on Transmitter Release

4 Prevention of synaptic transmission
Example: Tetrodotoxin, found in puffer fish, blocks voltage-gated Na^+ channels and prevents nerve conduction.

5 Alteration of synaptic transmitter release through calcium channel blockade
Example: Verapamil, a calcium channel blocker, inhibits transmitter release by reducing the influx of calcium ions that drives vesicles to release transmitter.

6 Alteration of transmitter release through modulation of presynaptic activity
Example: Caffeine competes with adenosine for presynaptic receptors, thus preventing its inhibitory effects.

7 Alteration of synaptic transmitter release through other mechanisms
Example: Amphetamine stimulates release of catecholamine transmitters, especially DA and NE. Botox (botulinum toxin) disrupts the proteins that allow the vesicles of motor neurons to release ACh, resulting in local paralysis.

C Effects on Transmitter Clearance

8 Inactivation of transmitter reuptake
Example: Cocaine and amphetamine inhibit reuptake mechanisms, thus prolonging synaptic activity. Certain antidepressants inhibit serotonin or norepinephrine reuptake.

9 Blockade of transmitter degradation
Example: Some drugs (e.g., monoamine oxidase [MAO] inhibitors) inhibit enzymes that normally break down neurotransmitter molecules in the axon terminal or in the synaptic cleft. As a result, transmitter remains active longer and to greater effect.

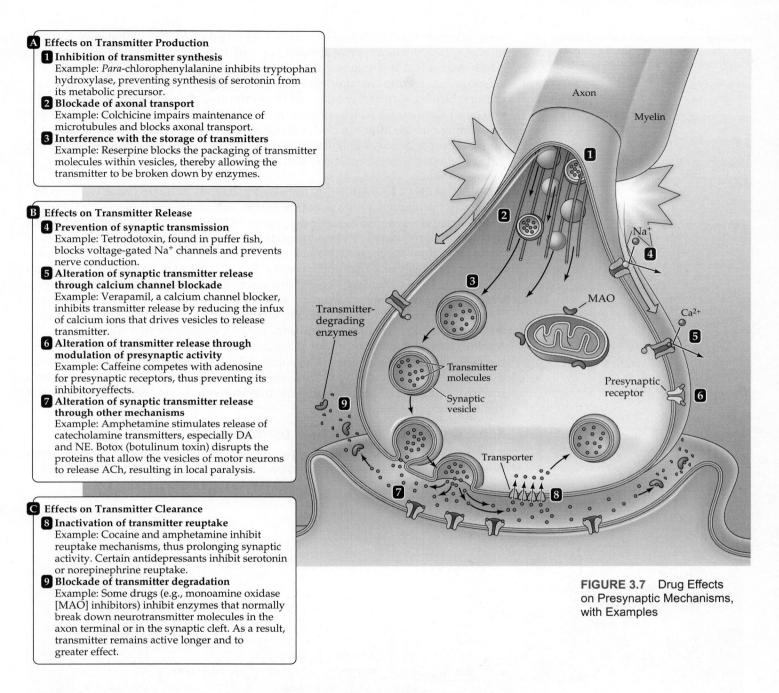

FIGURE 3.7 Drug Effects on Presynaptic Mechanisms, with Examples

that normally drives the release of transmitter into the synapse (**FIGURE 3.7B**). The active ingredient in Botox—botulinum toxin—specifically blocks ACh release from axon terminals near the injection site. The resulting local paralysis of underlying muscles reduces wrinkling of the overlying skin, but it may also interfere with the ability to produce normal facial expressions.

A different way to alter transmitter release is to modify the systems that the neuron normally uses to monitor and regulate its own transmitter release. For example, presynaptic neurons often use **autoreceptors** to monitor how much transmitter they have released; it's a kind of feedback system. Drugs that stimulate these receptors provide a false feedback signal, prompting the presynaptic cell to release less transmitter. Drugs that instead *block* autoreceptors prevent the presynaptic neuron from receiving its normal feedback, tricking the cell into releasing more transmitter than usual. Worldwide,

autoreceptor A receptor for a synaptic transmitter that is located in the presynaptic membrane and tells the axon terminal how much transmitter has been released.

caffeine   A compound found in coffee and other plants that exerts a stimulant action by blocking adenosine receptors.

we drink more than 2.2 billion cups of coffee every day, and the **caffeine** we get from all that coffee blocks a type of autoreceptor called the *adenosine receptor*. Adenosine, which is classified as a *neuromodulator,* is coreleased with the neuron's transmitter and acts to reduce further transmitter release. So, by blocking presynaptic adenosine receptors, caffeine *increases* the amount of neurotransmitter released, resulting in the enhanced alertness for which coffee is renowned (McLellan et al., 2016). Interestingly, consuming caffeine after a period of studying may improve memory consolidation in humans for some, but not all, learning tasks (Borota et al., 2014; Hussain and Cole, 2015), perhaps thanks to enhanced neural activity.

TRANSMITTER CLEARANCE   After action potentials have arrived at the axon terminals and prompted a release of transmitter substance, the transmitter is rapidly cleared from the synapse by several processes (**FIGURE 3.7C**). Obviously, getting rid of the used transmitter is an important step, because until it is gone, new releases of transmitter from the presynaptic side won't be able to have much extra effect. However, researchers think that under certain circumstances, neurons may be *too* good at clearing the used transmitter and that a significant lack of transmitter in certain synapses may contribute to disorders such as depression. As we'll see shortly, some important psychiatric drugs, called *reuptake inhibitors*, work by blocking the presynaptic system that normally reabsorbs transmitter molecules after their release; this blocking action allows transmitter molecules to stay a bit longer in the synaptic cleft, having a greater effect on the postsynaptic cell. Other drugs achieve a similar result by blocking the enzymes that normally break up molecules of neurotransmitter into inactive metabolites, again allowing the transmitter to accumulate, having a greater effect on the postsynaptic cell.

Some drugs alter postsynaptic processes

An alternate way for drugs to change synaptic transmission is by altering the postsynaptic systems that respond to the released neurotransmitter. As illustrated in **FIGURE 3.8**,

FIGURE 3.8   Drug Effects on Postsynaptic Mechanisms

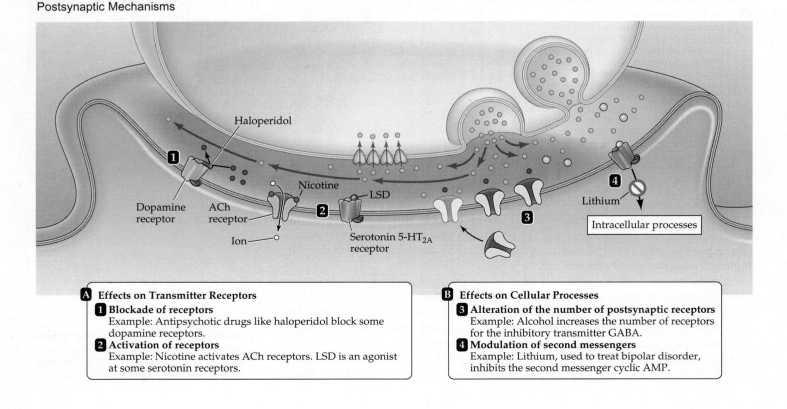

A **Effects on Transmitter Receptors**
  1 Blockade of receptors
   Example: Antipsychotic drugs like haloperidol block some dopamine receptors.
  2 Activation of receptors
   Example: Nicotine activates ACh receptors. LSD is an agonist at some serotonin receptors.

B **Effects on Cellular Processes**
  3 Alteration of the number of postsynaptic receptors
   Example: Alcohol increases the number of receptors for the inhibitory transmitter GABA.
  4 Modulation of second messengers
   Example: Lithium, used to treat bipolar disorder, inhibits the second messenger cyclic AMP.

there are two major classes of postsynaptic drug actions: (1) direct effects on transmitter receptors and (2) effects on cellular processes within the postsynaptic neuron.

TRANSMITTER RECEPTOR ACTIVATION   As we discussed earlier in the chapter, selective receptor antagonists bind directly to postsynaptic receptors and block them from being activated by their neurotransmitter (**FIGURE 3.8A**). The results may be immediate and dramatic. Curare, for example, blocks the nicotinic ACh receptors found on muscles, resulting in immediate paralysis of all skeletal muscles, including those used for breathing (which is why curare is an effective arrow poison).

Selective receptor *agonists* bind to specific receptors and activate them, mimicking the natural neurotransmitter at those receptors. These drugs are often very potent, with effects that vary depending on the particular types of receptors activated. LSD is an example, producing bizarre visual experiences through strong stimulation of a subtype of serotonin receptors (namely, 5-HT_{2A} receptors) found in visual cortex.

POSTSYNAPTIC INTRACELLULAR PROCESSES   When they bind to their matching receptors on postsynaptic membranes, neurotransmitters can stimulate a variety of changes within the postsynaptic cells, such as the activation of second messengers, the activation of genes, and the production of various proteins. These intracellular processes present additional targets for drug action (**FIGURE 3.8B**). For example, some drugs induce the postsynaptic cell to up-regulate its receptors, thus changing the sensitivity of the synapse. Other drugs cause a down-regulation in receptor density. Some drugs, like lithium chloride, directly alter second-messenger systems, with widespread effects in the brain. Future research will probably focus on drugs to selectively activate, alter, or block targeted genes within the DNA of neurons. These *genomic* effects could produce profound long-term changes in the structure and function of neurons.

3.5 Some Neuroactive Drugs Provide Relief from Mental Illness and Pain

THE ROAD AHEAD

In the next section we look at the major categories of neuroactive drugs used for clinical purposes. After reading this section, you should be able to:

3.5.1 Summarize the two major types of antipsychotic medications, and review their pharmacological actions.

3.5.2 Discuss the major types of actions of drugs for treating depression and anxiety, with examples.

3.5.3 Review the discovery of opiates, and their major actions in the brain. Using the opiate receptors as examples, discuss the significance of the discovery of orphan receptors in the brain.

Mental disorders have bedeviled people across the centuries. Historical accounts of sorcery, strange visions, and possession by demons no doubt reflect a misunderstanding of the symptoms of severe mental illness (the topic of Chapter 12) rather than supernatural events. But where the historical response to psychiatric illness was to lock away the afflicted, neuroscience breakthroughs of the last 70 years have revolutionized psychiatry and liberated millions from the purgatory of institutionalized care. In the sections that follow, we will briefly review some of the major categories of psychoactive drugs, based on how they affect behavior.

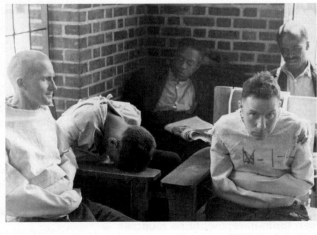

© Alfred Eisenstaedt/Time & Life Pictures/Getty Images

The Antipsychotic Revolution   The introduction of antipsychotic drugs relieved the suffering of millions of patients who had previously required hospitalization in psychiatric institutions like this one. Antipsychotics dramatically curb the striking hallucinations and delusions that are symptomatic of schizophrenia.

Antipsychotics relieve symptoms of schizophrenia

It's hard to believe now, but prior to the 1950s about half of all hospital beds were taken up by psychiatric patients (Menninger, 1948), and owing to its debilitating nature, a high proportion of these were people suffering from the delusions and hallucinations of schizophrenia. This awful situation was suddenly and dramatically improved by the development of a family of drugs now called **first-generation antipsychotics** (or *neuroleptics*). The first of these drugs, chlorpromazine (Thorazine), and successors like haloperidol (Haldol) and loxapine (Loxitane) all share one crucial feature: they act as selective antagonists of dopamine D_2 receptors in the brain. These drugs are so good at relieving *positive symptoms* of schizophrenia—emergent symptoms and behaviors that were previously absent, such as hallucinations and delusions—that a dopaminergic model of the disease became dominant (see Chapter 12). More recently, **second-generation antipsychotics** have been developed that have both dopaminergic and additional, nondopaminergic actions, especially the blockade of certain serotonin receptors. These drugs may be helpful in relieving symptoms that are resistant to first-generation antipsychotics—especially the *negative symptoms* that involve impairment or loss of a behavior, such as social withdrawal and blunted emotional responses—but early hopes that these drugs would generally outperform first-generation antipsychotics have not been borne out (Kane and Correll, 2010). Growing evidence that schizophrenia also involves transmitters other than the classic targets has since prompted an intense research effort aimed at developing third-generation antipsychotics, with novel targets like glutamate and oxytocin, but effective treatments remain elusive (M. C. Davis et al., 2014; O'Tuathaigh et al., 2017). So, although there has been progress in its treatment, schizophrenia remains a difficult, multifaceted disease and a major health problem, with little agreement regarding optimal treatment strategies (Correll et al., 2017).

Antidepressants reduce chronic mood problems

Disturbances of mood called *affective disorders* are among the most common of all psychiatric complaints (World Health Organization, 2001). In contrast to the antipsychotic drugs, which reduce synaptic activity by blocking receptors, effective **antidepressant** drugs act to *increase* synaptic transmission. Some of the earliest antidepressants were the **monoamine oxidase** (**MAO**) inhibitors, which, as their name suggests, block the enzyme responsible for breaking down monoamine transmitters such as dopamine, serotonin, and norepinephrine. This action allows transmitter molecules to accumulate in the synapses (see Figure 3.7, step 9), with an associated improvement in mood. A second generation of drugs, called the **tricyclic antidepressants** (an example is imipramine), likewise promote an accumulation of synaptic transmitter, by blocking the reuptake of transmitter molecules into the presynaptic terminal (see Figure 3.7, step 8). More recent generations of antidepressants also increase synaptic transmitter availability, but they focus on specific transmitters: **selective serotonin reuptake inhibitors** (**SSRIs**) like fluoxetine (Prozac) and citalopram (Celexa) are so named because they act specifically to block reuptake at serotonergic synapses. Related compounds called **serotonin-norepinephrine reuptake inhibitors** (**SNRIs**), like venlafaxine (Effexor), promote the accumulation of both serotonin and norepinephrine, by blocking reuptake of both, and have therapeutic applications that extend beyond depression to include anxiety disorders.

Anxiolytics combat anxiety

Severe anxiety, in the form of panic attacks, phobias (specific irrational fears), and generalized anxiety, can spiral out of control and become disabling; many millions of people are affected by anxiety disorders (see Chapter 12). Anything that reduces or *depresses* the excitability of neurons tends to counter these states, which explains some of the historical popularity of **depressants** like alcohol and opium. Unfortunately, these substances have a strong potential for intoxication and addiction, so they are not

first-generation antipsychotics Also called *neuroleptics*. Any of a class of antipsychotic drugs that alleviate symptoms of schizophrenia, typically by blocking dopamine receptors.

second-generation antipsychotic An antipsychotic drug that has actions other than or in addition to the D_2 receptor antagonism that characterizes first-generation antipsychotics.

antidepressant A drug that relieves the symptoms of depression.

monoamine oxidase (MAO) An enzyme that breaks down monoamine transmitters, thereby inactivating them.

tricyclic antidepressant An antidepressant that acts by increasing the synaptic accumulation of serotonin and norepinephrine.

selective serotonin reuptake inhibitor (SSRI) An antidepressant drug that blocks the reuptake of transmitter at serotonergic synapses.

serotonin-norepinephrine reuptake inhibitor (SNRI) Any of a class of drugs that promote the synaptic accumulation of serotonin and norepinephrine by blocking transmitter reuptake.

depressant A drug that reduces the excitability of neurons.

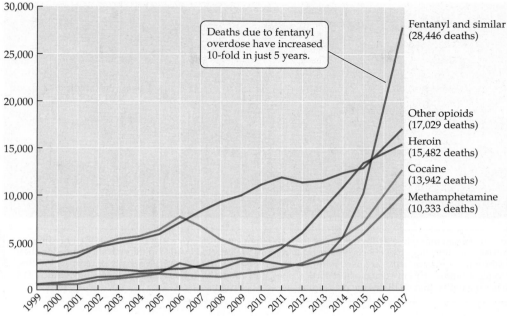

Deaths due to fentanyl overdose have increased 10-fold in just 5 years.

Fentanyl and similar (28,446 deaths)

Other opioids (17,029 deaths)

Heroin (15,482 deaths)

Cocaine (13,942 deaths)

Methamphetamine (10,333 deaths)

FIGURE 3.9 An Epidemic of Overdose Deaths (After NIDA [2017], based on data from Natl. Ctr. Hlth. Stat., CDC Wonder database, 2017.)

barbiturate An early anxiolytic drug and sleep aid that has depressant activity in the nervous system.

anxiolytic A drug that is used to combat anxiety.

benzodiazepine Any of a class of antianxiety drugs that are agonists of GABA$_A$ receptors in the central nervous system. One example is diazepam (Valium).

opium An extract of the opium poppy, *Papaver somniferum*. Drugs based on opium are potent painkillers.

morphine An opiate compound derived from the poppy flower.

analgesic Having painkilling properties.

heroin Diacetylmorphine, an artificially modified, very potent form of morphine.

opioid receptor A receptor that responds to endogenous opioids and/or exogenous opiates.

suitable for therapeutic use. **Barbiturate** drugs, such as phenobarbital, were originally developed to reduce anxiety, promote sleep, and avoid epileptic seizures. They are still used occasionally for those purposes, but they are also addictive and easy to overdose on, often fatally, as illustrated in Figure 3.6B.

Since the 1970s the most widely prescribed **anxiolytics** (antianxiety drugs) have been the **benzodiazepines**, which are both safer and more specific than the barbiturates (see Figure 3.6B), although they still carry some risk of addiction. Members of this class of drug, such as alprazolam (trade name Xanax) and lorazepam (Ativan), bind to specific sites on GABA$_A$ receptors and enhance the activity of GABA (R. W. Olsen, 2018). Because GABA$_A$ receptors are inhibitory, benzodiazepines help GABA to produce larger inhibitory postsynaptic potentials than GABA would produce alone. The net effect is a reduction in the excitability of neurons. The GABA$_A$ receptor is large and complex and contains multiple bindings sites through which drugs may act (Masiulis et al., 2019). Hormones that interact with GABA receptors, as well as drugs that subtly alter serotonergic neurotransmission, are examples of these novel anxiolytics (Belelli et al., 2018). Antidepressant drugs are often effective anxiolytics too. Unsurprisingly, given the high prevalence of anxiety disorders in society, the hunt for new antianxiety agents is an area of intense research effort.

Opiates have powerful painkilling effects

Opium, extracted from poppy flower seedpods, has been used by humans since at least the Stone Age. **Morphine**, the major active substance in opium, is a very effective **analgesic** (painkiller) that has brought relief from severe pain to many millions of people (see Chapter 5). Unfortunately, because it produces powerful feelings of euphoria, morphine also has a strong potential for addiction, as do close relatives like **heroin** (diacetylmorphine) and opiate painkillers like oxycodone (OxyContin) and fentanyl, a synthetic opiate that is 30 to 40 times stronger than heroin. Accidental opiate overdose is a rapidly growing epidemic: the fatal fentanyl overdose of the musician Prince in 2016 was just one of many thousands every year (**FIGURE 3.9**).

Opiates like morphine, heroin, and codeine bind to specific receptors— **opioid receptors**—that are concentrated in various regions of the brain. An

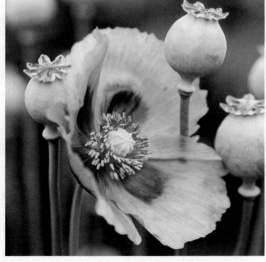

The Source of Opium and Morphine The opium poppy has a distinctive flower and seedpod. The bitter flavor and brain actions of opium may provide the poppy plant a defense against being eaten.

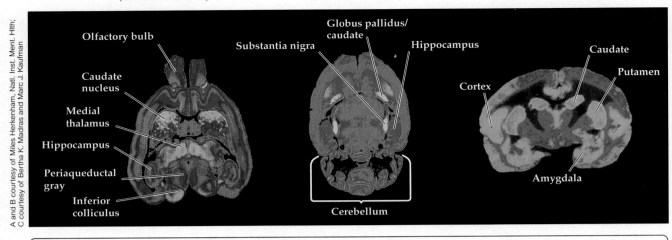

(A) Opioid binding in rat brain (horizontal section)

(B) Cannabinoid binding in rat brain (horizontal section)

(C) Cocaine binding in monkey brain (coronal section)

Maps of drug binding in the brain reveal that while drugs belonging to these major categories vary significantly in their binding patterns – explaining their widely varying subjective effects – some brain regions are affected by almost all such substances. In these *radioligand binding* studies, radioactive forms of drugs are used to highlight regions showing the highest density of receptor binding (warmer colors correspond to more binding). Many drugs affect cortical sites, and almost all will activate the mesolimbocortical DA pathway, terminating in the basal ganglia, that mediates the pleasurable aspects of drug use.

FIGURE 3.10 Recreational Drugs Bind to Varying Brain Sites

area within the midbrain called the **periaqueductal gray** (**FIGURE 3.10A**) contains a very high density of opioid receptors and is an especially important target because it is here that opiates exert much of their painkilling effects (see Chapter 5).

As we mentioned earlier in the chapter, we now know that the brain makes its own morphine-like compounds, called **endogenous opioids**. Researchers have identified three major families of these potent peptides: the *enkephalins*, from the Greek *en*, "in," and *kephale*, "head" (J. Hughes et al., 1975); the *endorphins*, a contraction of *endogenous morphine*; and the *dynorphins*, short for *dynamic endorphins*, in recognition of their potency and speed of action (see Table 3.1). There are also three main kinds of opioid receptors—delta (δ), kappa (κ), and mu (μ)—all of which are metabotropic receptors (see Table 3.2). Powerful drugs that block opioid receptors—naloxone (Narcan) is an example—can rapidly reverse the effects of opiates and rescue people from overdose. Opiate antagonists also block the rewarding aspects of drugs like heroin, so they can be helpful for treating addiction, as we discuss at the end of this chapter.

periaqueductal gray A midbrain region involved in pain perception.

endogenous opioid Any of a class of opium-like peptide transmitters that have been referred to as the body's own narcotics. The three kinds are enkephalins, endorphins, and dynorphins.

3.6 Some Neuroactive Drugs Are Used to Alter Conscious Experience

THE ROAD AHEAD

In addition to treating illness, humans seek out drugs for recreational use. After reading this section, you should be able to:

3.6.1 Identify the main active ingredients in cannabis, describe their sites of action in the brain, and discuss the effects of cannabinoids on behavior.

3.6.2 Compare and contrast the main families of stimulant drugs, and explain how they interact with neurons, their major effects, and risks they pose to human health.

3.6.3 Review the modes of action of alcohol in the brain, and discuss the prevalence and treatment of alcohol use disorders.

3.6.4 Define hallucinogenic drugs, and summarize the ways in which the major hallucinogens have shared or different actions in the brain, their major behavioral effects, and their potential therapeutic applications.

Whether to experience pleasurable sensations, to artificially increase vigor and wakefulness, or simply to satisfy curiosity, people have a long history of tinkering with their conscious experience of the world. Some of the most familiar types of drugs that modify consciousness include cannabinoids, stimulants, alcohol, and hallucinogens.

Cannabinoids have many effects

Cannabis and its related preparations, such as hashish, are derived from the *Cannabis sativa* plant, which has been widely cultivated and used by human societies for thousands of years (Russo, 2008). (The common alternative name *marijuana* is considered by some to have dubious, possibly racist origins; see Halperin, 2018.) Typically administered by smoking, by vaping, or via edible products such as cookies and candies, cannabis contains dozens of active ingredients, the best known of which are the compounds **delta-9-tetrahydrocannabinol** (**THC**), which is thought to produce the feeling of being "high" most closely associated with cannabis use, and **cannabidiol** (**CBD**), which appears to have anxiolytic effects as well as other medicinal actions (Boggs et al., 2018; Freeman et al., 2019). Cannabis use usually produces pleasant relaxation and mood alteration, although the drug can occasionally cause stimulation and paranoia instead.

Occasional use of cannabis seems to be mostly harmless, but as with other substances, heavy use can be harmful. For example, persistent heavy use (i.e., ongoing use of cannabis four or more times per week) may be associated with respiratory problems, addiction, cognitive decline, and psychiatric disorders (Meier et al., 2012; Curran et al., 2016). Adolescents who use cannabis appear to be at greater risk of subsequently developing schizophrenia (Marconi et al., 2016; H. J. Jones et al., 2018). However, it remains to be determined whether the cannabis use causes the illness, or conversely whether adolescents who are already experiencing symptoms of mental illness may be more drawn to cannabis use (J. Bourque et al., 2017).

As with opiates and benzodiazepines, researchers found that the brain contains specific **cannabinoid receptors** that mediate the effects of compounds like THC. Cannabinoid receptors are found in the substantia nigra, the hippocampus, the cerebellar cortex, and the cerebral cortex (**FIGURE 3.10B**) (Devane et al., 1988). Later research revealed that the brain makes several THC-like endogenous ligands for these receptors. The most studied of these **endocannabinoids** is **anandamide** (from the Sanskrit *ananda*, "bliss") (Devane et al., 1992), which produces some of the most familiar physiological and psychological effects of cannabis use, such as mood improvement, pain relief, lowered blood pressure, relief from nausea, improvements in the eye disease glaucoma, and so on. Cannabinoids are thus targets of an intense research effort aimed at developing drugs with some of the specific beneficial effects of cannabis.

The documented use of cannabis for recreational and medicinal purposes spans over 6,000 years, but for most of the twentieth century it was subject to widespread legal prohibition. More recently, however, the sale and use of cannabis products is being legalized increasingly in various U.S. states, nationwide in Canada, and to varying extents in other countries, and possession of cannabis for recreational or medical purposes has been "decriminalized" (i.e., tolerated while technically illegal) in many additional jurisdictions. It seems likely that the relaxation of cannabis laws will continue, so a fuller understanding of both the beneficial and adverse effects of cannabis, and potential for cannabis addiction, is a high priority for researchers (Zehra et al., 2018; Freeman et al., 2019).

Stimulants increase neural activity

Proper functioning of the nervous system involves a fine balance between excitatory and inhibitory influences. A **stimulant** is a drug that tips the balance toward the excitatory side, with an overall alerting, activating effect. People use many different naturally occurring and synthetic stimulants; familiar examples include nicotine, caffeine, amphetamine, and cocaine. Some stimulants act directly by increasing excitatory

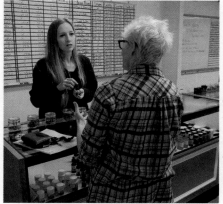

Relaxation   Cannabis laws are being relaxed in many jurisdictions. Legal access through licensed shops, like this one in California, acknowledges existing widespread use of cannabis for recreational and medicinal purposes and is expected to reduce criminal activity, but health risks remain for adolescents and heavy users.

cannabis   Also known as *marijuana*, although this name is considered pejorative. A psychoactive plant containing numerous active compounds in varying proportions.

delta-9-tetrahydrocannabinol (THC)   The major active ingredient in cannabis.

cannabidiol (CBD)   One of the two major types of active compounds found in cannabis. The other is THC.

cannabinoid receptor   A receptor that responds to endogenous and/or exogenous cannabinoids.

endocannabinoid   An endogenous ligand of cannabinoid receptors, thus an analog of cannabis that is produced by the brain.

anandamide   An endogenous substance that binds the cannabinoid receptor molecule.

stimulant   A drug that enhances the excitability of neurons.

synaptic potentials. Others act by blocking normal inhibitory processes: we've already seen that caffeine acts as a stimulant by blocking presynaptic adenosine receptors that monitor and inhibit transmitter release. Interestingly, people with attention deficit hyperactivity disorder (ADHD) often find that stimulants like methylphenidate (Ritalin) help them to focus, possibly because of changes in synaptic activity in the frontal lobes (Faraone, 2018). The stimulants thus form a large class of drugs that are exceptionally diverse in their behavioral effects, neurobiological modes of action, and potential for both benefit and harm.

NICOTINE   Tobacco is native to the Americas, where European explorers first encountered smoking; these explorers brought tobacco back to Europe with them. Tobacco use became much more widespread following technological innovations that made it easier to smoke, in the form of cigarettes (W. Bennett, 1983). Delivered to the large surface of the lungs, the **nicotine** from conventional or e-cigarettes enters the blood and brain much more rapidly than does nicotine from other tobacco products. Nicotine acts as a stimulant, increasing heart rate, blood pressure, digestive action, and alertness. In the short run, these effects make tobacco use pleasurable. But these alterations of body function, quite apart from the effects of tobacco tar on the lungs, make prolonged exposure to nicotine unhealthful. Smoking and nicotine exposure during development—even as early as in the womb, via the mother—can have a lasting impact on physiology and cognitive development, due to changes in the pubertal development of cholinergic and glutamatergic systems, and possible long-lasting modifications of neural function (Yuan et al., 2015; Rauschert et al., 2019).

The *nicotinic* ACh receptors didn't get their name by coincidence; it is through these receptors that the nicotine from tobacco exerts most of its effects in the body. Nicotinic receptors drive the contraction of skeletal muscles, and the activation of various visceral organs, but they are also found in high concentrations in the brain, including the cortex. This is one way in which nicotine enhances some aspects of cognitive performance. Nicotine also acts directly on nicotinic receptors within the ventral tegmental area to exert its rewarding/addicting effects (Durand-de Cuttoli et al., 2018). (We will discuss the ventral tegmental area in more detail when we discuss positive reward models later in this chapter.)

COCAINE   For hundreds of years, people in Bolivia, Colombia, and Peru have used the leaves of the coca shrub—either chewed or brewed as a tea—to increase endurance, alleviate hunger, and promote a sense of well-being. The use of coca leaves in this manner does not seem to cause problems. But processing and purifying an extract from this plant produces a much more potent and dangerous drug: **cocaine**.

First isolated in 1859, cocaine was added to beverages (such as Coca-Cola) and tonics for its stimulant qualities, and subsequently it was used as a local anesthetic (it is in the same chemical family as procaine) and as an antidepressant. But people soon discovered that the rapid hit resulting from snorting cocaine (see Table 3.3) has a stimulant effect that is powerful and pleasurable. Cocaine exerts its stimulant effects by blocking the reuptake of monoamine transmitters—especially dopamine and norepinephrine. This action causes transmitters to accumulate in synapses throughout much of the brain (**FIGURE 3.10C**), therefore boosting their effects.

Crack, a smokable form of cocaine that appeared in the mid-1980s, enters the blood and the brain even more rapidly and thus is even more addictive than cocaine powder. However it is consumed, cocaine is highly addictive. Furthermore, heavy cocaine use raises the risk of serious side effects like stroke, psychosis, loss of gray matter in the frontal lobes, and severe mood disturbances (Franklin et al., 2002; Crunelle et al., 2014). Cocaine causes changes in the structure and function of many regions of the brain (Hanlon et al., 2013), which contribute to high rates of relapse in people attempting to quit cocaine use. People who use cocaine along with other substances run the

nicotine   A compound found in plants, including tobacco, that acts as an agonist on a large class of cholinergic receptors.

cocaine   A drug of abuse, derived from the coca plant, that acts by enhancing catecholamine neurotransmission.

added risk of dual dependence, in which the interaction of two (or more) drugs produces another addictive state. For example, cocaine metabolized in the presence of ethanol (alcohol) yields an active metabolite called *cocaethylene*, to which the user may develop an additional addiction (Y. Liu et al., 2018).

AMPHETAMINE   The synthetic stimulant **amphetamine** ("speed") and its more potent relatives, like methamphetamine ("meth"), have a mode of action that superficially resembles that of cocaine, inducing an accumulation of the synaptic transmitters norepinephrine and dopamine. However, the mechanics of amphetamine's actions, involving two steps, are quite different from those of cocaine. First, amphetamine acts within axon terminals to cause a larger-than-normal release of neurotransmitter when the synapse is activated. Second, amphetamine then interferes with the clearance of the released transmitter by blocking its reuptake and metabolic breakdown. The result is that the affected synapses become unnaturally potent, having strong effects on behavior.

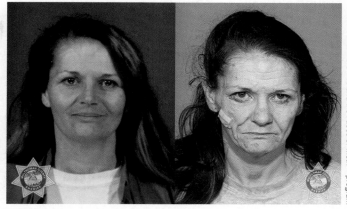

Faces of Meth   These before and after photos, taken just 2½ years apart, testify to the heavy toll taken by chronic methamphetamine abuse. Meth causes multiple severe problems such as motor disorders, cognitive impairment, psychosis, rapid changes in appearance due to accelerated tooth decay ("meth mouth"), skin pathology, and excessive weight loss.

Over the short term, amphetamine causes increased vigor and stamina, wakefulness, decreased appetite, and feelings of euphoria. For these reasons, amphetamine has historically been used in military applications and other settings where intense sustained effort is required. However, the quality of the work being performed may suffer, and the costs of amphetamine use soon outweigh the benefits. Addiction and tolerance to amphetamine and methamphetamine develop rapidly, requiring ever-larger doses that lead to sleeplessness, severe weight loss, and general deterioration of mental and physical condition.

Prolonged use of amphetamine or methamphetamine may lead to symptoms that resemble those of schizophrenia: compulsive, agitated behavior and irrational suspiciousness. Users may neglect their diet and basic hygiene, aging rapidly. Users also experience a variety of peripheral effects, like high blood pressure, tremor, dizziness, sweating, rapid breathing, and nausea. And worst of all, people who chronically abuse meth often display symptoms of brain damage long after they quit using the drug (Moratalla et al., 2017; Wu et al., 2018). As we'll discuss a little later in the chapter, increased activation of the mesolimbocortical dopaminergic reward system of the brain appears to be crucial for the rewarding aspects of drug use.

Amphetamine-like stimulants called *cathinones* are released when the African shrub **khat** (or *qat*, pronounced "cot") is chewed. Many types of synthetic cathinones—known collectively as "bath salts"—have been developed and marketed in recent years (Baumann et al., 2018). These new designer drugs, especially *mephedrone* ("plant food" or "meow meow"), have shown rapid growth in popularity despite the potential for damaging effects on the brain, muscular system, and kidneys (Zawilska, 2014; C. M. White et al., 2016).

Alcohol acts as both a stimulant and a depressant

The most widely consumed psychoactive drug, alcohol, is easily produced by the fermentation of fruit or grains. Taken in moderation (perhaps one or two drinks per day at most), alcohol is probably harmless or maybe even beneficial to the health of adults (e.g., Katsiki et al., 2014; Scarmeas et al., 2018). *Heavy* alcohol consumption is very damaging and linked to a multitude of serious diseases (O'Keefe et al., 2014; Bell et al., 2017).

Alcohol has a biphasic effect on the nervous system: at first it acts as a stimulant, and then it has a more prolonged depressant phase. (Remember, the word *depressant* relates to a depression or inhibition of neural activity, not an effect on mood.) This complex action is thought to be the result of alcohol's effects on several different

amphetamine   A molecule that resembles the structure of the catecholamine transmitters and enhances their activity.

khat   Also spelled *qat*. An African shrub that, when chewed, acts as a stimulant.

FIGURE 3.11 Abnormal Brain Development in Fetal Alcohol Spectrum Disorder

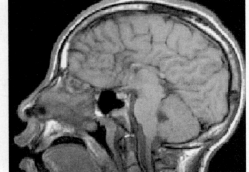

(A) Healthy infant   Corpus callosum   (B) Infant with fetal alcohol spectrum disorder

Both images courtesy of E. Riley

Compared to MRI images of a healthy infant's brain…

…the MRI of an infant affected by fetal alcohol spectrum disorder—caused by heavy consumption of alcohol by the mother during pregnancy—shows extensive abnormality, including reduced gray matter, complete absence of the corpus callosum, abnormal organization of the brain, and characteristic deformities of the head and face.

neurotransmitter systems, such as glutamate and GABA (Roberto and Varodavan, 2017). Like the anxiety-reducing benzodiazepines we discussed earlier, alcohol inhibits neural excitability in multiple brain regions via an action on GABA receptors, resulting in the social disinhibition, poor motor control, and sensory disturbances that we call *drunkenness* (Harrison et al., 2017). Alcohol additionally activates dopamine-mediated reward systems of the brain, accounting for some of the pleasurable aspects of drinking.

Chronic abuse of alcohol damages or destroys nerve cells in many regions of the brain. Heavy drinking by expectant mothers can cause grievous permanent damage to the developing fetus, termed **fetal alcohol spectrum disorder** (**FASD**), which in the most severe cases is characterized by facial deformities and stunted brain growth, sometimes including the absence of the corpus callosum that normally connects the two hemispheres of the brain (**FIGURE 3.11**). Furthermore, although it was previously thought that low levels of alcohol consumption were safe during pregnancy, as few as one or two drinks per week may be associated with lower fetal weight and preterm birth (Mamluk et al., 2017), changes in craniofacial development (Muggli et al., 2017), and later behavioral problems (Murray et al., 2016). Such findings, combined with a paucity of information on the impact of light drinking on other aspects of fetal health, such as cognitive function, and clear evidence of fetal risks from alcohol in studies with lab animals (Valenzuela et al., 2012), encourage an abundance of caution: the Centers for Disease Control and Prevention (CDC) currently advises that there is no known safe level of alcohol use in pregnancy (CDC, 2016). In adults, chronic alcohol abuse is associated with pathological changes in white matter pathways, widespread cortical atrophy, and damage of the diencephalon and cerebellum (de la Monte and Kril, 2014), resulting in a host of behavioral symptoms including cognitive decline, memory impairment, and movement disorders. Happily, some of the anatomical changes associated with chronic alcoholism may be reversible with abstinence. In humans recovering from alcoholism, MRI studies show increased volumes of gray matter throughout multiple cortical regions, along with improvements in subcortical sites like the thalamus, amygdala, and cerebellum, within days of giving up alcohol (Cardenas et al., 2007) (**FIGURE 3.12**), along with at least partial reversal of alcohol-induced atrophy of white matter pathways (Zahr and Pfefferbaum, 2017). Even in the absence of clear-cut alcoholism, periodic binge drinking, which is defined as four (female) or five (male) or more drinks on a single occasion by the Substance Abuse and Mental Health Services Administration (SAMHSA, 2018) and is a

fetal alcohol spectrum disorder (FASD) A family of developmental disorders that vary in severity, resulting from fetal exposure to alcohol consumed by the mother. Severe cases, associated with high levels of alcohol abuse by the mother, include characteristic intellectual disability and facial abnormalities.

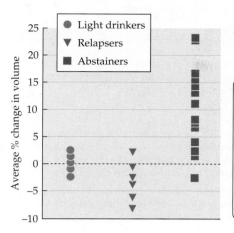

FIGURE 3.12 Immediate Changes in Brain Volume in Recovering Alcoholics (After V. A. Cardenas et al. 2007. *NeuroImage* 34: 879–887.)

After just one week of abstinence, the average volume of several brain regions was noticeably increased in a group of alcoholics, compared with alcoholic and nonalcoholic control groups. It's not yet clear how much cognitive improvement accompanies these changes, but the results clearly illustrate the potential benefits of reduced intake in heavy drinkers.

common mode of alcohol use in young people, can harm the brains and alter the behavior of adolescents in ways that last into adulthood (Crews et al., 2016).

Hallucinogens alter sensory perceptions

Humans have long prized **hallucinogens** (also called *psychedelics* or *entheogens*), substances that produce powerful sensory alterations, often finding the resultant experiences to have deep spiritual or psychological meaning. The effects of lysergic acid diethylamide (LSD, or *acid*) and related substances like mescaline (from the peyote cactus) and muscarine and psilocybin (both from mushrooms) are predominantly visual, producing bizarre and mysterious sensory experiences, but the term *hallucinogen* is really a misnomer: a hallucination is a novel perception that takes place in the absence of sensory stimulation (hearing voices, or seeing something that isn't there), but drugs in this category mostly alter or distort *existing* perceptions (mainly visual in nature). Users may see fantastic images (**FIGURE 3.13**), often with intense colors, but often they are aware that these strangely altered perceptions are not real events.

Hallucinogenic agents are diverse in their neural actions. Whereas muscarine affects the ACh system, mescaline acts via noradrenergic and serotonergic systems.

hallucinogen Also called *psychedelics* or *entheogens*. A drug that alters sensory perception and produces peculiar experiences.

These images are portraits produced by a professional artist just after taking LSD (leftmost drawing) and then at three successive time points as the drug took effect. The model for all four drawings is the same man (the researcher, in fact).

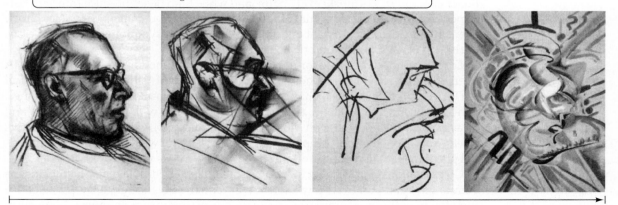

20 minutes   Time   3 hours

FIGURE 3.13 Perceptual Alterations with LSD

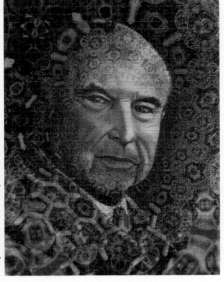

Art by Wes Black, courtesy of www.blotterart.com

The Father of LSD   Albert Hofmann discovered LSD by accidentally taking some in 1943, and he devoted the rest of his career to studying it. A prohibited drug in most jurisdictions, LSD is distributed on colorful blotter paper. This example, picturing Hofmann and the LSD molecule, is made up of 1,036 individual doses, or "hits."

TABLE 3.4 Possible Clinical Applications for Hallucinogens

Drug name and date of discovery	Action in brain
Psilocybin/psilocin (*Psilocybe* mushroom) (according to archaeological evidence, used in prehistory)	Is a partial agonist of 5-HT receptors, especially 5-HT$_{2A}$ receptors that occur in high density in visual cortex. Modifies activity of frontal and occipital cortex.
Lysergic acid diethylamide (LSD) (1938)	Activates many subtypes of monoamine receptors, especially DA and 5-HT, resulting in heightened activity in many cortical regions, especially frontal, cingulate, and occipital cortex.
Ketamine (1962)	Has widespread effects in the brain, especially blockade of NMDA receptors, and stimulates opioid and ACh receptors.
3,4-Methylenedioxymeth-amphetamine (MDMA) (1912/1970s)	Stimulates release of monoamine transmitters and the prosocial hormone oxytocin.

The herb *Salvia divinorum* is unusual among hallucinogens because it acts on the opioid kappa receptor. But research with LSD and related drugs suggests that perhaps the most important shared neural action of hallucinogens is the stimulation of serotonin receptors. Discovered by Albert Hofmann in the 1940s, **LSD** (lysergic acid diethylamide, or more simply *acid*) structurally resembles serotonin. Even in tiny doses, LSD strongly activates serotonin 5-HT$_{2A}$ receptors that are found in especially heavy concentrations in the visual cortex. Other hallucinogens, such as mescaline and psilocybin, share this action. Research with psilocybin has also demonstrated disinhibition of emotion-processing regions in the limbic system (Carhart-Harris et al., 2012), perhaps accounting for some of the drug's emotional, mystical qualities. In addition to their impressive perceptual effects, LSD, psilocybin, and other hallucinogens can produce mood changes, introspective states, and feelings of creativity that have led to renewed interest in the possibility of using hallucinogens to treat specific psychiatric disorders, including depression, anxiety, and obsessive-compulsive disorder (Kyzar et al., 2017).

Ketamine (known as *Special K*) is already in widespread use in medical settings as a component of anesthesia but also has pronounced hallucinogenic properties. Acting principally (but not exclusively) to block NMDA receptors, ketamine increases activity in the prefrontal cortex and hippocampus and produces feelings of depersonalization and detachment from reality. Ketamine increases activity in the prefrontal cortex (Breier et al., 1997; Zorumski et al., 2016), and while high doses produce transient hallucinogenic effects and occasional psychotic symptoms in volunteers, low doses have a potent and rapid antidepressant effect that may help ease symptoms in resistant cases (Carlson et al., 2013; Williams and Schatzberg, 2016).

Ecstasy is the street name for the hallucinogenic amphetamine derivative **MDMA** (3,4-methylenedioxymethamphetamine). Like LSD, MDMA stimulates visual cortical 5-HT$_{2A}$ receptors, but it also changes the levels of dopamine and certain hormones, such as prolactin and oxytocin, that have been associated with prosocial feelings and behaviors. Exactly how these physiological actions of MDMA account for its subjective effects—positive emotions, empathy, euphoria, a sense of well-being, and colorful visual phenomena—remains uncertain.

Complications due to hallucinogen use are quite varied. The major hallucinogens seem to have comparatively low addiction potential. LSD has relatively few negative side effects (although some users report long-lasting visual changes). Long-term MDMA use may cause problems with mood and cognitive performance (Sumnall and Cole, 2005; Parrott, 2013) and long-lasting changes in patterns of brain activation,

LSD   Also called *acid*. Lysergic acid diethylamide, a hallucinogenic drug.

MDMA   Also called *Ecstasy* or *Molly*. 3,4-Methylenedioxymethamphetamine, a drug of abuse.

Recreational use	Possible clinical application
Users of "shrooms" often report spiritual experiences and feelings of transcendence, along with intense visual experiences and alterations in the perception of time. The exact effects are strongly influenced by the expectations and surroundings of the user.	Recent studies suggest that psilocybin—administered in controlled settings—can offer substantial and enduring improvements in the symptoms of obsessive-compulsive disorder (OCD), cluster headache (a type of migraine), treatment-resistant depression, and debilitating anxiety and anguish (as in a sample of terminal cancer patients) (Grob et al., 2011; Schindler et al., 2015; Carhart-Harris et al., 2016).
"Acid" produces pronounced perceptual changes that resemble hallucinations. Intense colors in geometric patterns, novel visual objects, and an altered sense of time are common.	LSD may be an effective treatment for alcoholism and other addictions and may also be an effective treatment for some types of debilitating anxiety (Gasser et al., 2014; Bogenschutz and Johnson, 2016).
"Special K" creates a detached, trancelike state, in keeping with its routine medical use as an anesthetic. It may also produce hallucinogenic perceptual alterations.	Recent experiments have revealed a potent antidepressant effect of ketamine at lower doses, even in cases that resist other types of treatments (Williams and Schatzberg, 2016).
Users of "Ecstasy" experience intense visual phenomena, empathy, strongly prosocial feelings, and euphoria.	MDMA treatment may reduce symptoms of post-traumatic stress disorder (PTSD), especially in combination with conventional psychotherapy, but concerns remain regarding drug safety (Parrott, 2014; Sessa, 2017).

even at low doses (de Win et al., 2008). However, short-term MDMA treatment is also being investigated as a possible treatment for persistent post-traumatic stress disorder (Feduccia et al., 2019). The neural actions, recreational properties, and possible psychiatric uses of some of the major hallucinogens are summarized in **TABLE 3.4**.

HOW'S IT GOING ?

1. Compare and contrast the three major categories of presynaptic effects of psychoactive drugs. Give examples of each kind of action. (*Hint*: The words *production*, *release*, and *clearance* will be important for your discussion.)

2. Compare and contrast the main postsynaptic actions of psychotropic drugs, with examples. Be sure to distinguish between actions at receptors and actions within the postsynaptic neuron.

3. At least four general categories of psychoactive drugs are used to relieve disorders. Describe these categories, and give some examples of each class of drugs. Be sure to discuss the modes of action of the drugs you cite.

4. Identify and discuss the major categories of drugs that people use to alter their consciousness. In what ways are the major categories similar, and in what ways do they differ? What are some of the threats to health that these compounds present?

5. Discuss the renewed scientific interest in the therapeutic use of hallucinogens. How might they help in psychiatric disorders?

3.7 Substance Abuse and Addiction Are Global Social Problems

THE ROAD AHEAD

In the final section of the chapter we turn to the urgent public health problem posed by substance abuse. By the end of this section, you should be able to:

3.7.1 Provide a formal definition of substance abuse, and distinguish between mild, moderate, and severe forms.

3.7.2 Summarize the major theoretical models of substance abuse.

3.7.3 Describe some individual differences that affect susceptibility to addiction.

3.7.4 Review leading categories of treatments for addiction, briefly explaining the logic of each.

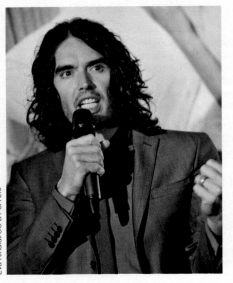

Eva Rinaldi/CC BY-SA 2.0

Feeding the Monkey Addiction exerts a powerful grip on the lives of people from all walks of life, leading them to go to sometimes extreme lengths to obtain larger and more frequent doses. Author and entertainer Russell Brand has documented his personal descent into addiction, and road to recovery, in several books and documentaries.

The habitual use of drugs to alter consciousness can be costly to the user and to society. Governments attempt to minimize these costs by controlling (or preventing) the production and distribution of designated drugs, but the division of drugs into licit and illicit categories is largely a matter of historical accident. Some classes of drugs—the opiates, for example—span both categories, being both useful medicines and harmful drugs of abuse. And some substances, like tobacco, are legal only because they have been cultivated for centuries and are backed by powerful economic interests. In terms of illness, death, lost productivity, and sheer human misery, some of the legal drugs may be the worst offenders. Just one example reveals the extent of the problem: in the United States each year, more men and women die of smoking-related lung cancer than of colon, breast, and prostate cancers *combined*. In addition to the personal impact of so much illness and early death, there are dire social costs: huge expenses for medical and social services; millions of hours lost in the workplace; elevated rates of crime associated with illicit drugs; and scores of children who are damaged by their parents' substance abuse behavior, in the uterine environment as well as in the childhood home. Males are more likely than females to engage in substance abuse, but it is unclear whether this sex difference is related to biological differences between the sexes or to differences in social influences on males versus females.

For medical purposes, addiction is defined as "substance use disorder" (SUD) in the *Diagnostic and Statistical Manual of Mental Disorders*, fifth edition (*DSM-5*; American Psychiatric Association, 2013). SUD can take multiple forms, and it varies in severity from mild to severe. The *DSM-5* criteria for a diagnosis of alcohol use disorder appear in **TABLE 3.5**; about 7% of adults in the USA (approximately 17 million people) currently meet these criteria (SAMSHA, 2018). Identical criteria are used for diagnosis of all other types of substance use disorders, including opioids like heroin,

---

TABLE 3.5 *DSM-5* **Diagnostic Criteria for Alcohol Use Disorder**

A problematic pattern of alcohol use leading to clinically significant impairment or distress, as manifested by at least two of the following, occurring within a 12-month period:

1. Alcohol is often taken in larger amounts or over a longer period than was intended.

2. There is a persistent desire or unsuccessful efforts to cut down or control alcohol use.

3. A great deal of time is spent in activities necessary to obtain alcohol, use alcohol, or recover from its effects.

4. Craving, or a strong desire or urge to use alcohol.

5. Recurrent alcohol use resulting in a failure to fulfill major role obligations at work, school, or home.

6. Continued alcohol use despite having persistent or recurrent social or interpersonal problems caused or exacerbated by the effects of alcohol.

7. Important social, occupational, or recreational activities are given up or reduced because of alcohol use.

8. Recurrent alcohol use in situations in which it is physically hazardous.

9. Alcohol use is continued despite knowledge of having a persistent or recurrent physical or psychological problem that is likely to have been caused or exacerbated by alcohol.

10. Tolerance, as defined by either of the following:
    a. A need for markedly increased amounts of alcohol to achieve intoxication or desired effect.
    b. A markedly diminished effect with continued use of the same amount of alcohol.

11. Withdrawal, as manifested by either of the following:
    a. The characteristic withdrawal syndrome for alcohol [listed elsewhere in *DSM-5* as an alcohol-induced disorder].
    b. Alcohol (or a closely related substance, such as a benzodiazepine) is taken to relieve or avoid withdrawal symptoms.

stimulants like cocaine and meth, tobacco, cannabis, hallucinogens, and so on. Almost everyone will meet some of the criteria some of the time; a diagnosis of a specific substance use disorder requires more-sustained problems and a pattern of use that interferes with normal daily functioning. A mild substance use disorder is diagnosed if two or three of the listed criteria are met. People meeting four or five criteria are classified as having moderate substance use disorder, and severe substance use disorder is diagnosed in cases where six or more of the criteria are met. In the discussion that follows, we will look at some of the most prevalent perspectives on addiction: what it is, where it comes from, how it can be treated. Some of these models stem from social forces; others are more deeply rooted in scientific observations and theories. But for any model of drug abuse, the challenge is to come up with a single account that can explain the addicting power of substances as seemingly dissimilar as cocaine (a stimulant), heroin (an analgesic and euphoriant), and alcohol (largely a sedative). We will focus primarily on addiction to cocaine, the opiate drugs (such as morphine and heroin), nicotine, and alcohol because these substances have been studied the most thoroughly. According to the 2016 National Survey on Drug Use and Health, some 20.1 million people in the United States alone have substance-related disorders (SAMHSA, 2017). Worldwide, the number is probably in the hundreds of millions. Sex differences are evident in multiple aspects of drug abuse and dependence (Becker et al., 2017), but although historically men have been more likely than women to engage in substance abuse, in young people rates are now roughly equivalent for the sexes (SAMHSA, 2017).

Competing models of substance abuse have been proposed

Any comprehensive model of substance abuse has to answer several difficult questions: What social and environmental factors cause someone to start abusing a substance? What factors cause the person to continue abusing? What physiological mechanisms make a substance rewarding? What is addiction, physiologically and behaviorally, and why is it so hard to quit? Four major models attempt to answer at least some of these questions:

1. The *moral model* blames substance abuse on weakness of character and a lack of self-control. Proponents of this view may apply exhortation, peer pressure, and/or religious intervention in an attempt to curb abusive practices. These approaches have historically had limited success, probably because they aren't founded in a scientific framework that addresses the neurobiological roots of addiction. The temperance movement that commenced in the early 1800s did seem to reduce alcohol consumption for a time, but despite good intentions, high hopes, and multibillion-dollar budgets, there remains little evidence that modern morality-based campaigns—Project D.A.R.E., for example—have a substantial effect on rates of drug abuse (S. L. West and O'Neil, 2004; Vincus et al., 2010).

2. The *disease model* takes the view that the person who abuses drugs requires medical treatment rather than moral exhortation or punishment. The problem is that substance abuse is not like any other disease we know about. We generally reserve the term *disease* for cases involving a physical abnormality, and no such condition has been found in the case of drug addiction (although some people are genetically more susceptible to addiction than others). Furthermore, the disease model offers no clue about how addiction initially arises. Nevertheless, this model continues to appeal to many, and much research is focused on looking for pathological states that create addiction after initial exposure to a drug.

3. The *physical dependence model* argues that people keep taking drugs in order to avoid unpleasant **withdrawal symptoms**. The specific withdrawal symptoms depend on the drug, but they are often the opposite of the effects produced by the drug itself. For example, withdrawal from morphine causes irritability, a

withdrawal symptom An uncomfortable symptom that arises when a person stops taking a drug that they have used frequently, especially at high doses.

A drug's rewarding properties and addictive potential are reflected in the number of lever presses performed to receive a dose. Lab animals will press the lever thousands of times to receive a single small dose of highly addictive compounds like cocaine and methamphetamine.

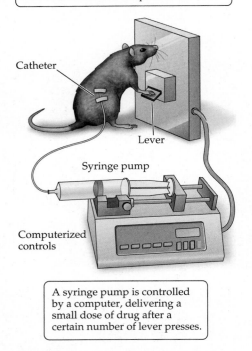

A syringe pump is controlled by a computer, delivering a small dose of drug after a certain number of lever presses.

FIGURE 3.14 Experimental Setup for Drug Self-Administration

dysphoria Unpleasant feelings; the opposite of euphoria.

nucleus accumbens A region of the forebrain that receives dopaminergic innervation from the ventral tegmental area, often associated with reward and pleasurable sensations.

insula A region of cortex lying below the surface, within the lateral sulcus, of the frontal, temporal, and parietal lobes.

racing heart, and waves of goose bumps (that's where the term *cold turkey* comes from—the skin looks like the skin of a plucked turkey). And of course, the opposite of the euphoria caused by many drugs is **dysphoria**: strongly negative feelings that can be rapidly relieved by administration of the withdrawn drug. So the model does a good job of explaining why addicts will go to great lengths to obtain the drug they are addicted to, but it has an important shortcoming: the model is mute on how the addiction becomes established in the first place. Why do some people, but not all, start to abuse a drug before physical dependence (tolerance) has developed? And how is it that some people can become addicted to some drugs even in the absence of clear physical withdrawal symptoms? A striking example is cocaine, which is powerfully addictive and produces intense drug craving, yet cocaine withdrawal is not accompanied by the shaking and vomiting and other physical symptoms that are seen during withdrawal from equally addictive substances like heroin.

4. The *positive reward model* proposes that people get started with drug abuse, and become addicted, because the abused drug provides powerful reinforcement. Using an apparatus that allows animals to administer drugs to themselves (**FIGURE 3.14**), researchers have collected plenty of evidence for this view. Laboratory animals will quickly learn to press a lever repeatedly in order to receive a small dose of an addictive drug like cocaine or morphine (T. Thompson and Schuster, 1964; McKim, 1991). We can infer that the more lever presses animals will perform for a single dose, or the smaller the dose that will support the lever-pressing behavior, the more rewarding and addictive the drug must be. For example, it turns out that animals will self-administer doses of morphine that are so low that no signs of physical dependence ever develop (Schuster, 1970). Animals will also furiously press a lever to self-administer tiny doses of cocaine and other stimulants (Pickens and Thompson, 1968; Koob, 1995; Tanda et al., 2000). In fact, cocaine supports some of the highest rates of lever pressing ever recorded.

Experiments using drug self-administration suggest that, by itself, the physical dependence model is inadequate to explain drug addiction, although physical dependence and tolerance may contribute to drug hunger. The more comprehensive view of drug self-administration interprets it as a behavior controlled by a powerful pattern of positive and negative rewards (a variant of operant conditioning theory; see Chapter 13), without the need to implicate a disease process.

Many—but not all—addictive drugs cause the release of dopamine in the **nucleus accumbens**, just as occurs with more conventional rewards, such as food, sex, and gambling (Nutt et al., 2015; Volkow et al., 2017). As we mentioned previously, dopamine released from axons originating in the ventral tegmental area (VTA), part of the mesolimbocortical dopaminergic pathway illustrated in Figure 3.4, has been widely implicated in the perception of reward (**FIGURE 3.15**). If the dopaminergic pathway from the VTA to the nucleus accumbens serves as a reward system for a wide variety of experiences, then the addictive power of drugs may come from their extra strong stimulation of this pathway. When the drug activates this system, providing an abnormally powerful reward, the user learns to associate the drug-taking behavior with that pleasure and begins seeking out drugs more and more until life's other pleasures fade into the background. If natural activities like conversation, food, and even sex no longer provide appreciable reward, addicts may seek drugs as the only source of pleasure available to them.

Tucked deep within the folds of the frontal cortex, the **insula** (Latin for "island"; **FIGURE 3.16**) likewise appears to play an important role in addiction, craving, and pleasure. For example, people with damage to the left insula reportedly lose their urge to smoke tobacco and are able to effortlessly quit smoking (Naqvi et al., 2007), and addiction to numerous substances is associated with abnormalities of the insula (Mackey et al., 2018). It is thought that through its rich interconnections with prefrontal and sensory cortex and the VTA, the insula interacts with several large brain networks to mediate multiple features of addiction (Droutman et al., 2015; Ibrahim et al., 2019). Interestingly, abnormality of the insula is also evident in people whose compulsive use of social media resembles addiction (Turel et al., 2018).

Not everyone who uses an addictive drug becomes addicted, of course. For example, most hospitalized patients treated with opiates for pain relief do not go on to abuse opiates after their pain has resolved. However, modern prescription painkillers are highly effective at activating the dopamine reward system, so the use of these drugs outside of medical contexts carries a high risk of addiction. The individual and environmental factors that account for differential susceptibility are the subject of active investigation (Karch, 2006). Some of the major risk factors include biological factors (being male, heritable tendencies to addiction), poor family life, personality factors (poor emotional control), and environmental factors (living in a neighborhood with high rates of addiction). Simply returning to a neighborhood where drugs were previously used can trigger drug craving in an addict (Ciccocioppo et al., 2004); this *cue-induced drug use* is thought to rely on long-lasting associations that involve remodeling of the brain's reward circuitry (M. E. Wolf, 2016; J. Wang et al., 2018). Let's conclude the chapter considering strategies to treat addiction in Signs and Symptoms, next.

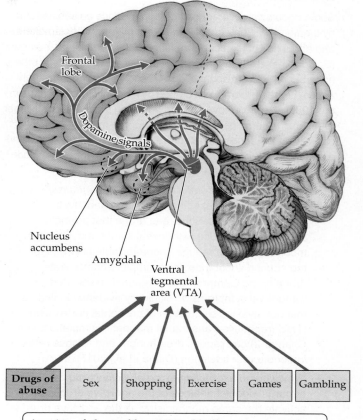

FIGURE 3.15 A Neural Pathway Implicated in Drug Abuse (After H. O. Pettit and J. B. Justice Jr. 1991. *Brain Res.* 539: 93.)

Frontal lobe

Dopamine signals

Nucleus accumbens

Amygdala

Ventral tegmental area (VTA)

| Drugs of abuse | Sex | Shopping | Exercise | Games | Gambling |

A variety of pleasurable activities, like the ones suggested here, probably activate the dopaminergic pathway that produces rewarding sensations. Drugs of abuse powerfully activate this system and may eclipse other sources of pleasure.

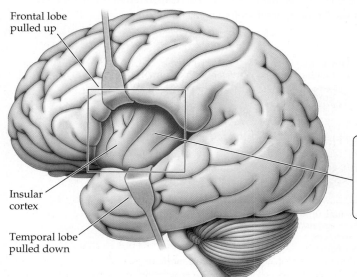

Frontal lobe pulled up

Insular cortex

Temporal lobe pulled down

Buried deep within the frontal lobe, changes in insular cortex are associated with the development of drug craving. Shrinkage of the left insula is observed in individuals addicted to various substances.

FIGURE 3.16 The Insula and Addiction

Medical Interventions for Substance Abuse

Some people can overcome their dependence on substances by themselves. For example, the great majority of ex-smokers, and about half of ex-alcoholics, appear to have quit on their own (S. Cohen et al., 1989; Institute of Medicine, 1990). Many others have benefited from counseling and social interventions such as the 12-step program developed by Alcoholics Anonymous in the 1930s. However, overcoming addiction may require stronger measures in some cases, especially for the most powerfully addictive substances. An intensive research effort has identified a variety of medicines that can help lessen the grip of addiction through the following strategies:

- *Lessening the discomfort of withdrawal and drug craving*   Benzodiazepines and other sedatives, anti-nausea medications, and drugs that promote sleep all help reduce withdrawal symptoms. Other medications help reduce uncomfortable cravings for the abused substance; for example, acamprosate (trade name Campral) eases alcohol-associated withdrawal symptoms. Preliminary evidence indicates that noninvasive stimulation of prefrontal cortex using rTMS (repetitive transcranial magnetic stimulation; see Chapter 2) can reduce drug hunger and relapse rates in people with addiction (Diana et al., 2017).

- *Providing an alternative to the addictive drug*   Agonist or partial agonist analogs of the addictive drug weakly activate the same mechanisms as the addictive drug, to help wean the individual. For example, the opioid receptor agonist methadone reduces heroin appetite; nicotine patches work in a similar fashion to reduce cravings for cigarettes.

- *Directly blocking the actions of the addictive drug*   Specific receptor antagonists can prevent an abused drug from interacting with its receptors. For example, the opiate receptor antagonist naloxone (Narcan) blocks heroin's actions, but it also may produce harsh withdrawal symptoms.

- *Altering metabolism of the addictive drug*   Changing the breakdown of a drug can reduce or reverse its rewarding properties. Disulfiram (Antabuse) changes alcohol metabolism such that a nausea-inducing metabolite (acetaldehyde) accumulates.

- *Blocking the brain's reward circuitry*   When a person takes medicine (e.g., dopamine receptor blockers) to blunt the activity of the mesolimbocortical dopamine reward system, the addictive drugs lose their pleasurable qualities (but at the cost of a general loss of pleasurable feelings, called *anhedonia*).

- *Immunization to render the drug ineffective*   Vaccines against such drugs as cocaine, heroin, and methamphetamine have been developed and are being tested (Hicks et al., 2011; Nguyen et al., 2017). Here the strategy is to prompt the individual's immune system to produce antibodies that remove the targeted drugs from circulation before they ever reach the brain (**FIGURE 3.17**).

The economic impact of substance abuse—the costs of law enforcement, medical care, and lost productivity—exceeds $700 billion per year in the USA alone (National Institute on Drug Abuse, 2017). The social costs of abuse and addiction, furthermore, are incalculable. Unfortunately, no single approach so far appears to be uniformly effective, and rates of relapse remain high. Research breakthroughs are therefore badly needed.

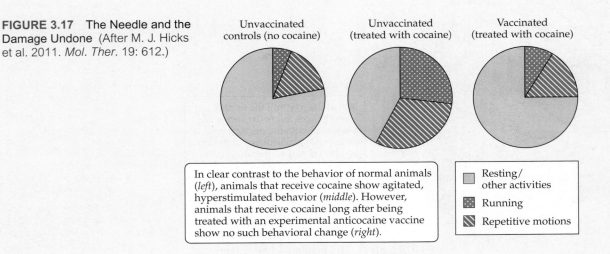

FIGURE 3.17   The Needle and the Damage Undone (After M. J. Hicks et al. 2011. *Mol. Ther.* 19: 612.)

Unvaccinated controls (no cocaine)

Unvaccinated (treated with cocaine)

Vaccinated (treated with cocaine)

In clear contrast to the behavior of normal animals (*left*), animals that receive cocaine show agitated, hyperstimulated behavior (*middle*). However, animals that receive cocaine long after being treated with an experimental anticocaine vaccine show no such behavioral change (*right*).

- Resting/ other activities
- Running
- Repetitive motions

HOW'S IT GOING ❓

1. Define substance abuse. How prevalent is drug abuse in the population?
2. Summarize the major models of drug abuse and addiction, highlighting the strengths and shortcomings of each perspective.
3. Describe an experimental setup for measuring the rewarding properties of a drug.
4. Provide a survey of the anatomical system that mediates reward. What happens when this system is activated? What are some triggers that can activate the system, and how does activity of the reward system relate to drug addiction?
5. Provide a thorough overview of medical approaches and interventions in substance abuse.

Recommended Reading

Advokat, C. D., Comaty, J. E., and Julien, R. M. (2014). *Julien's Primer of Drug Action* (13th ed.). New York, NY: Worth.

Erickson, C. K. (2018). *The Science of Addiction: From Neurobiology to Treatment* (2nd ed.). New York, NY: Norton.

Grilly, D. M., and Salamone, J. (2011). *Drugs, Brain and Behavior* (6th ed.). Boston, MA: Allyn & Bacon.

Karch, S. B., and Drummer, O. (2015). *Karch's Pathology of Drug Abuse* (5th ed.). Boca Raton, FL: CRC Press.

Meyer, J. S., and Quenzer, L. F. (2018). *Psychopharmacology: Drugs, the Brain, and Behavior* (3rd ed.). Sunderland, MA: Oxford University Press/Sinauer.

Nestler, E., Hyman, S., and Malenka, R. (2014). *Molecular Neuropharmacology* (3rd ed.). New York, NY: McGraw-Hill.

Nutt, D. (2012). *Drugs without the Hot Air.* Cambridge, UK: UIT Cambridge.

Thombs, D. L., and Osborn, C. J. (2013). *Introduction to Addictive Behaviors* (4th ed.). New York, NY: Guilford Press.

3 • VISUAL SUMMARY

You should be able to relate each summary to the adjacent illustration, including structures and processes. The online version of this **Visual Summary** includes links to figures, animations, and activities that will help you consolidate the material.

1 The function of the classical **synapse** is to communicate information from a **presynaptic** neuron to a postsynaptic cell. It does so by converting an electrical signal—the action potential—into secretion of a **neurotransmitter** that crosses to the postsynaptic cell and alters that cell's functioning. Review **Figure 3.1**, **Animation 3.2**

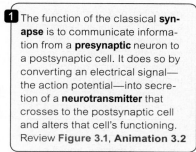

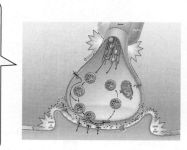

2 Neurotransmitters exert their effects via **neurotransmitter receptors**; these are also the site of action for many psychoactive drugs. Most transmitters have several different subtypes of receptors, which may be individually targeted by drugs. A given neurotransmitter may normally bind several different subtypes of receptors. Review **Figure 3.2**, **Table 3.2**

3 The major categories of neurotransmitters are **amine**, **amino acid**, **peptide**, and soluble **gas neurotransmitters**. Neurotransmitter systems form complex, overlapping patterns of projections throughout the brain. Review **Figures 3.3** and **3.4**, **Table 3.1**, **Animation 3.3**, **Activity 3.1**

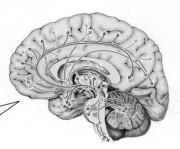

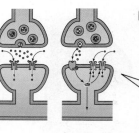

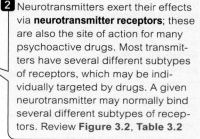

4 Drugs classified as **agonists** activate transmitter pathways, and **antagonists** block transmitter pathways. Repeated exposure to drugs may cause a compensatory **down-regulation** (decrease) or **up-regulation** (increase) in the number of receptors. Changes in receptor density are one mechanism of **drug tolerance**. Review **Figure 3.5**, **Animation 3.4**

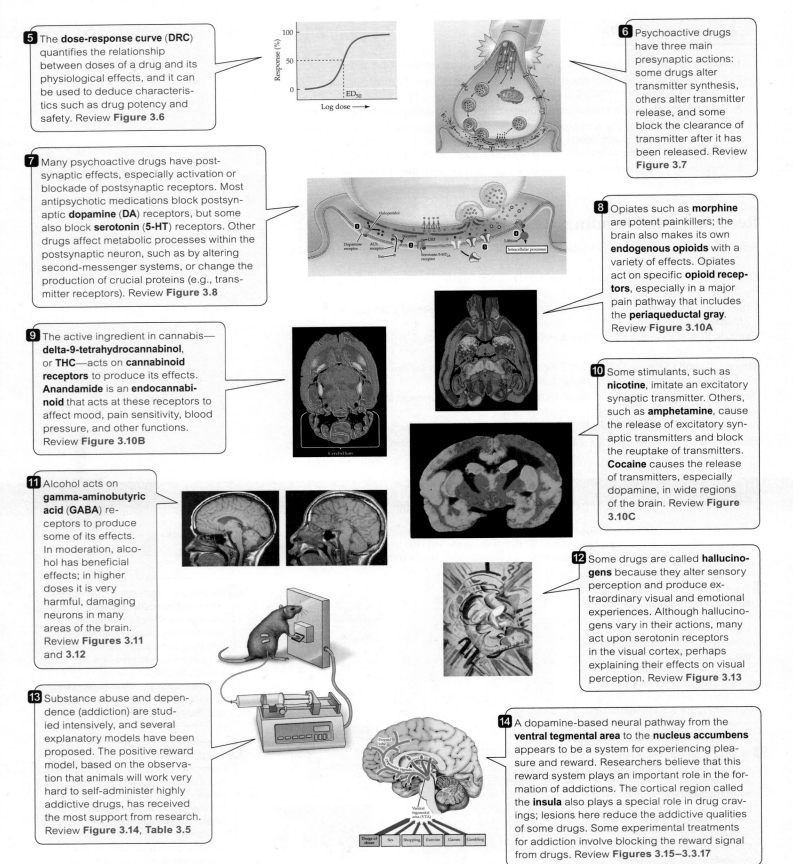

5 The **dose-response curve** (**DRC**) quantifies the relationship between doses of a drug and its physiological effects, and it can be used to deduce characteristics such as drug potency and safety. Review **Figure 3.6**

6 Psychoactive drugs have three main presynaptic actions: some drugs alter transmitter synthesis, others alter transmitter release, and some block the clearance of transmitter after it has been released. Review **Figure 3.7**

7 Many psychoactive drugs have post-synaptic effects, especially activation or blockade of postsynaptic receptors. Most antipsychotic medications block postsynaptic **dopamine** (**DA**) receptors, but some also block **serotonin** (**5-HT**) receptors. Other drugs affect metabolic processes within the postsynaptic neuron, such as by altering second-messenger systems, or change the production of crucial proteins (e.g., transmitter receptors). Review **Figure 3.8**

8 Opiates such as **morphine** are potent painkillers; the brain also makes its own **endogenous opioids** with a variety of effects. Opiates act on specific **opioid receptors**, especially in a major pain pathway that includes the **periaqueductal gray**. Review **Figure 3.10A**

9 The active ingredient in cannabis—**delta-9-tetrahydrocannabinol**, or **THC**—acts on **cannabinoid receptors** to produce its effects. **Anandamide** is an **endocannabinoid** that acts at these receptors to affect mood, pain sensitivity, blood pressure, and other functions. Review **Figure 3.10B**

10 Some stimulants, such as **nicotine**, imitate an excitatory synaptic transmitter. Others, such as **amphetamine**, cause the release of excitatory synaptic transmitters and block the reuptake of transmitters. **Cocaine** causes the release of transmitters, especially dopamine, in wide regions of the brain. Review **Figure 3.10C**

11 Alcohol acts on **gamma-aminobutyric acid** (**GABA**) receptors to produce some of its effects. In moderation, alcohol has beneficial effects; in higher doses it is very harmful, damaging neurons in many areas of the brain. Review **Figures 3.11** and **3.12**

12 Some drugs are called **hallucinogens** because they alter sensory perception and produce extraordinary visual and emotional experiences. Although hallucinogens vary in their actions, many act upon serotonin receptors in the visual cortex, perhaps explaining their effects on visual perception. Review **Figure 3.13**

13 Substance abuse and dependence (addiction) are studied intensively, and several explanatory models have been proposed. The positive reward model, based on the observation that animals will work very hard to self-administer highly addictive drugs, has received the most support from research. Review **Figure 3.14**, **Table 3.5**

14 A dopamine-based neural pathway from the **ventral tegmental area** to the **nucleus accumbens** appears to be a system for experiencing pleasure and reward. Researchers believe that this reward system plays an important role in the formation of addictions. The cortical region called the **insula** also plays a special role in drug cravings; lesions here reduce the addictive qualities of some drugs. Some experimental treatments for addiction involve blocking the reward signal from drugs. Review **Figures 3.15–3.3.17**

The Mind's Machine digital resources include additional videos, flashcards, and other study tools.

4 Development of the Brain

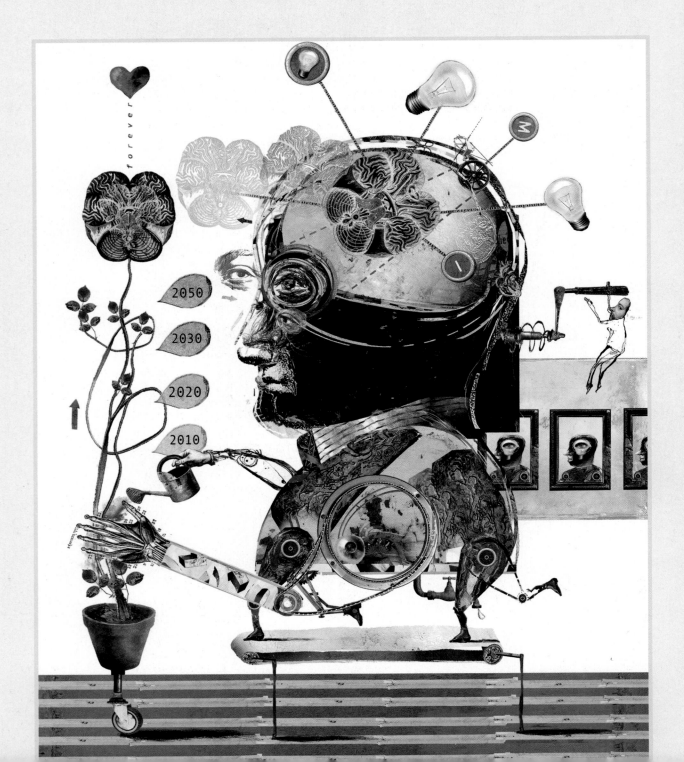

Overcoming Blindness

As a 3-year-old, Michael May was injured by a chemical explosion that destroyed his left eye and damaged the surface of his right eye so badly that he was blind. He could tell whether it was day or night, but otherwise he couldn't see anything. An early attempt to restore his sight with corneal transplants failed, but Michael seemed undaunted. He learned to play Ping-Pong using his hearing alone (but only on the table at his parents' house, where he learned to interpret the sound cues). Michael also enjoyed riding a bicycle, but his parents made him stop after he crashed first his brother's bike and then his sister's.

As an adult, Michael became a champion skier, marrying his instructor and raising two sons. He also started his own company, making equipment to help blind people navigate on their own. Then, when Michael was 46, technical advances made it possible to restore vision in his right eye. As soon as the bandages were removed, he could see his wife's blue eyes and blond hair. But even years later, he could not recognize her face unless she spoke to him, or recognize three-dimensional objects like cubes or spheres unless they were moving. Michael could still ski, but he found that he had to close his eyes to avoid falling over. On the slopes, seeing was more distracting than helpful.

The doctors could tell that images were focusing properly on Michael's retina, so why was his vision so poor?

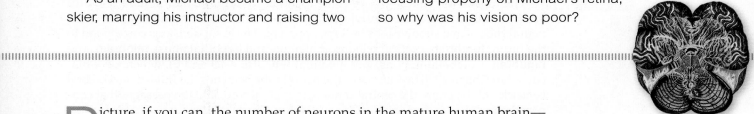

Picture, if you can, the number of neurons in the mature human brain—more than 80 billion (Herculano-Houzel, 2012). There are many types of neurons, each forming a vast array of hundreds or thousands of connections. More than 100 trillion synapses are formed to guide our thoughts and behavior! Yet each of us began as a single microscopic cell, the fertilized egg. How can one cell divide and grow to form one of the most complicated machines on Earth, perhaps in the universe? No one can answer that question in detail, but in this chapter we'll learn the basic processes at work in the extraordinary developing brain.

See Video 4.1:
Understanding Blindness
and the Brain

**View Animation 4.2:
Brain Explorer
View Activity 4.1:
Development of the Nervous System**

4.1 Growth and Development of the Brain Are Orderly Processes

THE ROAD AHEAD

In the first part of the chapter, we describe brains in terms of their progress from a single fertilized egg to a machine containing billions of neurons with an incredible number of connections. Learning this material should allow you to:

4.1.1 List the six stages of cellular processes needed for brain development.

4.1.2 Describe the two phases of brain development characterized by the loss of structures.

4.1.3 Identify the basic mechanism that directs each developing neuron to take on the appropriate structure and function.

4.1.4 Discuss the significance of generating new neurons in adulthood.

Within 12 hours after a human egg is fertilized, the single cell begins dividing, forming a small mass of homogeneous cells, like a cluster of grapes, that is a mere 200 micrometers in diameter. Within a week the emerging human embryo shows three distinct cell layers (**FIGURE 4.1A**)—the beginnings of all the tissues of the body. The nervous system develops from the outermost layer, called the **ectoderm** (from the Greek *ektos*, "out," and *derma*, "skin"). As the cell layers thicken, they grow to form a groove that will become the midline and then the neural groove. At the head end of this, a thickened collection of cells forms (**FIGURE 4.1B**).

The tops of the neural groove come together to form the **neural tube** (**FIGURE 4.1C**), the beginning of the central nervous system (CNS). At the anterior part of the neural tube, three subdivisions become apparent. These subdivisions correspond to the future **forebrain** (cortical regions, thalamus, and hypothalamus), **midbrain**, and **hindbrain** (cerebellum, pons, and medulla) (**FIGURE 4.1D** and **E**), which were discussed in Chapter 1. The interior of the neural tube becomes the fluid-filled cerebral ventricles of the brain, the central canal of the spinal cord, and the passages that connect them.

By the end of the eighth week, the human embryo shows the rudimentary beginnings of most body organs. The rapid development of the brain is reflected in the fact that by this time the head is half the total size of the embryo! The developing human is called an **embryo** during the first 10 weeks after fertilization and a **fetus** thereafter.

Development of the nervous system can be divided into six distinct stages

From a cellular viewpoint it is useful to consider brain development as a sequence of six distinct stages. The six stages proceed at different rates and times in different parts of the nervous system. Some of the stages may overlap even within a region:

1. *Neurogenesis,* the mitotic division of nonneuronal cells to produce neurons
2. *Cell migration,* the massive movements of nerve cells or their precursors to establish distinct nerve cell populations (nuclei in the CNS, layers of the cerebral cortex, and so on)
3. *Cell differentiation,* the refining of cells into distinctive types of neurons or glial cells
4. *Synaptogenesis,* the establishment of synaptic connections as axons and dendrites grow
5. *Neuronal cell death,* the selective death of many nerve cells
6. *Synapse rearrangement,* the loss of some synapses and the development of others, to refine synaptic connections, which extends throughout our lifespan

ectoderm   The outer cellular layer of the developing embryo, giving rise to the skin and the nervous system.

neural tube   An embryonic structure with subdivisions that correspond to the future forebrain, midbrain, and hindbrain.

forebrain   The front division of the brain, which in the mature vertebrate contains the cerebral hemispheres, the thalamus, and the hypothalamus.

midbrain   The middle division of the brain.

hindbrain   The rear division of the brain, which in the mature vertebrate contains the cerebellum, pons, and medulla.

embryo   The earliest stage in a developing animal.

fetus   A developing individual after the embryo stage.

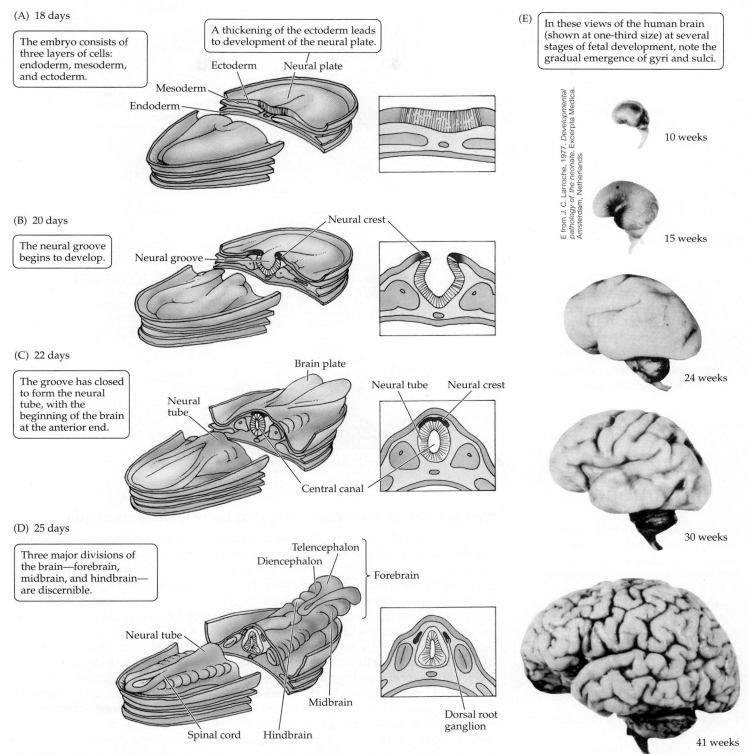

(A) 18 days

The embryo consists of three layers of cells: endoderm, mesoderm, and ectoderm.

A thickening of the ectoderm leads to development of the neural plate.

Ectoderm

Neural plate

Mesoderm

Endoderm

(B) 20 days

The neural groove begins to develop.

Neural crest

Neural groove

(C) 22 days

The groove has closed to form the neural tube, with the beginning of the brain at the anterior end.

Brain plate

Neural tube

Neural tube   Neural crest

Central canal

(D) 25 days

Three major divisions of the brain—forebrain, midbrain, and hindbrain—are discernible.

Telencephalon

Diencephalon

Forebrain

Neural tube

Midbrain

Dorsal root ganglion

Spinal cord   Hindbrain

(E)

In these views of the human brain (shown at one-third size) at several stages of fetal development, note the gradual emergence of gyri and sulci.

E from J. C. Larroche, 1977. *Developmental pathology of the neonate.* Excerpta Medica. Amsterdam, Netherlands

10 weeks

15 weeks

24 weeks

30 weeks

41 weeks

FIGURE 4.1   Development of the Nervous System in the Human Embryo and Fetus

Humans are unique among primates in showing dramatic brain growth after birth, as illustrated by **FIGURE 4.2** on the next page.

View Animation 4.3:
Stages of Neuronal Development

FIGURE 4.2   Fetal-like Rapid Development of the Brain outside the Womb (After B. Bogin, 1997. *Yearb. Phys. Anthropol.* 40: 63.)

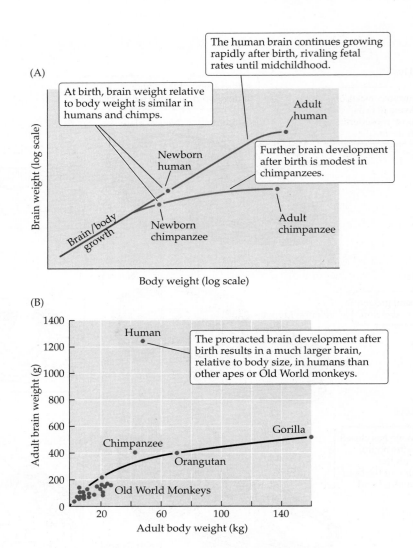

(A)

The human brain continues growing rapidly after birth, rivaling fetal rates until midchildhood.

At birth, brain weight relative to body weight is similar in humans and chimps.

Adult human

Newborn human

Further brain development after birth is modest in chimpanzees.

Brain weight (log scale)

Newborn chimpanzee

Adult chimpanzee

Brain/body growth

Body weight (log scale)

(B)

The protracted brain development after birth results in a much larger brain, relative to body size, in humans than other apes or Old World monkeys.

Human

Chimpanzee

Gorilla

Orangutan

Old World Monkeys

Adult brain weight (g)

Adult body weight (kg)

See Video 4.4:
Migration of a Neuron along a Radial Glial Cell

neurogenesis   The mitotic division of nonneuronal cells to produce neurons.

mitosis   The process of division of somatic cells that involves duplication of DNA.

ventricular zone   Also called *ependymal layer*. A region lining the cerebral ventricles that displays mitosis, providing neurons early in development and glial cells throughout life.

cell migration   The movement of cells from site of origin to final location.

gene expression   The process by which a cell makes an mRNA transcript of a particular gene.

cell differentiation   The developmental stage in which cells acquire distinctive characteristics, such as those of neurons, as a result of expressing particular genes.

synaptogenesis   The establishment of synaptic connections as axons and dendrites grow.

Cell proliferation produces cells that become neurons or glia

The production of neurons is called **neurogenesis**. Neurons themselves do not divide, but the cells that will give rise to neurons begin as a single layer of cells along the inner surface of the neural tube. These cells divide in a process called **mitosis**, which takes place within the **ventricular zone** inside the neural tube (**FIGURE 4.3A**). Eventually, some cells leave the ventricular zone and begin transforming into either neurons or glial cells. As the nervous system grows, **cell migration** follows, as the cells move over relatively long distances to fill out the brain (**FIGURE 4.3B**).

Newly arrived cells in the brain bear no more resemblance to mature nerve cells than they do to the cells of other organs. Once the cells reach their destinations, however, **gene expression** begins, that is, the cells begin to use, or express, particular genes. This means that each type of cell makes use of a particular subset of genes to make the particular proteins that type of cell needs. This process of **cell differentiation** enables cells to acquire the distinctive appearance and functions of neurons characteristic of their particular regions (**FIGURE 4.3C**). Once they take on the characteristics of neurons, they begin making synaptic connections with one another, in the process of **synaptogenesis** (**FIGURE 4.3D**).

The particular fate of a differentiating cell depends on where in the brain the cell happens to be and what the cell's neighbors are doing. Cells in the developing brain are constantly sending chemical signals to one another, each shaping the development of the other. This is the hallmark of vertebrate development: cells sort themselves out

FIGURE 4.3 The Six Stages of Neural Development

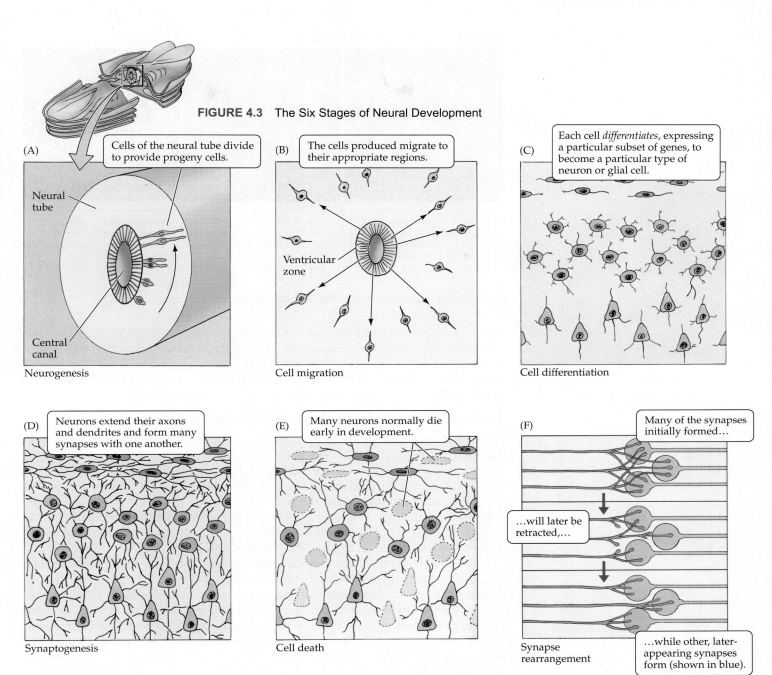

(A) Cells of the neural tube divide to provide progeny cells.

Neural tube

Central canal

Neurogenesis

(B) The cells produced migrate to their appropriate regions.

Ventricular zone

Cell migration

(C) Each cell *differentiates*, expressing a particular subset of genes, to become a particular type of neuron or glial cell.

Cell differentiation

(D) Neurons extend their axons and dendrites and form many synapses with one another.

Synaptogenesis

(E) Many neurons normally die early in development.

Cell death

(F) Many of the synapses initially formed…

…will later be retracted,…

…while other, later-appearing synapses form (shown in blue).

Synapse rearrangement

via **cell-cell interactions**, taking on fates that are appropriate in the context of what neighboring cells are doing. When the negotiations are all over, if things go properly, a new person is formed with all the types of cells in the brain that they need to live.

This system of cell-cell interactions determining how brain cells develop has an important consequence: If cells that have not yet differentiated extensively can be obtained and placed in a particular brain region, they can differentiate in an appropriate way and become properly integrated. Such undifferentiated cells, called **stem cells**, are present throughout embryonic tissues, so they can be gathered from umbilical cord blood, miscarried embryos, or unused embryos produced during in vitro fertilization. It may even be possible someday to take cells from adult tissue and, by treating them

cell-cell interaction The general process during development in which one cell affects the differentiation of other, usually neighboring, cells.

stem cell A cell that is undifferentiated and therefore can take on the fate of any cell that a donor organism can produce.

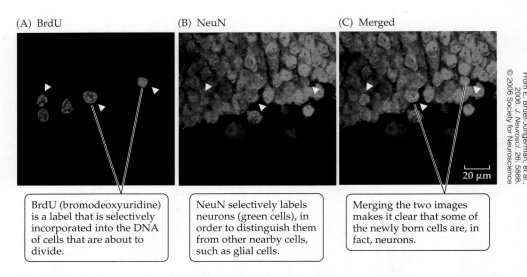

(A) BrdU

(B) NeuN

(C) Merged

20 µm

BrdU (bromodeoxyuridine) is a label that is selectively incorporated into the DNA of cells that are about to divide.

NeuN selectively labels neurons (green cells), in order to distinguish them from other nearby cells, such as glial cells.

Merging the two images makes it clear that some of the newly born cells are, in fact, neurons.

FIGURE 4.4   Neurogenesis in the Dentate Gyrus

with various factors in a dish, transform them into stem cells (Dulak et al., 2015). It is hoped that placing stem cells in areas of brain degeneration, such as loss of myelin in multiple sclerosis (see Chapter 2) or loss of dopaminergic neurons in Parkinson's disease (see Chapter 5), might reverse such degeneration as the implanted cells differentiate to fill in for the missing components (Y. K. Wang et al., 2018).

In the adult brain, newly born neurons aid learning

At birth, mammals have already produced most of the neurons they will ever have. The postnatal increase of human brain weight (see Figure 4.2) is due primarily to growth in the size of neurons, branching of dendrites, elaboration of synapses, increase in myelin, and addition of glial cells. But research has shown that we are also capable of **adult neurogenesis**, the generation of new neurons in adulthood, especially in the dentate gyrus of the hippocampal formation (**FIGURE 4.4**) (Anacker et al., 2018; Boldrini et al., 2018). By one estimate, 700 new neurons are produced every day in the adult human hippocampus (Spalding et al., 2013).

Indeed, although the new neurons acquired in adulthood represent just a tiny minority of the total, there's reason to think they matter (Snyder, 2019). In experimental animals, the birth and/or survival of new neurons is enhanced by factors like exercise, environmental enrichment, and training (Opendak and Gould, 2015). Neurogenesis appears to enhance various forms of hippocampus-dependent learning, such as spatial memory and fear conditioning, in some (but not all) studies (Kee et al., 2007). Mice with a genetic manipulation that turns off neurogenesis in the brains of adults showed a marked impairment in spatial learning with little effect on other behaviors (C. L. Zhang et al., 2008).

So by studying this chapter, you may be giving your brain a few more neurons to use on exam day! Physical exercise also boosts neurogenesis in rats—an effect that can be blocked by stressors such as social isolation (Stranahan et al., 2006)—so invest in exercise and a network of friends too.

The death of many neurons is a normal part of development

As strange as it may seem, cell death is a crucial phase of brain development (**FIGURE 4.3E**). This developmental stage is not unique to the nervous system. Naturally occurring **cell death**, also called *apoptosis* (from the Greek *apo*, "away from," and *ptosis*, "act of falling"), is evident as a kind of sculpting process in the emergence of other tissues in both animals and plants.

adult neurogenesis   The creation of new neurons in the brain of an adult.

cell death   Also called *apoptosis*. The developmental process during which "surplus" cells die.

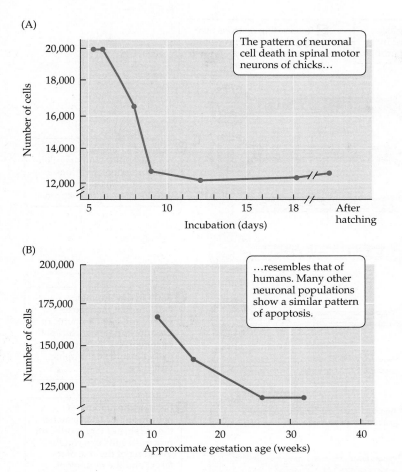

FIGURE 4.5 Many Neurons Die during Normal Early Development (Part A after V. Hamburger, 1975. *J. Comp. Neurol.* 160: 535; B after N. G. Forger and S. M. Breedlove, 1987. *J. Comp. Neurol.* 264: 118.)

The number of neurons that die during early development is quite large. In some regions of the brain and spinal cord, *most* of the young nerve cells die during prenatal development. In 1958, Viktor Hamburger (1900–2001) first described naturally occurring neuronal cell death in chicks, in which nearly half the originally produced spinal motor neurons die before the chick hatches. A similar loss of spinal motor neurons was later reported in developing humans (**FIGURE 4.5**).

These cells are not dying because of a defect. Rather, these cells die as a consequence of complex interactions with surrounding cells, so they are actively "committing suicide." Your chromosomes carry *death genes*—genes that are expressed only when a cell undergoes apoptosis (Yamaguchi and Miura, 2015). Genetically interfering with death genes in fetal mice causes them to grow brains that are too large to fit in the skull (Depaepe et al., 2005), so we can see how vital it is that some cells die.

Neurons compete for connections to target structures (other nerve cells or end organs, such as muscle). Cells that make adequate synapses remain; those without a place to form synaptic connections die. Apparently the cells compete not just for synaptic sites, but for a chemical that the target structure makes and releases. Neurons that receive enough of the chemical survive; those that do not, die. Such target-derived chemicals are called **neurotrophic factors** (or simply *trophic factors*) because they act as if they "feed" the neurons to help them survive (in Greek, *trophe* means "nourishment") (**FIGURE 4.6**). That same competition for neurotrophic factors probably also controls the next phase of development, when an enormous proliferation of synapses is followed by a careful pruning, as we'll see next.

neurotrophic factor Also called simply *trophic factor*. A target-derived chemical that acts as if it "feeds" certain neurons to help them survive.

FIGURE 4.6 A Model for the Action of Neurotrophic Factors

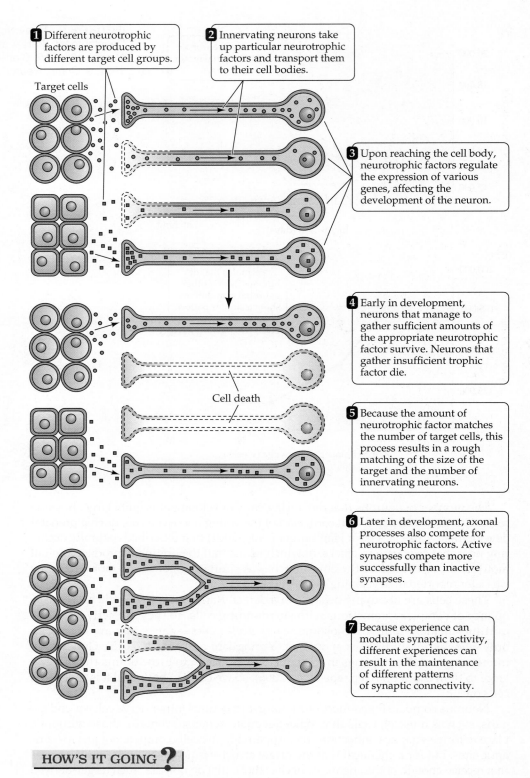

1 Different neurotrophic factors are produced by different target cell groups.

2 Innervating neurons take up particular neurotrophic factors and transport them to their cell bodies.

Target cells

3 Upon reaching the cell body, neurotrophic factors regulate the expression of various genes, affecting the development of the neuron.

4 Early in development, neurons that manage to gather sufficient amounts of the appropriate neurotrophic factor survive. Neurons that gather insufficient trophic factor die.

Cell death

5 Because the amount of neurotrophic factor matches the number of target cells, this process results in a rough matching of the size of the target and the number of innervating neurons.

6 Later in development, axonal processes also compete for neurotrophic factors. Active synapses compete more successfully than inactive synapses.

7 Because experience can modulate synaptic activity, different experiences can result in the maintenance of different patterns of synaptic connectivity.

HOW'S IT GOING ?

1. What six stages of cellular processes take place in the developing brain?
2. What is cell differentiation, and what guides this process in each cell in the developing brain?
3. What two classes of brain structures undergo loss during development?
4. What are neurotrophic factors, and what role do they play in brain development?

4.2 An Explosion of Synapse Formation Is Followed by Synapse Rearrangement

THE ROAD AHEAD

Now we describe the lifelong process by which synapses are lost and gained in the brain. Learning this material should allow you to:

4.2.1 Describe the process of synapse rearrangement, and offer evidence that a net loss of synapses may be adaptive.

4.2.2 Describe studies showing that visual experience early in life is required to develop normal vision.

Before birth and after, neurons in the human cortex grow ever longer and more elaborate dendrites, each jammed with synapses. As we noted earlier, this massive increase in dendrites and synapses is responsible for most of the increase in brain size after birth (**FIGURE 4.7**). But just as not all the neurons produced by a developing individual are kept into adulthood, some of the synapses formed early in development are later retracted. Some original synapses are lost, and many, many new synapses are formed (**FIGURE 4.3F**). This **synapse rearrangement**, or *synaptic remodeling*, typically takes place after the period of cell death.

For example, as we learned already, about half of the spinal motor neurons that form die later (see Figure 4.5). By the end of the cell death period, each surviving motor neuron innervates many muscle fibers, and every muscle fiber is innervated by several motor neurons. But later the surviving motor neurons retract many of their axon collaterals, until each muscle fiber comes to be innervated by only one motor neuron. Again, which synaptic connections are retained, and which new connections are formed, is thought to depend on competition for trophic factors during development (see Figure 4.6) and/or competition between Hebbian synapses (see Figure 13.22).

synapse rearrangement   Also called *synaptic remodeling*. The loss of some synapses and the development of others.

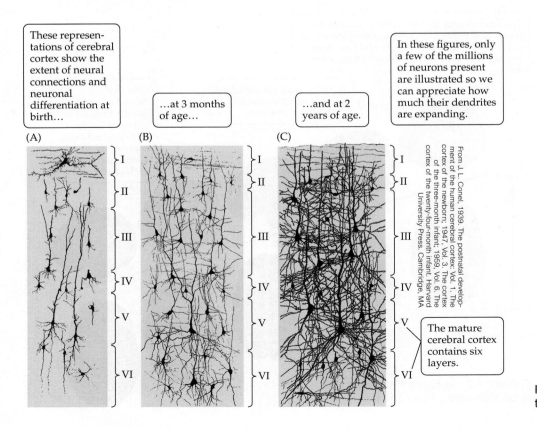

These representations of cerebral cortex show the extent of neural connections and neuronal differentiation at birth…

…at 3 months of age…

…and at 2 years of age.

In these figures, only a few of the millions of neurons present are illustrated so we can appreciate how much their dendrites are expanding.

(A)   (B)   (C)

From J. L. Conel, 1939. The postnatal development of the human cerebral cortex: Vol. 1. The cortex of the newborn; 1947, Vol. 3. The cortex of the three-month infant; 1959, Vol. 6. The cortex of the twenty-four-month infant. Harvard University Press, Cambridge, MA

The mature cerebral cortex contains six layers.

FIGURE 4.7   Cerebral Cortex Tissue in the Early Development of Humans

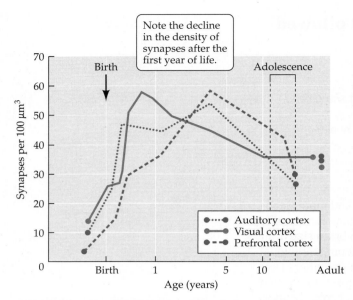

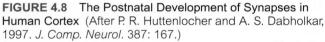

FIGURE 4.8 The Postnatal Development of Synapses in Human Cortex (After P. R. Huttenlocher and A. S. Dabholkar, 1997. *J. Comp. Neurol.* 387: 167.)

Similar events have been documented in several neural regions, including the cerebellum, the brainstem, the visual cortex, and the autonomic nervous system (Lichtman and Purves, 1980). In human cerebral cortex there is a net loss of synapses from late childhood until midadolescence (**FIGURE 4.8**). This synaptic remodeling is evident in thinning of the cortical gray matter as pruning of dendrites and axon terminals progresses. The thinning process continues in a caudal–rostral (posterior–anterior) direction during maturation (**FIGURE 4.9**), so prefrontal cortex matures last (Gogtay et al., 2004). Since prefrontal cortex is important for inhibiting behavior (see Chapter 14), this delayed brain maturation may contribute to teenagers' impulsivity and relative lack of control (Paus et al., 2008).

What determines which synapses are kept and which are lost? Although we don't know all the factors, one important influence is neural activity. One theory is that active synapses take up some neurotrophic factor that maintains the synapse, while inactive synapses get too little trophic factor to remain stable (see Figure 4.6). Intellectual stimulation probably contributes, as suggested by the fact that teenagers with the highest IQ show an especially prolonged period of cortical thinning (P. Shaw et al., 2006). Another stage of brain development, the formation of myelin sheaths for axons, is discussed in **A STEP FURTHER 4.1**, on the website.

Retaining too many synapses can impair intellectual development

One syndrome indicates that the loss of synapses actually helps the brain function better. The most frequent inherited cause of **intellectual disability**, a significant limitation in intellectual functioning and adaptive behavior, is **fragile X syndrome**

intellectual disability A disability characterized by significant limitations in intellectual functioning and adaptive behavior.

fragile X syndrome A condition that is a frequent cause of inherited intellectual disability and is produced by a fragile site on the X chromosome that seems prone to breaking because the DNA there is unstable.

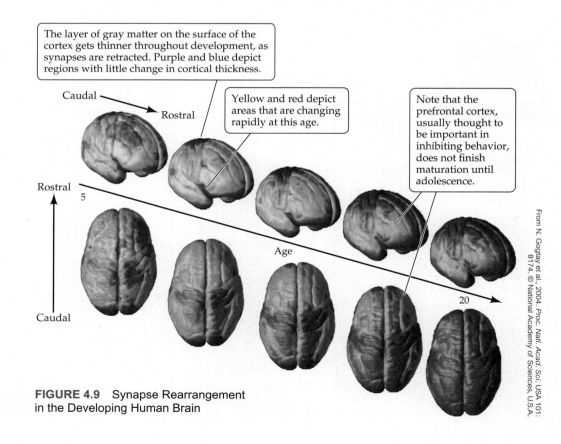

FIGURE 4.9 Synapse Rearrangement in the Developing Human Brain

From N. Gogtay et al., 2004. *Proc. Natl. Acad. Sci. USA* 101: 8174. © National Academy of Sciences, U.S.A.

(**FIGURE 4.10**). Researchers have found that some people are born with an X chromosome that is prone to breaking because the DNA at one site is unstable (Lyons et al., 2015). A person with this condition has a modified facial appearance, including elongation of the face, large prominent ears, and a prominent chin. A wide range of cognitive effects—from mild to severe impairment—are associated with the syndrome. Cortical neurons from the brains of people with fragile X syndrome, as well as mice genetically engineered to have this syndrome, possess an *excess* of small, immature dendritic spines (Bagni and Greenough, 2005). These findings suggest that the syndrome affects mental development by blocking the normal elimination of synapses after birth (see Figure 7.9).

We'll run into lifelong synaptic rearrangement repeatedly in this book. In Chapter 5 we'll see that regions of cerebral cortex that process touch information undergo synapse rearrangement throughout life, and in Chapter 13 we'll find that learning and memory happen through the strengthening and weakening of existing synapses or through synapse rearrangement. Next we'll consider another example of synaptic rearrangement, in the visual system, where experience is crucial for proper development.

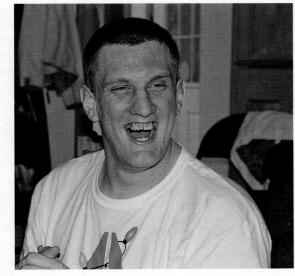

FIGURE 4.10   Too Many Synapses? A man with fragile X syndrome.

Visual deprivation can lead to blindness

Some people do not see forms clearly with one of their eyes, even though the eye is intact and a sharp image is focused on the retina. Such impairments of vision are known as **amblyopia** (from the Greek *amblys*, "dull," and *ops*, "eye"). Some people with this disorder have an eye that is turned inward (are cross-eyed) or outward. Children born with such a misalignment see a double image rather than a single fused image. By the time an untreated person reaches the age of 7 or 8, pattern vision in the deviated eye is almost completely suppressed. If the eyes are realigned during childhood, the person learns to fuse the two images and has good depth perception. But if realignment is done in adulthood, it's too late to restore acute vision to the turned eye.

Much of what we know about the causes of amblyopia comes from visual deprivation experiments with lab animals, in which the eyelids are reversibly sutured shut or the animal is fitted with frosted contact lenses, thereby preventing focused images on the retina. These experiments have revealed startling changes related to disuse of the visual system in early life. **Binocular deprivation**, depriving animals of sight in both eyes, produces structural changes in visual cortical neurons: a loss of dendritic spines and a reduction in synapses. If such deprivation is maintained for several weeks during development, when the animal's eyes are opened, it will be blind. Although light enters its eyes, and the cells of the eyes send messages to the brain, the brain seems to ignore the messages, and the animal is unable to detect visual stimuli. If the deprivation lasts long enough, the animal is *never* able to recover eyesight. Thus, early visual experience is crucial for the proper development of vision, and there is a **sensitive period** during which these manipulations of experience can exert long-lasting effects on the system (**FIGURE 4.11**). These effects are most extensive during the early period of synaptic development in the visual cortex. After the sensitive period, the manipulations have little or no effect.

amblyopia   Reduced visual acuity of one eye that is not caused by optical or retinal impairments.

binocular deprivation   Depriving both eyes of form vision, as by sealing the eyelids.

sensitive period   The period during development in which an organism can be permanently altered by a particular experience or treatment.

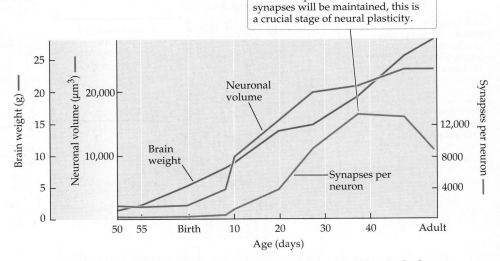

FIGURE 4.11   Brain Development in the Visual Cortex of Cats (After B. G. Cragg, 1975. *J. Comp. Neurol.* 160: 147–166.)

monocular deprivation Depriving one eye of light.

ocular dominance histogram A graph that portrays the strength of response of a brain neuron to stimuli presented to either the left eye or the right eye.

Depriving only one eye of light during the developmental sensitive period—**monocular deprivation**—produces profound structural and functional changes in the thalamus and visual cortex and permanently impairs vision in the deprived eye. The effect of visual deprivation can be illustrated graphically by an **ocular dominance histogram**, which portrays the strength of response of a brain neuron to stimuli presented to either the left or the right eye. Normally, most cortical neurons (except those in layer IV) are excited equally by light presented to either eye (**FIGURE 4.12A**). Keeping one eye closed or covered in development results in a striking shift from the normal graph; most cortical neurons now respond only to input from the nondeprived eye

FIGURE 4.12 Ocular Dominance Histograms (A and C after D. H. Hubel and T. N. Wiesel, 1965. *J. Neurophysiol.* 28: 1041; B after T. N. Wiesel and D. H. Hubel, 1965. *J. Neurophysiol.* 28: 1029.)

The numbers along the *x*-axis represent a gradation in response: Cells that respond *only* to stimulation of the opposite eye are class 1 cells. Cells that respond *mainly* to stimulation of the opposite eye are class 2. Cells that respond equally to either eye are class 4. Cell that respond only to stimulation of the eye on the same side are class 7, and so on.

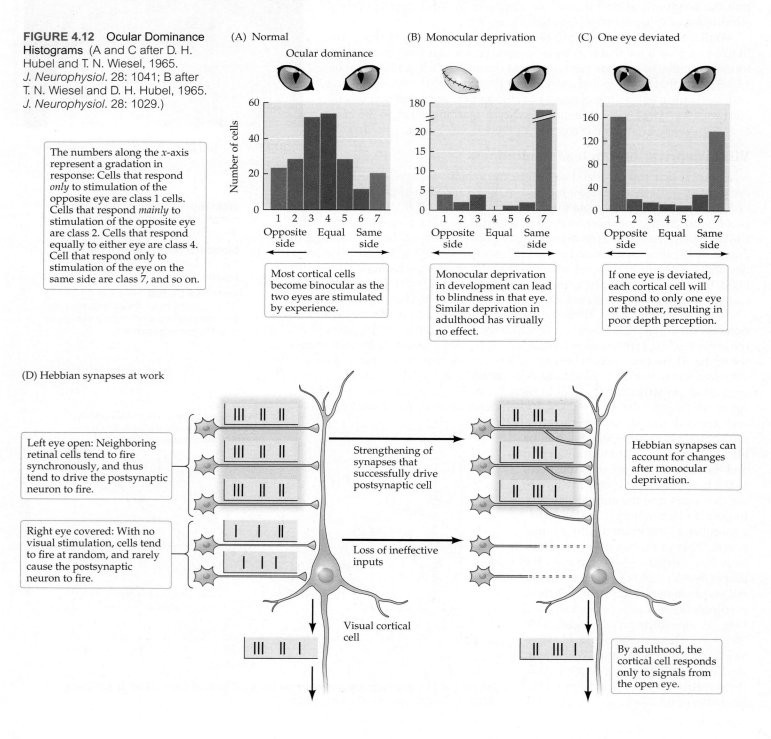

(A) Normal

Ocular dominance

Most cortical cells become binocular as the two eyes are stimulated by experience.

(B) Monocular deprivation

Monocular deprivation in development can lead to blindness in that eye. Similar deprivation in adulthood has virually no effect.

(C) One eye deviated

If one eye is deviated, each cortical cell will respond to only one eye or the other, resulting in poor depth perception.

(D) Hebbian synapses at work

Left eye open: Neighboring retinal cells tend to fire synchronously, and thus tend to drive the postsynaptic neuron to fire.

Right eye covered: With no visual stimulation, cells tend to fire at random, and rarely cause the postsynaptic neuron to fire.

Strengthening of synapses that successfully drive postsynaptic cell

Loss of ineffective inputs

Hebbian synapses can account for changes after monocular deprivation.

Visual cortical cell

By adulthood, the cortical cell responds only to signals from the open eye.

(**FIGURE 4.12B**). In cats the critical period for this effect is the first 4 months of life. In rhesus monkeys the sensitive period extends to age 6 months. After these ages, visual deprivation has little effect.

During early development, synapses are rearranged in the visual cortex, and axons representing input from each eye "compete" for synaptic places. Active, effective synapses predominate over inactive synapses. Thus, if one eye is "silenced," synapses carrying information from that eye are retracted while synapses driven by the other eye are maintained. Donald O. Hebb (1949) proposed that effective synapses (those that successfully drive the postsynaptic cell) might grow stronger at the expense of ineffective synapses. Thus, synapses that grow stronger or weaker depending on their effectiveness in driving their target cell are known as **Hebbian synapses** (**FIGURE 4.12D**). In Chapter 13 we will learn about a particular neurotransmitter receptor, the *NMDA receptor*, that causes synapses to act like Hebbian synapses, and likely plays a role in learning and memory (see Figure 13.22).

Researchers offer a similar explanation for amblyopia produced by misalignment of the eyes. Hubel and Wiesel (1965) produced an animal replica of this human condition by surgically causing the eyes to diverge in kittens. The ocular dominance histogram of these animals reveals that the normal binocular sensitivity of visual cortical cells is greatly reduced (**FIGURE 4.12C**). A much larger proportion of visual cortical cells is excited by stimulation of either the right or the left eye in these animals than in control animals. The reason for this effect is that after surgery, visual stimuli falling on the misaligned eyes no longer provide simultaneous, convergent input to the cells of the visual cortex.

Neurotrophic factors may be playing a role in experience-driven synapse rearrangement. For example, if the postsynaptic cells are making a limited supply of a neurotrophic factor, and if active synapses take up more of the factor than inactive synapses do, then perhaps the inactive axons retract for lack of neurotrophic factor. Brain-derived neurotrophic factor (BDNF) has been implicated as a neurotrophic factor being competed for in the mammalian visual cortex (Sansevero et al., 2019). So perhaps ineffective synapses wither for lack of neurotrophic support. In **A STEP FURTHER 4.2** on the website, you can learn how mouse whiskers compete for synapses in the cortex.

Early exposure to visual patterns helps fine-tune connections in the visual system

Human disorders have also proven that early experience is crucial for vision. Babies born with cataracts (cloudy lenses) in industrialized countries usually have them removed a few months after birth and will have good vision. But if such a child grows up with the cataracts in place, removing them in adulthood is much less effective; the adults acquire the use of vision slowly (Ostrovsky et al., 2009) and to only a limited extent (Bower, 2003). Early visual experience is known to be especially crucial for learning to perceive faces, because infants with cataracts that occlude vision for just the first 6 months of life are impaired at recognizing faces even 9 years later (Le Grand et al., 2001). These experience-dependent effects are probably mediated by synapse rearrangement within the visual cortex (Ruthazer et al., 2003) like that seen in kittens.

Why does Michael May, whom we met at the start of the chapter, have such poor vision despite the clear images entering his eye? Had the accident happened to him as an adult, the surgery to let light back into his eye would have restored normal vision. But, like a kitten growing up with opaque contact lenses, Michael was deprived of form vision, beginning while he was a child and lasting for 40 years. So, synaptic connections within his developing visual cortex were not strengthened by the patterns of light moving across the retina, and in the absence of patterned stimulation, synapses between the eye and the brain languished and disappeared.

In one sense, Michael was lucky that his blindness came as late as it did. He had normal form vision for the first 3½ years of his life, and that stimulation may have been sufficient to maintain some synapses that would otherwise have been lost. These

Hebbian synapse A synapse that is strengthened when it successfully drives the postsynaptic cell.

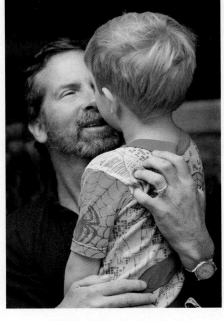

Learning to See Michael May finds it particularly difficult to recognize faces by sight alone.

© Florence Low

4.13 What Do I See?
(After E. Huber et al. 2015.
Psychol. Sci. 26: 393.)

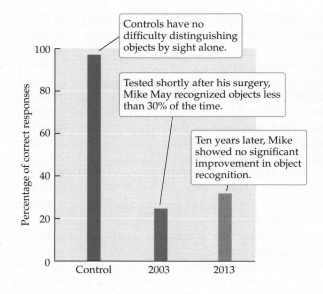

Controls have no difficulty distinguishing objects by sight alone.

Tested shortly after his surgery, Mike May recognized objects less than 30% of the time.

Ten years later, Mike showed no significant improvement in object recognition.

Despite having the damage to his eye surgically corrected as an adult, Michael May was rather poor at distinguishing between basic objects, like spheres versus cubes. When retested 10 years later, there was no significant improvement in his ability to distinguish objects by sight alone.

y-axis: Percentage of correct responses (0, 20, 40, 60, 80, 100)
x-axis: Control, 2003, 2013

residual synapses are probably what allow him to make any sense whatsoever of his vision. Yet, despite more than a decade of visual experience as an adult, Michael still has problems distinguishing three-dimensional objects or faces (**FIGURE 4.13**) (Huber et al., 2015). Other people who gain vision for the first time as adults have similar difficulties recognizing objects and faces (Gregory and Wallace, 1963; Sikl et al., 2013).

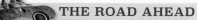

HOW'S IT GOING ?

1. What is the evidence that early visual experience is important for being able to see?
2. What's an ocular dominance histogram, and what manipulation(s) can alter it in cats?
3. What is a Hebbian synapse, and how might such synapses affect development of the visual system?

4.3 Experience Can Affect Brain Development by Altering Gene Expression

THE ROAD AHEAD

In this section we discuss how experience can affect the way genes work. Learning this material should allow you to:

4.3.1 Describe how the environment can regulate gene expression and how experience and genes interact to affect behavior.

4.3.2 Define epigenetic changes, and explain how they might play a role in the interaction of genes and the environment.

4.3.3 Describe the mechanism by which rodent dams can alter their offspring's lifelong stress response.

Many factors shape the form, arrangements, and connections of the developing brain. One influence is genes, which direct the production of every protein the cell can make. An individual who has inherited an altered gene will make an altered protein, which will affect every cell that uses that protein. Thus, every neuronal structure, and therefore every behavior, can be altered by changes in the relevant gene(s). It is useful to think of genes as *intrinsic* factors—that is, factors that originate within the developing cell itself. All other influences we can consider *extrinsic*—originating outside of the developing cell.

Genotype is fixed at birth, but phenotype changes throughout life

Two terms help illustrate how these intrinsic and extrinsic factors interact. The sum of all the intrinsic, genetic information that an individual has is its **genotype**. The sum of all the anatomical, physiological and behavioral characteristics that make up an individual is its **phenotype**. Your genotype was determined at the moment of fertilization and remains the same throughout your life. But your phenotype changes constantly, as you grow up and grow old and even, in a tiny way, as you take each breath. In other words, phenotype is determined by the interaction of genotype and extrinsic factors, including experience. Thus, as we'll see, individuals who have identical genotypes do not have identical phenotypes, because they have not received identical extrinsic influences. And since their nervous system phenotypes are somewhat different, they do not behave exactly the same.

Several hundred different genetic disorders affect the metabolism of proteins, carbohydrates, or lipids, having a profound impact on the developing brain. Characteristically, the genetic defect is the absence of a particular enzyme that controls a critical biochemical step in the synthesis or breakdown of a vital body product.

An example is **phenylketonuria** (**PKU**), a heritable disorder of protein metabolism that at one time resulted in many people with intellectual disability. About one out of 100 persons is a carrier; one in 10,000 births produces an affected victim. The basic defect is the absence of an enzyme necessary to metabolize phenylalanine, an amino acid that is present in many foods. As a result, the brain is damaged by an enormous buildup of phenylalanine, which becomes toxic.

The discovery of PKU marked the first time that an inherited error of metabolism was associated with intellectual disability. These days, the level of phenylalanine in the blood is measured in children a few days after birth. Early detection is important because brain impairment can be prevented simply by reducing phenylalanine in the diet. Such dietary control of PKU is critical during the early years of life (L. Bernstein et al., 2017). Note this important example of the interaction of genes and the environment in PKU: the dysfunctional gene causes intellectual disability only in the presence of phenylalanine. Reducing phenylalanine consumption reduces or prevents this effect of the gene.

PKU illustrates one reason why, despite the importance of genes for nervous system development, understanding the genotype alone could never enable an understanding of the developing brain. Knowing that a baby is born with PKU doesn't tell you anything about how that child's brain will develop unless you also know something about the child's diet. Another reason why genes alone cannot tell the whole story is that experience can affect the activity of genes, as we discuss next.

Experience regulates gene expression in the developing and mature brain

Genetically identical animals, called **clones**, used to be known mainly in science fiction and horror films. But life imitates art. In pigs, genetically identical clones show as much variation in behavior and temperament as do normal siblings (G. S. Archer et al., 2003), and genetically identical mice raised in different laboratories behave very differently on a variety of tests (Finch and Kirkwood, 2000). If genes are so important to the developing nervous system, how can genetically identical individuals differ in their behavior?

Recall that although nearly all of the cells in your body have a complete copy of your genotype, each cell uses only a small subset of those genes at any one time. We mentioned earlier that when a cell uses a particular gene to make a particular protein, we say the cell has *expressed* that gene. **Epigenetics** is the study of factors that affect gene expression without making any changes in the nucleotide sequence of the genes. The same protein is produced, but the *amount* of protein can vary considerably, which leads to variation in brain development. We'll consider two factors that may affect gene expression next.

genotype   All the genetic information that one specific individual has inherited.

phenotype   The sum of an individual's physical characteristics at one particular time.

phenylketonuria   An inherited disorder in which the absence of an enzyme leads to a toxic buildup of phenylalanine metabolites, causing intellectual disability.

clones   Asexually produced organisms that are genetically identical.

epigenetics   The study of factors that affect gene expression without making any changes in the nucleotide sequence of the genes themselves.

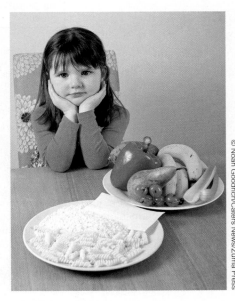

© Noah Goodrich/Caters News/Zuma Press

Be Careful What You Eat   Millie Lonergan, who has phenylketonuria, eats fruit and protein-free rice and pasta (without cheese) for a diet low in phenylalanine.

RESEARCHERS AT WORK |||||||||||||||||||||||||||||||||||||||||||||||||||||||||||||||||||||||||||||||||||||||||||||||||||||||||||||||||||

Maternal care affects mouse behaviors

■ Hypothesis

The behavior of genetically identical male mice can be affected by the prenatal environment and/or the mothering they receive after birth.

■ Experiment

Take genetically identical mouse embryos of the Black6 strain, and implant them into the womb of a foster mother of either their own strain or another strain (the albino Balb strain). After birth, transfer half the males to be raised by either a Black6 female or a Balb female. When the males grow up, measure their behavior on tests in which Black6 and Balb mice normally differ.

■ Result

Males of the Black6 strain carried and raised by mothers from the albino strain show significant differences in several behaviors (Francis et al., 2003), including maze running and measures of anxiety (**Figure 4.14**).

■ Conclusion

Since the various males are genetically identical to one another, their different behaviors must be due to the effect of different prenatal environments and postnatal experiences, such as the mothering they received, on how those genes are expressed.

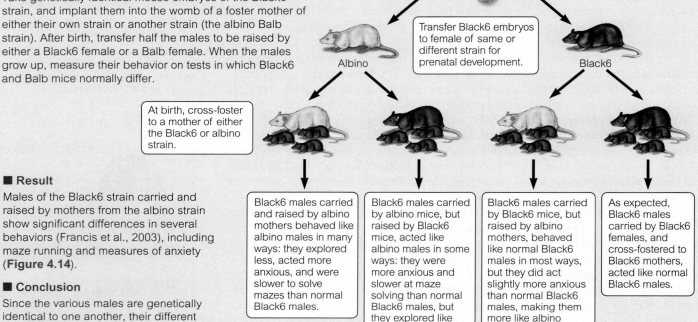

FIGURE 4.14 Epigenetic Effects on Mouse Behavior (After D. D. Francis et al., 2003. *Nat. Neurosci.* 6: 445.)

Gene expression in the brain can be affected by mothering

One particular influence of mothering on gene expression has been well document-ed. **Methylation** is a chemical modification of DNA that does not affect the nucleotide sequence of a gene but makes that gene less likely to be expressed. Rodent pups pro-vided with inattentive mothers, or subjected to interruptions in maternal care, secrete more glucocorticoids in response to stress as adults (T. Y. Zhang and Meaney, 2010). Poor maternal care produces this heightened stress hormone response by inducing methylation of the glucocorticoid receptor gene in the brain, making the pups hyper-responsive to stress for the rest of their lives (**FIGURE 4.15**).

A similar mechanism may apply to humans, because this same gene is also more likely to be methylated in the postmortem brains of suicide victims than of controls, *but only in those victims who were subjected to childhood abuse*. Suicide victims who did not suffer childhood abuse were no more likely to have the gene methylated than were controls (McGowan et al., 2009). These results suggest that methylation of the gene in abused children may make them hyperresponsive to stress as adults—a con-dition that may lead them to take their own lives. This is a powerful demonstration

methylation A chemical modification of DNA that does not affect the nucleotide sequence of a gene but makes that gene less likely to be expressed.

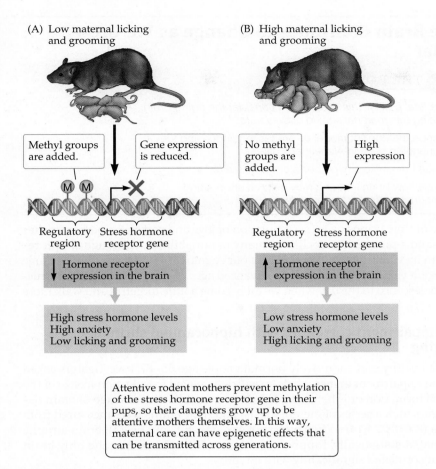

(A) Low maternal licking and grooming

Methyl groups are added.

Gene expression is reduced.

Regulatory region   Stress hormone receptor gene

↓ Hormone receptor expression in the brain

High stress hormone levels
High anxiety
Low licking and grooming

(B) High maternal licking and grooming

No methyl groups are added.

High expression

Regulatory region   Stress hormone receptor gene

↑ Hormone receptor expression in the brain

Low stress hormone levels
Low anxiety
High licking and grooming

Attentive rodent mothers prevent methylation of the stress hormone receptor gene in their pups, so their daughters grow up to be attentive mothers themselves. In this way, maternal care can have epigenetic effects that can be transmitted across generations.

FIGURE 4.15 Early Experience Imprints Genes to Affect the Stress Response in Adulthood (After D. A. Hackman et al., 2010. *Nat. Rev. Neurosci.* 11: 651.)

of epigenetic influences on behavior. Other developmental disorders are also influenced by both genes and the environment, as we discuss in **A STEP FURTHER 4.3**, on the website.

Taken together, these studies lead us to the conclusion that the incredible intelligence of the adult human is due not only to the inheritance of genes provided us by natural selection, but also to the effect of the environment and experience that determines where and when those genes are expressed in the brain, especially in development. Thus, the tremendous, fetal-like development of the human brain after birth (see Figure 4.2) is molded by experience and social guidance. We wish we could tell you that once your brain has been sharpened by experience (including what you gain by reading this book), you will remain brilliant forever. Sadly, development continues relentlessly toward old age. Just as our faces and bodies weaken and fade, the brain also declines, the depressing topic that concludes this chapter.

HOW'S IT GOING ?

1. Compare changes in genotype and phenotype in an individual during development and aging.
2. How does PKU illustrate an interaction between genes and the environment?
3. Describe two demonstrations of epigenetic effects on development.

4.4 The Brain Continues to Change as We Grow Older

THE ROAD AHEAD

In the final part of this chapter, we consider the aging brain. Learning this material should allow you to:

4.4.1 Describe the current model of processes underlying the degeneration seen in Alzheimer's disease.

4.4.2 Critique the amyloid hypothesis of Alzheimer's.

4.4.3 Discuss how brain imaging may help us understand the mechanism(s) of Alzheimer's.

The passage of time brings us an accumulation of joys and sorrows—perhaps riches and fame—and a progressive decline in many of our abilities. Although slower responses seem inevitable with aging, many of our cognitive abilities show little change during the adult years, until we reach an advanced age. What happens to brain structure from adolescence to the day when we all become a little forgetful and walk more hesitantly?

Memory impairment correlates with hippocampal shrinkage during aging

In a study of healthy and cognitively normal people age 55–87, investigators asked whether mild impairment in memory is specifically related to reduction in size of the hippocampal formation or is better explained by generalized shrinkage of brain tissue. Volunteers took a series of memory tests, and their brains were measured from MRI images (**FIGURE 4.16**). When effects of sex, age, IQ, and overall brain atrophy were eliminated statistically, hippocampal formation volume was the only brain measure that correlated significantly with memory.

PET scans of elderly people reveal that cerebral metabolism normally remains almost constant as we age. This stability is in marked contrast to the dramatic decline of brain activity in Alzheimer's disease, which we will consider next.

Alzheimer's disease is associated with a decline in cerebral metabolism

The population of elderly people in the United States is increasing dramatically. Most people reaching an advanced age lead happy, productive lives, although at a slower pace than they did in their earlier years. In a growing number of elderly people,

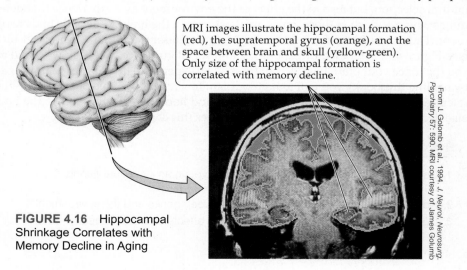

MRI images illustrate the hippocampal formation (red), the supratemporal gyrus (orange), and the space between brain and skull (yellow-green). Only size of the hippocampal formation is correlated with memory decline.

FIGURE 4.16 Hippocampal Shrinkage Correlates with Memory Decline in Aging

From J. Golomb et al., 1994. *J. Neurol. Neurosurg. Psychiatry* 57: 590. MRI courtesy of James Golumb

however, age has brought a particular agony: the disorder called **Alzheimer's disease**, named after Alois Alzheimer (1864–1915), the neurologist who first described a type of **dementia** (drastic failure of cognitive ability, including memory failure and loss of orientation).

Nearly 6 million Americans suffer from Alzheimer's disease, and the progressive aging of our population means that these ranks will continue to swell (Alzheimer's Association, 2019). This disorder is found worldwide with almost no geographic differences. The frequency of Alzheimer's increases with aging up to age 85–90, but people who reach that age *without* symptoms become increasingly *less* likely ever to develop them (Breitner et al., 1999; Y. Zhao et al., 2018). This last finding indicates that Alzheimer's is in fact a disease, and not simply the result of wear and tear in the brain. The fact that remaining physically and mentally active reduces the risk of developing Alzheimer's disease (Gallagher et al., 2019) also refutes the notion that brains simply "wear out" with age. Extensive use of the brain makes Alzheimer's *less* likely.

Alzheimer's disease begins as a loss of memory of recent events. Eventually this memory impairment becomes all-encompassing, so extensive that people with Alzheimer's cannot maintain any form of conversation, because both context and prior information are rapidly lost. They cannot answer simple questions such as, What year is it? Who is the president of the United States? or Where are you now? Cognitive decline is progressive and relentless. In time, people with Alzheimer's become disoriented and easily lose themselves even in familiar surroundings.

Observations of the brains of people with Alzheimer's reveal striking *cortical atrophy* (shrinkage), especially in the frontal, temporal, and parietal areas. PET scans show marked reduction of metabolism in posterior parietal cortex and some portions of the temporal lobe (see Figure 1.18E) (Teipel et al., 2016). The brains of individuals with Alzheimer's also reveal progressive changes at the cellular level (**FIGURE 4.17**):

- Strange patches termed **amyloid plaques** appear in cortex, the hippocampus, and associated limbic system sites. The plaques are formed by the buildup of a substance called **beta-amyloid** (Selkoe and Hardy, 2016), which is how amyloid plaques got their name.

Alzheimer's disease   A form of dementia that may appear in middle age but is more frequent among the aged.

dementia   Drastic failure of cognitive ability, including memory failure and disorientation.

amyloid plaque   Also called *senile plaque*. A small area of the brain that has abnormal cellular and chemical patterns. Amyloid plaques correlate with dementia.

beta-amyloid   A protein that accumulates in amyloid plaques in Alzheimer's disease.

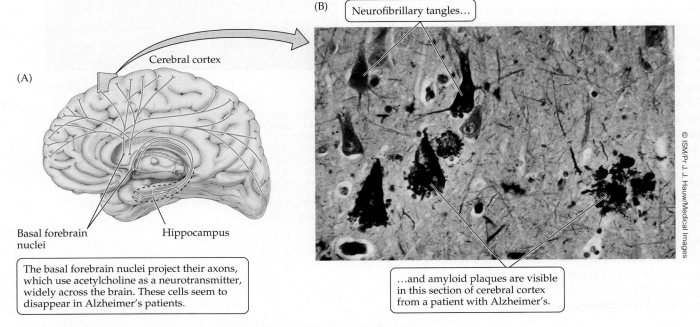

(A)

Cerebral cortex

(B)

Neurofibrillary tangles…

Basal forebrain nuclei

Hippocampus

The basal forebrain nuclei project their axons, which use acetylcholine as a neurotransmitter, widely across the brain. These cells seem to disappear in Alzheimer's patients.

…and amyloid plaques are visible in this section of cerebral cortex from a patient with Alzheimer's.

© ISM/Pr-J. J. Hauw/Medical Images

FIGURE 4.17   People with Alzheimer's Show Structural Changes in the Brain

- Some cells show abnormalities called **neurofibrillary tangles**, which are abnormal whorls of neurofilaments that form a tangled array inside the cell. The number of neurofibrillary tangles is directly related to the magnitude of cognitive impairment, and they are probably a secondary response to amyloid plaques.

- People with Alzheimer's gradually lose many neurons in the basal forebrain, which make the transmitter acetylcholine (ACh). Drugs that boost ACh signaling may reduce some of the symptoms of Alzheimer's for a time.

neurofibrillary tangle   An abnormal whorl of neurofilaments within nerve cells that is seen in Alzheimer's disease.

One hypothesis about how these processes are related to each other is offered in **A STEP FURTHER 4.4**, on the website. Perhaps measuring beta-amyloid will help future Alzheimer's research, as Signs & Symptoms discusses next.

SIGNS & SYMPTOMS

Imaging Alzheimer's Plaques

At present, the only surefire diagnosis for Alzheimer's is post-mortem examination of the brain revealing amyloid plaques and neurofibrillary tangles. But one innovative approach is to inject the dye Pittsburgh Blue (PiB), which has an affinity for beta-amyloid (Sheikh-Bahaei et al., 2018). Then a PET scan determines how much of the dye accumulates in the brain. The brain of virtually every person diagnosed with Alzheimer's accumulates the dye, as do the brains of many elderly people showing mild cognitive impairment (**FIGURE 4.18**). A meta-analysis of findings from thousands of participants confirmed that levels of amyloid, as revealed by PiB imaging, indeed correlated with who would develop Alzheimer's (Ossenkoppele et al., 2015). One important implication of this finding is that now it will be easier to track the effectiveness of various therapies for Alzheimer's.

One treatment strategy is to develop drugs that interfere with enzymes that favor beta-amyloid production (O. Singer et al., 2005; Yu et al., 2015). However, there is increasing skepticism about whether beta-amyloid actually *causes* the symptoms of Alzheimer's, or whether the accumulating amyloid is the result of something the brain is doing to *avoid* the symptoms of Alzheimer's (Makin, 2018). In that case, interfering with amyloid production would not help, and might even exacerbate the disease. Supporting that gloomy idea, several manipulations in mice that successfully interfered with amyloid accumulation provided no behavioral benefit.

In the meantime, and in keeping with the repeated theme of this chapter—that genes and experience interact—there is good evidence that physical activity (Ngandu et al., 2015), mental activity (Gates and Sachdev, 2014), and adequate sleep (Gelber et al., 2015) can postpone the appearance of Alzheimer's disease. So unless you want to pin your hopes on medical miracles in the future, the best way to avoid suffering from Alzheimer's is to remain physically and mentally active. Perhaps you should consider a career in neuroscience research…

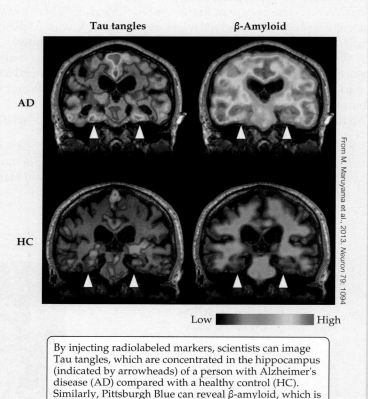

From M. Maruyama et al., 2013. *Neuron* 79: 1094

By injecting radiolabeled markers, scientists can image Tau tangles, which are concentrated in the hippocampus (indicated by arrowheads) of a person with Alzheimer's disease (AD) compared with a healthy control (HC). Similarly, Pittsburgh Blue can reveal β-amyloid, which is abundant throughout the brain of a person with AD.

FIGURE 4.18   Imaging Tau Tangles and Amyloid Plaques in the Brain

HOW'S IT GOING ?

1. What is Alzheimer's disease, and how is it diagnosed?
2. Why is beta-amyloid a suspected cause of Alzheimer's?
3. Although genes clearly influence the risk of Alzheimer's, what environmental factors can postpone its onset?

Recommended Reading

Barresi, M. J. F., and Gilbert, S. F. (2019). *Developmental Biology* (12th ed.). Sunderland, MA: Oxford University Press/Sinauer.

Breedlove, S. M. (2017). *Foundations of Neural Development.* Sunderland, MA: Oxford University Press/Sinauer.

Marcus, G. (2008). *The Birth of the Mind: How a Tiny Number of Genes Creates the Complexities of Human Thought.* New York, NY: Basic Books.

4 • VISUAL SUMMARY

You should be able to relate each summary to the adjacent illustration, including structures and processes. The online version of this **Visual Summary** includes links to figures, animations, and activities that will help you consolidate the material.

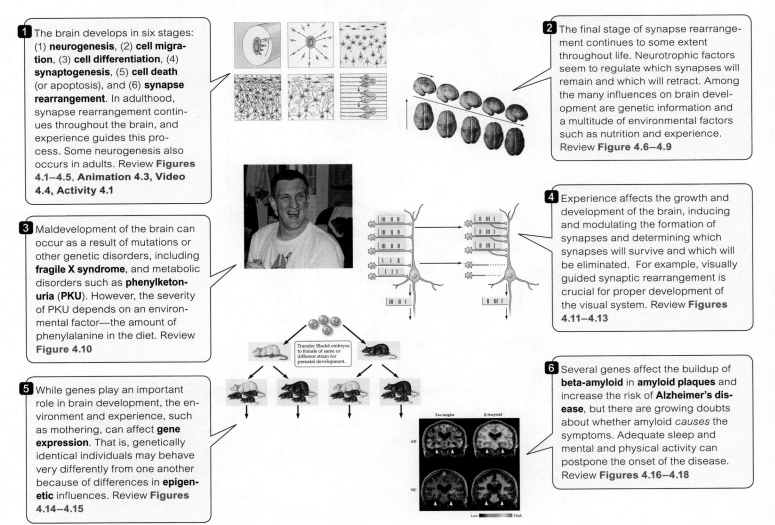

1 The brain develops in six stages: (1) **neurogenesis**, (2) **cell migration**, (3) **cell differentiation**, (4) **synaptogenesis**, (5) **cell death** (or apoptosis), and (6) **synapse rearrangement**. In adulthood, synapse rearrangement continues throughout the brain, and experience guides this process. Some neurogenesis also occurs in adults. Review **Figures 4.1–4.5, Animation 4.3, Video 4.4, Activity 4.1**

2 The final stage of synapse rearrangement continues to some extent throughout life. Neurotrophic factors seem to regulate which synapses will remain and which will retract. Among the many influences on brain development are genetic information and a multitude of environmental factors such as nutrition and experience. Review **Figure 4.6–4.9**

3 Maldevelopment of the brain can occur as a result of mutations or other genetic disorders, including **fragile X syndrome**, and metabolic disorders such as **phenylketonuria (PKU)**. However, the severity of PKU depends on an environmental factor—the amount of phenylalanine in the diet. Review **Figure 4.10**

4 Experience affects the growth and development of the brain, inducing and modulating the formation of synapses and determining which synapses will survive and which will be eliminated. For example, visually guided synaptic rearrangement is crucial for proper development of the visual system. Review **Figures 4.11–4.13**

5 While genes play an important role in brain development, the environment and experience, such as mothering, can affect **gene expression**. That is, genetically identical individuals may behave very differently from one another because of differences in **epigenetic** influences. Review **Figures 4.14–4.15**

6 Several genes affect the buildup of **beta-amyloid** in **amyloid plaques** and increase the risk of **Alzheimer's disease**, but there are growing doubts about whether amyloid *causes* the symptoms. Adequate sleep and mental and physical activity can postpone the onset of the disease. Review **Figures 4.16–4.18**

The Mind's Machine digital resources include additional videos, flashcards, and other study tools.

5 The Sensorimotor System

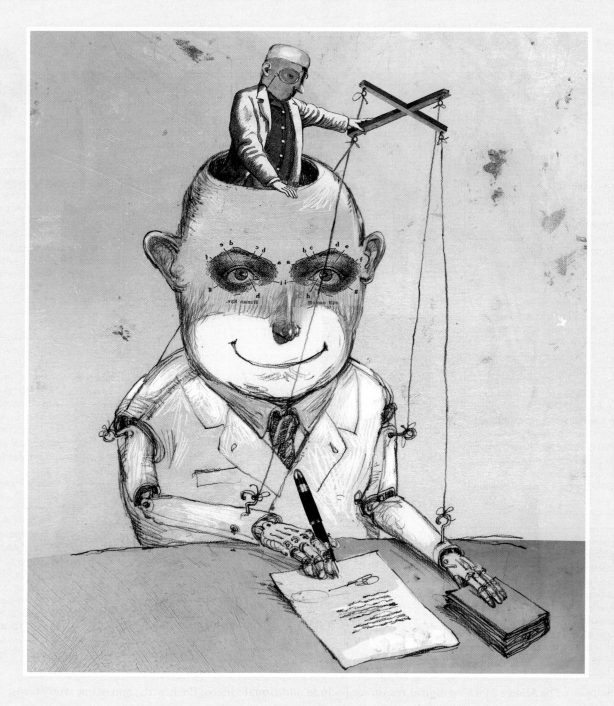

What You See Is What You Get

Ian Waterman had a perfectly ordinary life until he caught a viral infection at age 19. For reasons no one understands, the infection targeted a very specific set of nerves sending information from his body to his brain. Ian can still feel pain or deep pressure, as well as warm and cool surfaces on his skin, but he has no sensation of light touch below his neck. What's more, although Ian can still move all of his muscles, he receives no information about muscle activity or body position (Cole, 1995, 2016). You might think this deficiency wouldn't cause any problem, because you've probably never thought much about your "body sense"; it's not even one of the five senses that people talk about, is it?

In fact, however, the loss of this information was devastating. Ian couldn't walk across a room without falling down, and he couldn't walk up or down stairs. The few other people suffering a loss like this spent the rest of their lives in wheelchairs. But Ian was a young and determined person, so he started teaching himself how to walk using another source of feedback about his body: his vision. Now, as long as the lights are on, Ian can carefully watch his moving body to judge which motor commands to send out to keep walking. If the lights go out, however, Ian collapses, and he has learned that in that circumstance he just has to lie where he is until the lights come on again. He has so finely honed this ability to guide movements with vision that if asked to point repeatedly to the same location in the air, he does so more accurately than control participants do. Still, it's a mental drain to have to watch and attend constantly to his body just to do everyday tasks.

Today Ian has a good job and an active, independent life, but he is always vigilant. Lying in bed, he has to be very careful to remain calm, tethering his limbs with the covers to prevent them from flailing about.

And the lights are always on at Ian's house.

E very individual of every species is immersed in a sea of environmental cues that signal opportunities and hazards. Molecules in the air are sensed as odors—of food, or mates, or smoke. Vibrations traveling through air are perceived as sounds, ranging from infant cries to the roar of a predator (or a waterfall). Light reflected from surfaces is used to create a visual representation of the world.

We open this chapter by considering basic principles of sensory processing, using the sense of touch to illustrate some of the major concepts. We then take a closer look at an unpleasant but crucial sense: pain. To conclude the chapter, we turn our attention to the integration of sensory inputs to guide our movement: the streamlined system that allows us to interact with our environment.

**See Video 5.1:
Sensory Systems**

5.1 Sensory Processing and the Somatosensory System

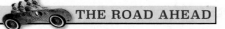

THE ROAD AHEAD

The first portion of the chapter covers the general principles that apply to all sensory systems, using touch as an example. Reading this material should allow you to:

5.1.1 Understand the concepts of labeled lines and sensory transduction.

5.1.2 Describe several different types of receptors in the skin and the stimuli they detect.

5.1.3 Relate the concepts of receptive fields and sensory adaptation.

5.1.4 Describe the neural pathway for the system reporting touch information from the body.

Because species differ in the environmental features they must sense for survival, evolution has endowed each species with its own unique set of capabilities. Bats are specially equipped to detect their own ultrasonic cries, which we humans are unable to hear. Some snakes have infrared-sensing organs in their faces that allow them to "see" heat sources (like a warm, tasty mouse) in the dark. Some of the impressive array of sensory modalities that animals possess are listed in **TABLE 5.1**.

Receptor cells detect various forms of energy

All animals have sensory organs containing **receptor cells** that sense some forms of energy—called **stimuli**—but not others. So in a way, receptor cells act as filters, ignoring the environmental background and converting the key stimuli into the language of the nervous system: electrical signals. Information from sensory receptors floods the brain in an unending barrage of action potentials traveling along millions of axons, and our brains must make sense of it all. What type of stimulus was that, where did it come from, how intense was it, etc. Of course, different kinds of energy—light, sound, touch, and so on—need different sensory organs to convert them into neural activity, just as taking a photograph requires a camera, not a microphone. There is tremendous diversity in sensory organs across the animal kingdom; for example, the eye is just one type of sensory organ, yet it is found in a dazzling array of sizes, shapes, and forms, reflecting the varying survival needs of different animals. Likewise, the specific auditory abilities of species reflect their unique ecological pressures (**FIGURE 5.1**).

Although the end product of sensory receptors—action potentials—is the same for all the different sensory modalities, the brain recognizes the modalities as separate and distinct because the action potentials for each sense are carried in separate nerve tracts. This is the concept of **labeled lines**: particular neurons that are, right from the outset, labeled for distinctive sensory experiences. Action potentials in one line signal a sound, activity in another line signals a smell, and activity in other lines signals touch. And there are labeled lines within general sensory categories too; for example, we can distinguish different types of touch because our skin contains a variety of receptors and uses some lines to signal

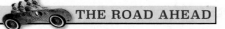
View Animation 5.2: Brain Explorer

receptor cell A specialized cell that responds to a particular energy or substance in the internal or external environment and converts this energy into a change in the electrical potential across its membrane.

stimulus A physical event that triggers a sensory response.

labeled lines The concept that each nerve input to the brain reports only a particular type of information.

TABLE 5.1 Classification of Sensory Systems

System type	Modality	Sensed stimuli
Mechanical	Touch	Contact with body surface
	Pain	Tissue damage
	Hearing	Sound vibrations in air or water
	Vestibular	Head movement and orientation
	Joint	Position and movement
	Muscle	Tension
Light	Vision	Photons, from light sources or reflected from surfaces
Thermal	Cold	Decrease in skin temperature
	Warmth	Increase in skin temperature
Chemical	Smell	Odorant chemicals in air
	Taste	Substances in contact with the tongue or other taste receptors
	Vomeronasal	Pheromones in air or water
Electrical	Electroreception	Differences in density of electrical currents
Magnetic	Magnetoreception	Magnetic fields for orientation

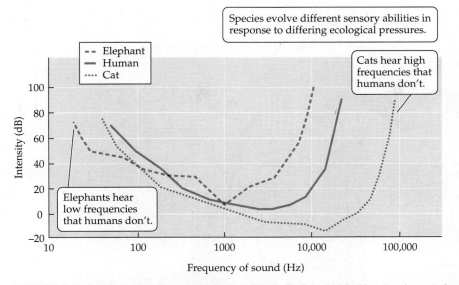

Species evolve different sensory abilities in response to differing ecological pressures.

Cats hear high frequencies that humans don't.

Elephants hear low frequencies that humans don't.

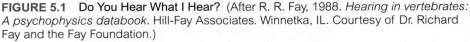

FIGURE 5.1   Do You Hear What I Hear? (After R. R. Fay, 1988. *Hearing in vertebrates: A psychophysics databook*. Hill-Fay Associates. Winnetka, IL. Courtesy of Dr. Richard Fay and the Fay Foundation.)

light touch, others to signal vibration, and yet other lines to signal stretching of the skin (**FIGURE 5.2**).

Receptor cells convert sensory signals into electrical activity

The structure of a receptor cell determines the particular kind of energy or chemical to which it will respond. And although a wide variety of cellular mechanisms are used to detect different stimuli, the outcome is always the same: an electrical change in the receptor, called a **receptor potential** (or *generator potential*), that resembles the

receptor potential   Also called *generator potential*. A local change in the resting potential of a receptor cell in response to stimuli, which may initiate an action potential.

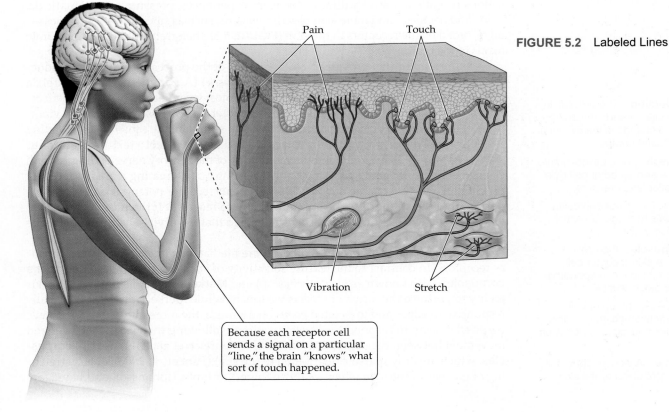

FIGURE 5.2   Labeled Lines

Pain

Touch

Vibration

Stretch

Because each receptor cell sends a signal on a particular "line," the brain "knows" what sort of touch happened.

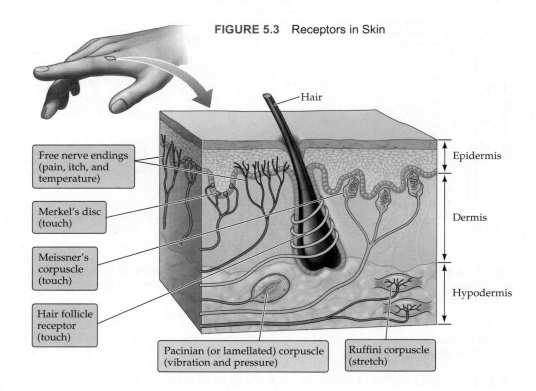

FIGURE 5.3 Receptors in Skin

Hair

Free nerve endings (pain, itch, and temperature)

Merkel's disc (touch)

Meissner's corpuscle (touch)

Hair follicle receptor (touch)

Pacinian (or lamellated) corpuscle (vibration and pressure)

Ruffini corpuscle (stretch)

Epidermis

Dermis

Hypodermis

sensory transduction   The process in which a receptor cell converts the energy in a stimulus into a change in the electrical potential across its membrane.

Pacinian corpuscle   Also called *lamellated corpuscle*. A skin receptor cell type that detects vibration and pressure.

threshold   Here, the stimulus intensity that is just adequate to trigger an action potential in a sensory cell.

Meissner's corpuscle   Also called *tactile corpuscle*. A skin receptor cell type that detects light touch, responding especially to changes in stimuli.

Merkel's disc   A skin receptor cell type that detects light touch, responding especially to edges and isolated points on a surface.

Ruffini corpuscle   A skin receptor cell type that detects stretching of the skin.

excitatory postsynaptic potentials we discussed in Chapter 3. Converting the signal in this way—from environmental stimuli into action potentials that our brain can understand—is called **sensory transduction**.

Our skin contains a rich array of receptors that transduce different forms of energy to provide our sense of touch. But touch is not just touch. Careful studies of skin sensations reveal qualitatively different sensory experiences: pressure, vibration, tickle, "pins and needles," and more-complex dimensions, such as smoothness or wetness—all recorded by the receptors in the skin (**FIGURE 5.3**), then transmitted along separate axons to the brain.

A skin receptor that provides a clear example of the process of sensory transduction is the **Pacinian corpuscle** (or *lamellated corpuscle*) (A. Zimmerman et al., 2014), a tiny onion-like structure embedded in the innermost layer of the skin that selectively responds to vibration and pressure. Acting as a filter, the corpuscle allows only vibrations of more than about 200 cycles per second to stimulate the sensory nerve ending inside it; this type of stimulation is what's created when we feel a texture against our skin (see Figure 5.3). By stretching the membrane of the sensory nerve ending, stimuli cause mechanically gated sodium channels to pop open, creating a graded receptor potential (**FIGURE 5.4**). The amplitude (size) of this receptor potential is directly proportional to the strength of the stimulus that was received. If the receptor potential exceeds **threshold**, action potentials are generated that travel via sensory nerves to the spinal cord.

Other dimensions of the sense of touch are mediated by their own unique sensory receptors. In contrast to the texture sensitivity of Pacinian corpuscles, **Meissner's corpuscles** (also known as *tactile corpuscles*) and **Merkel's discs** mediate most of our ability to perceive the forms of objects we touch. While Merkel's discs are especially responsive to edges and to isolated *points* on a surface, the more numerous Meissner's corpuscles seem to respond to *changes* in stimuli, allowing them to detect localized movement between the skin and a surface (Heidenreich et al., 2011). **Ruffini corpuscles**, which are only sparsely distributed in the skin (Pare et al., 2003), detect stretching of patches of the skin when we move fingers or limbs (Johansson and Flanagan,

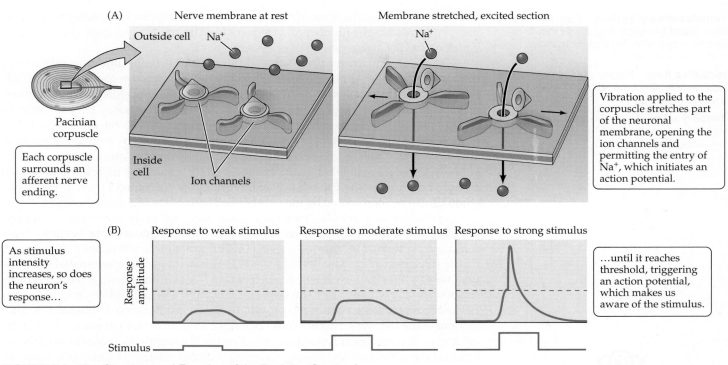

(A) Nerve membrane at rest

Outside cell   Na⁺

Pacinian corpuscle

Each corpuscle surrounds an afferent nerve ending.

Inside cell   Ion channels

Membrane stretched, excited section

Na⁺

Vibration applied to the corpuscle stretches part of the neuronal membrane, opening the ion channels and permitting the entry of Na⁺, which initiates an action potential.

(B)

As stimulus intensity increases, so does the neuron's response…

Response amplitude

Response to weak stimulus   Response to moderate stimulus   Response to strong stimulus

…until it reaches threshold, triggering an action potential, which makes us aware of the stimulus.

Stimulus

FIGURE 5.4   The Structure and Function of the Pacinian Corpuscle

2009). Finally, pain, itch, heat, and cold stimuli are detected by **free nerve endings** in the skin (see Figure 5.3), which we'll return to a little later in the chapter. All of these sensory receptors are found in their highest concentrations in regions of the skin where our sense of touch is finest (fingertips, tongue, and lips).

View Activity 5.1: Receptors in Skin

HOW'S IT GOING ?

1. Discuss the relationship between the ecology of a species and its sensory capabilities.
2. What are labeled lines? What do they transmit?
3. Give a general explanation of sensory transduction. What is a receptor potential?
4. Identify and describe four sensory receptors found in the skin.

Sensory information processing is selective and analytical

Many people assume that the sensory systems simply capture an accurate snapshot of stimulation and transmit it to the brain—in other words, that the sensory systems provide an uncolored window on the world. But neuroscientists realize that the sensory organs and pathways convey only limited—*even distorted*—information to the brain. A good deal of selection and analysis takes place along sensory pathways, before the information ever reaches the brain. So the brain ultimately receives a highly filtered representation of the external world, in which stimuli that are critical for survival are strongly emphasized at the expense of less important stimuli. This processing and filtering is seen in several aspects of sensory transduction, including stimulus coding and processing across receptive fields, as well as in adaptation and active suppression by the brain, which we discuss next.

Sensory events are encoded as streams of action potentials

We've already seen that the nervous system uses labeled lines to identify the *type* of stimulus that is encountered. But how do sensory neurons tell the brain about the *intensity* or *location* of a stimulus? Because the action potentials produced by a sensory

free nerve ending   An axon that terminates in the skin and has no specialized cell associated with it. Free nerve endings detect pain or itch, or changes in temperature.

somatosensory system A set of specialized receptors and neural mechanisms responsible for body sensations such as touch and pain.

receptive field The stimulus region and features that affect the activity of a cell in a sensory system.

sensory adaptation The progressive loss of receptor response as stimulation is maintained.

View Animation 5.3:
Somatosensory Receptive Fields

neuron always have the same size and duration, the intensity of a sensory stimulus must be *encoded* in the number and frequency of the action potentials, the rhythm in which clusters of action potentials occur, and so on.

We can respond to amazingly small differences in stimulus intensity, over a wide range of intensities. Although a single sensory receptor neuron could simply encode the intensity of a stimulus in the frequency of action potentials that the cell produces, only a very limited range of intensities could be represented this way, because neurons can fire only so fast (up to maybe 1,200 action potentials per second, and probably less in most neurons). Some sensory systems solve this problem by employing multiple sensory receptor cells, each specializing in just one part of the overall range of intensities, to cover the whole range. As the strength of a stimulus increases, additional sensory neurons sensitive to the higher intensities are "recruited"; thus, intensity of a stimulus can be represented by the number and thresholds of activated cells.

The position of a stimulus, either outside or inside the body, is likewise an important piece of information. Some sensory systems—the **somatosensory system** ("body sensation" system), for example—reveal this information by the position of receptors on the sensory surface. Thanks to labeled lines that uniquely convey spatial information, we can directly encode which patch of skin that darn mosquito is biting, in order to know exactly where to aim the slap. Similarly, in the visual system an object's spatial location determines which receptors in the eye are stimulated. In bilateral receptor systems—the two eyes, two ears, and two nostrils—differences in stimulation of the left and right receptors are encoded, providing the brain with additional cues to the location of the stimulus (this type of processing is discussed in more detail in Chapter 6).

Neurons at all levels of the visual and the touch pathways—from the surface sheet of receptors all the way up to the cerebral cortex—are arranged in an orderly, maplike manner. The map at each level is not exact, but it does reflect both spatial positions and receptor density. More cells are allocated to the spatial representation of sensitive, densely innervated sites, like the lips, than to sites that are less sensitive, such as the skin of the back. Each cell in the sensory map thus preferentially responds to a particular type of stimulus occurring in a particular place, as we'll see next.

Sensory neurons respond to stimuli falling in their receptive fields

The **receptive field** of a sensory neuron consists of a region of space in which a stimulus will alter that neuron's firing rate. To determine this receptive field, investigators record the neuron's electrical responses to a variety of stimuli to see what makes the activity of that cell change from its resting rate. For example, which patch of skin must we stimulate to change the activity of one particular touch receptor? Experiments show that these somatosensory receptive fields are shaped like doughnuts, with either an excitatory center and an inhibitory surround (**FIGURE 5.5**), or an inhibitory center and an excitatory surround. Such somatosensory receptive fields make it easier to detect edges on the objects we feel. Receptive fields differ in size and shape and in the quality of stimulation that activates them. For example, some neurons respond preferentially to light touch, while others fire most rapidly in response to painful stimuli, and still others respond to cooling.

Experiments tracing sensory information along the pathway from the receptor cell to the brain show that neurons at every level will respond to particular stimuli, so each of these cells has its own receptive field. But as each successive neuron performs additional processing, the receptive fields change considerably, as we will see later in this chapter and in Chapter 6 and Chapter 7.

RECEPTORS MAY SHOW ADAPTATION TO UNCHANGING STIMULI **Sensory adaptation** is the progressive decrease in a receptor's response to sustained stimulation (**FIGURE 5.6**). This process allows us to ignore unimportant events. By not noticing the touch of our clothes on our skin, the buzz of overhead lights, and other stimuli that are unchanging, our sensory systems avoid overload and can remain vigilant for

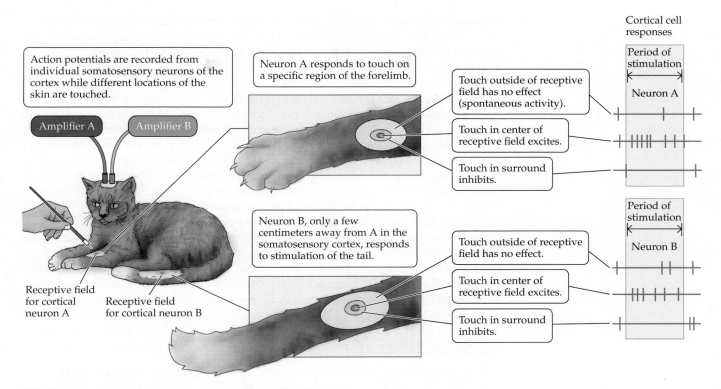

FIGURE 5.5 Identifying Somatosensory Receptive Fields

critical events. Neuroscientists distinguish between **phasic receptors**, which display this sort of adaptation, and **tonic receptors**, which show little or no adaptation and thus can signal the duration of a stimulus. (As each of us knows all too well, pain sensors are often tonic receptors, maintaining a high level of activity to help us avoid further injury.)

The process of adaptation illustrates the principle we referred to earlier in our discussion of selection and analysis: sensory systems often shift *away from accurate portrayal* of the external world. In some mechanical receptors, such as the Pacinian

phasic receptor A receptor in which the frequency of action potentials drops rapidly as stimulation is maintained.

tonic receptor A receptor in which the frequency of action potentials declines slowly or not at all as stimulation is maintained.

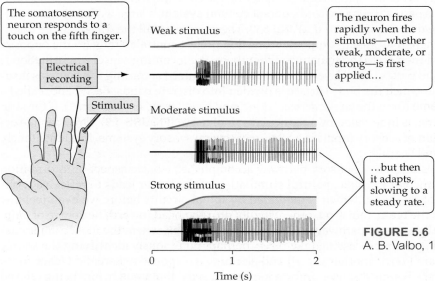

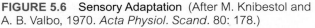

FIGURE 5.6 **Sensory Adaptation** (After M. Knibestol and A. B. Valbo, 1970. *Acta Physiol. Scand.* 80: 178.)

corpuscle described earlier, adaptation develops from the elasticity of the receptor cell itself. When the corpuscle (which is a separate, accessory structure) is removed, the uncovered sensory nerve fiber does not adapt, but continues discharging action potentials in response to a constant stimulus.

SOMETIMES WE NEED RECEPTORS TO BE QUIET We've already noted that survival depends more on sensitivity to important *changes* than on exact reporting of stimuli. To maintain such sensitivity, we need to suppress unneeded or unimportant sensory activity. As we just discussed, adaptation is one way in which sensory activity is controlled, and we are equipped with two additional suppression systems.

One way to suppress sensory activity is simply to physically prevent the stimuli from reaching the sensors. Closing the eyelids provides this function in the visual system; in the auditory system, tiny middle-ear muscles reduce the intensity of sounds that reach the inner ear. A second kind of suppression of sensory inputs is entirely neural in nature. In many sensory and pain pathways, reciprocal neural connections descend from the brain to synapse on lower sensory levels, where they can then inhibit activity in the ascending sensory axons. This **central modulation of sensory information**, whereby the brain actively controls the information it receives, is a feature of many sensory and pain pathways. Such modulation helps the brain attend to some stimuli more than others.

HOW'S IT GOING ❓

1. In general terms, explain how a sensory event is encoded in action potentials in sensory fibers.
2. Why do some receptor cells respond only to strong stimuli?
3. Describe receptive fields and how scientists detect them.
4. Name and briefly describe a couple of processes that change a sensory neuron's response to stimuli.

Successive levels of the CNS process sensory information

Sensory information travels from the sensory surface to the highest levels of the brain, and each sensory system—such as touch, vision, or hearing—has its own distinctive pathway from the periphery to successively higher levels of the spinal cord and/or brain. For example, the somatosensory touch receptors that we've been discussing send their axons—eventually bundled into sensory nerves—from the skin to the dorsal (rear) part of the spinal cord. On entering the cord, the somatosensory projections ascend as part of the spinal cord's **dorsal column system**, a large wedge of white matter in the dorsal spinal cord (**FIGURE 5.7**). These axons go all the way up to the brainstem, where they synapse onto neurons that project contralaterally (to the opposite side) and then go to the thalamus. From there, the incoming sensory information is directed to cortex. At all levels, the inputs are organized according to a somatosensory map in which the body surface is divided into discrete bands. Each band, called a **dermatome** (from the Greek *derma*, "skin," and *tome*, "part" or "segment"), is the strip of skin that is innervated by a particular spinal nerve (**FIGURE 5.8**). This maplike organization of sensory inputs is a feature of several sensory systems, including touch, vision, and hearing.

Each station in a sensory pathway accomplishes a basic aspect of information processing. For example, painful stimulation of the finger leads to reflexive withdrawal of the hand, which is mediated by spinal circuits before we even feel any pain. At the brainstem level, other circuits turn the head toward the source of pain. Eventually, sensory pathways reach the cerebral cortex, where the most complex aspects of sensory processing take place, perhaps consciously identifying the source of the pain (darn, another sliver!) and planning a response (where did I leave those tweezers?). For most senses, information reaches the **thalamus** before being relayed

central modulation of sensory information The process in which higher brain centers, such as the cortex and thalamus, suppress some sources of sensory information and amplify others.

dorsal column system A somatosensory system that delivers most touch stimuli to the brain via the dorsal columns of spinal white matter.

dermatome A strip of skin innervated by a particular spinal nerve.

thalamus The brain regions at the top of the brainstem that trade information with the cortex.

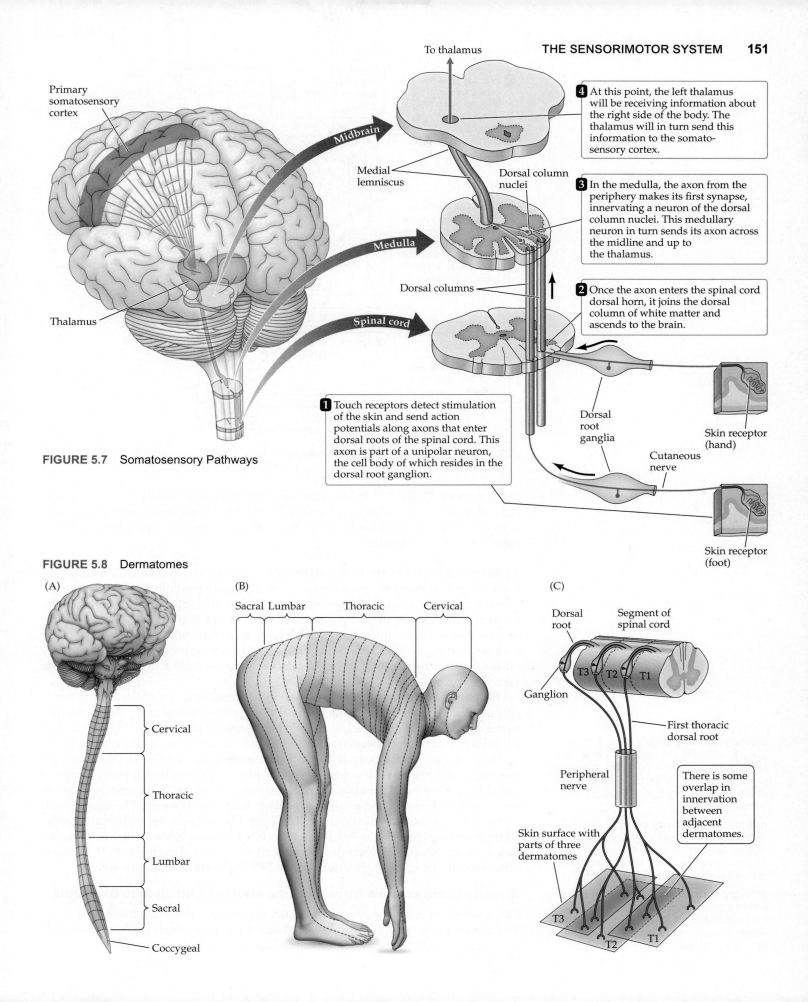

To thalamus

Primary
somatosensory
cortex

Midbrain

Medial
lemniscus

Thalamus

Medulla

Dorsal column
nuclei

Dorsal columns

Spinal cord

Dorsal
root
ganglia

Cutaneous
nerve

Skin receptor
(hand)

Skin receptor
(foot)

4 At this point, the left thalamus
will be receiving information about
the right side of the body. The
thalamus will in turn send this
information to the somatosensory cortex.

3 In the medulla, the axon from the
periphery makes its first synapse,
innervating a neuron of the dorsal
column nuclei. This medullary
neuron in turn sends its axon across
the midline and up to
the thalamus.

2 Once the axon enters the spinal cord
dorsal horn, it joins the dorsal
column of white matter and
ascends to the brain.

1 Touch receptors detect stimulation
of the skin and send action
potentials along axons that enter
dorsal roots of the spinal cord. This
axon is part of a unipolar neuron,
the cell body of which resides in the
dorsal root ganglion.

FIGURE 5.7 Somatosensory Pathways

FIGURE 5.8 Dermatomes

(A)

Cervical

Thoracic

Lumbar

Sacral

Coccygeal

(B)

Sacral Lumbar   Thoracic   Cervical

(C)

Dorsal
root

Segment of
spinal cord

Ganglion

T3 T2 T1

First thoracic
dorsal root

Peripheral
nerve

Skin surface with
parts of three
dermatomes

There is some
overlap in
innervation
between
adjacent
dermatomes.

T3

T2 T1

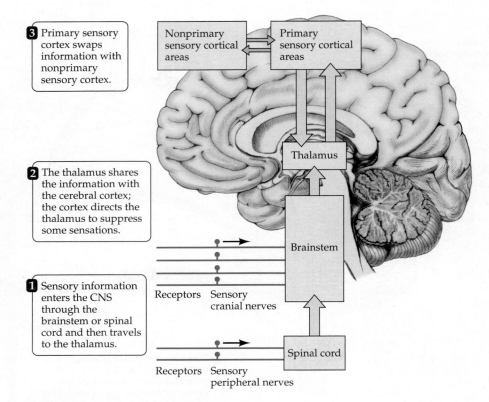

3 Primary sensory cortex swaps information with nonprimary sensory cortex.

2 The thalamus shares the information with the cerebral cortex; the cortex directs the thalamus to suppress some sensations.

1 Sensory information enters the CNS through the brainstem or spinal cord and then travels to the thalamus.

FIGURE 5.9   Levels of Sensory Processing

to the cortex (**FIGURE 5.9**). Information about each sensory modality is sent to a separate division of the thalamus. One way for the brain to suppress particular stimuli is for the cortex to direct the thalamus to emphasize some sensory information and suppress other information.

SENSORY CORTEX IS HIGHLY ORGANIZED   Researchers have identified a region designated as **primary sensory cortex** for each sensory modality—primary somatosensory cortex, primary auditory cortex, and so on—that is generally the initial destination of sensory inputs to the cortex. However, other cortical regions may receive and process the same information, often in collaboration with the primary sensory cortex; sensibly enough (pardon the pun), we call these regions **nonprimary sensory cortex** (see Figure 5.9). Each cortical sensory region processes different aspects of our perceptual experiences.

Primary somatosensory cortex (also called *somatosensory 1* or *S1*) of each hemisphere is located in the postcentral gyrus, the long strip of tissue that lies just posterior to the central sulcus dividing the parietal lobe from the frontal lobe (**FIGURE 5.10A**). S1 receives touch information from the opposite side of the body. The cells in S1 are arranged as a map of the body (**FIGURE 5.10B**), but it is a very unusual, distorted map: the size of each region on the map is proportional to the density of sensory receptors found in that region of the skin. Parts of the body where we are especially sensitive to touch (like the hand and fingers) have large representations in S1 compared with less sensitive areas (like the shoulder). This proportional mapping is illustrated in the strange-looking character in **FIGURE 5.10C**, called a *sensory homunculus,* in whom the size of each body part reflects the proportion of S1 devoted to that part. We discuss other aspects of cortical organization in **A STEP FURTHER 5.1**, on the website.

Sensory brain regions influence one another and change over time

Often the use of one sensory system influences perception from another sensory system. For example, humans detect a visual signal more accurately if it is accompanied by a sound from the same part of space (Hillyard et al., 2016).

primary sensory cortex   For a given sensory modality, the region of cortex that receives most of the information about that modality from the thalamus (or, in the case of olfaction, directly from the secondary sensory neurons).

nonprimary sensory cortex   Also called *secondary sensory cortex.* For a given sensory modality, the cortical regions receiving direct projections from primary sensory cortex for that modality.

primary somatosensory cortex   Also called *somatosensory 1* or *S1.* Primarily the postcentral gyrus of the parietal lobe, where sensory inputs from the body surface are mapped.

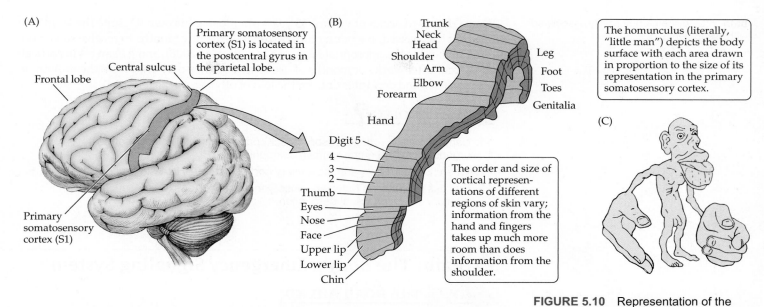

FIGURE 5.10 Representation of the Body Surface in Somatosensory Cortex

Many sensory areas in the brain—called *association areas*—process a mixture of inputs from different modalities. Some "visual" cells, for instance, also respond to auditory or touch stimuli. The convergence of information from different sensory systems on these **polymodal neurons** allows different sensory systems to interact (B. E. Stein and Stanford, 2008). And for a few people, a stimulus in one sensory modality may evoke an additional perception in another sensory modality, as when seeing a number evokes a color, or music literally becomes a matter of taste, where each note has both a sound and a flavor (Beeli et al., 2005). This condition is known as **synesthesia**. For more information and an example of synesthesia, see **A STEP FURTHER 5.2**, on the website.

At one time, most researchers thought that sensory regions of cortex were fixed early in life. Now, however, we know that cortical maps are highly plastic, changing considerably as a result of experience (D. T. Blake et al., 2006). For example, two artists born without arms who used their toes extensively had distinct maps of each toe, unlike control participants (Dempsey-Jones et al., 2019). Professional musicians who play stringed instruments have expanded cortical representations of their left fingers, presumably because they use these fingers to depress the strings for precisely the right notes (Münte et al., 2002). Brain imaging also reveals cortical reorganization in people who lose a hand in adulthood (**FIGURE 5.11**). One man received a transplanted hand

polymodal neuron A neuron upon which information from more than one sensory system converges.

synesthesia A condition in which stimuli in one modality evoke the involuntary experience of an additional sensation in another modality.

(A)

Normally, the hand region of S1 lies between the regions representing the upper arm and the face.

Face
Hand
Arm
Central sulcus

(B)

After the loss of one hand, the cortical regions representing the upper arm and face expand, taking over the cortical region previously representing the missing hand.

Region formerly stimulated by receptors in the hand now responds to touch on face or arm.

FIGURE 5.11 Plasticity in Somatosensory Cortex (After T. T. Yang et al., 1994. *NeuroReport* 5: 701.)

pain   The discomfort normally associated with tissue damage.

(from a deceased accident victim) 35 years after losing his own. Despite the length of time that had passed, his brain reorganized in just a few months to receive sensation from the hand in the appropriate part of S1 (Frey et al., 2008). Some changes in cortical maps occur after weeks or months of use or disuse; they may arise from the growth of new synapses and dendrites or from the loss of others.

HOW'S IT GOING ❓

1. Name the main somatosensory (touch) pathway to the brain, describe its organization, and name its main components.
2. Where is the primary somatosensory cortex located? How is it organized?
3. Discuss interactions between sensory modalities—for example, effects of auditory inputs on visual perception.

5.2 Pain: The Body's Emergency Signaling System

THE ROAD AHEAD

This next section describes the system bringing us the unpleasant but adaptive sensation of pain. Studying this material should enable you to:

5.2.1 List and describe the three separate components of pain experience.

5.2.2 Describe the neuronal receptor cells that detect painful stimuli and the molecular receptor proteins they use.

5.2.3 Trace the neuronal pathway that transmits pain information from the periphery to the brain, as well as the neuronal pathway by which the brain can modulate pain.

5.2.4 Discuss the various methods for controlling pain, including advantages and disadvantages of each.

One important aspect of body sensation is at best a mixed blessing. The International Association for the Study of Pain defines **pain** as "an unpleasant sensory and emotional experience associated with actual or potential tissue damage, or described in terms of such damage." Pain forcefully guides our behavior in several ways that minimize the risk to our bodies (Melzack et al., 2001). Immediate, short-term pain causes us to withdraw from the source, often reflexively, thus preventing further damage. Longer-lasting pain encourages behaviors, such as sleep, inactivity, grooming, feeding, and drinking, that promote recuperation. And the pain-related social communication—grimacing, groaning, shrieking, and the rest of the miserable lineup—provides a warning to kin and elicits caregiving behaviors from them, including grooming, defending, and feeding.

Learning, experience, emotion, and culture all affect our perception of pain in striking ways, and these factors may strongly influence people's descriptions of pain, ranging from an apparent absence of pain in badly injured soldiers and athletes, to the anguish of a child with a paper cut. A widely used quantitative measure of pain perception—the McGill Pain Questionnaire (Main, 2016)—asks people to select words that tap three different dimensions of pain:

1. The *sensory-discriminative* dimension (e.g., throbbing, gnawing, shooting)
2. The *motivational-affective* (emotional) dimension (e.g., tiring, sickening, fearful)
3. An overall *cognitive-evaluative* dimension (e.g., no pain, mild, excruciating)

Researchers found that people use different constellations of descriptors in various forms of pain: tooth pain is described differently from arthritic pain, which in turn is

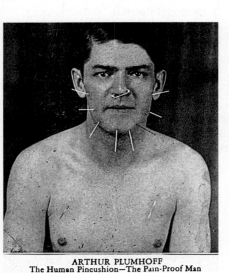

ARTHUR PLUMHOFF
The Human Pincushion—The Pain-Proof Man

Doesn't That Hurt?   Although it might seem like a blessing, people with congenital insensitivity to pain, like the "Human Pincushion" pictured here, tend to die young as a consequence of repeated body injuries.

© Chronicle/Alamy Stock Photo

described differently from menstrual pain. This more detailed analysis provides better information for the diagnosis and treatment of illness.

A discrete pain pathway projects from body to brain

Most tissues of the body (but not all) contain receptors specialized for detecting painful stimuli. These receptors are particularly well studied in the skin; in this section we discuss some features of these receptors, along with the peripheral and CNS pathways that mediate pain.

PERIPHERAL RECEPTORS GET THE INITIAL MESSAGE   When tissue is injured, the affected cells release chemicals that activate nearby pain receptors, called **nociceptors**, on free nerve endings specialized to detect damage. These chemicals also cause inflammation (**FIGURE 5.12**). Many different substances in injured tissue—serotonin, histamine, and various enzymes and peptides, to name just a few—can stimulate these nociceptors. Different nociceptors respond to various stimuli, such as pain and/or changes in temperature.

Identification of the nociceptor that detects *physical* damage was aided through careful study of the family of a Pakistani boy who died in tragic circumstances—performing dangerous pranks because he could feel no pain. Scientists isolated a mutation in a gene (called *SCN9A*) that appears to be responsible for his congenital insensitivity to pain (CIP). Children with CIP require constant monitoring to prevent them from poking out their eyes or pulling out their teeth (Oppenheim, 2006). The *SCN9A* gene encodes a sodium channel expressed in free nerve endings that serve as nociceptors (J. J. Cox et al., 2006), offering a new target for developing high-potency pain medication.

Some free nerve endings detect temperature changes. Studies of capsaicin, the chemical that makes chili peppers spicy hot, helped reveal the receptor that signals sudden increases in temperature (this action is the reason spicy food seems to *burn*)

nociceptor   A receptor that responds to stimuli that produce tissue damage or pose the threat of damage.

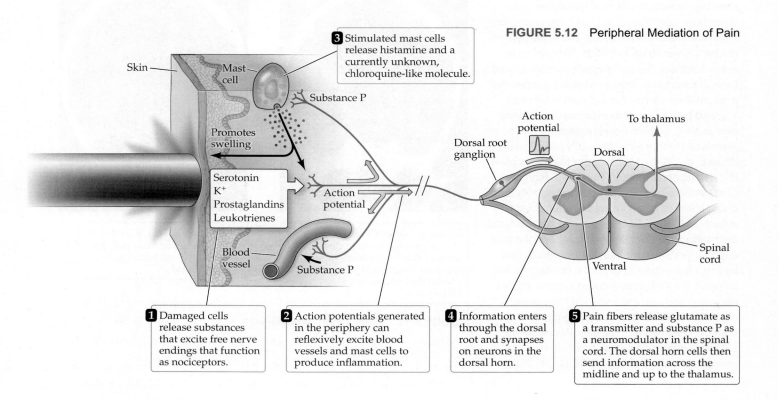

FIGURE 5.12   Peripheral Mediation of Pain

3 Stimulated mast cells release histamine and a currently unknown, chloroquine-like molecule.

Skin

Mast cell

Substance P

Promotes swelling

Serotonin
K⁺
Prostaglandins
Leukotrienes

Action potential

Blood vessel

Substance P

Action potential

Dorsal root ganglion

Action potential

To thalamus

Dorsal

Ventral

Spinal cord

1 Damaged cells release substances that excite free nerve endings that function as nociceptors.

2 Action potentials generated in the periphery can reflexively excite blood vessels and mast cells to produce inflammation.

4 Information enters through the dorsal root and synapses on neurons in the dorsal horn.

5 Pain fibers release glutamate as a transmitter and substance P as a neuromodulator in the spinal cord. The dorsal horn cells then send information across the midline and up to the thalamus.

(C. Moore et al., 2018). This receptor, with the not-so-spicy name *transient receptor potential vanilloid type 1* (*TRPV1*, or just *vanilloid receptor 1*), belongs to a larger family of proteins called *transient receptor potential (TRP) ion channels*. Mice lacking the gene for TRPV1 still respond to mechanosensory pain, but not to mild heat or capsaicin (Caterina et al., 2000).

TRPV1's normal job is to report a rise in temperature to warn us of danger, so chili peppers cleverly evolved capsaicin to ward off mammalian predators—by falsely signaling burning heat. A related receptor, **transient receptor potential type M3 (TRPM3)**, detects even higher temperatures than does TRPV1, but it does *not* respond to capsaicin (Vriens and Voets, 2018). TRPM3 receptors are found on **A delta (Aδ) fibers**, which are large-diameter, myelinated axons. Because of the relatively large axon diameter and myelination, action potentials in these fibers reach the spinal cord very quickly. In contrast, the nerve fibers that possess TRPV1 receptors consist of thin, unmyelinated fibers called **C fibers**. So, when you burn your hand on that hot pan, the initial sharp pain you feel is conducted by the fat A delta fibers activated by their TRPM3 receptors, and the long-lasting dull ache that follows arises from slower C fibers and their TRPV1 receptors. Other members of the TRP family of receptors detect coolness as well as constituents of spices like oregano, cloves, garlic, and wasabi (Jordt et al., 2004; Bautista et al., 2007; Salazar et al., 2008), but their relation to pain receptors remains a delicious mystery (sorry). Stimulating your TRPV1 receptor too much can be hazardous to your health, as we see in Signs & Symptoms next.

transient receptor potential type M3 (TRPM3) A receptor, found in some free nerve endings, that opens its channel in response to rising temperatures.

A delta (Aδ) fiber A moderately large, myelinated, and therefore fast-conducting axon that usually transmits pain information.

C fiber A small, unmyelinated axon that conducts pain information slowly and adapts slowly.

SIGNS & SYMPTOMS ||||||||||||||||||||||||||||||||||||||||||||||||||||||||||||||||||||||||||||||||||||||||||||||||||||||||||||

A Professional Eater Meets His Match

The 34-year-old man was a professional eater, entering contests to see how quickly he could down huge quantities of food. He'd been moderately successful in this pursuit, but a chili pepper contest proved to be too much. After eating an entire "Carolina Reaper" pepper, purposely bred to be 6 times hotter than a habanero pepper, the man suffered dry heaves and pain in his neck followed by a series of thunderclap headaches: excruciating, sudden-onset headaches that peak in a minute before subsiding, only to return (Boddhula et al., 2018). MRI scans of the man's brain showed no abnormalities, but a CAT scan of blood vessels revealed that several arteries supplying his brain had narrowed to a remarkable extent (**FIGURE 5.13A**), which may have caused the headaches. Over the next few days, the man suffered several more thunderclap headaches lasting a few seconds. Once the headaches had stopped, the CAT scan showed that the arteries supplying his brain had expanded to a more normal size (**FIGURE 5.13B**). The gentleman may have gotten off lightly. People have suffered severe, even fatal, heart attacks after eating superhot chili peppers (N. Davis, 2018).

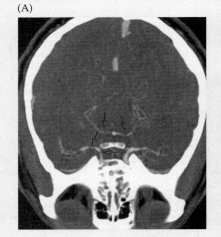

(A) (B)

From S. K. Boddhula et al., 2018, *BMJ Case Reports*, Courtesy of Kulothungan Gunasekaran

Eating an entire "Carolina Reaper" chili pepper appeared to close off some of the blood vessels supplying this man's brain, which may have caused the sudden, severe headaches he suffered.

Five weeks later, after the headaches had stopped, the blood vessels were much less constricted.

FIGURE 5.13   Thunderclap Headache

Special neural pathways carry pain information to the brain

Nerve fibers carrying information about pain and temperature send their axons to enter the dorsal horns of the spinal cord, where they synapse onto spinal neurons that project across the midline to the opposite side and then up toward the thalamus of the brain, forming the **anterolateral system** (or *spinothalamic system*) (**FIGURE 5.14**). This projection is distinct from the somatosensory system that we discussed earlier (the dorsal column system; see Figure 5.7), but as in that system, each hemisphere receives its inputs from the contralateral side of the body. Within the spinal cord, the arriving pain fibers release the excitatory transmitter glutamate along with a peptide, **substance P**, that selectively boosts pain signals and remodels pain pathway neurons (Zieglgänsberger, 2019). Mice lacking substance P cannot feel intense pain, but they still feel mild pain (Hökfelt et al., 2001).

Pain information is eventually integrated in the **cingulate cortex**, part of the limbic system we mentioned in Chapter 1 (see Figure 1.14B). The extent of activation in the cingulate (as well as in somatosensory) cortex correlates with how much discomfort different people report in response to the same mildly painful stimulus (Coghill et al., 2003). Different subregions of the cingulate cortex seem to mediate emotional

anterolateral system Also called *spinothalamic system*. A somatosensory system that carries most of the pain information from the body to the brain.

substance P A peptide transmitter that is involved in pain transmission.

cingulate cortex Also called *cingulum*. A region of medial cerebral cortex that lies dorsal to the corpus callosum.

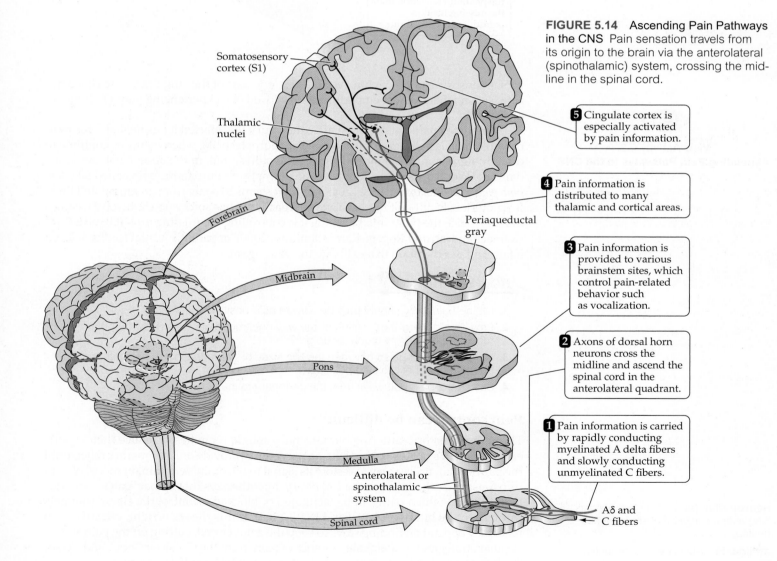

FIGURE 5.14 Ascending Pain Pathways in the CNS Pain sensation travels from its origin to the brain via the anterolateral (spinothalamic) system, crossing the midline in the spinal cord.

5 Cingulate cortex is especially activated by pain information.

4 Pain information is distributed to many thalamic and cortical areas.

3 Pain information is provided to various brainstem sites, which control pain-related behavior such as vocalization.

2 Axons of dorsal horn neurons cross the midline and ascend the spinal cord in the anterolateral quadrant.

1 Pain information is carried by rapidly conducting myelinated A delta fibers and slowly conducting unmyelinated C fibers.

Somatosensory cortex (S1)

Thalamic nuclei

Forebrain

Midbrain

Pons

Medulla

Spinal cord

Periaqueductal gray

Anterolateral or spinothalamic system

Aδ and C fibers

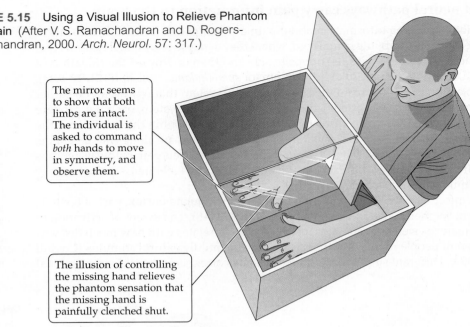

FIGURE 5.15 Using a Visual Illusion to Relieve Phantom Limb Pain (After V. S. Ramachandran and D. Rogers-Ramachandran, 2000. *Arch. Neurol.* 57: 317.)

The mirror seems to show that both limbs are intact. The individual is asked to command *both* hands to move in symmetry, and observe them.

The illusion of controlling the missing hand relieves the phantom sensation that the missing hand is painfully clenched shut.

View Activity 5.2: Ascending Pain Pathways in the CNS

versus sensory aspects of pain (Vogt, 2005); one part of the cingulate cortex becomes active even when we just empathize with a loved one experiencing pain (T. Singer et al., 2004).

Sometimes pain persists long after the injury that started it has healed. This **neuropathic pain** is a disagreeable example of neuroplasticity, where neurons continue to directly signal pain, and indeed *amplify* the pain signal, in the absence of any tissue damage (Woolf and Salter, 2000). In one example of neuropathic pain called *phantom limb pain*, patients experience great pain that seems to come from an amputated limb. It is notoriously difficult to treat. One approach that has some success involves using a mirror to trick the brain into believing it is controlling the missing limb (**FIGURE 5.15**) (Ramachandran and Rogers-Ramachandran, 2000); apparently, visual feedback (even if false) allows the brain to recalibrate the pain signal.

HOW'S IT GOING ?

1. Define *pain*. Why should pain be viewed as a positive adaptation?
2. Provide a general explanation of the way pain receptors work. How do pain receptors differ from touch receptors?
3. Name and distinguish between the two sizes of fibers that carry pain information from the periphery to the spinal cord.
4. Sketch the pain pathways from the periphery to the cortex.

Pain control can be difficult

Throughout history, suffering humans have sought remedies to reduce their experience of pain. It's not easy; even cutting nerves may provide only temporary relief, until the pain system finds a way to restore its signal to the brain. A dominant model of pain transmission, called the *gate control theory*, hypothesizes that spinal "gates"—modulation sites at which pain can be facilitated or blocked—control the signal that gets through to the brain (Melzack and Wall, 1965). If this theory is right, effective pain relief may depend on finding ways to keep the gates closed, cutting off the pain signal. Popular strategies for **analgesia** (absence of pain; from the Greek *an*, "not," and *algesis*, "feeling of pain") fall into four general categories, which we'll discuss next.

neuropathic pain   Pain that persists long after the injury that started it has healed.

analgesia   Absence of or reduction in pain.

Analgesic drugs are highly effective

The opiates (opium-related drugs, like morphine) have been known for centuries to relieve pain sensations. Along with brain-derived painkillers such as the **endorphins** and other endogenous opioids, opiate drugs bind to specific receptors in the brain to reduce pain (see Chapter 4). Researchers have found that this action is especially pronounced in the brainstem region called the *periaqueductal gray* (see Figure 5.14); one possibility is that the brainstem system activates the pain-gating mechanism of the spinal cord via descending projections, thereby blocking the transmission of pain signals. Similar benefits can be obtained by (carefully!) injecting opiates directly into the spinal cord; this is called an *epidural* or *intrathecal* injection.

Although people sometimes become addicted to painkillers, that is usually not true of people who are using them to treat severe pain; in fact, the danger of addiction from the use of morphine to relieve surgical pain has been vastly exaggerated and is estimated to be less than 1% (Brownlee and Schrof, 1997). Unfortunately, those few who do become addicted face a very real danger of death by overdose (Volkow et al., 2018); an opioid epidemic has been made worse by the development of extremely potent opioids such as OxyContin and fentanyl, resulting in more and more deaths (see Figure 3.9). If given in time, opioid antagonists like **naloxone** (Narcan) can save addicts' lives, so more and more public safety officers carry the drug.

Of course, there are other painkilling drugs, but none are as effective as the opiates. Over-the-counter medications like aspirin and acetaminophen (Tylenol) act via non-opiate mechanisms (especially the cyclooxygenase enzymes COX-1 and COX-2) to reduce pain and inflammation. Cannabis reduces pain by stimulating endogenous cannabinoid receptors (CB_1 receptors) in the spinal cord and in the brain (Agarwal et al., 2007; Pernía-Andrade et al., 2009).

Electrical stimulation can sometimes relieve pain

In **transcutaneous electrical nerve stimulation** (**TENS**), mild electrical stimulation is applied to nerves around the injury sites to relieve pain. The exact mechanism of this pain relief is not clear, but one possibility is that TENS closes the spinal "gate" for pain that Melzack and Wall (1965) described. Recall, for example, the last time you stubbed your toe. In addition to expelling a string of expletives, you may have vigorously rubbed the injured area, bringing a little relief. TENS is a more efficient way of stimulating those adjacent nerves, and it may bring dramatic relief lasting for hours (Vance et al., 2014). We know that TENS acts at least in part by releasing endogenous opioids, because administration of the opioid antagonist naloxone partially blocks this analgesic action (Gonçalves et al., 2014).

Placebos effectively control pain in some people, but not all

In some people, simply believing that they are receiving a proven treatment can effectively relieve pain. In a classic example of this **placebo effect**, when participants who had just had their wisdom teeth extracted were given morphine or a placebo, fully a third of those receiving the placebo experienced pain relief (J. D. Levine et al., 1978). But when the placebo was coadministered with a drug that blocks opioid receptors (naloxone), the participants did not experience the benefits of the placebo effect. This latter finding strongly implies that placebos work by activating the brain's endogenous opioid system. In fact, functional brain imaging indicates that opioids and placebos activate the same brain regions (Petrovic et al., 2002; D. J. Scott et al., 2008). For reasons unknown, some people consistently experience relief from placebos while others do not (**FIGURE 5.16**).

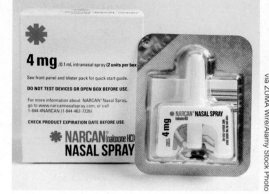

Life Saver   Naloxone is sometimes called the "Lazarus drug" for its ability to revive people dying of a narcotic overdose in less than a minute.

endorphin   One of three kinds of endogenous opioids.

naloxone   A potent antagonist of opiates that is often administered to people who have taken drug overdoses.

transcutaneous electrical nerve stimulation (TENS)   The delivery of electrical pulses through electrodes attached to the skin, which excite nerves that supply the region to which pain is referred.

placebo effect   Relief of a symptom, such as pain, that results following a treatment that is known to be ineffective or inert.

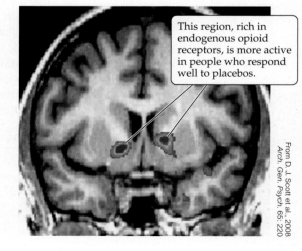

This region, rich in endogenous opioid receptors, is more active in people who respond well to placebos.

FIGURE 5.16   Placebos Affect Opioid Systems in the Brain

TABLE 5.2 Types of Pain Relief

Type	Mechanism
PSYCHOGENIC	
Placebo	May activate endorphin-mediated pain control system
Hypnosis	Alters brain's perception of pain
Stress	Uses both opioid and non-opioid mechanisms
Cognitive (learning, coping strategies)	May activate endorphin-mediated pain control system
PHARMACOLOGICAL	
Opiates	Bind to opioid receptors in periaqueductal gray and spinal cord
Spinal block	Blocks pain signals in spinal cord
Anti-inflammatory drugs	Block chemical inflammatory signals at the site of injury (see Figure 5.12)
Cannabinoids	Act in nociceptor endings, spinal cord, and brain
STIMULATION	
TENS/mechanical	On large fibers, blocks or alters pain signal to brain
Acupuncture	Activates endogenous opioids and/or placebo-like effect, possibly modulating effect on activity of peripheral pain pathways
Central gray	Electrically activates endorphin-mediated pain control systems, blocking pain signal in spinal cord

Activation of endogenous opioids relieves pain

acupuncture The insertion of needles at designated points on the skin to alleviate pain or neurological malfunction.

Although the ancient pain-relieving technique **acupuncture** remains very popular, only a minority of people using acupuncture achieve lasting relief from chronic pain. In those people for whom acupuncture is effective, a release of endorphins may be an important part of the process, since treatment with naloxone often blocks acupuncture's effectiveness (Staud and Price, 2006). Acupuncture thus resembles placebos in this regard. Although many rules govern needle placement in acupuncture, systematic research indicates that the placement of the needles actually has little to do with its effects on pain (Linde et al., 2009). The *expectation* that the needles will relieve pain appears to be the important factor, presumably inducing a release of endogenous opioids.

Likewise, stressful life events can produce significant analgesia; for example, tales abound of gravely wounded soldiers who feel no pain for some time after their injuries occur (Bowman, 1997). Research in animals indicates that stress activates both an opioid-dependent form of analgesia, which can be blocked by naloxone, and another, non-opioid analgesia system that has not yet been characterized (but may rely on endocannabinoids) (A. G. Hohmann et al., 2005). These endogenous analgesic systems allow a wounded individual to fight or escape rather than be overwhelmed with pain.

Pain relief remains a major challenge for neuroscience research. Chronic pain can have dramatic effects on the brain: for example, the prefrontal cortex in people with chronic back pain shrinks much faster than normal, as if the patients are rapidly aging (Apkarian et al., 2004). The wide range of pain relief strategies (summarized in **TABLE 5.2**), some of which reflect desperation in the face of great anguish, testifies to the elusive nature of pain. As we learn more about how the brain controls pain, we can hope for better, safer analgesics in the future.

> **HOW'S IT GOING** ❓
>
> 1. What is the most effective pharmacological method of pain control? How and where do these drugs work in the brain?
> 2. How is TENS thought to work to control pain?
> 3. Compare and contrast placebos and acupuncture for pain. Discuss the possibility that they act on the same neural system.

5.3 Movement and the Motor System

THE ROAD AHEAD

This chapter concludes with the system that enables the brain to move the body, allowing us to interact with the world. Learning this information means you can:

5.3.1 Discuss the importance of motor planning and sensory feedback in controlling behavior.

5.3.2 Trace the pathways by which the brain sends commands to individual muscles.

5.3.3 Distinguish between the two main types of sensory feedback from muscles to the nervous system.

5.3.4 Discuss the interaction of various cortical and subcortical brain regions in regulating behavior.

5.3.5 Describe the behavioral symptoms and underlying pathology of two major motor disorders.

Our apparently effortless adult motor abilities—such as reaching out and picking up an object, walking across the room, sipping a cup of coffee—require complex muscular systems with constant feedback from the body. Ian, whom we met at the beginning of the chapter, knows this all too well. Our survey of motor control starts with a discussion of a theoretical framework for studying motor behavior, followed by a tour of the anatomy and pathology of movement.

When you think about it, *all* behavior must involve **movements**—contractions of muscles that provide our sole means of interacting with the world around us. Early discoveries suggested that **reflexes**—simple, unvarying, and unlearned responses to sensory stimuli such as touch, pressure, and pain—might be the basic units of behavior. It was thought that more-complex behaviors, or **acts**, such as getting dressed, walking, or speaking a sentence, might result from simply connecting together different reflexes, the sensation from one reflex triggering the next.

The flaws of this perspective soon became apparent: for most acts we have a *plan* in which several units (arm movements, leg movements, speech sounds) are placed in a larger pattern (the intended complete act), and they are not always produced in the same (or even the correct) order. So, researchers realized that acts require a **motor plan** (or *motor program*), a complex set of commands to muscles that is established *before* an act occurs. Feedback from movements informs and fine-tunes the motor program as the execution is unfolding, but the basic sequence of movements is planned. Examples of behaviors that exhibit this kind of internal plan range from highly skilled acts, such as piano playing, to the simple escape behaviors of animals such as crayfish.

Researchers can track the simple movements that make up an act by recording the electrical activity of muscles as they contract—a technique called **electromyography** (**EMG**)—and the moment-to-moment positions of the body. The EMG recordings in **FIGURE 5.17** show that a person pulling a lever will adjust his legs just

movement A single relocation of a body part, usually resulting from a brief muscle contraction. It is less complex than an act.

reflex A simple, highly stereotyped, and unlearned response to a particular stimulus (e.g., an eye blink in response to a puff of air).

act Complex behavior, as distinct from a simple movement.

motor plan Also called *motor program*. A plan for a series of muscular contractions, established in the nervous system prior to its execution.

electromyography (EMG)
The electrical recording of muscle activity.

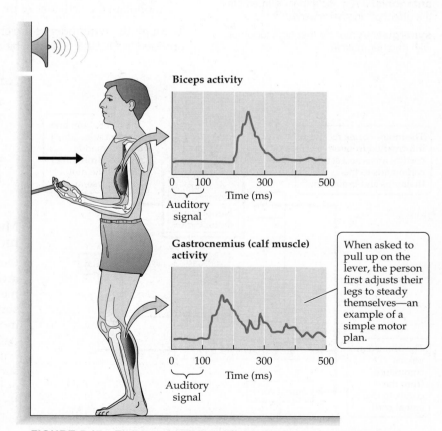

FIGURE 5.17 Electromyography (After D. Purves et al., 2001. *Neuroscience* [2nd ed.]. Oxford University Press/Sinauer. Sunderland, MA.)

before moving his arm—an example of motor planning. Motor plans resemble engineering concepts that are applied to the operation of machines. In designing machines, engineers commonly have two goals: (1) accuracy, to prevent or minimize error; and (2) speed, to complete a task quickly and efficiently. Improvements in one goal usually come at some cost to the other goal; in other words, there is a trade-off between speed and accuracy, and this trade-off is also apparent in motor planning by the nervous system.

The neuromuscular system consists of the muscles of the body plus a collection of brain mechanisms and nerves that prepare and execute motor plans and obtain feedback information from the sensory system for use in error correction. The system is organized according to a distinct hierarchy:

1. The *skeletal system* and the muscles attached to it determine which movements are possible.

2. The *spinal cord* controls skeletal muscles in response to motor commands from the brain or, in the case of simple reflexes, in direct response to sensory inputs.

3. The *brainstem* integrates motor commands from higher levels of the brain and transmits them to the spinal cord. It also relays sensory information about the body from the spinal cord to the forebrain.

4. Some of the main commands for action are initiated in the *primary motor cortex*.

5. Areas adjacent to the primary motor cortex, *nonprimary motor cortex*, provide an additional source of motor commands, acting indirectly via primary motor cortex and through direct connections to lower levels of the motor hierarchy. At the very top of the movement hierarchy is the prefrontal cortex, which is crucial to the formulation of behavioral plans.

6. Other brain regions—the *cerebellum* and *basal ganglia*, via the *thalamus*—modulate the activities of the other parts of the control system.

Through the remainder of the chapter we'll look at the elements of this hierarchy, as outlined in **FIGURE 5.18**, in a bit more detail.

antagonist   A muscle that counteracts the effect of another muscle.

synergist   A muscle that acts together with another muscle.

HOW'S IT GOING ?

1. Distinguish among reflexes, movements, and acts.
2. Discuss the importance of sensory feedback for the control of movements. How are speed and accuracy related, in the context of movement control?
3. What is a motor plan?
4. Identify the six major levels of the motor control hierarchy.

Muscles and the skeleton work together to move the body

Our skeleton, like those of other species with bones, is articulated with joints that vary in their planes of movement—ranging from "universal" joints, like the hip or shoulder, to joints that act more like hinges and move mostly in one direction, such as the elbow or knee. Around a joint, different muscles, connected to the bones by tendons, are arranged in a reciprocal fashion such that when one muscle group contracts, it stretches the other group; that is, the muscles are **antagonists**. Some groups of muscles, called **synergists**, may work together to move a limb in one direction. A simple example of muscle action around a joint is shown in **FIGURE 5.19**. The movement of a limb is determined by the degree and rate of contraction in some muscles and relaxation

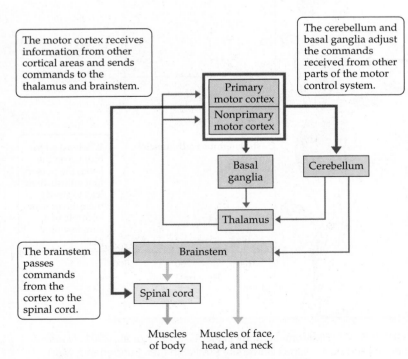

The motor cortex receives information from other cortical areas and sends commands to the thalamus and brainstem.

The cerebellum and basal ganglia adjust the commands received from other parts of the motor control system.

Primary motor cortex

Nonprimary motor cortex

Basal ganglia

Cerebellum

Thalamus

The brainstem passes commands from the cortex to the spinal cord.

Brainstem

Spinal cord

Muscles of body

Muscles of face, head, and neck

FIGURE 5.18   The Hierarchy of Movement Control

in others, or we can lock a limb in position by contracting opposing muscles at the same time.

The muscles that we use for movement of the skeleton are called *skeletal muscles*. Because they have a striped appearance on microscopic examination, due to overlapping layers of contractile proteins called *myosin* and *actin*, skeletal muscles are said to be made of *striate muscle*. (*Smooth muscle*, which has a different appearance and is found in visceral organs and blood vessels, is not generally involved in voluntary behavior, so we will not concern ourselves with it here.) Contraction of the muscle increases the overlap of the actin and myosin filaments within *muscle fibers*, and as these filaments slide past each other, the muscle fiber shortens. Most muscles consist of a specific mixture of two types of fibers: *slow-twitch fibers* that contract with relatively low intensity but fatigue slowly, and *fast-twitch fibers* that contract strongly but fatigue quickly. Through training, endurance athletes enhance the slow-twitch properties of their muscles (Putman et al., 2004).

Muscles contract because **motor neurons** (or *motoneurons*) of the spinal cord and brainstem (see Figure 1.7 and Figure 1.8) send action potentials along their axons and axon collaterals to terminate at specialized synapses, called **neuromuscular junctions**, that are found on muscle fibers (**FIGURE 5.20**). The production of an action potential by a motor neuron triggers a release of the neurotransmitter **acetylcholine (ACh)** at all of the

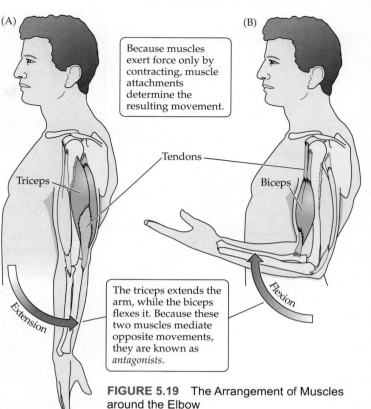

Because muscles exert force only by contracting, muscle attachments determine the resulting movement.

Tendons

Triceps

Biceps

The triceps extends the arm, while the biceps flexes it. Because these two muscles mediate opposite movements, they are known as *antagonists*.

Extension

Flexion

FIGURE 5.19   The Arrangement of Muscles around the Elbow

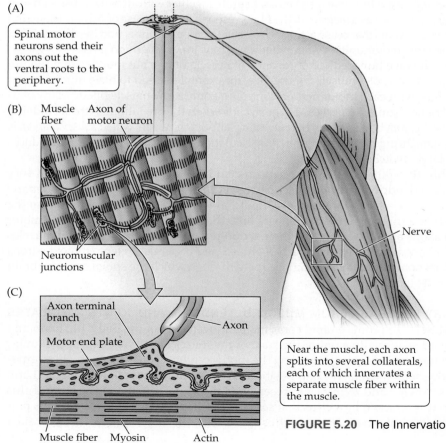

(A)

Spinal motor neurons send their axons out the ventral roots to the periphery.

(B) Muscle fiber   Axon of motor neuron

Neuromuscular junctions

(C)

Axon terminal branch

Motor end plate

Axon

Muscle fiber   Myosin   Actin

Nerve

Near the muscle, each axon splits into several collaterals, each of which innervates a separate muscle fiber within the muscle.

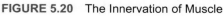

FIGURE 5.20   The Innervation of Muscle

motor neuron   Also called *motoneuron*. A neuron that transmits neural messages to muscles (or glands).

neuromuscular junction   The region where the motor neuron terminal meets its target muscle fiber. It is the point where the nerve transmits its message to the muscle fiber.

acetylcholine (ACh)   A neurotransmitter that is produced and released by the autonomic nervous system, by motor neurons, and by neurons throughout the brain.

FIGURE 5.21   Muscle Receptors

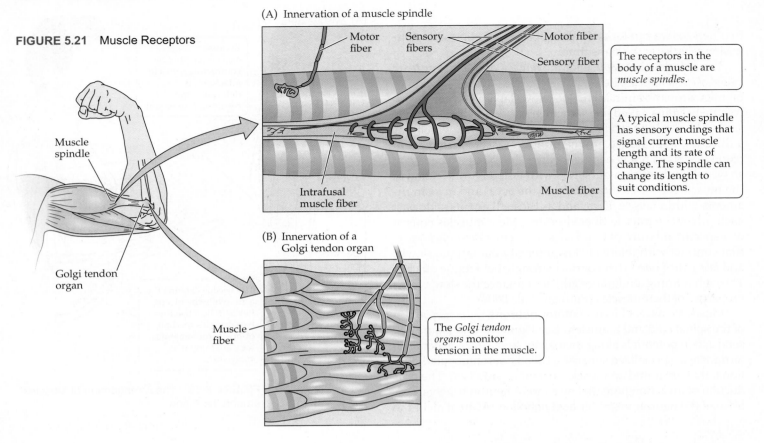

(A) Innervation of a muscle spindle

Motor fiber

Sensory fibers

Motor fiber

Sensory fiber

Intrafusal muscle fiber

Muscle fiber

> The receptors in the body of a muscle are *muscle spindles*.

> A typical muscle spindle has sensory endings that signal current muscle length and its rate of change. The spindle can change its length to suit conditions.

Muscle spindle

Golgi tendon organ

(B) Innervation of a Golgi tendon organ

Muscle fiber

> The *Golgi tendon organs* monitor tension in the muscle.

motor neuron's axon terminals. The motor neuron, together with all of the muscle fibers it innervates, is known as a *motor unit*; the fibers respond to the release of ACh by triggering the molecular events that cause actin and myosin to produce contraction (see Figure 5.20).

Some large motor units—where motor neurons innervate thigh muscle, for example—may involve hundreds or thousands of muscle fibers. But muscles that require more precise control—muscles of the face, for example—tend to have much smaller motor units, with each motor neuron controlling only a few muscle fibers. Many people experience "jumping nerves" in the eyelids when they're fatigued (from studying neuroscience, maybe). This tiny but incredibly annoying twitch, called a *fasciculation*, is actually a misfiring facial motor unit. A fasciculation in the thigh, in contrast, produces a much larger twitch.

Within the spinal cord, motor neurons tend to have large cell bodies and very widespread dendritic fields because they receive and integrate inputs from so many different sources—incoming sensory inputs, as well as descending signals from the brain—that form thousands of synapses onto the motor neurons. Virtually all motor neuron axons are myelinated, so their action potentials reach their target muscles quickly. In a somewhat dramatic turn of phrase, neuroscientists refer to motor neurons as the **final common pathway**: the sole route through which the spinal cord and brain can control our many muscles.

SENSORY FEEDBACK FROM MUSCLES, TENDONS, AND JOINTS REGULATES MOVEMENT   To produce rapid coordinated movements of the body, the brain and spinal cord continually monitor the state of the muscles, the positions of the limbs, and the instructions being issued by the motor centers. This collection of information about body movements and positions is called **proprioception** (from the Latin *proprius*, "own," and *recipere*, "to receive"). Ian, whom we met at the start of this chapter, was attacked by a virus that selectively killed proprioceptive axons; his predicament illustrates how important this "sixth sense" is for movement. Let's consider

final common pathway   The motor neurons of the brain and spinal cord, so called because they receive and integrate all motor signals from the brain to direct movement.

proprioception   Body sense; information about the position and movement of the body.

two proprioceptors—muscle spindles and Golgi tendon organs—that monitor muscle length and muscle tension.

The **muscle spindle** is basically a capsule, buried within the other fibers of the muscle, that contains a special kind of muscle fiber called an **intrafusal fiber** (from the Latin *intra*, "within," and *fusus*, "spindle") (**FIGURE 5.21A**). When a muscle is stretched beyond its relaxed state, so it is lengthened—imagine someone handing you a heavy book, causing your arm to bend downward and lengthening the biceps muscle— sensory endings within the spindle fiber become excited and trigger action potentials in sensory nerves. This proprioceptive signal informs the spinal cord and brain about the extent and rate of change in the length of the muscle, and therefore about the load being imposed. Interestingly, a special motor neuron controls the length of the intra- fusal fiber, adjusting it according to the movements being planned by the brain—in a sense, calibrating the muscle spindle to the *expected* limb position.

While muscle spindles respond primarily to *length*, the other proprioceptive recep- tors for muscle—**Golgi tendon organs**—are especially sensitive to the *tension* of the muscle as it shortens. Loads that are strong enough to stretch the tough tendon are sensed by the nerve endings of the Golgi tendon organ that weave through the tendon (**FIGURE 5.21B**). It takes a pretty strong load to stretch a tendon to this degree, so it makes sense that the primary function of Golgi tendon organs is to monitor the force of muscle contractions, providing a second source of sensory information about the muscles (**FIGURE 5.22**). This arrangement makes the Golgi tendon organs useful in another important way: they detect overloads that threaten to tear muscles and ten- dons, and they can cause a reflexive relaxation of the affected muscles, protecting the muscles (and causing you to drop that book). Another familiar example of a stretch re- flex is the knee-jerk (or patellar) reflex that we discussed in Chapter 2 (see Figure 2.14).

Classic studies in physiology emphasized the importance of information from muscle spindles and Golgi tendon organs for controlling movement. Mott (1895) and

muscle spindle   A muscle receptor that lies parallel to a muscle and sends impuls- es to the central nervous system when the muscle is lengthened.

intrafusal fiber   Any of the small muscle fibers that lie within each muscle spindle.

Golgi tendon organ   A type of receptor found within tendons that sends impulses to the central nervous system when a muscle contracts.

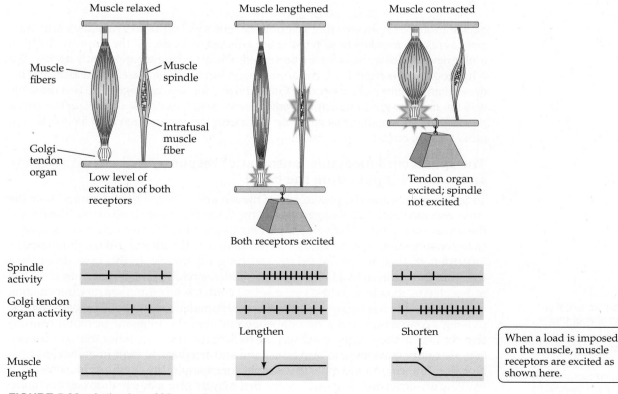

FIGURE 5.22   Activation of Muscle Receptors

View Animation 5.4:
The Stretch Reflex Circuit

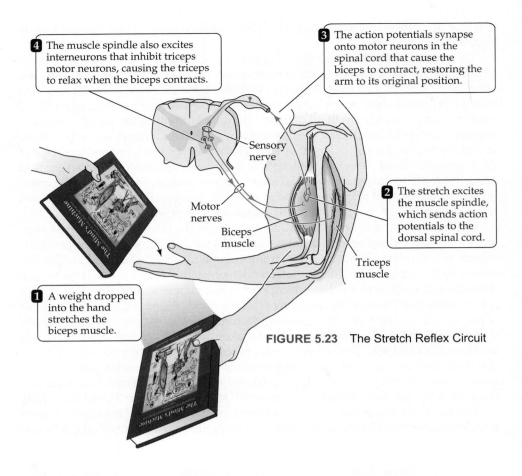

4 The muscle spindle also excites interneurons that inhibit triceps motor neurons, causing the triceps to relax when the biceps contracts.

3 The action potentials synapse onto motor neurons in the spinal cord that cause the biceps to contract, restoring the arm to its original position.

Sensory nerve

Motor nerves

Biceps muscle

2 The stretch excites the muscle spindle, which sends action potentials to the dorsal spinal cord.

Triceps muscle

1 A weight dropped into the hand stretches the biceps muscle.

FIGURE 5.23 The Stretch Reflex Circuit

Sherrington (1898) showed that severing the sensory fibers from a monkey's arm muscles causes the monkey to stop using the affected limb, even if the connections from motor neurons to the muscles are preserved. The arm dangles, apparently useless. But if the good arm is restrained, the animal soon learns to use the affected arm, and indeed it can become quite dexterous (Taub, 1976). Monkeys manage to do this the same way Ian does, by guiding their movements with visual feedback about how the arm is moving. In fact, we all supplement our proprioceptive information with feedback from other sensory channels, like vision.

The spinal cord mediates "automatic" responses and receives inputs from the brain

To really understand the physiology of movement, we need to understand how the "final common pathway" is controlled by the CNS. The lowest level of this hierarchy is the spinal cord, where relatively simple circuits produce reflexive behavioral responses to sensory stimuli. A straightforward example is the **stretch reflex**, illustrated in **FIGURE 5.23**, that can be elicited by stretching any muscle. In this case, dropping a load into the outstretched hand causes a sudden stretch of the biceps muscle, which is detected by muscle spindles. In the spinal cord, the incoming sensory information from the spindles has two immediate effects: it stimulates motor neurons of the biceps, causing a contraction, and it simultaneously inhibits the antagonistic motor neurons that connect to the triceps muscle on the back of the arm. The reflex thus generates a compensatory movement to bring the hand and arm back to their intended position. Not all spinal circuits are quite this simple; for example, the rhythmic movements of walking are governed by spinal circuits that may involve many neurons across multiple spinal segments.

stretch reflex The contraction of a muscle in response to stretch of that muscle.

pyramidal system Also called *corticospinal system*. The motor system that includes neurons within the cerebral cortex and their axons, which form the pyramidal tract.

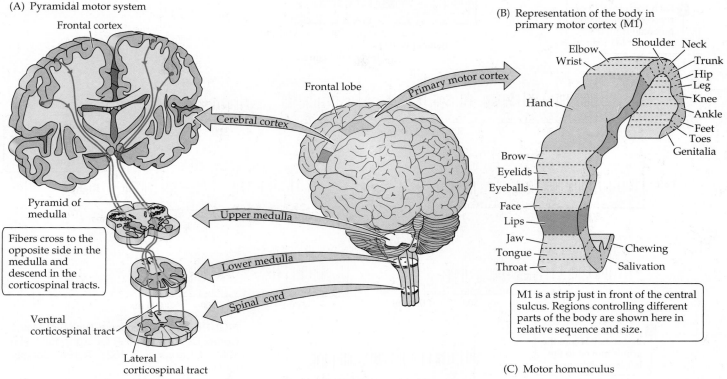

(A) Pyramidal motor system

Frontal cortex

Frontal lobe

Primary motor cortex

Cerebral cortex

Pyramid of medulla

Upper medulla

Fibers cross to the opposite side in the medulla and descend in the corticospinal tracts.

Lower medulla

Spinal cord

Ventral corticospinal tract

Lateral corticospinal tract

(B) Representation of the body in primary motor cortex (M1)

Elbow   Shoulder   Neck
Wrist   Trunk
                     Hip
Hand   Leg
                     Knee
                     Ankle
                     Feet
Brow   Toes
Eyelids   Genitalia
Eyeballs
Face
Lips
Jaw   Chewing
Tongue
Throat   Salivation

M1 is a strip just in front of the central sulcus. Regions controlling different parts of the body are shown here in relative sequence and size.

FIGURE 5.24   The Pyramidal System and Primary Motor Cortex (B after C. N. Prudente et al., 2015. *J. Neurosci.* 35: 9163.)

(C) Motor homunculus

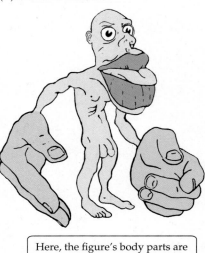

Here, the figure's body parts are proportional to the amount of motor cortex devoted to the corresponding muscles, although this sort of mapping oversimplifies the organization of the motor cortex.

Although muscles of the head are controlled *directly* by the brain, via the cranial nerves (see Figure 1.7), the muscles of the rest of the body are ultimately controlled by commands from the brain and spinal cord via the somatic nerves. The brain sends these commands through two major pathways: the pyramidal system and the extrapyramidal system. The **pyramidal system** (or *corticospinal system*) consists of neuronal cell bodies within the frontal cortex and their axons, which pass through the brainstem, forming the pyramidal tract to the spinal cord (**FIGURE 5.24A**). In a cross section of the medulla, the tract is a wedge-shaped anterior protuberance (pyramid) on each side of the midline. Because the left and right pyramidal tracts each cross over to the other side, the right cortex controls the left side of the body while the left cortex controls the right. Lesions anywhere in the pyramidal tract will cause paralysis in the muscles controlled by the damaged neurons. Many of the axons of the pyramidal tract originate from neurons in the primary motor cortex (M1), which consists mainly of the precentral gyrus, just anterior to the central sulcus (**FIGURE 5.24B**). We will return to the topic of motor cortex a little later.

Many other axon pathways run from the forebrain to the brainstem and spinal cord. Because these tracts are outside the pyramids of the medulla, they and their connections are lumped together as the **extrapyramidal system**. In general, lesions of the extrapyramidal system do not prevent the movement of individual joints and limbs, but they do interfere with spinal reflexes, usually exaggerating them, and they interfere with systems that regulate and fine-tune motor behavior. Many of these extrapyramidal projections pass to the spinal cord via specialized motor regions (the reticular formation and red nucleus) of the midbrain and brainstem; as we'll see shortly, the basal ganglia are an important point of origin for extrapyramidal projections.

Spinal injuries due to vehicular accidents, violence, falls, and sports injuries are all too common, and they often cause heartbreaking disabilities. Because the spinal cord

extrapyramidal system   A motor system that includes the basal ganglia and some closely related brainstem structures. Axons of this system pass into the spinal cord outside the pyramids of the medulla.

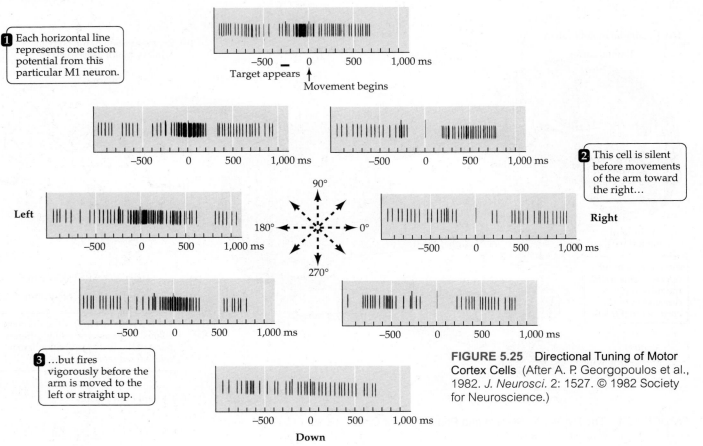

❶ Each horizontal line represents one action potential from this particular M1 neuron.

Up

−500   0   500   1,000 ms

Target appears ↑ Movement begins

90°

180° ← → 0°

270°

Left

Right

❷ This cell is silent before movements of the arm toward the right…

❸ …but fires vigorously before the arm is moved to the left or straight up.

Down

FIGURE 5.25   Directional Tuning of Motor Cortex Cells (After A. P. Georgopoulos et al., 1982. *J. Neurosci.* 2: 1527. © 1982 Society for Neuroscience.)

carries all of the instructions from the brain to the muscles, an injury that completely severs the cord results in immediate and permanent paralysis below the level of injury. Depending on the extent of destruction of the spinal cord below the injury site, spinal reflexes may or may not be lost as well (in fact, reflexes may become *stronger* because of the loss of descending inhibition from the brain). Over 250,000 people in the United States have spinal cord injuries (Richards et al., 2017), and thousands more occur each year, mostly in young people. Although much remains to be discovered, the hope of reconnecting the injured spinal cord no longer seems far-fetched, as discussed in **A STEP FURTHER 5.3**, on the website.

Motor cortex plans and executes movements—and more

The **primary motor cortex** of humans—**M1**—is a major source of axons forming the pyramidal tract. Like S1, the primary somatosensory cortex that we discussed earlier in the chapter, M1 occupies a single large cortical gyrus: the **precentral gyrus**, located immediately in front of the central sulcus (M1 is thus a part of the frontal lobe; see Figure 5.24B). And like S1, M1 is organized as a map of the contralateral side of the body. So, electrical stimulation of a discrete region of the left M1 will cause movement in the corresponding region of the right side of the body. Once again, the map is distorted, in the sense that the parts of the body that we control most precisely—hands, lips, tongue—are overrepresented in M1. **FIGURE 5.24C** shows the *motor homunculus*, a figure drawn using the body proportions represented in M1. But although the M1 map helps us understand the basic organization of motor cortex, recent research indicates that the map is really an oversimplification. The mapping of individual body regions in M1 isn't nearly as clear-cut and discrete as traditional M1 maps suggest. In fact, there is a fair bit of intermingling of body regions in the map, because many body parts coordinate with one another across regions of M1 (Rathelot and Strick, 2006).

primary motor cortex (M1) The apparent executive region for the initiation of movement. It is primarily the precentral gyrus.

precentral gyrus The strip of frontal cortex, just in front of the central sulcus, that is crucial for motor control.

(A) Before training

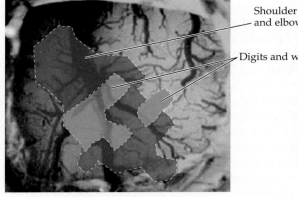

This map illustrates forelimb control in a rat's motor cortex, prior to training.

(B) After training

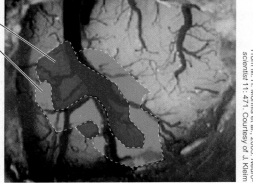

Shoulder and elbow

Digits and wrist

From M. H. Monfils et al., 2005. Neuro-scientist 11: 471. Courtesy of J. Kleim

After 10 days of training on a task requiring precise reaching and grasping, the representation of the digits and wrist (green) has expanded into areas previously associated with the shoulder and elbow (blue).

FIGURE 5.26   Motor Learning Causes Remapping of Motor Cortex

By recording from M1 neurons in monkeys making arm movements, we can eavesdrop on the commands originating there (**FIGURE 5.25**). Many M1 cells change their firing rates according to the direction of the movement, but for any one cell, discharge rates are highest in one particular direction. Only by averaging the activity of hundreds of M1 neurons at once can we predict the direction of arm movements with reasonable accuracy. But of course, *millions* of M1 neurons are available, so in principle a larger sampling would provide a more accurate prediction.

Motor representations in M1 are not static; they change as a result of training. For example, M1 is wider in piano players, especially in the hand area, than in nonmusicians. The younger the musician was at the start of musical training, the larger the gyrus is in adulthood (Amunts et al., 1997), so this expansion of M1 seems to be in response to the experience of musical training. Studies using transcranial magnetic stimulation (TMS) (see Chapter 1) to noninvasively stimulate cortical neurons have shown that the movements produced by a patch of M1 may change with repeated use or as a result of motor learning. In rats, this cortical plasticity associated with motor learning has been directly observed by means of sophisticated mapping of the motor cortex before and after extended training of a new skill (Monfils et al., 2005) (**FIGURE 5.26**).

Just anterior to M1 are cortical regions, collectively known as **nonprimary motor cortex**, that make additional crucial contributions to motor control. Nonprimary motor systems can contribute to behavior directly, through communication with lower levels of the motor hierarchy in the brainstem and spinal cord systems, as well as indirectly, through M1. The traditional account of nonprimary motor cortex emphasizes two main regions: the **supplementary motor area** (**SMA**), which lies mainly on the medial aspect of the hemisphere, and the **premotor cortex**, which is anterior to the primary motor cortex (**FIGURE 5.27**).

nonprimary motor cortex   Frontal lobe regions adjacent to the primary motor cortex that contribute to motor control and modulate the activity of the primary motor cortex.

supplementary motor area (SMA)   A region of nonprimary motor cortex that receives input from the basal ganglia and modulates the activity of the primary motor cortex.

premotor cortex   A region of nonprimary motor cortex just anterior to the primary motor cortex.

FIGURE 5.27   Human Motor Cortical Areas

(A) Lateral view

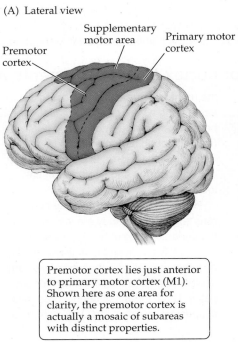

Premotor cortex

Supplementary motor area

Primary motor cortex

Premotor cortex lies just anterior to primary motor cortex (M1). Shown here as one area for clarity, the premotor cortex is actually a mosaic of subareas with distinct properties.

(B) Medial view

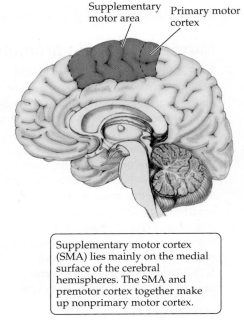

Supplementary motor area

Primary motor cortex

Supplementary motor cortex (SMA) lies mainly on the medial surface of the cerebral hemispheres. The SMA and premotor cortex together make up nonprimary motor cortex.

plegia Paralysis; the loss of the ability to move.

paresis Muscular weakness, often the result of damage to motor cortex.

apraxia An impairment in the ability to carry out complex movements, even though there is no muscle paralysis.

mirror neuron A neuron that is active both when an individual makes a particular movement and when that individual sees another individual make the same movement.

The SMA seems important for the *initiation* of movement sequences, especially when they're being executed according to an internal preprogrammed plan (Tanji, 2001). In contrast, the premotor cortex seems to be activated when motor sequences are guided by *external* events (Svoboda and Li, 2018). However, evidence is mounting that premotor cortex is not a single system, but really a mosaic of different units, controlling groups of motor behaviors that cluster together into major categories: defensive movements, feeding behavior, and so on (Graziano, 2006; Graziano and Aflalo, 2007). This organization suggests that motor and premotor areas mostly map *behaviors*, rather than mapping specific *movements*, as in M1.

Strokes or other injuries in motor areas of the cortex result in **plegia** (paralysis) or **paresis** (weakness) of voluntary movements, usually on the contralateral side of the body (*hemiplegia* or *hemiparesis*). Damage to nonmotor zones of the cerebral cortex, such as some regions of parietal or frontal association cortex, produces more-complicated changes in motor control, such as **apraxia** (from the Greek *a*, "not," and *praxis*, "action"), the inability to carry out complex movements even though paralysis or weakness is not evident and language comprehension and motivation are intact. There are several subtypes of apraxia, but in general it's as though the patient is unable to work out the sequence of movements required to perform a desired behavior—a high-level motor-programming problem.

HOW'S IT GOING ❓

1. Describe the arrangement of muscles and joints that allows movement.
2. Briefly describe the main components of a motor unit.
3. Define *proprioception*. Explain how two specialized sensors in muscle provide feedback about the muscle's current state.
4. Provide a summary of the path taken by motor fibers innervating the skeletal musculature—from the level of the brain, through the spinal cord, to the muscle targets.
5. Where is primary motor cortex located, and how is it organized?
6. Distinguish between the pyramidal and extrapyramidal systems.
7. What are some of the contributions of nonprimary motor cortex?

RESEARCHERS AT WORK ||||||||||||||||||||||||||||||||||||||||||||||||||||||||||||||||||||||||||||||||||||||||||||||||||||||||||||||||

Mirror neurons in premotor cortex track movements in others

A subregion of premotor cortex (called *F5*) may contain a population of remarkable neurons that seem to fulfill two functions. These neurons fire shortly before a monkey makes a very particular movement of the hand and arm to reach for an object; different neurons fire during different reaching movements. The data thus suggest that these neurons trigger specific movements. But these neurons also seem to fire whenever the monkey sees *another* monkey (or a human) make that same movement (**FIGURE 5.28**). These cells are called **mirror neurons** because they fire as though

the monkey were imagining doing the same thing as the other individual. Mirror neurons are also found in adult humans (Buccino et al., 2004) and children (Lepage and Theoret, 2006), both in the premotor cortex and in other cortical locations.

Because the activity of these neurons suggests that they are important in the understanding of other individuals' actions (Rizzolatti and Craighero, 2004), an intriguing notion is that mirror neurons could be part of a neural system for empathy. Thus, there has been a great deal of speculation about the function of mirror

neurons in the imitating behavior of human infants, the evolution of language, and other behavior (Gallese and Sinigaglia, 2011). Some have speculated that people with autism spectrum disorder, which is characterized by a failure to anticipate other people's thinking and actions, may have a deficit in mirror neuron activity (J. H. Williams et al., 2006). Note, however, that the specific functions ascribed to mirror neurons remain somewhat controversial (Caramazza et al., 2014).

RESEARCHERS AT WORK (*continued*) |||||||||||||||||||||||||||||||||||||||||||||||||||||||||||||||||||

■ Question

The researchers hypothesized that neurons of the premotor cortex, in a ventral subregion called F5, encode specific and detailed movements rather than muscle contractions.

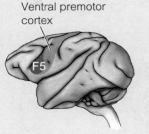

Ventral premotor cortex

F5

■ Experiment

The activity of single F5 neurons was recorded while the monkey made reaching movements.

■ Result

The neurons fired shortly before the monkey made a specific movement, in accordance with the initial hypothesis. But to the experimenters' surprise, the neurons also became active when the monkey simply watched an experimenter perform the same movement, as if the monkey was *imagining* making the movement.

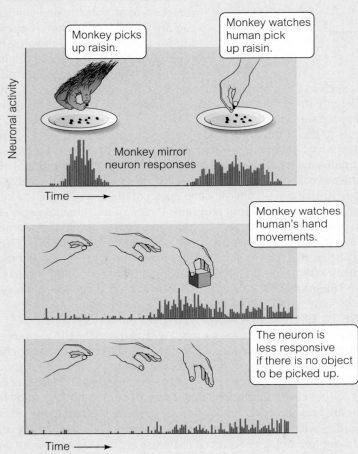

Monkey picks up raisin.

Monkey watches human pick up raisin.

Neuronal activity

Monkey mirror neuron responses

Time ⟶

Monkey watches human's hand movements.

The neuron is less responsive if there is no object to be picked up.

Time ⟶

■ Conclusion

These "mirror neurons" may be part of a system for analyzing the behavior of others (Umilta et al., 2001).

FIGURE 5.28   Mirror Neurons (After M. A. Umilta et al., 2001. *Neuron* 31: 155.)

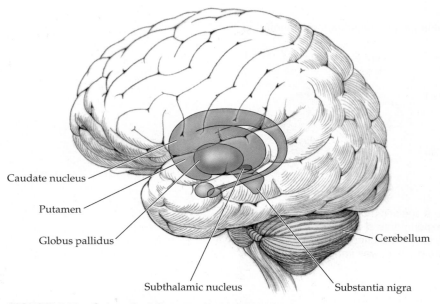

Caudate nucleus

Putamen

Globus pallidus

Subthalamic nucleus

Cerebellum

Substantia nigra

FIGURE 5.29   Subcortical Systems Involved in Movement

View Activity 5.3:
Subcortical Systems Involved
in Movement

basal ganglia   A group of forebrain nuclei, including caudate nucleus, globus pallidus, and putamen, found deep within the cerebral hemispheres.

cerebellum   A structure located at the back of the brain, dorsal to the pons, that is involved in the central regulation of movement and in some forms of learning.

ataxia   A loss of movement coordination, often caused by disease of the cerebellum.

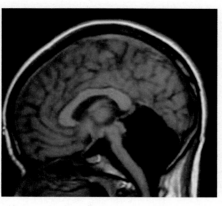

From F. Yu et al., 2015. *Brain* 138: e353

FIGURE 5.30   A Woman without a Cerebellum

Extrapyramidal systems regulate and fine-tune motor commands

Earlier we noted that extrapyramidal projections—the motor fibers outside the pyramidal tracts—are especially important in modulation and ongoing control of movement. Two of the most important sources of extrapyramidal fibers are the basal ganglia and the cerebellum.

As we saw in Chapter 1, the **basal ganglia** are a group of several interconnected forebrain nuclei (especially the caudate nucleus, putamen, and globus pallidus), with strong inputs from the substantia nigra and the subthalamic nucleus. The basal ganglia receive inputs, via the thalamus, from wide expanses of the cortex forming a loop from the cortex through the basal ganglia and thalamus and back to the cortex (**FIGURE 5.29**). The basal ganglia help control the amplitude and direction of movement, and changes in activity in regions of the basal ganglia appear to be important for the initiation of movement. Much of the motor function of the basal ganglia appears to be the modulation of activity started by other brain circuits, such as the motor pathways of the cortex (see Figure 5.24). The basal ganglia are especially important for movements performed by memory, in contrast to those guided by sensory control.

Inputs to the **cerebellum** come both from sensory sources and from other brain motor systems. Sensory inputs include the muscle and joint receptors and the vestibular, somatosensory, visual, and auditory systems. Both pyramidal and nonpyramidal pathways contribute inputs to the cerebellum and in turn receive outputs—all of which are inhibitory—from the deep nuclei of the cerebellum. The cerebellum helps establish and fine-tune neural programs for *skilled* movements, especially the kinds of rapid, repeated movements that become automatic. Remarkably, some people appear to be born without a cerebellum, yet develop normal motor skills (**FIGURE 5.30**), presumably because of the great plasticity of the brain during development. In addition to its role in motor function, the cerebellum is also crucial for some types of learning (Katz and Steinmetz, 2002), as we'll discuss in more detail in Chapter 13.

DAMAGE TO EXTRAPYRAMIDAL SYSTEMS IMPAIRS MOVEMENT   Different constellations of symptoms are associated with damage to the various extrapyramidal motor structures. The exact consequences of cerebellar damage depend on the part of the cerebellum that has been damaged, but common motor symptoms include characteristic abnormalities of gait and posture, especially **ataxia** (loss of coordination) of the legs. Other cerebellar lesions may cause **decomposition of movement** (in which gestures are broken up into individual segments instead of being executed smoothly) or difficulties with gaze and visual tracking of objects. The anatomy of the cerebellum and the symptomatology of cerebellar disease are discussed in more detail in **A STEP FURTHER 5.4**, on the website.

Two diseases that target the basal ganglia reveal important aspects of extrapyramidal contributions to motor control. Patients with **Parkinson's disease** show progressive degeneration of dopamine-containing cells in the **substantia nigra**. Loss of these neurons, which project to the caudate nucleus and putamen, is associated with a cluster of symptoms that are all too familiar: slow movement, tremors of the hands and face while at rest, a rigid bearing, and diminished facial expressions. Patients who have Parkinson's show few spontaneous actions and have great difficulty in all motor efforts, no matter how routine. Exercise can slow the progression of Parkinson's, and studies indicate that dance therapy, using music to encourage movement, helps patients with Parkinson's (Kalyani et al., 2019).

Whereas damage to the basal ganglia in Parkinson's disease *reduces* movement, other kinds of basal ganglia disorders cause the opposite: *excessive* movement. The first symptoms of **Huntington's disease** are subtle behavioral changes: clumsiness, and twitches in the fingers and face. Subtlety is rapidly lost as the illness progresses; a continuing stream of involuntary jerks engulfs the entire body. Aimless movements of the eyes, jerky leg movements, and writhing of the body make even routine activity a major challenge, exacerbated in later stages of the disease by intellectual deterioration. The neuroanatomical basis of this disorder is widespread destruction of the basal ganglia, including the caudate nucleus and the putamen (rather than just the substantia nigra, which greatly reduces movement in Parkinson's).

Although much remains to be discovered, there is more reason than ever to look forward to the introduction of effective treatments for motor disorders. Scientists are learning more and more about what goes wrong in Parkinson's and Huntington's diseases, and their continuing research efforts may pave the way to new therapies.

HOW'S IT GOING ❓

1. What are mirror neurons, and what is their significance?
2. What are the symptoms of Parkinson's disease, and what brain changes cause it?
3. What are the symptoms of Huntington's disease, and what brain changes cause it?
4. Children of people with Huntington's disease have a fifty-fifty chance of inheriting the gene causing it. If you had a parent with Huntington's, would you want to take the test to see if you carry the disease?

Recommended Reading

Ballantyne, J. C., Fishman, S. M., and Rathmell, J. P. (Eds.). (2018). *Bonica's Management of Pain* (5th ed.). Philadelphia, PA: Lippincott.

Cole, J. (2016). *Losing Touch: A Man without His Body*. Oxford, UK: Oxford University Press.

Cytowic, R. E. (2018). *Synesthesia.* Cambridge, MA: MIT Press.

McMahon, C., Koltzenberg, M., Tracey, I., and Turk, D. C. (2013). *Wall and Melzack's Textbook of Pain* (6th ed.). Philadelphia, PA: Saunders.

Purves, D., Augustine, G. J., Fitzpatrick, D., Hall, W., et al. (Eds.). (2017). *Neuroscience* (6th ed.). Sunderland, MA: Oxford University Press/Sinauer. (See Unit III: "Movement and Its Central Control," Chapters 16–21.)

Turk, D. C., and Gatchel, R. J. (Eds.). (2018). *Psychological Approaches to Pain Management: A Practitioner's Handbook* (3rd ed.). New York, NY: Guilford Press.

Walsh, R. A., de Bie, R. M., and Fox, S. H. (2017). *Movement Disorders: What Do I Do Now?* (2nd ed.). New York, NY: Oxford University Press.

Wolfe, J. M., Kluender, J. R., Levi, D. M., Bartoshuk, L. M., et al. (2021). *Sensation & Perception* (6th ed.). Sunderland, MA: Oxford University Press/Sinauer.

decomposition of movement
Difficulty of movement in which gestures are broken up into individual segments instead of being executed smoothly. It is a symptom of cerebellar lesions.

Parkinson's disease A degenerative neurological disorder, characterized by tremors at rest, muscular rigidity, and reduction in voluntary movement, caused by loss of the dopaminergic neurons of the substantia nigra.

substantia nigra A brainstem structure that is a major source of dopaminergic projections to the basal ganglia.

Huntington's disease A genetic disorder, with onset in middle age, in which the destruction of basal ganglia results in a syndrome of abrupt, involuntary writhing movements and changes in mental functioning.

You should be able to relate each summary to the adjacent illustration, including structures and processes. The online version of this **Visual Summary** includes links to figures, animations, and activities that will help you consolidate the material.

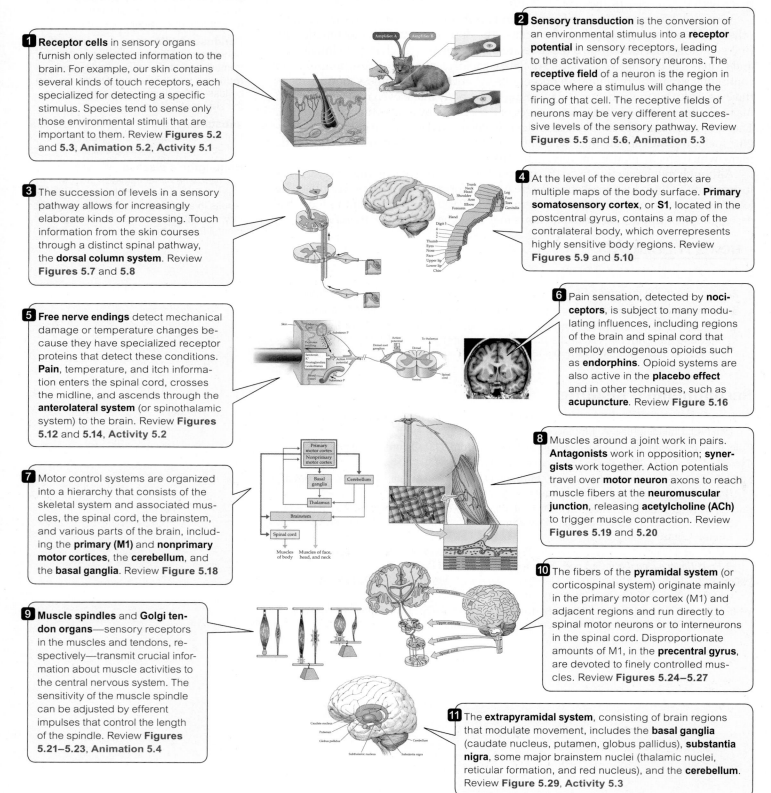

1 **Receptor cells** in sensory organs furnish only selected information to the brain. For example, our skin contains several kinds of touch receptors, each specialized for detecting a specific stimulus. Species tend to sense only those environmental stimuli that are important to them. Review **Figures 5.2** and **5.3**, **Animation 5.2**, **Activity 5.1**

2 **Sensory transduction** is the conversion of an environmental stimulus into a **receptor potential** in sensory receptors, leading to the activation of sensory neurons. The **receptive field** of a neuron is the region in space where a stimulus will change the firing of that cell. The receptive fields of neurons may be very different at successive levels of the sensory pathway. Review **Figures 5.5** and **5.6**, **Animation 5.3**

3 The succession of levels in a sensory pathway allows for increasingly elaborate kinds of processing. Touch information from the skin courses through a distinct spinal pathway, the **dorsal column system**. Review **Figures 5.7** and **5.8**

4 At the level of the cerebral cortex are multiple maps of the body surface. **Primary somatosensory cortex**, or **S1**, located in the postcentral gyrus, contains a map of the contralateral body, which overrepresents highly sensitive body regions. Review **Figures 5.9** and **5.10**

5 **Free nerve endings** detect mechanical damage or temperature changes because they have specialized receptor proteins that detect these conditions. **Pain**, temperature, and itch information enters the spinal cord, crosses the midline, and ascends through the **anterolateral system** (or spinothalamic system) to the brain. Review **Figures 5.12** and **5.14**, **Activity 5.2**

6 Pain sensation, detected by **nociceptors**, is subject to many modulating influences, including regions of the brain and spinal cord that employ endogenous opioids such as **endorphins**. Opioid systems are also active in the **placebo effect** and in other techniques, such as **acupuncture**. Review **Figure 5.16**

7 Motor control systems are organized into a hierarchy that consists of the skeletal system and associated muscles, the spinal cord, the brainstem, and various parts of the brain, including the **primary (M1)** and **nonprimary motor cortices**, the **cerebellum**, and the **basal ganglia**. Review **Figure 5.18**

8 Muscles around a joint work in pairs. **Antagonists** work in opposition; **synergists** work together. Action potentials travel over **motor neuron** axons to reach muscle fibers at the **neuromuscular junction**, releasing **acetylcholine (ACh)** to trigger muscle contraction. Review **Figures 5.19** and **5.20**

9 **Muscle spindles** and **Golgi tendon organs**—sensory receptors in the muscles and tendons, respectively—transmit crucial information about muscle activities to the central nervous system. The sensitivity of the muscle spindle can be adjusted by efferent impulses that control the length of the spindle. Review **Figures 5.21–5.23**, **Animation 5.4**

10 The fibers of the **pyramidal system** (or corticospinal system) originate mainly in the primary motor cortex (M1) and adjacent regions and run directly to spinal motor neurons or to interneurons in the spinal cord. Disproportionate amounts of M1, in the **precentral gyrus**, are devoted to finely controlled muscles. Review **Figures 5.24–5.27**

11 The **extrapyramidal system**, consisting of brain regions that modulate movement, includes the **basal ganglia** (caudate nucleus, putamen, globus pallidus), **substantia nigra**, some major brainstem nuclei (thalamic nuclei, reticular formation, and red nucleus), and the **cerebellum**. Review **Figure 5.29**, **Activity 5.3**

6 Hearing, Balance, Taste, and Smell

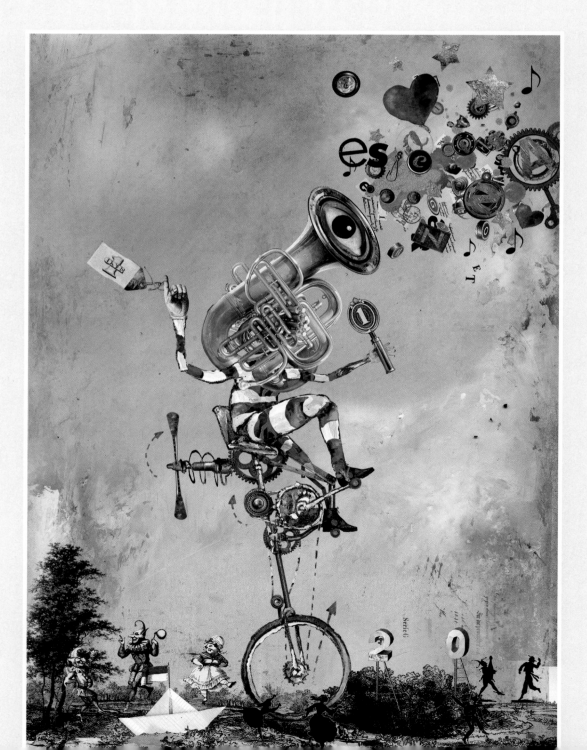

Hold the Phone

It's like a classic horror movie scene: a scientist using amazing technology in an attempt to reanimate parts of dead bodies, seeking out nature's secrets. But when the young Hungarian engineer Georg von Békésy started experimenting with cadavers in the 1920s, he was not trying to create life. He was seeking to answer a practical question: Why are human ears so much more sensitive than most microphones? Békésy thought that learning how the human ear works might allow him to make a better microphone for his employer, the Hungarian phone company. He gathered cadavers from local hospitals and came up with a clever dissection that would reveal the inner ear without destroying it. (His work was not always appreciated by his fellow engineers; they didn't like finding their drill press full of human bone dust in the morning.)

Bringing his background in physics to bear, Békésy devised exquisitely precise physical models and biophysical experiments that let him measure extremely brief, minuscule movements in the inner ear. His subsequent discoveries provided us with the key to understanding how we translate a stream of auditory data—sounds—into neural activity that the brain can understand.

In the end, Békésy did not come up with a better microphone, but his discoveries have helped restore hearing to thousands of people who once were deaf, as we'll see in this chapter.

Your existence is directly attributable to the keen senses possessed by your distant ancestors—senses that enabled them to find food and mates and to avoid predators and other dangers. In this chapter we consider some of the incredible sensors that let us monitor important signals from distant sources, especially sounds (by audition) and smells (by olfaction). We also discuss related systems for detecting position and movement of the body (the vestibular system, related to the auditory system) and tastes of foods (the gustatory or taste sense, which like olfaction is a chemical sense). We begin with hearing, because audition evolved from special mechanical receptors related to the touch system that we discussed in Chapter 5.

See Video 6.1: Inside the Ear

6.1 Hearing: Pressure Waves in the Air Are Perceived as Sound

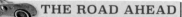

 THE ROAD AHEAD

The first part of the chapter is concerned with the structure and function of the ear, especially the inner ear, which gives us our sense of hearing. After reading this section, you should be able to:

6.1.1 Explain how the external ear and middle ear capture and concentrate sound energy and convey it to the inner ear.

6.1.2 Sketch the anatomy of the middle and inner ears, highlighting the location of sensorineural components.

6.1.3 Explain how vibrations travel through the cochlea and how they are converted into neural activity.

6.1.4 Describe the process by which the organ of Corti encodes the frequencies of sounds.

6.1.5 Summarize the neural projections between the cochlea and brain.

6.1.6 Identify the principal auditory pathways and structures of the brain, and describe the integration of signals from the left and right ears.

6.1.7 Describe the orderly map of frequencies found at each level of the auditory system.

View Animation 6.2:
Brain Explorer

The Ears Have It   The external ears, or pinnae, of mammals come in a variety of shapes, each adapted to a particular ecological niche. Many mammals can move their ears to direct them toward a particular sound. In such cases, the brain must account for the position of the ear to judge where a particular sound came from. (Fennec fox [top left]; whispering bat [top right]; sea otter [bottom left]; chimpanzee [bottom right].)

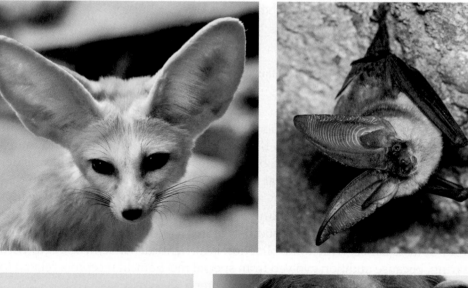

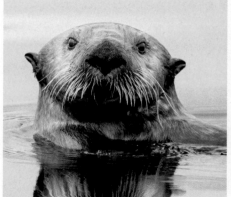

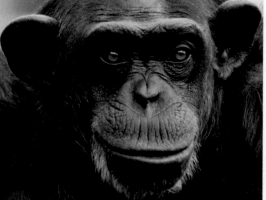

decibel (dB)   A measure of sound intensity, perceived as loudness.

hertz (Hz)   Cycles per second, as of an auditory stimulus. Hertz is a measure of frequency.

transduction   The conversion of one form of energy to another.

© iStock.com/wrangel

© A.S. Floru/Shutterstock.com

© iStock.com/Ken-Canning

© bierchen/Shutterstock.com

Hearing is vital for the survival of most animals. Humans can produce an impressive variety of vocalizations—from barely audible murmurs to soaring flights of song—but we especially rely on speech sounds for our social relations and for the transmission of knowledge between individuals. Across the animal kingdom, species produce and perceive sounds in wildly different ways, shaped by their unique evolutionary history. Birds sing and crickets chirp in order to attract mates, while monkeys grunt and screech and burble to signal comfort, danger, and pleasure. Owls and bats exploit the directional property of sound to locate prey and avoid obstacles in the dark, because unlike light, sound can be detected in the darkest night, or even around a corner.

How does energy transmitted through air become the speech, music, and other sounds we hear? Your auditory system detects changes in the vibration of air molecules that are caused by sound sources: it senses both the *intensity* of sounds, measured in **decibels (dB)** and perceived as *loudness*, and their *frequency*, measured in cycles per second, or **hertz (Hz)**, and perceived as *pitch*. **BOX 6.1** describes some of the basic properties of sound that are relevant to our discussion of hearing. The outer ear directs sound into the inner parts of the ear, where the mechanical force of sound is **transduced** into neural activity: the action potentials that inform the brain. Your ears are incredibly sensitive

pure tone   A tone with a single frequency of vibration.

amplitude   Also called *intensity*. The force that sound exerts per unit area, which we experience as loudness.

frequency   The number of cycles per second in a sound wave, measured in hertz.

fundamental   The predominant frequency of an auditory tone.

harmonic   A multiple of a particular frequency called the *fundamental*.

timbre   The characteristic sound quality of a musical instrument, as determined by the relative intensities of its various harmonics.

BOX 6.1   **The Basics of Sound**

We perceive a repetitive pattern of local increases and decreases in air pressure as sound. Usually this oscillation is caused by a vibrating object, such as a loudspeaker or a person's larynx during speaking. A single alternation of compression and expansion of air is called one *cycle*.

The figure illustrates the oscillations in pressure produced by a vibrating loudspeaker. Because the sound produced by the loudspeaker here has only one frequency of vibration, it is called a **pure tone** and can be represented by a sine wave. A pure tone is described physically in terms of two measures:

Amplitude   Also called *intensity*, this is usually measured as sound pressure in dynes per square centimeter (dyn/cm^2). Our perception of amplitude is termed *loudness*, expressed as decibels (dB). The decibel scale is logarithmic: one decibel is the threshold for human hearing, a whisper is about 20 dB, and a departing jetliner a couple of hundred feet overhead—a sound a million times as intense—is about 120 dB.

Frequency   This is the number of cycles per second, measured in hertz (Hz). So, middle A on a piano has a frequency of 440 Hz. Our perception of frequency is termed *pitch*.

Most sounds are more complicated than a pure tone. For example, a sound made by a musical instrument contains a **fundamental** frequency and **harmonics**. The fundamental is the basic frequency, and the harmonics are multiples of the fundamental. For example, if the fundamental is 440 Hz, the harmonics are 880 Hz, 1,320 Hz, 1,760 Hz, and so on. When different instruments play the same note, the notes differ in the relative intensities of the various harmonics and there are subtle qualitative differences between instruments in the way they commence, shape, and sustain the sound; these differences are what give each instrument its characteristic voice, or **timbre**.

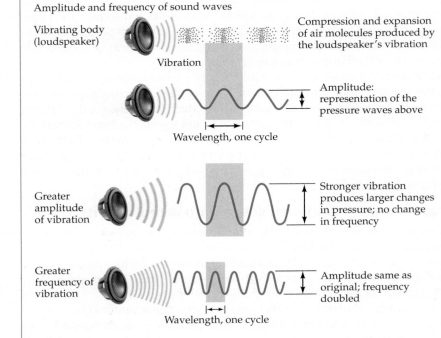

Amplitude and frequency of sound waves

Vibrating body (loudspeaker) — Vibration — Compression and expansion of air molecules produced by the loudspeaker's vibration

Amplitude: representation of the pressure waves above

Wavelength, one cycle

Greater amplitude of vibration — Stronger vibration produces larger changes in pressure; no change in frequency

Greater frequency of vibration — Amplitude same as original; frequency doubled

Wavelength, one cycle

pinna   The external part of the ear.

ear canal   Also called *auditory canal*. The tube leading from the pinna to the tympanic membrane.

inner ear   The cochlea and vestibular apparatus.

middle ear   The cavity between the tympanic membrane and the cochlea.

tympanic membrane   Also called *eardrum*. The partition between the external ear and the middle ear.

ossicles   Three small bones (incus, malleus, and stapes) that transmit vibration across the middle ear, from the tympanic membrane to the oval window.

oval window   The opening from the middle ear to the inner ear.

cochlea   A snail-shaped structure in the inner ear canal that contains the primary receptor cells for hearing.

scala vestibuli   Also called *vestibular canal*. One of three principal canals running along the length of the cochlea.

scala media   Also called *middle canal*. The central of the three spiraling canals inside the cochlea, situated between the vestibular canal and the tympanic canal.

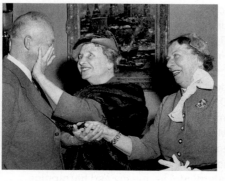

A Touching Moment   Helen Keller, who was both blind and deaf, said, "Blindness deprives you of contact with things; deafness deprives you of contact with people"—a poignant reminder of the importance of speech for our social lives. Here, Keller (center, accompanied by her aide and interpreter, Polly Thompson) communicates with U.S. President Dwight Eisenhower by feeling Eisenhower's face as he speaks and makes facial expressions. Rather than living in sensory and social isolation, Keller honed her intact senses to such a degree that she was able to become a noted teacher and writer.

organs; in fact, one of the main jobs of your powers of attention is to filter out the constant barrage of unimportant little noises that your ears detect (see Chapter 14).

The external ear captures, focuses, and filters sound

The oddly shaped fleshy objects that most people call *ears* are properly known as **pinnae** (singular *pinna*). Aside from their occasional utility as handles and jewelry hangers, the pinnae funnel sound waves into the second part of the external ear: the **ear canal** (or *auditory canal*). The pinna is a distinctly mammalian characteristic, and mammals show a wide array of ear shapes and sizes. Furthermore, although only a minority of humans can move their ears—and even then only enough to entertain children—many other mammals deftly shape and swivel their pinnae to help locate the source of a sound. Animals with exceptional auditory localization abilities, such as bats, may have especially mobile ears.

The "ridges and valleys" of the pinna modify the character of sound that reaches the middle ear. Some frequencies of sound are enhanced; others are suppressed. For example, the shape of the human ear especially increases the reception of sounds between 2,000 and 5,000 Hz—a frequency range that is important for speech perception. The shape of the external ear—and, in many species, the direction in which it is being pointed—provides additional cues about the direction and distance of the source of a sound, as we will discuss later in this chapter.

The middle ear concentrates sound energies

A collection of tiny structures made of membrane, muscle, and bone—essentially a tiny biological microphone—links the ear canal to the neural receptor cells of the **inner ear** (**FIGURE 6.1A**). This **middle ear** (**FIGURE 6.1B**) consists of the taut **tympanic membrane** (*eardrum*) sealing the end of the ear canal plus a chain of tiny bones, called **ossicles**, that mechanically couple the tympanic membrane to the inner ear at a specialized patch of membrane called the **oval window**. These ossicles, the smallest bones in the body, are called the *malleus* (Latin for "hammer"), the *incus* (Latin for "anvil"), and the *stapes* (Latin for "stirrup").

Sound waves in the air strike the tympanic membrane and cause it to vibrate with the same frequency as the sound; as a result, the ossicles start moving too. Because of how they are attached to the eardrum, the ossicles concentrate and amplify the vibrations, focusing the pressures collected from the relatively large tympanic membrane onto the small oval window. This amplification is crucial for converting vibrations in air into movements of fluid in the inner ear, as we'll see shortly.

The middle ear is equipped with the equivalent of a volume control, which helps protect against the damaging forces of extremely loud noises. Two tiny muscles—the tensor tympani and the stapedius (see Figure 6.1B)—attach to the ends of the chain of ossicles. Within 200 milliseconds of the arrival of a loud sound, the brain signals the muscles to contract, which stiffens the chain of ossicles and reduces the effectiveness of the sounds. Interestingly, the middle-ear muscles activate just before we produce self-made sounds like speech or coughing, which is why we don't perceive our own sounds as distractingly loud.

The cochlea converts vibrational energy into neural activity

The part of the inner ear that ultimately converts vibrations from sound into neural activity—the coiled, fluid-filled **cochlea** (from the Greek *kochlos*, "snail")—is a marvel of miniaturization (**FIGURES 6.1C** and **D**). In an adult human, the cochlea measures only about 9 millimeters in diameter at its widest point—roughly the size of a pea. Fully unrolled, the human cochlea would be about 35–40 millimeters long.

The cochlea is a spiral of three parallel canals: (1) the **scala vestibuli** (also called the *vestibular canal*), (2) the **scala media** (*middle canal*), and (3) the **scala tympani** (*tympanic canal*). The scala media contains the receptor system, called the **organ of Corti**, that converts vibration (from sound) into neural activity (see Figure 6.1D). It consists

(A) Structures of the ear

FIGURE 6.1 External and Internal Structures of the Human Ear

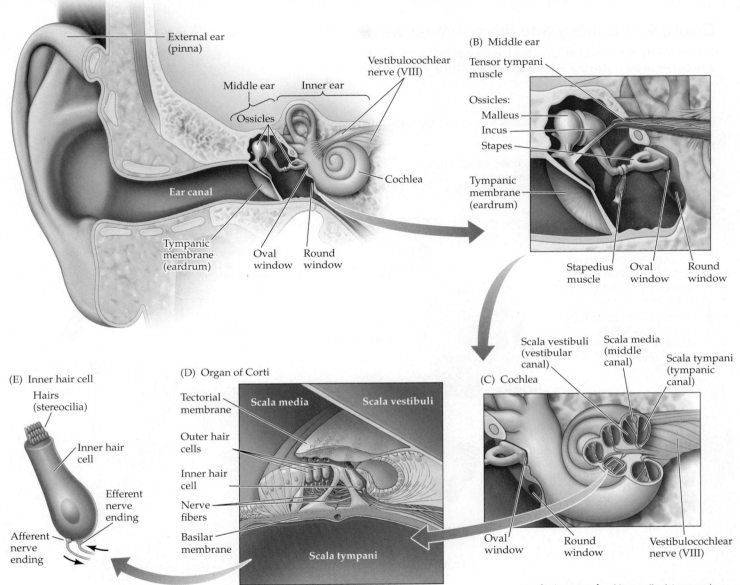

(B) Middle ear

(E) Inner hair cell

(D) Organ of Corti

(C) Cochlea

scala tympani Also called *tympanic canal*. One of three principal canals running along the length of the cochlea.

organ of Corti A structure in the inner ear that lies on the basilar membrane of the cochlea and contains the hair cells and terminations of the auditory nerve.

hair cell One of the receptor cells for hearing in the cochlea, named for the stereocilia that protrude from the top of the cell and transduce vibrational energy in the cochlea into neural activity.

basilar membrane A membrane in the cochlea that contains the principal structures involved in auditory transduction.

tectorial membrane A gelatinous membrane located atop the organ of Corti.

of three main structures: (1) the auditory sensory cells, called **hair cells** (**FIGURE 6.1E**), which bridge between the **basilar membrane** and the overlying **tectorial membrane**; (2) an elaborate framework of supporting cells; and (3) the auditory nerve terminals that transmit neural signals to and from the brain.

When the ossicles transmit vibrations from the tympanic membrane to the oval window, waves or ripples are created in the fluid of the scala vestibuli, which in turn cause the basilar membrane to ripple, like shaking out a rug. A crucial feature of the basilar membrane is that it is tapered—it's much wider at the apex of the cochlea than at the base. Thanks to this taper, each successive location along the basilar membrane shows its strongest response to a different frequency of sound. High frequencies have their greatest effects near the base, where the basilar membrane is narrow and comparatively stiff; low-frequency sounds produce a larger response near the apex, where the basilar membrane is wider and floppier, as we'll see next. (Yoon et al., 2011).

RESEARCHERS AT WORK

Georg von Békésy and the cochlear wave

The discovery of the mechanics of the basilar membrane garnered a Nobel Prize for Georg von Békésy in 1961 (**FIGURE 6.2**).

View Animation 6.3:
Sound Transduction

FIGURE 6.2   Deformation of the Basilar Membrane Encodes Sound Frequencies

■ **Hypothesis**

That sound waves of different frequencies cause ripples at different places on the basilar membrane.

■ **Experiment**

I.   Open a human cochlea (from a cadaver) and add a reflective fluid.

II. Bounce intense flash of light off the basilar membrane during vibration at the oval window.

III. Record the displacement of reflective fluid to measure movement of basilar membrane.

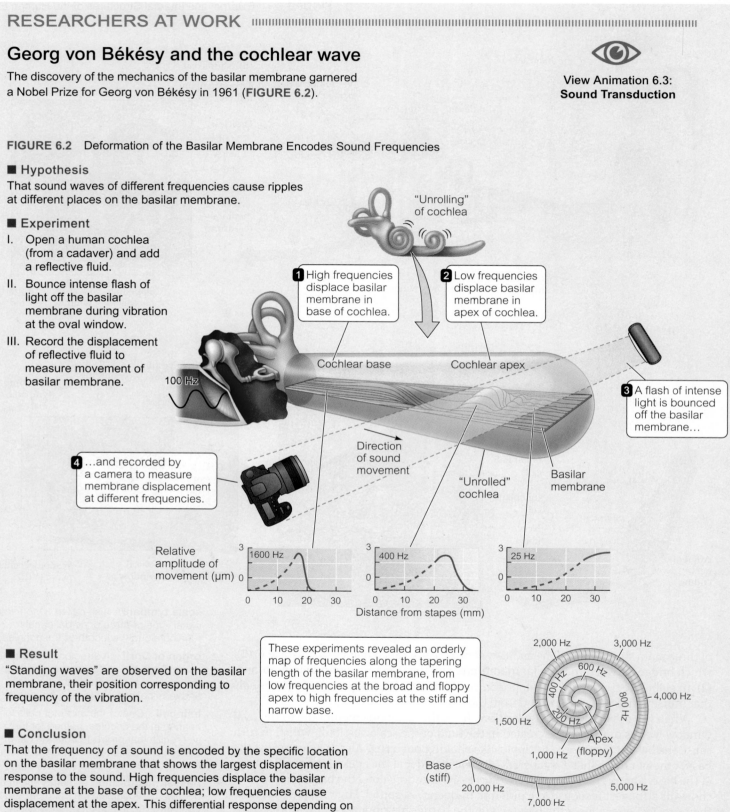

"Unrolling" of cochlea

1 High frequencies displace basilar membrane in base of cochlea.

2 Low frequencies displace basilar membrane in apex of cochlea.

Cochlear base

Cochlear apex

3 A flash of intense light is bounced off the basilar membrane…

100 Hz

4 …and recorded by a camera to measure membrane displacement at different frequencies.

Direction of sound movement

"Unrolled" cochlea

Basilar membrane

Relative amplitude of movement (μm)

1600 Hz

400 Hz

25 Hz

Distance from stapes (mm)

■ **Result**

"Standing waves" are observed on the basilar membrane, their position corresponding to frequency of the vibration.

These experiments revealed an orderly map of frequencies along the tapering length of the basilar membrane, from low frequencies at the broad and floppy apex to high frequencies at the stiff and narrow base.

2,000 Hz   3,000 Hz

600 Hz

400 Hz   800 Hz   4,000 Hz

200 Hz

1,500 Hz

Apex (floppy)

1,000 Hz

Base (stiff)

20,000 Hz   5,000 Hz

7,000 Hz

■ **Conclusion**

That the frequency of a sound is encoded by the specific location on the basilar membrane that shows the largest displacement in response to the sound. High frequencies displace the basilar membrane at the base of the cochlea; low frequencies cause displacement at the apex. This differential response depending on location along the membrane has become known as *place coding*.

The hair cells transduce movements of the basilar membrane into electrical signals

The rippling of the basilar membrane is converted into neural activity through the actions of the hair cells. Each hair cell features a sloping brush of minuscule hairs called **stereocilia** (singular *stereocilium*) on its upper surface. In Figure 6.1D you'll notice that, although the bases of hair cells are implanted in the basilar membrane, the stereocilia nestle into hollows in the tectorial membrane that lies above. The hair cells—and especially the stereocilia themselves—thus form a mechanical bridge between the two membranes that is forced to bend when sounds cause the basilar membrane to ripple.

Even a tiny bend of the stereocilia produces a large and rapid depolarization of the hair cells. This depolarization results from the operation of a special type of large and nonselective ion channel found on stereocilia. Like spring-loaded trapdoors, these channels are mechanically popped open as stereocilia bend (Hudspeth et al., 2000), allowing an inrush of potassium (K^+) and calcium (Ca^{2+}) ions. Just as we saw in neurons (in Chapter 2), this depolarization leads to a rapid influx of Ca^{2+} at the base of the hair cell, which in turn causes synaptic vesicles there to fuse with the presynaptic membrane and release neurotransmitter, stimulating adjacent nerve fibers. The stereocilia channels snap shut again in a fraction of a millisecond as the hair cell sways back. This ability to rapidly switch on and off allows hair cells to accurately track the rapid oscillations of the basilar membrane with exquisite sensitivity.

In the human cochlea, the hair cells are organized into a single row of about 3,500 **inner hair cells** (**IHCs**, called *inner* because they are closer to the central axis of the coiled cochlea) and about 12,000 **outer hair cells** (**OHCs**) in three rows (see Figure 6.1D). Fibers of the **vestibulocochlear nerve** (cranial nerve VIII) contact the bases of the hair cells (see Figure 6.1E). Some of these fibers do indeed convey sound information to the brain, but the neural connections of the cochlea are a little more complicated than this. In fact, there are four kinds of neural connections with hair cells, each relying on a different neurotransmitter (Goutman et al., 2015), as you can see in **FIGURE 6.3**.

The fibers are distinguished as follows:

1. *IHC afferents* convey to the brain the action potentials that provide the perception of sounds. IHC afferents make up about 95% of the fibers leading to the brain.

2. *IHC efferents* lead from the brain to the IHCs. They allow the brain to control the responsiveness of IHCs.

3. *OHC afferents* convey information to the brain about the mechanical state of the basilar membrane, but not the perception of sounds themselves.

4. *OHC efferents* from the brain enable it to activate a remarkable property of OHCs, making them change their length almost instantaneously (Zheng et al., 2000; He et al., 2014). Through this electromechanical action, the brain continually modifies the stiffness of regions of the basilar membrane, resulting in both sharpened tuning and pronounced amplification (Hudspeth, 2014). Evidence is mounting

stereocilium   A tiny bristle that protrudes from a hair cell in the auditory or vestibular system.

inner hair cell (IHC)   One of the two types of receptor cells for hearing in the cochlea. Compared with outer hair cells, IHCs are positioned closer to the central axis of the coiled cochlea.

outer hair cell (OHC)   One of the two types of receptor cells for hearing in the cochlea. Compared with inner hair cells, OHCs are positioned farther from the central axis of the coiled cochlea.

vestibulocochlear nerve   Cranial nerve VIII, which runs from the cochlea to the brainstem auditory nuclei.

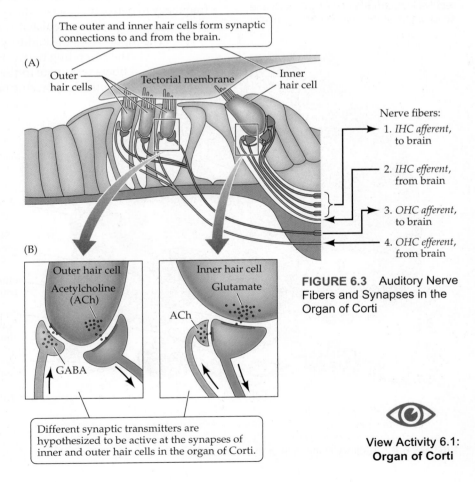

The outer and inner hair cells form synaptic connections to and from the brain.

(A)

Outer hair cells

Tectorial membrane

Inner hair cell

Nerve fibers:
1. *IHC afferent*, to brain
2. *IHC efferent*, from brain
3. *OHC afferent*, to brain
4. *OHC efferent*, from brain

(B)

Outer hair cell
Acetylcholine (ACh)
GABA

Inner hair cell
Glutamate
ACh

Different synaptic transmitters are hypothesized to be active at the synapses of inner and outer hair cells in the organ of Corti.

FIGURE 6.3   Auditory Nerve Fibers and Synapses in the Organ of Corti

View Activity 6.1: Organ of Corti

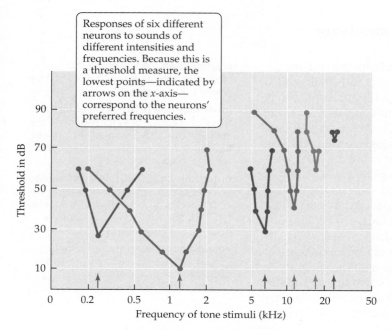

Responses of six different neurons to sounds of different intensities and frequencies. Because this is a threshold measure, the lowest points—indicated by arrows on the *x*-axis—correspond to the neurons' preferred frequencies.

FIGURE 6.4 Tuning Curves of Auditory Nerve Cells (After N. Y.-S. Kiang et al., 1965. *Discharge patterns of single fibers in the cat's auditory nerve*. MIT Press. Cambridge, MA.)

cochlear nuclei Brainstem nuclei that receive input from auditory hair cells and send output to the superior olivary nuclei.

that a complementary process also modifies the local stiffness of the tectorial membrane (see Figure 6.3A), further improving the tuning and amplification of the organ of Corti (Sellon et al., 2019).

Now that the inner ear has transduced the vibrations from sound into trains of action potentials, the auditory signals must leave the cochlea and enter the brain.

Auditory signals run from cochlea to cortex

On each side of your head, about 30,000–50,000 auditory axons from the cochlea make up the auditory part of the vestibulocochlear nerve (cranial nerve VIII), and most of these afferent fibers carry information from the IHCs (each of which stimulates several nerve fibers) to the brain. If we record from these IHC afferents, we find that each one has a maximum sensitivity to sound of a particular frequency but will also respond to neighboring frequencies if the sound is loud enough. For example, the auditory neuron whose responses are shown in red in **FIGURE 6.4** has its best frequency at 1,200 Hz (1.2 kHz)—that is, it is sensitive to even a very weak tone at 1,200 Hz—but for sounds that are 20 dB louder, the cell will respond to frequencies from 500 to 1,800 Hz. We call this the cell's *tuning curve*. If the brain received a signal from only one such fiber, it would not be able to tell whether the stimulus was a weak tone of 1,200 Hz or a stronger tone of 500 or 1,800 Hz, or any frequency in between. Instead, the brain analyzes the activity from thousands of such units simultaneously to calculate the intensity and frequency of each sound.

The inputs from the auditory nerves are distributed to both sides of the brain via the ascending network shown in **FIGURE 6.5**. First, the auditory nerve fibers terminate in the (sensibly named) **cochlear nuclei**, where some initial processing occurs. Output from the cochlear nuclei primarily

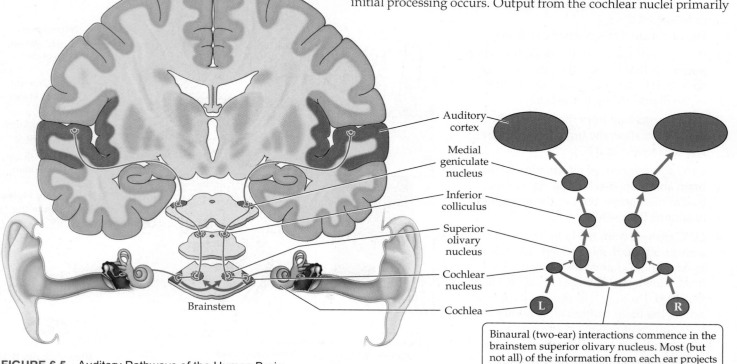

FIGURE 6.5   Auditory Pathways of the Human Brain

Auditory cortex

Medial geniculate nucleus

Inferior colliculus

Superior olivary nucleus

Cochlear nucleus

Cochlea

Brainstem

L

R

Binaural (two-ear) interactions commence in the brainstem superior olivary nucleus. Most (but not all) of the information from each ear projects to the cortex on the opposite side of the brain, depicted by the blended colors in this schematic.

projects to the **superior olivary nuclei**, each of which receives inputs from both right and left cochlear nuclei. This bilateral input makes the superior olivary nucleus the first brain site at which binaural (two-ear) processing occurs. As you might expect, this mechanism plays a key role in localizing sounds by comparing the two ears, as we'll discuss shortly.

The superior olivary nuclei pass information derived from both ears to the **inferior colliculi**, which are the primary auditory centers of the midbrain. Outputs of the inferior colliculi go to the **medial geniculate nuclei** of the thalamus. Outputs from the medial geniculate nuclei extend to several auditory cortical areas.

The neurons within all levels of the auditory system, from cochlea to auditory cortex, display **tonotopic organization**; that is, they are internally arranged according to an orderly map of sound frequencies (*topos* is Greek for "place") from low frequency (sounds that we perceive as lower pitched or "bass") to high frequency (perceived as higher pitched or "treble"). Furthermore, at the higher levels of the auditory system, auditory neurons are not only excited by specific frequencies, but also inhibited by neighboring frequencies, resulting in much sharper tuning of the frequency responses of these cells. This precision helps us discriminate tiny differences in the frequencies of sounds.

Brain-imaging studies in humans confirm that many sounds (tones, noises, and so on) activate the **primary auditory cortex** (**A1**), which is located on the upper surface of the temporal lobes (**FIGURE 6.6A**). Speech sounds produce similar activation, but they also activate other, more specialized auditory areas (**FIGURE 6.6B**). Interestingly, at least some of these regions are activated in hearing people when they try to lip-read—that is, to understand someone by watching that person's lips without auditory cues (Calvert et al., 1997; L. E. Bernstein et al., 2002). This suggests that the auditory cortex integrates other, nonauditory, information with sounds. (The organization of auditory cortical areas in other species is described in **A STEP FURTHER 6.1**, on the website.)

superior olivary nuclei Brainstem nuclei that receive input from both right and left cochlear nuclei and provide the first binaural analysis of auditory information.

inferior colliculi Paired gray matter structures of the dorsal midbrain that process auditory information.

medial geniculate nucleus Either of two nuclei—left and right—in the thalamus that receive input from the inferior colliculi and send output to the auditory cortex.

tonotopic organization The organization of auditory neurons according to an orderly map of stimulus frequency, from low to high.

primary auditory cortex Also called *A1*. The cortical region, located on the superior surface of the temporal lobe, that processes complex sounds transmitted from lower auditory pathways.

View Animation 6.4: Mapping Auditory Frequencies

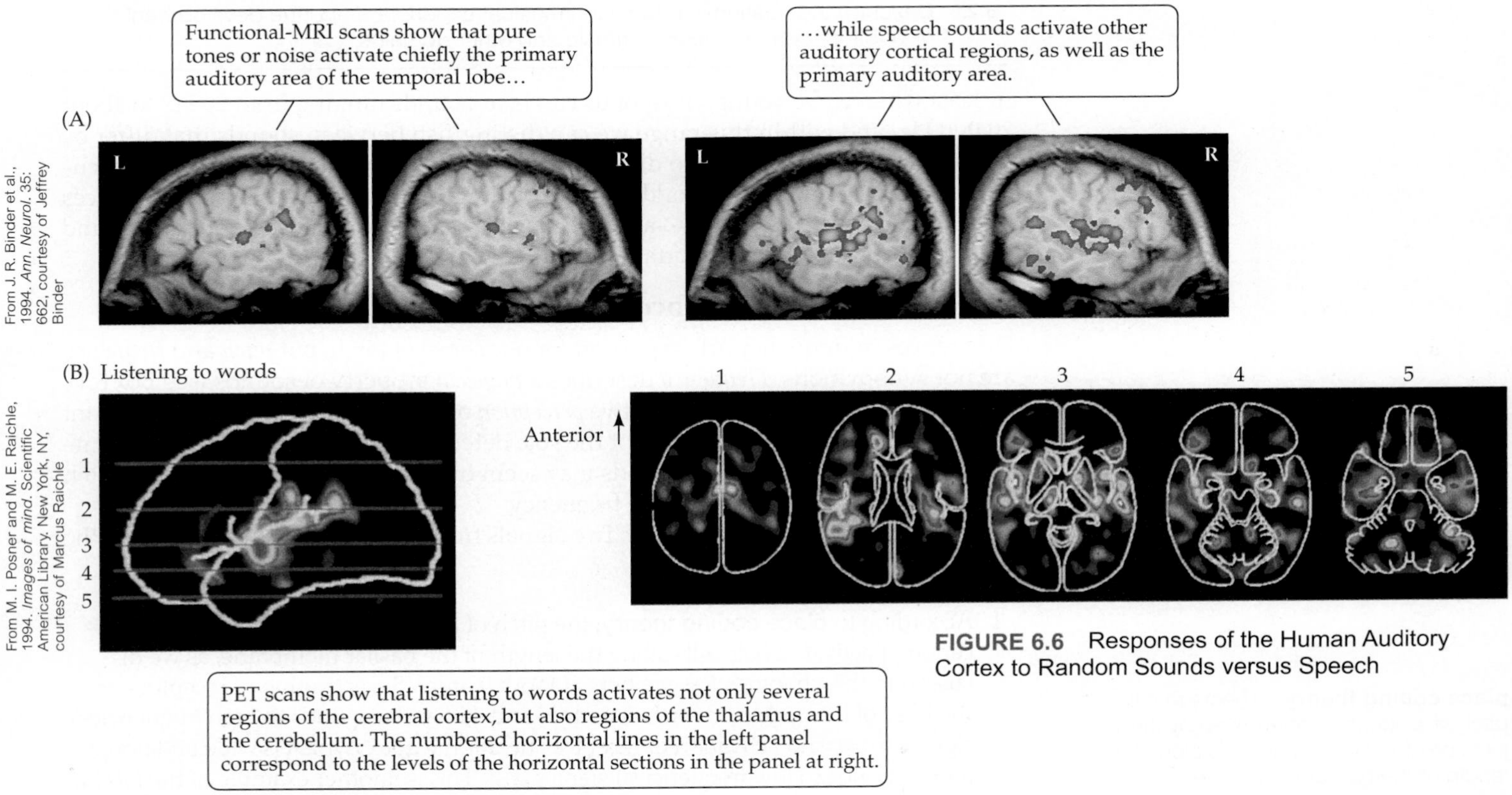

FIGURE 6.6 Responses of the Human Auditory Cortex to Random Sounds versus Speech

HOW'S IT GOING ❓

1. Identify the major components of the external ear. What does the external ear do?

2. Identify the three ossicles, and explain their function. To what structures do the ossicles connect, and how is their action moderated?

3. Provide a brief description of the organ of Corti, naming the components that are most important for the perception of sound.

4. Explain how the movement of hair cells transduces sound waves into action potentials. Compare and contrast the functions of inner hair cells and outer hair cells.

5. Sketch the major anatomical components of the auditory projections in the brain. Where does binaural processing first occur? What is tonotopic organization? What kind of processing does auditory cortex perform?

6.2 Specialized Neural Systems Extract Information from Auditory Signals

THE ROAD AHEAD

Higher levels of the auditory system process different features of the sounds captured by the ears. After reading this section, you should be able to:

6.2.1 Explain the relationship between frequency and pitch, and discuss the ranges of frequencies perceived by humans and other species.

6.2.2 Describe the two major ways in which frequency information is encoded.

6.2.3 Explain the principal features of sound that the nervous system uses for sound localization.

6.2.4 Discuss the functions of auditory cortex, from an ecological perspective.

6.2.5 Evaluate the importance of experience in the development and tuning of the auditory system, throughout the life span.

6.2.6 Describe the relationship between musical experience and the development of auditory competencies in music and other domains.

At least when we're young, most of us can hear sounds ranging from 20 Hz to about 20,000 Hz, and within this range we can distinguish between sounds that differ by just a few hertz. Our ability to discern many frequencies simultaneously, and accurately identify where in the world they are coming from, helps us to define the spaces and sound emitters around us—acoustical objects as varied as insects and tubas—and identify the ones that are important for our daily lives.

The pitch of sounds is encoded in two complementary ways

Differences in frequency are important for our sense of pitch, but *pitch* and *frequency* are not synonymous. *Frequency* describes a *physical* property of sounds (see Box 6.1), but *pitch* relates solely to our subjective *perception* of those sounds. This is an important distinction because frequency is not the sole determinant of perceived pitch; at some frequencies, higher-intensity sounds may seem higher pitched, and changes in pitch do not precisely parallel changes in frequency.

How do we distinguish pitches? Two signals from the cochlea appear to inform the brain about the pitch of sounds:

1. According to **place coding theory**, the pitch of a sound is determined by the location of activated hair cells along the length of the basilar membrane, as we discussed in this chapter's Researchers at Work feature. So, activation of receptors near the base of the cochlea (which is narrow and stiff and responds to high frequencies) signals *treble*, and activation of receptors nearer the apex (which is wide and floppy and responds to low frequencies) signals *bass*. This is another example of the *labeled*

place coding theory   Theory that the pitch of a sound is determined by the location of activated hair cells along the length of the basilar membrane.

lines we discussed in Chapter 5—each neuron fires in response to its particular favorite frequency.

2. A complementary account called **temporal coding theory** proposes that the frequency of auditory stimuli is encoded in the rate of firing of auditory neurons. According to this model, the frequency of action potentials produced by the neuron is directly mathematically related to the number of cycles per second (i.e., hertz) of the sound. For example, a 500 Hz sound might cause some auditory neurons to fire 500 action potentials per second. Encoding sound frequency within *volleys* of action potentials averaged across a number of neurons with similar tunings provides the brain with a reliable additional source of pitch information.

Experimental evidence indicates that we rely on both of these processes to discriminate the pitch of sounds. Temporal coding is most evident at lower frequencies, up to about 4,000 Hz: auditory neurons can fire a maximum of only about 1,000 action potentials per second, but to some extent they can encode sound frequencies that are multiples of the action potential frequency. Beyond about 4,000 Hz, however, this encoding becomes impossible, and pitch discrimination relies on place coding of pitch along the basilar membrane.

Mammalian species employ a huge range of frequencies in their vocalizations, from **infrasound** (less than 20 Hz) in elephants and whales to **ultrasound** (greater than 20,000 Hz) in bats and porpoises and many other species (the ghost-faced bat emits vocalizations at an incredible 160,000 Hz). These sounds have been shaped by evolution to serve special purposes. For example, many species of bats analyze the reflected echoes of their ultrasonic vocalizations to navigate and hunt in the dark. At the other end of the spectrum, elephants emit ultra-low-frequency alarm calls that are so powerful that they travel partly through the ground and are detected seismically by other elephants (O'Connell-Rodwell, 2007; Herbst et al., 2012) and yet are so nuanced that the elephants can distinguish human-related threats from bee-related threats (Soltis et al., 2014) and can use their "rumbles" to identify potential mates (Stoeger and Baotic, 2017).

Brainstem systems compare the ears to localize sounds

Being able to quickly identify where a sound is coming from—whether it is the crack of a twig under a predator's foot, or the sweet tones of a would-be mate—is a matter of great evolutionary significance. So it's no surprise that we are remarkably good at locating a sound source (our accuracy is about ±1 degree horizontally around the head, and many animals do even better). The auditory system accomplishes this feat by analyzing two kinds of binaural cues that signal the location of a sound source:

1. **Interaural intensity differences (IIDs)** result from comparison of the *intensity* of the sound—the physical property that we perceive as *loudness*—at the left and right ears (*interaural* means "between the two ears"). Depending on the species—and the placement and characteristics of their pinnae—intensity differences occur because one ear is pointed more directly toward the sound source or because the head casts a sound shadow (**FIGURE 6.7A**), preventing sounds originating on one side (called *off-axis sounds*) from reaching both ears with equal loudness. The head shadow (or sound shadow) effect is most pronounced for higher-frequency sounds (**FIGURE 6.7B**).

2. **Interaural temporal differences (ITDs)** are differences between the two ears in the *time of arrival* of sounds. They arise because one ear is always a little closer to an off-axis sound than the other ear is. Two kinds of temporal (time) differences are present in a sound: *onset disparity*, which is the difference between the two ears in hearing the beginning of the sound; and *ongoing phase disparity*, which is the continuing mismatch between the two ears in the time of arrival of all the peaks and troughs that make up the sound wave, as illustrated in **FIGURE 6.7C**.

temporal coding theory Theory that the pitch of a sound is determined by the rate of firing of auditory neurons.

infrasound Very-low-frequency sound, generally below the 20 Hz threshold for human hearing.

ultrasound Very-high-frequency sound, generally beyond 20,000 Hz, which is the upper bound for a young adult human.

interaural intensity difference (IID) A perceived difference in loudness between the two ears, which the nervous system can use to localize a sound source.

interaural temporal difference (ITD) A difference between the two ears in the time of arrival of a sound, which the nervous system can use to localize a sound source.

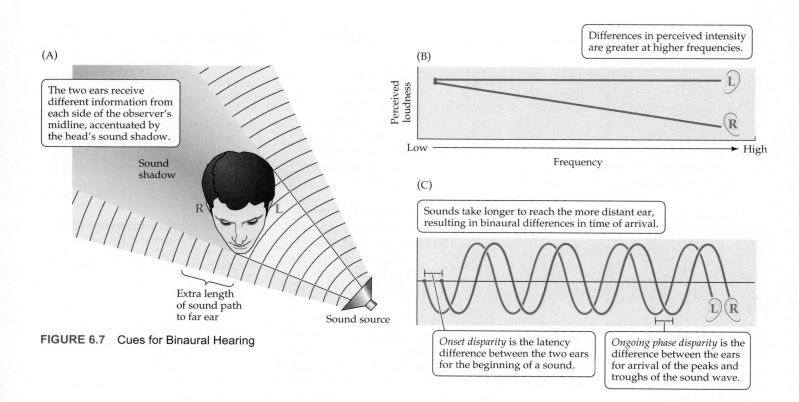

(A)

The two ears receive different information from each side of the observer's midline, accentuated by the head's sound shadow.

Sound shadow

R   L

Extra length of sound path to far ear

Sound source

FIGURE 6.7 Cues for Binaural Hearing

(B)

Differences in perceived intensity are greater at higher frequencies.

Perceived loudness

L

R

Low ——————————————→ High

Frequency

(C)

Sounds take longer to reach the more distant ear, resulting in binaural differences in time of arrival.

L R

Onset disparity is the latency difference between the two ears for the beginning of a sound.

Ongoing phase disparity is the difference between the ears for arrival of the peaks and troughs of the sound wave.

Both types of cues are employed in sound localization. At low frequencies, though, no matter where sounds are presented horizontally around the head, there are virtually no intensity differences between the ears. For these frequencies, differences in times of arrival are the principal cues for sound localization (and at very low frequencies, neither cue is much help; this is why you can place the subwoofer of an audio system anywhere you want within a room). At higher frequencies, however, the sound shadow cast by the head produces significant binaural intensity differences. Of course, we can't perceive which types of processing we're relying on for any given sound; in general, we are aware of the results of neural processing but not the processing itself. (You can learn about brain mechanisms of auditory localization in **A STEP FURTHER 6.2**, on the website.)

The structure of the external ear provides yet another localization cue. As we mentioned earlier, the hills and valleys of the external ear selectively reinforce some frequencies in a complex sound and diminish others. This process is known as **spectral filtering**, and the frequencies that are affected depend on the angle at which the sound arrives at those peaks and valleys (Kulkarni and Colburn, 1998; Zonooz et al., 2019). That angle varies, of course, depending on where the sound comes from; these spectral cues provide critical information about the vertical localization (or elevation) of a sound source. Without them, you would have a hard time knowing whether a sound from straight in front of you came from the ground or from the treetops. The various binaural and spectral cues used for sound localization converge and are integrated in the inferior colliculus (Slee and Young, 2014).

The auditory cortex processes complex sound

In some sensory areas of the brain, lesions cause the loss of basic perceptions. For example, lesions of visual cortex result in blind spots, as we will discuss in Chapter 7. But the auditory cortex is different: researchers have long known that simple pure tones can be heard even after the entire auditory cortex has been surgically removed (Neff and Casseday, 1977). So if the auditory cortex is not involved in basic auditory perception, then what does it do? The auditory cortex seems to be specialized for the

spectral filtering The process by which the hills and valleys of the external ear alter the amplitude of some, but not all, frequencies in a sound.

detection of more-complex "biologically relevant" sounds, of the sort we mentioned earlier—vocalizations of animals, footsteps, snaps, crackles, and pops—containing many frequencies and complex patterns (Theunissen and Elie, 2014). In other words, the auditory cortex evolved to process the sounds of everyday life.

The unique capabilities of the auditory cortex result from a sensitivity that is fine-tuned by experience as we grow (Kandler et al., 2009). Human infants have diverse hearing capabilities at birth, but their hearing for complex speech sounds in particular becomes more precise and rapid through exposure to the speech of their families and other people. Newborns can distinguish all the different sounds that are made in any human language. But as they develop, they get better and better at distinguishing sounds in the language(s) they hear, and worse at distinguishing sounds that occur in other languages. Similarly, early experience with binaural hearing, compared with equivalent monaural (one-eared) hearing, has a significant effect on the ability of children to localize sound sources later in life (W. D. Beggs and Foreman, 1980). Studies with lab animals confirm that experience with sounds of a particular frequency can cause a rapid retuning of auditory neurons (**FIGURE 6.8**; N. M. Weinberger, 1998; Fritz et al., 2003). (You can learn about the role of experience in auditory localization in owls in **A STEP FURTHER 6.3**, on the website). Later in life, aging takes a steady toll on our hearing, gradually impairing auditory cortex neurons and reducing our ability to distinguish between sounds that occur simultaneously (Overton and Recanzone, 2016; Recanzone, 2018). So it turns out there's a good reason why grandparents find it so difficult to follow a conversation in a noisy restaurant.

Music also shapes the responses of auditory cortex. It might not surprise you to learn that the auditory cortex of trained musicians shows a bigger response to musical sounds than does the same cortex in nonmusicians. After all, when two people differ in any skill, their brains must be different in some way, and maybe people born with brains that are more responsive to complex sounds are also more likely to become musicians. The surprising part is that the extent to which a musician's brain is extra sensitive to musical notes is correlated with the age at which they began their serious training in music: the earlier the training began, the bigger the difference in auditory cortex in adulthood (Pantev et al., 1998). Kids who receive intensive musical education also show enhanced speech perception later in life (Weiss and Bidelman, 2015; Intartaglia et al., 2017). Findings like these show that early musical training alters the functioning of auditory cortex later in an enduring manner. By adulthood, the portion of primary auditory cortex where music is first processed, called *Heschl's gyrus*, is more than twice as large in professional musicians as in nonmusicians, and more than twice as strongly activated by music (P. Schneider et al., 2002). And in addition to the effects of early musical experience on auditory structures, cortical regions that process music are reportedly influenced by the brain's mesolimbic reward system (see Chapter 3) to attach a reward value to music that is new to us (Salimpoor et al., 2015; Gold et al., 2019).

So, to what extent is music perception inborn? Some people show a lifelong inability to discern tunes or sing, called **amusia**. Amusia is associated with subtly abnormal function in the right frontal lobe and impoverished connectivity between frontal and

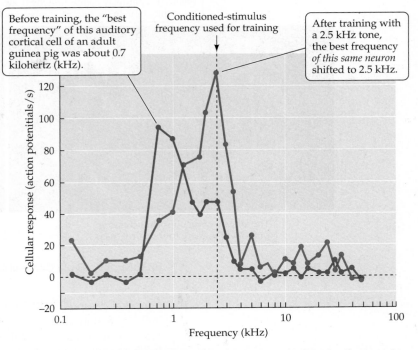

FIGURE 6.8 Long-Term Retention of a Trained Shift in the Tuning of an Auditory Receptive Field (After N. M. Weinberger, 1998. *Neurobiol. of Learn. Mem.* 70: 226.)

amusia A disorder characterized by the inability to discern tunes accurately or to sing.

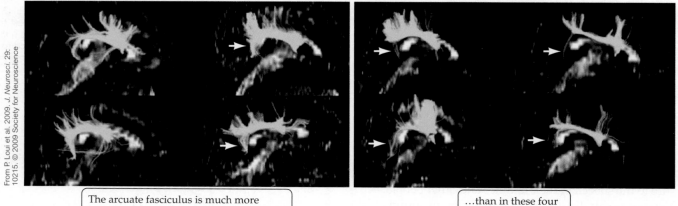

Diffusion tensor imaging (DTI) of axon projections reveals the arcuate fasciculus (yellow), a pathway connecting the frontal cortex, which is active during pitch discrimination, to the temporal lobe, where auditory processing begins (arrows).

From P. Loui et al. 2009. *J. Neurosci.* 29: 10215. © 2009 Society for Neuroscience

The arcuate fasciculus is much more prominent in these four control cases...

...than in these four people with amusia.

FIGURE 6.9 Brain Connections in People with Amusia

temporal cortex (**FIGURE 6.9**) (K. L. Hyde et al., 2006; Loui et al., 2009). The result is an inability to consciously access pitch information, even though cortical pitch-processing systems are intact (Zendel et al., 2015). Interestingly, studies of people with amusia indicate that when listening to music, we process pitch and rhythm quite separately (K. L. Hyde and Peretz, 2004). If you're worried about your own ability to carry a tune, the National Institutes of Health (NIH) provides an online test of pitch perception at www.nidcd.nih.gov/tunestest/test-your-sense-pitch.

6.3 Hearing Loss Is a Widespread Problem

THE ROAD AHEAD

Next we consider the main causes of auditory dysfunction. After reading this section, you should be able to:

6.3.1 Define and distinguish between hearing loss and deafness.

6.3.2 Describe and contrast the three major categories of hearing loss.

6.3.3 Identify potentially harmful noise intensities, and discuss the ways in which noise damages the auditory system.

6.3.4 Summarize and evaluate methods for treating each form of hearing loss.

Disorders of hearing, including **hearing loss** (defined as a moderate to severe decrease in sensitivity to sound) and **deafness** (defined as hearing loss so profound that speech cannot be perceived even with the use of hearing aids), affect about 15% of the population: some 37.5 million people in the United States alone (Blackwell et al., 2014). By now, you may have anticipated that there are three kinds of problems that can prevent sound waves in the air from being transformed into conscious auditory perceptions: problems with sound waves reaching the cochlea, trouble converting sound waves into action potentials, and dysfunction of brain regions that process sound (**FIGURE 6.10**):

1. Before anything even happens in the nervous system, the ear may fail to convert the sound vibrations in air into waves of fluid within the cochlea. This form of hearing loss, called **conduction deafness** (**FIGURE 6.10A**), often comes about when the ossicles of the middle ear become fused together and vibrations of the eardrum can no longer be conveyed to the oval window of the cochlea.

hearing loss Decreased sensitivity to sound, in varying degrees.

deafness Hearing loss so profound that speech perception is lost.

conduction deafness A hearing impairment in which the ears fail to convert sound vibrations in air into waves of fluid in the cochlea. It is associated with defects of the external ear or middle ear.

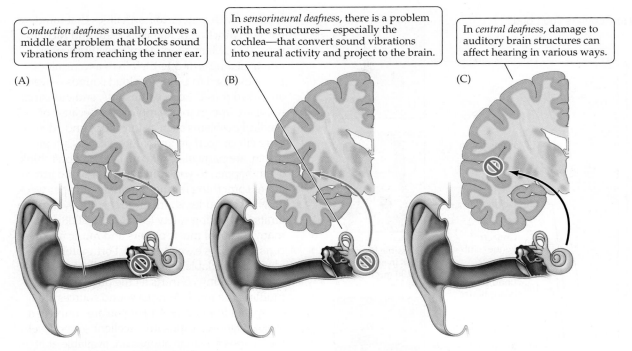

Conduction deafness usually involves a middle ear problem that blocks sound vibrations from reaching the inner ear.

In *sensorineural deafness*, there is a problem with the structures— especially the cochlea—that convert sound vibrations into neural activity and project to the brain.

In *central deafness*, damage to auditory brain structures can affect hearing in various ways.

(A) (B) (C)

FIGURE 6.10 Types of Hearing Loss

2. Even if vibrations are successfully conducted to the cochlea, the sensory apparatus of the cochlea—the organ of Corti, and the hair cells it contains—may fail to convert the ripples created in the basilar membrane into the volleys of action potentials that ordinarily inform the brain about sounds. This form of hearing loss, termed **sensorineural deafness** (**FIGURE 6.10B**), is most often the result of permanent damage or destruction of hair cells by any of a variety of causes (**FIGURE 6.11**). Some people

sensorineural deafness A hearing impairment most often caused by the permanent damage or destruction of hair cells or by interruption of the vestibulocochlear nerve that carries auditory information to the brain.

(A) Normal cochlea

In a normal cochlea, hair cells line the organ of Corti throughout its length, but exposure to excessively loud sounds can have rapid destructive effects. After exposure to excessive noise, a long section of the sound-damaged cochlea is completely missing its hair cells, resulting in deafness from the corresponding frequencies.

(B) Severe noise damage

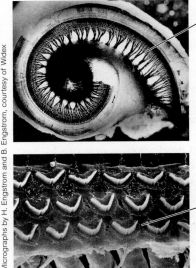
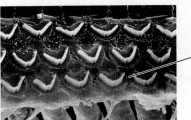

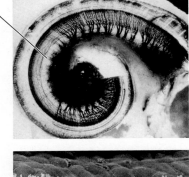
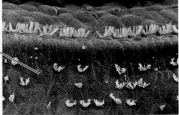

Electron microscopy reveals that the orderly rows of stereocilia found in the organ of Corti in a normal cochlea are crushed and flattened by excessive noise exposure, like trees blown down in a windstorm.

FIGURE 6.11 The Destructive Effects of Loud Noise

FIGURE 6.12 How Loud Is Too Loud?

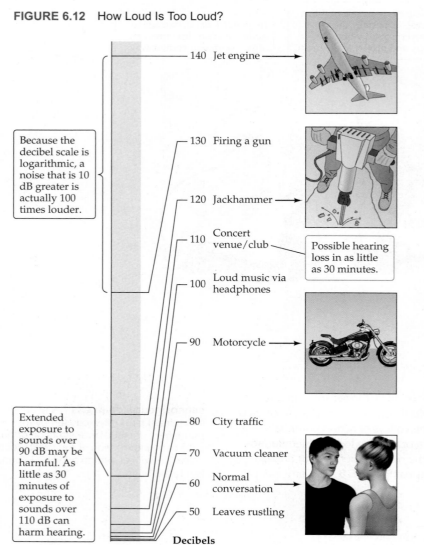

Because the decibel scale is logarithmic, a noise that is 10 dB greater is actually 100 times louder.

- 140 Jet engine
- 130 Firing a gun
- 120 Jackhammer
- 110 Concert venue/club
- 100 Loud music via headphones
- 90 Motorcycle
- 80 City traffic
- 70 Vacuum cleaner
- 60 Normal conversation
- 50 Leaves rustling

Decibels

Possible hearing loss in as little as 30 minutes.

Extended exposure to sounds over 90 dB may be harmful. As little as 30 minutes of exposure to sounds over 110 dB can harm hearing.

tinnitus A sensation of noises or ringing in the ears not caused by external sound.

central deafness A hearing impairment in which the auditory areas of the brain fail to process and interpret action potentials from sound stimuli in meaningful ways, usually as a consequence of damage in auditory brain areas.

word deafness A form of central deafness that is characterized by the specific inability to hear words although other sounds can be detected.

cortical deafness A form of central deafness, caused by damage to both sides of the auditory cortex, that is characterized by difficulty in recognizing all complex sounds, whether verbal or nonverbal.

are born with genetic abnormalities that interfere with the function of hair cells (Petit and Richardson, 2009). Many more people acquire sensorineural deafness during their lives as a result of being exposed to extremely loud sounds—overamplified music, nearby gunshots, and industrial noise are important examples—or because of medical problems such as infections and adverse drug effects (certain antibiotics, such as streptomycin, are particularly *ototoxic*). If you don't think it can happen to you, think again. Anyone listening to something for more than 5 hours per week at 89 dB or louder is already exceeding workplace limits for hearing safety (SCENIHR, 2008), yet many personal music players and music at concerts and clubs exceed 100 dB. Fortunately, earplugs are available that attenuate all frequencies equally, making concerts a little quieter without muffling the music. Various sound sources are compared in **FIGURE 6.12**; if you are concerned about your own exposure, excellent sound level meter apps for smartphones are available at little or no cost (including one from the National Institute for Occupational Safety and Health (NIOSH) at www.cdc.gov/niosh/topics/noise/app. html). Long-term exposure to loud sounds can cause lasting hearing problems ranging from a persistent ringing in the ears, called **tinnitus** (Zenner et al., 2017), to a permanent profound loss of hearing for the frequencies being listened to at such high volumes.

3. For the action potentials sent from the cochlea to be of any use, the auditory areas of the brain must process and interpret them in meaningful ways. **Central deafness** (**FIGURE 6.10C**) occurs when auditory brain areas are damaged by, for example, strokes, tumors, or traumatic injuries. As you might expect from our earlier discussion of auditory processing in the brain, this type of deafness almost never involves a simple loss of auditory sensitivity. Afflicted individuals can often hear a normal range of pure tones but are impaired in the perception of complex, behaviorally relevant sounds. An example in humans is **word deafness**: selective trouble with speech sounds despite normal speech and normal hearing for nonverbal sounds. In **cortical deafness**—a rare syndrome involving bilateral lesions of auditory cortex—patients have more-complete impairment, struggling to recognize all complex sounds, whether verbal or nonverbal.

Although there are few treatments available for central deafness, we can use electronic prostheses to restore the auditory stimulation that is missing in conduction or sensorineural deafness. We discuss these approaches in Signs & Symptoms, next.

SIGNS & SYMPTOMS ||||||||||||||||||||||||||||||||||||||||||||||||||||||||||||||||||||||||||||||||||||||||||||||||||||||

(A)

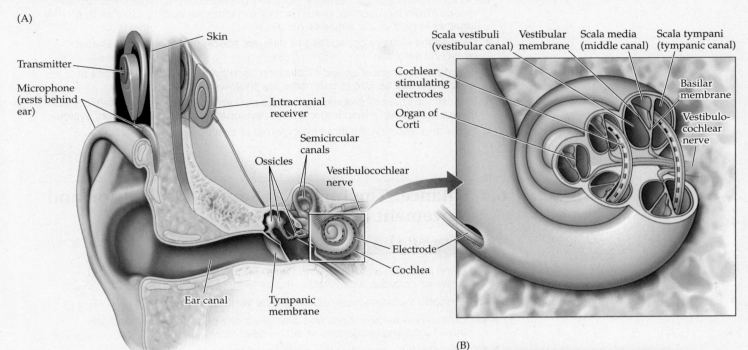

(B)

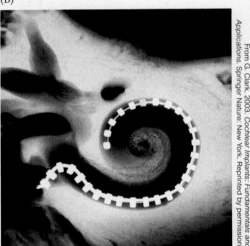

From G. Clark. 2003. Cochlear Implants: Fundamentals and Applications. Springer Nature: New York. Reprinted by permission.

FIGURE 6.13 Cochlear Implants Provide Hearing in Some Deaf People

Restoring Auditory Stimulation in Deafness

People with conduction deafness use hearing aids that employ electronic amplification to deliver louder sounds to the impaired—but still functional—auditory system, and it is sometimes possible to surgically free up the fused ossicles or replace them with Teflon prosthetics and thus restore the transmission of sound vibrations to the cochlea. But sensorineural deafness presents a much thornier problem because neural elements have been destroyed (or were absent from birth). Can new hair cells be grown? Although fishes and amphibians produce new hair cells throughout life, mammals traditionally have long been viewed as incapable of regenerating hair cells. This conclusion may have been too hasty, however (Géléoc and Holt, 2014). Using several different strategies, researchers have succeeded in inducing the birth of new hair cells in cochlear tissues of lab animals (Li et al., 2015), so there is reason to hope that an effective restorative therapy for deafness may be available someday.

For now, treatments for sensorineural deafness focus on the use of prostheses. Implantable devices called **cochlear implants** can detect sounds and then directly stimulate the auditory nerve fibers of the cochlea, bypassing the ossicles and hair cells altogether and offering partial restoration of hearing even in cases of complete sensorineural deafness (**FIGURE 6.13**). You may have had doubts about the value of Békésy's work with cadavers that we described at the start of this chapter. If so, consider this: the cochlear implants that have brought hearing to thousands of deaf people work by reproducing the phenomena Békésy discovered. In other words, the device

sends information about low frequencies to electrodes stimulating nerves at the apex of the cochlea and sends information about high frequencies to electrodes stimulating nerves at the base. As you might predict from our discussion of the importance of experience in shaping auditory responsiveness, the earlier in life these devices are implanted, the better the person will be able to understand complex sounds, especially speech (Geers et al., 2017). So in a sense, the success of these implants is due to the cleverness of the brain.

cochlear implant An implantable device that detects sounds and selectively stimulates nerves in different regions of the cochlea.

1. Compare and contrast the two important signals about pitch that the brain receives from the cochlea: place coding and temporal coding. How do they work together to give us our sense of pitch?

2. Discuss the sensory capabilities of different species as adaptations shaped by natural selection.

3. Provide an account of sound localization, identifying the several sources of information that we use to determine the source of a sound.

4. Discuss the types of processing that are performed by primary auditory cortex. Is experience with sound important for development of cortical auditory systems?

5. Name and describe the three major forms of deafness.

6.4   Balance: The Inner Ear Senses the Position and Movement of the Head

THE ROAD AHEAD

In the next section we look at the inner ear system that gives us our sense of balance. After reading this section, you should be able to:

6.4.1 Describe the anatomical features of the vestibular system.

6.4.2 Explain how accelerations and changes in the position of the head are transduced into sequences of action potentials.

6.4.3 Describe the vestibular projections to the brainstem, and summarize the functional importance of these projections.

6.4.4 Discuss some of the consequences of vestibular dysfunction or abnormal vestibular stimulation.

Without our sense of balance, it would be a challenge to simply stand on two feet. When you use an elevator, you clearly sense that your body is rising or falling, despite the sameness of your surroundings. When you turn your head, take a tight curve in your car, or bounce through the seas in a boat, your continual awareness of motion allows you to plan further movements and anticipate changes in perception due to movement of your head. And of course, too much of this sort of stimulation can make you lose your lunch.

Like hearing, our sense of balance is the product of the inner ear, relying on several small structures that adjoin the cochlea and are known collectively as the **vestibular system** (from the Latin *vestibulum*, "entrance hall," reflecting the fact that the system lies in hollow spaces in the temporal bone). In fact, it is generally accepted that the auditory organ evolved from the vestibular system, although the ossicles probably evolved from parts of the jaw. The most obvious components of the vestibular system are the three fluid-filled **semicircular canals**, plus two bulbs called the *saccule* and the *utricle* that are located near the ends of the semicircular canals (**FIGURE 6.14A**). Notice that the three canals are oriented in the three different planes in which the head can rotate (**FIGURE 6.14B**)—nodding up and down (technically known as *pitch*), shaking from side to side (*yaw*), and tilting left or right (*roll*).

The receptors of the vestibular system are hair cells—just like the ones in the cochlea—whose bending ultimately produces action potentials. The cilia of these hair cells are embedded in a gelatinous mass inside an enlarged chamber called the **ampulla** (plural *ampullae*) that lies at the base of each semicircular canal (see Figure 6.14B). Movement of the head in one axis sets up a flow of the fluid in the semicircular canal that lies in the same plane, bending the stereocilia in that particular ampulla and signaling the brain that the head has moved. Working together, the three semicircular canals accurately track the movement of the head. The utricle and saccule each contain an *otolithic membrane* (a gelatinous sheet studded with tiny crystals; *otolith* literally means "ear stone") that, thanks to its mass, lags slightly when

vestibular system The sensory system that detects balance. It consists of several small inner-ear structures that adjoin the cochlea.

semicircular canal Any one of the three fluid-filled tubes in the inner ear that are part of the vestibular system. Each of the tubes, which are at right angles to each other, detects angular acceleration in a particular direction.

ampulla An enlarged region of each semicircular canal that contains the receptor cells (hair cells) of the vestibular system.

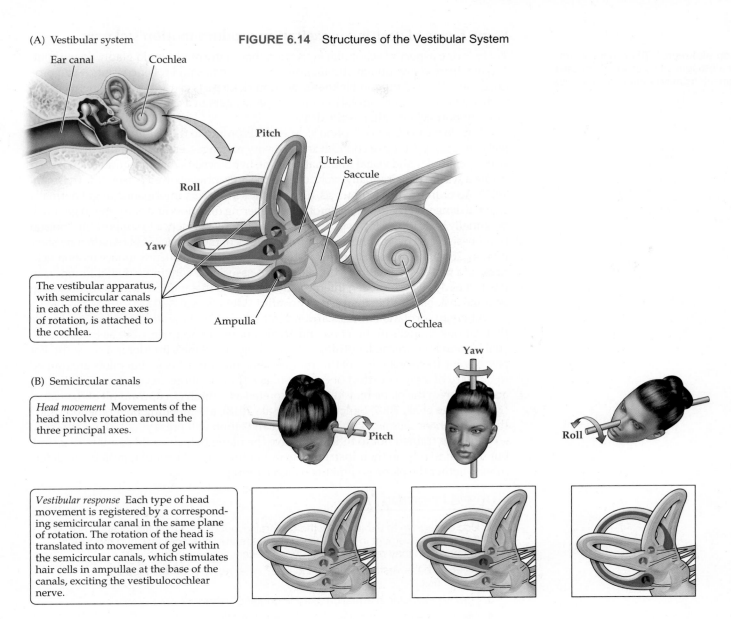

(A) Vestibular system

FIGURE 6.14 Structures of the Vestibular System

Ear canal

Cochlea

Pitch

Utricle

Saccule

Roll

Yaw

The vestibular apparatus, with semicircular canals in each of the three axes of rotation, is attached to the cochlea.

Ampulla

Cochlea

Yaw

Pitch

Roll

(B) Semicircular canals

Head movement Movements of the head involve rotation around the three principal axes.

Vestibular response Each type of head movement is registered by a corresponding semicircular canal in the same plane of rotation. The rotation of the head is translated into movement of gel within the semicircular canals, which stimulates hair cells in ampullae at the base of the canals, exciting the vestibulocochlear nerve.

the head moves. This bends nearby hair cells, stimulating them to track straight-line acceleration and deceleration—the final signals that the brain needs in order to calculate the position and movement of the body in three-dimensional space. Nerve fibers leading from these hair cells to the brain make up the vestibular part of the vestibulocochlear nerve (cranial nerve VIII).

Vestibular information is crucial for planning body movements, maintaining balance against gravity, and smoothly directing sensory organs like the eyes and ears toward specific locations, even when our bodies are themselves in motion. So, it's no surprise that the nerve pathways from the vestibular system have strong connections to brain regions responsible for the planning and control of movement. On entering the brainstem, many of the vestibular fibers terminate in the **vestibular nuclei**, while some fibers project directly to the cerebellum to aid in motor programming there. Outputs from the vestibular nuclei project in a complex manner to motor areas throughout the brain, including motor nuclei of the eye muscles, the thalamus, and the cerebral cortex.

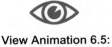

View Animation 6.5: The Vestibular System

vestibular nuclei Brainstem nuclei that receive information from the vestibular organs through cranial nerve VIII (the vestibulocochlear nerve).

motion sickness The experience of nausea brought on by unnatural passive movement, as may occur in a car or boat.

Some forms of vestibular excitation produce motion sickness

There is one aspect of vestibular activation that many of us would gladly do without. Too much strong vestibular stimulation—think of boats and roller coasters—can produce the misery of **motion sickness**. Motion sickness is caused by movements of the body that we cannot control. For example, passengers in a car are more likely to suffer from motion sickness than is the driver.

Why do we experience motion sickness? According to the *sensory conflict theory,* we feel bad when we receive contradictory sensory messages, especially a discrepancy between vestibular and visual information. One hypothesis is that the stimulation is activating a system that originally evolved to rid the body of swallowed poison (M. Treisman, 1977). According to this hypothesis, discrepancies in sensory information might normally signal a dangerous neurological problem, triggering dizziness and vomiting to get rid of potentially toxic food. However, there is little objective evidence to support the "poison hypothesis," and overall the evolutionary origins of motion sickness remain a mystery (Oman, 2012). The observation that virtual reality devices frequently induce motion sickness, and that susceptibility to this sickness is associated with individual differences in pre-test body sway, has been interpreted as evidence that motion sickness results from postural instability rather than sensory conflict (Munafo et al., 2017).

When an airplane bounces around in turbulence, the vestibular system signals that various changes in direction and accelerations are occurring, but as far as the visual system is concerned, nothing is happening; the plane's interior is a constant. For passengers, the worst effect of this may be some motion sickness, but pilots are trained to be wary of a second effect of this mismatch. In conditions of very low visibility, an acceleration of the plane may be misinterpreted as a climb (an upward tilt of the plane) (MacNeilage et al., 2007; Sánchez-Tena et al., 2018), a compelling phenomenon called the *somatogravic illusion.* Both acceleration and climb will press you back in your seat, so pilots are trained not to reflexively dive the plane (which could result in disaster), but instead to rely on their instruments rather than their vestibular systems to determine whether the plane is climbing or accelerating.

HOW'S IT GOING ❓

1. Use a diagram to explain how the general layout of the vestibular system allows it to track movement in three axes. Where are the receptors for head movement located? Do they resemble other types of sensory receptors?
2. Where are the vestibular nuclei located? What nerve provides inputs to these nuclei?
3. How is vestibular information used in ongoing behavior?
4. Discuss the role of the vestibular system in motion sickness.

6.5 Taste: Chemicals in Foods Are Perceived as Tastes

THE ROAD AHEAD

We now turn our attention to the specialized sensors that gives us our sense of taste. After reading this section, you should be able to:

6.5.1 Describe the structure, function, and distribution of the papillae on the tongue.

6.5.2 Summarize the structure of taste buds, and discuss their relationship to papillae.

6.5.3 Describe the basic tastes and the distribution of taste sensitivity across the surface of the tongue.

6.5.4 Describe the specialized cellular mechanisms through which taste cells transduce each of the major tastes.

6.5.5 Trace the neural projection of gustatory information to the brainstem and higher-order systems.

Delicious foods, poisons, dangerous adversaries, and fertile mates—these are just a few of the sources of chemical signals in the environment. Being able to detect these signals is vital for survival and reproduction throughout the animal kingdom.

Most people derive great pleasure from eating delicious food, and because we recognize many substances by their distinct flavors, we tend to think that we can discriminate many tastes. In reality, though, humans detect only a small number of basic tastes; the huge variety of sensations aroused by different foods are actually **flavors** rather than simple tastes, and they rely on the sense of smell as well as taste. (To appreciate the importance of smell to flavor, block your nose while eating first a little bit of raw potato and then some apple: without the sense of smell, you can't tell them apart!)

Scientists are in broad agreement that we possess at least five basic **tastes**: salty, sour, sweet, bitter, and umami. (*Umami*, Japanese for "delicious taste," is the term for the savory, meaty taste that is characteristic of gravy or soy sauce.) These tastes are determined genetically, as we will see shortly, but there is considerable genetic variation across the globe in both the strength and pleasurable qualities of the basic tastes (Pirastu et al., 2016). Further, the hunt continues for additional basic tastes. For example, studies suggest that humans may possess a primary fat taste (Mattes, 2011); another candidate, called *kokumi*, is described as the full-bodied, thick, mouth-filling quality of some foods (S. C. Brennan et al., 2014). But no matter how many basic tastes we are eventually shown to possess, it is clear that evolution shaped them to help us find nutritious food and avoid toxins.

Tastes excite specialized receptor cells on the tongue

Many people think that the many little bumps on their tongues are **taste buds**, but they aren't. They are actually **papillae** (singular *papilla*) (**FIGURE 6.15**), tiny lumps of tissue that increase the surface area of the tongue.

flavor   The sense of taste combined with the sense of smell.

taste   Any of the five basic sensations detected by the tongue—sweet, salty, sour, bitter, and umami.

taste bud   A cluster of 50–150 cells that detects tastes. Taste buds are found in papillae.

papilla   A small bump that projects from the surface of the tongue. Papillae contain most of the taste receptor cells.

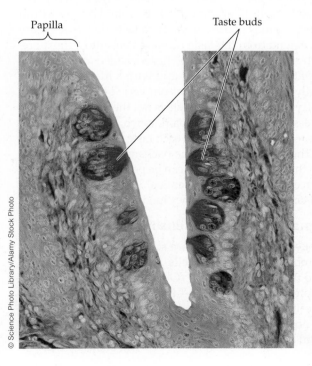

Papilla

Taste buds

© Science Photo Library/Alamy Stock Photo

FIGURE 6.15   A Cross Section of the Tongue

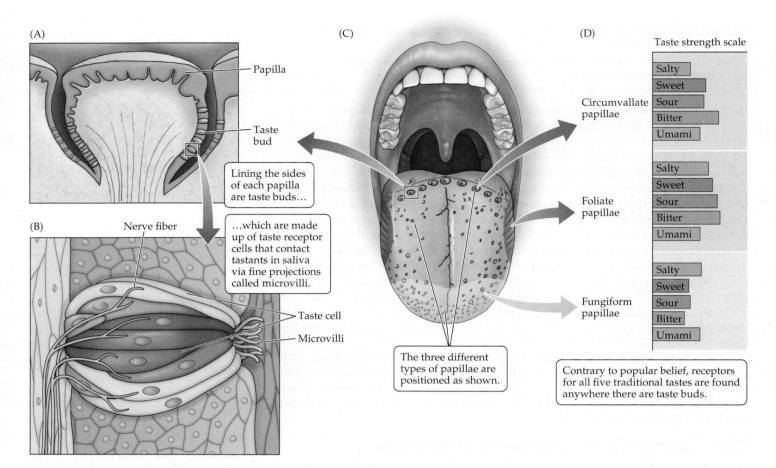

FIGURE 6.16 Taste Buds and Taste Receptor Cells (Part A after S. K. McLaughlin et al., 1994. *Physiol. Behav.* 56: 1157; C and D after L. M. Bartoshuk in D. Chadwick et al., 1993. *The Molecular Basis of Smell and Taste Transduction.* Wiley. New York.)

Labels in figure:
- Papilla
- Taste bud
- Lining the sides of each papilla are taste buds…
- …which are made up of taste receptor cells that contact tastants in saliva via fine projections called microvilli.
- Nerve fiber
- Taste cell
- Microvilli
- The three different types of papillae are positioned as shown.
- Taste strength scale
- Circumvallate papillae
- Foliate papillae
- Fungiform papillae
- Salty, Sweet, Sour, Bitter, Umami
- Contrary to popular belief, receptors for all five traditional tastes are found anywhere there are taste buds.

View Activity 6.2:
Taste Buds and Taste Receptor Cells

There are three kinds of papillae—*circumvallate, foliate,* and *fungiform* papillae—occurring in different locations on the tongue (**FIGURE 6.16**). Taste buds, each consisting of a cluster of 50–150 taste receptor cells (**FIGURE 6.16B**), are found buried within the walls of the papillae (a single papilla may house several such taste buds; see Figure 6.15). Fine fibers, called *microvilli*, extend from the taste receptor cells into a tiny pore, where they come into contact with substances that can be tasted, called *tastants*. Each taste cell is sensitive to just one of the five basic tastes, and with a life span of only 10–14 days, taste cells are constantly being replaced. But as our varied experience with hot drinks, frozen flagpoles, or spicy foods informs us, taste is not the only sensory capability of the tongue. It also possesses sensory cells for pain, touch, and temperature.

You may have seen maps of the tongue indicating that each taste is perceived mainly in one region (sweet at the tip of the tongue, bitter at the back, and so on), but these maps are based on an enduring myth. All five basic tastes can be perceived anywhere on the tongue where there are taste receptors (Chandrashekar et al., 2006). Those areas do not differ greatly in the strength of taste sensations that they mediate (**FIGURE 6.16D**).

The five basic tastes are signaled by specific sensors on taste cells

The tastes salty and sour are evoked when taste cells are stimulated by simple ions acting on ion channels in the membranes of the taste cells. Sweet, bitter, and umami tastes are perceived by specialized receptor molecules—G protein–coupled receptors (GPCRs), as we discussed in Chapter 3 (see Figure 3.2)—that use second messengers to change the activity of the taste cell. Researchers have also discovered taste receptors in numerous tissues of the body—not just the tongue (**FIGURE 6.17**)—where they serve functions unrelated to conventional taste, such as the control of appetite and digestion (Behrens and Meyerhof, 2019).

SALTY   Taste cells apparently sense salt (NaCl) in several different ways, which are not yet completely understood. As you might guess, one kind of salt sensor simply relies on sodium (Na⁺) channels, just like the ones we have seen in previous chapters. In this case, sodium ions (Na⁺) from salty food enter taste cells via sodium channels in the cell membrane, causing a depolarization of the cell and release of neurotransmitter. We know that this is a crucial mechanism for perceiving saltiness, because blocking the sodium channels with a drug reduces salt discrimination—though it does not eliminate it (Chandrashekar et al., 2010). This system also seems to be responsible for the appetizing qualities of moderate concentrations of salt in food. However, research indicates that taste cells are also sensitive to the other ion that is liberated when salt dissolves: chloride (Cl⁻). This parallel salt-sensing system seems to mediate the aversive properties of *high* concentrations of salt. Because drugs that block chloride-selective ion channels have little effect on the Cl⁻ sensitivity of the tongue, researchers believe that Cl⁻ transduction by taste cells involves a different, as-yet-unknown mechanism (Roebber et al., 2019). Depolarization of the salt-sensitive taste cells ultimately causes them to release neurotransmitters that stimulate afferent neurons that relay the information to the brain.

SOUR   Acids in food taste sour—the more acidic the food, the more sour it tastes—but no one knows exactly how sour tastants are detected. Researchers think that the protons (H⁺, also called *hydrogen ions*) that all acids release may interact with special acid-sensing ion channels (like the ionotropic receptors in Chapter 2 and Chapter 3) to change the polarity of taste cells and alter transmitter release. It seems that all sour-sensitive taste cells contain a particular type of ion channel protein and share an inward flow of protons that depolarizes the cell (A. L. Huang et al., 2006; Bushman et al., 2015). Interestingly, the same sensor appears to detect the sensation and taste of carbonation in drinks (Chandrashekar et al., 2009) and prompts thirsty animals to drink (Zocchi et al., 2017).

SWEET   The receptors for sweet, bitter, and umami tastes are more like metabotropic receptors than ionotropic receptors (see Figure 3.2) because tastant molecules bind to a complex receptor protein on the taste cell's surface that activates a second messenger within the cell. These receptors are made up of simpler proteins belonging to two families—designated **T1R** and **T2R**—that are combined in various ways.

When two members of the T1R family—T1R2 and T1R3—combine (*heterodimerize*), they make a receptor that selectively detects sweet tastants (Nelson et al., 2001). Mice engineered to lack either T1R2 or T1R3 are insensitive to sweet tastes (Zhao et al., 2003). And if you've spent any time around cats, you may be aware that they couldn't care less about sweets. It turns out that in all cats, from tabbies to tigers, the gene that encodes T1R2 is disabled, so their sweet receptors don't work (X. Li et al., 2009).

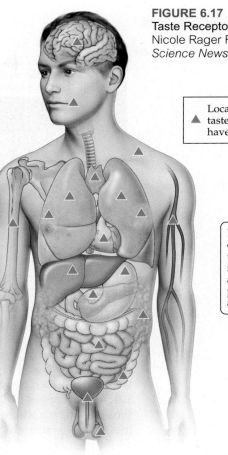

FIGURE 6.17   Body Tissues Expressing Taste Receptors (After an illustration by Nicole Rager Fuller in R. Ehrenberg, 2010. *Science News* 177: 22–25.)

▲ Locations in which taste-related components have been found.

By searching for the molecular components of the known taste receptors, researchers found taste-like sensors in a surprising variety of tissues, performing functions that are as yet unknown.

T1R   A family of taste receptor proteins that, when particular members bind together, form taste receptors for sweet flavors and umami flavors.

T2R   A family of bitter taste receptors.

FIGURE 6.18 It's All a Matter of Taste Buds

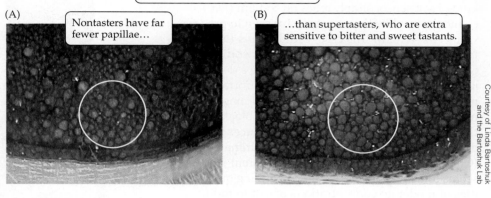

Certain substances that taste unpleasantly bitter to most people can't be tasted at all by some people.

(A) Nontasters have far fewer papillae…

(B) …than supertasters, who are extra sensitive to bitter and sweet tastants.

Courtesy of Linda Bartoshuk and the Bartoshuk Lab

BITTER In nature, bitter tastes often signal the presence of toxins, so it's not surprising that a high sensitivity to different kinds of bitter tastes has evolved (Lush, 1989), although individuals vary significantly in their taste sensitivity (**FIGURE 6.18**). Members of the T2R family of receptor proteins appear to function as bitter receptors (Chandrashekar et al., 2000; Behrens and Meyerhof, 2018). The T2R family has about 30 members, and this large number may reflect the wide variety of bitter substances encountered in the environment, as well as the adaptive importance of being able to detect and avoid them. Interestingly, each bitter-sensing taste cell produces most or all of the different types of T2R bitter receptors (Adler et al., 2000). So bitter-sensing taste cells exhibit broadly tuned sensitivity to *any* bitter-tasting substances (Brasser et al., 2005)—just what you'd expect in a sensory system that has evolved to act as a poison detector.

UMAMI The fifth basic taste, **umami**—the meaty, savory flavor—is detected by at least two kinds of receptors. One of these is a variant of the metabotropic glutamate receptor (Chaudhari et al., 2000; Maruyama et al., 2006) and most likely responds to the amino acid glutamate, which is found in high concentrations in meats, cheeses, kombu, and other savory foodstuffs (that's why MSG—monosodium *glutamate*—is used as a "flavor enhancer"). The second probable umami receptor, a heterodimer of T1R1 and T1R3 proteins, responds to most of the dietary amino acids (Nelson et al., 2002). Given this receptor's similarity to the T1R2+T1R3 sweet receptor, there is reason to suppose that receptors for things that taste good may have shared evolutionary origins. Consider the taste abilities of birds that, just like their house cat enemies, lack the T1R2 gene and thus ordinarily can't taste sweet. How then do hummingbirds sense the nectar they need for survival? It appears that evolution repurposed the hummingbird T1R1+T1R3 umami receptor into a new class of sweet receptor (Baldwin et al., 2014), allowing hummingbirds to thrive and spread.

Taste information is transmitted to several parts of the brain

Taste projections of the **gustatory system** (from the Latin *gustare*, "to taste") extend from the tongue to several brainstem nuclei, then to the thalamus, and ultimately to gustatory regions of the somatosensory cortex (**FIGURE 6.19**). Because there are only five basic tastes, and because each taste cell detects just one of the five, the encoding of taste perception could be quite straightforward, with the brain simply monitoring which specific axons are active in order to determine which tastes are present (Chandrashekar et al., 2006). In such a simple arrangement—as we noted earlier, it is sometimes called a *labeled-line system*—there is no need to analyze complex patterns of activity across multiple kinds of taste receptors (called *pattern coding*). Experimental evidence seemingly supports the conclusion that taste is a labeled-line system: selectively inactivating taste

umami One of the five basic tastes—the meaty, savory flavor. (The other four tastes are salty, sour, sweet, and bitter.)

gustatory system The sensory system that detects taste.

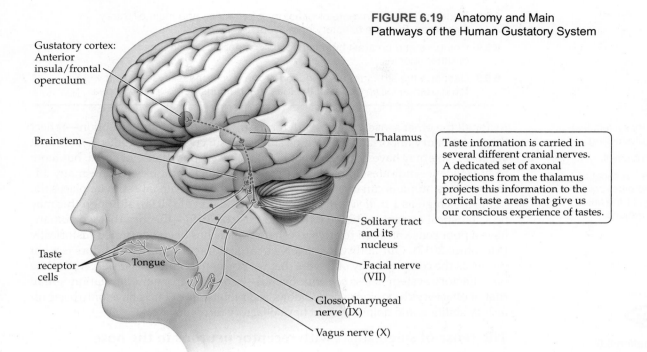

FIGURE 6.19 Anatomy and Main Pathways of the Human Gustatory System

Gustatory cortex:
Anterior insula/frontal operculum

Brainstem

Thalamus

Taste receptor cells

Tongue

Solitary tract and its nucleus

Facial nerve (VII)

Glossopharyngeal nerve (IX)

Vagus nerve (X)

> Taste information is carried in several different cranial nerves. A dedicated set of axonal projections from the thalamus projects this information to the cortical taste areas that give us our conscious experience of tastes.

cells that express receptors for just one of the five tastes tends to completely eradicate sensitivity to that one taste while leaving the other four tastes unaffected (Huang et al., 2006). However, the same manipulation can also be viewed as knocking out one-fifth of any pattern of activity that would be normally present. From this perspective, the pattern-coding account cannot be ruled out. A precise understanding of the way in which the brain encodes taste information thus awaits future developments.

HOW'S IT GOING ?

1. What are the five basic tastes?
2. Generate a map of the human tongue, showing how sensitive each region is to the five basic tastes.
3. Compare and contrast taste buds and papillae.
4. Identify the cellular mechanisms underlying each of the five tastes. Discuss the evolution of taste sensitivity: How do these five tastes help us survive?

6.6 Smell: Chemicals in the Air Elicit Odor Sensations

THE ROAD AHEAD

Finally we turn our attention to the specialized sensory system that samples chemicals in the air: our sense of smell. After reading this section, you should be able to:

6.6.1 Describe the main structures of the olfactory system, with a focus on the cells and projections of the olfactory epithelium.

6.6.2 Explain the process of olfactory transduction, and discuss the function and variety of olfactory receptors that have been discovered.

olfaction The sensory system that detects smell; the act of smelling.

odor The sensation of smell.

olfactory epithelium A sheet of olfactory receptors and other cells that lines the dorsal portion of the nasal cavities and adjacent regions.

View Animation 6.6:
The Human Olfactory System

As for all the other senses, species differences in **olfaction**—odor perception—reflect the evolutionary importance of various smells for survival and reproduction (Bear et al., 2016). You may have been told that humans have a poor sense of smell, but more recent evidence indicates otherwise. Although we don't know exactly how many different **odors** humans can *discriminate* between—a controversial estimate places the number as high as 1 *trillion* different odors (Bushdid et al., 2014), although this may be a statistical overestimation (Gerkin and Castro, 2015)—the idea that we humans have a poor sense of smell relative to other animals has been overstated historically (McGann, 2017). Our ability to perceive a large number of different odors is what produces the complex array of flavors that we normally think of as tastes. And while our olfactory system is less *sensitive* overall—requires stronger stimulation—than that of olfactory champions such as dogs and rabbits, most birds have only basic olfactory abilities, and dolphins don't have olfactory receptors at all.

The sense of smell starts with receptor neurons in the nose

In humans (and most other mammals), a sheet of cells called the **olfactory epithelium** lines part of the nasal cavities. Within the 5–10 square centimeters of olfactory epithelium that we possess, three types of cells are found (**FIGURE 6.20**): supporting cells, basal cells, and about 6 million olfactory receptor neurons. For comparison, dogs have 100–300 million olfactory receptor neurons, which explains their ability to detect odors at extremely low concentrations—as low as 2 parts per trillion (King, 2013), which is like tasting a pinch of sugar dissolved in a billion cups of tea!

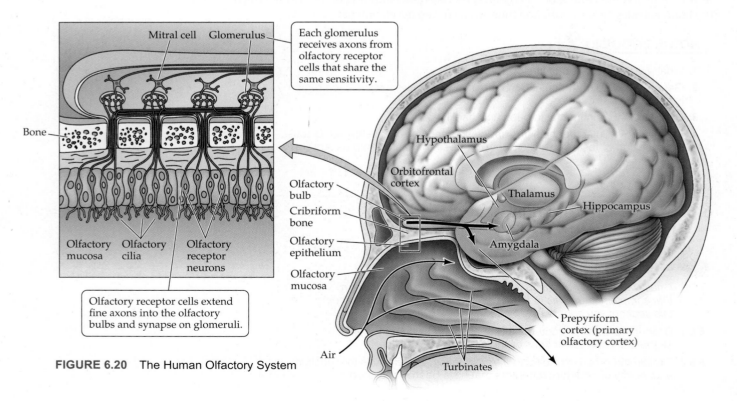

FIGURE 6.20 The Human Olfactory System

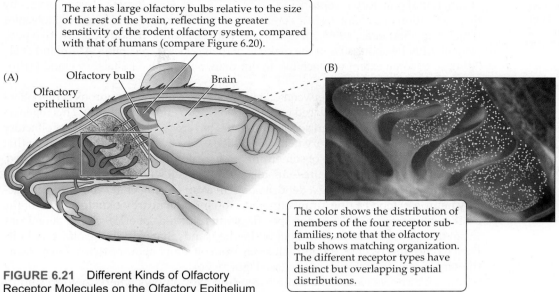

The rat has large olfactory bulbs relative to the size of the rest of the brain, reflecting the greater sensitivity of the rodent olfactory system, compared with that of humans (compare Figure 6.20).

(A)

Olfactory bulb   Brain

Olfactory epithelium

(B)

Courtesy of Robert Vassar

The color shows the distribution of members of the four receptor subfamilies; note that the olfactory bulb shows matching organization. The different receptor types have distinct but overlapping spatial distributions.

FIGURE 6.21   Different Kinds of Olfactory Receptor Molecules on the Olfactory Epithelium (Part A after R. Vassar et al., 1993. *Cell* 74: 309.)

Each olfactory receptor cell is a complete neuron, with a long, slender apical dendrite that divides into branches (cilia) that extend into the moist mucosal surface. Substances that we can smell from the air that we inhale or sniff, called *odorants*, dissolve into the mucosal layer and interact with receptors studding the dendritic cilia of the olfactory neurons (Mohrhardt et al., 2018). Like the metabotropic receptors found on neurons, the olfactory receptor proteins are a variety of G protein–coupled receptors (GPCRs), employing a second-messenger system to respond to the presence of odorants. However, despite these similarities, olfactory neurons differ from the neurons of the brain in several ways.

One way in which olfactory neurons are distinct from their cousins in the brain relates to the production of receptors: there is an incredible diversity of olfactory receptor protein subtypes. So, while there may be up to a dozen or so subtypes of receptors for a given neurotransmitter in the brain, there are hundreds or even thousands of subtypes within the family of odorant receptors, depending on the species under study. The Nobel Prize–winning discovery of the genes encoding this odorant receptor superfamily (Buck and Axel, 1991) provided one of the most important advances in the history of olfaction research.

Mice have about 2 million olfactory receptor neurons, each of which expresses only one of about 1,000 different receptor proteins. These receptor proteins can be divided into four different subfamilies of about 250 receptors each (Mori et al., 1999). Within each subfamily, members have similar structure and presumably recognize chemically similar odorants. Receptors of different subfamilies are expressed in separate bands of olfactory neurons within the olfactory epithelium (**FIGURE 6.21**) (Coleman et al., 2019). By comparison, humans make a total of about 400 different kinds of functional olfactory receptor proteins. That's still a large number, but in our case, it looks like hundreds of additional olfactory receptor genes have become nonfunctional during the course of evolution (Olender et al., 2008), suggesting that the substances they detected ceased to be important to our ancestors' survival and reproduction. And in a curious parallel to the discovery of taste receptors throughout the body, it turns out that some of the tongue's taste cells possess functional olfactory receptors (Malik et al., 2019), perhaps reflecting the great importance of flavors to our species. Whatever turns out to be the actual number of odors humans can distinguish, our ability to discriminate thousands, millions, or perhaps billions of odors using just 400 kinds

olfactory bulb An anterior projection of the brain that terminates in the upper nasal passages and, through small openings in the skull, provides receptors for smell.

glomerulus A complex arbor of dendrites from a group of olfactory cells.

of functional olfactory receptors indicates that we must recognize most odorants by their activation of a characteristic combination of different kinds of receptor molecules (Duchamp-Viret et al., 1999), an example of pattern coding. In addition, any two people will differ by about 30% in the makeup of their olfactory receptors (Mainland et al., 2014), so to some extent we each live in our own, personalized olfactory world (Trimmer et al., 2019).

Another big difference between olfactory neurons and brain neurons is that olfactory neurons die and are replaced in adulthood (Lledo and Valley, 2018). This regenerative capacity is most likely an adaptation to the hazardous environment that olfactory neurons inhabit. If an olfactory neuron is killed—say, by the virus that gave you that darn head cold, or by a whiff of something toxic while you were cleaning out the shed, or by some other misadventure—an adjacent basal cell will soon differentiate into a neuron and begin extending a dendrite and an axon (Leung et al., 2007). Each olfactory neuron extends a fine, unmyelinated axon into the nearby **olfactory bulb** of the brain, where it terminates on one specific **glomerulus**—a spherical clump of neurons (from the Latin *glomus*, "ball")—out of the thousands that exist in the olfactory bulb. Each glomerulus receives inputs exclusively from olfactory neurons that are expressing the same type of olfactory receptor (see Figure 6.20).

No one knows exactly how the extending axon knows where to go to find its specific glomerulus, or how it knows where to form synapses within the glomerulus after it arrives. One possibility is that olfactory receptor proteins that are found on the axons of these cells (as well as on the dendrites) guide the axons to their corresponding glomeruli (Barnea et al., 2004; Imai et al., 2009). But whatever may be the exact mechanisms of neuroplasticity in these cells, better understanding of the process of olfactory neurogenesis may someday help us develop methods for restoring damaged regions of the brain and spinal cord.

Olfactory information projects from the olfactory bulbs to several brain regions

Having received information from multiple olfactory neurons all expressing the same type of olfactory receptor, the glomerulus then actively tunes and sharpens the neural activity associated with the corresponding odorants (Aungst et al., 2003). The glomeruli are organized within the olfactory bulb according to an orderly, topographic map of smells, with neighboring glomeruli receiving inputs from receptors that are closely related. And, as Figure 6.21 shows, the spatial organization of glomeruli within the olfactory bulbs reflects the segregation of the four receptor protein subfamilies in the olfactory epithelium (Mori et al., 1999). This glomerular organization is established during a critical period in early life, after which it becomes fixed (Tsai and Barnea, 2014), resulting in an "olfactotopic" map that is maintained within the olfactory projections throughout the brain.

Olfactory information is conveyed to the brain via the axons of *mitral cells* (see Figure 6.20), which extend from the glomeruli in the olfactory bulbs to various regions of the forebrain; smell is the only sensory modality that synapses directly in the cortex rather than having to pass through the thalamus. Important targets for olfactory inputs include the hypothalamus, the amygdala, and the prepyriform cortex (**FIGURE 6.22**). These limbic structures are closely involved in memory and emotion, which may help explain the potency of odors in evoking nostalgic memories of childhood (M. Larsson and Willander, 2009).

Many vertebrates possess a vomeronasal system

Though many perfumers have tried to create one, there is no perfume for humans that is as alluring as the natural scents that other species use to find possible mates. The majority of terrestrial vertebrates—mammals, amphibians, and reptiles—possess a secondary chemical detection system that is specialized for detecting such

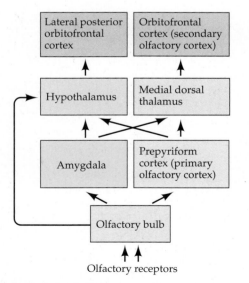

FIGURE 6.22 Components of the Brain's Olfactory System

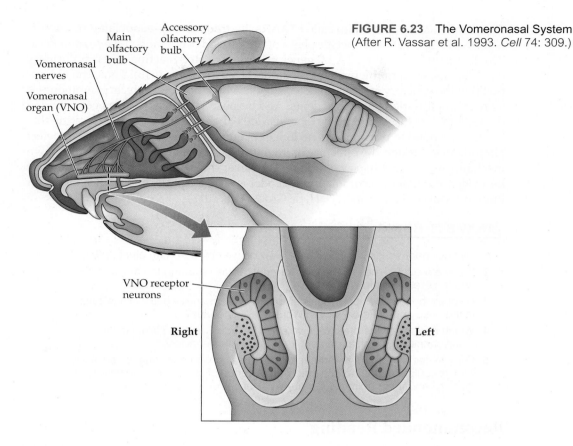

FIGURE 6.23 The Vomeronasal System
(After R. Vassar et al. 1993. *Cell* 74: 309.)

Main olfactory bulb

Accessory olfactory bulb

Vomeronasal nerves

Vomeronasal organ (VNO)

VNO receptor neurons

Right

Left

pheromones. The system is called the *vomeronasal system* (**FIGURE 6.23**), and its receptors are found in the **vomeronasal organ** (**VNO**), near the olfactory epithelium.

In rodents, the sensory neurons of the VNO make hundreds of different vomeronasal receptor proteins, forming two large families of GPCRs called *V1R* and *V2R* (Dulac and Torello, 2003). These receptors are extremely sensitive, able to detect very low levels of the pheromone signals—such as sex hormone metabolites and signals of genetic relatedness—that are released by other individuals (Leinders-Zufall et al., 2000; Loconto et al., 2003). From the VNO, information is transmitted to the accessory olfactory bulb (adjacent to the main olfactory bulb), which projects to the medial amygdala and hypothalamus, structures that play crucial roles in governing emotional and sexual behaviors and in regulating hormone secretion. Hamsters and mice can distinguish relatives from nonrelatives just by smell (Mateo and Johnston, 2000; Isles et al., 2001), allowing these animals to optimize their reproductive activities. In parallel, dedicated mechanisms in olfactory cortex activate fear and stress responses to predator odor signals, helping the animal to avoid their toothy source (Kondoh et al., 2016).

Do humans communicate via pheromones? Studies reporting pheromone-like phenomena in humans attract plenty of media attention because of the apparent link to our evolutionary past. Well-known examples include the report that simple exposure to each other's bodily odors can shift women's menstrual cycles (Stern and McClintock, 1998) and a report that exposure to female tears causes reductions in testosterone and sexual arousal in men (Gelstein et al., 2011). However, the VNO is either vestigial or absent in humans, and almost all of our V1R and V2R receptor genes have become nonfunctional "pseudogenes" over evolutionary time (Lübke and Pause, 2015). So, if humans do communicate through pheromones, it is most likely accomplished using the main olfactory epithelium, and not the VNO. In mice, receptors in

pheromone A chemical signal that is released outside the body of an animal and affects other members of the same species.

vomeronasal organ (VNO) A collection of specialized receptor cells, near to but separate from the olfactory epithelium, that detect pheromones and send electrical signals to the accessory olfactory bulb in the brain.

trace amine–associated receptor (TAAR)   Any one of a family of probable pheromone receptors produced by neurons in the main olfactory epithelium.

the main olfactory epithelium called **TAARs**, for **trace amine–associated receptors**, reportedly respond to sex-specific pheromones instead of odorants (Liberles and Buck, 2006), and mice with their TAAR genes knocked out stop reacting to certain urinary odor signals, even in the urine of predators (Dewan et al., 2013). Thus, the old notion that the olfactory epithelium detects odors while the VNO detects pheromones is an oversimplification, even in rodents. And because TAARs have also been found in the human olfactory epithelium (Liberles, 2009), behavioral evidence indicating that humans respond to pheromones no longer presents a paradox. If rodents can detect pheromones through the olfactory epithelium, using TAARs or other yet-unknown mechanisms, then perhaps we can too. Whatever the details of the mechanism may be, evidence is rapidly accumulating that odor is an ecologically important channel for human social communication (J. H. de Groot et al., 2017).

HOW'S IT GOING ❓

1. Discuss odor sensitivity in humans. How do we compare with other species?
2. Provide a brief sketch of the olfactory epithelium, showing the major cell types and their relationships to the brain.
3. Discuss the genetics of odor receptors, as well as their spatial organization in the nose and olfactory bulbs. What is a glomerulus?
4. Which regions of the brain receive strong olfactory inputs? What is the significance of this arrangement for an animal's behavior?
5. Discuss the structures and receptors associated with pheromone sensitivity, and speculate about the ecological importance of pheromone sensitivity in humans and other animals. Are humans sensitive to pheromones?

Recommended Reading

Doty, R. L. (2015). *Handbook of Olfaction and Gustation* (3rd ed.). New York, NY: Wiley-Blackwell.

Hawkes, C. H. (2018). *Smell and Taste Disorders*. Cambridge, UK: Cambridge University Press.

Horowitz, S. S. (2012). *The Universal Sense: How Hearing Shapes the Mind*. London, UK: Bloomsbury.

Musiek, F. E., and Baran, J. A. (2018). *The Auditory System: Anatomy, Physiology, and Clinical Correlates* (2nd ed.). San Diego, CA: Plural.

Palmer, A., and Rees, A. (2010). *Oxford Handbook of Auditory Science*. Oxford, UK: Oxford University Press.

Wolfe, J. M., Kluender, K. R., Levi, D. M., Bartoshuk, L. M., et al. (2021). *Sensation & Perception* (6th ed.). Sunderland, MA: Oxford University Press/Sinauer.

Wyatt, T. D. (2014). *Pheromones and Animal Behavior: Chemical Signals and Signatures* (2nd ed.). Cambridge, UK: Cambridge University Press.

Yost, W. A. (2013). *Fundamentals of Hearing* (5th ed.). San Diego, CA: Academic Press.

You should be able to relate each summary to the adjacent illustration, including structures and processes. The online version of this **Visual Summary** includes links to figures, animations, and activities that will help you consolidate the material.

1 The **pinna** (external ear) captures, focuses, and filters sound. The sound arriving at the **tympanic membrane** (eardrum) is focused by the three **ossicles** of the **middle ear** onto the **oval window** to stimulate the fluid-filled **inner ear** (specifically, the cochlea). Review **Figure 6.1**, **Animations 6.2** and **6.3**

2 Sound arriving at the oval window causes traveling waves to sweep along the **basilar membrane** of the **cochlea**. For sounds of high **frequency**, the largest displacement of the basilar membrane is at the base of the cochlea, near the oval window; for low-frequency sounds, the largest amplitude is near the apex of the cochlea. Review **Figure 6.2**, **Box 6.1**

3 Movement of the **stereocilia** of the **hair cells** causes the opening and closing of ion channels, thereby **transducing** mechanical movement into changes in electrical potential. The hair cell then releases neurotransmitter to simulate the nerve cell endings that contact them. Review **Figure 6.3**

4 The **organ of Corti** has both **inner hair cells** (**IHCs**, about 3,500 in humans) and **outer hair cells** (**OHCs**, about 12,000 in humans). The inner hair cells convey most of the information about sounds. The outer hair cells change their length under the control of the brain, amplifying the movements of the basilar membrane in response to sound and sharpening the frequency tuning of the cochlea. Review **Figure 6.3**, **Activity 6.1**

5 Afferents from the inner hair cells transmit auditory information to the **cochlear nuclei** of the brainstem. Cochlear neurons project bilaterally to the **superior olivary nucleus**, which in turn innervates the **inferior colliculus**. From there auditory information is relayed to the **medial geniculate nucleus** and then the **primary auditory cortex** in the temporal lobe. Review **Figure 6.5**, **Animation 6.4**

6 Auditory localization depends on differences in the sounds arriving at the two ears. For low-frequency sounds, **interaural temporal differences** (differences in time of arrival at the two ears) are especially important. For high-frequency sounds, **interaural intensity differences** are especially important, and **spectral filtering** provides cues about elevation. Review **Figure 6.7**

7 Primary auditory cortex is specialized for processing complex, biologically important sounds, rather than **pure tones**. Experiences with sound early in life can influence later auditory localization and the responses of neurons in auditory pathways. Experiences later in life can also lead to changes in the responses of auditory neurons. Review **Figures 6.8** and **6.9**

8 **Conduction deafness** consists of impairments in the transmission of sound through the external or middle ear to the cochlea. **Sensorineural deafness** arises in the cochlea, often because of the destruction of hair cells, or in the auditory nerve. **Central deafness** stems from brain damage. Review **Figure 6.10**

9 Some forms of deafness may be alleviated by direct electrical stimulation of the auditory nerve by a **cochlear implant**. Genetic manipulations can induce new hair cell growth in laboratory animals, raising hope of a gene therapy for sensorineural deafness. Review **Figure 6.13**

10 The receptors of the **vestibular system** that detect movement of the head lie within the inner ear next to the cochlea. In mammals the vestibular system consists of three **semicircular canals** plus the utricle and the saccule. The semicircular canals use hair cells to detect rotation of the body in three planes, and the utricle and saccule sense static positions and linear accelerations. Review **Figure 6.14**, **Animation 6.5**

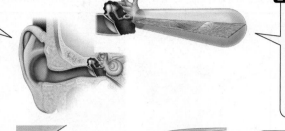

Pitch

Roll

Yaw

Yaw

11 Humans detect only five main **tastes**—salty, sour, sweet, bitter, and **umami**—using taste receptor cells located in clusters called **taste buds**. Taste cells extend fine filaments into the taste pore of each bud, where tastants come into contact with them. The taste buds are situated on small projections from the surface of the tongue called **papillae**. The tastes of salty and sour are evoked primarily by the movement of ions (usually from food) through ion channels in the membranes of taste cells. Sweet, umami, and bitter tastes are perceived by specialized G protein–coupled receptors (GPCRs) belonging to the **T1R** and **T2R** families. Taste receptors are also expressed in tissues elsewhere in the body. Review **Figures 6.16** and **6.17**, **Activity 6.2**

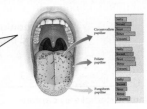

12 Each taste cell transmits information via cranial nerves to brainstem nuclei. This **gustatory system** extends from the taste receptor cells through brainstem nuclei to the thalamus and then to the cerebral cortex. Each taste axon responds most strongly to one category of tastes, providing a labeled line to the brain. Review **Figure 6.19**

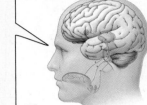

13 In contrast to being able to detect only a few tastes, humans can detect a huge number of different **odors**. Olfactory receptor neurons extend dendrites in the **olfactory epithelium** that express olfactory receptor proteins. The fine, unmyelinated axons of olfactory neurons project to the **olfactory bulbs** and synapse within **glomeruli**. If an olfactory receptor cell dies, an adjacent cell will replace it. Review **Figure 6.20**, **Animation 6.6**

14 There is a large family of odor receptor molecules, each of which utilizes G proteins and second messengers. Large subfamilies of receptors are synthesized in distinct bands of the olfactory epithelium. Review **Figure 6.21**

15 Outputs from the olfactory bulb extend to prepyriform cortex, amygdala, and hypothalamus, among other brain regions. Olfactory projections to the cortex maintain a stereotyped olfactory map of slightly overlapping projections from the glomeruli. Review **Figure 6.22**

16 The **vomeronasal organ** (**VNO**) contains receptors to detect pheromones released from other individuals of the species. These receptors transmit signals to the accessory olfactory bulb, which in turn communicates with the amygdala. **Pheromones** can also be detected by specialized receptors in the main olfactory epithelium. Review **Figure 6.23**

The Mind's Machine digital resources include additional videos, flashcards, and other study tools.

7 Vision
From Eye to Brain

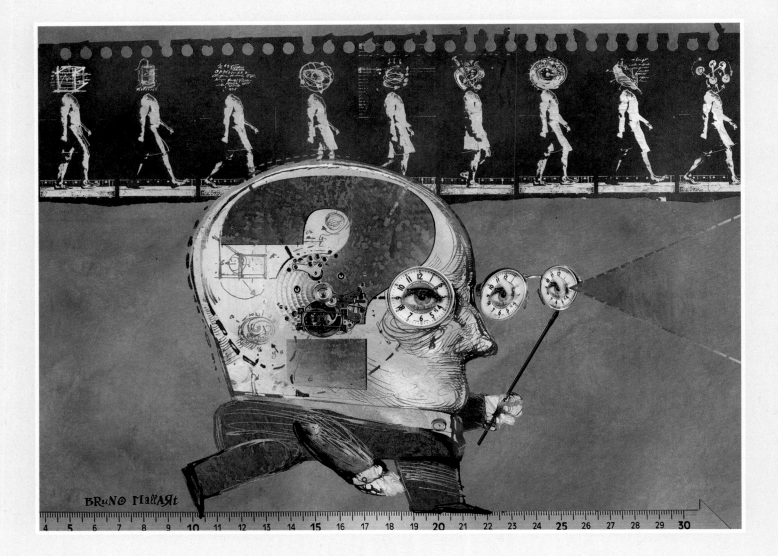

BRuNO MallARt

When Seeing Isn't Seeing

It was cold in the bathroom, so the young woman turned on a small heater before she got in the shower. She didn't know that the heater was malfunctioning, filling the room with deadly, odorless carbon monoxide gas. Her husband found her unconscious on the floor and called for an ambulance to rush her to the emergency room. When she regained consciousness, "D.F." seemed to have gotten off lightly, avoiding what could have been a fatal accident. She could understand the doctors' questions and reply sensibly, move all her limbs, and perceive touch on her skin. But something was wrong with her sight.

D.F. had lost the ability to identify things that she viewed. Even the faces of family members had become unfamiliar. More than a decade later, D.F. still could not recognize commonplace objects, yet she was not entirely blind. If you showed her a flashlight, she could tell you that it was made of shiny aluminum with some red plastic, but she didn't recognize it ("Is it a kitchen utensil?"). Without telling her what it was, if you asked her to pick it up, her hand moved directly to grasp the flashlight exactly as one normally does. Shown a slot in a piece of plastic, D.F. could not tell you whether the slot was oriented vertically, horizontally, or diagonally; but if you handed her a disk and asked her to put it through the slot, she invariably turned the disk so that it went smoothly through (Ganel and Goodale, 2019).

Could D.F. see or not?

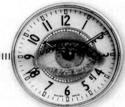

Many species rely on vision to find food and mates, avoid predators, and locate shelter. However, the sheer volume of visual information poses a serious problem.

Viewing the surrounding world has been compared to drinking from a waterfall. How does the visual system avoid being overwhelmed by the flood of information entering the eyes? One answer is that each species evolved visual capabilities that are tailored to that species' particular lifestyle. Most nocturnal species have better night vision than do animals that are active during the day, like us. Most rodent species, such as rats and mice, which live in tunnels and close quarters, have poor vision for distant objects, while daytime hunters like hawks have incredibly keen distance vision. Birds and bees can detect ultraviolet light, allowing them to see patterns in flowers that we cannot. But even within our limits of sight, we humans process a remarkable amount of visual information, which keeps about one-third of our cerebral cortex busy analyzing it.

See Video 7.1:
Object Recognition

7.1 The Vision Pathway Extends from the Eye to the Brain

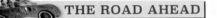 **THE ROAD AHEAD**

To begin this chapter, you'll learn how light entering the eye affects the firing of neurons and how that visual information reaches the brain. By the end of this section, you should be able to:

7.1.1 Describe how a visual scene is projected onto the back of the eyes.

7.1.2 Identify the major types of neurons there, which detect and analyze light.

7.1.3 Explain how we are able to detect visual images over a very broad range of illumination.

7.1.4 Describe the orderly mapping of information from a visual scene projecting into the brain.

View Animation 7.2:
Brain Explorer
View Activity 7.1:
The Structure of the Eye

retina The receptive surface inside the eye that contains photoreceptors and other neurons.

transduction The conversion of one form of energy to another, such as from light to neuronal activity.

cornea The transparent outer layer of the eye, whose curvature is fixed. The cornea bends light rays and is primarily responsible for forming the image on the retina.

refraction The bending of light rays by a change in the density of a medium, such as the cornea and the lens of the eyes.

lens A structure in the eye that helps focus an image on the retina.

ciliary muscle One of the muscles that control the shape of the lens inside the eye, focusing an image on the retina.

accommodation The process by which the ciliary muscles adjust the lens to bring nearby objects into focus.

The eye is an elaborate structure that captures light at the front and projects detailed images of the external world onto a layer of neurons at the back. That layer of neurons, called the **retina**, turns the light into neural signals in a process called **transduction**. So, good vision requires an accurate optical image focused on the retina. In other words, light from a point on a target object must end up as a point of light—rather than a blur—on the retina.

To produce this sharply focused optical image, the eye has many of the features of a camera, starting with the transparent outer layer of the eye, called the **cornea** (**FIGURE 7.1**). Light travels in a straight line until it encounters a change in the density of the medium, such as when it moves from air into water, which causes light rays to bend. This bending of light rays, called **refraction**, is the basis of such instruments as eyeglasses, telescopes, and microscopes. The curvature of the cornea, which does not change shape, refracts light rays and is primarily responsible for focusing on the retina. Light passing through the cornea is further refracted by the **lens**, which changes its shape to fine-tune that image on the retina.

The change in the shape of the lens is controlled by the **ciliary muscles** inside the eye. Contraction of the ciliary muscles alters the focal distance of the eye, causing nearer images to come into focus on the retina; this process is called **accommodation**.

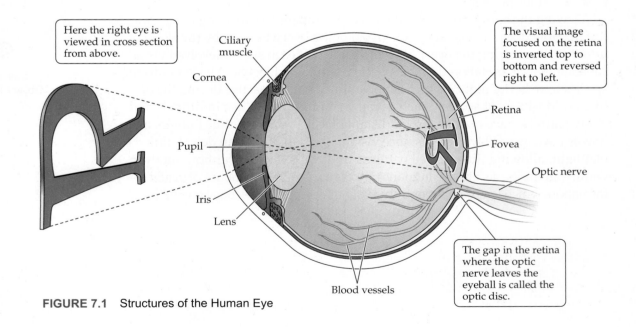

Here the right eye is viewed in cross section from above.

The visual image focused on the retina is inverted top to bottom and reversed right to left.

Ciliary muscle

Cornea

Pupil

Iris

Lens

Retina

Fovea

Optic nerve

The gap in the retina where the optic nerve leaves the eyeball is called the optic disc.

Blood vessels

FIGURE 7.1   Structures of the Human Eye

As mammals age, their lenses become less elastic and therefore less able to bring nearby objects into focus (we call this *farsightedness*). Aging humans correct this problem either by holding books and menus farther away from their eyes, or by wearing reading glasses. In contrast, the most common vision problem in young people is **myopia** (*nearsightedness*), which is difficulty seeing *distant* objects. Myopia develops if the eyeball is too long, causing the cornea and lens to focus images in front of the retina rather than on it (**FIGURE 7.2**). Distance vision can be restored in such cases by lenses that correct refraction of the visual image so that it is on the retina.

If you've ever played around with a magnifying glass, you've probably noticed that if you hold the lens at arm's length, you can see a clearly focused image of a distant scene through the glass but that scene is upside down and reversed. Like a magnifying glass, the biconvex (bulging on both sides) shape of the lens of the eye causes the visual scene that is focused on the retina to be upside down and reversed compared with the real world (see Figure 7.1).

Movement of the eyes is controlled by the **extraocular muscles**, three pairs of muscles that extend from the outside of the eyeball to the bony socket of the eye. Fixing your gaze on still or moving targets requires delicate control of these muscles to anchor the visual image on the retina. Let's talk about how that sharply focused visual image is processed in the retina.

Visual processing begins in the retina

The first stages of visual information processing occur in the retina, the receptive surface inside the back of the eye. The retina is only 200–300 micrometers thick—as thick as 2–3 sheets of paper—but it contains several types of cells in distinct layers (**FIGURE 7.3A**). Sensory neurons that detect light are called **photoreceptors**. There are two types of photoreceptors in the retina, called **rods** and **cones**, reflecting their respective shapes (**FIGURE 7.3B**). Cones come in several different varieties, which respond differently to light of varying wavelengths, providing us with color vision (as described later in the chapter). Rods respond to visible light of almost any wavelength.

Both rod and cone photoreceptors release neurotransmitter molecules into synapses on the **bipolar cells**, controlling their activity. The bipolar cells, in turn, connect with **ganglion cells**. The axons of the ganglion cells form the **optic nerve**, which carries information to the brain. Two additional types of cells—**horizontal cells** and **amacrine cells**—are especially significant in interactions within the retina. The horizontal cells make contacts among the receptor cells and bipolar cells; the amacrine cells contact both the bipolar cells and the ganglion cells.

Interestingly, the rods, cones, bipolar cells, and horizontal cells generate only graded, local potentials; they do not produce action potentials. Unlike most neurons, these cells affect each other through the *graded* release of neurotransmitters in response to *graded* changes in electrical potentials. The ganglion cells, on the other hand, conduct action potentials in the same way that most other neurons do. From the receptor cells to the ganglion cells, enormous amounts of data converge and are compressed; the human eye contains about 100 million rods and 4 million cones, but there are only 1 million ganglion cells to transmit all that information to the brain. Thus, a great deal of information processing is done inside the eye, as the input of over 100 million photoreceptors is compressed into the action potentials of 1 million ganglion cell axons.

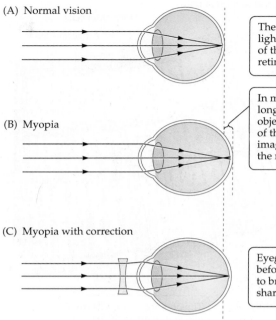

(A) Normal vision

> The cornea and lens refract light to focus a sharp image of the outside world on the retina.

(B) Myopia

> In myopia, the eyeball is too long, so images from distant objects are in focus in front of the retina. In this case, the image that actually reaches the retina is blurred.

(C) Myopia with correction

> Eyeglasses refract the light before it reaches the cornea to bring the image into sharp focus on the retina.

FIGURE 7.2 Focusing Images on the Retina

myopia Nearsightedness; the inability to focus the retinal image of objects that are far away.

extraocular muscle One of the muscles attached to the eyeball that controls its position and movements.

photoreceptor A neural cell in the retina that responds to light.

rod A photoreceptor cell in the retina that is most active at low levels of light.

cone Any of several classes of photoreceptor cells in the retina that are responsible for color vision.

bipolar cell An interneuron in the retina that receives information from rods and cones and passes the information to retinal ganglion cells.

ganglion cell Any of a class of cells in the retina whose axons form the optic nerve.

optic nerve Cranial nerve II; the collection of ganglion cell axons that extends from the retina to the brain.

horizontal cell A specialized retinal cell that contacts both photoreceptors and bipolar cells.

amacrine cell A specialized retinal cell that contacts both bipolar cells and ganglion cells and is especially significant in inhibitory interactions within the retina.

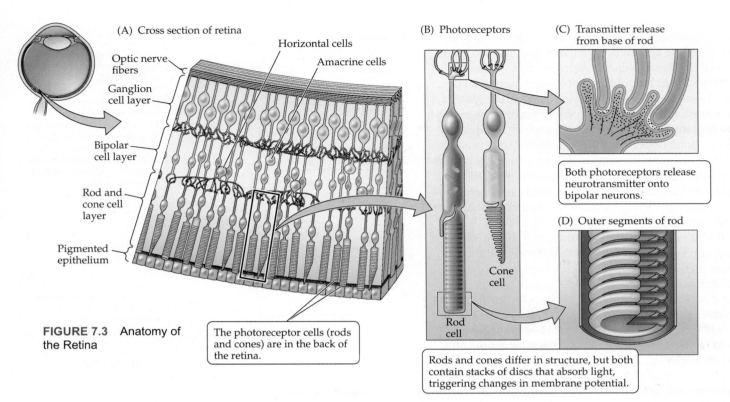

(A) Cross section of retina

Optic nerve fibers

Ganglion cell layer

Bipolar cell layer

Rod and cone cell layer

Pigmented epithelium

Horizontal cells

Amacrine cells

FIGURE 7.3 Anatomy of the Retina

The photoreceptor cells (rods and cones) are in the back of the retina.

(B) Photoreceptors

(C) Transmitter release from base of rod

Both photoreceptors release neurotransmitter onto bipolar neurons.

(D) Outer segments of rod

Cone cell

Rod cell

Rods and cones differ in structure, but both contain stacks of discs that absorb light, triggering changes in membrane potential.

scotopic system A system in the retina that operates at low levels of light and involves the rods.

convergence The phenomenon of neural connections in which many cells send signals to a single cell.

photopic system A system in the retina that operates at high levels of light, shows sensitivity to color, and involves the cones.

rhodopsin The photopigment in rods that responds to light.

The two different populations of photoreceptors (rods and cones) provide input to two different functional systems in the retina. A rod-based system, called the **scotopic system** (from the Greek *skotos*, "darkness," and *ops*, "eye"), is very sensitive and thus works especially well in low light—we use rod vision to detect objects in dim light—but it is insensitive to color. That's why in the darkness of night, when only our rods can detect light, we can't tell colors apart. There is a lot of **convergence** in the scotopic system because the information from many rods *converges* onto each ganglion cell.

The other system uses cones, which are less sensitive than rods (i.e., they have a higher threshold before they respond), and therefore it requires more light to function. This **photopic system** (which, like the term *photon*, gets its name from the Greek *phos*, "light") shows differential sensitivity to wavelengths, enabling our color vision. Compared with the scotopic system, the photopic system has less convergence, with some ganglion cells reporting information from only a single cone. At moderate levels of illumination, both the rods and the cones function, and some ganglion cells receive input from both types of receptors. **TABLE 7.1** summarizes the characteristics of the photopic and scotopic systems.

Photoreceptors respond to light by releasing less neurotransmitter

Rods and cones owe their extraordinary sensitivity to their unusual structure and biochemistry (**FIGURE 7.3B–D**). Each of these cells contains a stack of discs, which is where light particles are detected. Because light is reflected in many directions by the various parts of the eye, only a fraction of the light that strikes the cornea actually reaches the retina. The stacking of the discs increases the probability that one of them will capture the light particles that make it to the retina.

The light particles, called *quanta* or *photons*, that strike the discs are captured by special photopigment receptor molecules. In the rods this photopigment is **rhodopsin** (from the Greek *rhodon*, "rose," and *opsis*, "vision"). Cones use similar photopigments, as we'll see later. Curiously enough, photoreceptors in the dark continually release neurotransmitter onto bipolar cells. When light hits photopigment in the photoreceptor, it triggers a cascade of chemical reactions that *hyperpolarize* the cell, causing the

Table 7.1 Properties of the Human Photopic and Scotopic Visual Systems

Property	Photopic system	Scotopic system
Receptors	Cones	Rods
Approximate number of receptors per eye	4 million	100 million
Photopigments	Three classes of cone opsins; the basis of color vision	Rhodopsin
Sensitivity	Low; needs relatively strong stimulation; used for day vision	High; can be stimulated by weak light intensity; used for night vision
Location in retina	Concentrated in and near fovea; present less densely throughout the retina	Outside fovea
Receptive-field size and visual acuity	Small in fovea, so acuity is high; larger outside fovea	Larger, so acuity is lower
Response time	Relatively rapid	Slow

cell to release *less* neurotransmitter onto bipolar cells (**FIGURE 7.4**). You can learn the details of this process in **A STEP FURTHER 7.1**, on the website. It may seem puzzling that light causes photoreceptors to release *less* neurotransmitter, but remember that the visual system responds to *changes* in light. Either an increase or a decrease in the intensity of light can stimulate the visual system, and hyperpolarization is just as much a neural signal as depolarization is.

This change of potential in photoreceptors is the initial electrical signal in the visual pathway. Stimulation of rhodopsin by light hyperpolarizes the rods, just as light stimulation of the cone pigments hyperpolarizes them. For both rods and cones, the size of the hyperpolarizing photoreceptor potential determines how much less transmitter will be released (see Figure 7.4). Another important feature of photoreceptors is that their sensitivity to light is constantly changing, as discussed next.

Different mechanisms enable the eyes to work over a wide range of light intensities

Our visual system must respond to stimuli of vastly different intensities: a very bright light is about 10 billion times as intense as the weakest lights we can see. One way the visual system deals with this large range of intensities is by adjusting the size of the **pupil**, which is an opening in the colorful disc called the **iris** (see Figure 7.1). In Chapter 1 we mentioned that dilation (opening) of the pupils is controlled by the sympathetic division of the autonomic system and that constriction is triggered by the parasympathetic division. Because usually both divisions are active, pupil size reflects a balance of influences. Drugs that block acetylcholine

pupil The opening, formed by the iris, that allows light to enter the eye.

iris The circular structure of the eye that provides an opening to form the pupil.

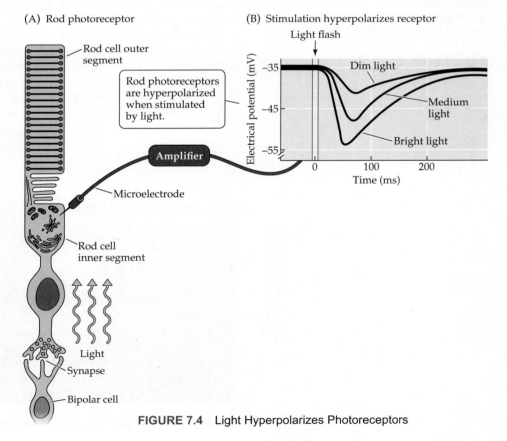

(A) Rod photoreceptor

Rod cell outer segment

Rod photoreceptors are hyperpolarized when stimulated by light.

Amplifier

Microelectrode

Rod cell inner segment

Light

Synapse

Bipolar cell

(B) Stimulation hyperpolarizes receptor

Light flash

Dim light

Medium light

Bright light

FIGURE 7.4 Light Hyperpolarizes Photoreceptors

(A) Bright illumination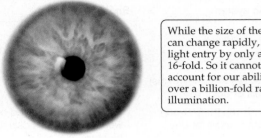

(B) Dark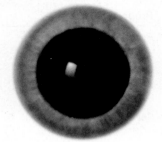

> While the size of the pupil can change rapidly, it affects light entry by only about 16-fold. So it cannot possibly account for our ability to see over a billion-fold range of illumination.

FIGURE 7.5 The Iris Controls the Size of the Pupil Opening

transmission in the parasympathetic synapses onto muscles controlling the iris relax them, opening the pupil widely. One drug that has this effect—belladonna—got its name (Italian for "beautiful woman") because it was thought to make a woman more beautiful by giving her the wide-open pupils of an attentive person. Other drugs, such as morphine, constrict the pupils.

In bright light, the pupil contracts quickly to admit only about one-sixteenth as much light as when illumination is dim (**FIGURE 7.5**). Although rapid, the 16-fold difference in light controlled by the pupil doesn't come close to accounting for the *billion*-fold range of visual sensitivity (**FIGURE 7.6**). Another mechanism for handling different light intensities is **range fractionation**, the handling of different intensities by different receptors—some with low thresholds (rods) and others with high thresholds (cones) (see Figure 7.5). But the main reason we can see over such a vast range of light is **photoreceptor adaptation**: each photoreceptor constantly adjusts its sensitivity to match the average level of ambient illumination, over a tremendous range. Thus, the visual system is concerned with *differences*, or changes, in brightness—not with the absolute level of illumination.

At any given time, a photoreceptor operates over a range of intensities of about a hundred-fold; that is, it is completely depolarized by a stimulus about one-tenth the ambient level of illumination, and a light 10 times more intense than the ambient level will completely hyperpolarize it. The receptors constantly shift their whole range of response to work around the prevailing level of illumination. Further adaptation, controlled by neural circuits, occurs in the brain.

range fractionation The means by which sensory systems cover a wide range of intensity values, as each sensory receptor cell specializes in just one part of the overall range of intensities.

photoreceptor adaptation The tendency of rods and cones to adjust their light sensitivity to match current levels of illumination.

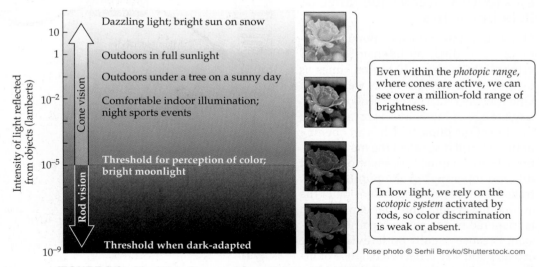

FIGURE 7.6 The Wide Range of Sensitivity to Light Intensity

Acuity is best in foveal vision

The whole area that you can see without moving your head or eyes is called your **visual field**. **Visual acuity**, commonly known as the *sharpness* of vision, is especially fine in the center of the visual field and falls off rapidly toward the periphery. That's why when we want to look at something closely, we center our gaze on the object of interest.

The fine structure of the retina explains why our acuity is best in the center of the visual field, called the **fovea** (**FIGURE 7.7A**). Notice how much more densely packed cones are in the fovea, where acuity is highest (**FIGURE 7.7B**), than in other parts of the retina. The fovea has an especially dense concentration of cones, absorbing so much light that the region looks dark in the photo (Figure 7.7A). That is one reason visual acuity is so high in this region. People differ in their concentrations of cones (Legras et al., 2018), and this variation may be related to individual differences in visual acuity. Species differences in visual acuity also reflect the density of cones in the fovea. For example, hawks, whose acuity is much greater than that of humans, have much narrower and more densely packed cones in the fovea than we do. Acuity is reduced in the periphery of the retina in part because both rods and cones are larger there.

The rods show a different distribution from the cones: they are absent in the fovea but more numerous than cones in the periphery of the retina (see Figure 7.7A). This is

visual field The whole area that you can see without moving your head or eyes.

visual acuity Sharpness of vision.

fovea The central portion of the retina, which is packed with the highest density of photoreceptors and is the center of our gaze.

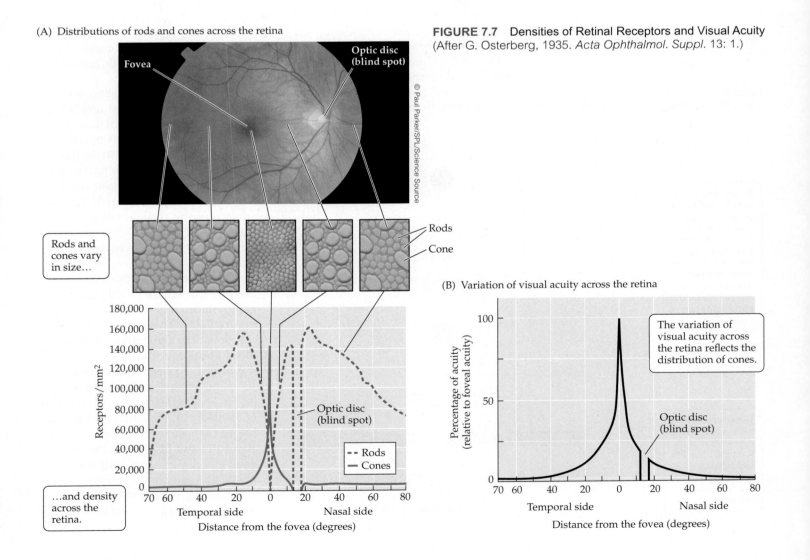

(A) Distributions of rods and cones across the retina

FIGURE 7.7 Densities of Retinal Receptors and Visual Acuity (After G. Osterberg, 1935. *Acta Ophthalmol. Suppl.* 13: 1.)

(B) Variation of visual acuity across the retina

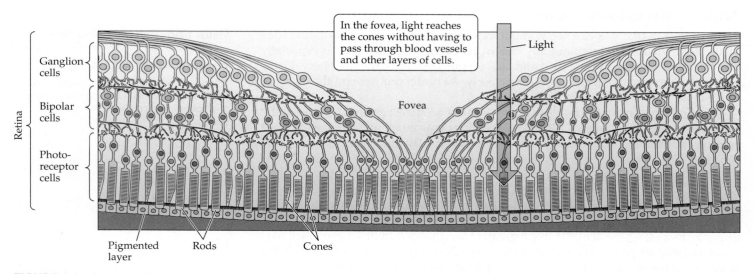

In the fovea, light reaches the cones without having to pass through blood vessels and other layers of cells.

Light

Fovea

Retina

Ganglion cells

Bipolar cells

Photo-receptor cells

Pigmented layer

Rods

Cones

FIGURE 7.8   An Unobstructed View

why, if you want to see a dim star, you do best to search for it a little off to the side of your center of gaze. Not only are rods more sensitive than cones to dim light, but as we mentioned earlier, input from many rods converges on each ganglion cell in the scotopic system, further increasing the system's sensitivity to weak stimuli. But that greater convergence of rods comes at the cost of diminished acuity compared with the fovea. Rods provide high sensitivity with limited acuity; cones provide high acuity with limited sensitivity. Thus, really fine vision requires good lighting.

In addition to the tight packing of cones in the fovea, another reason acuity is greater there than elsewhere on the retina is that in this region light reaches the cones directly, without having to pass through other layers of cells and blood vessels (**FIGURE 7.8**). In the rest of the retina, many light particles hit those upper layers without reaching the photoreceptors. This is why the surface of the retina is depressed at the fovea (see Figure 7.1A), giving the structure its name (*fovea* means "pit" in Latin).

The **optic disc**, to the nasal side of the fovea, is where blood vessels and ganglion cell axons leave the eye (see Figure 7.7A). There are no photoreceptors at the optic disc, so there is a **blind spot** here that we normally do not notice. You can locate your blind spot, and experience firsthand some of its interesting features, with the help of **FIGURE 7.9**. The blind spot is much bigger than we usually appreciate; it is about 10 times larger than the image of a full moon, yet we typically don't even notice it! Again, brain systems "fill in" the missing information so that we perceive an uninterrupted visual scene.

optic disc   The region of the retina that is devoid of photoreceptors because ganglion cell axons and blood vessels exit the eyeball there.

blind spot   The portion of the visual field from which light falls on the optic disc.

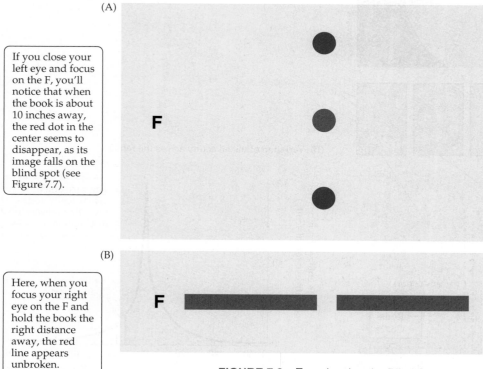

(A)

If you close your left eye and focus on the F, you'll notice that when the book is about 10 inches away, the red dot in the center seems to disappear, as its image falls on the blind spot (see Figure 7.7).

F

(B)

Here, when you focus your right eye on the F and hold the book the right distance away, the red line appears unbroken.

F

FIGURE 7.9   Experiencing the Blind Spot

Before we consider how information is processed at different levels of the visual system, we need to describe the pathway from the eye to the cortex, which we'll discuss next.

HOW'S IT GOING ❓

1. Describe how structures of the eye refract light to focus an image on the retina.
2. How do the photopic and scotopic visual systems differ?
3. How are we able to discriminate differences in light over such a wide range of illumination?
4. Why is our vision so much more acute at the fovea than it is elsewhere?

Neural signals travel from the retina to several brain regions

The ganglion cells in each eye produce action potentials that are conducted along their axons to send visual information to the brain. These axons make up the optic nerve (also known as *cranial nerve II*), which brings visual information into the brain, eventually reaching the **occipital cortex** at the back of the brain.

In vertebrates, many of the axons of each optic nerve cross to the opposite cerebral hemisphere. The optic nerves cross the midline at the **optic chiasm** (named for the Greek letter χ [chi] because of its crossover shape). Proportionally more axons cross the midline in prey animals, such as rabbits, that have laterally placed eyes with little overlap in their fields of vision (**FIGURE 7.10**). This arrangement gives a prey animal an especially wide field of view (good for spotting threats) at the cost of poor depth perception (which predators gain by comparing the overlapping visual fields of their front-facing eyes).

In humans, axons from the half of the retina toward your nose (the *nasal hemiretina*) cross over to the opposite side of the brain. The half of the retina toward your temple (the *temporal hemiretina*) projects its axons to its own side of the brain. The result of these projections is that the right hemisphere of the brain "sees" the left side of the visual field, and the left hemisphere "sees" the right side of the visual field

occipital cortex   Also called *visual cortex*. The cortex of the occipital lobe of the brain, corresponding to the visual area of the cortex.

optic chiasm   The point at which parts of the two optic nerves cross the midline.

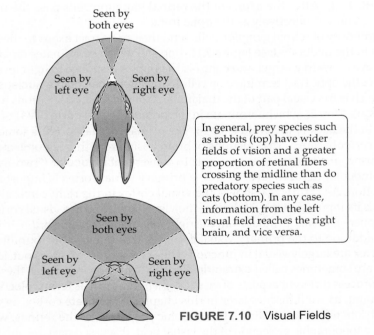

In general, prey species such as rabbits (top) have wider fields of vision and a greater proportion of retinal fibers crossing the midline than do predatory species such as cats (bottom). In any case, information from the left visual field reaches the right brain, and vice versa.

FIGURE 7.10   Visual Fields

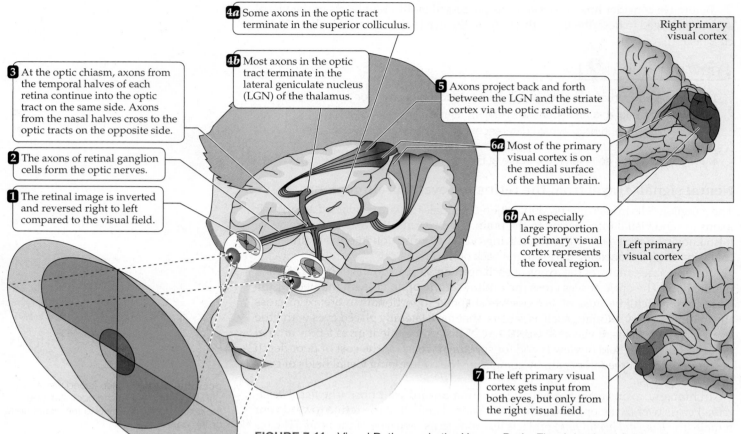

4a Some axons in the optic tract terminate in the superior colliculus.

4b Most axons in the optic tract terminate in the lateral geniculate nucleus (LGN) of the thalamus.

3 At the optic chiasm, axons from the temporal halves of each retina continue into the optic tract on the same side. Axons from the nasal halves cross to the optic tracts on the opposite side.

5 Axons project back and forth between the LGN and the striate cortex via the optic radiations.

2 The axons of retinal ganglion cells form the optic nerves.

6a Most of the primary visual cortex is on the medial surface of the human brain.

1 The retinal image is inverted and reversed right to left compared to the visual field.

6b An especially large proportion of primary visual cortex represents the foveal region.

Right primary visual cortex

Left primary visual cortex

7 The left primary visual cortex gets input from both eyes, but only from the right visual field.

FIGURE 7.11 **Visual Pathways in the Human Brain** The right visual field, which falls on parts of both retinas, projects to the left cerebral hemisphere. Similarly, the left visual field projects to both eyes and then to the right cerebral hemisphere.

View Animation 7.3:
Visual Pathways in the Human Brain

optic tract The axons of retinal ganglion cells after they have passed the optic chiasm. Most of these axons terminate in the lateral geniculate nucleus.

lateral geniculate nucleus (LGN) The part of the thalamus that receives information from the optic tract and sends it to visual areas in the occipital cortex.

optic radiation Axons from the lateral geniculate nucleus that terminate in the primary visual areas of the occipital cortex.

primary visual cortex (V1) Also called *striate cortex* or *area 17*. The region of the occipital cortex where most visual information first arrives.

binocular Referring to two-eyed processes.

extrastriate cortex Visual cortex outside of the primary visual (striate) cortex.

(**FIGURE 7.11**). After the axons of the retinal ganglion cells pass the optic chiasm, they are known collectively as the **optic tract**.

A minority of retinal ganglion cells send their optic tract axons to the superior colliculus in the midbrain (see Figure 7.11, step 4a), which coordinates rapid movements of the eyes toward a target and controls the pupil's response to light levels. But most axons of the optic tract terminate on cells in the **lateral geniculate nucleus** (LGN) (step 4b), which is the visual part of the thalamus. Axons of the LGN neurons form the **optic radiations** (step 5), which terminate in the **primary visual cortex** (**V1**) of the occipital cortex at the back of the brain (step 6). The primary visual cortex is sometimes called *striate cortex* because cross sections of brain tissue from this region feature a prominent stripe, or *striation*, corresponding to convergent **binocular** ("two-eyed") inputs. This binocular input to layer IV of the primary visual cortex is important for depth perception. As Figure 7.11 shows, the visual cortex in the right cerebral hemisphere receives its input from the left half of the visual field, and the visual cortex in the left hemisphere receives its input from the right half of the visual field.

In addition to the primary visual cortex (V1), numerous surrounding regions of the cortex are largely visual in function. These visual cortical areas outside the striate cortex are sometimes called **extrastriate cortex**. Working in parallel, these cortical regions process different aspects of visual perception, such as form, color, location, and movement, as we'll discuss later in this chapter. The striate cortex, as well as most extrastriate regions, contains a topographic projection of the retinas, which means there's a topographic projection of the visual field, discussed next.

The retina projects to the brain in a topographic fashion

The retina represents a two-dimensional map of the visual field. As this information courses through the brain, the point-to-point correspondence between neighboring parts of visual space is maintained, forming a maplike projection (see Figure 7.11). Much of this **topographic projection** of visual space is devoted to the foveal region (**FIGURE 7.12A**). Human V1 is located mainly on the medial surface of the cortex (**FIGURE 7.12B**; see also Figure 7.11). About half of the human V1 is devoted to the fovea and the retinal region just around the fovea, even though this represents a tiny fraction of the total retina. This disproportionate representation does not mean that our spatial perception is distorted. Rather, this representation makes possible the great acuity in the central part of the visual field. In other words, another reason why our vision is so much more acute in the foveal region is that we devote proportionally more brain regions to analyzing information from that region.

Because of the orderly mapping of the visual field (known as *retinotopic mapping*) at the various levels of the visual system, damage to parts of the visual system can be diagnosed from perceptual defects within the visual field. And if we know the site of injury in the visual pathway, we can predict the location of such a perceptual gap, or **scotoma**, in the visual field. Although the word *scotoma* comes from the Greek *skotos*, meaning "darkness," a scotoma is not perceived as a dark patch in the visual field; rather, it is a spot where nothing can be perceived, and usually rigorous testing is required to demonstrate its existence. As with the blind spots we all have, people may not be aware of scotomas that arise.

topographic projection   A mapping that preserves the point-to-point correspondence between neighboring parts of space. For example, a topographic projection extends from the retina to the cortex.

scotoma   A region of blindness within the visual fields, caused by injury to the visual pathway or brain.

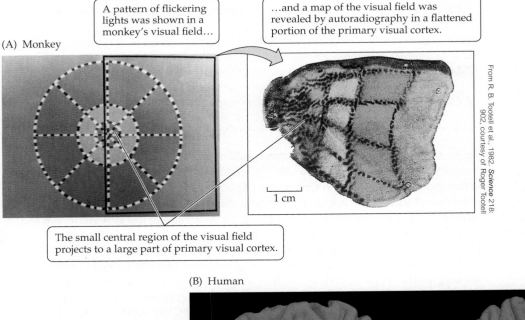

(A) Monkey

A pattern of flickering lights was shown in a monkey's visual field…

…and a map of the visual field was revealed by autoradiography in a flattened portion of the primary visual cortex.

1 cm

From R. B. Tooell et al., 1982. *Science* 218: 902, courtesy of Roger Tooell

The small central region of the visual field projects to a large part of primary visual cortex.

(B) Human

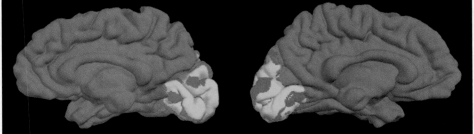

Maps of human visual cortex from fMRI show primary visual cortex as the innermost yellow region in each of these medial views.

From R. B. H. Tooell et al., 1998. *Proc. Natl. Acad. Sci. U.S.A.* 95: 811. © National Academy of Sciences, U.S.A.

FIGURE 7.12   Location of the Primary Visual Cortex

Within a scotoma, a person cannot *consciously* perceive visual cues, but some visual discrimination in this region may still be possible; this paradoxical phenomenon has been called **blindsight**. People with blindsight say they cannot see, but when asked to *guess* whether a stimulus is present, they're correct more often than could be expected by chance alone, or they may walk down a corridor strewn with objects without running into them (De Gelder et al., 2008).

HOW'S IT GOING ❓

1. Describe the path of information from the left visual field to the right side of the brain.
2. Name the structures that carry information from the eye to the brain.
3. Why is the proportion of primary visual cortex devoted to the fovea so large compared with other parts of the retina?

7.2 Neurons at Different Levels of the Visual System Have Very Different Receptive Fields

THE ROAD AHEAD

This next section describes how neurons in the retina and brain respond to light that enters the eye. Reading this section should enable you to:

7.2.1 Describe the kinds of light stimuli that best excite or inhibit neurons in the retina, LGN, and striate and extrastriate cortex.

7.2.2 Understand why our perception of light and dark is not a simple function of how much light strikes the eye.

7.2.3 Explain how simple receptive fields of the retina can be combined to produce more-complex receptive fields in V1.

7.2.4 Contrast hierarchical models of visual processing with a spatial-frequency model.

7.2.5 Identify extrastriate brain regions specialized to detect complex forms and motion.

blindsight The paradoxical phenomenon whereby, within a scotoma, a person cannot *consciously* perceive visual cues but may still be able to make some visual discrimination.

receptive field The stimulus region and features that affect the activity of a cell in a sensory system.

on-center bipolar cell A retinal bipolar cell that is excited by light in the center of its receptive field.

off-center bipolar cell A retinal bipolar cell that is inhibited by light in the center of its receptive field.

on-center ganglion cell A retinal ganglion cell that is activated when light is presented to the center, rather than the periphery, of the cell's receptive field.

off-center ganglion cell A retinal ganglion cell that is activated when light is presented to the periphery, rather than the center, of the cell's receptive field.

As we noted in Chapter 5, the **receptive field** of a sensory cell consists of the stimulus features that excite or inhibit the cell. Understanding the receptive fields of cells in the visual system begins with the response of photoreceptors. At rest, both rod and cone photoreceptors steadily release the synaptic neurotransmitter glutamate. Light always hyperpolarizes the photoreceptors, causing them to release *less* glutamate. But the responses of the bipolar cells that receive this glutamate differ, depending on the type of glutamate receptor they possess.

One group of bipolar cells consists of **on-center bipolar cells**. Glutamate is *inhibitory* to this type of cell, so light on the on-center bipolar cell's receptive field (which would cause the photoreceptor to release *less* glutamate) would *excite* this bipolar cell (think of taking the brakes off a system) (**FIGURE 7.13A**). The second group consists of **off-center bipolar cells**. Glutamate is *excitatory* to off-center bipolar cells, so shining light on this cell's receptive field (which causes the photoreceptor to release less glutamate) would *inhibit* this bipolar cell. It's called an *off-center bipolar cell* because turning *off* a light in the center of its receptive field excites it (**FIGURE 7.13B**).

Bipolar cells also release glutamate, which always depolarizes ganglion cells. Therefore, when light is turned on, on-center bipolar cells depolarize (excite) **on-center ganglion cells**; when light is turned off, off-center bipolar cells depolarize (excite) **off-center ganglion cells** (see Figure 7.13). The stimulated on-center and

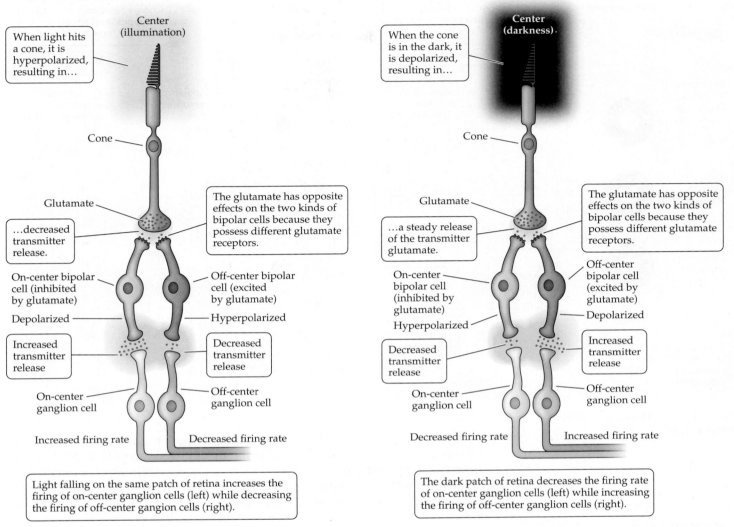

(A) On-center receptive fields

Center (illumination)

When light hits a cone, it is hyperpolarized, resulting in…

Cone

Glutamate

…decreased transmitter release.

The glutamate has opposite effects on the two kinds of bipolar cells because they possess different glutamate receptors.

On-center bipolar cell (inhibited by glutamate)

Off-center bipolar cell (excited by glutamate)

Depolarized

Hyperpolarized

Increased transmitter release

Decreased transmitter release

On-center ganglion cell

Off-center ganglion cell

Increased firing rate

Decreased firing rate

Light falling on the same patch of retina increases the firing of on-center ganglion cells (left) while decreasing the firing of off-center gangion cells (right).

(B) Off-center receptive fields

Center (darkness)

When the cone is in the dark, it is depolarized, resulting in…

Cone

Glutamate

…a steady release of the transmitter glutamate.

The glutamate has opposite effects on the two kinds of bipolar cells because they possess different glutamate receptors.

On-center bipolar cell (inhibited by glutamate)

Off-center bipolar cell (excited by glutamate)

Hyperpolarized

Depolarized

Decreased transmitter release

Increased transmitter release

On-center ganglion cell

Off-center ganglion cell

Decreased firing rate

Increased firing rate

The dark patch of retina decreases the firing rate of on-center ganglion cells (left) while increasing the firing of off-center ganglion cells (right).

FIGURE 7.13   Connections of Cones to Bipolar Cells (After D. Purves et al., 2001. *Neuroscience* [2nd ed.]. Oxford University Press/Sinauer. Sunderland, MA.)

off-center ganglion cells then fire nerve impulses and report "light" or "dark" to higher visual centers.

Neurons in the retina and the LGN have concentric receptive fields

Recordings from single ganglion cells show that in addition to the on- or off-center portion we've just discussed, their receptive fields also include a ring around that center, which is called a *surround* because it surrounds the central patch. Thus the entire receptive field of a bipolar cell is *concentric*, consisting of a roughly circular central area and the ringlike area surrounding it. Through various retinal connections, the photoreceptors in the central area and those in the ring surrounding it tend to have opposite effects on the next cells in the circuit. Thus, both bipolar cells and ganglion cells have two basic types of retinal receptive fields: **on-center/off-surround** and **off-center/on-surround**. These antagonistic effects of the center and its surround explain why uniform illumination of the entire receptive field has little effect on ganglion cell activity, compared with a well-placed small spot of light within the cell's receptive field. Neurons in the LGN, which are stimulated by retinal ganglion cells, also have these concentric on-center/off-surround or off-center/on-surround receptive fields, as shown in **FIGURE 7.14.**

on-center/off-surround Referring to a concentric receptive field in which stimulation of the center excites the cell of interest while stimulation of the surround inhibits it.

off-center/on-surround Referring to a concentric receptive field in which stimulation of the center inhibits the cell of interest while stimulation of the surround excites it.

Each retinal bipolar cell and ganglion cell has a concentric receptive field, with antagonistic center and surround. Bipolar cells respond with changes in local membrane potentials, while ganglion cells respond with action potentials.

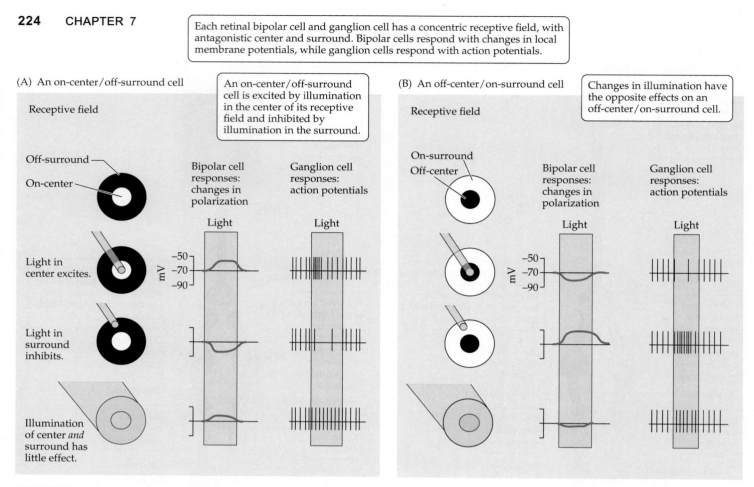

(A) An on-center/off-surround cell

An on-center/off-surround cell is excited by illumination in the center of its receptive field and inhibited by illumination in the surround.

(B) An off-center/on-surround cell

Changes in illumination have the opposite effects on an off-center/on-surround cell.

FIGURE 7.14   Receptive Fields of Retinal Cells

To understand why the effect of light falling on the surround of a firing ganglion cell is opposite to the effect of light falling in the center, we need to understand the concept of **lateral inhibition**, in which sensory receptor cells inhibit the reporting of information from neighboring receptor cells. As illustrated in **FIGURE 7.15**, the bipolar cells that relay information from photoreceptors to ganglion cells also inhibit one another. So when one bipolar cell is active, it inhibits its neighbors.

Because of this lateral inhibition, the ganglion cells stimulated by the right-hand edge of each dark band in **FIGURE 7.16A** are inhibited by the neighboring photoreceptors stimulated by the lighter band next door. Thus, ganglion cells stimulated by the right edge of each bar report receiving less light than they actually do (i.e., that edge looks darker to us). Conversely, the left edge of each bar appears lighter than the rest of the bar.

Again, in **FIGURE 7.16B** two indicated patches, which clearly differ in the brightness we perceive, *reflect the same amount of light*. If you use your pinkie to cover the edge where the two tiles meet, you'll see that the two patches are the same shade of gray. How are such puzzling effects produced? Although the contrast effect in Figure 7.16A is determined, at least in part, by lateral inhibition among adjacent retinal cells, the entire areas indicated in Figure 7.16B, not just the edges, appear different, so the effect must be produced higher in the visual system. One explanation is that we are accustomed to light sources coming from overhead (such as the sun, or a room light), so our brain assumes that the upper patch must actually be darker than the lower patch, because the upper one should be receiving more light than the lower one.

The important point is that our *visual experience is not a simple reporting of the physical properties of light*. Rather, our perception of light versus dark is created by the brain in response to many factors, including surrounding stimuli. For example, if you read this book in bright sunlight, the black ink reflects far more light to your eyes than the blank parts of the page do indoors. Yet, whether you're in sunlight or indoors, you perceive the ink as black and the blank parts as white. Later in the chapter we'll find

lateral inhibition   The phenomenon by which interconnected neurons inhibit their neighbors, producing contrast at the edges of regions.

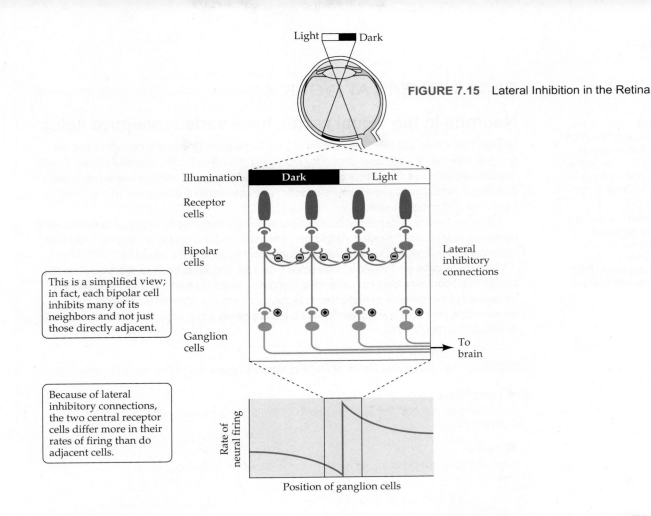

FIGURE 7.15   Lateral Inhibition in the Retina

Light ☐ Dark

Illumination | Dark | Light

Receptor cells

Bipolar cells

Lateral inhibitory connections

This is a simplified view; in fact, each bipolar cell inhibits many of its neighbors and not just those directly adjacent.

Ganglion cells

To brain

Because of lateral inhibitory connections, the two central receptor cells differ more in their rates of firing than do adjacent cells.

Rate of neural firing

Position of ganglion cells

that our experience of color is also created by the visual system, not a simple reporting of the wavelengths of light, and is very sensitive to nearby stimuli.

View Animation 7.4: Receptive Fields in the Retina

HOW'S IT GOING ?

1. Given that all photoreceptors are hyperpolarized by light, how can the same photoreceptor excite some bipolar cells while inhibiting others?

2. What is a receptive field, and what two kinds of receptive fields are displayed by retinal ganglion cells?

3. Describe lateral inhibition in the retina and how it can sharpen our vision yet make us susceptible to the optical illusion we experience in Figure 7.16A.

(A)

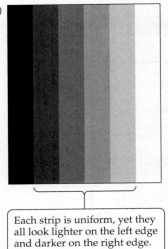

Each strip is uniform, yet they all look lighter on the left edge and darker on the right edge.

(B)

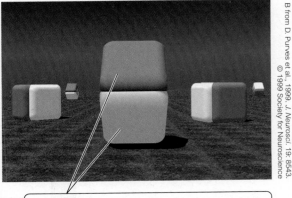

Of the two indicated patches, the upper one looks darker, even though they are in fact the same shade of gray. If you don't believe this, use your finger to cover up the line where they meet. See?

FIGURE 7.16   The Effect of Context on the Perception of Brightness

simple cortical cell Also called *bar detector* or *edge detector*. A cell in the visual cortex that responds best to an edge or a bar that has a particular width, as well as a particular orientation and location in the visual field.

complex cortical cell A cell in the visual cortex that responds best to a bar of a particular size and orientation anywhere within a particular area of the visual field and that needs movement to make it respond actively.

RESEARCHERS AT WORK |||||||||||||||||||||||||||||||||||||||||||||||||||||||||||||

Neurons in the visual cortex have varied receptive fields

Neurons from the LGN send their axons to cells in the primary visual cortex (V1), but the *spots* of light that are effective stimuli for LGN cells (**FIGURE 7.17A**; see also Figure 7.14A) are not very effective for cortical cells. In 1959, David Hubel and Torsten Wiesel reported that visual cortical cells require more-specific, elongated stimuli than those that activate LGN cells and ganglion cells.

Hubel and Wiesel categorized cortical cells according to the types of stimuli that produced maximum responses. So-called **simple cortical cells** respond best to an edge or a bar that has a particular width and a particular orientation and location in the visual field (**FIGURE 7.17B**). These cells are therefore sometimes called *bar detectors* or *edge detectors*. Like the simple cells, **complex cortical cells** have elongated receptive fields, but they also require *movement* of the stimulus to make them respond actively. For some of these cells, any movement in their field is sufficient; others are more demanding, requiring motion in a specific direction (**FIGURE 7.17C**).

FIGURE 7.17 Receptive Fields of Cells at Various Levels in the Cat Visual System

■ **Hypothesis**

Cells at higher levels of the visual system respond to progressively more complex stimuli.

■ **Test**

Compare receptive fields of neurons at each level, and see how they relate to one another.

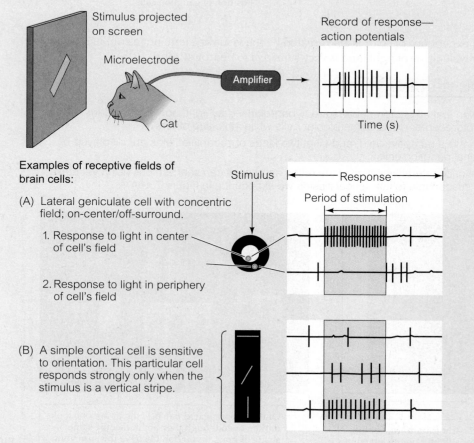

Stimulus projected on screen

Microelectrode

Amplifier

Cat

Record of response— action potentials

Time (s)

Examples of receptive fields of brain cells:

(A) Lateral geniculate cell with concentric field; on-center/off-surround.

1. Response to light in center of cell's field

2. Response to light in periphery of cell's field

Stimulus

Response

Period of stimulation

(B) A simple cortical cell is sensitive to orientation. This particular cell responds strongly only when the stimulus is a vertical stripe.

RESEARCHERS AT WORK (*continued*) |||||||||||||||||||||||||||||||||||||||||||||||||||||||||||||||||||||||||||||||

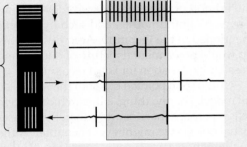

(C) A complex cortical cell is also sensitive to motion. This particular cell responds strongly only when the stimulus moves down. It responds weakly to upward motion and does not respond at all to sideways motion.

■ **Result**

(A) Visual cells in the LGN have concentric receptive fields.

(B) Visual cells in the cerebral cortex may show orientation specificity or respond only to motion, or…

(C) …they may respond only to motion in a particular direction.

■ **Conclusion**

Neurons at each level of the visual system combine input from neurons at lower levels to make progressively more complex receptive fields. Thus, retinal and LGN neurons respond best to spots of light on the retina, while cortical cells respond best to lines of particular orientation, or lines that move in a particular direction.

Spatial-frequency analysis is unintuitive but efficient

Hubel and Wiesel's theoretical model of visual analysis can be described as hierarchical; that is, more-complex receptive fields are built up from inputs of simpler ones. For example, a simple cortical cell can be thought of as receiving input from a row of LGN cells (**FIGURE 7.18A**), and a complex cortical cell can be thought of as receiving input from a row of simple cortical cells. (**FIGURE 7.18B**)

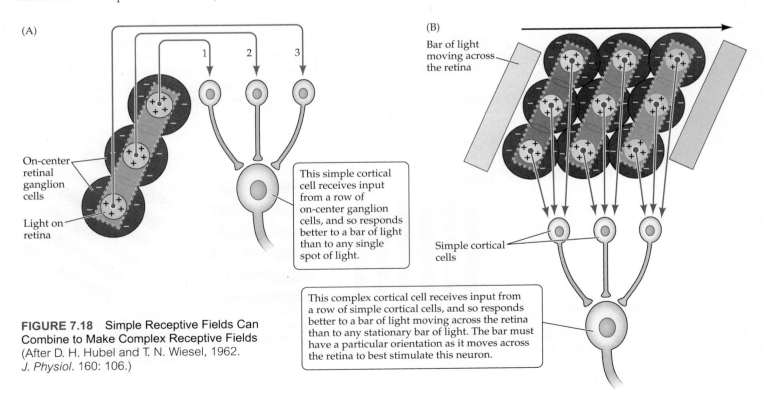

(A)

On-center retinal ganglion cells

Light on retina

This simple cortical cell receives input from a row of on-center ganglion cells, and so responds better to a bar of light than to any single spot of light.

(B)

Bar of light moving across the retina

Simple cortical cells

This complex cortical cell receives input from a row of simple cortical cells, and so responds better to a bar of light moving across the retina than to any stationary bar of light. The bar must have a particular orientation as it moves across the retina to best stimulate this neuron.

FIGURE 7.18 Simple Receptive Fields Can Combine to Make Complex Receptive Fields (After D. H. Hubel and T. N. Wiesel, 1962. *J. Physiol.* 160: 106.)

spatial-frequency model A model of visual perception that emphasizes the analysis of the different spatial frequencies present in various orientations and in various parts of a visual scene.

Other theorists extrapolated from this hierarchical model, suggesting that higher-order circuits of cells could detect any possible form. Thus it was suggested that, by integration of enough successive levels of analysis, a neuron might respond only to a person's grandmother, and such hypothetical "grandmother cells" were frequently mentioned in the literature. According to this view, whenever such a cell was excited, up would pop a mental picture of one's grandmother. This hypothesis was given as a possible explanation for facial recognition.

Critics soon pointed out both theoretical and empirical problems with the hierarchical model. For one thing, a hierarchical system like this would require a *vast* number of cells—perhaps more neurons than the cortex possesses—in order to account for all the visual objects we might ever encounter. Although some neurons are indeed activated by the sight of very specific faces (e.g., "Halle Berry neurons" were found, which were activated by photos of that actress) in both humans (Pedreira et al., 2010) and monkeys (Freiwald et al., 2009), these neurons do not respond to specific features of the face, as we would expect if they were built up from feature detectors. Rather, they respond only when the *whole face* or most of the face is presented (Freiwald et al., 2009).

Confronted with the inadequacies of the hierarchical model, scientists proposed an alternative account of vision, known as the **spatial-frequency model** (F. W. Campbell and Robson, 1968), that is more powerful but less intuitive. This model proposes that the visual system analyzes the number of cycles of light-dark (or color) patches in any stimulus. Some cycles are narrow, others broad. Some cycles of light-dark are oriented vertically, others horizontally, and others somewhere in between. If cortical neurons are indeed optimized to detect light-dark cycles, then they should respond to repeating bars of light, as in the examples shown in **FIGURE 7.19**, even better than to a single bar of light. And that's precisely what researchers found (R. L. De Valois and De Valois, 1988).

The idea that the visual system processes spatial-frequency information was revolutionary because it led to entirely different conceptions of how the visual system might work. The idea suggests that, rather than specifically detecting such seminaturalistic features as bars and edges, the system is breaking down complex stimuli into their individual spatial-frequency components (Kauffmann et al., 2015). In such a system, we might require a view of the whole face, which includes the low-frequency components, for recognition. This could explain why "Halle Berry neurons" do not respond to small portions of a face, because such snippets contain only high-frequency components. The spatial-frequency approach has proven useful in the analysis of many aspects of human pattern vision, and it provides the basis of high-definition television (HDTV). If you would like to know more about how the spatial-frequency model works, see **A STEP FURTHER 7.2**, on the website.

View Animation 7.5: Spatial Frequencies

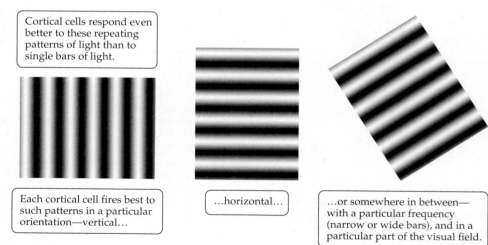

Cortical cells respond even better to these repeating patterns of light than to single bars of light.

Each cortical cell fires best to such patterns in a particular orientation—vertical…

…horizontal…

…or somewhere in between—with a particular frequency (narrow or wide bars), and in a particular part of the visual field.

FIGURE 7.19 Examples of Spatial Frequencies in Vision The brain combines information about all these spatial frequencies to give us our perception of the scene.

Neurons in the visual cortex beyond area V1 have complex receptive fields and help identify forms

Area V1 represents only a small fraction of the total amount of cortex that is devoted to vision. From area V1, axons extend to cortical areas involved in the perception of form: V2, V4, and the inferior temporal area (**FIGURE 7.20A–C**). The receptive fields of the cells in many of these extrastriate visual areas are even more complex than those of area V1.

The visual areas of the human brain (**FIGURE 7.20D**) have been less thoroughly mapped than those of the monkey brain, and mainly by neuroimaging (the spatial resolution of which is not as fine as that of the electrophysiological recording used in the monkey brain), but the general layout appears similar in the two species, especially for V1 (Tootell et al., 2003).

An astonishing proportion of primate cortex analyzes visual information. The areas that are largely or entirely visual in function occupy over half of the surface of the macaque cortex (Van Essen et al., 2001) and about 30% of human cortex (Tootell et al., 2003). We will discuss only a few of the main visual cortical areas and their functions.

Area V2 is adjacent to V1, and many of its cells have receptive fields similar to those of V1 cells. Many V2 cells can respond to illusory contours, such as the boundaries of

FIGURE 7.20 Main Visual Areas in Monkey and Human Brains (Parts A–C after D. J. Felleman and D. C. Van Essen, 1991. *Cereb. Cortex* 1: 1.)

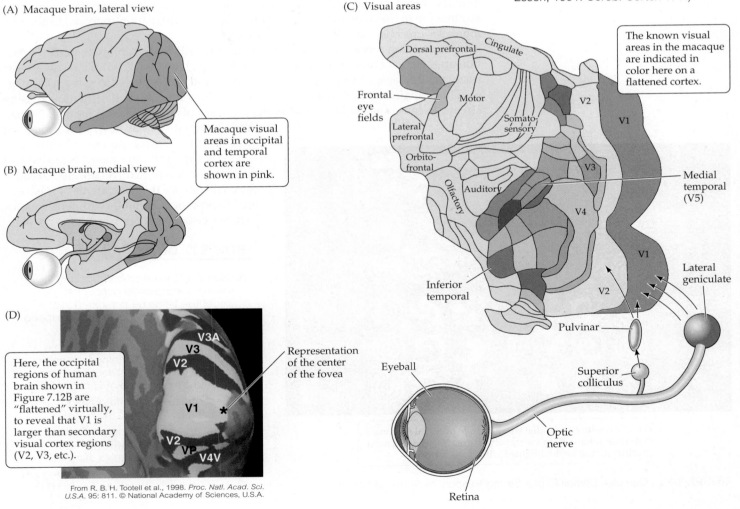

(A) Macaque brain, lateral view

Macaque visual areas in occipital and temporal cortex are shown in pink.

(B) Macaque brain, medial view

(D)

Here, the occipital regions of human brain shown in Figure 7.12B are "flattened" virtually, to reveal that V1 is larger than secondary visual cortex regions (V2, V3, etc.).

V3A
V3
V2
V1 *
V2
VP
V4V

Representation of the center of the fovea

From R. B. H. Tootell et al., 1998. *Proc. Natl. Acad. Sci. U.S.A.* 95: 811. © National Academy of Sciences, U.S.A.

(C) Visual areas

The known visual areas in the macaque are indicated in color here on a flattened cortex.

Dorsal prefrontal — Cingulate
Frontal eye fields
Motor
Lateral prefrontal
Somato-sensory
Orbito-frontal
Olfactory
Auditory
V2
V1
V3
V4
Medial temporal (V5)
Inferior temporal
V1
V2
Pulvinar
Lateral geniculate
Eyeball
Superior colliculus
Optic nerve
Retina

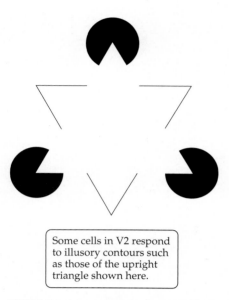

> Some cells in V2 respond to illusory contours such as those of the upright triangle shown here.

FIGURE 7.21 A Geometric Figure with "Illusory" or "Subjective" Contours

the upright triangle in **FIGURE 7.21**. Clearly, such cells respond to complex relations among the parts of their receptive fields.

Area V4 cells generally give their strongest responses to the frequency gratings that we discussed earlier (see Figure 7.19). However, some V4 cells give even stronger responses to concentric and radial stimuli, such as those in **FIGURE 7.22** (Roe et al., 2012). Area V4 also has many cells that respond most strongly to color differences, as we will see later when we discuss color vision.

The prefrontal cortex also contains a restricted region of neurons that are activated by faces (Dinh et al., 2018). These findings indicate that a pathway mediating visual recognition extends from V1 through temporal cortex to the prefrontal cortex. Later we'll see that this pathway was damaged in D.F., the woman described at the start of the chapter.

Visual perception of motion is analyzed by a special system that includes cortical area V5

In area V5 (also called the *medial temporal area* or *area MT*; see Figure 7.20C) of monkeys, neurons respond to moving visual stimuli, indicating that they are specialized for the perception of motion and its direction. Imaging studies show that moving stimuli also evoke responses in human area V5.

Experimental lesions of area V5 in monkeys trained to report the direction of perceived motion impaired their performance, at least temporarily. Conversely, electrically *stimulating* an area of V5 that normally responds to stimuli moving up caused monkeys to report that dots on the screen were moving up even when they were actually moving to the right. In other words, the electrical stimulation appeared to alter the monkeys' *experience* of visual motion (Zeki, 2015).

One striking report described a woman who had lost the ability to perceive motion after a stroke damaged her area V5 (Zihl and Heywood, 2015). The woman was unable to perceive continuous motion and saw only separate, successive still images. This impairment led to many problems in daily life. She had difficulty crossing streets, because she could not follow the positions of automobiles in motion: "When I'm looking at the car at first, it seems far away. But then when I want to cross the road, suddenly the car is very near." She also had difficulty following conversations, because she could not see the movements of speakers' lips. Except for her inability to perceive motion, her visual perception appeared normal.

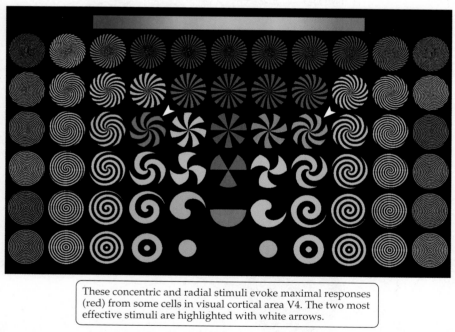

From J. L. Gallant et al., 1993. *Science* 259: 100, courtesy of Jack Gallant

> These concentric and radial stimuli evoke maximal responses (red) from some cells in visual cortical area V4. The two most effective stimuli are highlighted with white arrows.

FIGURE 7.22 Complex Stimuli Evoke Strong Responses in Visual Cortex

HOW'S IT GOING ?

1. How could information from LGN neurons with simple concentric receptive fields be combined in a cortical cell such that it would respond best to a line of light?

2. How could information from simple cortical cells be combined in another cortical cell so that it would respond best to a moving line of light?

3. Describe the spatial-frequency hypothesis of vision.

4. What are some examples of visual receptive fields outside of V1 that respond to very complex stimuli?

5. What kind of stimuli affect the firing of neurons in V5 (also called *area MT*)?

7.3 Color Vision Depends on Integrating Information from the Retinal Cones

THE ROAD AHEAD

For most people, color is a striking aspect of vision. In this portion of the chapter, you'll learn how our brain uses input from three different types of cones to construct our experience of color. By the end of this section, you should:

7.3.1 Know the physical properties of light that make objects appear colored.

7.3.2 Realize that our perception of color does *not* simply reflect those properties of light.

7.3.3 Be able to discuss the two major theories of how the visual system can detect colors.

7.3.4 Understand how comparing the activity of two or more types of cones informs us about color.

7.3.5 Understand why men are more likely than women to have difficulty distinguishing colors.

For most of us, the visible world has several distinguishable hues: blue, green, yellow, red, and their intermediates. These hues appear different because every light particle, or photon, vibrates as it travels across space, behaving like a sinusoidal wave. Photons vary in the frequency of vibration and therefore the **wavelength** (the distance between two adjacent peaks of the wave) of the light, and we can detect some of these differences, perceiving faster-vibrating (thus shorter-wavelength) photons as blue and green, and slower-vibrating (longer-wavelength) photons as more orange and red. The human visual system responds only to particles whose wavelengths lie within a very narrow section of the total electromagnetic range, from about 400 to 700 nanometers (nm) (**FIGURE 7.23**). If particles have shorter or longer wavelengths than this narrow range, we no longer call them photons but give them names like X-rays or radio waves. The color of an object depends on which wavelengths of light it absorbs versus which wavelengths it reflects. Our eyes detect the reflected wavelengths to distinguish different colors, as illustrated in **FIGURE 7.24**.

wavelength The length between two peaks in a repeated stimulus such as a wave, light, or sound.

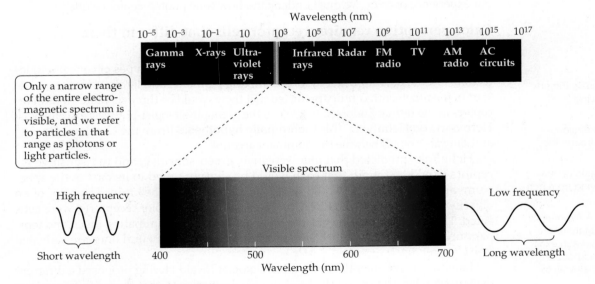

FIGURE 7.23 The Wavelengths of Light

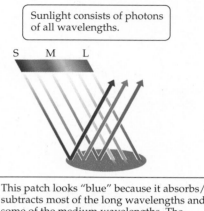

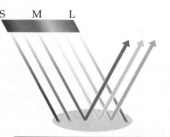

This patch looks "blue" because it absorbs/subtracts most of the long wavelengths and some of the medium wavelengths. The short- and medium-wavelength light that is reflected to the eye appears blue.

This patch looks "yellow" because it reflects best in the middle range of wavelengths and absorbs the other wavelengths.

Mix the two pigments together, and what you have left when each has absorbed its wavelengths are some remaining medium wavelengths that look "green."

FIGURE 7.24 Colored Objects Reflect Different Wavelengths of Light

brightness One of three basic dimensions of light perception, varying from dark to light.

hue One of three basic dimensions of light perception, varying through the spectrum from violet to red.

saturation One of three basic dimensions of light perception, varying from rich to pale.

trichromatic hypothesis A hypothesis of color perception stating that there are three different types of cones, each excited by a different region of the spectrum and each having a separate pathway to the brain.

There are three dimensions of color perception:

1. **Brightness**, which varies from dark to light
2. **Hue**, which varies continuously through blue, green, yellow, orange, and red (and is what most people mean when they use the term *color*)
3. **Saturation**, which varies from rich, full colors to gray; for example, rich red through pink to gray as saturation decreases

It is important to understand that the perception of a particular hue is *not* a simple function of the wavelength of light. For example, a patch reflecting light of a particular wavelength is perceived as various different hues, depending on several factors, including the intensity of illumination, prior exposure to a different stimulus, and the surrounding field.

As illumination fades, the blues in a painting or a rug appear more prominent and the reds appear duller, even though the wavelength distribution in the light reflecting off those objects has not changed. In addition, the hue perceived at a particular point is strongly affected by the pattern of wavelengths and intensities in other parts of the visual field, as **FIGURE 7.25** illustrates. To understand how the visual system creates our experience of color, we must understand how cone photoreceptors work.

Color perception requires receptor cells that differ in their sensitivities to different wavelengths

The first stage of color detection is accomplished by different types of cone photodetectors. On the basis of observations of mixing pigments and lights, scientists at the start of the nineteenth century predicted that there would be three separate kinds of receptors in the retina. Endorsed in 1852 by the great physiologist-physicist-psychologist Hermann von Helmholtz, this **trichromatic hypothesis** (from the Greek *tri*, "three," and *chroma*, "color") became the dominant account.

Helmholtz predicted that blue-sensitive, green-sensitive, and red-sensitive receptors would be found, that each would be sharply tuned to its part of the spectrum, and that each type would have a separate path to the brain. The color of an object would be recognized, then, on the basis of which color receptor(s) were activated. This system would be like the mechanisms for discriminating touch and temperature on the basis of which skin receptors and labeled neural lines are activated (see Chapter 5).

Later in the nineteenth century, physiologist Ewald Hering proposed a different explanation. He argued, on the basis of visual experience, that there are *four* unique

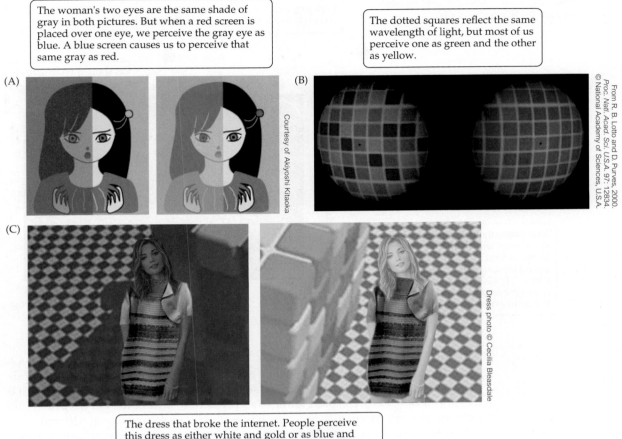

The woman's two eyes are the same shade of gray in both pictures. But when a red screen is placed over one eye, we perceive the gray eye as blue. A blue screen causes us to perceive that same gray as red.

(A)

Courtesy of Akiyoshi Kitaoka

The dotted squares reflect the same wavelength of light, but most of us perceive one as green and the other as yellow.

(B)

From R. B. Lotto and D. Purves, 2000. *Proc. Natl. Acad. Sci. USA* 97: 12834. © National Academy of Sciences, U.S.A.

(C)

Dress photo © Cecilia Bleasdale

The dress that broke the internet. People perceive this dress as either white and gold or as blue and black, depending on how they interpret the lighting of the scene. If you cut a rectangle 2 cm x 1 cm out of a sheet of paper and place the opening over the dress, you'll see it's the same color in the two panels.

FIGURE 7.25 Color Perception

hues (blue, green, yellow, red) and three *opposed pairs of colors*—blue versus yellow, green versus red, and black versus white—and that three physiological processes with opposed positive and negative values must therefore be the basis of color vision. As we will see, both this **opponent-process hypothesis** and the trichromatic hypothesis are encompassed in current color vision theory, but neither of the old hypotheses is sufficient by itself.

Measurements of photopigments in cones have borne out the trichromatic hypothesis in part. Each cone of the human retina has one of three classes of pigments (each pigment has a name, but we'll just refer to them as *opsins*). The response of the cone depends on which wavelength of light its pigment absorbs to start the process depicted in Figure 7.4. These pigments do not, however, have the narrow spectral distributions that Helmholtz predicted.

Despite what you may have heard in other classes (or even read in other textbooks!), the human visual system does *not* have receptors that are sensitive to only narrow parts of the visible spectrum, such as "red" cones and "green" cones; instead, the receptor pigments exhibit broad sensitivities that substantially overlap. In fact, two of the three retinal cone pigments show some response to light of almost *any* wavelength. The pigments have different *peaks* of sensitivity, but even the peaks are not as far apart as Helmholtz predicted, and those peaks don't always correspond to a

opponent-process hypothesis
A hypothesis of color perception stating that different systems produce opposite responses to light of different wavelengths.

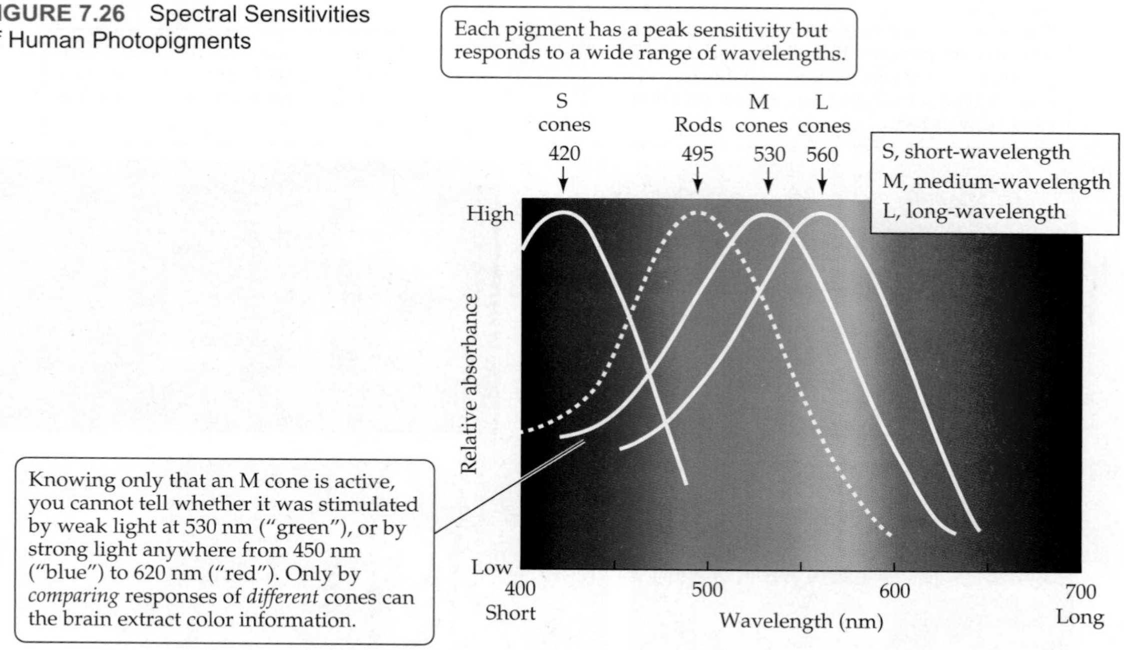

FIGURE 7.26 Spectral Sensitivities of Human Photopigments

Each pigment has a peak sensitivity but responds to a wide range of wavelengths.

S, short-wavelength
M, medium-wavelength
L, long-wavelength

Knowing only that an M cone is active, you cannot tell whether it was stimulated by weak light at 530 nm ("green"), or by strong light anywhere from 450 nm ("blue") to 620 nm ("red"). Only by *comparing* responses of *different* cones can the brain extract color information.

particular color. As **FIGURE 7.26** shows, the cone pigment peaks occur at about 420 nm (in the part of the spectrum where we usually see violet under daylight conditions), about 530 nm (where most of us see green), and about 560 nm (where most of us see yellow-green). Despite Helmholtz's prediction, *none* of the curves peak in the long-wavelength part of the spectrum, where most of us see red (about 630 nm).

Under ordinary conditions, almost any object, no matter what color it is, stimulates at least two kinds of cones, thus ensuring high visual acuity and good perception of form. It is the subsequent processing performed by the nervous system, comparing the *differences* in activation across cones, that extracts color information about the light falling on the retina. Thus, certain ganglion cells and certain neurons at higher stations in the visual system are color-specific, even though the photoreceptors are not. In a similar manner, photoreceptors are not form-specific (they respond to single points of light), but form is detected later in the system, by comparison of the outputs of different receptors.

Because the cones are not color detectors, the most appropriate brief names for them can be taken from their peak areas of wavelength sensitivity: *short* (S) for the receptor with peak sensitivity at about 420 nm, *medium* (M) for 530 nm, and *long* (L) for 560 nm (see Figure 7.26). There are typically twice as many L as M receptors, but the ratio varies across individuals (**FIGURE 7.27A,B**). There are far fewer S cones, which explains why acuity is much lower with short-wavelength illumination (blue light) than in the other parts of the visible spectrum. In some insects, including bees, the short-wavelength receptors respond to ultraviolet wavelengths that we humans cannot see. This ability permits bees to see color patterns in flowers that are invisible to us (**FIGURE 7.28**). Most birds have not three but four different types of cones, and they can also detect ultraviolet light (Osorio and Vorobyev, 2008).

The genes for wavelength-sensitive pigments in the retina have been analyzed, and the similarities in structure of the three genes suggest that they are all derived from a common ancestral gene (Carvalho et al., 2017). In addition, the genes for the medium- and long-wavelength pigments occupy adjacent positions on the X chromosome and are much more similar to each other than either is to the gene for the short-wavelength pigment on chromosome 7. Probably our primate ancestors had only one photopigment gene on the X chromosome, which became duplicated. Then

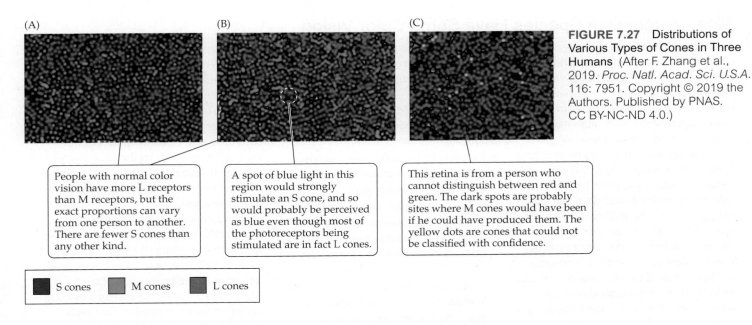

(A)

People with normal color vision have more L receptors than M receptors, but the exact proportions can vary from one person to another. There are fewer S cones than any other kind.

(B)

A spot of blue light in this region would strongly stimulate an S cone, and so would probably be perceived as blue even though most of the photoreceptors being stimulated are in fact L cones.

(C)

This retina is from a person who cannot distinguish between red and green. The dark spots are probably sites where M cones would have been if he could have produced them. The yellow dots are cones that could not be classified with confidence.

FIGURE 7.27 Distributions of Various Types of Cones in Three Humans (After F. Zhang et al., 2019. *Proc. Natl. Acad. Sci. U.S.A.* 116: 7951. Copyright © 2019 the Authors. Published by PNAS. CC BY-NC-ND 4.0.)

■ S cones ■ M cones ■ L cones

mutations caused the two genes to become more and more different, until their responses to various wavelengths of light were no longer the same. Thus, our ancestors went from having only two cone pigments (one on the X chromosome and the S pigment on chromosome 7) to three, with an associated improvement in color vision.

This evolution of a third photopigment may have happened recently (in evolutionary terms); for example, most South American monkeys have only a single longer-wavelength pigment. The fact that the genes for the M and L pigments are on the X chromosome also explains why defects of red-green color vision are much more frequent in human males (about 8%) than in human females (about 0.5%). Because males have only one X chromosome, mutations in the genes for the M and L pigments can impair color vision (**FIGURE 7.27C**). But if a female has defective photopigment genes on one of her two X chromosomes, normal copies of the genes on her other X chromosome can compensate. Even though the term *color blindness* is commonly used, most people with impaired color vision are able to distinguish some hues. Complete color blindness can be caused by brain lesions or by the congenital absence of *any* cones, but in humans it is extremely rare. Likewise, even those mammalian species with weak color vision can discriminate some colors, as we discuss in Signs & Symptoms next.

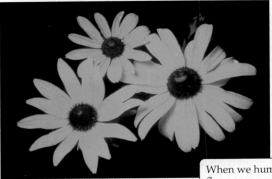

When we humans look at flowers, we cannot see the reflected ultraviolet light…

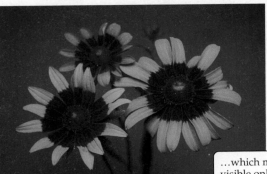

Courtesy of Thomas Eisner

…which may reveal patterns visible only to animals, like birds and bees, that detect light in that range.

FIGURE 7.28 How Flowers Look to the Birds and the Bees

Most Mammalian Species Have Some Color Vision

Animals exhibit different degrees of color vision. Many species of birds, fishes, and insects have excellent color vision. Humans and Old World monkeys also have an excellent ability to discriminate wavelengths. Many other mammals (e.g., cats) cannot discriminate wavelengths very well, but most mammals have at least some degree of color vision. Although only certain primates have good *tri*chromatic color vision (vision based on *three* classes of cone photopigments), most mammalian species have at least *di*chromatic color vision (based on *two* classes of cone pigments). Most so-called color-blind (actually color-*deficient*) people have dichromatic vision and can distinguish short-wavelength stimuli (blue) from long-wavelength stimuli (not blue) (**FIGURE 7.29**).

When a gene carrying a third photopigment was introduced into photoreceptors of adult male squirrel monkeys with such dichromatic vision, they soon displayed excellent trichromatic vision (Mancuso et al., 2009). Likewise, introducing photopigment genes in mice enabled them to discriminate colors they normally cannot see (G. H. Jacobs et al., 2007), so it may be possible to correct dichromatic vision in humans.

There is a continuum of color vision capabilities, including at least four categories among mammalian species:

1. Excellent trichromatic color vision is found in diurnal primates such as humans and rhesus monkeys.

2. Robust dichromatic color vision is found in species that have two kinds of cone photopigments and a reasonably large population of cones, for example the dog and the pig.

3. Feeble dichromatic color vision occurs in species that have two kinds of cone pigments but very few cones, such as the cat and the coati.

4. Minimal color vision is possessed by species that have only a single kind of cone pigment and must compare activity of rods and cones to discriminate wavelength, such as the owl monkey and raccoon.

Among those species of South American monkeys that are generally dichromats, some females are actually trichromatic. Why? Because the gene encoding one photopigment is on the X chromosome. Since females have two X chromosomes, if the two chromosomes carry *different* genes for the photopigment, then the female possesses a total of three different kinds of cones and therefore has trichromatic vision.

Interestingly, a woman may carry slightly different genes for the long-wavelength photopigment on her two X chromosomes (Jordan et al., 2010) and therefore have *four* different kinds of cones. Such "tetrachromats" tend to be very good at discriminating colors and very sensitive to clashing colors. It's interesting to speculate on whether such women have a different experience of, for example, green than those of us who are trichromats and dichromats. We will take up the question of our subjective experience of color again in Chapter 14.

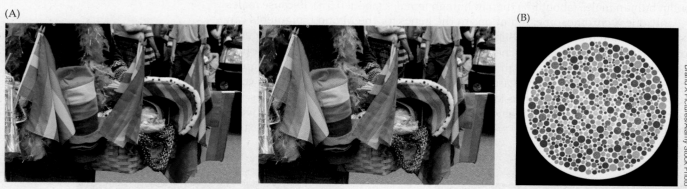

(A) (B)

Photo by David McIntyre; simulation created using software from Vischeck [www.vischeck.com]

Brand X Pictures/Alamy Stock Photo

FIGURE 7.29 Simulating Color Blindness (A) The photograph on the right has been adjusted to simulate the experience of the most common form of color blindness in humans, which is the absence of cones sensitive to medium-wavelength light (M cones). For such individuals, the world's colors consist of blue (detected by short-wavelength photopigment encoded on the seventh chromosome) and not blue (detected by the long-wavelength photopigment encoded on the X chromosome). (B) In a typical test for color vision, dichromats may have a difficult time detecting the numerals displayed in figures like this.

Some retinal ganglion cells and LGN cells show spectral opponency

Monkeys discriminate colors about as well as humans do. Recordings made from monkeys reveal that most ganglion cells and LGN cells are excited and fire in response to some wavelengths and are inhibited by other wavelengths. **FIGURE 7.30A** shows the response of one such LGN cell as a light centered on its receptive field changes from one wavelength to another. Firing is stimulated by wavelengths above 600 nm,

spectrally opponent cell Also called *color-opponent cell*. A visual system neuron that has opposite firing responses to different regions of the spectrum.

where the L cones are most sensitive; it is inhibited at shorter wavelengths, where the L cones are less sensitive than the M cones. A cell exhibiting this response pattern is therefore called a *plus L/minus M cell* (+L/–M). This is an example of a **spectrally opponent cell** (or *color-opponent cell*) because two regions of the spectrum have opposite effects on the cell's rate of firing. Figure 7.30 shows the responses of the four main kinds of spectrally opponent cells.

Each spectrally opponent ganglion cell receives input from two or three different kinds of cones through bipolar cells. The connections from at least one type of cone are excitatory, and those from at least one other type are inhibitory. The spectrally opponent ganglion cells thus record the *difference* in stimulation of different types of cones. For example, a +M/–L cell responds to the difference in the excitation of M and L cones.

The peaks of the *sensitivity* curves of the M and L cones are not very different (see Figure 7.26). However, whereas the M-minus-L *difference* curve (**FIGURE 7.30B**) shows a clear peak at about 500 nm (in the green part of the spectrum), the L-minus-M difference function (see Figure 7.28A) shows a peak at about 650 nm (in the red part of the spectrum). Thus, +M/–L and +L/–M cells yield distinctly different neural response curves. LGN cells that are excited by the L and M cells but inhibited by S cells—that is, +(L+M)/–S cells—peak in the red range (**FIGURE 7.30C**), while cells excited by S but inhibited by L and M—that is, +S/–(L+M) cells—peak in the blue-violet range (**FIGURE 7.30D**).

Spectrally opponent neurons are the second stage in the system for color perception, but they still cannot be called *color cells*, because (1) they send their outputs into many higher circuits—for detection of form, depth, and movement, as well as hue; and (2) their peak wavelength sensitivities do not correspond precisely to the wavelengths that we see as the principal hues. The brightness detectors receive stimulation from both M and L cones (+M/+L); the darkness detectors are inhibited by those same cones (–M/–L).

In the monkey LGN, 70–80% of the cells are spectrally opponent; in the cat, very few spectrally opponent cells are found—only about 1%. This difference explains why monkeys so easily distinguish between colors and it's so difficult to train cats to discriminate even large differences in color.

Some visual cortical cells and regions appear to be specialized for color perception

In the cortex, spectral information is used for various kinds of information processing. Forms are segregated from their background by differences in color or intensity (or both). The most important role that color plays in our perception is to denote which parts of a complex image belong to one object and which belong to another. Some animals use displays of brightly colored body parts to call attention to themselves, but color can also be used as camouflage.

Some spectrally opponent cortical cells contribute to the perception of color, providing the third stage of the color vision

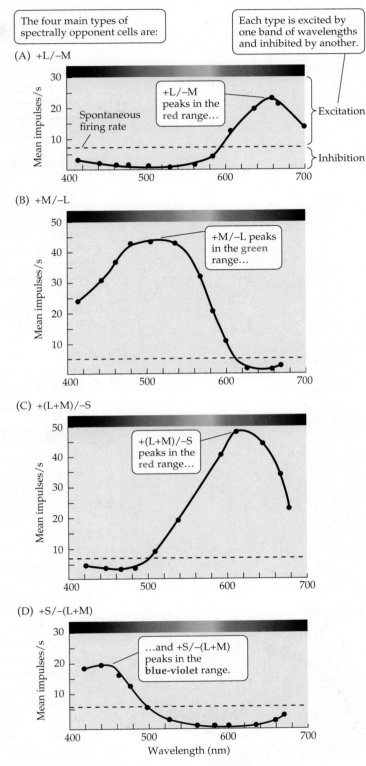

FIGURE 7.30 Responses by the Four Main Types of Spectrally Opponent Cells in Monkey LGN (After R. L. De Valois and K. K. De Valois, 1993. *Vision Res.* 33: 1053.)

system. These cells are not just responding to the differences between two types of cones, as retinal ganglion cells and LGN cells do. Rather, they are responding to differences in colors that we *perceive*; in other words, they are perceptually opponent, as predicted by Hering: red versus green, blue versus yellow, and black versus white (R. L. De Valois and De Valois, 1993). The spectral responses of these cells correspond to the wavelengths of the principal hues specified by human observers, and their characteristics also help explain other color phenomena.

Visual cortical region V4 is particularly rich in color-sensitive cells; each of these cells truly responds best to a particular hue, including the four that Hering postulated (blue, green, yellow, red). V4 cells respond best if the color outside the receptive field is different from the color preferred inside the receptive field (Roe et al., 2012).

HOW'S IT GOING ❓

1. What two main hypotheses were developed to explain our ability to discriminate colors? Which aspects of the visual system appear to match each hypothesis?
2. Describe some examples in which our perception of color is not simply the detection of particular wavelengths of light.
3. Why do we label cones as S cones, M cones, and L cones rather than blue, green, and red cones?
4. Why are men more likely than women to have difficulty distinguishing some colors?
5. Why is it a good idea to make life rafts yellow if they are to be detected on a blue sea?

7.4 What versus Where: Cortical Visual Areas Are Organized into Two Streams

THE ROAD AHEAD

Vision is so crucial for us primates that we devote lots of brain space to analyzing visual stimuli and work hard to correct vision deficiencies. After reading this final section of the chapter, you should be able to:

7.4.1 Identify the major streams of visual processing that deal with what a stimulus is, and where it is.

7.4.2 Understand why D.F. can use vision to guide her movements but not to recognize objects.

7.4.3 Describe the underlying causes of nearsightedness and how it can be avoided.

7.4.4 Understand the role of visual experience in sharpening vision, especially in children.

Mortimer Mishkin and Leslie Ungerleider (1982) proposed that primates have two main visual processing streams, both originating in primary visual cortex: a ventral processing stream responsible for visually *identifying* objects, and a dorsal stream responsible for appreciating the spatial *location* of objects and for visually guiding our movement toward them (**FIGURE 7.31**). They called these processing streams, respectively, the *what* and *where* streams.

PET studies, as well as brain lesions in patients, indicate that the human brain possesses *what* and *where* visual processing streams similar to those that have been found in monkeys. The two streams are not completely separate, because there are normally many cross connections between them. In the ventral stream, including regions of the occipitotemporal, inferior temporal, and inferior frontal areas, information about faces becomes more specific as the stream proceeds farther forward. In Chapter 15, we'll

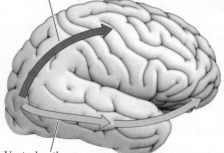

Dorsal pathway

Ventral pathway

FIGURE 7.31 Parallel Processing Pathways in the Visual System

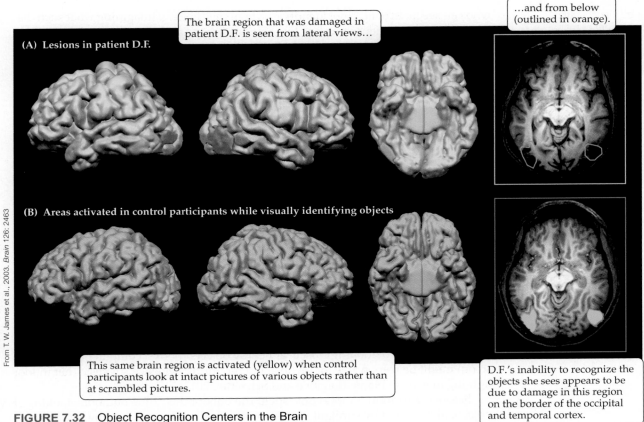

(A) Lesions in patient D.F.

The brain region that was damaged in patient D.F. is seen from lateral views…

…and from below (outlined in orange).

(B) Areas activated in control participants while visually identifying objects

This same brain region is activated (yellow) when control participants look at intact pictures of various objects rather than at scrambled pictures.

D.F.'s inability to recognize the objects she sees appears to be due to damage in this region on the border of the occipital and temporal cortex.

From T. W. James et al., 2003. *Brain* 126: 2463

FIGURE 7.32 Object Recognition Centers in the Brain

discuss a portion of the ventral stream, the fusiform gyrus, that is specialized to identify faces.

Discovery of these separate visual cortical streams helps us understand the case of patient D.F., described at the start of this chapter. Recall that, as a result of carbon monoxide poisoning, D.F. lost the ability to perceive faces and objects but retained the ability to reach and grasp objects under visual control. D.F.'s visual ventral (*what*) stream appears to have been devastated, but her dorsal (*where*) stream seems unimpaired. An opposite kind of dissociation had already been reported: damage to the dorsal parietal cortex often results in **optic ataxia**, in which patients have difficulty using vision to reach for and grasp objects, yet some of these patients can still identify objects correctly (R. A. Andersen et al., 2014). We'll discuss optic ataxia again in Chapter 14.

High-resolution MRI of D.F.'s brain (**FIGURE 7.32A**) reveals diffuse damage concentrated in the ventrolateral occipital cortex (T. W. James et al., 2003). Throughout the brain there is evidence of atrophy, indicated by shrunken gyri and enlarged sulci. **FIGURE 7.32B** shows the area activated in fMRI recordings when healthy participants viewed pictures of objects; it corresponds to D.F.'s lateral occipital lesion. When D.F. reached for and grasped objects, her fMRI activation in the parietal lobe was similar to that of control participants, indicating that her dorsal stream is largely intact. D.F.'s intact dorsal pathway not only tells her where objects are, but also guides her movements to use these objects properly (Ganel and Goodale, 2019).

It is still puzzling that one part of D.F. knows exactly how to grasp a pencil held in front of her, yet another part of her—the part that talks to you—has no idea whether the object she's holding is a pencil, a ruler, or a bouquet of flowers. This condition is reminiscent of the cortical damage that causes blindsight, mentioned earlier: people with such damage report being unable to see, but they show evidence that they can. In Chapter 14 we'll learn about other people who can see only one thing at a time, or

optic ataxia Spatial disorientation in which the patient is unable to accurately reach for objects using visual guidance.

amblyopia Reduced visual acuity that is not caused by optical or retinal impairments.

who can see faces but cannot identify to whom they belong. Imagining what such disjointed visual experience must be like helps us appreciate how effortlessly our brains usually bind together information with our marvelous sense of sight.

Visual neuroscience can be applied to alleviate some visual deficiencies

Vision is so important that many investigators have sought ways to prevent its impairment, to improve inadequate vision, and to restore sight to the blind. In the United States, half a million people are blind. Recent medical advances have reduced some causes of blindness but have increased blindness from other causes. For example, medical advances permit people with diabetes to live longer, but because we don't know how to prevent blindness associated with diabetes, there are more people alive today with diabetes-induced blindness. In the discussion that follows, we will first consider ways of avoiding the impairment of vision. Then we will take up ways of improving an impaired visual system.

REDUCING VISUAL IMPAIRMENT   Studies of the development of vision show that the incidence of myopia (nearsightedness) can be reduced. Myopia develops if the eyeball is too long, causing the eye to focus images in front of the retina rather than on the retina (see Figure 7.2). As a result, distant objects appear blurred. Considerable evidence suggests that the reason some children develop myopia is that certain environmental factors cause the eyeball to grow excessively. Previously it was thought that the modern habit of looking closely at nearby objects (books, computer screens, and so on) might be responsible for myopia, but mounting evidence suggests that indoor lighting may be to blame (Lagrèze and Schaeffel, 2017).

Before civilization, most people spent the bulk of their time outdoors, looking at objects illuminated by sunlight. But with the advent of indoor lighting, we've come to spend a lot of time looking at things with light that, while containing many wavelengths, does not exactly match the composition of sunlight. Several studies found that children with myopia spend less time outdoors than do other children, but that correlation could be caused by genes that favor both myopia and indoor activities, like reading. Indeed, the advent of public schools in various nations is accompanied by increased rates of myopia. However, one of these studies focused on people of Chinese origin who lived in either Singapore, where crowded conditions mean that people spend little time outdoors, or Sydney, Australia. Even though these populations should be genetically similar, 30% of the Chinese children living in Singapore, who averaged only 30 minutes a day outdoors, were myopic, versus only 3% of those living in Sydney, who averaged 2 hours a day outdoors (Rose et al., 2008). What's more, in these populations myopia correlates much more strongly with time spent indoors than with time spent reading.

Of course, too much sunlight can be a bad thing, especially for our skin. So almost all children in Australia wear hats to shield their faces when outdoors, yet they still benefit from being outdoors in terms of avoiding myopia. Likewise, there's no evidence that wearing sunglasses blocks the benefit of light from the sun. The next challenge will be to determine what it is about indoor lighting, as opposed to sunlight, that encourages the eyeball to grow excessively in children, leading to myopia.

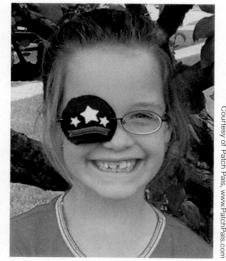

Hey There, You with the Stars over Your Eye   As a treatment for amblyopia, this girl is wearing a patch over her "good" eye—the one she has been relying on while ignoring information from her other, "weak" eye. Increased visual experience through the weak eye will strengthen its influence on the cortex.

Courtesy of Patch Pals, www.PatchPals.com

EXERCISING VISION   The misalignment of the two eyes (*lazy eye*) can lead to a condition called **amblyopia**, in which acuity is poor in one eye, even though the eye and retina are normal. If the two eyes are not aligned properly during the first few years of life, the primary visual cortex of the child tends to suppress the information arriving from one eye, and that eye becomes functionally blind (see Figure 4.12B). Studies of the development of vision in children and other animals show that most cases of amblyopia are avoidable.

The balance of the eye muscles can be surgically adjusted to bring the two eyes into better alignment. Alternatively, if the weak eye is given regular practice, with the good eye covered, vision can be preserved in both eyes. Attempts to alleviate amblyopia by training alone, however, have produced mixed results. The optimal treatment appears to be a combination of both surgical correction *and* eye patches and visual exercises (Pediatric Eye Disease Investigator Group, 2005).

SIGNS & SYMPTOMS

Macular Degeneration Is the Leading Cause of Vision Loss as We Age

Macular degeneration is a visual impairment caused by damage to the retina. The most common type, "dry" macular degeneration, is caused by atrophy of the retinal pigmented epithelium (see Figure 7.3), resulting in death of overlying photoreceptors. In the more severe, "wet" macular degeneration, abnormal growth of retinal capillaries leads to detachment of the retina and/or death of photoreceptors. The damage is mostly restricted to the fovea, but because visual acuity is poor for the rest of the retina, vision is quite impaired (**FIGURE 7.33**). An NIH-conducted trial (Age-Related Eye Disease Study [AREDS]) found that supplemental vitamins and antioxidants could slow the disease only slightly (Evans and Lawrenson, 2017).

(A) Normal vision

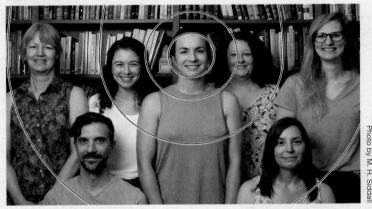

Photo by M. H. Siddall

(B) Vision with macular degeneration

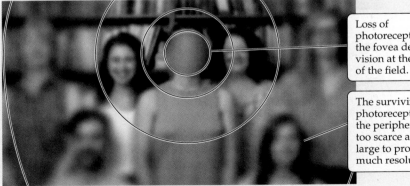

Loss of photoreceptors in the fovea degrades vision at the center of the field.

The surviving photoreceptors in the periphery are too scarce and too large to provide much resolution.

FIGURE 7.33 Simulating Visual Experience with Macular Degeneration (After D. J. Marmor & M. F. Marmor, 2010. *Arch. Ophthalmol.* 128: 117.)

HOW'S IT GOING ❓

1. What are the two main streams of visual processing in the cortex, and what aspects of vision does each stream support?
2. Describe D.F.'s symptoms, and relate them to the brain damage revealed by MRIs.
3. What is the evidence that indoor lighting may cause myopia in children?
4. Why does degeneration of the fovea impair acuity in the whole visual field?

Recommended Reading

Gregory, R. L. (2015). *Eye and Brain: The Psychology of Seeing* (5th ed.). Princeton, NJ: Princeton University Press.

Ings, S. (2008). *A Natural History of Seeing: The Art and Science of Vision.* New York, NY: Norton.

Masland, R. (2020). *We Know It When We See It: What the Neurobiology of Vision Tells Us about How We Think.* New York, NY: Basic Books.

Purves, D., and Lotto, R. B. (2011). *Why We See What We Do Redux: A Wholly Empirical Theory of Vision.* Sunderland, MA: Oxford University Press/Sinauer.

Wolfe, J. M., Kluender, K. R., Levi, D. M., Bartoshuk, L. M., et al. (2021). *Sensation & Perception* (6th ed.). Sunderland, MA: Oxford University Press/Sinauer.

7 • VISUAL SUMMARY

You should be able to relate each summary to the adjacent illustration, including structures and processes. The online version of this **Visual Summary** includes links to figures, animations, and activities that will help you consolidate the material.

1 Light is bent, or **refracted**, by the transparent outer layer of the eye, the **cornea**, focusing an image on the **retina** in the back of the eye. We vary the thickness of the **lens** to fine-tune the image. The refracted light forms an image on the retina that is upside down and reversed. Review **Figures 7.1** and **7.2**, **Animation 7.2**, **Activity 7.1**

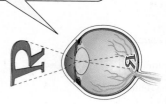

2 The retina contains two different types of **photoreceptors** to detect light forming the focused image. **Rods** are very sensitive, working even in very low light, and they respond to light of any **wavelength**. Rods drive the **scotopic system**, which can work in dim light. Each of the three different types of **cones** responds better to some wavelengths of light than others, allowing us to detect colors. The cones provide information for the **photopic system**, which requires more light to function. Photoreceptors **adapt** to function across a wide range of light intensities. Review **Figures 7.3–7.6**, **Table 7.1**

3 The retina consists of layers of neurons, with the photoreceptors in the very back stimulating **bipolar cells**, which stimulate **ganglion cells**. The ganglion cells of the retina project their axons to the brain via the **optic nerve**. **Amacrine cells** and **horizontal cells** communicate across the retina, using processes such as **lateral inhibition** to analyze **brightness**. Review **Figures 7.3**, **7.14**, and **7.15**

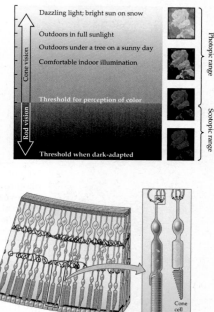

4 The center of our **visual field** lands on the **fovea**, the portion of the retina with the greatest density of photoreceptors, an absence of overlying cell layers, and more direct synaptic connections to ganglion cells, providing us with our greatest **visual acuity** (sharpness of vision). Cones are concentrated in the fovea, and rods are concentrated in the peripheral retina, so our peripheral vision is best for seeing dim objects, but it provides no color information. Review **Figures 7.7–7.9**

5 The left visual field falls on the nasal hemiretina of the left eye and the temporal hemiretina of the right eye. Only nasal retinal ganglion cells of each eye send their axons across the midline, forming the **optic chiasm**, so the left visual field projects to the right hemisphere, and the right visual field projects to the left hemisphere. Review **Figures 7.11** and **7.12**, **Animation 7.3**

7 The **receptive fields** of bipolar cells and ganglion cells consist of a circular center and a surround that have opposing effects: either **on-center/off-surround** or **off-center/on-surround**. Review **Figures 7.13** and **7.14**, **Animation 7.4**

9 Rods detect light using a pigment called **rhodopsin**. Our detection of hue (color) depends on the three different cone photopigments (opsins). Each cone responds to a wide range of wavelengths, not just a single color. Our perception of hue results from the relative activity of each type of cone. One way of assessing this relative activity is by retinal connections that yield **spectrally opponent** neurons. Review **Figures 7.23–7.30**

6 Most ganglion cells of the retina synapse on neurons in the **lateral geniculate nucleus** (**LGN**) of the thalamus. The LGN neurons send axons to synapse on neurons in layer IV of the **primary visual cortex** (**V1**) in the **occipital cortex**. V1 sends information to many different cortical areas, called **extrastriate cortex** (nearly one-third of the human cortex), to further analyze visual information. Review **Figures 7.11** and **7.20**

8 Receptive fields of cells at successively higher levels in the visual cortex change in two main ways: (1) they become larger (occupy larger parts of the visual field), and (2) they require increasingly specific stimuli to evoke responses. For example, they respond best to a bar of light at a particular angle or to bars that move in a particular direction. Review **Figures 7.17–7.22**, **Animation 7.5**

10 Visual cortical areas are organized into two main streams: a ventral *what* stream that serves in the recognition of faces and objects, and a dorsal *where* stream that serves in location and visuomotor skills. Review **Figures 7.31** and **7.32**

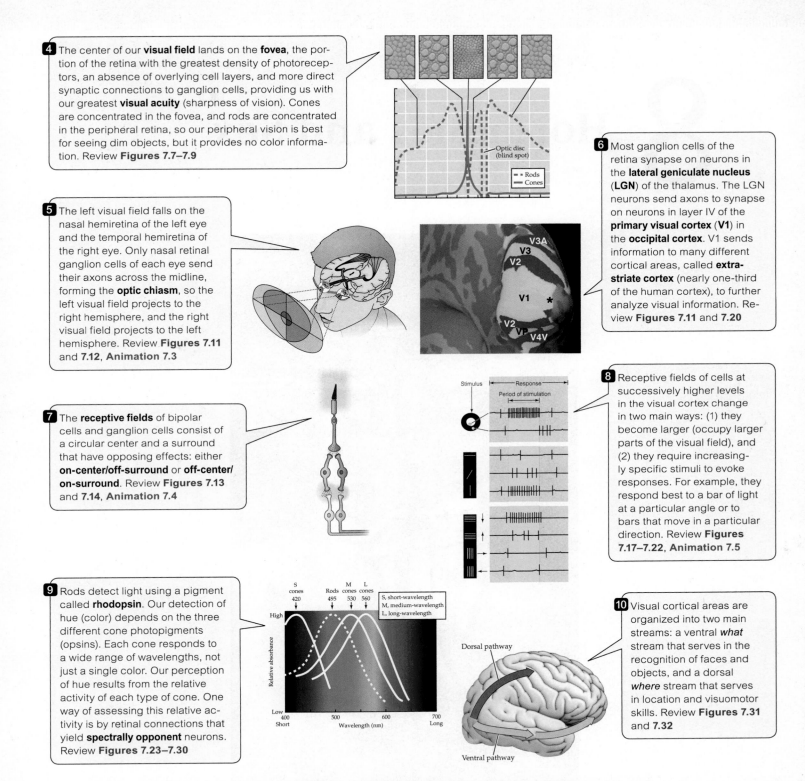

The Mind's Machine digital resources include additional videos, flashcards, and other study tools.

8 Hormones and Sex

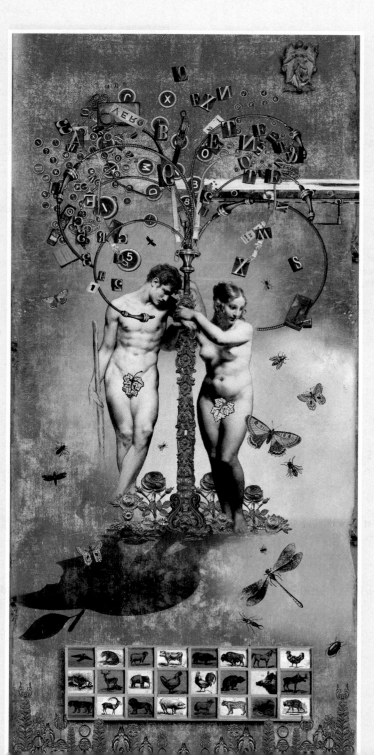

Genitals and Gender: What Makes Us Male and Female?

No aspects of biology are more impressive or humbling than the making of a baby; it is a developmental ballet of staggering complexity and critical timing. Given the countless processes that must unfold perfectly and in precisely the right order, it is a marvel that, in most cases, development proceeds without a hitch. Inevitably, though, there are times when a crucial part of the program is derailed along the way and a baby is born with a heartbreaking deformity.

Such is the case with **cloacal exstrophy**, which occurs in about one in 400,000 human births, characterized by an incomplete closing of the abdomen that leaves the bladder and intestines exposed. A genetic male with this condition is typically born with normal testes but a very short, split penis or no penis at all. Surgery is required to close up the abdomen, but it isn't really possible to surgically fashion a normal penis, so the parents are faced with a dilemma. Is it better to raise the child as a boy without a penis, despite the emotional costs of the deformity? Or is it better to assign the child to the female gender, surgically remove the testes and fashion female-looking genitals, and then raise the child as a girl? Which would you choose?

Arguments for each course of action boil down to different opinions about the extent to which our gender is shaped through nurturing and socialization, rather than biological factors. In other words, we need to consider the larger question of why men and women behave differently. Is it because as boys and girls they were treated differently and trained to grow into their gender roles, or do the forces that provide a fetus with testes or ovaries also induce the developing brain to take on a masculine or feminine form? In an age where many people reject the notion of only two genders, do biological factors have any say in gender identity?

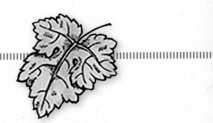

In this chapter we'll discuss research that informs us about this long-standing question: How do biological and social forces combine to direct development in male-typical and female-typical ways? First, we'll learn how hormones can affect the brain to influence behavior. Then we will explore how hormones act on different parts of the brain to influence sexual behavior and parental behavior in particular. That will take us to the question of how the fetus normally develops into either a male or a female form, not just in terms of the body, but also in terms of the brain and behavior. We'll see that not everyone fits neatly into the binary categories in terms of either body structures or behavior. In animals, prenatal hormones have a tremendous influence on the brain and sexual behaviors. We'll close by reviewing growing evidence that those same prenatal hormones also affect our development into men, women, or other, as well as our sexual orientation.

See Video 8.1:
Gender

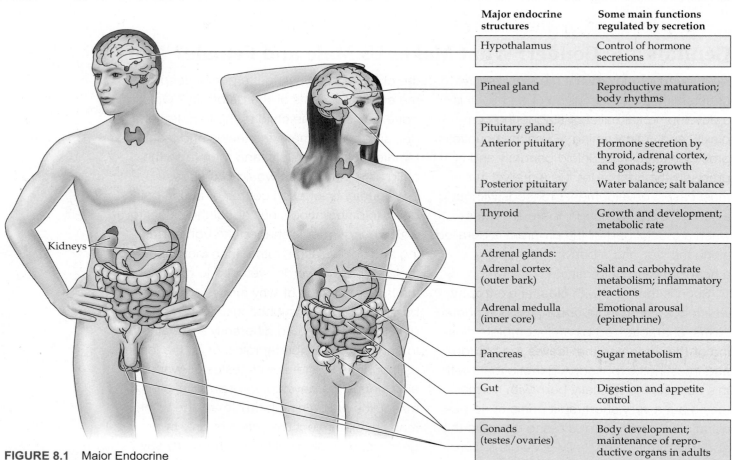

Major endocrine structures	Some main functions regulated by secretion
Hypothalamus	Control of hormone secretions
Pineal gland	Reproductive maturation; body rhythms
Pituitary gland:	
Anterior pituitary	Hormone secretion by thyroid, adrenal cortex, and gonads; growth
Posterior pituitary	Water balance; salt balance
Thyroid	Growth and development; metabolic rate
Adrenal glands:	
Adrenal cortex (outer bark)	Salt and carbohydrate metabolism; inflammatory reactions
Adrenal medulla (inner core)	Emotional arousal (epinephrine)
Pancreas	Sugar metabolism
Gut	Digestion and appetite control
Gonads (testes/ovaries)	Body development; maintenance of reproductive organs in adults

FIGURE 8.1 Major Endocrine Glands and Their Functions

View Activity 8.1:
Major Endocrine Glands

cloacal exstrophy A rare medical condition in which individuals are born with an incompletely sealed lower abdomen.

hormone A chemical, usually secreted by an endocrine gland, that is conveyed by the bloodstream and regulates target organs or tissues.

endocrine gland A gland that secretes hormones into the bloodstream to act on distant targets.

castration Removal of the gonads, usually the testes.

8.1 Hormones Act in a Great Variety of Ways throughout the Body

THE ROAD AHEAD

The chapter begins by considering the way the chemical signals called hormones coordinate action in different parts of the body. After reading this material, you should be able to:

8.1.1 Distinguish the different classes of chemical signaling, from neurotransmitters to hormones and pheromones.

8.1.2 Contrast the mechanisms of action of peptide and amine hormones versus steroid hormones.

8.1.3 Contrast the modes of hormone release from the posterior pituitary versus the anterior pituitary.

8.1.4 Explain how the brain regulates circulating levels of hormone.

8.1.5 Give examples of the interaction of hormonal and neuronal communication in controlling behavior.

Hormones are chemicals secreted by one group of cells and carried through the bloodstream to other parts of the body, where they act on specific target tissues to produce physiological effects. Most hormones are produced by **endocrine glands** (from the Greek *endon*, "within," and *krinein*, "to secrete"), so called because they release their hormones *within* the body (**FIGURE 8.1**). Endocrine glands are sometimes contrasted with *exocrine glands* (tear glands, salivary glands, sweat glands), which use ducts to secrete fluid *outside* the body.

Our current understanding of hormones developed in stages

Without knowing that hormones exist, ancient civilizations nevertheless noted their consequences. In the fourth century BCE, Aristotle described the effects of **castration** (removal of the testes) in chickens and compared them with the effects in eunuchs (castrated men). But learning that these effects were due to the loss of chemical signals coming from the testes would not happen until 1849, when German physician Arnold Berthold (1803–1861) conducted the first endocrinology experiment. Aristotle had reported that when roosters are castrated as juveniles, they fail to develop normal reproductive behavior and secondary sexual characteristics, such as the rooster's comb, in adulthood. Berthold observed, however, that returning one testis back into the body cavity of the young birds allowed them to develop normal male anatomy and behavior. In adulthood, these animals showed the usual male sexual behaviors—mounting hens, fighting, and crowing (**FIGURE 8.2**). Because no nerves had reestablished contact with the transplanted testis, the organ could not be communicating to the brain through nerves. Berthold (1849) concluded that the testes release a chemical into the blood that affects both male behavior and male body structures.

Today we know that the testes make and release the hormone testosterone to exert these effects.

Although Berthold didn't know it, experiments like this also illustrate another principle of hormone action. If he had waited until the castrated chicks were adults before returning their testes, Berthold would have seen little effect. The testosterone must be present *early* in life to have such dramatic effects on the body and behavior. We'll return to this point later in this chapter. For now, let's see how hormones fit into the grand scheme of chemical signaling by the body.

FIGURE 8.2 Berthold's (1849) Experiment Demonstrated the Importance of Hormones for Behavior

■ **Question**

Male chicks that are castrated grow up to have small wattles and combs, and they show little interest in mounting hens, fighting, or crowing. What causes these changes—the loss of a nerve connection between the testes and the body, or the loss of a chemical signal released from the testes?

■ **Experiment**

Berthold removed the testes from their normal position but then reimplanted them elsewhere in the abdomen, disconnected from normal innervation.

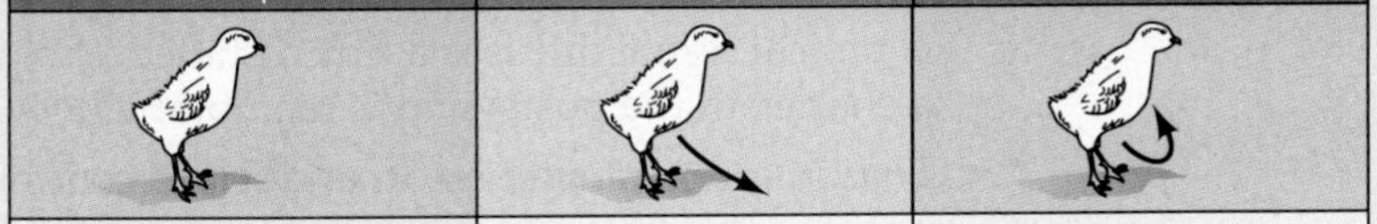

Group 1	Group 2	Group 3
Left undisturbed, young roosters grow up to have large red wattles and combs, to mount and mate with hens readily, and to fight one another and crow loudly.	Males whose testes were removed during development displayed neither the appearance nor the behavior of normal roosters as adults.	However, if one of the testes was reimplanted into the abdominal cavity immediately after its removal, the rooster developed normal wattles and normal behavior.

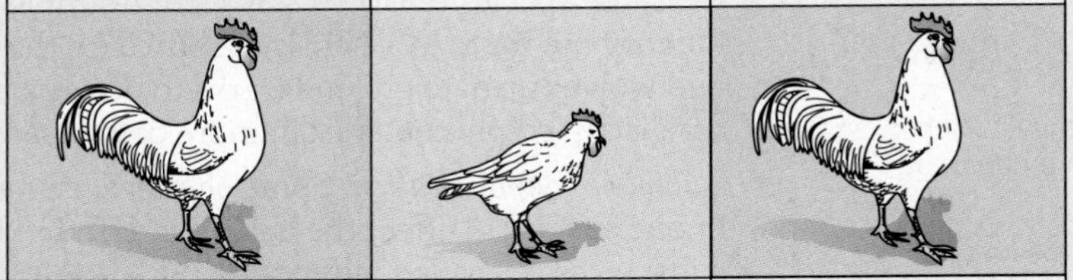

	Group 1	Group 2	Group 3
Comb and wattles:	Large	Small	Large
Mount hens?	Yes	No	Yes
Aggressive?	Yes	No	Yes
Crowing?	Normal	Weak	Normal

■ **Outcome**

The animals with the reimplanted testes grew up to look and act like normal males. Berthold reasoned that the testes must have secreted a signal, which today we would call a hormone, that has widespread effects on the body and brain. Today we know that the hormone is testosterone.

(A) Neural function (synaptic transmission)

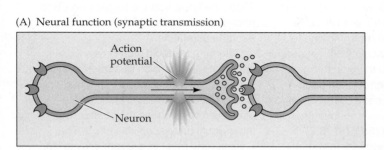

(B) Endocrine function

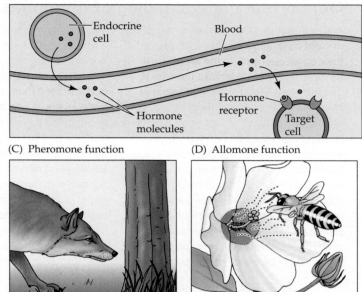

FIGURE 8.3 Chemical Communication Systems

View Animation 8.2:
Brain Explorer

View Animation 8.3:
Chemical Communication Systems

synapse The cellular location at which information is transmitted from a neuron to another cell.

endocrine Referring to glands that release chemicals to the interior of the body. These glands secrete the principal hormones used by the body.

pheromone A chemical signal that is released outside the body of an animal and affects other members of the same species.

allomone A chemical signal that is released outside the body by one species and affects the behavior of other species.

Hormones are one of several types of chemical communication

People had long suspected that special substances circulate to carry messages through the body, but as we discussed above, it wasn't until the nineteenth century that details of chemical communication began to emerge. We can compare hormonal communication with other methods of chemical signaling:

- *Synaptic communication* Communication via **synapses** was described in Chapter 2 and Chapter 3. In typical synaptic transmission, the released chemical signal diffuses a tiny distance across the synaptic cleft and causes a change in the postsynaptic membrane (**FIGURE 8.3A**).

- *Endocrine communication* In **endocrine** communication, our topic for this chapter, the chemical signal is a hormone released into the bloodstream to selectively affect distant target organs (**FIGURE 8.3B**).

- *Pheromone communication* Chemicals can be used for communication not only within an individual, but also *between* individuals. **Pheromones** are chemicals that are released outside the body to affect other individuals of the same species (**FIGURE 8.3C**). For example, ants produce pheromones that identify the route to a rich food source (to the annoyance of picnickers). Dogs and wolves urinate on landmarks to designate their territory. In Chapter 6 we discussed pheromones in more detail (see Figure 6.23).

- *Allomone communication* Some chemical signals are released by members of one species to affect the behavior of individuals of *another* species. These substances are called **allomones** (**FIGURE 8.3D**). Flowers exude scented allomones to attract insects and birds in order to distribute pollen. And the bolas spider—nature's femme fatale—releases a moth sex pheromone to lure male moths to their doom (Haynes et al., 2002).

Let's review the basic types of hormones and how they influence cells.

Hormones can be classified by chemical structure

Most hormones fall into one of three categories: peptide hormones, amine hormones, or steroid hormones. Peptides are simply small protein molecules, so, like any other

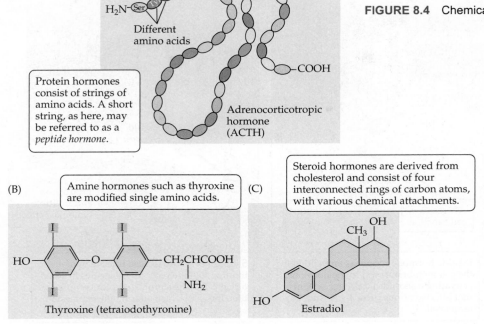

FIGURE 8.4 Chemical Structures of the Three Main Hormone Types

(A) Protein hormone

H₂N—Ser—Ser—Ser

Different amino acids

Protein hormones consist of strings of amino acids. A short string, as here, may be referred to as a *peptide hormone*.

—COOH

Adrenocorticotropic hormone (ACTH)

(B) Amine hormones such as thyroxine are modified single amino acids.

Thyroxine (tetraiodothyronine)

(C) Steroid hormones are derived from cholesterol and consist of four interconnected rings of carbon atoms, with various chemical attachments.

Estradiol

peptide hormone   Also called *protein hormone*. A hormone that consists of a string of amino acids.

amine hormone   Also called *monoamine hormone*. A hormone composed of a single amino acid that has been modified into a related molecule, such as melatonin or epinephrine.

steroid hormone   Any of a class of hormones, each of which is composed of four interconnected rings of carbon atoms.

protein, a molecule of **peptide hormone** is made up of a short string of amino acids (**FIGURE 8.4A**). Different peptide hormones consist of different combinations of amino acids. **Amine hormones** are smaller and simpler, consisting of a modified version of a single amino acid (hence their alias, *monoamine hormones*) (**FIGURE 8.4B**). The amine hormone melatonin is discussed in **A STEP FURTHER 8.1**, on the website.

Steroid hormones are derived from cholesterol and thus share its structure of four rings of carbon atoms (**FIGURE 8.4C**). Different steroid hormones vary in the number and kinds of atoms attached to the rings. Because steroids dissolve readily in lipids, they can pass through membranes easily (recall from Chapter 1 that cell membranes consist of a lipid bilayer). **TABLE 8.1** gives examples of each class of hormones.

The distinction between peptide or amine hormones and steroid hormones is important because the different types of hormones interact with different types of receptors, as we discuss next.

Hormones act on a wide variety of cellular mechanisms

Let's look briefly at two aspects of hormone activity: first the mechanisms of hormone action, then the types of changes that hormones cause in target cells, including neurons. The three classes of hormones exert their influences on target organs in two different ways.

PEPTIDE AND AMINE HORMONES   Peptide and amine hormones bind to specific receptor proteins *on the surface* of the target cell and activate chemical signals inside the

TABLE 8.1 Examples of Major Classes of Hormones

Class	Hormone
Peptide hormones	Adrenocorticotropic hormone (ACTH)
	Follicle-stimulating hormone (FSH)
	Luteinizing hormone (LH)
	Thyroid-stimulating hormone (TSH)
	Growth hormone (GH)
	Prolactin
	Insulin
	Glucagon
	Oxytocin
	Vasopressin (arginine vasopressin, AVP; antidiuretic hormone, ADH)
	Releasing hormones, such as:
	Corticotropin-releasing hormone (CRH)
	Gonadotropin-releasing hormone (GnRH)
Amine hormones	Epinephrine (adrenaline)
	Norepinephrine (NE)
	Thyroid hormones (e.g., thyroxine)
	Melatonin
Steroid hormones	Estrogens (e.g., estradiol)
	Progestins (e.g., progesterone)
	Androgens (e.g., testosterone, dihydrotestosterone)
	Glucocorticoids (e.g., cortisol)
	Mineralocorticoids (e.g., aldosterone)

FIGURE 8.5 Two Main Mechanisms of Hormone Action

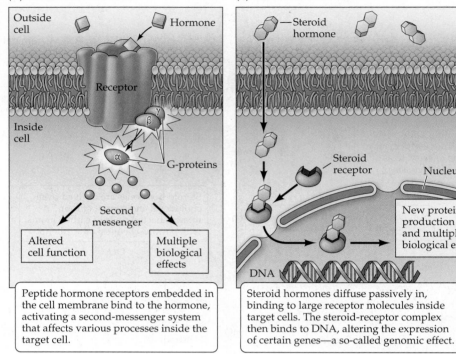

(A) Protein hormone action

Outside cell

Hormone

Receptor

Inside cell

γ
β

α

G-proteins

Second messenger

Altered cell function

Multiple biological effects

Peptide hormone receptors embedded in the cell membrane bind to the hormone, activating a second-messenger system that affects various processes inside the target cell.

(B) Steroid hormone action

Steroid hormone

Steroid receptor

Nucleus

New protein production and multiple biological effects

DNA

Steroid hormones diffuse passively in, binding to large receptor molecules inside target cells. The steroid-receptor complex then binds to DNA, altering the expression of certain genes—a so-called genomic effect.

cell that are called **second messengers** (see Chapter 3) (**FIGURE 8.5A**). What determines whether a cell responds to a particular peptide hormone? Receptors are highly specific, so only those cells that produce the appropriate receptor proteins for a hormone can respond to that hormone. As we saw with neurotransmitter receptors in Chapter 2 and Chapter 3, the receptor protein spans the cellular membrane. The specific effect of the hormone depends in large part on the receptor it activates. Peptide and amine hormones usually act relatively rapidly, within seconds to minutes. (Although rapid for a hormone, this action is much slower than neural activity.)

STEROID HORMONES   We mentioned earlier that steroid hormones easily pass through cell membranes, so their receptors are generally located *inside* the target cell. Different classes of steroids have their own specific receptors; for example, estrogens selectively interact with estrogen receptors, and androgens like testosterone bind to androgen receptors. When a steroid molecule and a receptor molecule combine, the steroid-receptor complex enters the nucleus of the cell and binds to the DNA, controlling the expression of specific genes (**FIGURE 8.5B**), increasing or decreasing the rate of protein production (see the Appendix). Because they involve multiple steps and the synthesis of large new molecules, steroid hormones are typically slower acting than peptide or amine hormones. Steroid effects may take hours, days, or even years to fully unfold.

   We can study where a steroid hormone is active by injecting radioactively tagged molecules of the steroid and observing where they accumulate. For example, tagged estrogens accumulate not only in the uterus (as you might expect), but also in the nuclei of some neurons throughout the hypothalamus. Because neurons that produce hormone receptors are found in only a limited number of brain regions, we can begin to learn how hormones affect behavior by finding those brain sites and asking what happens when the hormone arrives there. This strategy for learning about hormones and behavior is discussed in **BOX 8.1**.

Hormones can have different effects on different target organs

Virtually all hormones, whether peptide or steroid, act on more than one target organ. What's more, a given hormone may have one type of effect on one organ, and a quite different effect on another organ. This means hormones often act to coordinate

second messenger   A slow-acting substance in a target cell that amplifies the effects of synaptic or hormonal activity and regulates activity within the target cell.

knockout organism   An individual in which a particular gene has been disabled by an experimenter.

autoradiography   A technique that shows the distribution of radioactive chemicals in tissues.

Box 8.1 Techniques of Behavioral Endocrinology

To establish that a particular hormone affects behavior, investigators usually begin with an experiment like that of Arnold Berthold (see Figure 8.2): observing the behavior of the intact animal and then removing the endocrine gland and looking for a change in behavior. Modern scientists have many options to understand that basic finding. Let's imagine that we're investigating a particular effect of hormones on behavior to see how we might proceed.

First we carefully observe the behavior of several individuals, to classify and quantify the different types of behavior and to place them in the context of other individuals. For example, most adult male rats will try to mount and copulate with females placed in their cages. If its testes are removed, the male rat will eventually stop copulating with females. We know that one of the hormones produced by the testes is testosterone. Is it the loss of testosterone that causes the loss of male copulatory behavior?

To explore this question, we inject some testosterone into castrated males and observe whether the copulatory behavior returns. (It does.) Another way to ask whether a steroid hormone is affecting a particular behavior is to examine the behavior of animals that lack the receptors for that steroid. We can delete the gene for a given hormone receptor, making a **knockout organism** (so called because the targeted gene has been "knocked out"), and ask which behaviors are different in the receptor knockouts versus normal animals.

What does testosterone do to facilitate sexual behavior? One step toward answering this question is to determine which parts of the brain are normally affected by this hormone.

First we might inject a castrated animal with radioactively labeled testosterone and wait for the hormone to accumulate in the brain regions that have receptors

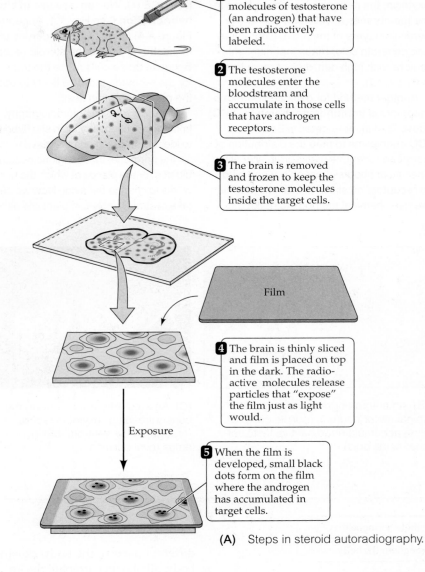

1 A rat is injected with molecules of testosterone (an androgen) that have been radioactively labeled.

2 The testosterone molecules enter the bloodstream and accumulate in those cells that have androgen receptors.

3 The brain is removed and frozen to keep the testosterone molecules inside the target cells.

Film

4 The brain is thinly sliced and film is placed on top in the dark. The radioactive molecules release particles that "expose" the film just as light would.

Exposure

5 When the film is developed, small black dots form on the film where the androgen has accumulated in target cells.

(A) Steps in steroid autoradiography.

for the hormone. Then we could sacrifice the animal, remove the brain, freeze it, cut thin sections from it, and place the thin sections on photographic film. Radioactive emissions from the tissue would expose the film, revealing which brain regions accumulated the labeled testosterone. This method is known as **autoradiography** because the tissue "takes its own picture" with radioactivity (**FIGURE A**).

When the labeled hormone is a steroid like testosterone, the radioactivity accumulates in the nuclei of neurons and leaves small black specks on the overlying

(Continued)

Box 8.1   (continued)

film (**FIGURE B**). When the radiolabeled hormone is a peptide hormone such as oxytocin, the radioactivity accumulates in the membranes of cells and appears in particular layers of the brain. Computers can generate color maps that highlight regions with high densities of receptors (**FIGURE C**).

Another method for detecting hormone receptors is **immunocytochemistry (ICC)** (described in more detail in Box 1.1). ICC enables us to map the distribution of hormone receptors in the brain. We allow specific antibodies to seek out and bind to receptors on slices of brain tissue, then we use chemical methods to make the

antibodies visible, leaving a dark color in the spherical nuclei of target brain cells (**FIGURE D**). We can also use **in situ hybridization** (see Box 1.1, Appendix Figure A.4) to look for the neurons that make the mRNA for the steroid receptor. Because these cells make the transcript for the receptor, they are likely to possess the receptor protein itself.

Once we've used autoradiography, immunocytochemistry, or in situ hybridization to identify brain regions that have receptors for the hormone, those regions become candidates for the places at which the hormone works to change behavior. Now we can take castrated males, implant tiny pellets of

testosterone into one of those brain regions, and see whether the behavior is restored.

It turns out that such implants can restore male sexual behavior in rats only if they are placed in the medial preoptic area (mPOA) of the hypothalamus. So far, we've found that testosterone does something to the mPOA to permit individual males to display sexual behavior. Now we can examine the mPOA in detail to learn which changes in the anatomy, physiology, or protein production of this region are caused by testosterone. And with that, we have more or less caught up to present-day scientists who work on this very question.

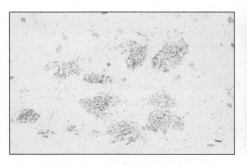

(B) An autoradiogram showing that spinal motor neurons (purple cell profiles) accumulate radioactive testosterone (small dots).

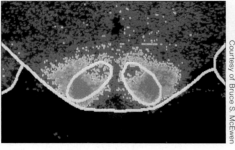

Courtesy of Bruce S. McEwen

(C) An autoradiogram showing the concentration of oxytocin receptors (orange) in the ventromedial hypothalamus (oval outlines).

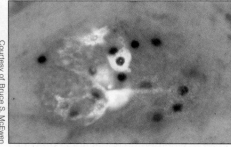

Courtesy of Cynthia L. Jordan (Michigan State University)

(D) Immunocytochemistry revealing cells with nuclei that contain androgen receptors (dark circles), to which testosterone can bind. The cell bodies of these neurons have been labeled with two different tracers, one white and the other red.

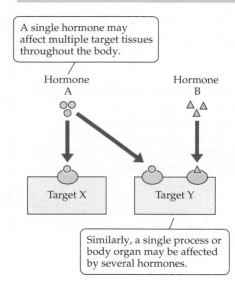

A single hormone may affect multiple target tissues throughout the body.

Hormone A

Hormone B

Target X

Target Y

Similarly, a single process or body organ may be affected by several hormones.

FIGURE 8.6   The Multiplicity of Hormone Action

different parts of the body, causing diverse changes to several different parts of the body, all of which prepare the animal for a particular activity. For example, the testes secrete testosterone, which acts in the testes themselves to drive sperm production but also acts to masculinize the body in diverse ways, favoring muscle development and, in humans, beard growth (**FIGURE 8.6**). In this and numerous other cases we'll discuss, the same hormone also acts on the brain—in the case of testosterone, to promote sexual behavior and aggression in many animal species.

How can the same hormone cause many different responses in different organs? First, often more than one receptor responds to a given hormone. For example, there are at least two different subtypes of receptors for estrogens, and for other hormones there may be four or more. In addition, sometimes the same receptor, in response to the same hormone, will have a different effect because the target cell uses different second messengers to respond differently.

As we'll see later, the brain maintains strict control over most hormone secretions, which means, among other things, that the brain has receptors to detect almost all hormones, in order to monitor their release.

HOW'S IT GOING

1. What are hormones, and how do they act?
2. Describe Berthold's experiment with young roosters, and explain how it indicated hormonal effects.
3. Compare and contrast the mechanisms by which peptide/amine hormones versus steroid hormones act on cells.
4. Why are hormones effective for coordinating different changes in different parts of the body?

Each endocrine gland secretes specific hormones

Now we'll discuss the specific hormones that endocrine glands secrete. To cover all the hormones would require an entire book, so we will consider only some of the main endocrine glands. **A STEP FURTHER 8.2**, on the website, gives a fuller (though far from complete) listing of hormones and their functions. Hormones involved in thirst and hunger are discussed in Chapter 9.

We begin with the pituitary because it regulates so many other endocrine glands. Resting in a socket in the base of the skull, the **pituitary gland** is about the size of a garden pea, weighing about 1 gram (see Figure 8.1). The hypothalamus sits just above the pituitary and is connected to the gland by a slender thread called the **pituitary stalk**. The term *pituitary* comes from the Latin *pituita*, "mucus," reflecting the outmoded belief that waste products dripped down from the brain into the pituitary, which then secreted them out through the nose. (If this were true, you could literally sneeze some of your brains out!) Because the pituitary regulates most other endocrine glands, it is sometimes referred to as the *master gland*. But the pituitary is itself enslaved by the hypothalamus above it, as we'll see.

To understand how the pituitary works, we need to consider a special category of cells that are something of a blend of neuronal cells and endocrine cells, called **neuroendocrine cells**. On the one hand, neuroendocrine cells receive synaptic input from other neurons and, if they are excited past threshold, produce action potentials. But unlike regular neurons, which release a neurotransmitter into a synapse when they fire, neuroendocrine cells release a hormone into the bloodstream (**FIGURE 8.7**).

To understand the pivotal role of such neuroendocrine cells in hormone release from the pituitary, we need to consider separately the two parts of the pituitary: the *anterior pituitary* and the *posterior pituitary*. The mechanism of hormone release is simpler in the posterior pituitary, so let's discuss that first.

immunocytochemistry (ICC) A method for detecting a particular protein in tissues in which an antibody recognizes and binds to the protein and then chemical methods are used to leave a visible reaction product around each antibody.

in situ hybridization A method for detecting particular RNA transcripts in tissue sections by providing a nucleotide probe that is complementary to, and will therefore hybridize with, the transcript of interest.

pituitary gland A small, complex endocrine gland located in a socket at the base of the skull.

pituitary stalk A thin piece of tissue that connects the pituitary gland to the hypothalamus.

neuroendocrine cell A neuron that releases hormones into local or general circulation.

View Animation 8.4:
Mechanisms of Hormone Action

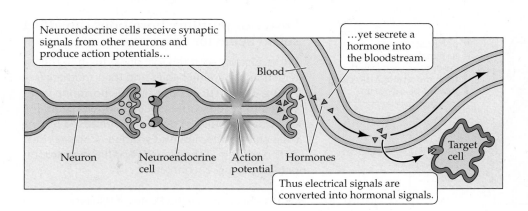

FIGURE 8.7 Neuroendocrine Cells Are the Interface between Neurons and Endocrine Glands

The posterior pituitary releases two hormones directly into the bloodstream

While the **posterior pituitary** releases hormones, the organ itself does not make them. Rather, the hormones are manufactured by neuroendocrine cells in two hypothalamic regions: the *supraoptic* and *paraventricular nuclei*. These neuroendocrine cells transport hormones down their axons, which extend through the pituitary stalk to terminate in the posterior pituitary. When the hypothalamic neuroendocrine cells are excited by synaptic input, they produce action potentials that travel down the axons and release hormone directly onto capillaries (small blood vessels) in the posterior pituitary, sending the hormone into circulation immediately (**FIGURE 8.8**).

In this fashion, the neuroendocrine cells in the hypothalamus produce and release two peptide hormones from the posterior pituitary: **oxytocin** and **vasopressin**. Some of the signals that activate the nerve cells of the supraoptic and paraventricular nuclei are related to thirst and water regulation; vasopressin is involved in these interactions, which will be discussed in Chapter 9. Oxytocin is involved in many aspects of reproductive and parental behavior. One of its functions is to stimulate contractions of the uterus in childbirth. Injections of oxytocin (or a synthetic version) are frequently used in hospitals to induce or accelerate labor and delivery.

Oxytocin also triggers the **milk letdown reflex**, the contraction of mammary gland cells that ejects milk into the breast ducts. This reflex exemplifies the reciprocal relationship between behavior and hormone release. When an infant first begins to suckle, the arrival of milk at the nipple is delayed by 30–60 seconds. This delay is caused by the sequence of steps that precedes letdown. Stimulation of the nipple activates receptors in the skin, which transmit this information through a chain of neurons and synapses to hypothalamic cells that contain oxytocin. Once these neuroendocrine cells have been sufficiently stimulated, they produce action potentials that travel down their axons to the posterior pituitary, where they release oxytocin into the bloodstream. The oxytocin reaches muscle tissue in the mammary glands, and the muscle contracts to make milk available at the nipple (**FIGURE 8.9**).

For mothers, this reflex response to suckling frequently becomes conditioned to baby cries, so milk appears promptly at the start of nursing. Because the mother is conditioned to release oxytocin *before* the suckling begins, sometimes the cries of *someone else's* baby in public may trigger an inconvenient release of milk.

Posterior pituitary hormones can affect social behavior

We've already seen the role of oxytocin in the interaction of nursing babies and their mothers (see Figure 8.9). It turns out that this hormone is involved in several other social behaviors too. For one thing, a pulse of oxytocin is released during orgasm in both men and women (Caruso et al., 2017), adding to the pleasurable feelings accompanying sexual encounters.

posterior pituitary The rear division of the pituitary gland.

oxytocin A peptide hormone, released from the posterior pituitary, that triggers milk letdown in the nursing female and is also associated with a variety of complex behaviors.

vasopressin Also called *arginine vasopressin* or *antidiuretic hormone*. A peptide hormone from the posterior pituitary that promotes water conservation and increases blood pressure.

milk letdown reflex The reflexive release of milk by the mammary glands of a nursing female in response to suckling or to stimuli associated with suckling.

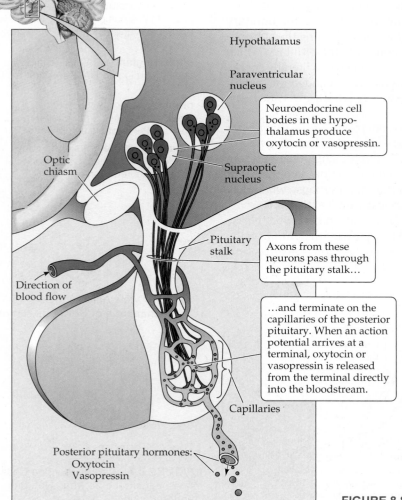

Hypothalamus

Paraventricular nucleus

Neuroendocrine cell bodies in the hypothalamus produce oxytocin or vasopressin.

Supraoptic nucleus

Optic chiasm

Pituitary stalk

Axons from these neurons pass through the pituitary stalk…

Direction of blood flow

…and terminate on the capillaries of the posterior pituitary. When an action potential arrives at a terminal, oxytocin or vasopressin is released from the terminal directly into the bloodstream.

Capillaries

Posterior pituitary hormones: Oxytocin Vasopressin

FIGURE 8.8 Hormone Secretion by the Posterior Pituitary

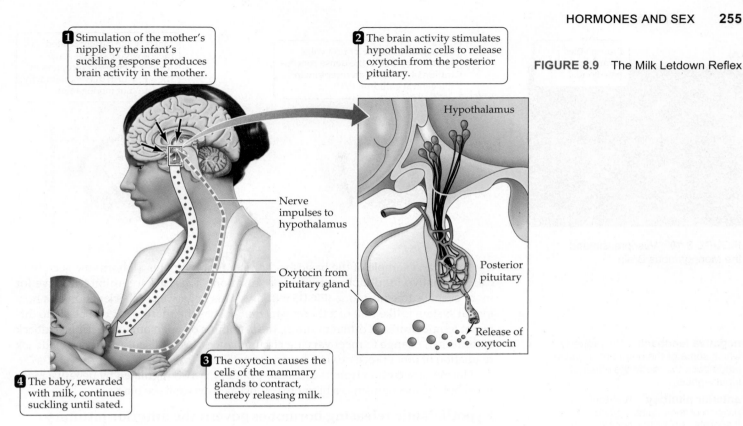

1 Stimulation of the mother's nipple by the infant's suckling response produces brain activity in the mother.

2 The brain activity stimulates hypothalamic cells to release oxytocin from the posterior pituitary.

FIGURE 8.9   The Milk Letdown Reflex

Hypothalamus

Nerve impulses to hypothalamus

Oxytocin from pituitary gland

Posterior pituitary

Release of oxytocin

3 The oxytocin causes the cells of the mammary glands to contract, thereby releasing milk.

4 The baby, rewarded with milk, continues suckling until sated.

In nonhuman animals, oxytocin and vasopressin facilitate many social processes (Lim and Young, 2006). Rodents given supplementary doses of oxytocin spend more time in physical contact with one another (Carter, 2017). Male mice that have the oxytocin gene knocked out and are therefore unable to produce the hormone display social amnesia: they seem unable to recognize the scents of female mice that they have met before (Ferguson et al., 2000). These oxytocin knockout males can be cured of their social amnesia with brain infusions of oxytocin (Winslow and Insel, 2002).

In prairie voles (*Microtus ochrogaster*), couples form stable **pair-bonds**, and oxytocin infusions in the brains of females help them bond to their mates. In *male* prairie voles, it is vasopressin rather than oxytocin that facilitates the formation of a preference for a specific female partner. In fact, the distribution of vasopressin receptors in the brains of male prairie voles may be what makes them monogamous. Supporting this idea is the finding that the closely related meadow voles (*Microtus pennsylvanicus*), which do not form pair-bonds and instead have multiple mating partners, have far fewer vasopressin receptors in certain brain regions than prairie voles have (Lim et al., 2004). Thus, oxytocin and vasopressin regulate a range of social behaviors, and natural selection appears to alter the social behaviors of a species by changing the brain distribution of receptors for the peptides (Donaldson and Young, 2008) (**FIGURE 8.10**).

Feedback control mechanisms regulate the secretion of hormones

All hormone release is carefully controlled by the brain, which monitors internal and external cues to decide whether and how much hormone should be released. Brain regulation of posterior pituitary hormone release is readily understood because the neuroendocrine cells secrete hormone only when they are excited synaptically. For example, sensory information from a child's suckling at the breast reaches the brain and excites hypothalamic neuroendocrine cells, which fire action potentials and release oxytocin. Once the baby is satisfied, the suckling stops, so the brain stops exciting the neuroendocrine cells and oxytocin release ceases.

pair-bond   A durable and exclusive relationship between two individuals.

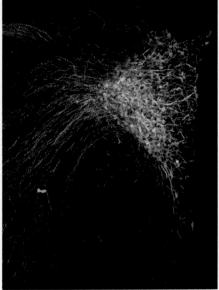

Image by Vicky Tobin and Mike Ludwig, Center for Integrative Physiology, University of Edinburgh

Peptide Hormones in the Hypothalamus This section of the paraventricular nucleus reveals cells that make oxytocin (red) or vasopressin (green), hormones that are released from the posterior pituitary.

(A)

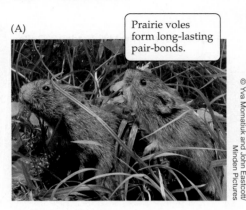

Prairie voles form long-lasting pair-bonds.

© Yva Momatiuk and John Eastcott/ Minden Pictures

FIGURE 8.10 Vasopressin and the Monogamous Brain

(B)

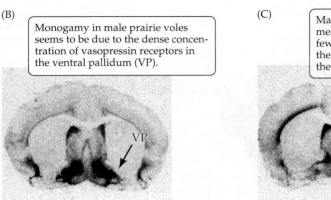

Monogamy in male prairie voles seems to be due to the dense concentration of vasopressin receptors in the ventral pallidum (VP).

VP

(C)

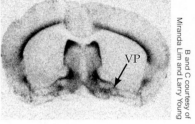

Males of the closely related meadow vole species have fewer vasopressin receptors in the VP, which may explain why they are not monogamous.

VP

B and C courtesy of Miranda Lim and Larry Young

negative feedback   The property by which some of the output of a system feeds back to reduce the effect of input signals.

anterior pituitary   The front division of the pituitary gland. It secretes tropic hormones.

tropic hormone   Any of a class of anterior pituitary hormones that affect the secretion of hormones by other endocrine glands.

This is an example of the basic mechanism that regulates all hormone secretion, called **negative feedback**: output of the hormone *feeds back* to inhibit the drive for more of that same hormone (**FIGURE 8.11A**). This negative feedback action of a hormonal system is like that of a thermostat, and just as the thermostat can be set to different temperatures at different times, the set points of a person's endocrine feedback systems can change to meet varying circumstances. We'll discuss negative feedback regulation of other processes in Chapter 9 (see Figure 9.1).

Hormone secretion from the *anterior* pituitary is also regulated by negative feedback, but the mechanism is a bit more complicated, as we'll see next.

Hypothalamic releasing hormones govern the anterior pituitary

The **anterior pituitary** consists of many different endocrine cells, each secreting a different peptide hormone. So, unlike the posterior half of the pituitary, the anterior pituitary actually synthesizes the hormones it releases. The anterior pituitary hormones are called **tropic hormones**. (The *o* in *tropic* is pronounced "oh"; there is nothing

View Animation 8.5:
The Hypothalamus and Endocrine Function

(A) Brain regulation

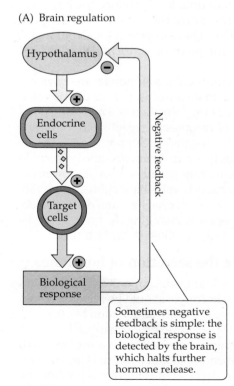

Sometimes negative feedback is simple: the biological response is detected by the brain, which halts further hormone release.

(B) Brain and pituitary regulation

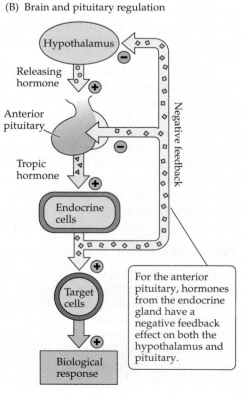

For the anterior pituitary, hormones from the endocrine gland have a negative feedback effect on both the hypothalamus and pituitary.

FIGURE 8.11 Endocrine Feedback Loops

"tropical" about these hormones.) The term *tropic* means "directed toward," and each tropic hormone acts on a different endocrine gland, such as the thyroid or ovaries, as if the tropic hormone were directed toward that gland. Actually, the tropic hormone travels throughout the bloodstream, reaching *all* glands, but only the *target* glands have the appropriate receptors to respond to it. Once the tropic hormone reaches a target gland, it drives the gland to produce its own hormone. For example, one anterior pituitary tropic hormone acts on the thyroid gland to make it secrete thyroid hormones.

To regulate secretions of tropic hormones from the anterior pituitary, the hypothalamus uses another whole set of peptide hormones, called **releasing hormones**. The cells that synthesize the different releasing hormones are neuroendocrine cells residing in various regions of the hypothalamus (**FIGURE 8.11B**). The axons of these neuroendocrine cells converge on the **median eminence**, just above the pituitary stalk. This region contains a profusion of blood vessels that form the **hypothalamic-pituitary portal system**. Here, in response to inputs from the rest of the brain, the axon terminals of the hypothalamic neuroendocrine cells secrete their releasing hormones into the *local* bloodstream (**FIGURE 8.12**). Blood carries the various releasing hormones only a very short distance, into the anterior pituitary. The rate at which releasing hormones arrive at the anterior pituitary controls the rate at which the anterior pituitary cells, in turn, release their tropic hormones into the *general* circulation. These tropic hormones then regulate the activity of major endocrine organs throughout the body. Thus, the brain's releasing hormones affect the anterior pituitary's tropic hormones, which affect the release of hormones from endocrine glands.

releasing hormone Any of a class of hormones, produced in the hypothalamus, that traverse the hypothalamic-pituitary portal system to control the pituitary's release of tropic hormones.

median eminence A midline feature on the base of the brain that marks the point at which the pituitary stalk exits the hypothalamus to connect to the pituitary. The median eminence contains one end of the hypothalamic-pituitary portal system.

hypothalamic-pituitary portal system An elaborate bed of blood vessels leading from the hypothalamus to the anterior pituitary.

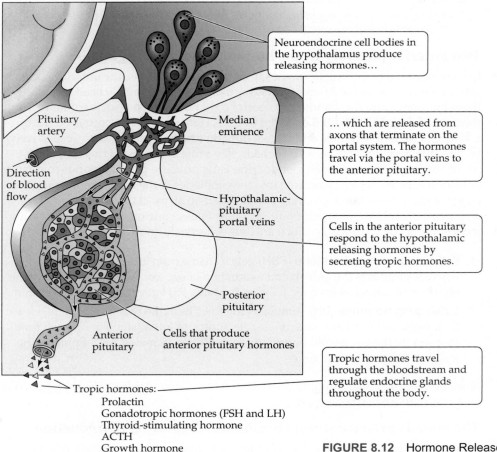

Neuroendocrine cell bodies in the hypothalamus produce releasing hormones…

Pituitary artery

Median eminence

Direction of blood flow

… which are released from axons that terminate on the portal system. The hormones travel via the portal veins to the anterior pituitary.

Hypothalamic-pituitary portal veins

Cells in the anterior pituitary respond to the hypothalamic releasing hormones by secreting tropic hormones.

Posterior pituitary

Anterior pituitary

Cells that produce anterior pituitary hormones

Tropic hormones travel through the bloodstream and regulate endocrine glands throughout the body.

Tropic hormones:
Prolactin
Gonadotropic hormones (FSH and LH)
Thyroid-stimulating hormone
ACTH
Growth hormone

FIGURE 8.12 Hormone Release by the Anterior Pituitary

The hypothalamic neuroendocrine cells that synthesize the releasing hormones are themselves subject to two kinds of influences. First, they are directly affected by *circulating messages*, such as other hormones, especially hormones that were secreted in response to tropic hormones (see Figure 8.11B). This hormone sensitivity of the hypothalamic neurons is an important part of the negative feedback we mentioned earlier, because typically the hormones secreted from an endocrine gland feed back to inhibit the secretion of releasing hormones and tropic hormones. Negative feedback in this case goes from the hormone of the endocrine gland to both the hypothalamus and the anterior pituitary.

Second, the hypothalamic neuroendocrine cells that provide releasing hormones also receive *synaptic inputs* (either excitatory or inhibitory) from many other brain regions. As a result, the release of hormones by the anterior pituitary is coordinated with ongoing events, such as time of day, time of the year, safety of the individual, and so on. For example, if a child is living in stressful, abusive conditions, the brain monitors these conditions and reduces the production of releasing hormones that stimulate the anterior pituitary secretion of **growth hormone** (**GH**), as we discuss in **A STEP FURTHER 8.3**, on the website.

Thus, the hypothalamic-releasing-hormone system exerts high-level control over endocrine organs throughout the body, translating brain activity into hormonal action. Cutting the pituitary stalk interrupts the portal blood vessels and the flow of releasing hormones, leading to profound atrophy of the pituitary, as well as major hormonal disruptions.

HOW'S IT GOING ?

1. How do hormones and behaviors interact in the milk letdown reflex?
2. How are hormones released from the posterior pituitary?
3. Describe the system regulating hormone release from the anterior pituitary, and explain how that system controls other endocrine glands.

Two anterior pituitary tropic hormones act on the gonads

Driven by various releasing hormones from the hypothalamus, the anterior pituitary gland secretes at least six different tropic hormones. We don't really need to go into all these hormones and the glands they control right now, but you can learn more about them in **A STEP FURTHER 8.4**, on the website. Here we will concentrate on the tropic hormones that affect male and female **gonads** (the *testes* and *ovaries*, respectively), because the hormones produced by gonads play a role in the rest of this chapter.

In the hypothalamus, neuroendocrine cells produce **gonadotropin-releasing hormone** (**GnRH**), which is secreted into the capillaries of the median eminence, traveling via the hypothalamic-pituitary portal system to arrive at the anterior pituitary. In response to this GnRH, anterior pituitary cells release one or both of the tropic hormones that act on the gonads, which are thus collectively known as **gonadotropins**:

1. **Follicle-stimulating hormone** (**FSH**) gets its name from its actions in the ovary, where it stimulates the growth and maturation of egg-containing **follicles** and the secretion of estrogens from the follicles. In males, FSH governs sperm production.
2. **Luteinizing hormone** (**LH**) stimulates the follicles of the ovary to rupture, release their eggs, and form into structures called **corpora lutea** (singular *corpus luteum*) that secrete the sex steroid hormone progesterone. In males, LH stimulates the testes to produce testosterone.

Since both of the gonadotropins drive the release of gonadal steroids, we'll turn our attention to those hormones next.

The gonads produce steroid hormones, regulating reproduction

Almost all aspects of reproductive behavior, including mating and parental behaviors, depend on hormones, as we'll see later in this chapter. Each ovary or testis consists of

growth hormone (GH)   Also called *somatotropin* or *somatotropic hormone*. A tropic hormone, secreted by the anterior pituitary, that promotes the growth of cells and tissues.

gonad   Any of the sexual organs (ovaries in females, testes in males) that produce gametes for reproduction.

gonadotropin-releasing hormone (GnRH)   A hypothalamic hormone that controls the release of luteinizing hormone and follicle-stimulating hormone from the pituitary.

gonadotropin   An anterior pituitary tropic hormone that stimulates the cells of the gonads to produce sex steroids and gametes.

follicle-stimulating hormone (FSH)   A gonadotropin, named for its actions on ovarian follicles.

follicle   The structure of the ovary that contains an immature ovum (egg).

luteinizing hormone (LH)   A gonadotropin, named for its stimulatory effects on the ovarian corpora lutea.

corpus luteum   The structure that forms from the collapsed ovarian follicle after ovulation. The corpora lutea are a major source of progesterone.

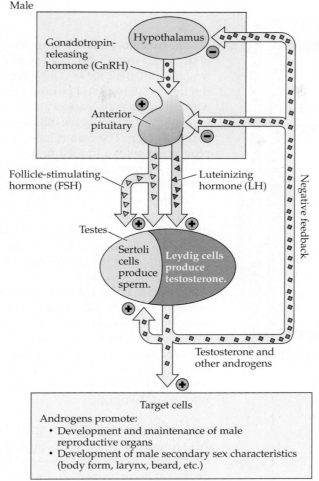

FIGURE 8.13 Gonadal Hormone Regulation in Males

Male

Gonadotropin-releasing hormone (GnRH)

Hypothalamus

Anterior pituitary

Follicle-stimulating hormone (FSH)

Luteinizing hormone (LH)

Negative feedback

Testes

Sertoli cells produce sperm.

Leydig cells produce testosterone.

Testosterone and other androgens

Target cells

Androgens promote:
• Development and maintenance of male reproductive organs
• Development of male secondary sex characteristics (body form, larynx, beard, etc.)

two different subcompartments—one to produce hormones (the sex steroids we mentioned earlier) and another to produce *gametes* (eggs or sperm). The gonadal hormones are critical for triggering both reproductive behavior controlled by the brain, and gamete production.

THE TESTES Within the **testes** (singular *testis*) are Sertoli cells, which produce sperm, and Leydig cells, which produce and secrete the steroid **testosterone**. Testosterone and other male hormones are called **androgens** (from the Greek *andro,* "man," and *gennan,* "to produce").

Testosterone controls a wide range of bodily changes that become visible at puberty, including changes in voice, hair growth, and genital size. In species that breed only in certain seasons of the year, testosterone has especially marked effects on appearance and behavior—for example, the antlers and fighting between males that are displayed by many species of deer. **FIGURE 8.13** summarizes the regulation of testosterone secretion.

THE OVARIES The paired female gonads, the **ovaries**, also produce both the mature gametes—called *ova* (singular *ovum*) or *eggs*—and sex steroid hormones. However, hormone secretion is more complicated in ovaries than in testes. Ovarian hormones are produced in cycles, the duration of which varies with the species. Human ovarian cycles last about 4 weeks; rat cycles last only 4 days.

The ovary produces two major classes of steroid hormones: **progestins** (from the Latin *pro,* "favoring," and *gestare,* "to bear," because these hormones help to maintain pregnancy) and **estrogens** (from the Latin *oestrus,* "frenzy"—*estrus* is the scientific term for the periodic sexual receptivity of females in many species). The most important naturally occurring estrogen is **estradiol** (specifically, 17-beta-estradiol). The primary progestin is **progesterone**.

testes The male gonads, which produce sperm and androgenic steroid hormones.

testosterone A hormone, produced by male gonads, that controls a variety of bodily changes that become visible at puberty. It is one of a class of hormones called *androgens.*

androgen Any of a class of hormones that includes testosterone and similar steroids.

ovaries The female gonads, which produce eggs (ova) for reproduction.

progestin Any of a major class of steroid hormones that are produced by the ovary, including progesterone.

estrogen Any of a class of steroid hormones, including estradiol, produced by female gonads.

estradiol Formally called *17-beta-estradiol.* The primary type of estrogen secreted by the ovary.

progesterone The primary type of progestin secreted by the ovary.

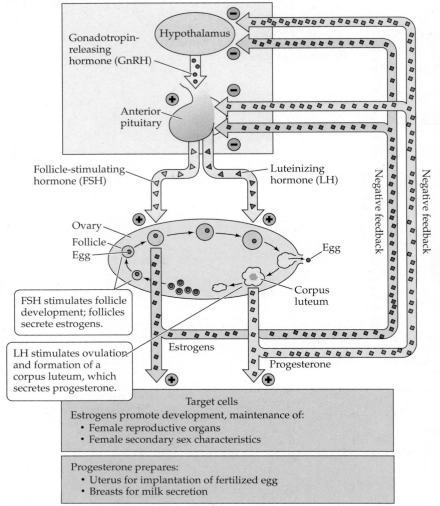

Female

Gonadotropin-releasing hormone (GnRH)

Hypothalamus

Anterior pituitary

Follicle-stimulating hormone (FSH)

Luteinizing hormone (LH)

Negative feedback

Negative feedback

Ovary

Follicle

Egg

Egg

Corpus luteum

FSH stimulates follicle development; follicles secrete estrogens.

LH stimulates ovulation and formation of a corpus luteum, which secretes progesterone.

Estrogens

Progesterone

Target cells

Estrogens promote development, maintenance of:
• Female reproductive organs
• Female secondary sex characteristics

Progesterone prepares:
• Uterus for implantation of fertilized egg
• Breasts for milk secretion

FIGURE 8.14 Gonadal Hormone Regulation in Females

ovulatory cycle The periodic occurrence of ovulation in females.

The **ovulatory cycle** begins when FSH stimulates ovarian follicles to grow and secrete estrogens (**FIGURE 8.14**). The estrogens induce the hypothalamus and pituitary to release LH, which triggers the release of an egg from a follicle (ovulation) and causes the follicle to develop as a corpus luteum. The corpus luteum then secretes progesterone for a limited time to maintain the uterus for pregnancy. If the female does not become pregnant, the cycle starts over again.

Estrogens may improve aspects of cognitive functioning (Ycaza Herrera and Mather, 2015), although this topic is still debated (Dohanich, 2003; Sherwin, 2009; Korol and Pisani, 2015). Estrogens may also protect the brain from some of the effects of stress and stroke (S. Suzuki et al., 2009; Petrone et al., 2014). For these reasons and others, estrogen replacement therapy has been a popular postmenopausal treatment, but the possibility that these treatments increase the risk of serious diseases like cancer and heart disease (Turgeon et al., 2004; Prentice, 2014) makes the decision of whether to take the hormones difficult for postmenopausal women.

RELATIONS AMONG GONADAL HORMONES
All steroid hormones—including androgens, estrogens, and progestins—are based on the chemical structure of cholesterol (see Figure 8.4C). Glands manufacture steroid hormones by using enzymes to modify cholesterol, step by step, into different steroids. For example, ovaries first convert cholesterol into progestins, and then they convert those progestins into androgens, which are then converted into estrogens.

Different organs—and the two sexes—differ in the *relative* amounts of gonadal steroids that they produce. For example, whereas the testes convert only a relatively small proportion of testosterone into estradiol, the ovaries convert most of the testosterone they make into estradiol. What's important to understand is that *no steroid is found exclusively in either males or females.*

Hormonal and neural systems interact to produce integrated responses

The endocrine system and the nervous system work together, each affecting the other, seamlessly integrating various body systems to produce adaptive responses to the environment. So, for example, if our sensory system tells us that a stimulus calls for action—perhaps that faint buzzing sound you're hearing turns out to be coming from a nest of angry wasps—hormones can be released to provide energy to fuel appropriate behaviors (sprinting away, yelling, cursing maybe).

Four kinds of signals are possible between neurons and endocrine cells: neural-to-neural, neural-to-endocrine, endocrine-to-endocrine, and endocrine-to-neural. All four types are illustrated in the courtship behavior of the ringdove. The visual processing that occurs when a male dove sees an attractive female involves neural-to-neural transmission (**FIGURE 8.15**, step 1). The details of the particular visual stimulus—namely, an opportunity to mate—activate a neural-to-endocrine link (step 2), which causes neuroendocrine cells in the male's hypothalamus to secrete GnRH.

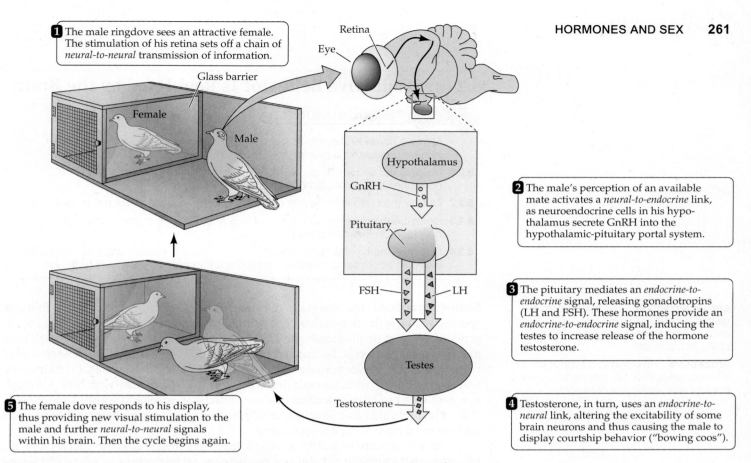

1 The male ringdove sees an attractive female. The stimulation of his retina sets off a chain of *neural-to-neural* transmission of information.

Glass barrier

Female

Male

Retina

Eye

Hypothalamus

GnRH

Pituitary

FSH   LH

Testes

Testosterone

2 The male's perception of an available mate activates a *neural-to-endocrine* link, as neuroendocrine cells in his hypothalamus secrete GnRH into the hypothalamic-pituitary portal system.

3 The pituitary mediates an *endocrine-to-endocrine* signal, releasing gonadotropins (LH and FSH). These hormones provide an *endocrine-to-endocrine* signal, inducing the testes to increase release of the hormone testosterone.

4 Testosterone, in turn, uses an *endocrine-to-neural* link, altering the excitability of some brain neurons and thus causing the male to display courtship behavior ("bowing coos").

5 The female dove responds to his display, thus providing new visual stimulation to the male and further *neural-to-neural* signals within his brain. Then the cycle begins again.

FIGURE 8.15   Four Kinds of Signals between the Nervous System and the Endocrine System

The GnRH provides an endocrine-to-endocrine signal (step 3), stimulating the pituitary to release gonadotropins, which induce the testes to release more testosterone. Testosterone in turn alters the excitability of neurons in the male's brain through an endocrine-to-neural link (step 4), causing the male to display courtship behavior. The female dove responds to this display (step 5), thus providing new visual stimulation to the male, which triggers another cycle of signaling in him.

The interactions between endocrine activity and behavior are cyclical, as depicted by the circle schema in **FIGURE 8.16**. The levels of circulating hormones can be altered by experience, which in turn can affect future behavior and future experience. For example, men supporting a candidate in a presidential election will produce more testosterone if their candidate wins, and less if their preferred candidate loses (Stanton et al., 2009), which may in turn affect their future behavior and future experience. Physical stresses, pain, and unpleasant emotional situations trigger the release of steroids from the adrenal gland (see Chapter 11).

Conversely, each of these hormonal events will affect the brain, shaping behavior, which will once more affect the person's future hormone production, and so on. It will be important to keep in mind these interactions between hormones and behavior as we consider reproductive behavior in the next section.

HOW'S IT GOING ❓

1. Describe the role of the hypothalamus and the anterior pituitary in regulating gonadal hormones.

2. What hormones are found in birth control pills, and how do they prevent pregnancy?

3. Describe the interplay of neural and hormonal signaling in the human milk letdown reflex and the male ringdove's courtship behavior.

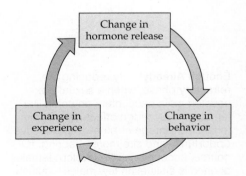

Change in hormone release

Change in behavior

Change in experience

FIGURE 8.16   The Reciprocal Relations between Hormones and Behavior

8.2 Reproductive Behavior Is Regulated by the Brain

THE ROAD AHEAD

Now we consider the role of hormones in regulating reproductive behavior, including maternal behavior. Integrating this material should allow you to:

8.2.1 Discuss the sequence of mating behaviors in animals and the role of hormones in regulating those behaviors.

8.2.2 Outline the brain regions that control sexual behavior in male and female rats.

8.2.3 Describe the maternal behaviors of rats and the roles of experience versus hormones in facilitating them.

8.2.4 Describe the typical sequence of sexual arousal in women and men, and offer a critical appraisal of whether hormones influence human sexual behavior.

sexual attraction The first step in the mating behavior of many animals, in which animals emit stimuli that attract members of the opposite sex.

proceptive Referring to a state in which a female advertises her readiness to mate through species-typical behaviors.

Sexual attraction is the first stage in bringing males and females together. In many species, sexual attraction is closely synchronized with physiological readiness to reproduce. Most male mammals are attracted by particular female odors, which tend to reflect estrogen levels. Because estrogen secretion is associated with the release of eggs, this means female sexual attractiveness peaks alongside fertility. Of course, the female may find a particular male unattractive and refuse to mate with him. Although apparent rape has been described in some nonhuman species (Thornhill and Palmer, 2000; Maggioncalda and Sapolsky, 2002), for most species copulation is not possible without the female's active cooperation.

If the animals are mutually attracted, they may progress to the species-specific behaviors that establish, maintain, or promote sexual interaction. A female displaying these behaviors is said to be **proceptive**: she may approach males, remain close to them, or show alternating approach and retreat behaviors. Proceptive female rats typically exhibit "ear wiggling" and a hopping and darting gait to induce a male to mount. Male behaviors usually consist of staying near the females. In many mammals, the male may sniff around the female's face and vagina. Male birds may engage in elaborate songs or nest-building behaviors, as illustrated for the ringdove in Figure 8.14.

Enough Already! By reducing the refractory phase, when a sexually exhausted male encounters an unfamiliar female, the Coolidge effect permits him to take advantage of a new reproductive opportunity and sire more offspring. (Of course, encountering 24 lovelorn females at once is a situation few males—guinea pig or otherwise—could even dream of.)

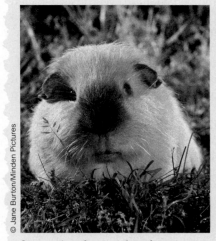

© Jane Burton/Minden Pictures

Sooty enjoyed two nights of passion among 24 females.

Guinea pig Don Juan sires 43 offspring in 2 nights

PONTYPRIDD, WALES, 1 DECEMBER 2000

HAVING ESCAPED from captivity at Little Friend's Farm earlier this year, a male guinea pig named Sooty chose to re-enter captivity immediately—in the nearby cage housing 24 females. Two months later he is now the father of 43 offspring.

According to his owner, Carol Feehan, Sooty was missing for two whole days before the staff checked the females' pen. "We did a head count and found 25 guinea pigs," she told the press. "Sooty was fast asleep in the corner.

"He was absolutely shattered. We put him back in his cage and he slept for two days."

The pair may then progress to **copulation**, also known as *coitus*. In many vertebrates, including all mammals, copulation involves one or more **intromissions**, in which the male inserts his penis into the female's **vagina**, followed by a variable amount of stimulation, usually through pelvic thrusting. When stimulation reaches a threshold level, the male **ejaculates** sperm-bearing **semen** into the female; the length of time required for ejaculation varies greatly between species.

After one bout of copulation, the animals will not mate again for a period of time, which is called the **refractory phase**. The refractory phase varies from minutes to months, depending on the species and circumstances. Many animals will resume mating sooner if they are provided with a new partner—a phenomenon known as the **Coolidge effect** (named after an old joke about U.S. President Calvin Coolidge [Google it]).

The female is often the one to choose whether copulation will take place; when she is willing to copulate, she is said to be **sexually receptive**, in heat, or in **estrus**. In some species, the female may show proceptive behaviors days before she will participate in copulation itself. In most (but not all) species, females are receptive only when mating is likely to produce offspring. Most species are seasonal breeders, with females that are receptive only during the breeding season; some—such as Pacific salmon, octopuses, and cicadas—reproduce only once, at the end of life.

Finally, reproductive behavior includes **postcopulatory behaviors**. These behaviors are especially varied, having been strongly shaped by diverse evolutionary pressures related to the different species' mating systems. For example, in some mammals, including dogs and southern grasshopper mice, the male's penis swells so much after ejaculation that he can't remove it from the female for a while. In species like these, where several males may copulate with an ovulating female in quick succession, this phenomenon, called *copulatory lock*, prevents other males from mating, at least for a while. Despite wild stories you may have heard or read, humans *never* experience copulatory lock; that urban myth started in 1884 when a physician submitted a fake report as a practical joke (Nation, 1973). For mammals and birds, postcopulatory behavior includes extensive parental behaviors to nurture the offspring, as we describe later in this chapter.

Copulation brings gametes together

All mammals, birds, and reptiles employ internal fertilization: the fusion of their **gametes**—**sperm** and **ovum**—within the female's body to form a **zygote**. Most of what we know about the copulatory behavior of mammals comes from studies of lab animals, especially rats. Like most other rodents, rats do not engage in lengthy courtship, nor do the partners tend to remain together after copulation. Rats are attracted to each other largely through odors. Female rats, like humans, are spontaneous ovulators; that is, even when left alone, they **ovulate** (release eggs from the ovary). For a few hours around the time of ovulation, the female rat seeks out a male and displays proceptive behaviors, including vocalizations at frequencies too high for humans to detect but audible to other rats.

These behaviors prompt the male to mount the female from the rear, grasp her flanks with his forelegs, and rhythmically thrust his hips against her rump. If she is receptive, the female adopts a stereotyped posture called **lordosis** (**FIGURE 8.17**), elevating her rump and moving her tail to one side to allow intromission. Once intromission has been achieved, the male rat makes a single deep thrust and then springs back off the female. During the next 6–7 minutes the male and female orchestrate seven to nine such intromissions; then, instead of springing away, the male raises the front half of his body up for a second or two while he ejaculates, then falls backward off the female.

FIGURE 8.17 Copulation in Rats (After S. A. Barnett, 1975. *The rat: A study in behavior.* University of Chicago Press. Chicago, IL.)

copulation Also called *coitus*. The transfer of sperm from a male to a female.

intromission Insertion of the penis into the vagina during copulation.

vagina The opening from the outside of the body to the cervix and uterus in females.

ejaculation The forceful expulsion of semen from the penis.

semen A mixture of fluid and sperm that is released during ejaculation.

refractory phase A period following copulation during which an individual does not recommence copulation.

Coolidge effect The propensity of an animal that appears sexually satisfied with a current partner to resume sexual activity when provided with a new partner.

sexually receptive Referring to the state in which an individual (in mammals, typically the female) is willing to copulate.

estrus The period during which female animals are sexually receptive.

postcopulatory behavior The final stage in mating behavior. Species-specific postcopulatory behaviors include rolling (in the cat) and grooming (in the rat).

gamete A sex cell (sperm or ovum) that contains only unpaired chromosomes and therefore has only half of the usual number of chromosomes.

sperm The gamete produced by males for the fertilization of eggs (ova).

ovum An egg, the female gamete.

zygote The fertilized egg.

ovulation The production and release of an egg (ovum).

lordosis A female receptive posture in four-legged animals in which the hindquarters are raised and the tail is turned to one side, facilitating intromission by the male.

The raised rump and deflected tail of the female (the lordosis posture) make intromission possible in rats.

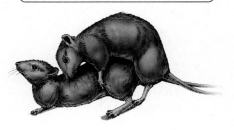

activational effect A temporary change in behavior resulting from the availability of a hormone to an adult animal.

After copulation, the male and female each groom their own genitalia, and the male pays little attention to the female for the next 5 minutes or so, until, often in response to the female's proceptive behaviors, the two engage in another bout of intromissions and ejaculation. The cycle may repeat five or six times in one mating session.

Gonadal steroids activate sexual behavior

Hormones play an important role in rat mating behaviors. Testosterone drives the male's interest in copulation: if he is castrated, he will stop ejaculating within a few weeks and will eventually stop mounting receptive females. Although testosterone disappears from the bloodstream within a few hours after castration, the hormone's effects on the nervous system take days or weeks to wane. Treating a castrated male with testosterone eventually restores mating behavior; if testosterone treatment is stopped, the mating behavior fades away again. This is an example of a hormone exerting an **activational effect**: the hormone transiently promotes certain behaviors. In normal development, the rise of androgen secretion at puberty activates masculine behavior in males. In female rats, estrogens secreted at the beginning of the ovulatory cycle facilitate proceptive behavior, and the subsequent production of progesterone increases proceptive behavior and activates receptivity (**FIGURE 8.18**). An adult female whose ovaries have been removed will show neither proceptive nor receptive behaviors. However, 2 days of estrogen treatment followed by a single injection of progesterone will, about 6 hours later, make the female rat proceptive and receptive for a few hours. Only the correct combination of estrogens and progesterone will fully activate copulatory behaviors in female rats. Because steroids activate sexual behavior, you might wonder if individual differences in hormone levels account for differences in mating vigor, the subject of Researchers at Work, next.

Next we'll discuss how steroid hormones affect the brain to activate mating behavior.

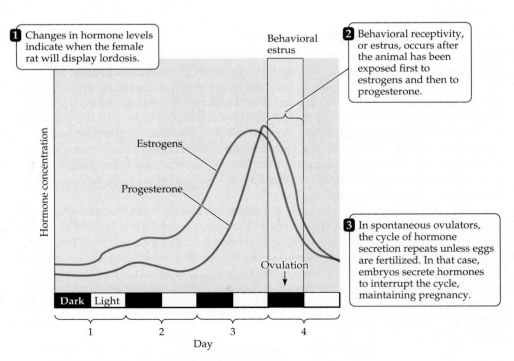

FIGURE 8.18   The Ovulatory Cycle of Rats

RESEARCHERS AT WORK ||||||||||||||||||||||||||||||||||||||||||||||||||||||

Individual differences in mating behavior

Although individual male rats and guinea pigs differ considerably in how eagerly they will mate, blood levels of testosterone clearly are *not* responsible for these differences. For one thing, animals displaying different levels of sexual vigor do not show reliable differences in blood levels of testosterone. Furthermore, when these males are castrated and subsequently all treated with exactly the same dose of testosterone, their precastration differences in sexual activity persist (**FIGURE 8.19**).

FIGURE 8.19 Androgens Permit Male Copulatory Behavior (After J. A. Grunt & W. C. Young, 1953. *J. Comp. Physiol. Psychol.* 46: 138.)

■ **Hypothesis**

Individual differences in the vigor with which male guinea pigs mate are caused by differences in testosterone secretion.

■ **Test**

Classify individual males by mating vigor, then castrate and provide them all with the same dose of testosterone.

■ **Result**

A few weeks after castration, all males stopped mating. But when provided the same dose of testosterone, males returned to their previous levels of mating vigor. Giving a higher dose of testosterone did not eliminate these differences.

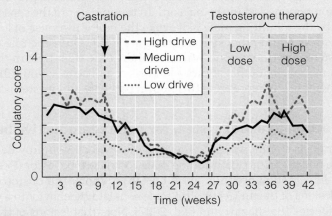

■ **Conclusion**

Although androgens—especially testosterone—are important for activating normal male sexual function, individual differences in sexual activity are not determined by differences in androgen levels.

Furthermore, it turns out that a very small amount of testosterone—one-tenth the amount normally produced by the animals—is enough to fully maintain the mating behavior of male rats (Damassa et al., 1977). Thus, since all male rats make more testosterone than is required to maintain their copulatory behavior, some other factor, which we can call drive, must differ across individual males.

HOW'S IT GOING ?

1. What are the stages of reproductive behavior?
2. Describe a typical mating session of laboratory rats.
3. Describe the activational effects of gonadal steroids on mating behaviors in male and female rodents.
4. How do we know whether differences in testosterone secretion are responsible for individual differences in male mating vigor?

Estrogen and progesterone act on a lordosis circuit that spans from brain to muscle

Although most of what we know about the neural circuitry of sexual behavior comes from studies of rats, steroid receptors are found in the same specific brain regions across a wide variety of vertebrate species. Steroid-sensitive regions include the cortex, brainstem nuclei, medial amygdala, hypothalamus, and many others. We'll see that the hypothalamus plays a particularly important role in regulating copulatory behavior.

Scientists exploited the steroid sensitivity of the rat lordosis response to map the neural circuitry that controls this behavior (Pfaff et al., 2018). Using steroid autoradiography (see Box 8.1), investigators identified hypothalamic nuclei containing many estrogen- and progesterone-sensitive neurons. In particular, the **ventromedial hypothalamus** (**VMH**) is crucial for lordosis, because lesions there abolish the response. Furthermore, tiny quantities of estradiol implanted directly into the brain can induce receptivity in females, but only when the hormone is placed in the VMH (Sakuma, 2015).

One action of estrogen treatment is to cause dendrites of VMH neurons to grow and become more complex (Ferri et al., 2014). Another important action of estrogens is to stimulate the production of progesterone receptors so that the animal will become more responsive to that hormone. Progesterone receptors in turn help mediate the lordosis reflex (Mani et al., 2000).

The VMH sends axons to the **periaqueductal gray** region of the midbrain, where again, lesions greatly diminish lordosis. The intact periaqueductal gray neurons project to other brain regions and the spinal cord. In the spinal cord the sensory information provided by the mounting male will evoke the motor response of lordosis when the female's estrogen and progesterone levels are right. Thus, the role of the VMH is to monitor steroid hormone concentrations and, at the right time in the ovulatory cycle, enable a neural circuit that allows a lordosis response to a mounting male. **FIGURE 8.20B** schematically represents this neural pathway and its steroid-responsive components.

Androgens act on a neural system for male reproductive behavior

As with the lordosis circuit, mapping the sites of steroid action provided important clues about the neural circuitry controlling male copulatory behavior (**FIGURE 8.20A**). The hypothalamic **medial preoptic area** (**mPOA**) is chock-full of steroid-sensitive neurons, and lesions of the mPOA abolish male copulatory behavior in a wide variety of vertebrate species (Balthazart and Ball, 2007). Note that lesions of the mPOA do not interfere with males' *motivation* for females; males will still press a bar to gain access to a receptive female, but they seem unable to commence mounting. Furthermore, mating can be reinstated in castrated males by small implants of testosterone in the mPOA, but not in other brain regions. Thus, the mPOA seems to provide "higher-order" control of male copulatory behaviors.

The mPOA coordinates copulatory behavior by sending axons to the ventral midbrain (which innervates several brain regions to coordinate mounting behaviors) and, via a multisynaptic pathway, to the spinal cord (Hamson and Watson, 2004), which mediates various genital reflexes, such as ejaculation. Brainstem projections of serotonergic fibers to the spinal cord normally hold the penile erection reflex in check (Hull et al., 2004). Antidepressant drugs that boost serotonergic activity in the brain—for example, selective serotonin reuptake inhibitors like Prozac (see Chapter 12)—can produce side effects that include difficulty achieving erection, ejaculation, and/or orgasm, probably by enhancing serotonergic inhibition of the spinal cord. (If you're wondering, the drug sildenafil, better known as Viagra, acts directly on tissue in the penis, not in the spinal cord or brain, to promote erection [Mitidieri et al., 2020].)

ventromedial hypothalamus (VMH) A hypothalamic region involved in sexual behaviors, eating, and aggression.

periaqueductal gray A midbrain region involved in pain perception.

medial preoptic area (mPOA) A region of the anterior hypothalamus implicated in the control of many behaviors, including sexual behavior, gonadotropin secretion, and thermoregulation.

vomeronasal organ (VNO) A collection of specialized receptor cells, near to but separate from the olfactory epithelium, that detects pheromones and sends electrical signals to the accessory olfactory bulb in the brain.

medial amygdala A portion of the amygdala that receives olfactory and pheromonal information.

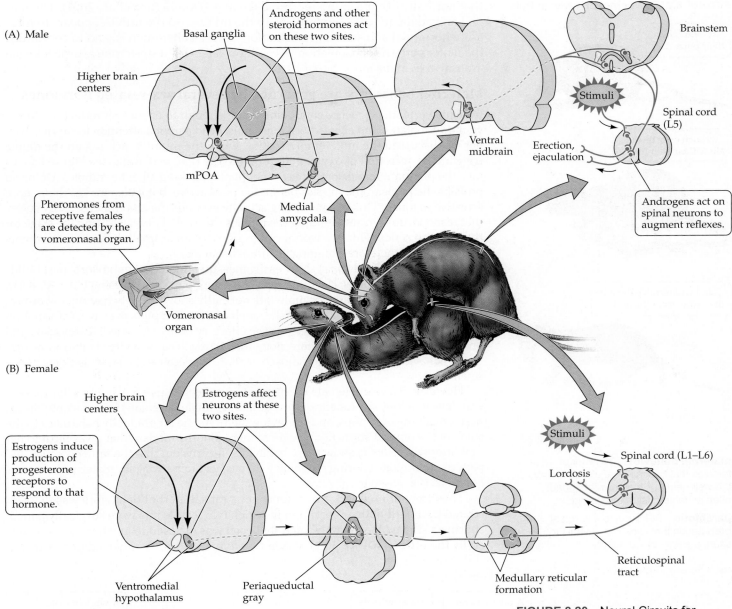

(A) Male

Basal ganglia

Higher brain centers

Androgens and other steroid hormones act on these two sites.

Brainstem

Stimuli

mPOA

Spinal cord (L5)

Ventral midbrain

Erection, ejaculation

Medial amygdala

Androgens act on spinal neurons to augment reflexes.

Pheromones from receptive females are detected by the vomeronasal organ.

Vomeronasal organ

(B) Female

Higher brain centers

Estrogens affect neurons at these two sites.

Stimuli

Estrogens induce production of progesterone receptors to respond to that hormone.

Spinal cord (L1–L6)

Lordosis

Ventromedial hypothalamus

Periaqueductal gray

Medullary reticular formation

Reticulospinal tract

FIGURE 8.20 Neural Circuits for Reproduction in Rodents (After D. W. Pfaff, 1980. *Estrogens and brain function: Neural analysis of a hormone-controlled mammalian reproductive behavior*. Springer-Verlag. New York, NY.)

We can also learn about male copulatory mechanisms by tracing a sensory system that boosts male arousal in rodents: the vomeronasal system. The **vomeronasal organ**, or **VNO** (see Chapter 9), consists of specialized receptor cells near to, but separate from, the olfactory epithelium. These sensory cells detect chemicals called *pheromones* (see Figure 8.3C and Chapter 6) that are released by other individuals. For example, receptive female rats release pheromones that male rats find arousing, as evidenced by penile erections. (You can learn more about the role of pheromones in reproductive behavior in **A STEP FURTHER 8.5**, on the website.)

Vomeronasal receptor neurons send their axons to the brain's accessory olfactory bulb. The accessory olfactory bulb in turn projects to the **medial amygdala**, which in rats depends on adult circulating levels of sex steroids to maintain a masculine form and function (Cooke et al., 2003). Lesions here will abolish the penile erections

FIGURE 8.21 Maternal Behavior in Rats

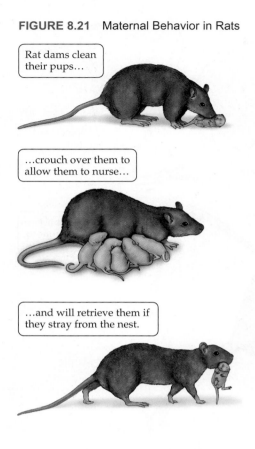

Rat dams clean their pups…

…crouch over them to allow them to nurse…

…and will retrieve them if they stray from the nest.

maternal behavior Behavior of adult females that has the goal of enhancing the well-being of their own offspring, often at some cost to the parents.

parabiotic Referring to a surgical preparation that joins two animals to share a single blood supply.

that normally occur around receptive females (Dominguez et al., 2001). The medial amygdala, in turn, sends axons to the mPOA. So the mPOA appears to integrate hormonal and sensory information, such as pheromones, and to coordinate the motor patterns of copulation. We will see later that testosterone activates sexual arousal in humans too.

Maternal behaviors are governed by several sex-related hormones

In many vertebrate species, copulation is not enough to ensure reproduction. Many young vertebrates, and all newborn mammals, need parental attention to survive. Earlier we discussed the milk letdown reflex, when the infant's suckling on the nipple triggers the secretion of oxytocin to promote the release of milk (see Figure 8.9). In rats, the pregnant female prepares for her pups by licking all of her nipples. Doing so probably helps clean the nipples before the pups arrive, but it also makes them more sensitive to touch. This self-grooming actually expands the amount of sensory cortex that responds to skin surrounding the nipples (Xerri et al., 1994), setting the stage for the letdown reflex. This is a wonderful example of an animal's behavior altering its own brain and therefore changing its future behavior.

Rat mothers (called *dams*) show easily measured **maternal behaviors**: nest building, crouching over pups, cleaning pups, retrieving pups, and nursing (**FIGURE 8.21**). Neither virgin female rats nor male rats normally show these behaviors toward rat pups. In fact, a virgin female finds the smell of newborn pups aversive. Information about the odor from pups projects via the olfactory bulb to the medial amygdala and on to the VMH. Lesions anywhere along that path will cause a virgin rat to show maternal behavior right away (Holschbach et al., 2018) because she no longer detects the smell.

However, if a virgin female is exposed to newborn pups a few hours a day for several days in a row, she (or almost any adult rat—male or female) will start building a nest, crouching over pups, and retrieving them. As the rat gradually habituates to the smell of the pups, it starts taking care of them. But the rat dam that gives birth to her first litter will *instantly* show these behaviors. It turns out that the rather complicated pattern of hormones during pregnancy shapes her brain to display maternal behaviors *before* she is exposed to the pups.

The effect of pregnancy hormones on a rat's maternal behaviors was demonstrated by a **parabiotic** preparation in which two female rats were surgically joined, sharing a single blood supply, such that each was exposed to any hormones secreted by the other (**FIGURE 8.22**). When two female rats are connected in this way, if

FIGURE 8.22 Parabiotic Exchange Facilitates Maternal Behavior (After J. Terkel and J. S. Rosenblatt, 1972. *J. Comp. Physiol. Psychol.* 80: 365.)

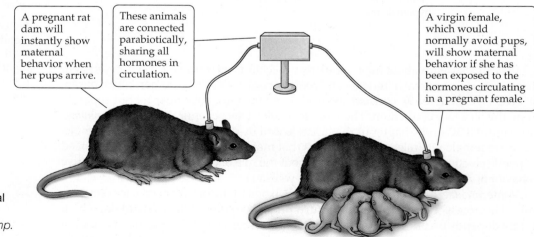

A pregnant rat dam will instantly show maternal behavior when her pups arrive.

These animals are connected parabiotically, sharing all hormones in circulation.

A virgin female, which would normally avoid pups, will show maternal behavior if she has been exposed to the hormones circulating in a pregnant female.

one is pregnant, then at the end of her pregnancy the other female, that was never pregnant but was exposed to the pregnant rat's hormones, will also immediately show maternal behavior (Bridges, 2015). Which hormone is responsible for promoting maternal behavior? No single hormone alone can do it; the combination of several hormones, including estrogens, progesterone, oxytocin, and prolactin, is required.

There is a growing realization that parenting behaviors shape the brains of male and female rodents (Kinsley and Lambert, 2006; Franssen et al., 2011). There is ample evidence that the hormones of pregnancy also prepare human mothers to nurture their newborns (Fleming et al., 2002). Compared with other women, mothers who have recently given birth are better at distinguishing odors from different newborns, and they can even recognize odors from their own newborn. This increased ability to discriminate odors correlates with hormone levels after delivery (Almanza-Sepulveda et al., 2020). Pregnancy may also have long-lasting effects on brain structure and cognitive processing in women (Henry and Sherwin, 2012; Hoekzema et al., 2017).

The hallmark of human sexual behavior is diversity

How much of what we've described so far about sexual behavior in animals is relevant to human sexuality? Until the 1940s, when biology professor Alfred Kinsey began to ask friends and colleagues about their sexual histories, there was virtually no scientific study of human sexual behavior. Kinsey constructed a standardized set of questions and procedures to get information. Eventually, he and his collaborators published extensive surveys, based on tens of thousands of respondents, on the sexual behavior of American males (Kinsey et al., 1948) and females (Kinsey et al., 1953).

Controversial in their time, these surveys indicated that nearly all men masturbated, that college-educated people were more likely to engage in oral sex than were non-college-educated people, that many people had at one time or another engaged in homosexual behaviors, and that a stable proportion of the population preferred same-sex partners.

Another way to investigate human sexual behavior is to make behavioral and physiological observations of people engaged in sexual intercourse or masturbation, but the squeamishness of the general public impeded such research for many years. Finally, after Kinsey's surveys were published, physician William Masters and psychologist Virginia Johnson began a large, famous project of this kind (Masters et al., 1994), documenting the impressively diverse sexuality of humans.

Among most mammalian species, including most nonhuman primates, the male mounts the female from the rear; but among humans, face-to-face postures are most common. A great variety of coital positions have been described, and many couples vary their positions from session to session or even within a session. It is this variety in reproductive behaviors, rather than differences in reproductive anatomy, that distinguishes human sexuality from that of most other species.

Unlike other animals, humans can report their subjective reactions to sexual behavior—specifically **orgasm**, the brief, extremely pleasurable sensations experienced by most men during ejaculation and by most women during copulation. In the original conceptual model of human sexuality, Masters and Johnson summarized the typical response patterns of both men and women as consisting of four phases: increasing excitement, plateau, orgasm, and resolution.

During the excitement phase, the **phallus**—the **penis** in men, the **clitoris** in women—becomes engorged with blood, making it erect. In women, parasympathetic activity during the excitement phase causes changes in vaginal blood vessels, producing lubricating fluids that facilitate intromission. Stimulation of the penis, clitoris, and vagina during rhythmic thrusting accompanying intromission may lead to orgasm. In both men and women, orgasm is accompanied by waves of contractions

orgasm The climax of sexual behavior, marked by extremely pleasurable sensations.

phallus The clitoris or penis.

penis The male phallus.

clitoris The female phallus.

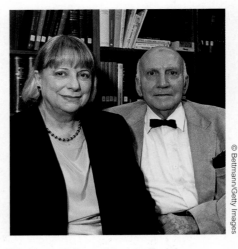

Masters of Sex Virginia E. Johnson and William H. Masters.

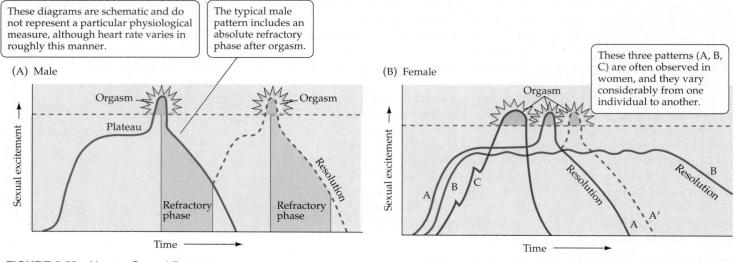

These diagrams are schematic and do not represent a particular physiological measure, although heart rate varies in roughly this manner.

The typical male pattern includes an absolute refractory phase after orgasm.

These three patterns (A, B, C) are often observed in women, and they vary considerably from one individual to another.

(A) Male

(B) Female

FIGURE 8.23 Human Sexual Response Cycles (After W. H. Masters and V. E. Johnson, 1966. *Human sexual response.* Little, Brown. Boston, MA.)

of genital muscles (mediating ejaculation in men and contractions of the uterus and vaginal opening in women) (**FIGURE 8.23A**).

In spite of some basic similarities, the sexual responses of men and women differ in important ways. For one thing, women show a much greater variety of commonly observed copulatory sequences. Whereas men have only one basic pattern, captured by the linear model of Masters and Johnson (see Figure 8.23A), women have at least three typical patterns (**FIGURE 8.23B**). Another important aspect of human sexuality is that most men, but not most women, have an absolute refractory phase following orgasm (also illustrated in Figure 8.23A). That is, most men cannot achieve full erection and another orgasm until some time has elapsed—the length of time varying from minutes to hours, depending on individual differences and other factors. Many women, on the other hand, can have multiple orgasms in rapid succession. Functional imaging of the brains of men and women during sexual activity suggests that, although the brain circuitry associated with orgasm itself is quite similar between the sexes, substantially different networks are active in men's and women's brains during sexual activity *prior* to orgasm (Georgiadis et al., 2009).

Taking a broader perspective on sexuality reveals additional distinctions between men and women (Peplau, 2003). Basic sex drive seems to be greater in men, reflected in more frequent masturbation, sexual fantasies, and pursuit of sexual contacts. Emotional components and cognitive factors play a stronger role in women's sex lives than in men's. While Masters and Johnson simply adapted the linear model of male sexuality to women, the more modern perspective views women's sexuality as a cycle, governed in large measure by emotional factors (Basson, 2001, 2008). According to this model, emotional intimacy and desire (more than physiological arousal) are crucial in the initiation of sexual responses, and following a sexual encounter, a combination of both emotional and physical satisfaction affects the likelihood of subsequent sexual activity.

Although male and female sexuality may bear the imprint of our evolutionary history, on an individual basis it is also shaped by sociocultural pressures and experience. Sexual therapy, for example, usually consists of helping the person to relax, to recognize the sensations associated with coitus, and to learn the behaviors that produce the desired effects in both partners. Masturbation during adolescence, rather than being harmful as suggested in previous times, may help avoid sexual problems in adulthood. As with other behaviors, practice, practice, practice helps. Of course, it is also important to one's health to take precautions (such as using condoms) to avoid contracting sexually transmitted infections.

Hormones play only a permissive role in human sexual behavior

We have already seen that a little bit of testosterone must be in circulation to activate male-typical mating behavior in rodents. The same relation seems to hold for human males. For example, boys who fail to produce testosterone at puberty show little interest in dating unless they receive androgen treatments. These males, as well as men who have lost their testes as a result of cancer or accident, made it possible to conduct experiments showing that testosterone indeed stimulates sexual interest and activity in men, as well as a sense of heightened energy.

Recall that, in rodents, *additional* testosterone has no effect on the vigor of mating. Consequently, there is no correlation between the amount of androgens produced by an individual male and his tendency to copulate. In humans, too, just a little testosterone is sufficient to restore behavior fully, and there is no correlation between circulating androgen levels and sexual activity among men who have at least *some* androgen.

Some women experience sexual dysfunction after menopause, reporting decreased sexual desire and difficulty achieving comfortable coitus. There are many possible reasons for such a change, including several hormonal changes. Providing postmenopausal women with low doses of both estrogens and androgens can have beneficial effects on the genital experience of sex and also on women's sexual interest (Sherwin, 2002; Basson, 2008).

Now that we've discussed some of the unique aspects of male and female sexuality, let's look at some of the developmental processes that cause the growing individual to take on male-typical or female-typical forms and functions in the first place.

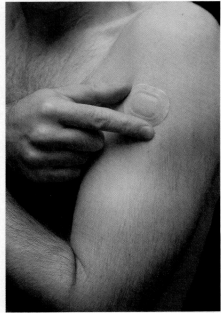

Photo by David McIntyre

Testosterone Patches   These patches can revive libido in men who have lost their testes through accident or disease.

HOW'S IT GOING ❓

1. What brain regions appear to be involved in male and female sexual behaviors?
2. Compare and contrast the maternal behavior of a female rat that has just been pregnant with that of a naive female. What factor is responsible for the differences?
3. Compare and contrast the patterns of sexual arousal in men and women.
4. What are the effects of gonadal steroids on human sexual behavior?

8.3 Genetic and Hormonal Mechanisms Guide the Development of Masculine and Feminine Structures

THE ROAD AHEAD

Now we take up the question of how developing females and males come to differ. Reading this final section of the chapter should allow you to:

8.3.1 Describe the chain of molecular and hormonal events that sculpt the mammalian fetus into a male or female form.

8.3.2 Identify several differences of sexual development that affect that process.

8.3.3 Explain the organizational hypothesis of how sex differences in animal behavior arise.

8.3.4 Describe the role of hormones in the development of two prominent sexual dimorphisms in neuronal structure.

8.3.5 Critically discuss the extent to which prenatal hormones influence sex differences in human behavior, including sexual orientation.

A persistent bias in biomedical science has resulted in males being studied exclusively in most cases, on the assumption that female ovulatory cycles would introduce more variability and that whatever was found in males would hold true for both sexes.

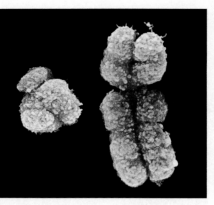

Mammalian Sex Chromosomes The Y chromosome (*left*) is much shorter than the X (*right*) because it carries far fewer genes. But one of those genes, *SRY*, is critical for masculine development.

sexual differentiation The process by which individuals develop either male-like or female-like bodies and behavior.

indifferent gonads The undifferentiated gonads of the early mammalian fetus, which will eventually develop into either testes or ovaries.

SRY gene A gene on the Y chromosome that directs the developing gonads to become testes. The name *SRY* stands for **s**ex-determining **r**egion on the **Y** chromosome.

genital tubercle In the early fetus, a "bump" between the legs that can develop into either a clitoris or a penis.

wolffian duct A duct system in the embryo that will develop into male reproductive structures (epididymis, vas deferens, and seminal vesicle) if androgens are present.

müllerian duct A duct system in the embryo that will develop into female reproductive structures (oviducts, uterus, and upper vagina) in the absence of AMH.

anti-müllerian hormone (AMH) A peptide hormone secreted by the fetal testes that inhibits müllerian duct development.

dihydrotestosterone (DHT) The 5-alpha-reduced metabolite of testosterone. DHT is a potent androgen that is principally responsible for the masculinization of the external genitalia in mammals.

However, analysis of the animal literature revealed that in fact there is more variability in males than females (Prendergast et al., 2014), and many biomedical "facts" established in men do not hold for women (Cahill, 2014). For example, heart attacks in women tend to produce symptoms that are very different from those symptoms, derived from observations of men, that were the only ones publicized until recent years. The fatality rate of COVID-19 infections is higher in men than in women. In the USA, the National Institutes of Health (NIH) require grant applicants to either include both sexes or provide a sound rationale for excluding one sex (Sandberg et al., 2015).

Sex chromosomes direct sexual differentiation of the gonads

Sexual differentiation is the process by which individuals develop either male or female bodies and behaviors. In mammals, this process begins before birth and continues into adulthood. In mammals, every egg carries an X chromosome from the mother; fusion with an X- or Y-bearing sperm is the key event in establishing the course of subsequent sexual differentiation of the body. With rare exceptions, mammals that receive an X chromosome from the father will become females with an XX sex chromosome complement; those that receive the father's Y chromosome will become XY males. The first major effect of sex chromosomes is on the gonads. Very early in development, each individual has a pair of **indifferent gonads**, glands that vaguely resemble both testes and ovaries. During the first month of gestation in humans, differential genetic instructions determine whether the indifferent gonads begin changing into ovaries or testes.

In mammals, the Y chromosome contains the **SRY gene** (for **s**ex-determining **r**egion on the **Y** chromosome), which is responsible for the development of testes. If an individual has a Y chromosome, the cells of the indifferent gonad begin making the Sry protein, inducing the organ to develop into a testis.

In XX individuals (or XY individuals with a dysfunctional *SRY* gene), no Sry protein is produced, and the indifferent gonad becomes an ovary. This early event of forming either testes or ovaries has a domino effect, setting off a chain of actions that usually results in either a male or a female.

Gonadal hormones direct sexual differentiation of the body

For all mammals, including humans, the gonads secrete hormones to direct sexual differentiation of the body. Fetal ovaries produce very little hormone, but fetal testes produce several hormones. If other embryonic cells are exposed to the testicular hormones, they begin developing masculine characters; if the cells are not exposed to testicular hormones, they develop feminine characters.

We can chart masculine or feminine development by examining the structures that connect the gonads to the outside of the body: these are quite different in adult males and females, but at the embryonic stage all individuals have the precursor tissues of both systems. The early fetus has a **genital tubercle** (a "bump" between the legs) that can form either a clitoris or a penis, as well as two sets of ducts that connect the tubercle to the indifferent gonads: the **wolffian ducts** and the **müllerian ducts** (**FIGURE 8.24A**). In females, the müllerian ducts develop into the oviducts (or *fallopian tubes*), uterus, and inner vagina (**FIGURES 8.24B** and **C** *right*), and only a remnant of the wolffian ducts remains. In males, hormones secreted by the testes orchestrate the converse outcome: each wolffian duct develops into an epididymis, vas deferens, and seminal vesicle (see Figure 8.24B and C *left*), while the müllerian ducts shrink to mere remnants.

The system is masculinized by two testicular secretions: testosterone, which promotes development of the wolffian system; and **anti-müllerian hormone** (**AMH**), which causes regression of the müllerian system. In the absence of testosterone and AMH, the genital tract develops in a feminine pattern, in which the wolffian ducts regress and the müllerian ducts develop into components of the female internal reproductive tract.

Testosterone masculinizes other structures too, acting on exterior tissues to form a scrotum and penis. These effects are aided by the local conversion of testosterone into a more potent androgen, **dihydrotestosterone** (**DHT**), promoted by an enzyme

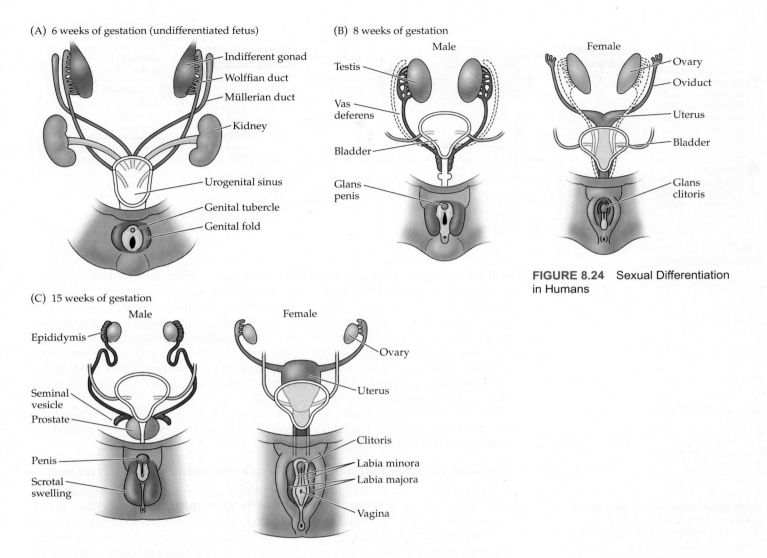

(A) 6 weeks of gestation (undifferentiated fetus)

- Indifferent gonad
- Wolffian duct
- Müllerian duct
- Kidney
- Urogenital sinus
- Genital tubercle
- Genital fold

(B) 8 weeks of gestation

Male

- Testis
- Vas deferens
- Bladder
- Glans penis

Female

- Ovary
- Oviduct
- Uterus
- Bladder
- Glans clitoris

FIGURE 8.24   Sexual Differentiation in Humans

(C) 15 weeks of gestation

Male

- Epididymis
- Seminal vesicle
- Prostate
- Penis
- Scrotal swelling

Female

- Ovary
- Uterus
- Clitoris
- Labia minora
- Labia majora
- Vagina

that is found in the genital skin, **5-alpha-reductase**. We'll see later that without the local production of DHT, testosterone alone is able to masculinize the genitalia only partially. If androgens are absent altogether, the genital tissues grow into the female labia and clitoris.

Changes in sexual differentiation processes result in predictable changes in development

Some people have only one sex chromosome: a single X (embryos containing only a single Y chromosome do not survive). This genetic makeup results in **Turner's syndrome**, in which an apparent female has underdeveloped but recognizable ovaries, as you might expect because no *SRY* gene is available. In general, unless the indifferent gonad becomes a testis and begins secreting hormones, mammalian fetuses develop as females in most respects. So the sex chromosomes determine the sex of the gonad, and gonadal hormones then drive sexual differentiation of the rest of the body (**FIGURE 8.25**).

Congenital adrenal hyperplasia (**CAH**) causes developing girls to be exposed to excess androgens before birth. In CAH, the adrenal glands produce considerable amounts of androgens, somewhere between those of normal females and males, so the newborn often has an **intersex** appearance: a phallus that is intermediate in size between a normal clitoris and a normal penis, and skin folds that resemble both labia

5-alpha-reductase   An enzyme that converts testosterone into dihydrotestosterone (DHT).

Turner's syndrome   A condition, seen in individuals carrying a single X chromosome but no other sex chromosome, in which an apparent female has underdeveloped but recognizable ovaries.

congenital adrenal hyperplasia (CAH) Any of several genetic mutations that can cause a female fetus to be exposed to adrenal androgens, resulting in partial masculinization at birth.

intersex   Referring to an individual with atypical genital development and sexual differentiation, whose genitalia are generally intermediate in form between typical male and typical female genitalia.

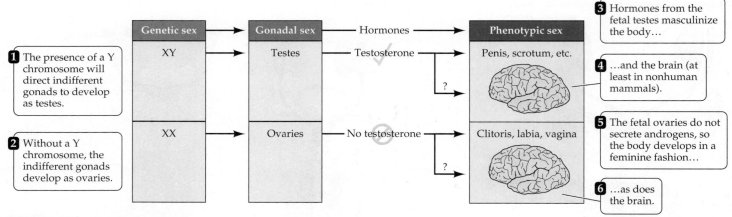

FIGURE 8.25 The Sequence of Sexual Differentiation

and scrotum (**FIGURE 8.26**). Such babies are usually recognizable at birth because, even in severe cases in which penis and scrotum appear well formed, no testes are present inside the "scrotum"; instead, these individuals have normal abdominal ovaries. Once born, children with CAH are given medicine to prevent further androgen production. There is controversy, however, over whether the best course of action for the parents of girls with CAH is to opt for immediate surgical modification of the genitalia or to wait until adulthood, when the CAH-affected individuals can decide for themselves whether to have surgery that is purely cosmetic (Hughes et al., 2006; Human Rights Watch, 2017).

In spotted hyenas, females are always exposed to prenatal androgens, resulting in highly masculinized genitalia. You can read about these fascinating animals in **A STEP FURTHER 8.6**, on the website.

Reduced androgen signaling can block masculinization of the body

The importance of androgens for masculine sexual differentiation is illustrated by the condition known as **androgen insensitivity syndrome** (**AIS**). AIS results when an XY zygote inherits a dysfunctional gene for the androgen receptor, so the embryo's tissues cannot respond to androgenic hormones like testosterone. The gonads of people with AIS develop as normal testes (as directed by Sry), and the testes produce AMH (which inhibits müllerian duct structures) and plenty of testosterone.

However, in the absence of working androgen receptors, the wolffian ducts fail to develop and the external genital tissue forms labia and a clitoris. At puberty, women

androgen insensitivity syndrome (AIS) A syndrome caused by an androgen receptor gene mutation that renders tissues insensitive to androgenic hormones like testosterone. Affected XY individuals are phenotypic females, but they have internal testes and regressed internal genital structures.

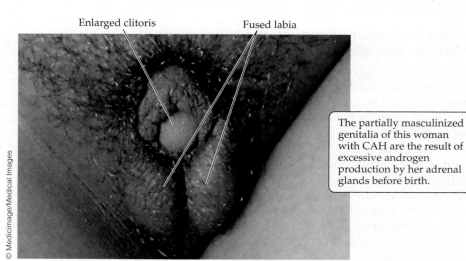

Enlarged clitoris   Fused labia

The partially masculinized genitalia of this woman with CAH are the result of excessive androgen production by her adrenal glands before birth.

© Medicimage/Medical Images

FIGURE 8.26 An Intersex Phenotype

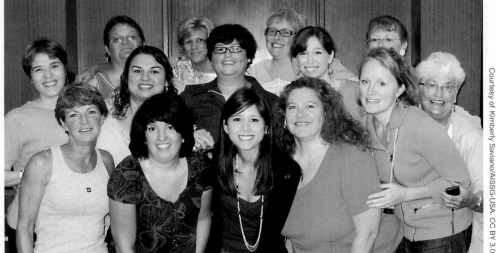

FIGURE 8.27   Women with AIS

with AIS develop breasts but fail to start menstruating, because neither ovaries nor uterus are present. Women with AIS are infertile, but otherwise they look like other women (**FIGURE 8.27**) and behave like other women.

Babies are occasionally born with a rare genetic mutation that disables 5-alpha-reductase, the enzyme that converts testosterone to DHT. An XY individual with this condition will develop testes and normal male internal reproductive structures (because testosterone and AMH function normally), but the external genitalia will fail to masculinize fully. The reason for this failure is that the genital epithelium, which normally possesses 5-alpha-reductase, is unable to amplify the androgenic signal by converting testosterone to the more active DHT. Consequently, the phallus is only slightly masculinized and resembles a large clitoris, and the genital folds resemble labia, although they contain the testes. Usually there is no vaginal opening (**FIGURE 8.28**).

(A) Newborn

(B) Adolescent

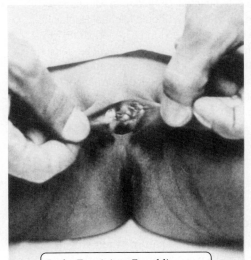

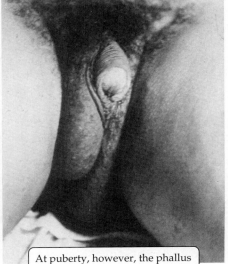

In the Dominican Republic, some individuals, called *guevedoces*, are born with ambiguous genitalia and are raised as girls.

At puberty, however, the phallus grows into a recognizable penis, and the individuals begin acting like young men.

FIGURE 8.28   *Guevedoces*

guevedoces Literally "eggs at 12" (in Spanish). A nickname for individuals who are raised as girls but at puberty change appearance and begin behaving as boys.

A particular village in the Dominican Republic is home to several families that carry the mutation causing 5-alpha-reductase deficiency. Children born with this appearance seem to be regarded as girls in the way they are dressed and raised (Imperato-McGinley, 2002). At puberty, however, the testes increase androgen production, and the external genitalia become more fully masculinized. The phallus grows into a small but recognizable penis; the body develops narrow hips and a muscular build, without breasts; and the individuals begin acting like young men. The villagers have nicknamed such individuals **guevedoces**, meaning "eggs (testes) at 12 (years)." These men never develop beards, but they usually have girlfriends, indicating that they are sexually interested in women. We will discuss the sexual behavior of *guevedoces*, as well as women with CAH or AIS, later.

SIGNS & SYMPTOMS ||||||||||||||||||||||||||||||||||||||||||||||||||||||||||||||||

Defining an Athlete's Sex

Raised as a girl, Olympic runner Mokgadi Caster Semenya naturally enough considers herself a woman. But after the South African athlete blew away the competition in a women's 800-meter race, rumors began circulating that she might have an intersex condition like AIS or CAH, giving her an unfair advantage. Olympic officials investigated and cleared her to compete, enabling Caster to win gold medals in 2012 and 2016. For the sake of her privacy, details about Caster's examination were never released, but she apparently has higher levels of circulating androgen than most women (Padawer, 2016), so the question of whether Caster and other women with "hyperandrogenism" should be allowed to compete as women continues. The International Association of Athletics Federations ruled that Caster and other women with "hyperandrogenism" (Chiu, 2018) should not compete as women in certain events unless they reduce their androgen levels either through surgery (e.g., removing testes in cases of AIS) or through drugs to suppress androgen production.

Most efforts to regulate sports events have centered on *preventing* athletes from taking drugs to enhance their performance ("doping"), but now we are in the strange position of *requiring* athletes to take drugs, or even to have surgery, as a prerequisite for competition. As others have pointed out, every elite athlete is very unusual in some regard, otherwise they wouldn't be elite athletes. Should men with especially high testosterone be disqualified from competition? Should Michael Phelps be excluded from swim competitions because his arms are so long (Dreger, 2018)? In Caster's case, we can identify a particular factor, testosterone, that *might* be helping her compete (G. Huang and Basaria, 2018), but the other women runners doubtless have some physiological advantage that contributes to their performance; the difference is we don't happen to know what their physiological advantage is. As we've seen in this chapter, many people are a mixture of masculine and feminine features, so who gets to decide whether a person is a "real" woman or man? Caster made her position clear in an interview: "I just want to be me. I was born this way. I don't want any changes."

Caster Semenya Growing up, the South African athlete considered herself female, but questions were raised about whether she should be allowed to compete among women.

How should we define sex—by genes, gonads, genitals?

Most humans are either male or female, and whether we examine their chromosomes, gonads, external genitalia, or internal structures, we see a consistent pattern: each one is either feminine or masculine in character. But as the various syndromes we've been discussing demonstrate, different physical features in a single person can be either masculine or feminine, so from a scientific perspective, legal efforts to categorize all people as either male or female are doomed. Women with androgen insensitivity have male XY sex chromosomes and internal testes, and like most males they do not have oviducts or a uterus. But they do have a vagina and breasts, and in most respects their behavior is typical of females: they dress like females, they are attracted to and marry males, and perhaps most important, even after they learn the details of their condition, they strongly identify themselves as women (Hines, 2011). They are males in some respects, but females in others. If laws define marriage as only between a man and a woman, whom should these individuals be allowed to marry? How about XY individuals with 5-alpha-reductase deficiency, born and raised as girls—with birth certificates to prove it? Should they be restricted to marrying men, even if, at 12 years of age, they sprout a penis?

This recognition that a single individual may be masculine in some regards and feminine in others is especially important as we consider hormonal effects on the brain, next.

organizational effect A permanent alteration of the nervous system, and thus permanent change in behavior, resulting from the action of a steroid hormone on an animal early in its development.

sensitive period The period during development in which an organism can be permanently altered by a particular experience or treatment.

neonatal Referring to newborns.

HOW'S IT GOING ❓

1. Describe the process of fetal sexual differentiation in males and females, especially the role of hormones.
2. What might be the advantage of having a single signal, such as androgens, masculinize the entire body?
3. What are some of the syndromes that can affect sexual differentiation, and what do they tell us about the problems of defining a person's gender?

👁

View Animation 8.6: Organizational Effects of Testosterone

RESEARCHERS AT WORK ||||||||||||||||||||||||||||||||||||||||||||||||||||||||||||||||||||||||||||||||||||||||||||||||||||||||||||||||

Gonadal hormones direct sexual differentiation of behavior and the brain

As scientists began discovering that testicular hormones direct masculine development of the fetal body, behavioral researchers found evidence for a similar influence on the fetal brain. A female guinea pig, like most other rodents, normally displays the lordosis posture in response to male mounting (see Figure 8.16) for only a short period around the time of ovulation, when her fertility is highest. If a male mounts her at other times, she does not show lordosis. Experimenters can induce female rodents to display lordosis by injecting them with ovarian steroids in the sequence they normally follow during ovulation—giving the animals estrogens for a few days and then progesterone (see Figure 8.17). A few hours after the progesterone injection, the female will display lordosis in response to male mounting.

Phoenix et al. (1959) exposed female guinea pigs to testosterone in utero. As adults, these females did *not* show lordosis. Even if their ovaries were removed and they were given the steroid regimen that reliably activated lordosis in normal females, these fetally androgenized females did not show lordosis. From these data the researchers inferred that the same testicular steroids that masculinize the genitalia during early development also masculinize the developing brain. In other words, they proposed that the brain was just one more target tissue that is masculinized by androgens acting early in life (see Figure 8.24). This type of lasting change due to steroid exposure is known as an **organizational effect**.

A steroid has an organizational effect only when present during a specific **sensitive period**, generally in early development. Unlike the transient nature that characterizes the activational effects of hormones, which we discussed earlier, the organizational effects of hormones tend to be permanent (**FIGURES 8.29A–C**). The exact boundaries of the sensitive period of development depend on which behavior and which species are being studied. For rats, androgens given during the **neonatal** period (just after birth) can affect later behavior. Guinea pigs, however, must be exposed to androgens *before* birth for adult lordosis behavior to be affected. In mammals, puberty can be viewed as a second sensitive period; for example, steroid exposure during puberty causes the addition of new cells (an organizational effect) to sex-related brain regions of rats (Schulz and Sisk, 2016).

(Continued)

RESEARCHERS AT WORK (*continued*) ||||||||||||||||||||||||||||||||||||||||||||||||||||||||||||||||||||||||||||||||||||||||||||||||||||

FIGURE 8.29 Organizational Effects of Testosterone on Rodent Behavior (After C. H. Phoenix et al., 1959. *Endocrinology* 65: 369.)

■ **Hypothesis**

Early in life, androgens organize the brain, and therefore adult behavior, in a masculine fashion.

■ **Test**

Manipulate androgen exposure in genetic male and female rodents early in life, then ask whether hormones in adulthood can elicit male and/or female behaviors.

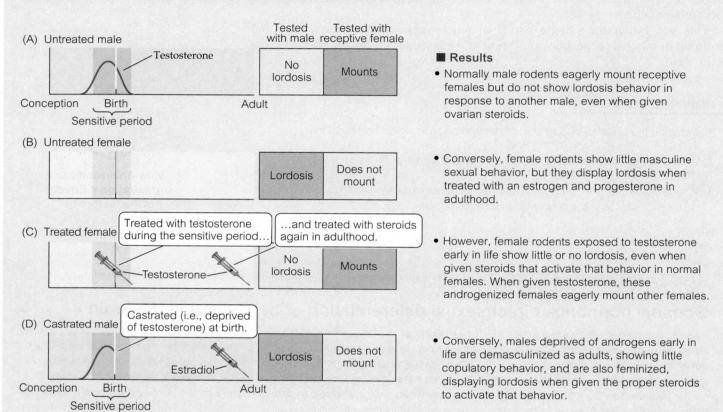

■ **Results**

- Normally male rodents eagerly mount receptive females but do not show lordosis behavior in response to another male, even when given ovarian steroids.

- Conversely, female rodents show little masculine sexual behavior, but they display lordosis when treated with an estrogen and progesterone in adulthood.

- However, female rodents exposed to testosterone early in life show little or no lordosis, even when given steroids that activate that behavior in normal females. When given testosterone, these androgenized females eagerly mount other females.

- Conversely, males deprived of androgens early in life are demasculinized as adults, showing little copulatory behavior, and are also feminized, displaying lordosis when given the proper steroids to activate that behavior.

■ **Conclusion**

When the developing brain is exposed to androgens, the animal's brain is organized in a masculine fashion, so, as an adult, it is more likely to show male-like behaviors, and less likely to show female-like behaviors.

Early testicular secretions result in masculine behavior in adulthood

What has come to be called the *organizational hypothesis* provides a unitary explanation for sexual differentiation: that a single steroid signal (androgen) diffuses through all tissues, masculinizing the body, the brain, and behavior (see Figure 8.24). From this point of view the nervous system is just another type of tissue listening for the androgenic signal that will instruct it to organize itself in a masculine fashion. If the nervous system does not detect androgens, it will organize itself in a mostly feminine fashion.

What was demonstrated originally for the lordosis behavior of guinea pigs has been observed in a variety of vertebrate species and for many behaviors. Exposing female rat pups to testosterone either just before birth or during the first 10 days after birth greatly reduces their lordosis responsiveness as adults. This explains the observation that adult male rats show very little lordosis, even when given estrogens and progesterone. Conversely, male rats that are castrated during the first week of life readily display lordosis responses in adulthood if injected with estrogens and progesterone (**FIGURE 8.29D**). In rats, many behaviors conform to the organizational hypothesis: animals exposed to androgens early in life behave like males, whereas animals not exposed to androgens early in life behave like females.

In most cases, full masculine behavior requires androgens both during development (to organize the nervous system to enable the later behavior) and in adulthood (to activate that behavior). Only animals exposed to androgen both in development and in adulthood show fully masculine behavior.

Several regions of the nervous system display prominent sexual dimorphism

The fact that male and female rats behave differently means that their brains must be different in some way, and according to the organizational hypothesis this difference results primarily from androgenic masculinization of the developing brain. Scientists soon found many sex differences in the brain, including differences in the number, size, and shape of neurons. Darwin coined a term, **sexual dimorphism**, to describe the condition in which males and females show pronounced sex differences in structure. In all species studied so far, androgens are responsible for the sexual dimorphism seen in the brain: androgens masculinize the brain region, and the absence of androgens leads to a female-typical brain anatomy. We'll discuss two well-studied models.

THE PREOPTIC AREA (POA) OF RATS   Roger Gorski examined the POA of the hypothalamus in rats because of the earlier reports that the number of synapses in this region was different in males and females and because lesions of the POA disrupt ovulatory cycles in female rats and, as we mentioned earlier, reduce copulatory behavior in males. Sure enough, he found a nucleus within the POA that has a much larger volume in males than in females (Gorski, 2002).

This nucleus, dubbed the **sexually dimorphic nucleus of the POA (SDN-POA)**, is much more evident in male rats than in females (**FIGURE 8.30**). The SDN-POA conformed beautifully to the organizational hypothesis: males castrated at birth had much smaller SDN-POAs in adulthood, while females androgenized at birth had large, male-like SDN-POAs as adults. Castrating male rats in adulthood, however, did not alter the size of the SDN-POA. Thus, testicular androgens somehow alter the

sexual dimorphism   The condition in which males and females of the same species show pronounced sex differences in appearance.

sexually dimorphic nucleus of the preoptic area (SDN-POA)   A region of the preoptic area that is 5 to 6 times larger in volume in male than in female rats.

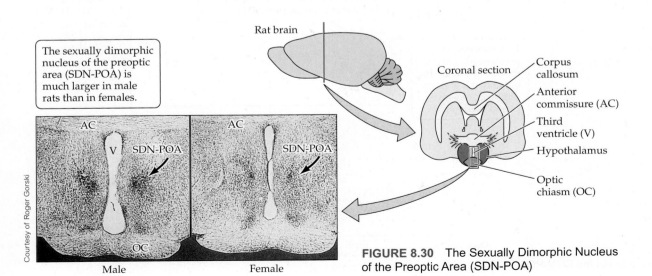

The sexually dimorphic nucleus of the preoptic area (SDN-POA) is much larger in male rats than in females.

Rat brain

Coronal section

Corpus callosum

Anterior commissure (AC)

Third ventricle (V)

Hypothalamus

Optic chiasm (OC)

AC

V   SDN-POA

Male

AC

SDN-POA

Female

Courtesy of Roger Gorski

FIGURE 8.30   The Sexually Dimorphic Nucleus of the Preoptic Area (SDN-POA)

development of the SDN-POA, resulting in a nucleus permanently larger in males than in females (**FIGURE 8.31**).

One quirk of sexual dimorphism in the brains of some lab species, including rodents, is that testosterone reaching the brain is converted into estrogens that act on estrogen receptors, not androgen receptors, to masculinize the SDN-POA and some other brain regions. For example, XY rats that are androgen-insensitive (like the people with AIS discussed earlier) have testes but a feminine exterior. These rats have a masculine SDN-POA because their estrogen receptors are normal. Androgen-insensitive rats also do not display lordosis in response to estrogens and progesterone, because the testosterone that they secreted early in life was converted to an *estrogen* in the brain and masculinized their behavior. Instead, the androgen-insensitive rats show normal male attraction to receptive females, with whom they may attempt to mate, despite the lack of a penis (Hamson et al., 2009). Estrogenic metabolites of testosterone do not seem to play a role in masculinizing the primate brain (Grumbach

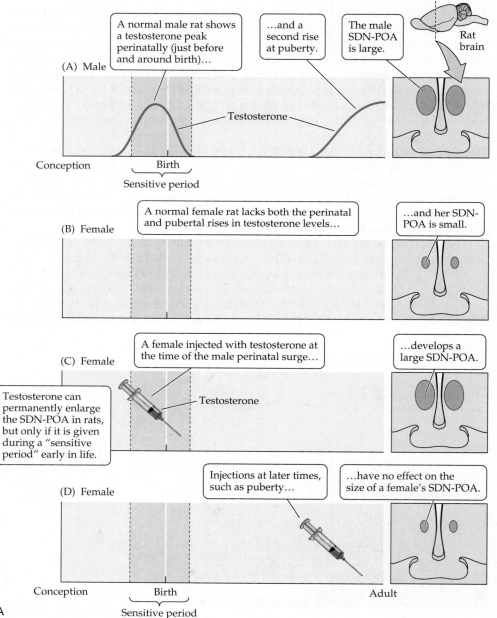

FIGURE 8.31 Organization of the SDN-POA

and Auchus, 1999), so we won't deal with that mechanism any further, but you can learn more about it in **A STEP FURTHER 8.7**, on the website.

THE SPINAL CORD IN MAMMALS   In rats, the bulbocavernosus (BC) muscles that surround the base of the penis are innervated by motor neurons in the **spinal nucleus of the bulbocavernosus (SNB)**. Male rats have about 200 SNB cells, but females have far fewer motor neurons in this region of the spinal cord.

On the day before birth, female rats have BC muscles attached to the base of the clitoris that are nearly as large as the BC muscles of males and that are innervated by motor neurons in the SNB region. In the days just before and after birth, however, many SNB cells die, especially in females, and the BC muscles of females die (**FIGURE 8.32**).

spinal nucleus of the bulbocavernosus (SNB)   A group of motor neurons in the spinal cord of rats that innervate muscles controlling the penis.

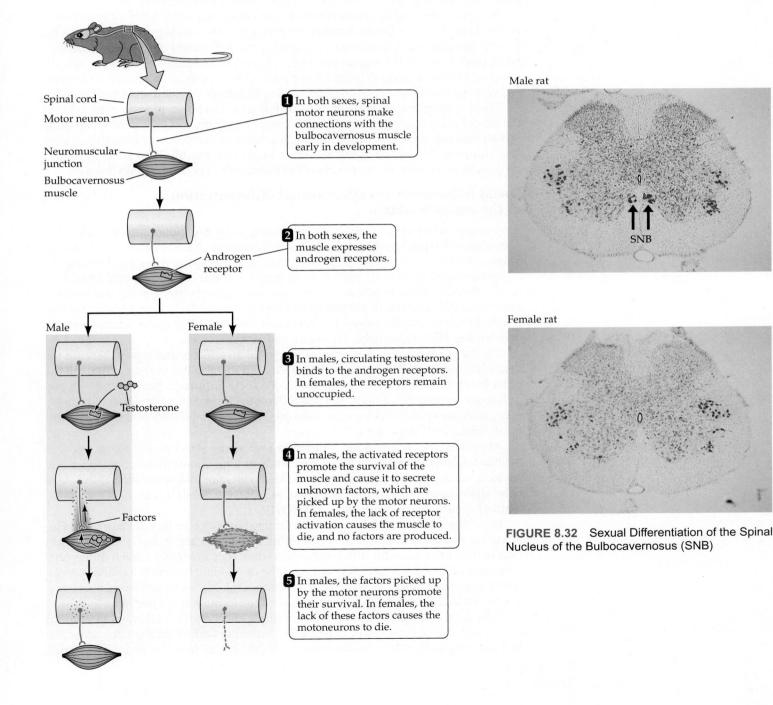

1 In both sexes, spinal motor neurons make connections with the bulbocavernosus muscle early in development.

2 In both sexes, the muscle expresses androgen receptors.

3 In males, circulating testosterone binds to the androgen receptors. In females, the receptors remain unoccupied.

4 In males, the activated receptors promote the survival of the muscle and cause it to secrete unknown factors, which are picked up by the motor neurons. In females, the lack of receptor activation causes the muscle to die, and no factors are produced.

5 In males, the factors picked up by the motor neurons promote their survival. In females, the lack of these factors causes the motoneurons to die.

Spinal cord
Motor neuron
Neuromuscular junction
Bulbocavernosus muscle
Androgen receptor
Male
Female
Testosterone
Factors

Male rat
SNB

Female rat

FIGURE 8.32   Sexual Differentiation of the Spinal Nucleus of the Bulbocavernosus (SNB)

Onuf's nucleus   The human homolog of the spinal nucleus of the bulbocavernosus (SNB) in rats.

A single injection of androgens delivered to a newborn female rat permanently spares some SNB motor neurons and their muscles. Castration of newborn males, accompanied by prenatal blockade of androgen receptors, causes the BC muscles and SNB motor neurons to die as in females. The system also dies in newborn androgen-insensitive rats, so estrogens seem to be unimportant for masculine development of the SNB.

Androgens act on the BC muscles to prevent their demise, and this sparing of the muscles causes the innervating SNB motor neurons to survive (J. A. Morris et al., 2004). Thus the developmental rescue of SNB motor neurons is accomplished indirectly as a consequence of actions on muscle. Adult SNB neurons contain androgen receptors and retain androgen sensitivity throughout life. In adulthood, androgen acts directly on the neurons to cause them to grow (Watson et al., 2001) and to express genes that help new spinal connections to form (Monks and Watson, 2001).

In nonrodents, the BC motor neurons are found in a slightly different spinal location and are known as **Onuf's nucleus**. Surprisingly, most female mammals retain a BC muscle into adulthood; in women, for example, the bulbocavernosus (or *constrictor vestibuli*) helps constrict the vaginal opening. But, as in rodents, the system is sexually dimorphic. Men have larger BC muscles and more Onuf's motor neurons than do women, probably because of androgen exposure during fetal development (Forger et al., 2018).

These systems and several others all demonstrate the power of androgens to affect the gender of the brain. By controlling the amount and timing of testosterone exposure, researchers can make the various brain structures as masculine or feminine as they like. However, despite the crucial role of androgens in masculinizing sexually dimorphic nuclei in the nervous system, there's evidence that experience affects them too.

Social influences also affect sexual differentiation of the nervous system

Environmental factors of many sorts, including social experience, can modulate the masculinization produced by steroids. The development of the SNB offers a classic example. Celia Moore et al. (1992) noticed that rat dams spend more time licking the anogenital regions of male pups than of females. If the dam is anosmic (unable to smell), she licks all the pups less and does not distinguish between males and females. Males raised by anosmic mothers thus receive less anogenital licking, and remarkably, fewer of their SNB cells survive the period around birth. The dam's stimulation of a male's anogenital region helps to masculinize his spinal cord.

On the one hand, this masculinization is still an effect of androgens, because the dam identifies male pups by detecting androgen metabolites in their urine. On the other hand, this effect is clearly the result of a social influence: the dam treats a pup differently because he's a male, and this differential treatment masculinizes his developing nervous system. Perhaps this example illustrates the futility of trying to distinguish "biological" from "social" influences.

Attention from the dam has a different organizing effect on female rat pups. In adulthood, females that were licked frequently as pups show enhanced estrogen and oxytocin sensitivity in brain regions associated with maternal behavior, and they tend to be attentive mothers themselves. Females that were licked less as pups are less attentive mothers later (Champagne et al., 2001).

What about humans? (No, no, not the licking part—the social influence part.) Humans are at least as sensitive to social influences as rats are. In every culture, most people treat boys and girls differently, even when they are infants. Such differential treatment undoubtedly has some effect on the developing human brain and contributes to later sex differences in behavior. Of course, this is a social influence, but testosterone instigated the influence when it induced the formation of a penis.

If prenatal androgens have even a very subtle effect on the fetal brain, then adults interacting with a baby might detect such differences and treat the baby differently. Thus, originally subtle sex differences might be magnified by social experience, especially early in life. Such interactions of steroidal and social influences are probably the norm in the sexual differentiation of human behavior. So does fetal testosterone play a role in masculinizing human behavior? Let's examine that question by zeroing in on human sexual orientation, the final topic of this chapter.

HOW'S IT GOING ?

1. How does exposure to androgens early in life masculinize the brain and spinal cord in rats?
2. Why is it difficult to distinguish between social and biological influences on sexual differentiation?

Do fetal hormones masculinize human behaviors in adulthood?

As with rats and other animals, the fact that men and women behave differently implies that something about them, probably something about their brains, must also be different. Indeed, many parts of the brain are different between men and women (**FIGURE 8.33**). But are these sexual dimorphisms in the human brain caused by prenatal exposure to hormones, as in other animals, or by social influences? In other words, does prenatal exposure to steroids affect the adult behavior of humans? This is a tricky problem because although prenatal androgens may act on the human brain, they certainly act on the rest of the body too.

For example, recall that people with androgen insensitivity syndrome (AIS) are usually raised as girls because their XY genotype is not discovered until puberty. We said earlier that women with androgen insensitivity tend to be very feminine, including being sexually attracted to men, and they often seek a family through adoption. Are they feminine because they received the social tutoring to be females, or because their brains, without androgen receptors, could not respond to testosterone? Their behavior is consistent with either hypothesis.

Females with congenital adrenal hyperplasia (CAH), who are exposed to androgens before birth, are much more likely to be described by their parents (and themselves) as tomboys than are other girls, and they exhibit enhanced spatial abilities on cognitive tests that usually favor males (Berenbaum, 2001). In adulthood, most women

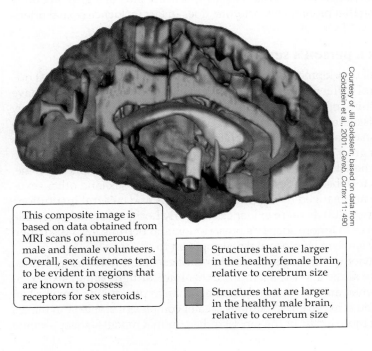

Courtesy of Jill Goldstein, based on data from Goldstein et al., 2001. *Cereb. Cortex* 11: 490

This composite image is based on data obtained from MRI scans of numerous male and female volunteers. Overall, sex differences tend to be evident in regions that are known to possess receptors for sex steroids.

Structures that are larger in the healthy female brain, relative to cerebrum size

Structures that are larger in the healthy male brain, relative to cerebrum size

FIGURE 8.33 Sexual Dimorphism in the Human Brain

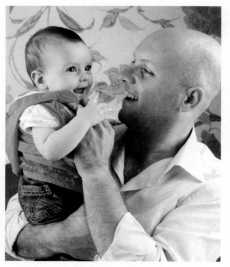

Training Girls to Be Verbal Adults tend to spend more time talking to a baby if they believe the baby is a girl (whether it actually is a girl or not) (Seavey et al., 1975).

with CAH describe themselves as heterosexual, but they are more likely than other women to report being lesbians. Interestingly, as females with CAH grow older, the proportion who report being lesbians increases (Meyer-Bahlburg, 2011), suggesting that they start off trying to follow the socially approved role of heterosexual female but then become more comfortable with a gay orientation later in life. Do women with CAH exhibit those behaviors because early androgens partially masculinized their brains? Or did their ambiguous genitalia cause parents and others to treat them differently from infancy?

The *guevedoces* of the Dominican Republic, who are raised as girls but grow a penis at puberty, behave like males as adults, dressing like men and seeking girlfriends. There are two competing explanations for why these people raised as girls later behave as men. First, prenatal testosterone may masculinize their brains; thus, despite being raised as girls, when they reach puberty, their brains lead them to seek out females for mates. This explanation suggests that the social influences of growing up—assigning oneself to a gender and mimicking role models of that gender, as well as gender-specific playing and dressing—are unimportant for later behavior and sexual orientation.

An alternative explanation is that early hormones have no effect—that the local culture simply recognizes and teaches children that some people can start out as girls and change to boys later. If so, then the social influences on gender role development might be completely different in this society from those in ours. Of course, a third option is that both mechanisms contribute to the final outcome.

At the opening of the chapter, we discussed the dilemma of cloacal exstrophy, in which genetic boys are born with functional testes but without penises. Historically in these cases, neonatal sex reassignment has been recommended on the assumption that unambiguously raising these children as girls, and surgically providing them with the appropriate external genitalia, could produce a more satisfactory outcome. In a long-term follow-up of 14 such cases, however, Reiner and Gearhart (2004) found that 8 of these "girls" eventually declared themselves to be boys, even though several were unaware that they had ever been operated on. Although this finding indicates that prenatal exposure to androgens strongly predisposes subsequent male gender identity, 5 of the remaining 6 cases were apparently content with their female identities, suggesting that socialization can also play a strong role. However, almost all of these teenagers, including those who felt comfortable as girls, reported being sexually attracted to girls. These reports are part of a growing body of evidence suggesting that prenatal testosterone does in fact influence sexual orientation in humans, as we'll see next.

What determines a person's sexual orientation?

There are two kinds of developmental influences that could shape human sexual orientation. Sociocultural influences instruct children about how they should behave when they grow up (think of all those charming princes wooing princesses in Disney movies). But, as we discussed in the previous section, differences in fetal exposure to testosterone could also organize developing brains to be attracted to females or males in adulthood. For that great majority of people who are heterosexual, there's no way to distinguish between these two influences, because they both favor the same outcome. Gay people provide a test, because people attracted to the same sex (and other sexual minorities) remain stigmatized by various social groups and cultural institutions (Herek and McLemore, 2013). Is there evidence that early hormones are responsible for causing some people to ignore society's prescription and become gay? If so, then maybe hormones play a role in heterosexual development too.

Homosexual behavior is certainly seen in other species—mountain sheep, swans, gulls, and dolphins, to name a few (Bagemihl, 1999). Interestingly, same-sex sexual behavior is more common among apes and monkeys than in prosimian primates like lemurs and lorises (Pfau et al., 2019), so perhaps greater complexity of the brain makes homosexual behavior more likely. In the most-studied animal model—sheep—some

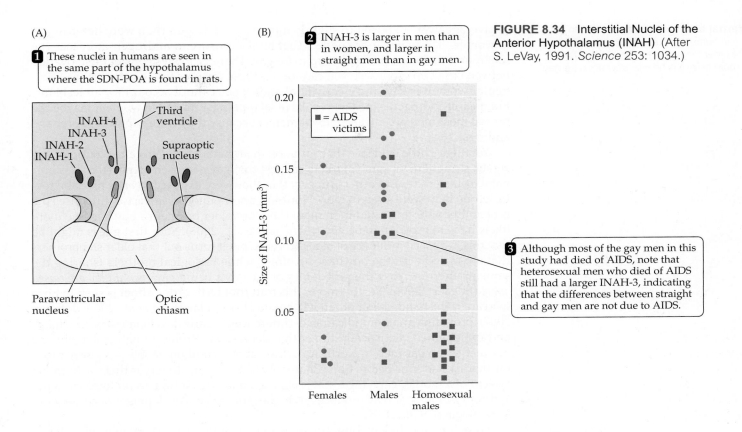

(A)

1 These nuclei in humans are seen in the same part of the hypothalamus where the SDN-POA is found in rats.

INAH-4
INAH-3
INAH-2
INAH-1

Third ventricle

Supraoptic nucleus

Paraventricular nucleus

Optic chiasm

(B)

2 INAH-3 is larger in men than in women, and larger in straight men than in gay men.

■ = AIDS victims

Size of INAH-3 (mm^3)

Females   Males   Homosexual males

3 Although most of the gay men in this study had died of AIDS, note that heterosexual men who died of AIDS still had a larger INAH-3, indicating that the differences between straight and gay men are not due to AIDS.

FIGURE 8.34 Interstitial Nuclei of the Anterior Hypothalamus (INAH) (After S. LeVay, 1991. *Science* 253: 1034.)

rams consistently refuse to mount females but prefer to mount other rams. There are differences in the POA of "gay" versus "straight" rams (Roselli et al., 2004), apparently organized by testosterone acting on the brain during fetal development (Roselli and Stormshak, 2009).

Simon LeVay (1991) performed postmortem examinations of the POA in humans and found a nucleus (the third interstitial nucleus of the anterior hypothalamus, or INAH-3) (**FIGURE 8.34A**) that is larger in men than in women, and larger in heterosexual men than in gay men (**FIGURE 8.34B**). All but one of the gay men in the study had died of AIDS, but the brain differences could not be due to AIDS pathology, because straight men with AIDS still had a significantly larger INAH-3 than did the gay men (Byne et al., 2001). To the press and the public, this finding sounded like strong evidence that sexual orientation is "built in." It's still possible, however, that early social experience affects the development of INAH-3 to determine later sexual orientation. Furthermore, sexual experiences as an adult could affect INAH-3 structure, so the smaller nucleus in some gay men may be the *result* of their gay orientation, rather than the *cause*, as LeVay himself was careful to point out.

In women, purported markers of exposure to androgen as a fetus—sounds emitted from the ears (McFadden, 2011), patterns of eye blinks (Rahman, 2005), and finger length patterns (**FIGURE 8.35**)—all indicate that lesbians,

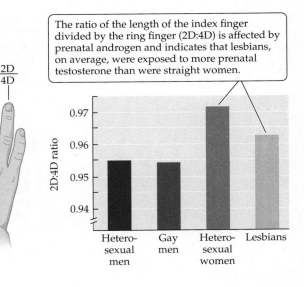

The ratio of the length of the index finger divided by the ring finger (2D:4D) is affected by prenatal androgen and indicates that lesbians, on average, were exposed to more prenatal testosterone than were straight women.

2D
4D

2D:4D ratio

Hetero-sexual men   Gay men   Hetero-sexual women   Lesbians

FIGURE 8.35 Bodily Indicators of Prenatal Androgen Note that these are group differences in averages; you cannot reliably determine an *individual's* orientation by examining digit ratios. (After T. J. Williams et al., 2000. *Nature* 404: 455.)

fraternal birth order effect   A phenomenon in human populations, such that the more older biological brothers a boy has, the more likely it is he will grow up to be gay.

on average, were exposed to slightly more fetal androgen than were heterosexual women. These findings suggest that fetal exposure to androgen increases the likelihood that a girl will grow up to be gay. There is always considerable overlap between the two groups, so you cannot use these features to predict whether a particular woman is gay, and clearly fetal androgens cannot account for all lesbians. But if early androgen exposure results in later being attracted to women, maybe the reason most men are attracted to women is because they were exposed to prenatal androgen.

Yet there's little evidence that variation in prenatal androgen can account for gay versus straight men; some markers suggest that gay men were exposed to less prenatal testosterone, and others suggest that they were exposed to *more* prenatal testosterone than were straight men. However, another nonsocial factor influences the probability of homosexuality in men: the more older brothers a boy has, the more likely he is to grow up to be gay (Blanchard et al., 2006). Your first guess might be that this is a social influence of older brothers, but it turns out that older stepbrothers that are raised with the boy have no effect, while biological brothers (sharing the same mother) increase the probability of the boy's being gay *even if they are raised apart* (Bogaert, 2006). Furthermore, this **fraternal birth order effect** is seen in boys who are right-handed, but not in left-handed boys (Blanchard et al., 2006; Bogaert, 2007), providing another indication of differences in early development between gay and straight men. Statistically, the birth order effect is strong enough that about one in every seven gay men in North America—about a million people—is gay because his mother had sons before him (Cantor et al., 2002). One theory is that the immune system of a mother carrying a son is exposed for the first time to proteins from the Y chromosome, so it may produce antibodies that affect development of subsequent sons (Bogaert et al., 2018).

From a political viewpoint, the question—whether sexual orientation is determined before birth or determined by early social influences—is irrelevant. Laws and prejudices against homosexuality are based primarily on religious views that it is a sin that some people "choose." But almost all gay and straight men report that, from the beginning, their interests and romantic attachments matched their adult orientation. So any social influence would have to be acting very early in life and without any conscious awareness (do you remember "choosing" whom to find attractive?). Furthermore, despite extensive efforts, no one has come up with a reliable way to change sexual orientation (Spitzer, 2012). These findings, added to evidence that older brothers and prenatal androgens affect the probability of being gay, have convinced most scientists that we do not choose our sexual orientation.

HOW'S IT GOING ❓

1. What does the sexual orientation of people with various syndromes of sexual differentiation suggest about hormonal influences on human sexual orientation?

2. If human sexual orientation were shown definitively to be influenced by prenatal factors such as hormones and the fraternal birth order effect, would you be more or less inclined to accept homosexuality?

Recommended Reading

Colapinto, J. (2006). *As Nature Made Him.* New York, NY: Harper Perennial.

Eugenides, J. (2002). *Middlesex: A Novel.* New York, NY: Farrar, Straus, and Giroux.

Komisaruk, B. R., and González-Mariscal, G. (2017). *Behavioral Neuroendocrinology.* Boca Raton, FL: CRC Press.

LeVay, S., Baldwin, J., and Baldwin, J. (2021). *Discovering Human Sexuality* (5th ed.). Sunderland, MA: Oxford University Press/Sinauer.

Nelson, R. J., and Kriegsfeld, L. J. (2016). *An Introduction to Behavioral Endocrinology* (5th ed.). Sunderland, MA: Oxford University Press/Sinauer.

Patisaul, H. B., and Belcher, S. M. (2017). *Endocrine Disruptors, Brain and Behavior.* New York, NY: Oxford University Press.

8 • VISUAL SUMMARY

You should be able to relate each summary to the adjacent illustration, including structures and processes. The online version of this **Visual Summary** includes links to figures, animations, and activities that will help you consolidate the material.

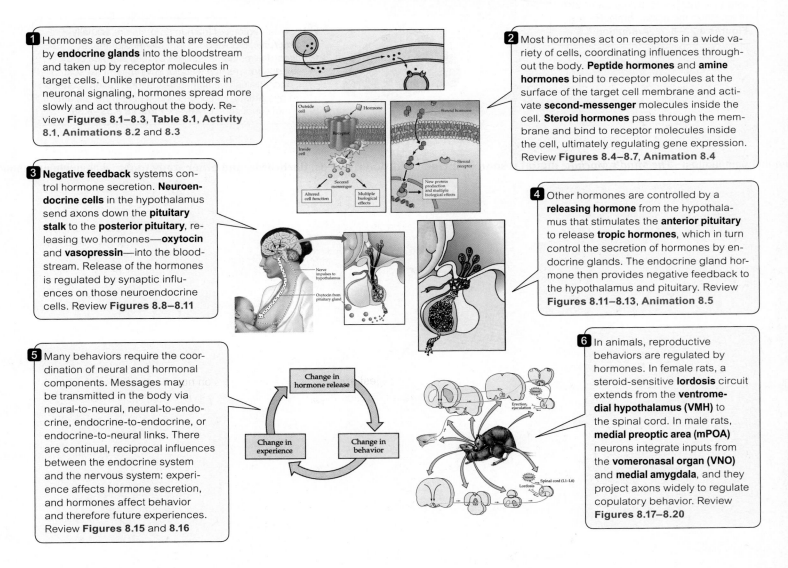

1 Hormones are chemicals that are secreted by **endocrine glands** into the bloodstream and taken up by receptor molecules in target cells. Unlike neurotransmitters in neuronal signaling, hormones spread more slowly and act throughout the body. Review **Figures 8.1–8.3**, **Table 8.1**, **Activity 8.1**, **Animations 8.2** and **8.3**

2 Most hormones act on receptors in a wide variety of cells, coordinating influences throughout the body. **Peptide hormones** and **amine hormones** bind to receptor molecules at the surface of the target cell membrane and activate **second-messenger** molecules inside the cell. **Steroid hormones** pass through the membrane and bind to receptor molecules inside the cell, ultimately regulating gene expression. Review **Figures 8.4–8.7**, **Animation 8.4**

3 **Negative feedback** systems control hormone secretion. **Neuroendocrine cells** in the hypothalamus send axons down the **pituitary stalk** to the **posterior pituitary**, releasing two hormones—**oxytocin** and **vasopressin**—into the bloodstream. Release of the hormones is regulated by synaptic influences on those neuroendocrine cells. Review **Figures 8.8–8.11**

4 Other hormones are controlled by a **releasing hormone** from the hypothalamus that stimulates the **anterior pituitary** to release **tropic hormones**, which in turn control the secretion of hormones by endocrine glands. The endocrine gland hormone then provides negative feedback to the hypothalamus and pituitary. Review **Figures 8.11–8.13**, **Animation 8.5**

5 Many behaviors require the coordination of neural and hormonal components. Messages may be transmitted in the body via neural-to-neural, neural-to-endocrine, endocrine-to-endocrine, or endocrine-to-neural links. There are continual, reciprocal influences between the endocrine system and the nervous system: experience affects hormone secretion, and hormones affect behavior and therefore future experiences. Review **Figures 8.15** and **8.16**

6 In animals, reproductive behaviors are regulated by hormones. In female rats, a steroid-sensitive **lordosis** circuit extends from the **ventromedial hypothalamus (VMH)** to the spinal cord. In male rats, **medial preoptic area (mPOA)** neurons integrate inputs from the **vomeronasal organ (VNO)** and **medial amygdala**, and they project axons widely to regulate copulatory behavior. Review **Figures 8.17–8.20**

7 In humans, very low levels of **testosterone** are required for either men or women to display a full interest in sex, but additional testosterone has no additional effect. In animals, hormones significantly influence **maternal behavior** by acting on the same brain regions that are important for sexual behavior (mPOA, VMH). Review **Figures 8.18** and **8.21–8.23**

9 In animals, **androgens** also organize the developing brain, masculinizing regions such as the **sexually dimorphic nucleus of the preoptic area (SDN-POA)** and the **spinal nucleus of the bulbocavernosus (SNB)**. There is evidence that prenatal androgens also masculinize the human brain. Review **Figures 8.29–8.32, Animation 8.6**

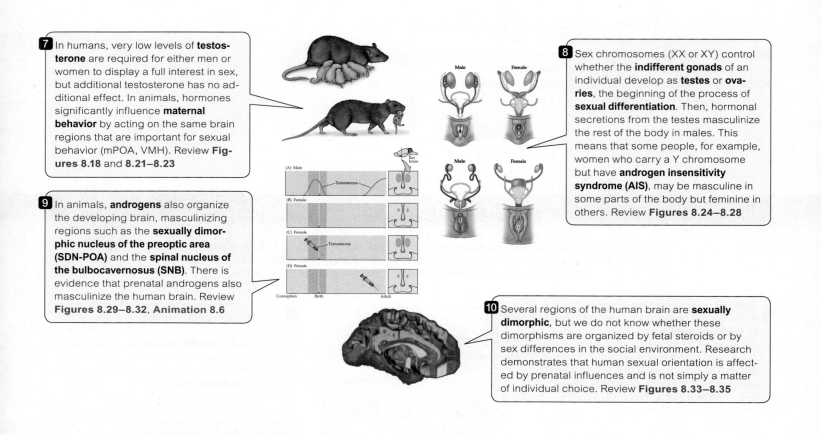

8 Sex chromosomes (XX or XY) control whether the **indifferent gonads** of an individual develop as **testes** or **ovaries**, the beginning of the process of **sexual differentiation**. Then, hormonal secretions from the testes masculinize the rest of the body in males. This means that some people, for example, women who carry a Y chromosome but have **androgen insensitivity syndrome (AIS)**, may be masculine in some parts of the body but feminine in others. Review **Figures 8.24–8.28**

10 Several regions of the human brain are **sexually dimorphic**, but we do not know whether these dimorphisms are organized by fetal steroids or by sex differences in the social environment. Research demonstrates that human sexual orientation is affected by prenatal influences and is not simply a matter of individual choice. Review **Figures 8.33–8.35**

The Mind's Machine digital resources include additional videos, flashcards, and other study tools.

9 Homeostasis: Active Regulation of the Internal Environment

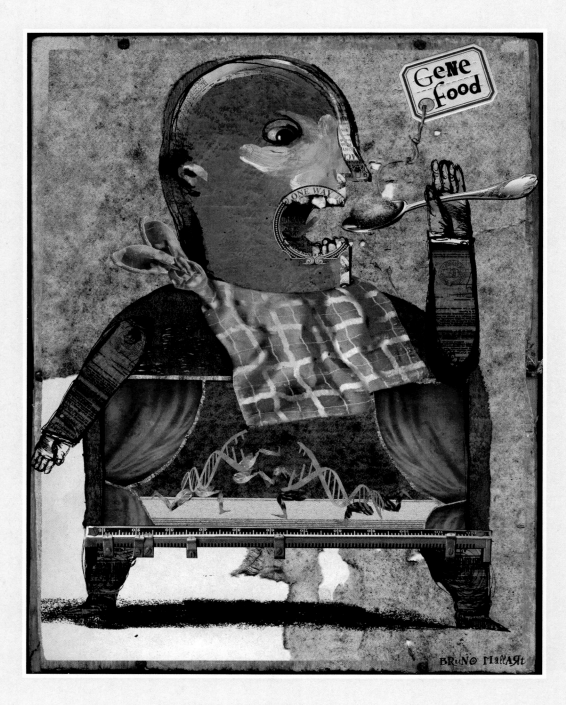

Harsh Reality TV

Introduced in 2004, the reality television show *The Biggest Loser* went on to become a huge prime-time hit. The premise of the show was simple enough—the contestant who lost the most weight during the season won—but the effort required from the contestants was immense. The biggest loser of them all in season 8 (2009) was Danny C. Through a punishing combination of near-starvation dieting and all-day exercise, Danny shed an incredible 239 pounds (108 kilograms), dropping from 430 pounds to a svelte 191 pounds in just 7 months. Other initially obese contestants similarly accomplished exceptional weight loss and delighted in revealing their new, slimmer silhouettes to their friends, families, and viewers.

Recognizing an unusual opportunity, a group of scientists followed Danny and other *Biggest Loser* contestants for 6 years following their weight loss: the longest-term study of its kind ever conducted (Fothergill et al., 2016). The results are discouraging. In the years after his appearance on the show, and despite exceptional ongoing efforts, Danny regained more than 100 pounds of the weight he had lost. In fact, all but one of the 14 contestants who were tracked in the study regained significant weight; some were even heavier after the show than they were before the contest started. The pattern of results confirms a common observation: it is very hard to keep the weight off after dieting. But what could explain the additional discovery that even after 6 long years of hard work, the metabolisms of these contestants still had not adjusted and instead strived to return them to their original obese state?

Millions of years of evolution have endowed our bodies with complex physiological mechanisms, and multiple backup systems, devoted to producing a stable internal environment, monitored and regulated by the brain at every stage. But in the context of modern society, some of these ancient systems are making trouble for us; obesity, for example, is reaching epidemic proportions and placing a severe burden on health care resources. The physiological and behavioral processes governing the internal environment, and their role when things go wrong, are our topic in this chapter.

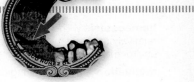

See Video 9.1:
Regaining the Weight

View Animation 9.2:
Brain Explorer

9.1 Homeostatic Systems Share Several Key Features

THE ROAD AHEAD

In the first part of the chapter, we use body temperature to explore the general principles of homeostasis. By the end of this section, you should be able to:

9.1.1 Define homeostasis and allostasis and their relationships to drive states.

9.1.2 Distinguish between endothermy and ectothermy, with examples, and discuss the pros and cons of each system.

9.1.3 Describe, with appropriate examples, how the engineering concepts of negative feedback and redundancy apply to homeostatic systems.

9.1.4 Discuss some of the ways in which animals use specialized behaviors to maintain a stable internal environment.

The bodies of many animals exhibit some degree of **homeostasis**: a relatively stable, balanced internal environment that is optimized for cellular activities. Variables such as acidity, saltiness, water level, oxygenation, temperature, and energy availability are closely monitored and controlled by elaborate physiological systems. Deviations from optimum states can affect **motivation**, the psychological process that induces or sustains a particular behavior, and the effect can escalate rapidly as the deviation worsens from a minor distraction (like the urge to take a couple of sips if water is handy) to an overwhelmingly powerful need (like the raging thirst of someone lost in the desert).

Because it is a relatively simple system, we'll start by using **thermoregulation**, the regulation of body temperature, to look at some important general concepts of homeostasis: negative feedback, redundancy, behavioral compensation, and the concept of allostasis. These topics will arise again when we talk about fluid balance, appetite, and body weight in the remainder of the chapter.

We mammals are **endotherms**, meaning that we make our own heat *inside* our bodies, using metabolism and muscular activity (and if our muscles aren't making enough heat, we can shiver them to make more). Endothermy gives us clear advantages over **ectotherms** (animals that get their heat mostly from *outside* the body—from the environment) by allowing us to roam more widely. Like endotherms, ectotherms such as lizards and snakes try to regulate their temperature within a range that is optimal for the functioning of their cells, but this means they need to stay near sources of warmth. Furthermore, the evolution of endothermy involved enhanced capacity for oxygen utilization, with the result that the muscles of mammals can work hard for longer periods of time: endothermic hares will always outrun ectothermic tortoises. (For more on the pros and cons of endothermy and ectothermy, see **A STEP FURTHER 9.1**, on the website.) So it's no surprise that we have dedicated systems for creating warmth and regulating our body temperature. The systems that govern body temperature operate according to several general principles common to almost all homeostatic systems.

Negative feedback allows precise control

The homeostatic mechanisms that regulate temperature, body fluids, and metabolism are primarily **negative feedback** systems, where deviation from a desired value, called the **set point**, triggers a compensatory action of the system. Restoring the desired value turns off the response (this is why it is called *negative* feedback). A simple analogy for this mechanism is a household thermostat (**FIGURE 9.1**): a temperature drop below the set point activates the thermostat, which turns on the heating system. The heat that is produced has a negative feedback effect on the thermostat, so it stops calling for heat. Most heating systems have at least a little bit of tolerance built in—otherwise the system would be going on and off too frequently—so there is generally a **set zone** rather than a rigid set point.

homeostasis   The maintenance of a relatively constant internal physiological environment.

motivation   The psychological process that induces or sustains a particular behavior.

thermoregulation   The active process of maintaining a relatively constant internal temperature through behavioral and physiological adjustments.

endotherm   An animal whose body temperature is regulated chiefly by internal metabolic processes.

ectotherm   An animal whose body temperature is regulated by, and whose heat comes mainly from, the environment.

negative feedback   The process whereby a system monitors its own output and reduces its activity when a set point is reached.

set point   The point of reference in a feedback system.

set zone   The optimal range of a variable that a negative feedback system tries to maintain.

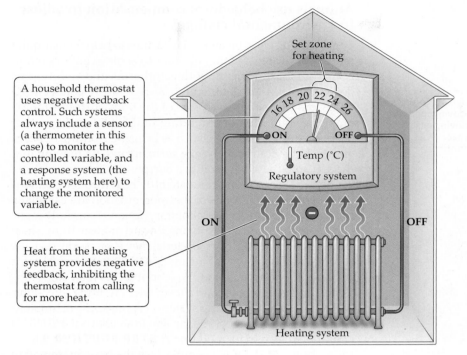

A household thermostat uses negative feedback control. Such systems always include a sensor (a thermometer in this case) to monitor the controlled variable, and a response system (the heating system here) to change the monitored variable.

Heat from the heating system provides negative feedback, inhibiting the thermostat from calling for more heat.

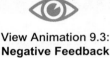

**View Animation 9.3:
Negative Feedback**

FIGURE 9.1   Negative Feedback

Just like a thermostat, your set zone for body temperature can be changed under certain circumstances. For example, your body temperature drops at night for much the same reason that people turn down their home thermostats at night: to conserve energy. Or your set zone may be temporarily elevated, producing a fever to help your body fight off an infection. But in either case there are narrow limits. Too hot, and proteins begin to lose their correct shape, link together, and malfunction (this modification of proteins is called *denaturing* or, if it is really hot, *cooking*), with lethal results if critical brain regions are compromised. If we are too cool, chemical reactions of the body occur too slowly; at very low body temperatures, ice crystals may disrupt cellular membranes, killing the cells.

Redundancy ensures critical needs are met

Just as engineers equip critical equipment with several backup systems, our bodies tend to have multiple mechanisms for monitoring our stores, conserving remaining supplies, obtaining new resources, and shedding excesses. Loss of function in one part of the system usually can be compensated for by the remaining parts. This redundancy attests to the importance of maintaining our inner environment, but it also complicates the lives of scientists who are trying to figure out exactly how the body normally regulates temperature, water balance, and food intake.

It has long been known that the hypothalamus senses and controls body temperature, but lesion experiments eventually showed that different hypothalamic sites control two separate thermoregulatory systems. Lesions in the preoptic area (POA) of rats impair physiological responses to cold, such as shivering and constriction of the blood vessels (Morrison, 2016), but did not interfere with such behaviors as pressing levers to control heating lamps or cooling fans. Lesions in the lateral hypothalamus of rats abolished behavioral regulation of temperature but did not affect the physiological responses (Van Zoeren and Stricker, 1977). This is a clear example of homeostatic redundancy: two different systems for regulating the same variable.

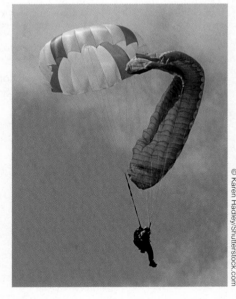

© Karen Hadley/Shutterstock.com

Redundancy   Engineers equip critical systems with multiple "fail-safe" redundancies—for example, skydivers generally carry a secondary parachute —so that a backup always protects the critical system (the skydiver, in this example). Multiple redundancy is a feature of many of the body's homeostatic systems, protecting the constant internal environment that is crucial for survival.

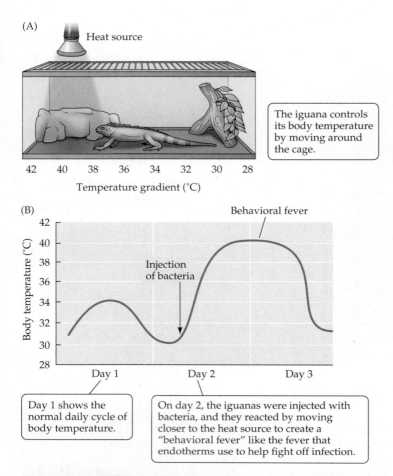

(A) Heat source

The iguana controls its body temperature by moving around the cage.

42 40 38 36 34 32 30 28

Temperature gradient (°C)

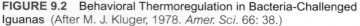

(B)

Behavioral fever

Injection of bacteria

Day 1 Day 2 Day 3

Day 1 shows the normal daily cycle of body temperature.

On day 2, the iguanas were injected with bacteria, and they reacted by moving closer to the heat source to create a "behavioral fever" like the fever that endotherms use to help fight off infection.

FIGURE 9.2 Behavioral Thermoregulation in Bacteria-Challenged Iguanas (After M. J. Kluger, 1978. *Amer. Sci.* 66: 38.)

allostasis The varying behavioral and physiological adjustments that an individual makes in order to maintain optimal (rather than unchanging) functioning of a regulated system in the face of changing environmental stressors.

Animals use behavioral compensation to adjust to environmental changes

Organisms also use behavioral measures to help them acquire more heat, water, or food, in order to achieve and maintain homeostasis. In general, both ectotherms and endotherms deploy three kinds of temperature-regulating behavior: (1) behaviors that change *exposure* of the body surface—for example, by huddling or extending limbs; (2) behaviors that change external *insulation*, such as by using clothing or nests; and (3) behaviors that change *surroundings*, by moving into the sun, into the shade, or into a burrow.

Because ectotherms generate little heat through metabolism, behavioral methods of thermoregulation are especially important to them. In the laboratory, iguanas carefully regulate their temperature by moving toward or away from a heat lamp, and when infected by bacteria, they even produce a fever through such behavioral means (**FIGURE 9.2**), which helps them fight off an infection. We endotherms instead use internal processes to generate a fever when fighting infections, which boosts our immune system response. Unfortunately, sometimes the body goes too far, as a fever above 104°F (40°C) does more harm than good (see **A STEP FURTHER 9.2**, on the website). **FIGURE 9.3** summarizes the basic mammalian thermoregulatory system: receptors in the skin, body core, and hypothalamus detect temperature and transmit that information to three neural regions (spinal cord, brainstem, and hypothalamus). If the body temperature moves outside the set zone, each of these neural regions can initiate physiological and behavioral responses to return it to the set zone.

A wide array of sensors continuously monitors the many internal and external threats to our physiological stability. At any given moment, depending on what's happening in the environment, simultaneous perturbations in multiple regulated systems cause varying degrees of physiological stress. Rather than defending a single set point, many physiological systems must continually shift their responses depending on the nature of the stressors and prior experience—for example, your heart rate and blood pressure are continually shifting to accommodate your current or anticipated activity level—a dynamic process termed **allostasis** (McEwen and Wingfield, 2010; McEwen, 2016). Allostatic adjustments are a normal part of dealing with the demands of daily life, but the heavy physiological burden on chronically stressed individuals puts them at risk of pathology due to allostatic overload.

View Animation 9.4:
Thermoregulation in Humans

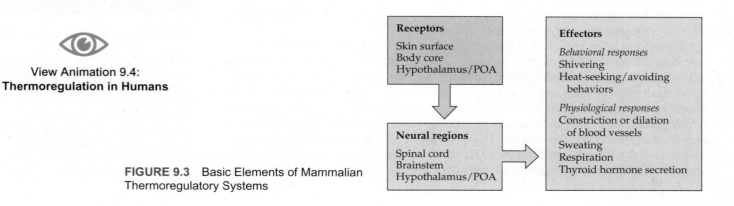

Receptors

Skin surface
Body core
Hypothalamus/POA

Neural regions

Spinal cord
Brainstem
Hypothalamus/POA

Effectors

Behavioral responses
Shivering
Heat-seeking/avoiding behaviors

Physiological responses
Constriction or dilation of blood vessels
Sweating
Respiration
Thyroid hormone secretion

FIGURE 9.3 Basic Elements of Mammalian Thermoregulatory Systems

HOW'S IT GOING ❓

1. Define homeostasis, and discuss its relation to the psychological concept of motivation. Why do homeostatic systems tend to have a set zone instead of a set point?
2. Distinguish between endotherms and ectotherms, and give a few examples of each.
3. Using examples, define and describe negative feedback as it applies to homeostasis.
4. Many homeostatic systems feature redundancy. What is it and why is it important?
5. Although the concept of homeostasis primarily relates to the physical internal environment, behavior can play an important role too. How?
6. Define allostasis. How does allostasis relate to homeostasis?

9.2 The Body's Water Is Actively Balanced between Two Major Compartments

THE ROAD AHEAD

In the next section, we discuss the processes that maintain an optimal balance of water and salt in the body. By the end of this section, you should be able to:

9.2.1 Describe the compartmentalization of fluids in the body.

9.2.2 Briefly define diffusion and osmosis.

9.2.3 Describe the semipermeable membrane, and explain its role in the movement of water between compartments.

9.2.4 Define and compare osmotic thirst and hypovolemic thirst and the sensors that monitor each type of fluid loss.

9.2.5 Discuss the importance of salt homeostasis in each type of thirst.

9.2.6 Give an overview of physiological responses to thirst, and tell how the brain gauges when to stop drinking.

Our homeostatic mechanisms are continually challenged by *obligatory losses*: the unavoidable expenditures of bodily resources that must then be regained from the external environment. Many body functions use up resources. Water (and some salt molecules), for example, are lost when we produce urine to get rid of waste molecules. We even lose water in our breath. Restoring expended water (and food) can take up much of an animal's waking life.

A precise balance of fluids and dissolved salts bathes the cells of the body and enables them to function. The composition of this fluid provides an echo of our evolutionary past. The first living organisms on Earth were single-celled inhabitants of the ancient oceans, and it was in these simple organisms that the fundamental processes of cellular life were established. When multicellular organisms evolved much later and began to exploit opportunities on land and in the air, they had no choice but to bring along with them the watery environment that their cells needed to survive. For this reason, most organisms evolved homeostatic systems that ensure that the composition of their body fluids closely resembles dilute seawater (Bourque, 2008) (**FIGURE 9.4**). Even relatively minor deviation from optimal water and salt balance can be lethal.

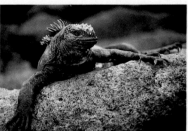

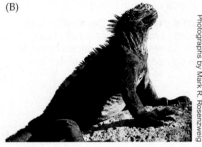

Behavioral Control of Body Temperature   (A) A Galápagos marine iguana, upon emerging from the cold sea, raises its body temperature by hugging a warm rock and lying broadside to the sun. (B) Once its temperature is sufficiently high, the iguana reduces its surface contact with the rock and faces the sun to minimize its exposure. These behaviors control body temperature.

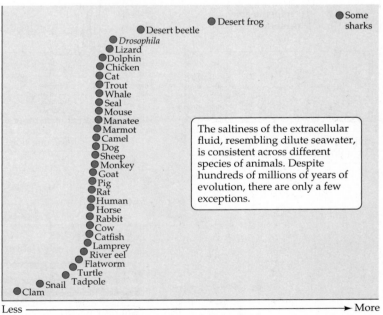

The saltiness of the extracellular fluid, resembling dilute seawater, is consistent across different species of animals. Despite hundreds of millions of years of evolution, there are only a few exceptions.

Less ——————————————→ More
Saltiness of extracellular fluid

FIGURE 9.4   Each Animal Contains a Tiny Sea   (After C. W. Bourque, 2008. *Nat. Rev. Neurosci.* 9: 519.)

intracellular compartment   The fluid of the body that is contained within cells.

extracellular compartment   The fluid of the body that exists outside the cells.

diffusion   The passive spread of solute molecules through a solvent until a uniform solute concentration is achieved.

osmosis   The passive movement of a solvent, usually water, through a semipermeable membrane until a uniform concentration of solute (often salt) is achieved on both sides of the membrane.

osmotic pressure   The tendency of a solvent to move across a membrane in order to equalize the concentration of solute on both sides of the membrane.

Scientists typically describe water balance by contrasting the inside versus the outside of our cells. Most of the water in the body is contained within our cells; this water is collectively referred to as the **intracellular compartment**. The fluid that is outside of our cells, called the **extracellular compartment**, is divided between the *interstitial fluid* (the fluid between cells) and *blood plasma* (the protein-rich fluid that carries red and white blood cells). Water is continually moving back and forth between these compartments, in and out of cells.

To understand the forces driving the movement of water, we must understand diffusion and osmosis. In **diffusion**, molecules of a substance, like salt (a *solute*), that are dissolved in a quantity of another substance, such as water (a *solvent*), will passively spread through the solvent because of the random jiggling and movement of the molecules until they are more or less uniformly distributed throughout it (see Figure 2.3). If we divide a container of water with a membrane that is impermeable to water and salt and then put salt in the water on one side, the salt molecules will diffuse only within the water on that side. If instead the membrane impedes salt molecules only a little, then the salt will distribute itself evenly within the water on the initial side but will also—more slowly—invade and distribute itself across the other side. A membrane that is permeable to some molecules but not others is referred to as *selectively permeable* or *semipermeable*. As we saw in Chapter 2, selective permeability of cell membranes is what lets neurons create and transmit electrical potentials.

Osmosis is the movement of water molecules that occurs so as to equalize the concentration of two solutions that are separated by a semipermeable membrane. This is the case we examine in **FIGURE 9.5**, where a semipermeable membrane that permits water to cross, *but not salt*, divides a tank into two sides. Adding extra salt to one side induces water molecules to move into the now-salty side until the concentrations of both solutions equalize. The physical force that pushes or pulls water across the membrane is called **osmotic pressure**.

FIGURE 9.5   Osmosis

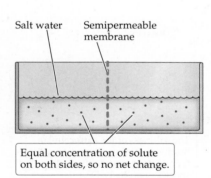

Salt water   Semipermeable membrane

Equal concentration of solute on both sides, so no net change.

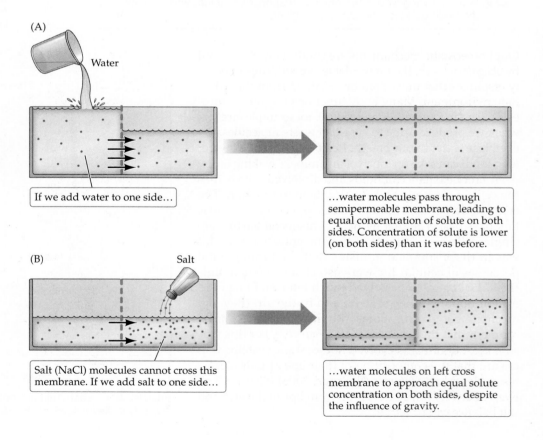

(A)

Water

If we add water to one side…

…water molecules pass through semipermeable membrane, leading to equal concentration of solute on both sides. Concentration of solute is lower (on both sides) than it was before.

(B)

Salt

Salt (NaCl) molecules cannot cross this membrane. If we add salt to one side…

…water molecules on left cross membrane to approach equal solute concentration on both sides, despite the influence of gravity.

Normally the concentration of salt (sodium chloride, or NaCl) in the extracellular fluid of mammals is about 0.9% (which means there's about 0.9 gram of NaCl for every 100 milliliters of water). A solution with this concentration of salt is called *physiological saline* or described as *isotonic*. Because water moves to produce uniform saltiness (see Figure 9.5), cells will lose water if placed in a saltier solution and will gain water in a less salty solution. If excessive, this movement of water will damage or kill the cell. The extracellular fluid serves as a *buffer*, a reservoir of isotonic fluid that provides and accepts water molecules, so cells can maintain proper internal conditions and prevent such damage. The nervous system uses two cues to ensure that the extracellular compartment has about the right amount of water and solute, as we'll see next.

osmotic thirst A desire to ingest fluids that is stimulated by high concentration of solute (like salt) in the extracellular compartment.

osmosensory neuron A specialized neuron that monitors the concentration of the extracellular fluid by measuring the movement of water into and out of the intracellular compartment.

Osmotic thirst occurs when the extracellular fluid becomes too salty

The brain contains a dedicated network that carefully monitors the quantity and concentration of the fluid in our bodies and triggers thirst to stimulate the intake of more water when needed (Zimmerman et al., 2017). Most of the time, we feel thirsty because of the obligatory water losses we mentioned earlier—through respiration, urination, and so on—in which more water is lost than salt. In this case, not only is the *volume* of the extracellular fluid *decreased*, but also the solute *concentration* of the extracellular fluid is *increased*. As a result of the increase in extracellular saltiness, water is pulled out of cells through osmosis and we experience **osmotic thirst** (**FIGURE 9.6A**). Another thing that can make the extracellular fluid more concentrated is eating a lot of salty food. Once again, water will be drawn out of cells through osmosis. This loss of intracellular water triggers osmotic thirst, and we want to drink water in order to return the extracellular fluid to a comfortable isotonic state.

Specialized **osmosensory neurons**—neurons that specifically monitor the concentration of the extracellular fluid—are found in numerous regions of the hypothalamus, including the preoptic area, the anterior hypothalamus, and the supraoptic nucleus. Osmosensory neurons are also found in the *organum vasculosum of the lamina terminalis (OVLT)*, one of a set of specialized brain structures, called the

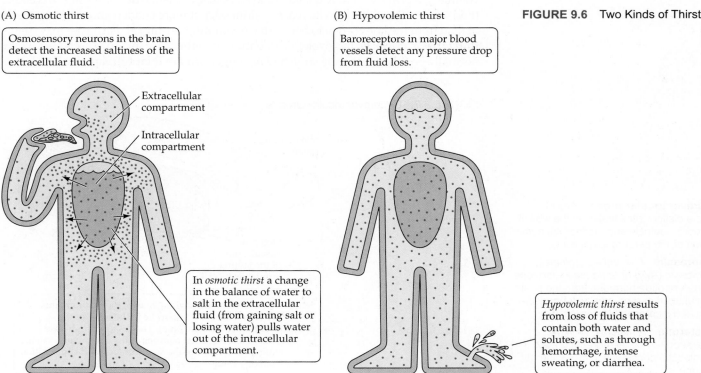

(A) Osmotic thirst

Osmosensory neurons in the brain detect the increased saltiness of the extracellular fluid.

Extracellular compartment

Intracellular compartment

In *osmotic thirst* a change in the balance of water to salt in the extracellular fluid (from gaining salt or losing water) pulls water out of the intracellular compartment.

(B) Hypovolemic thirst

Baroreceptors in major blood vessels detect any pressure drop from fluid loss.

Hypovolemic thirst results from loss of fluids that contain both water and solutes, such as through hemorrhage, intense sweating, or diarrhea.

FIGURE 9.6 Two Kinds of Thirst

circumventricular organs, that monitor the fluid balance of the body (**FIGURE 9.7**). Outputs from the circumventricular organs project to multiple cortical regions, including the insula and anterior cingulate cortex, leading to the conscious perception of thirst (Farrell et al., 2011; McKinley et al., 2019). One of the brain's primary thirst responses is increased release of the posterior pituitary hormone **vasopressin** (also called *arginine vasopressin* [*AVP*] or *antidiuretic hormone* [*ADH*]; *diuresis* refers to the production of urine), which acts on the kidneys to slow the production of urine by increasing the reabsorption of water.

Because osmotic forces are continually driving water into and out of cells, it is not enough to just control the intake of pure water; we must also regulate the intake and excretion of salt (NaCl). We cannot maintain water in the extracellular compartment without solutes; if the extracellular compartment contained pure water, osmotic pressure would drive it into the cells until they ruptured and died. In fact, the amount of water that we can retain is determined primarily by the number of Na^+ ions we possess. That's why thirst is quenched more effectively by very slightly salty drinks (like sports drinks) than by pure water. But saltier water, like seawater, has the reverse effect. Seawater is hypertonic (saltier than our body fluids), so just like eating salty food, drinking seawater causes ever-worsening osmotic thirst. Lacking the specialized salt-excreting organs that marine animals have evolved, we simply can't get rid of excess salt fast enough to survive on seawater.

Some Na^+ loss is inevitable, as during urination or sweating. When water is scarce, the body tries to conserve Na^+ in order to retain water. One way this is accomplished is through the release of the steroid hormone **aldosterone** from the adrenal glands. Aldosterone directly stimulates the kidneys to conserve Na^+, and it also contributes to the salt appetite that powerfully drives animals to find additional salt in their environments (de Kloet and Joëls, 2017).

Hypovolemic thirst is triggered by a loss of fluid volume

A second signal that triggers thirst involves not salt balance or osmosis, but rather a decrease in the overall volume of the extracellular fluid, called *hypovolemia* (literally "low volume"). Normal everyday obligatory losses cause moderate decreases in extracellular fluid volume (in addition to increased saltiness), but more sudden and dramatic losses of fluid from the body—due to hemorrhage, vomiting, sustained diarrhea—may trigger thirst that is *primarily* hypovolemic in nature. In either case, blood vessels that would normally be full and slightly stretched no longer contain their full capacity. The loss of

circumventricular organ Any of multiple distinct sites that lie in the wall of a cerebral ventricle and monitor the composition of the cerebrospinal fluid.

vasopressin Also called *arginine vasopressin* (*AVP*) or *antidiuretic hormone* (*ADH*). A peptide hormone from the posterior pituitary that promotes water conservation and increases blood pressure.

aldosterone A mineralocorticoid hormone, secreted by the adrenal cortex, that promotes the conservation of sodium by the kidneys.

FIGURE 9.7 Circumventricular Organs

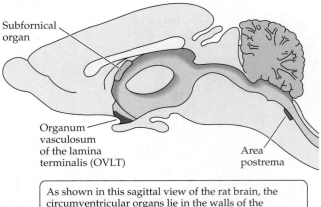

Subfornical organ

Organum vasculosum of the lamina terminalis (OVLT)

Area postrema

As shown in this sagittal view of the rat brain, the circumventricular organs lie in the walls of the ventricular system (blue). Thanks to a diminished blood-brain barrier, neurons of the circumventricular organs can monitor the concentration and composition of body fluids.

body fluids, and resultant decrease in extracellular volume and blood pressure, cause the individual to experience **hypovolemic thirst** (**FIGURE 9.6B**)—sometimes very powerfully, if the hemorrhage or other volume loss is severe enough. Note that a decrease in fluid volume from blood loss (or from severe diarrhea or vomiting) does not necessarily change the *concentration* of the extracellular fluid, because salts and other ions are lost along with the water (see Figure 9.6B).

The initial drop in extracellular volume is detected by pressure receptors, called **baroreceptors**, which are located in major blood vessels and in the heart. Reacting to the signal from the baroreceptors, the brain activates a variety of responses, such as thirst (to replace the lost water) and salt hunger (to replace the solutes that have been lost along with the water). Replacing the water without also replacing the salts would result in *hypotonic* (less salty than normal) extracellular fluid. The sympathetic nervous system also stimulates muscles in the artery walls to constrict, reducing the size of the vessels and partly compensating for the reduced volume.

Finally, several different organs respond by altering hormonal release. The heart decreases its secretion of **atrial natriuretic peptide** (**ANP**), which normally reduces blood pressure, inhibits drinking, and promotes the excretion of water and salt at the kidneys. The brain's posterior pituitary gland releases more vasopressin, and the kidneys trigger the production of **angiotensin II** (**AII**) from a precursor circulating in the bloodstream.

Angiotensin II has several water-conserving actions. By directly constricting blood vessels, AII increases blood pressure, ensuring that the brain and vital organs continue to receive essential materials for as long as possible. AII further stimulates the release of vasopressin and of aldosterone (discussed above) and acts directly on the brain, at the POA and at the circumventricular organs, to stimulate thirst and drinking behavior (Daniels and Marshall, 2012; Augustine et al., 2018) (**FIGURE 9.8**).

We don't stop drinking just because the throat and mouth are wet

Although plausible, the most obvious explanation of why we stop drinking—that we have dampened our previously dry throat and mouth—is insufficient. Classic research showed that thirsty animals allowed to drink water, but not *consume* water—because the water is diverted out of the esophagus before reaching the stomach—remain thirsty and continue drinking. However, researchers also know that a drink of water is more thirst quenching if taken by mouth than if infused directly into the stomach (N. E. Miller et al., 1957). So, provided that water actually reaches the stomach, oral sensations must play *some* role in reducing thirst. Further, although we stop drinking before most water has left the gastrointestinal tract and entered the extracellular compartment, gut neurons monitor the saltiness of the fluid in the stomach and intestine and communicate this information to the brain via the **vagus nerve** (Zimmerman et al., 2019). There, drinking behavior is governed by neurons within the *subfornical organ*—one of the circumventricular organs—and drinking is stopped in *anticipation* of correcting the extracellular volume and/or the concentration of solutes (Zimmerman et al., 2016; Augustine et al., 2018). Thus, experience may teach us how to gauge accurately whether we've ingested enough to counteract our thirst. Normally, all the signals—blood volume, solute concentration, moisture in the mouth, estimates of the amount of water we've ingested that's "on the way"—are in agreement, but the cessation of one signal alone will not stop thirst; in this way, animals ensure against dehydration.

hypovolemic thirst   A desire to ingest fluids that is stimulated by a reduction in volume of the extracellular fluid.

baroreceptor   A pressure receptor in the heart or a major artery that detects a change in blood pressure.

atrial natriuretic peptide (ANP) A hormone, secreted by the heart, that normally reduces blood pressure, inhibits drinking, and promotes the excretion of water and salt at the kidneys.

angiotensin II (AII)   A hormone produced in the blood by the action of renin and that may play a role in the control of thirst.

vagus nerve   Cranial nerve X, which transmits information between the brain and the viscera.

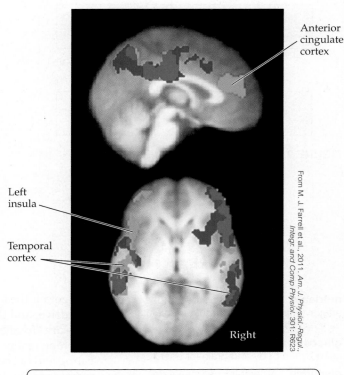

From M. J. Farrell et al., 2011, Am. J. Physiol.–Regul., Integr. and Comp. Physiol. 301: R623

These fMRI images show cortical regions selectively activated in thirsty subjects in green. Blue shows regions activated after drinking water, and red shows regions that are active in both states. Regions showing activation that is specific to strong thirst include the anterior cingulate (top) and the left insula (bottom), along with temporal regions.

FIGURE 9.8   Feeling Thirsty Patterns of brain activity in thirsty participants before and after drinking water.

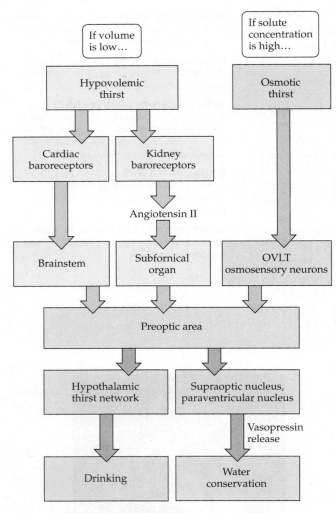

FIGURE 9.9 An Overview of Fluid Regulation

Thirst is a homeostatic signal that intrudes forcefully into consciousness, with associated strong activation of certain brain regions, particularly in the limbic system (Denton et al., 1999). The two types of thirst (osmotic and hypovolemic), the two fluid compartments (extracellular and intracellular), and the multiple redundant methods to conserve water make for a fairly complicated system that is not yet fully understood. The current conceptualization of this system is depicted in **FIGURE 9.9**. Our need to compensate for obligatory losses is also crucial to understanding energy regulation, as we'll see in the next section.

HOW'S IT GOING ?

1. After so many millions of years of evolution, why do we still have body fluids with composition resembling dilute seawater?
2. Briefly describe diffusion and osmosis, and define *osmotic pressure*. How do these relate to the composition of fluids in the intracellular versus extracellular compartments?
3. What is the normal concentration of salt in extracellular fluid? What happens to cells if the saltiness of the extracellular fluid increases or decreases?
4. Distinguish between hypovolemic and osmotic thirst, and identify the physiological sensors that detect each condition.
5. Why do we sometimes get hungry for salt?

9.3 Our Bodies Regulate Energy Balance and Nutrient Intake to Serve Current Needs and Prepare for Future Demands

THE ROAD AHEAD

We now turn to the topic of energy homeostasis. By the end of this section, you should be able to:

9.3.1 Define basal metabolism, and discuss its role in dieting and weight loss.

9.3.2 Discuss the importance of circulating glucose and bodily mechanisms of energy storage.

9.3.3 Summarize the relationship between insulin secretion and energy utilization by cells.

nutrients   Chemicals required for the effective functioning, growth, and maintenance of the body.

glucose   An important sugar molecule used by the body and brain for energy.

glycogen   A complex carbohydrate made by the combining of glucose molecules for a short-term store of energy.

insulin   A pancreatic hormone that lowers blood glucose, promotes energy storage, and facilitates glucose utilization by cells.

glucagon   A pancreatic hormone that converts glycogen to glucose and thus increases blood glucose.

Hunger for the food that we need to build, maintain, and fuel our bodies is a compelling drive, and the delicious flavors of foods provide powerful reward signals. Most of us are "foodies" to some extent, consuming "food porn," trying new recipes, and watching reality TV shows in which chefs try to outcook each other. The regulation of eating and of body energy, compared with regulation of drinking, involves even more redundancy and a more complex set of homeostatic mechanisms. The added complexity is due to the fact that the brain must monitor and regulate a wide range of **nutrients** (chemicals required for the effective functioning, growth, and maintenance of the body), including more than 20 amino acids (of which 9 *essential amino acids* cannot be synthesized by the body) and a variety of vitamins and minerals, as well as carbohydrates (sugars and starches) for energy. No animal can afford to run out of energy or nutrients, so we need systems to anticipate future needs and keep a reserve on hand (but not *too* much!). (For more information about the complexity and variation in the nutrient needs of different species, see **A STEP FURTHER 9.3**, on the website.)

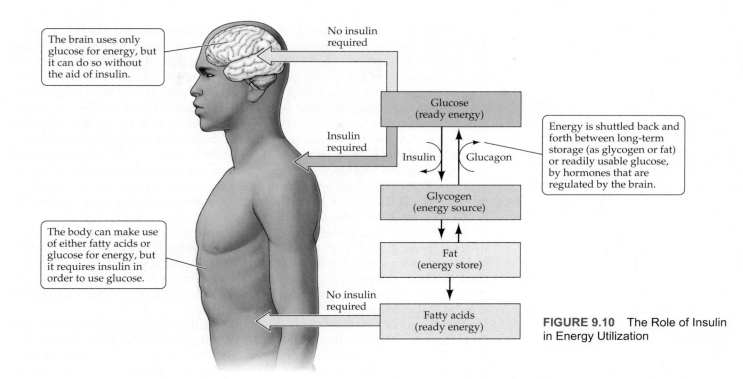

The brain uses only glucose for energy, but it can do so without the aid of insulin.

No insulin required

Insulin required

The body can make use of either fatty acids or glucose for energy, but it requires insulin in order to use glucose.

No insulin required

Glucose (ready energy)

Insulin   Glucagon

Energy is shuttled back and forth between long-term storage (as glycogen or fat) or readily usable glucose, by hormones that are regulated by the brain.

Glycogen (energy source)

Fat (energy store)

Fatty acids (ready energy)

FIGURE 9.10   The Role of Insulin in Energy Utilization

The principal fuel for the cells of the body is **glucose**, a simple sugar that is obtained through the breakdown of more-complex molecules. We need a steady supply of circulating glucose between meals, strictly maintained within an optimal range, and may also experience elevated demand for fuel at other times—for example, during intense physical activity—so several mechanisms have evolved for short- and long-term storage of excess fuel. For shorter-term storage, glucose can be converted into a more complex molecule called **glycogen** and stored as reserve fuel in several locations, notably the liver and skeletal muscles. This process, called *glycogenesis*, is promoted by the hormone **insulin**, which is synthesized and released by the pancreas. When blood glucose levels drop too low, a second pancreatic hormone, **glucagon**, converts glycogen back into glucose (a process called *glycogenolysis*; **FIGURE 9.10**). For longer-term storage, molecules of **lipid** (fat) from dietary sources or created from surplus sugars and other nutrients are stored in **adipose tissue** (commonly called *fat tissue*). Under conditions of prolonged food deprivation, body fat can be converted into glucose—a process called *gluconeogenesis*—and a secondary form of fuel, called **ketones**, which can similarly be utilized by the body and brain.

Only about 10–20% of the energy in food is used for active behavioral processes. The majority of food energy is spent on **basal metabolism**: the basic physiological processes of life, like heat production (the price we pay for endothermy), cellular activity, and maintenance of membrane potentials. Metabolism is under homeostatic control and can be adjusted to a surprising extent, but it is outside our conscious control. An all-too-familiar consequence of this metabolic flexibility is that the body tends to resist either losing or gaining weight following dietary changes (**FIGURE 9.11**).

lipid   A large molecule (frequently a fat) that consists of fatty acids and glycerol. Lipids are insoluble in water.

adipose tissue   Commonly called *fat tissue*. Tissue made up of fat cells.

ketone   An organic molecule, derived from the breakdown of fat, that can be used by cells as an energy source.

basal metabolism   The use of energy for processes such as heat production, maintenance of membrane potentials, and all the other basic life-sustaining functions of the body.

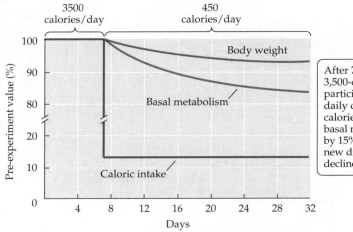

After 7 days on a rich 3,500-calorie diet, six obese participants reduced their daily calories by 87%, to 450 calories per day. However, basal metabolism also declined by 15%; so after 3 weeks on the new diet, body weight had declined by only 6%.

FIGURE 9.11   Why Losing Weight Is So Difficult   (After G. A. Bray, 1969. *Lancet* 2: 397.)

To the frustration of dieters everywhere, many studies show that a calorie-reduced diet prompts the body to reduce its basal metabolic rate, which in turn slows the loss of weight (C. K. Martin et al., 2007). Along with the other *Biggest Loser* contestants, Danny C., whom we met at the outset of the chapter, has learned the hard way that our brains and bodies vigorously defend our energy balance and body weight, even if we are obese. Due to a dramatic decrease in his basal metabolism following weight loss—a process called *metabolic adaptation*—Danny now needs to consume 800 fewer calories per day than the typical man, just to maintain his current 295-pound body weight. And to make matters worse, this metabolic adaptation is annoyingly persistent; even after 6 long years, the metabolisms of the other contestants also remained very low (**FIGURE 9.12**) as their brains continued to try to regain the lost weight (Fothergill et al., 2016). A major goal for researchers is thus to discover a way to reset the body's set point (or set zone) for energy storage.

An additional topic under debate is whether the concept of a set point, borrowed from engineering, really fits very well with observations from studying obesity, where body weight seems to drift steadily upward (Müller et al., 2018). Some researchers now think that body composition instead reflects a "settling point," where a complex set of physiological, behavioral, and social factors combine to determine body weight and resist radical losses or gains (Speakman et al., 2011).

Theories about how to best lose weight through dieting are endlessly popular topics in the mass media. Although it is counterintuitive, some evidence suggests that diets low in carbohydrates, and correspondingly high in fats and proteins, can help people lose weight and also may increase serum levels of "good" cholesterol while decreasing serum fats (G. D. Foster et al., 2003; Samaha et al., 2003). However, long-term studies will be required to establish the overall safety of low-carbohydrate diets.

The only certain way to lose weight is to decrease the number of calories taken in and/or increase the number of calories spent in physical activity, and for the weight loss to be permanent, these changes in diet and activity must be permanent too. As an added bonus, research with monkeys suggests that long-term restriction of caloric intake can slow the aging process and reduce the prevalence of disease (Colman et al., 2014; Mattson and Arumugam, 2018). And while the effects of caloric restriction on human aging remain to be established, researchers have reported that restricted food intake may have some beneficial effects on cognitive performance in elderly participants, at least over the short term (Witte et al., 2009; Prehn et al., 2017).

FIGURE 9.12 Metabolic Adaptation in the Biggest Losers (After E. Fothergill et al., 2016. *Obesity* 24: 1612.)

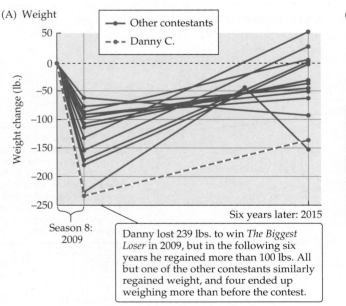

(A) Weight

Danny lost 239 lbs. to win *The Biggest Loser* in 2009, but in the following six years he regained more than 100 lbs. All but one of the other contestants similarly regained weight, and four ended up weighing more than before the contest.

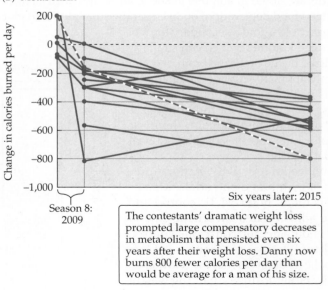

(B) Metabolism

The contestants' dramatic weight loss prompted large compensatory decreases in metabolism that persisted even six years after their weight loss. Danny now burns 800 fewer calories per day than would be average for a man of his size.

Insulin is essential for obtaining, storing, and using food energy

In addition to converting surplus glucose into glycogen, as we discussed earlier, insulin has another critical function: your body needs insulin to make any use of the circulating glucose (brain cells are an important exception; they can use glucose without the aid of insulin). That's because *glucose transporters*—the membrane-spanning proteins that most cells use to import glucose from the blood—need insulin in order to function properly. The disease **diabetes mellitus** results from a lack of insulin production (in the *type 1*, or *juvenile-onset*, variety of the disease) or from greatly reduced tissue sensitivity to insulin (*type 2*, or *adult-onset*, diabetes, which is often associated with obesity). Although the brain can still make use of glucose from the diet, the rest of the body cannot and is forced to use energy from fatty acids while glucose builds up in the blood, resulting in gradual severe damage to many tissues.

Insulin release around mealtimes is so important that it is triggered by several different mechanisms at different points in time. First comes the *cephalic phase* of insulin release, triggered by sights, smells, and tastes that we have learned to associate with food (*cephalic* means "of the head"). Then, during the *digestive phase,* food entering the digestive tract prompts an additional release of insulin. We now know that the digestive tract contains the same sort of sweet taste receptors as are found on the tongue, and it uses them to help regulate insulin release (Kokrashvili et al., 2009). Finally, during the *absorptive phase*, as digested food is absorbed into the bloodstream, specialized liver cells called **glucodetectors** detect the increase in circulating glucose and signal the pancreas to release still more insulin. The liver communicates with the pancreas via the nervous system. Information from glucodetectors in the liver travels via the vagus nerve to the *nucleus of the solitary tract* (*NST*) in the brainstem and is relayed to the hypothalamus (Maniscalco and Rinaman, 2018). This system informs the brain of circulating glucose levels and contributes to hunger, as we'll discuss shortly.

Given the crucial role of insulin in mobilizing and distributing food energy, and its fluctuations in association with feeding, it might seem an obvious candidate for signaling the brain to start or stop eating. Lowering an animal's blood insulin level does cause it to become hungry and eat a large meal, and injecting some insulin causes the animal to eat much less. But injecting a larger dose of insulin doesn't produce fully satiated animals; instead, they become hungry again and eat a large meal! The reason for this surprising result is that the high insulin levels direct much of the blood glucose into storage, which means that there is *less* glucose in circulation. The brain learns of this condition, called *hypoglycemia*, directly via glucodetectors, leading to a hunger response. And while it is certainly important, glucose can't be the sole appetite signal either, because people with untreated diabetes have very high levels of circulating glucose yet are constantly hungry. Somehow the brain integrates insulin and glucose

diabetes mellitus A condition, characterized by excessive glucose in the blood and urine and by reduced glucose utilization by body cells, that is caused by the failure of insulin to induce glucose absorption.

glucodetector A specialized type of liver cell that detects and informs the nervous system about levels of circulating glucose.

Not Too Sweet People with type 1 diabetes mellitus must receive insulin in order to utilize glucose. Taking insulin requires careful monitoring of blood glucose and, as shown here, self-administration via (A) daily injections or (B) drug pumps to infuse insulin throughout the day. Until the 1920s, when insulin was discovered as a result of experiments on dogs, this form of diabetes was a dreaded killer of children. (C) In an especially dramatic moment in science, three of the Canadian discoverers of insulin—Frederick Banting (right), Charles Best (left), and James Collip (not pictured)—went through a hospital ward full of dying diabetic children, injecting them with the newly purified hormone. By the time the last child had been injected, the first was already waking up from a diabetic coma. The discovery saved millions of lives and garnered a Nobel Prize in 1923.

(A)

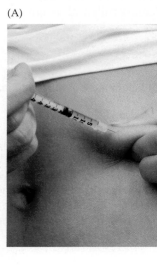

© Dmitry Lobanov/Shutterstock

(B)

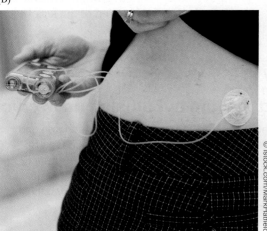

© istock.com/MarkHatfield

(C)

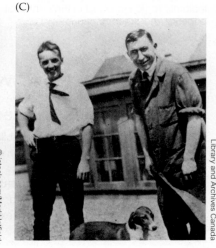

Library and Archives Canada

levels with other sources of information to decide whether to initiate eating. As we'll see next, this has become a central theme in research on appetite control—that the brain integrates many different signals rather than relying exclusively on any single signal to trigger hunger.

HOW'S IT GOING ?

1. Provide a review of how glucose is used, stored, and retrieved from storage. Be sure to identify the roles of pancreatic hormones in each step.
2. What is basal metabolism? How is it affected by homeostatic processes, and how does the homeostatic regulation of metabolism frustrate efforts to lose weight?
3. Define the types of diabetes mellitus, and discuss their causes. What are some of the ways that insulin release is normally controlled?
4. Discuss the evidence about whether blood levels of insulin and glucose directly control hunger.

9.4 The Hypothalamus Coordinates Multiple Systems That Control Hunger

THE ROAD AHEAD

There has been rapid progress in understanding the multiply redundant hypothalamic mechanisms for regulating appetite. After studying this section, you should be able to:

9.4.1 Summarize the historical evidence that hunger signals converge on the hypothalamus.

9.4.2 Identify and briefly describe the actions of major hormonal appetite signals.

9.4.3 Provide an overview of the hypothalamic appetite controller, including the organization of its neurons, and the signals it receives from the body.

9.4.4 Discuss some additional, redundant appetite signals.

9.4.5 Define the gut microbiome, and discuss some of the ways it may interact with the nervous system.

ventromedial hypothalamus (VMH) A hypothalamic region involved in eating and sexual behaviors.

lateral hypothalamus (LH) A hypothalamic region involved in the control of appetite and other functions.

Although no single brain region has exclusive control of appetite, decades of research in the twentieth century established that the hypothalamus is critically important for regulating metabolic rate, food intake, and body weight. In this classic research, scientists found that lesions in the hypothalamus of rats could induce either chronic hunger and massive weight gain, or chronic satiety (feeling full) and severe weight loss, depending on the location of the lesion.

RESEARCHERS AT WORK ||||||||||||||||||||||||||||||||||||||||||||||||||||||||||||||||||||||||||||||||||||||||||||||||||||

Lesion studies showed that the hypothalamus is crucial for appetite

Early researchers made discrete bilateral lesions in the hypothalamus—in either the **ventromedial hypothalamus (VMH)** or the **lateral hypothalamus (LH)**—of rats (**FIGURE 9.13**). After recovery, VMH-lesioned rats ate to excess and became obese (Hetherington and Ranson, 1940), leading researchers to suggest that the VMH is the *satiety center* of the brain (because the rats didn't show evidence of satiety once the VMH was gone). Rats with LH lesions, conversely, ceased eating and rapidly lost weight, suggesting that the LH acts as a *hunger center* (because rats who lost their LH stopped acting hungry) (Anand and Brobeck, 1951). So, an early model of feeding behavior featured the

VMH and LH acting in opposition to control appetite.

It soon became clear that this dual-center model of appetite was too simple. For one thing, although the VMH was identified as a satiety center, its destruction did not create out-of-control feeding machines. Instead, VMH-lesioned animals exhibited a period of rapid weight gain but then stabilized at a new, higher level. When obese VMH-lesioned animals were forced to either gain or lose weight through dietary manipulation, they returned to their new "normal" weight as soon as they were allowed to eat freely again. So, because VMH-lesioned rats experienced satiety, the VMH cannot be the sole satiety controller.

Similarly, although they initially stopped eating, LH-lesioned rats that were kept alive with a feeding tube soon resumed eating and drinking, and their body weight eventually stabilized at a new, lower level. As with the VMH-lesioned animals, LH-lesioned animals that were later forced to gain weight would swiftly return to their new, lower set point for body weight after they returned to eating at will (see Figure 9.13) (Keesey, 1980). Researchers thus realized that the hypothalamic system controlling feeding must involve multiple components that coordinate to establish a set point for metabolic fuels, monitor energy balance in the body, and trigger behavioral responses to meet the established energy goals, with a collective effect on body weight.

■ **Hypothesis**
The hypothalamus contains discrete systems for controlling hunger and satiety.

■ **Test**
Place small lesions in target areas within the hypothalamus.

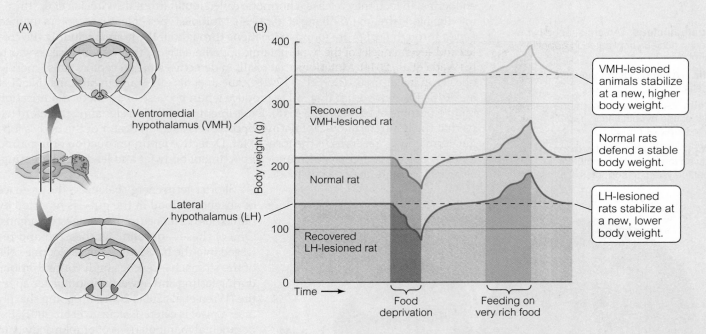

(A) Ventromedial hypothalamus (VMH)

Lateral hypothalamus (LH)

(B) Body weight (g) — 400, 300, 200, 100, 0

Recovered VMH-lesioned rat

Normal rat

Recovered LH-lesioned rat

Time →

Food deprivation

Feeding on very rich food

VMH-lesioned animals stabilize at a new, higher body weight.

Normal rats defend a stable body weight.

LH-lesioned rats stabilize at a new, lower body weight.

■ **Result**
Animals with lesions of the lateral hypothalamus (LH) decrease their food intake and rapidly lose weight, but they eventually stabilize at a new, lower weight. Following recovery, LH-lesioned animals forced to gain or lose weight return to the new lower weight when allowed to feed freely. Animals with lesions of the ventromedial hypothalamus (VMH) increase their food intake and rapidly gain weight, but they eventually stabilize at a new, higher weight. Following recovery, VMH-lesioned animals forced to gain or lose weight return to their new higher weight when allowed to feed freely.

■ **Conclusion**
The LH and VMH appear to play a role in appetite and body weight control, but because LH- and VMH-lesioned animals eventually show hunger and satiety, these two hypothalamic centers alone cannot constitute the entire appetite control system.

FIGURE 9.13 Lesion Studies Revealed That the Hypothalamus Is Involved in Appetite (After R. E. Keesey and P. C. Boyle, 1973. *J. Comp. Physiol. Psychol.* 84: 38 and D. Sclafani et al., 1976. *Physiol. Behav.* 16: 631.)

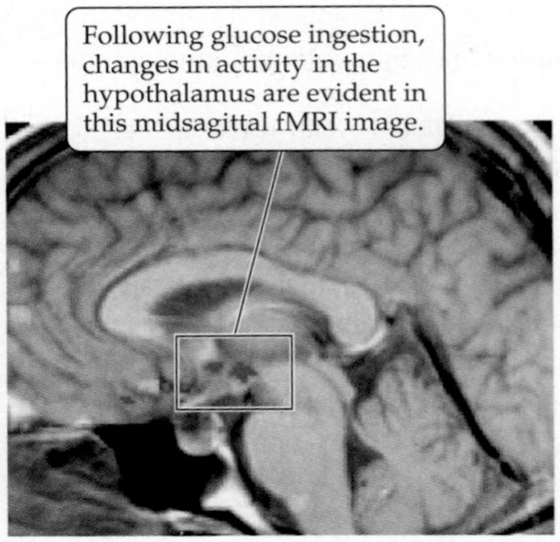

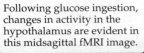

Following glucose ingestion, changes in activity in the hypothalamus are evident in this midsagittal fMRI image.

From Y. Liu et al., 2000. *Nature* 405: 1058

FIGURE 9.14   Sweet Spot

arcuate nucleus   An arc-shaped hypothalamic nucleus implicated in appetite control.

leptin   A peptide hormone released by fat cells.

ghrelin   A peptide gut hormone believed to act on the hypothalamic appetite system to increase hunger.

PYY$_{3\text{-}36}$ A peptide gut hormone believed to act on the hypothalamic appetite system to suppress appetite.

By demonstrating that the hypothalamus contains distinct components of an appetite control network, the early work on hunger and satiety provided a framework for subsequent research. For example, fMRI studies show that elevations in circulating glucose after a period of fasting produce large changes in the activity of the human hypothalamus (**FIGURE 9.14**), probably acting via hypothalamic glucodetector neurons that directly monitor blood levels of glucose (Parton et al., 2007). Today it is clear that the hypothalamic control of feeding is quite complicated and, as we will see shortly, exhibits considerable redundancy as a safety measure.

Hormones from the body drive a hypothalamic appetite controller

A spate of discoveries has sharpened our understanding of the hypothalamic control of appetite. This evidence indicates that a circuit within the **arcuate nucleus** of the hypothalamus is the key element in a highly specialized appetite network integrating peptide hormone signals from several sites in the body. One important source of information about energy stores is the pancreas; we have already discussed how the pancreatic hormone insulin signals the state of glucose circulating in the blood. Other information about energy balance—especially short-term and long-term reserves—comes in the form of hormonal secretions from elsewhere in the body, particularly the digestive organs and fat tissue.

You may be surprised to learn that the fat cells that make up adipose tissue are endocrine; in fact, they release a hormone called **leptin** (from the Greek *leptos*, "thin") into the bloodstream (Y. Zhang et al., 1994). Multiple types of leptin receptors (named *LepRa* through *LepRf*) are found in locations throughout the brain, including the cortex and several nuclei of the hypothalamic appetite network that we will discuss shortly (Wada et al., 2014). Mutations that result in defective leptin receptors cause morbid obesity in lab animals (Roh et al., 2018; Zabeau et al., 2019) and in humans (Niazi et al., 2018). Likewise, mice that fail to produce leptin because of a genetic modification rapidly become obese (**FIGURE 9.15**). Experiments with leptin signaling therefore tell us that the brain monitors circulating leptin levels as an indicator of the body's longer-term energy reserves in the form of fat. Defective leptin production or impaired leptin sensitivity causes a false underreporting of body fat and leads to overeating, especially of high-fat or sugary foods.

Shorter-term energy balance—the presence or absence of food in the gut—is reported by numerous hormones from the digestive organs. One of these—**ghrelin**, synthesized and released into the bloodstream by endocrine cells of the stomach—reaches high concentrations during fasting and powerfully stimulates appetite (Wren et al., 2000, 2001), dropping sharply after a meal is eaten (Nakazato et al., 2001). Experimental manipulations of ghrelin activity in the brains of hamsters alter their foraging and feeding behaviors, illustrating the importance of ghrelin for stimulating food intake (M. A. Thomas et al., 2016).

Conversely, several intestinal hormones are candidate satiety signals. For example, the actions of the awkwardly named intestinal peptide **PYY$_{3\text{-}36}$** may be the converse of ghrelin's actions, with PYY$_{3\text{-}36}$ spiking to higher levels on ingestion of a meal and providing an appetite-*suppressing* signal (Karra et al., 2009). Injections of ghrelin cause increased appetite and feeding in rats or humans, and injections

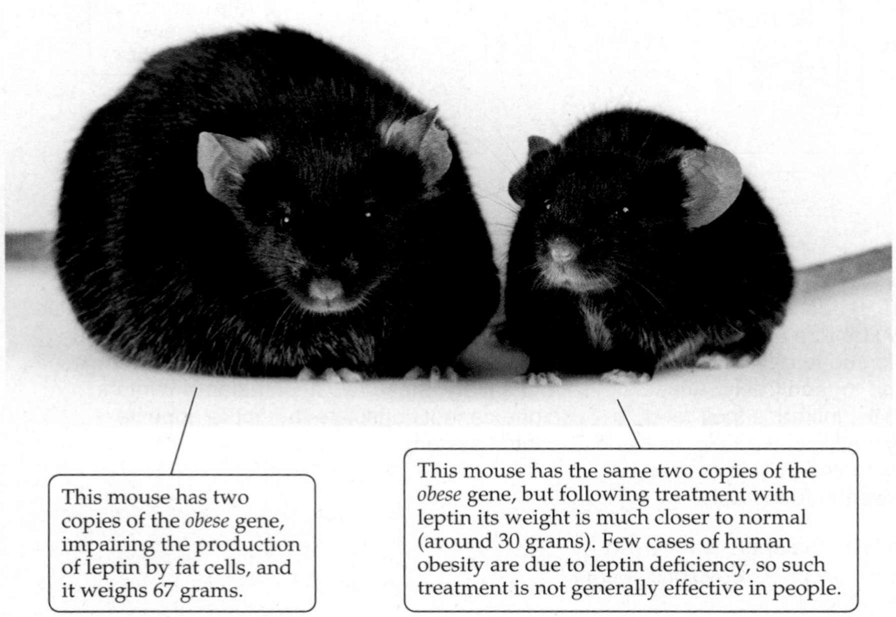

© Janson George/Shutterstock.com

This mouse has two copies of the *obese* gene, impairing the production of leptin by fat cells, and it weighs 67 grams.

This mouse has the same two copies of the *obese* gene, but following treatment with leptin its weight is much closer to normal (around 30 grams). Few cases of human obesity are due to leptin deficiency, so such treatment is not generally effective in people.

FIGURE 9.15   Inherited Obesity Can Be Overcome

of PYY$_{3-36}$ into the bloodstream or directly into the arcuate nucleus curb appetite (Chelikani et al., 2005; Baynes et al., 2006). Furthermore, ghrelin is chronically slightly elevated in obese people, and PYY$_{3-36}$ is chronically lowered—possibly causing continual hunger (English et al., 2002).

Like PYY$_{3-36}$, the intestinal hormone **glucagon-like peptide 1** (**GLP-1**) shows a rapid increase in secretion during a meal, especially if the meal is high in fats and carbohydrates. The release of GLP-1 is initially governed by a rapid autonomic neural mechanism, and then by the presence of nutrients in the intestinal tract (E. W. L. Sun et al., 2019). Receptors for GLP-1 are found in several brain regions implicated in food intake (Knudsen et al., 2016; Burmeister et al., 2017), mediating reductions in appetite and feeding, along with changes in the system that signals the rewarding aspects of food (Sekar et al., 2017; Yang et al., 2017). In addition, GLP-1 activity directly blocks the effects of ghrelin on metabolism and appetite (Abtahi et al., 2019).

The discoveries of PYY$_{3-36}$, ghrelin, and GLP-1 have provided important clues about the appetite control mystery, and these hormones converge on an appetite controller in the arcuate nucleus, so next we'll have a look at how that system seems to work.

A simplified (yes, really) view of the organization of the appetite control circuitry in the hypothalamus is illustrated in **FIGURE 9.16**. Within the arcuate nucleus, the system relies on two types of neurons with opposite effects. **POMC neurons** act as satiety

glucagon-like peptide 1 (GLP-1)
A peptide gut hormone believed to act on the hypothalamic appetite system to suppress appetite.

POMC neuron   A neuron, involved in the hypothalamic appetite control system, that produces both pro-opiomelanocortin and cocaine- and amphetamine-regulated transcript.

View Activity 9.1:
**An Appetite Controller
in the Hypothalamus**

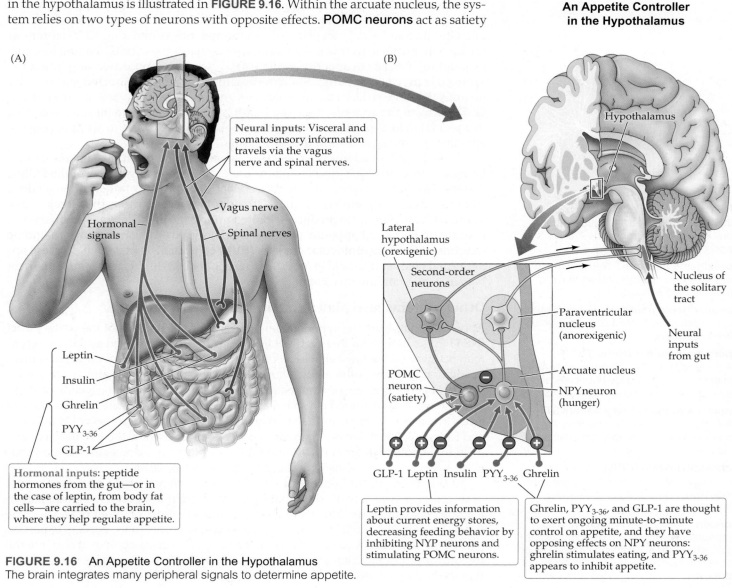

FIGURE 9.16   An Appetite Controller in the Hypothalamus
The brain integrates many peripheral signals to determine appetite.

neurons when activated, inhibiting appetite and increasing metabolism. However, neighboring **NPY neurons** act as hunger neurons when they are activated, stimulating appetite directly and also inhibiting the POMC neurons (thereby blocking satiety signals) and reducing metabolism. (In case you are wondering, these neurons get their names from the signaling compounds they produce: *pro-opiomelanocortin* in the case of POMC neurons, and *neuropeptide Y* for NPY neurons. POMC neurons also produce CART, short for *cocaine- and amphetamine-regulated transcript*, and NPY neurons also produce AgRP, short for *agouti-related peptide*. (These sorts of details are why graduate school takes so long.)

So how do the peripheral hormone signals interact with the arcuate-based appetite controller? As we've discussed, leptin levels (and to a lesser extent, insulin levels) in the blood convey information about the body's longer-term energy reserves, stored in fat cells. Leptin affects both types of arcuate appetite neurons, but in opposite ways. High circulating levels of leptin activate the POMC satiety neurons and simultaneously inhibit the NPY hunger neurons—so in both ways leptin is working to suppress hunger, and selective deletion of the leptin receptors on NPY neurons causes mice to rapidly become obese (Xu et al., 2018).

In contrast to leptin, the trio of gut hormones that we discussed earlier—ghrelin, PYY_{3-36}, and GLP-1—provide shorter-term, hour-to-hour hunger signals from the gut. Ghrelin and PYY_{3-36} act primarily on the appetite-stimulating NPY neurons of the arcuate nucleus. In this model, ghrelin stimulates these cells, leading to a corresponding increase in appetite, while PYY_{3-36} works in opposition, inhibiting the same cells to *reduce* appetite. Short-term effects on appetite exerted via the NPY neurons therefore reflect a balance between ghrelin and PYY_{3-36} activity. In contrast, GLP-1 acts on the appetite-reducing POMC cells of the arcuate nucleus, resulting in a reduction in appetite and food intake (Sekar et al., 2017), directly opposing the appetite-enhancing actions of the NPY system.

The net result of all this is a constant balancing act between the appetite-stimulating effects of the NPY system and the appetite-suppressing effects of the POMC system. Two nearby hypothalamic sites appear to be primary targets of projections from the arcuate appetite controller. **Orexigenic neurons** (from the Greek *orexis*, "appetite," and *genein*, "to produce"), located principally in the lateral hypothalamus, coordinate increased appetite and food intake signals. In contrast, **anorexigenic neurons** of the **paraventricular nucleus** (**PVN**) coordinate signals that decrease appetite and feeding (Garfield et al., 2015; Krashes et al., 2016) (refer to Figure 9.16B for help in understanding this circuit).

Other systems also play a role in hunger and satiety

Appetite signals from the hypothalamus converge on the **nucleus of the solitary tract** (**NST**) in the brainstem (see Figure 9.16B). The NST can be viewed as part of a common pathway for feeding behavior, receiving appetite signals from a variety of sources in addition to the hypothalamus. Thus, the sensation of hunger is affected by a wide variety of peripheral sensory inputs, such as oral stimulation and the feeling of stomach distension, transmitted via spinal and cranial nerves. Information about nutrient levels is conveyed directly from the body to the NST via the vagus nerve (Maniscalco and Rinaman, 2018). For example, various peptides released by the gut after feeding, including **cholecystokinin** (**CCK**) and GLP-1, act directly on receptors of the vagus nerve to alter appetite (Alhadeff et al., 2017; Huston et al., 2019).

In keeping with the concept of multiple redundancy that we discussed earlier in the chapter, a variety of additional signals and brain locations also participate in feeding behavior, either directly or through indirect effects on other processes. The peptide **orexin**, produced by neurons in the lateral hypothalamus, appears to participate in the subsequent control of feeding behavior. Direct injection of orexin into the hypothalamus of rats increases feeding. And it probably won't surprise you to learn that the brain's reward system is intimately involved with feeding. Activity of a circuit

NPY neuron A neuron in the hypothalamic appetite control system, that produces both neuropeptide Y and agouti-related peptide.

orexigenic neurons Neurons of the hypothalamic appetite system that promote feeding behavior.

anorexigenic neurons Neurons of the hypothalamic appetite system that inhibit feeding behavior.

paraventricular nucleus (PVN) A nucleus of the hypothalamus involved in the release of peptide hormones and in the control of feeding and other behaviors.

nucleus of the solitary tract (NST) A complicated brainstem nucleus that receives visceral and taste information via several cranial nerves.

cholecystokinin (CCK) A peptide hormone that is released by the gut after ingestion of food that is high in protein and/or fat.

orexin Also called *hypocretin*. A neuropeptide produced in the hypothalamus that is involved in switching between sleep states, in narcolepsy, and in the control of appetite.

including the amygdala and the dopamine-mediated reward system of the nucleus accumbens (see Chapter 3) is hypothesized to mediate pleasurable aspects of feeding (Volkow and Wise, 2005).

The **endocannabinoid** system (see Chapter 3) likewise has a potent effect in appetite and feeding. Endocannabinoids, such as anandamide, are endogenous substances that act much like the active ingredient in cannabis (*Cannabis sativa*) and, like cannabis, can potently stimulate hunger. Acting both in the brain and in the periphery, endocannabinoids might stimulate feeding by affecting the mesolimbic dopamine reward system. However, injection of anandamide into the hypothalamus also stimulates eating (C. D. Chapman et al., 2012), confirming that endocannabinoids act directly on hypothalamic appetite mechanisms, while inhibiting satiety signals from the gut (Di Marzo and Matias, 2005). Cannabinoid drugs may be useful for stimulating appetite and weight gain in people who are having trouble maintaining their body weight because of cancer or other diseases (Horn et al., 2019; J. Wang et al., 2019).

Hypothalamic feeding control must be strongly influenced by inputs from higher brain centers, but little is known about these mechanisms. During development, for example, our feeding patterns are increasingly influenced by social factors such as parental and peer group pressures. Understanding the nature of cortical influences on feeding mechanisms is a major challenge for the future. The list of participants in appetite regulation is long and growing longer, revealing overlapping and complex controls with a high degree of redundancy, as befits a behavioral function of such critical importance to health and survival. There is also growing evidence that gut bacteria regulate body weight, as we'll see in Signs & Symptoms next.

endocannabinoid   An endogenous ligand of cannabinoid receptors, thus a cannabis analog that is produced by the brain.

gut microbiota   The microorganisms that normally inhabit the digestive system.

microbiome   The collective term for a population of microorganisms.

enterotype   Each individual's personal composition of the gut microbiota.

fecal transplantation   A medical procedure in which gut microbiota, via fecal matter, are transplanted from a donor to a host.

SIGNS & SYMPTOMS ||||||||||||||||||||||||||||||||||||||||||||||||||||||||||||||||||||||||||||||||||||||||||||||||||||||||||||||||||||||||||||||||||||||||||||||||||||||||

Friends with Benefits

Most people know that the gut is normally inhabited by helpful bacteria, but the extent of that occupation may surprise you. You probably contain in the range of 2.5–5 pounds of gut microbes: trillions of individual organisms belonging to dozens (perhaps hundreds) of different species of bacteria, fungi, and viruses, making up more than half the contents of your large intestine (Guarner and Malagelada, 2003). Put another way, you have more gut microbes than body cells, and they weigh more than your brain. This huge population, known as the **gut microbiota** or, collectively, as the **microbiome**, normally provide a variety of beneficial actions in return for their comfortable lodgings.

Each of us possesses a distinct microbial **enterotype**—a personal combination of different species of microbiota—that researchers increasingly believe to be in extensive two-way communication with our brain via the vagus nerve and chemical signals (Bonaz et al., 2018; Cussotto et al., 2018). Your enterotype reflects the history of your gut, so substantial changes in your diet, or the use of antibiotics to treat infections, can change the composition and health of the microbiome, with varying consequences for health (David et al., 2014; Wilson et al., 2020). Preliminary evidence has tentatively linked the microbiome enterotype to such diverse domains as mood, stress, social behavior, and cognitive functioning (Sylvia and Demas, 2018; Tetel

et al., 2018) and also various neurological conditions, including autism, schizophrenia, bipolar disorder, and Parkinson's disease (Fung et al., 2017; Tremlett et al., 2017). But one of the areas where an effect of changes in the gut microbiota may be most evident is obesity.

Feeding antibiotics to young mice, even at relatively low doses, changes gut microbiota and circulating hormones, leading to weight gain (I. Cho et al., 2012). Similarly, two studies looking at almost 40,000 babies have found that human infants given antibiotics in their first 6 months were statistically more likely to be overweight at age 7 (Ajslev et al., 2011; Trasande et al., 2013). It remains to be seen how much adult obesity is accounted for by long-lasting changes to our enterotypes, but it is at least possible that early exposure to antibiotics—or even chlorinated drinking water (because the whole point of adding chlorine is to kill bacteria)—is making some of us fat (L. M. Cox and Blaser, 2015). What can we do about it?

Scientists hope to turn our new knowledge of the connection between the gut and brain into novel treatments, such as drugs based on metabolites secreted by specific gut bacteria (Suez and Elinav, 2017). Researchers have also been investigating the possible benefits of a nasty-sounding procedure: **fecal transplantation**. Yes, it is just what it sounds like: feces are collected from carefully screened donors, processed to create a liquid

(Continued)

SIGNS & SYMPTOMS *(continued)* ||||||||||||||||||||||||||||||||||||||||||||||||||||||||||||||||||||||||||||||||||||||||||||||||||||||||||||||||||||||||

suspension, and then passed through a catheter into the colon of the recipient (**FIGURE 9.17**), where the donor's healthy enterotype establishes itself. Transplantation is an effective treatment for certain dangerous gut infections and may be effective in various diseases, including inflammatory bowel disease and type 2 diabetes (F. Yu et al., 2019; Zou et al., 2020). Initial findings suggest that fecal transplants improve metabolic function and other digestive processes in obese people (Vrieze et al., 2012; Z. Zhang et al., 2019). Although research on the topic is in its infancy, we can hope that our tiny passengers can someday be coaxed to pay their way by supplying benefits like weight loss and better brain health. Each new discovery brings us closer to developing safe and effective treatments for obesity and eating disorders, as we discuss next.

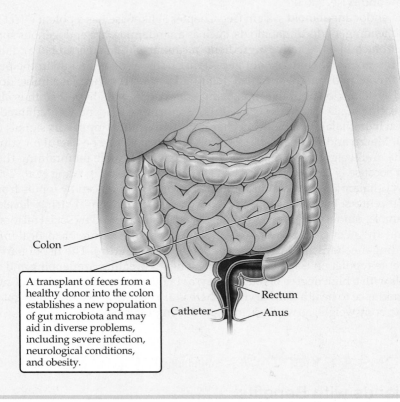

A transplant of feces from a healthy donor into the colon establishes a new population of gut microbiota and may aid in diverse problems, including severe infection, neurological conditions, and obesity.

FIGURE 9.17   Fecal Transplantation

HOW'S IT GOING ?

1. Review the early work implicating the LH and VMH in appetite control. Why did researchers abandon the view that the LH and VMH were the sole controllers of appetite and satiety?
2. Sketch or briefly describe the major components of the hypothalamic appetite controller, as currently understood.
3. Describe how the hypothalamic appetite controller functions during hunger, in contrast to just after a meal.
4. What is leptin? Discuss its origins in the body and its effects on feeding behavior.
5. What are some of the gut hormones that may be involved in appetite control, and what are they thought to do?
6. Briefly describe some of the additional (redundant) mechanisms of appetite control that supplement the hypothalamic appetite system. What is the basis of the increased appetite frequently experienced after use of cannabis?
7. Describe the makeup of the gut microbiome. What are some ways that the microbiome affects the brain and behavior?

9.5 Obesity and Eating Disorders Are Difficult to Treat

THE ROAD AHEAD

Problems with appetite, energy balance, and body weight are all too common. After reading this section, you will be able to:

9.5.1 Define overweight and obesity, with reference to BMI.

9.5.2 Describe and compare the various pharmacological and surgical approaches to treating obesity.

9.5.3 Discuss the symptoms, possible causes, and treatment of the major eating disorders: anorexia nervosa, bulimia, and binge eating disorder.

Unfortunately, effective treatments to aid weight loss have been elusive. In our modern world, with its plentiful calories and sedentary lifestyles, the multiple redundant systems for appetite and energy management that evolved in our distant ancestors work all too well in preventing weight loss. Obesity has certainly reached epidemic proportions: a majority of the adults in the United States are overweight as defined by body mass index (BMI) (**TABLE 9.1**)—about two-thirds—and about one in three qualify as obese (**FIGURE 9.18**) (Flegal et al., 2002). To date, no country has ever succeeded in reducing obesity to any significant degree (M. Ng et al., 2014), and it seems likely that future health care systems will be burdened by obesity-related disorders such as cardiovascular disease and diabetes. To make matters worse, parental obesity may program metabolic disadvantages in offspring via **epigenetic transmission** (S. F. Ng et al., 2010). As in adults, overweight and obesity in children (2–19 years old) has steadily increased in recent decades; more than 30% of children in the USA are now overweight or obese (E. A. O'Connor et al., 2017), in many cases leading to lifelong impacts on metabolic and behavioral aspects of energy homeostasis, and elevated risk of many associated diseases.

In Lewis Carroll's *Alice's Adventures in Wonderland,* Alice quaffs the contents of a small bottle in order to shrink. The quest for a real-life

TABLE 9.1 Body Mass Index (BMI)

Value	Body weight category
<15	Starvation
15–18.5	Underweight
18.5–25	Ideal weight
25–30	Overweight
30–40	Obese
>40	Morbidly obese

Note:
$$BMI = \frac{weight\ (kg)}{height \times height\ (m \times m)}$$
or
$$BMI = 703\ \frac{weight\ (lb)}{height \times height\ (in. \times in.)}$$

epigenetic transmission The passage from one individual to another of changes in the expression of targeted genes, without altering the sequence of nucleotides in the gene.

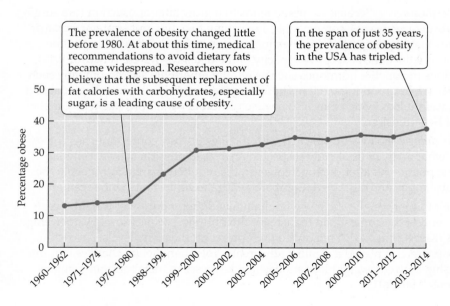

FIGURE 9.18 An Epidemic of Obesity (After Fryar et al., 2016. *Natl. Ctr. Hlth. Stat.* July 2016. www.cdc. gov/nchs/data/hestat/obesity_adult_13_14/obesity_ adult_13_14.htm.)

shrinking potion—but one that makes you thin rather than short—is the subject of intense scientific activity, and several major strategies or targets are emerging:

1. *Appetite control* Hopes are high that drugs designed to reset the hypothalamic appetite controller will be safe and potent obesity treatments. Alteration of leptin levels has not proven to be very effective (DePaoli, 2014). Drugs that directly interfere with endocannabinoid activity, which is normally regulated by leptin in the hypothalamus, effectively produce "anti-munchies"—the reverse of the hunger experienced by cannabis users (Thornton-Jones et al., 2006). However, significant mood problems (an "anti-high"?) also occur, so the search continues for drugs that can selectively modify the signaling systems in the arcuate appetite controller. Treatments that mimic other signaling hormones are promising, especially those that exploit the shorter-term satiety-signaling peptides from the gut. Simply spraying a PYY3-36 solution into the mouths of lab mice is apparently not aversive, yet it powerfully suppresses their appetite (Hurtado et al., 2013). The prescription anti-obesity drug Saxenda (liraglutide) suppresses appetite by mimicking the gut peptide hormone GLP-1 (glucagon-like peptide), which we discussed earlier (Halford et al., 2010).

2. *Increased metabolism* An alternative approach to treating obesity is to raise the body's metabolic rate and thus expend extra calories in the form of heat. For example, scientists are trying to design drugs that will mimic some of the metabolism-elevating actions of thyroid hormones without producing harmful side effects (Grover et al., 2003). Another promising approach involves inducing fat tissue to start burning stored energy faster than normal (Kajimura and Saito, 2014).

3. *Inhibition of fat tissue* A third way to treat obesity involves blocking the formation of new fat tissue. For example, in order for fat tissue to grow, it must be able to recruit and develop new blood vessels. Drugs that block this process inhibit weight gain in mice and may have similar anti-obesity benefits in humans (Tam et al., 2009).

4. *Reduced absorption* The anti-obesity medication orlistat (trade name Xenical) works by interfering with the digestion of fat. However, this approach has generally produced only modest weight loss, and it often causes intestinal discomfort.

5. *Reduced reward* A different perspective on treating obesity focuses on the rewarding properties of food. Not only is food delicious, but "comfort foods" also directly reduce circulating stress hormones, thereby providing another reward. Drugs that affect the brain's reward circuitry (see Chapter 4), reducing the rewarding properties of food, may promote weight loss (Volkow and Wise, 2005).

6. *Anti-obesity surgery* Because fat tissue tends to regrow after liposuction (the surgical removal of fat tissue), some people are turning to a different strategy: bariatric surgeries that bypass part of the intestinal tract or stomach, or install a gut liner, in order to reduce the absorptive capacity of the digestive system (**FIGURE 9.19**). Alterations in appetite hormones such as ghrelin reportedly also accompany such surgeries (D. E. Cummings, 2006). These surgeries can bring about substantial and lasting weight loss, which may also reverse comorbid conditions like type 2 diabetes and hypertension.

7. *Lifestyle changes* Follow-up research with the *Biggest Loser* contestants has confirmed what many of us already suspected: increased physical activity can help keep the pounds off after dieting. However, the required change may need to be very substantial, and sustained. Compared with the contestants who regained all of their former weight, the few who maintained their new lower weight 6 years after the end of the contest had to increase their physical activity level by an average of 160% (Kerns et al., 2017) relative to their pre-contest activity levels. At least in this group, exercise played a significantly greater role than dietary changes, but the relationship between weight loss and lasting decreases in metabolic rate remains mysterious (Hall, 2018).

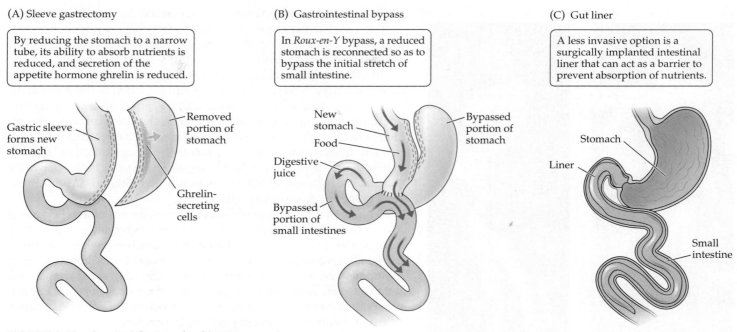

(A) Sleeve gastrectomy

By reducing the stomach to a narrow tube, its ability to absorb nutrients is reduced, and secretion of the appetite hormone ghrelin is reduced.

Gastric sleeve forms new stomach

Removed portion of stomach

Ghrelin-secreting cells

(B) Gastrointestinal bypass

In *Roux-en-Y* bypass, a reduced stomach is reconnected so as to bypass the initial stretch of small intestine.

New stomach

Food

Digestive juice

Bypassed portion of small intestines

Bypassed portion of stomach

(C) Gut liner

A less invasive option is a surgically implanted intestinal liner that can act as a barrier to prevent absorption of nutrients.

Stomach

Liner

Small intestine

FIGURE 9.19 Surgical Options for Obesity

Eating disorders can be life-threatening

Sometimes people shun food, despite having no apparent aversion to it. These people are usually young, become obsessed with their body weight, and become extremely thin—generally by eating very little and sometimes also by vomiting, taking laxatives, overexercising, or drinking large amounts of water to suppress appetite. This condition, which is more common in adolescent and adult women than in men, is called **anorexia nervosa**. The name of the disorder indicates (1) that the afflicted people have no appetite (*anorexia*) and (2) that the disorder originates in the nervous system (*nervosa*).

People with anorexia nervosa tend to think about food a good deal, and evidence suggests that they respond even *more* than healthy people to the presentation of food (Brooks et al., 2012). So, in a physiological sense their hunger may be normal or even exaggerated, but this hunger is somehow absent from their conscious perceptions and they refuse to eat. The idea that anorexia nervosa is primarily a nervous system disorder stems from this mismatch between physiology and cognition, as well as from the distorted body image of the people with anorexia (they may consider themselves fat when others see them as emaciated). There may also be abnormalities in the functioning of the dopamine-based reward system that signals pleasurable aspects of eating, persisting even after recovery (Kaye et al., 2009).

Anorexia nervosa is notoriously difficult to treat, because it appears to involve an unfortunate combination of genetic, endocrine, personality, cognitive, and environmental variables. One approach that is successful in some cases is a family-based treatment (sometimes termed *Maudsley therapy* after the hospital where it was introduced) that de-emphasizes the identification of causal factors and instead focuses on intensive, parent-led "refeeding" of the anorexic person (Le Grange, 2005; Kass et al., 2013).

Bulimia (or *bulimia nervosa*, from the Greek *boulimia*, "great hunger") is a related disorder. Like people with anorexia nervosa, people with bulimia may believe themselves to be fatter than they are, but they periodically gorge themselves, usually with "junk food," and then either vomit the food or take laxatives to avoid weight gain. Also like people with anorexia nervosa, people with bulimia may be obsessed with food and body weight, but not all of them become emaciated. And as in anorexia nervosa, bulimia can be deadly if the person's lack of nutrient reserves damages various organ systems and/or

anorexia nervosa A syndrome in which individuals severely deprive themselves of food.

bulimia Also called *bulimia nervosa*. A syndrome in which individuals periodically gorge themselves, usually with "junk food," and then either vomit or take laxatives to avoid weight gain.

(A) (B)

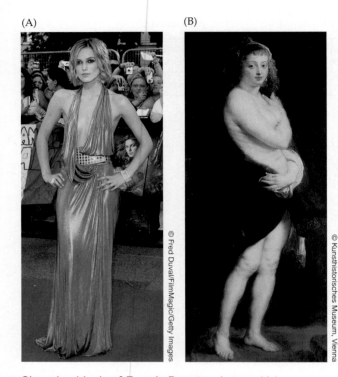

© Fred Duval/FilmMagic/Getty Images

© Kunsthistorisches Museum, Vienna

Changing Ideals of Female Beauty Actress Keira Knightley (A) exemplifies modern society's emphasis on thinness as an aspect of beauty, while *Helena Fourment as Aphrodite* (B), which Flemish painter Peter Paul Rubens painted of his wife circa 1630, illustrates the very different fashion of her era. This treatment of the female body as an object, subject to fluctuating cultural norms and whims of fashion, may play a role in the development of eating disorders such as anorexia nervosa and bulimia.

See Video 9.5:
Anorexia

binge eating The rapid intake of large quantities of food, often poor in nutritional value and high in calories.

leaves the body unable to battle otherwise mild diseases. Prompt interventions, such as cognitive behavioral therapy that focuses on overcoming distorted views of food and eating, can relieve bulimia and lessen the risk of relapse and serious health impacts (De Jong et al., 2018).

In **binge eating**, people spontaneously gorge themselves with far more food than is required to satisfy hunger, often to the point of illness. Such people are often obese, and the causes of the bingeing are not fully understood. In susceptible people, the strong pleasure associated with food activates opiate and dopaminergic reward mechanisms to such an extent that bingeing resembles drug addiction. Indeed, "binge eating disorder" is now a psychiatric diagnosis in the *Diagnostic and Statistical Manual of Mental Disorders*, 5th edition (*DSM-5*; American Psychiatric Association, 2013).

Despite the epidemic of obesity in our society, or perhaps because of it, our present culture emphasizes that women, especially young women, must be thin to be attractive. This cultural pressure is widely perceived as one of the causes of eating disorders. In earlier times, however, when plump women were considered the most beautiful, some women still fasted severely, showing all the hallmarks of anorexia nervosa. The origins of these disorders remain elusive, and to date, the available therapies help only a minority of people with eating disorders.

HOW'S IT GOING ❓

1. What proportion of adults in the United States are overweight or obese? How might homeostasis be part of the problem?
2. If you were designing drugs to combat obesity, what specific parts of the hypothalamic appetite controller might you target? Why?
3. Compare and contrast anorexia nervosa and bulimia. Are people with anorexia interested in food at all? Briefly discuss possible methods of treating anorexia.
4. Drawing on concepts covered in this chapter, discuss the likely contributions of cultural versus biological factors in various eating disorders.
5. Discuss nonpharmacological methods of weight reduction. Is surgery a good option?

Recommended Reading

Agras, W. S., and Robinson, A. (Eds.). (2018). *Oxford Handbook of Eating Disorders* (2nd ed.). New York, NY: Oxford University Press.

Anderson, S. C., Cryan, J. F., and Dinan, T. (2019). *The Psychobiotic Revolution: Mood, Food, and the New Science of the Gut-Brain Connection.* Washington, DC: National Geographic.

Brownell, K. D., and Walsh, B. T. (2017). *Eating Disorders and Obesity* (3rd ed.). New York, NY: Guilford Press.

DeSalle, R., and Perkins, S. L. (2015). *Welcome to the Microbiome: Getting to Know the Trillions of Bacteria and Other Microbes In, On, and Around You.* New Haven, CT: Yale University Press.

Logue, A. W. (2014). *The Psychology of Eating and Drinking* (4th ed.). New York, NY: Routledge.

Lustig, R. H. (2018). *The Hacking of the American Mind: The Science behind the Corporate Takeover of Our Bodies and Brains.* New York, NY: Avery.

McNab, B. K. (2012). *Extreme Measures: The Ecological Energetics of Birds and Mammals.* Chicago, IL: University of Chicago Press.

Schulkin, J. (Ed.). (2012). *Allostasis, Homeostasis, and the Costs of Physiological Adaptation.* Cambridge, UK: Cambridge University Press.

You should be able to relate each summary to the adjacent illustration, including structures and processes.
The online version of this **Visual Summary** includes links to figures, animations, and activities that will help you consolidate the material.

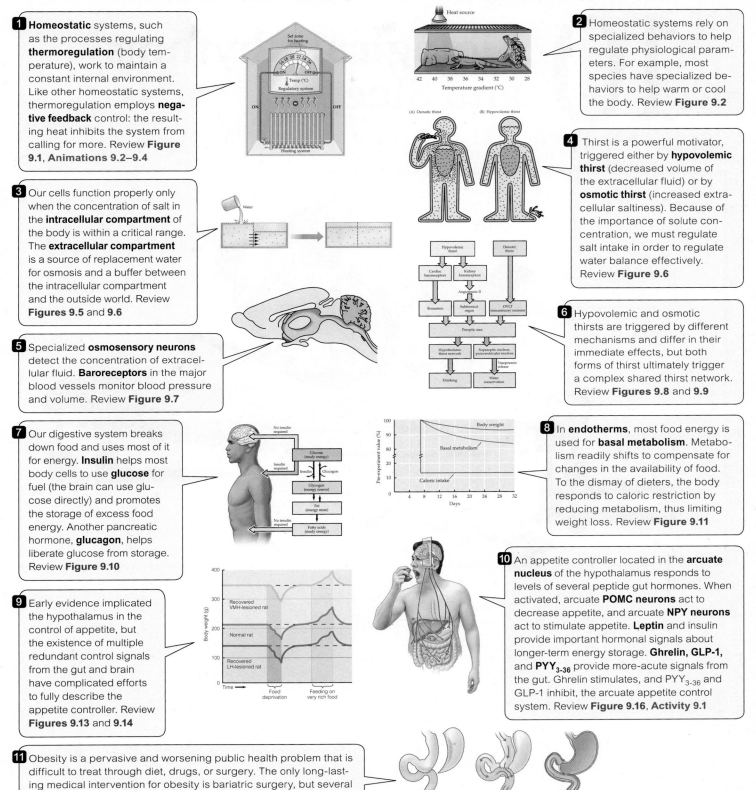

1 **Homeostatic** systems, such as the processes regulating **thermoregulation** (body temperature), work to maintain a constant internal environment. Like other homeostatic systems, thermoregulation employs **negative feedback** control: the resulting heat inhibits the system from calling for more. Review **Figure 9.1, Animations 9.2–9.4**

2 Homeostatic systems rely on specialized behaviors to help regulate physiological parameters. For example, most species have specialized behaviors to help warm or cool the body. Review **Figure 9.2**

3 Our cells function properly only when the concentration of salt in the **intracellular compartment** of the body is within a critical range. The **extracellular compartment** is a source of replacement water for osmosis and a buffer between the intracellular compartment and the outside world. Review **Figures 9.5** and **9.6**

4 Thirst is a powerful motivator, triggered either by **hypovolemic thirst** (decreased volume of the extracellular fluid) or by **osmotic thirst** (increased extracellular saltiness). Because of the importance of solute concentration, we must regulate salt intake in order to regulate water balance effectively. Review **Figure 9.6**

5 Specialized **osmosensory neurons** detect the concentration of extracellular fluid. **Baroreceptors** in the major blood vessels monitor blood pressure and volume. Review **Figure 9.7**

6 Hypovolemic and osmotic thirsts are triggered by different mechanisms and differ in their immediate effects, but both forms of thirst ultimately trigger a complex shared thirst network. Review **Figures 9.8** and **9.9**

7 Our digestive system breaks down food and uses most of it for energy. **Insulin** helps most body cells to use **glucose** for fuel (the brain can use glucose directly) and promotes the storage of excess food energy. Another pancreatic hormone, **glucagon**, helps liberate glucose from storage. Review **Figure 9.10**

8 In **endotherms**, most food energy is used for **basal metabolism**. Metabolism readily shifts to compensate for changes in the availability of food. To the dismay of dieters, the body responds to caloric restriction by reducing metabolism, thus limiting weight loss. Review **Figure 9.11**

9 Early evidence implicated the hypothalamus in the control of appetite, but the existence of multiple redundant control signals from the gut and brain have complicated efforts to fully describe the appetite controller. Review **Figures 9.13** and **9.14**

10 An appetite controller located in the **arcuate nucleus** of the hypothalamus responds to levels of several peptide gut hormones. When activated, arcuate **POMC neurons** act to decrease appetite, and arcuate **NPY neurons** act to stimulate appetite. **Leptin** and insulin provide important hormonal signals about longer-term energy storage. **Ghrelin, GLP-1, and PYY$_{3-36}$** provide more-acute signals from the gut. Ghrelin stimulates, and PYY$_{3-36}$ and GLP-1 inhibit, the arcuate appetite control system. Review **Figure 9.16, Activity 9.1**

11 Obesity is a pervasive and worsening public health problem that is difficult to treat through diet, drugs, or surgery. The only long-lasting medical intervention for obesity is bariatric surgery, but several drug strategies based on a new understanding of appetite control offer promise. Review **Figure 9.18** and **9.19, Video 9.5**

10 Biological Rhythms and Sleep

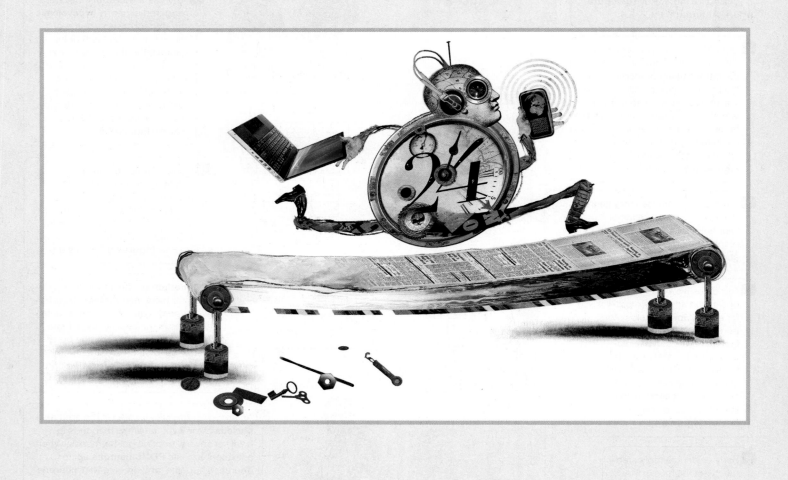

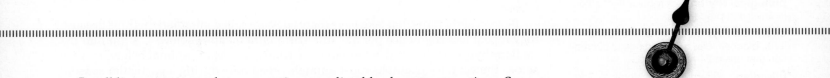

Don't Make Me Laugh

Adrian first became aware of his problem as an adult when he decided to sneak up on his mother working in the garden, thinking that surprising her would be funny. As Adrian expected, she was indeed startled; she, Adrian, and the rest of his family laughed. But then Adrian suddenly felt progressively weaker in his knees and back, slowly slumping until he was lying down, totally paralyzed, for 15–20 seconds. Several more instances of paralysis occurred in the following months, always when Adrian was doing something he thought would be funny. He would laugh and then slowly collapse to the floor, fully conscious but unable to move. During a visit to the zoo, a joke that he thought would amuse his daughters left Adrian slumped over the fence in front of the monkey enclosure, helpless. According to Adrian, the trigger is not laughing but doing something that he thinks is funny and would make others laugh. "I can sit and watch a comedian, I can laugh myself inside out without any effect at all. But if I were to say something that I felt was very funny to you, there's a good chance that I would end up on the floor" (Leschziner, 2019, p. 113).

What was happening to Adrian? By the end of this chapter, we'll know a lot more about sleep and what went wrong in Adrian's brain to cause these problems.

A ll living systems show repeating, predictable changes over time. Some rhythms, like brain potentials, are rapid; other rhythms, like annual hibernations, are slow. Daily rhythms, the topic of the start of this chapter, have an intriguing clocklike regularity and are seen in virtually every physiological measure, including body temperature and hormone secretion. The rest of the chapter concerns that familiar daily rhythm known as the *sleep-waking cycle*. By age 60, most humans have spent 20 years asleep (some, alas, on one side or the other of the classroom podium). We'll find that sleep is not a passive state of "nonwaking," but rather the interlocking of several different brain states. We'll conclude with a consideration of sleep disorders, as well as some tips on how to get the sleep you need.

**See Video 10.1:
Narcolepsy**

10.1 Biological Rhythms Organize Behavior

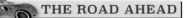 **THE ROAD AHEAD**

The start of the chapter reviews the evidence that the brain contains a biological clock to synchronize our behavior to the world around us. After reading this section, you should be able to:

10.1.1 Discuss the evidence that a tiny brain structure imposes a daily rhythm on behavior.

10.1.2 Describe the neural pathway by which information about daylight synchronizes that structure.

10.1.3 Understand how a molecular clock in brain neurons generates that daily rhythm.

10.1.4 Evaluate the evidence that later start times benefit high school students.

**View Animation 10.2:
Brain Explorer**

biological rhythm   A regular fluctuation in any living process.

circadian rhythm   A pattern of behavioral, biochemical, or physiological fluctuation that has a 24-hour period.

ultradian   Referring to a rhythmic biological event with a period shorter than a day, usually from several minutes to several hours long.

infradian   Referring to a rhythmic biological event with a period longer than a day.

Biological rhythms are regular fluctuations in any living process. Almost all physiological measures—hormone levels, body temperature, drug sensitivity—change over the course of the day in a repeating pattern. Because such rhythms last about a day, they are called **circadian rhythms** (from the Latin *circa*, "about," and *dies*, "day"). Circadian rhythms are by far the most studied of the biological rhythms, and they will be our major concern in this chapter.

Still, you should know that some biological rhythms are shorter than a day. Such rhythms are referred to as **ultradian** (because they repeat more than once per day; the Latin *ultra* means "beyond"), and they vary from several minutes to hours long. Ultradian rhythms are seen in such behaviors as bouts of activity, feeding, and hormone release.

Biological rhythms that take *more* than a day are called **infradian** rhythms because they repeat less than once per day (the Latin *infra* means "below"). A familiar infradian rhythm is the 28-day human menstrual cycle. Many animal behaviors vary across the year; for example, most animals breed only during a particular season. There's also growing evidence of annual rhythms in the onset of human behavioral disorders, such as depression (see Chapter 12). (By the way, despite the urban myth that cases of depression peak around the winter holiday season, in fact they peak in the spring.) You might think that breeding seasons in animals would be triggered by changes in temperatures or food availability, but experiments suggest that the duration of light each day is the real trigger: in the laboratory, animals exposed to short days and long nights (mimicking wintertime conditions) reliably change to the nonbreeding condition (**FIGURE 10.1**).

Circadian rhythms are generated by an endogenous clock

Humans and many other primates are diurnal—active during the day. But most other mammals, including most rodents, are nocturnal—active during dark periods. These circadian rhythms are extraordinarily precise: the beginning of activity may vary only a few minutes from one day to another. For humans equipped with watches and clocks, this regularity may seem uninteresting, but other animals achieve such remarkable regularity using only a built-in biological clock.

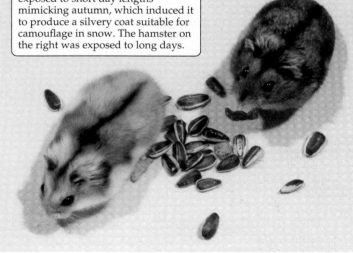

The Siberian hamster on the left was exposed to short day lengths mimicking autumn, which induced it to produce a silvery coat suitable for camouflage in snow. The hamster on the right was exposed to long days.

Photo by Carol D. Hegstrom

FIGURE 10.1   Winter Is Coming

(A)

(B)

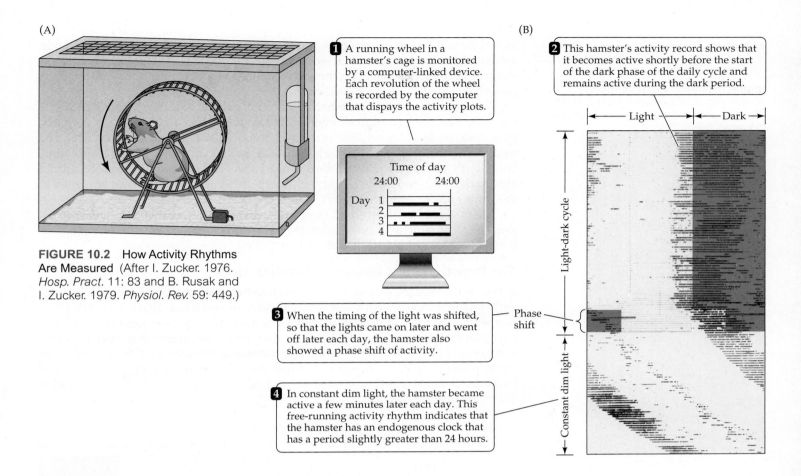

1 A running wheel in a hamster's cage is monitored by a computer-linked device. Each revolution of the wheel is recorded by the computer that dispays the activity plots.

Time of day

24:00   24:00

Day 1
     2
     3
     4

3 When the timing of the light was shifted, so that the lights came on later and went off later each day, the hamster also showed a phase shift of activity.

Phase shift

4 In constant dim light, the hamster became active a few minutes later each day. This free-running activity rhythm indicates that the hamster has an endogenous clock that has a period slightly greater than 24 hours.

2 This hamster's activity record shows that it becomes active shortly before the start of the dark phase of the daily cycle and remains active during the dark period.

Light   Dark

Light–dark cycle

Constant dim light

FIGURE 10.2 How Activity Rhythms Are Measured (After I. Zucker. 1976. *Hosp. Pract.* 11: 83 and B. Rusak and I. Zucker. 1979. *Physiol. Rev.* 59: 449.)

A favorite way to study circadian rhythms exploits rodents' love of running wheels. A switch attached to the wheel connects to a computer that registers each turn, revealing an activity rhythm as in **FIGURE 10.2A**. A hamster placed in a dimly lit room continues to show a daily rhythm in wheel running despite the absence of day versus night, suggesting that the animal has an internal clock. But even when the light is constantly dim, it is always possible that the animal detects other external cues (e.g., outside noises, temperature, barometric pressure—who knows?) signaling the time of day. Arguing for a biological clock, however, is the fact that in constant light or dark the circadian cycle is not *exactly* 24 hours: activity starts a few minutes later each day, so eventually the normally nocturnal hamster is active while it is daytime outside (**FIGURE 10.2B**, bottom). The animal is said to be **free-running**, maintaining its own personal cycle, which, in the absence of external cues, is a bit more than 24 hours long.

The free-running **period**, the time between two similar points of successive cycles (such as sunset to sunset), differs from one hamster to another. If two hamsters are placed in constant dim light next door to each other, eventually one may be active when the other is asleep—further evidence that they are not detecting some mysterious external cue. Rather, every animal has its own endogenous clock; periods vary from one individual to another.

Normally this internal clock is reset by light. If we expose a free-running nocturnal animal to periods of light and dark, the animal soon synchronizes its wheel running to start just before the dark period. The shift of activity produced by a synchronizing stimulus is referred to as a **phase shift** (see Figure 10.2B, middle), and the process of shifting the rhythm is called **entrainment**. Any cue that an animal uses to synchronize

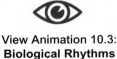

View Animation 10.3: Biological Rhythms

free-running   Referring to a rhythm of behavior shown by an animal deprived of external cues about time of day.

period   The interval of time between two similar points of successive cycles, such as sunset to sunset.

phase shift   A shift in the activity of a biological rhythm, typically provided by a synchronizing environmental stimulus, such as light.

entrainment   The process of synchronizing a biological rhythm to an environmental stimulus.

zeitgeber   Literally "time giver" (in German). The stimulus (usually the light-dark cycle) that entrains circadian rhythms.

suprachiasmatic nucleus (SCN)   A small region of the hypothalamus above the optic chiasm that is the location of a circadian clock.

its activity with the environment is called a **zeitgeber** (German for "time giver"). Light acts as a powerful zeitgeber, and we can easily manipulate it in the lab. Because light stimuli can entrain circadian rhythms, the endogenous clock must receive information about light and dark, as we'll confirm shortly.

We humans experience a mismatch of internal and external time when we fly from one time zone to another. Flying three time zones east (say, from California to New York) means that sunlight arrives 3 hours sooner than our brain expects. The next morning we'll probably have a hard time waking up at 7:00 AM New York time, because it's 4:00 AM California time. We need about one day per time zone to entrain after such travel, and in the meantime we experience jet lag, with symptoms such as insomnia and daytime fatigue.

The major value of circadian rhythms is obvious: they enable us to *anticipate* an event, such as sunrise or sunset, and to begin physiological and behavioral preparations *before* that event. Let's talk about how this circadian clock works.

The hypothalamus houses a circadian clock

Where is the biological clock that drives circadian rhythms, and how does it work? Early research showed that while removing various endocrine glands had little effect on the free-running rhythm of rats, large lesions of the hypothalamus interfered with circadian rhythms (Richter, 1967). It was subsequently discovered that lesions of a tiny subregion of the hypothalamus—the **suprachiasmatic nucleus** (**SCN**), named for its location above the optic chiasm—eliminate circadian rhythms of drinking and locomotor behavior (**FIGURE 10.3**) (Stephan and Zucker, 1972) and of hormone secretion (R. Y. Moore and Eichler, 1972).

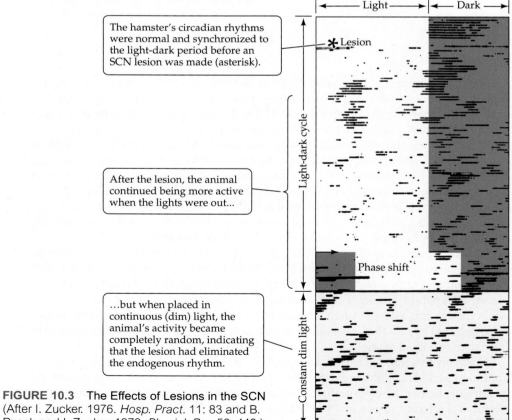

The hamster's circadian rhythms were normal and synchronized to the light-dark period before an SCN lesion was made (asterisk).

After the lesion, the animal continued being more active when the lights were out...

...but when placed in continuous (dim) light, the animal's activity became completely random, indicating that the lesion had eliminated the endogenous rhythm.

FIGURE 10.3   The Effects of Lesions in the SCN (After I. Zucker. 1976. *Hosp. Pract.* 11: 83 and B. Rusak and I. Zucker. 1979. *Physiol. Rev.* 59: 449.)

The clocklike nature of the SCN is also evident in its metabolic activity. If we take SCN cells out of the brain and put them in a dish (Yamazaki et al., 2000), their electrical activity continues to show a circadian rhythm for days or weeks. This striking evidence supports the idea that the SCN contains an endogenous clock. But even stronger proof that the SCN generates a circadian rhythm comes from transplanting the SCN from one animal to another, as we'll see next.

RESEARCHERS AT WORK

Transplants prove that the SCN produces a circadian rhythm

Ralph and Menaker (1988) found a male hamster that exhibited an unusually short free-running activity rhythm in constant conditions. Normally, hamsters free-run at a period slightly longer than 24 hours, but this male showed a free-running period of 22 hours. Half of his offspring also had a shorter circadian rhythm, indicating that he had a genetic mutation affecting the endogenous clock. Grandchildren inheriting two copies of this mutation had an even shorter period: 20 hours. The mutation was named *tau*, after the Greek symbol used by scientists to represent the period (duration) of cyclical processes. These hamsters entrained to a normal 24-hour light-dark cycle just fine; their abnormal endogenous circadian rhythm was revealed only in constant conditions.

Dramatic evidence that the SCN is a master clock was provided by transplant experiments (Ralph et al., 1990), as detailed in **FIGURE 10.4**.

Reciprocal transplants gave comparable results: the endogenous rhythm following the transplant was always that of the donor SCN, not the recipient, so the SCN must be driving the circadian rhythms. This remains the only known case of transplanting brain tissue from one individual to another in which the recipient subsequently displayed the donor's behavior!

FIGURE 10.4 Brain Transplants Prove That the SCN Contains a Clock

■ **Hypothesis**

The endogenous clock determining an individual hamster's circadian rhythm is in the suprachiasmatic nucleus (SCN).

■ **Test**

The SCN is lesioned in several normal hamsters, rendering them arrhythmic.

Adult hamsters receive SCN transplants from newborn hamsters. This hamster received an SCN from a mutant hamster with a period of about 20 hours.

■ **Alternative Outcomes**

- If the endogenous circadian rhythm is generated outside the SCN, then when the hamster recovers, it should return to its original period of just over 24 hours.
- If the endogenous circadian rhythm is controlled by the SCN, then when the adult hamster recovers, its period should match that of the donor—about 20 hours.

■ **Result**

When the adult hamster recovered, it did not show its original circadian rhythm of about 24 hours, but displayed a rhythm that matched that of its donor, about 20 hours.

■ **Conclusion**

Within the SCN itself there must be a mechanism that can drive a circadian rhythm in activity, and this biological clock is affected by mutation of the gene *tau*.

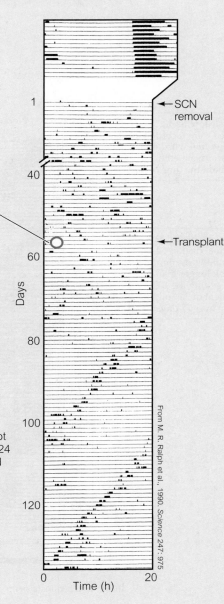

From M. R. Ralph et al., 1990. *Science* 247: 975

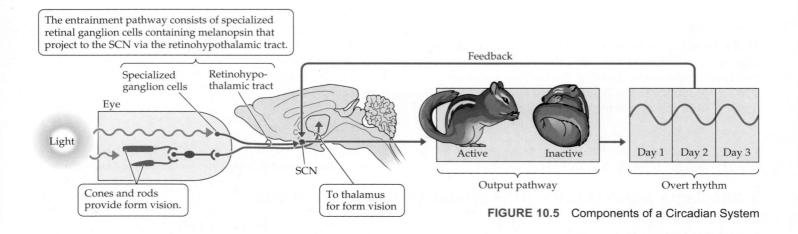

The entrainment pathway consists of specialized retinal ganglion cells containing melanopsin that project to the SCN via the retinohypothalamic tract.

Specialized ganglion cells

Retinohypo-thalamic tract

Eye

Light

Cones and rods provide form vision.

SCN

To thalamus for form vision

Feedback

Active

Inactive

Day 1 | Day 2 | Day 3

Output pathway

Overt rhythm

FIGURE 10.5 Components of a Circadian System

In mammals, light information from the eyes reaches the SCN directly

Most vertebrates have photoreceptors outside the eye that are part of the mechanism of light entrainment (Ekström and Meissl, 2003). For example, the pineal gland of some birds and amphibians is itself sensitive to light (Doyle and Menaker, 2007) and helps entrain circadian rhythms to light. Because the skull over the pineal is especially thin in some species, we can think of those species as having a primitive "third eye" in the back of the head. (Some elementary school teachers also seem to have an eye in the back of the head, but this has not been proven to be the pineal gland.) At night, the pineal gland secretes a hormone, **melatonin**, that informs the brain about day length. For more on the nocturnal secretion of melatonin, see A Step Further 8.1, on the website.

In mammals, however, cells in the eye tell the SCN when it is light out. Certain retinal ganglion cells send their axons along the **retinohypothalamic pathway**, veering out of the optic chiasm to synapse directly within the SCN. This short pathway carries information about light to the hypothalamus (R. Y. Moore, 2013) to entrain rhythms (**FIGURE 10.5**). Most of the retinal ganglion cells that extend their axons to the SCN do not rely on the traditional photoreceptors—rods and cones—to learn about light. Rather, these retinal ganglion cells themselves contain a special photopigment, called **melanopsin**, that makes them sensitive to light (Do et al., 2009). Transgenic mice that lack rods and cones, and so are blind in every other respect, will still entrain their behavior to light (Wee et al., 2002) if the specialized melanopsin-containing ganglion cells are present.

Unfortunately, those melanopsin-containing retinal ganglion cells appear to be absent or dysfunctional in most totally blind humans, because people who are blind often show a free-running circadian rhythm, with difficulties getting to sleep at night and staying awake during the day (Sack and Lewy, 2001). Taking melatonin at bedtime, thus mimicking the normal nightly release of the hormone from the pineal gland, helps sighted people to get to sleep (Burgess and Emens, 2018), and it also helps blind people to entrain to daylight. This result suggests that while humans rely primarily on light stimulation of the retinohypothalamic tract to the SCN in

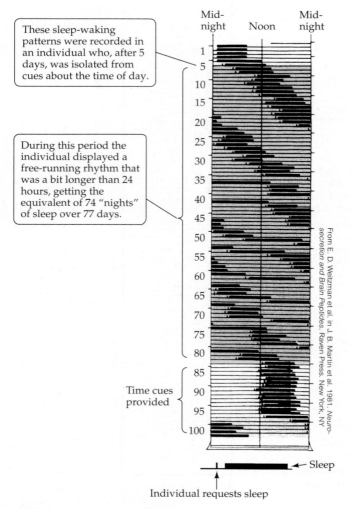

These sleep-waking patterns were recorded in an individual who, after 5 days, was isolated from cues about the time of day.

During this period the individual displayed a free-running rhythm that was a bit longer than 24 hours, getting the equivalent of 74 "nights" of sleep over 77 days.

Mid-night Noon Mid-night

Time cues provided

From E. D. Weitzman et al. in J. B. Martin et al. 1981. *Neuro-secretion and Brain Peptides.* Raven Press, New York, NY.

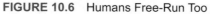
Sleep

Individual requests sleep

FIGURE 10.6 Humans Free-Run Too

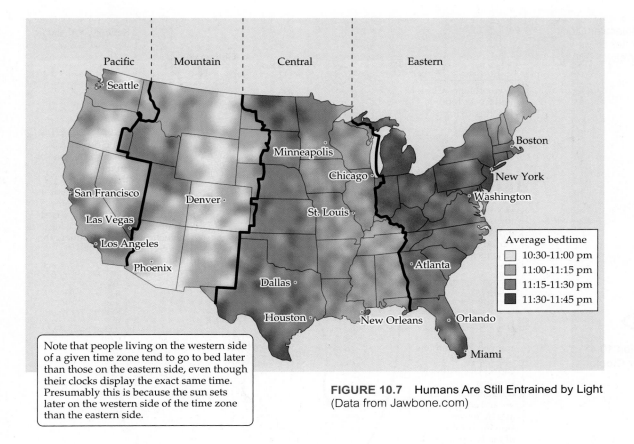

Note that people living on the western side of a given time zone tend to go to bed later than those on the eastern side, even though their clocks display the exact same time. Presumably this is because the sun sets later on the western side of the time zone than the eastern side.

FIGURE 10.7 Humans Are Still Entrained by Light (Data from Jawbone.com)

order to entrain to light, our brains have retained enough sensitivity to melatonin that we can use that cue in the absence of information about light.

Deprived of light cues, people free-run just like hamsters (Wever, 1979). Spending weeks in a cave with all cues to external time removed, they display a circadian rhythm of the sleep-waking cycle that slowly shifts from 24 to 25 hours (**FIGURE 10.6**), just as a hamster does (see Figure 10.2). Because the free-running period is greater than 24 hours, some people in these studies are surprised when they're told that the experiment has ended. They may have experienced only 74 sleep-waking cycles during a 77-day study.

Another way to detect the effect of daylight on human circadian rhythms is to examine when people go to sleep within a given time zone. Even though everyone's clocks/watches/phones report the same time, people in the western part of the time zone go to bed a bit later than those in the eastern part, presumably because the sun sets later in the western half (**FIGURE 10.7**).

Circadian rhythms have been genetically dissected in flies and mice

Genes that were found to affect circadian rhythms in the fruit fly *Drosophila melanogaster* (Belle and Allen, 2018) were later discovered to have differently named but similar-acting counterparts in mammals. This paved the way for understanding the molecular basis of the circadian clock. Neurons in the mammalian SCN make the proteins Clock and Cycle, which bind together to form a dimer (a pair of proteins attached to each other). The Clock/Cycle dimer then binds to the cell's DNA to promote the transcription of other genes, including one called *period* (*per*). The proteins made from these other genes go back to inhibit the action of Clock and Cycle, which started the whole process. Because those inhibitory proteins degrade with time, eventually the

melatonin An amine hormone that is secreted by the pineal gland at night, thereby signaling day length to the brain.

retinohypothalamic pathway The route by which specialized retinal ganglion cells send their axons to the suprachiasmatic nuclei.

melanopsin A photopigment found in those retinal ganglion cells that project to the suprachiasmatic nucleus.

FIGURE 10.8 A Molecular Clock in Flies and Mice (After S. M. Reppert and D. R. Weaver. 2002. *Nature* 418: 935.)

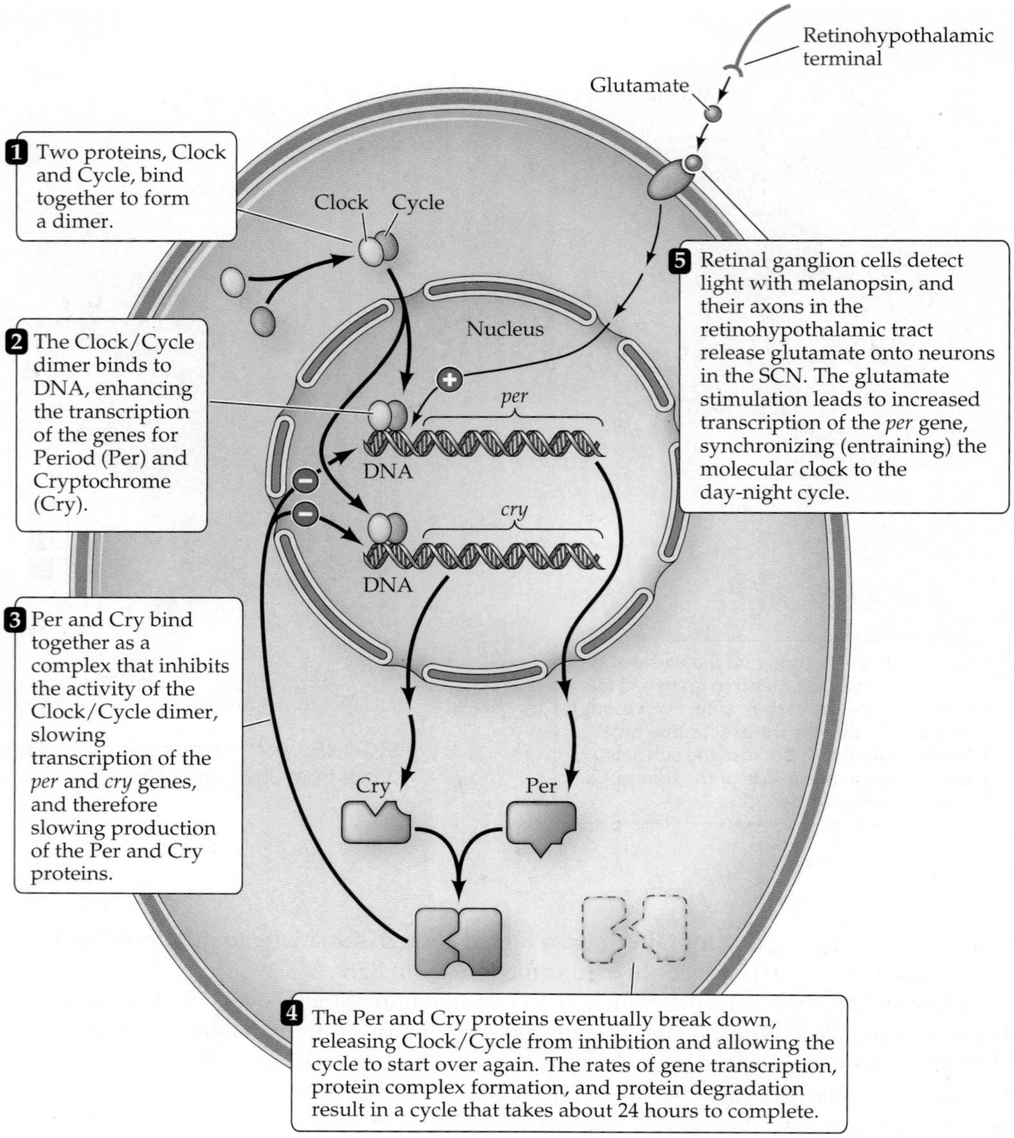

Retinohypothalamic terminal
Glutamate
1 Two proteins, Clock and Cycle, bind together to form a dimer.
Clock
Cycle
Nucleus
2 The Clock/Cycle dimer binds to DNA, enhancing the transcription of the genes for Period (Per) and Cryptochrome (Cry).
per
DNA
cry
DNA
5 Retinal ganglion cells detect light with melanopsin, and their axons in the retinohypothalamic tract release glutamate onto neurons in the SCN. The glutamate stimulation leads to increased transcription of the per gene, synchronizing (entraining) the molecular clock to the day-night cycle.
3 Per and Cry bind together as a complex that inhibits the activity of the Clock/Cycle dimer, slowing transcription of the per and cry genes, and therefore slowing production of the Per and Cry proteins.
Cry
Per
4 The Per and Cry proteins eventually break down, releasing Clock/Cycle from inhibition and allowing the cycle to start over again. The rates of gene transcription, protein complex formation, and protein degradation result in a cycle that takes about 24 hours to complete.

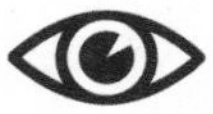

View Animation 10.4: A Molecular Clock

inhibition is lifted, starting the whole cycle over again (**FIGURE 10.8**). The entire cycle takes about 24 hours to complete, and it is this 24-hour molecular cycle that drives the 24-hour activity cycle of SCN cells. You can learn more about the molecular basis of the circadian clock in **A STEP FURTHER 10.1**, on the website.

One indication of the importance of the molecular clock in controlling circadian behavior is the effect of differences in the genes involved in the clock. We've already seen that hamsters with a mutation in *tau* have a free-running rhythm that is shorter than normal. Mice in which both copies of the *Clock* gene are disrupted show severe arrhythmicity under constant conditions (**FIGURE 10.9**). People who feel energetic in the morning ("larks") are likely to carry a different version of the *Clock* gene than "night owls" have (S. E. Jones et al., 2019). Different versions of other genes in the molecular clock are also associated with being a lark versus an owl in both humans (Blum et al., 2018) and mice (Pfeffer et al., 2015). Human night owls are at greater risk than larks for depression (R. G. Foster et al., 2013) and obesity (Roenneberg et al., 2012), perhaps because they are forced to adapt their natural sleep rhythm to fit into an early-bird society.

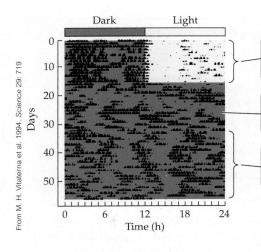

From M. H. Vitaterna et al. 1994. *Science* 29: 719

This homozygous *Clock/Clock* mouse showed a normal circadian rhythm when given light cues.

In constant dim light, it maintained an activity period of 27 hours for a few days but then lost circadian rhythmicity.

Note, however, that an ultradian rhythm (i.e., a rhythm that has a frequency of more than once a day) remains.

FIGURE 10.9 When the Endogenous Clock Goes Kaput

At puberty, most people shift their circadian rhythm of sleep, so they get up later in the day (**FIGURE 10.10**), basically acting more like night owls. Unfortunately, many school systems require students to come to school *earlier* in the day when they hit adolescence. When high schools shifted their morning start to after 8:30 AM, students showed improved academic performance, including (big surprise!) less sleeping in class, and a reduced incidence of depression (J. C. Lo et al., 2018). Plus, the student drivers had 70% fewer car crashes (Wahlstrom et al., 2014)!

Having covered some of the mechanisms that enforce our daily rhythms, we'll spend the rest of the chapter exploring that mysterious circadian behavior called *sleep*.

HOW'S IT GOING ❓

1. Give some examples of ultradian and infradian rhythms.
2. What are circadian rhythms, and how can they be studied and manipulated in lab animals?
3. Describe experiments that established which parts of the brain control circadian rhythms.
4. How does information about day and night reach the mammalian brain?
5. Describe in general terms how a molecular process in the brain cycles about every 24 hours.

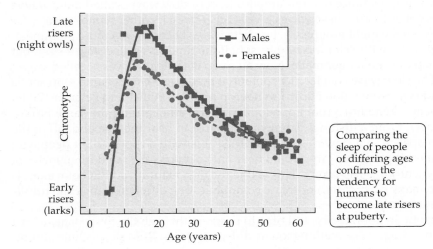

Comparing the sleep of people of differing ages confirms the tendency for humans to become late risers at puberty.

FIGURE 10.10 How I Hate to Get Out of Bed in the Morning! (After T. Roenneberg et al. 2004. *Curr. Biol.* 14: R1038.)

10.2 Sleep Is an Active Process

THE ROAD AHEAD

The next section concerns our most prominent circadian behavior: sleep. Studying this material should allow you to:

10.2.1 Describe the various stages of sleep and how they are distributed across the night.

10.2.2 Distinguish the types of mental activity typical of the two major classes of sleep.

Human sleep exhibits different stages

In the 1930s, experimenters found that brain potentials recorded from electrodes on the scalp by **electroencephalography** (**EEG**; see Figure 3.15A) provide a way to define, describe, and classify levels of arousal and states of sleep. In sleep studies, eye movements and muscle tension are monitored in addition to the EEG. Together, these measures led to the groundbreaking discovery that there are two distinct classes of sleep: **rapid-eye-movement** (**REM**) **sleep** (Aserinsky and Kleitman, 1953) and **non-REM sleep**.

What are the electrophysiological distinctions that define different sleep states? Let's begin with the pattern of EEG activity in the brain of a fully awake, alert person. It is a mixture of low-amplitude waves with many relatively fast frequencies (greater than 15–20 cycles per second, or hertz [Hz]). This pattern is sometimes referred to as *beta activity* or a **desynchronized EEG** (**FIGURE 10.11A**).

When you relax and close your eyes, a distinctive rhythm appears in the EEG, consisting of a regular oscillation at a frequency of 8–12 Hz, known as the **alpha rhythm**. As drowsiness sets in, the time spent in the alpha rhythm decreases, and the EEG shows waves of smaller amplitude and irregular frequency, as well as sharp waves called **vertex spikes**. This is the beginning of non-REM sleep, called **stage 1 sleep** (**FIGURE 10.11B**), which is accompanied by slowing of the heart rate and relaxation of the muscles; in addition, under the closed eyelids the eyes may roll about slowly. Stage 1 sleep usually lasts several minutes and gives way to **stage 2 sleep** (**FIGURE 10.11C**), which is defined by waves of 12–14 Hz called **sleep spindles** that occur in periodic bursts, and by **K complexes**. If awakened during these first two stages of sleep, many people deny that they have been asleep, even though they failed to respond to signals while in those stages.

Stage 2 sleep leads to (can you guess?) **stage 3 sleep** (**FIGURE 10.11D**), which is defined by the appearance of large-amplitude, *very* slow waves called **delta waves** (about one per second). These waves give stage 3 sleep its other name—*slow wave sleep* (SWS). As the night progresses, the delta waves become even more prominent. (Previously, SWS with delta waves at least half the time was called *stage 4 sleep*, but that distinction is no longer made. Now all sleep with delta waves is called *stage 3* or *SWS*.) The slow waves of electrical potential that give SWS its name represent a widespread synchronization of cortical neuron activity (Poulet and Petersen, 2008) that has been likened to a room of people who are all chanting the same phrase over and over. From a distance, you would be able to hear the rise and fall of the cadence of speech in a slow rhythm. Contrast this with a room full of people all saying something *different*. You would hear only a buzz—the rapid frequencies of many desynchronized speakers. This is like the desynchronized EEG of wakefulness, when many parts of the cortex are communicating different things and fulfilling different functions.

After about an hour, the typical time to progress through the SWS stage, with a brief return to stage 2—something totally different occurs: REM sleep. Quite abruptly, the EEG displays a pattern of small-amplitude, high-frequency activity similar in

---

electroencephalography (EEG)
The recording of gross electrical activity of the brain via large electrodes placed on the scalp.

rapid-eye-movement (REM) sleep
Also called *paradoxical sleep*. A stage of sleep characterized by small-amplitude, fast EEG waves, no postural tension, and rapid eye movements. *REM* rhymes with "gem."

non-REM sleep Sleep, divided into stages 1–3, that is defined by the presence of distinctive EEG activity that differs from that seen in REM sleep.

desynchronized EEG Also called *beta activity*. A pattern of EEG activity comprising a mix of many different high frequencies with low amplitude.

alpha rhythm A brain potential of 8–12 Hz that occurs during relaxed wakefulness.

vertex spike A sharp-wave EEG pattern that is seen during stage 1 sleep.

stage 1 sleep The initial stage of non-REM sleep, which is characterized by small-amplitude EEG waves of irregular frequency, slow heart rate, and reduced muscle tension.

stage 2 sleep A stage of sleep that is defined by bursts of EEG waves called *sleep spindles*.

sleep spindle A characteristic 12–14 Hz wave in the EEG of a person said to be in stage 2 sleep.

K complex A sharp, negative EEG potential that is seen in stage 2 sleep.

stage 3 sleep Also called *slow wave sleep* (SWS). A stage of non-REM sleep that is defined by the presence of large-amplitude, slow delta waves.

delta wave The slowest type of EEG wave, about 1 per second, characteristic of stage 3 sleep.

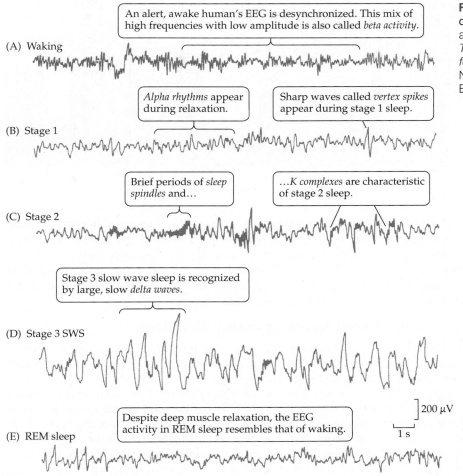

(A) Waking

An alert, awake human's EEG is desynchronized. This mix of high frequencies with low amplitude is also called *beta activity*.

(B) Stage 1

Alpha rhythms appear during relaxation.

Sharp waves called *vertex spikes* appear during stage 1 sleep.

(C) Stage 2

Brief periods of *sleep spindles* and…

…*K complexes* are characteristic of stage 2 sleep.

(D) Stage 3 SWS

Stage 3 slow wave sleep is recognized by large, slow *delta waves*.

(E) REM sleep

Despite deep muscle relaxation, the EEG activity in REM sleep resembles that of waking.

$200\ \mu V$

1 s

FIGURE 10.11 Electrophysiological Correlates of Sleep and Waking (After A. Rechtschaffen and A. Kales. 1968. *A Manual of Standardized Terminology, Techniques and Scoring System for Sleep Stages of Human Subjects.* U.S. NINDB, Neurological Information Network. Bethesda, MD.)

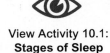

View Activity 10.1:
Stages of Sleep

many ways to the pattern of an awake individual (**FIGURE 10.11E**), except the eyes are darting rapidly about under their lids (the *r*apid *e*ye *m*ovements that give REM sleep its name). Aside from those muscles moving the eyes, all other skeletal muscles not only are relaxed, but show a complete absence of muscle tone, called *atonia*. The active-looking EEG coupled with deeply relaxed muscles is typical of REM sleep. If you see a cat sleeping in the sitting, sphinx position, it cannot be in REM sleep; in REM, it will be sprawled limply on the floor. For the same reason, a student sleeping while sitting upright in class cannot be in REM sleep.

This flaccid muscle state appears, despite intense brain activity, because during REM sleep, brainstem regions are profoundly inhibiting motor neurons. This seeming contradiction—the brain waves look awake, but the muscles are flaccid and unresponsive—is what gives REM sleep its other name: *paradoxical sleep*. Unlike SWS, REM sleep is accompanied by irregular breathing and pulse rate, as in wakefulness. During REM sleep we experience vivid dreams, as we'll discuss shortly.

The EEG portrait in Figure 10.11 shows that sleep consists of a complex series of brain states, not just an "inactive" period. The total sleep time of young adults usually ranges from 7 to 8 hours, about half of it in stage 2 sleep. REM sleep accounts for about 20% of total sleep. A typical night of adult human sleep shows repeating cycles approximately 90–110 minutes long, recurring four or five times in a night, reflecting a basic ultradian rest-activity cycle (Kaiser, 2013). These cycles change in a subtle but regular manner through the night. Stage 3 SWS, when we are most deeply asleep and the pituitary releases growth hormone, is more prominent early in the

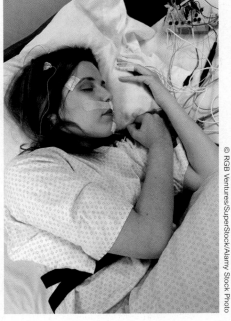

Wired for Sleep   Machines measure electrical activity across the various electrodes to monitor EEG, eye movements, and muscle tension across sleep stages.

FIGURE 10.12 A Typical Night of Sleep in a Young Adult (After A. Kales and J. Kales. 1970. *JAMA* 213: 2229.)

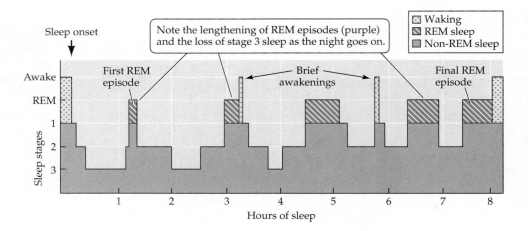

night (**FIGURE 10.12**), and then it tapers off as the night progresses. In contrast, REM sleep is more prominent in the later cycles of sleep. The first REM period is the shortest, while the last REM period, just before waking, may last up to 40 minutes. Brief arousals (yellow bars in Figure 10.12) occasionally occur immediately after a REM period, and the sleeper may shift posture at this time (Amici et al., 2014). **TABLE 10.1** compares the properties of REM and non-REM sleep.

We do our most vivid dreaming during REM sleep

We can record the EEGs of participants to monitor their sleep stages, awaken them at a particular stage (1, 2, 3, or REM), and question them about thoughts or perceptions they were having. Early studies of this sort suggested that dreams happen only during REM sleep, but we now know that dreams also occur in other sleep stages. What is distinctive about dreams during REM sleep is that they are characterized by visual imagery, whereas dreams during non-REM sleep are of a more "thinking" type. REM dreams are apt to include a story that involves odd perceptions and the sense that the dreamer "is there" experiencing sights, sounds, smells, and emotions (McNamara et al., 2010). People awakened from non-REM sleep report thinking about problems rather than seeing themselves in a mental movie. The dreams of these two states are so different that people can be trained to predict accurately whether a described dream occurred during REM sleep or SWS (Siclari et al., 2017).

TABLE 10.1 Properties of REM Sleep and Non-REM Sleep

Property	REM sleep	Non-REM sleep
AUTONOMIC ACTIVITIES		
Heart rate	Variable, with high burst	Slow decline
Respiration	Variable, with high burst	Slow decline
Brain temperature	Increased	Decreased
Cerebral blood flow	High	Reduced
SKELETAL MUSCULAR SYSTEM		
Postural tension	Eliminated	Progressively reduced
Knee-jerk reflex	Suppressed	Normal
Twitches	Increased	Reduced
Eye movements	Rapid, coordinated	Infrequent, slow, uncoordinated
COGNITIVE STATE		
Dream state	Vivid dreams, well organized	Vague thoughts
HORMONE SECRETION		
Growth hormone secretion	Low	High in SWS
NEURAL FIRING RATES		
Cerebral cortex activity	Increased firing rates	Many cells reduced

Almost everyone has terrifying dreams on occasion (Llewellyn and Hobson, 2015). **Nightmares** are defined as long, frightening dreams that awaken the sleeper. They are occasionally confused with **night terror**, which is a sudden arousal from stage 3 SWS marked by intense fear and autonomic activation. In night terror, the sleeper does not recall a vivid dream but may remember a sense of a crushing feeling on the chest, as though being suffocated. Night terrors are common in children during the early part of an evening's sleep.

Many medications, including antidepressants and drugs that control blood pressure, make nightmares more frequent (J. F. Pagel and Helfter, 2003), but nightmares are quite prevalent even without such influences. At least 25% of college students report having one or more nightmares per month. Have you had the common one, which Sigmund Freud had, of suddenly remembering that you're supposed to be taking a final exam that is already in progress?

As fascinating as they are, we still do not know what function, if any, is fulfilled by dreams. The activation-synthesis theory suggests our experiences in REM sleep are the more or less random results of which neurons happen to get activated (Hobson and Friston, 2012). The brain strings together these disparate activated elements into a more or less coherent story, a narrative. Later we'll discuss evidence that at least some other animals experience dreaming, which suggests that dreaming either fulfills an important function or is an unavoidable consequence of some other function of REM sleep.

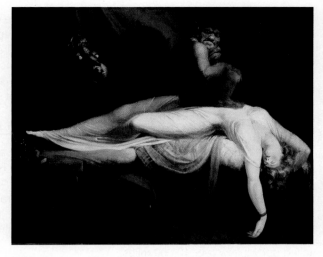

Night Terror   This 1781 painting by Henry Fuseli is called *The Nightmare*. It also aptly illustrates night terror, or even sleep paralysis, discussed later in the chapter, as the demon crushes the breath from his victim.

Different species provide clues about the evolution of sleep

With the aid of behavioral and EEG techniques, sleep has been studied in a wide assortment of mammals and, to a lesser extent, in reptiles, birds, and amphibians (Lesku et al., 2009; Hartse, 2011). Nearly all mammalian species that have been investigated thus far, including our most distant mammalian relatives, such as the platypus (Manger et al., 2002), display both REM sleep and SWS. Among the other vertebrates, birds display clear signs of both SWS and REM sleep, which indicates that REM sleep was present in an ancestor common to birds and mammals. The report of REM sleep in a reptile (Shein-Idelson et al., 2016) suggests that maybe it arose even earlier.

The absence of REM sleep in dolphins is probably a late adaptation that evolved when their land-dwelling ancestors took to the water, because they must come to the surface of the water to breathe. That requirement may be incompatible with the deep relaxation of muscles during REM sleep. Another dolphin adaptation to living in water is that only one side of the dolphin brain engages in SWS at a time (Lyamin et al., 2008). It's as if one whole hemisphere is asleep while the other is awake (**FIGURE 10.13**). During these periods of "unilateral sleep," the animals continue to come up to

nightmare   A long, frightening dream that awakens the sleeper from REM sleep.

night terror   A sudden arousal from stage 3 sleep that is marked by intense fear and autonomic activation.

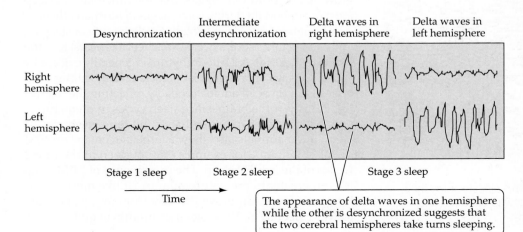

FIGURE 10.13   Sleep in Marine Mammals   (After L. M. Mukhametov in A. Borbély and J. L. Valatx. 1984. *Experimental Brain Research: Suppl. 8. Sleep Mechanisms*. Springer-Verlag. Berlin, Germany.)

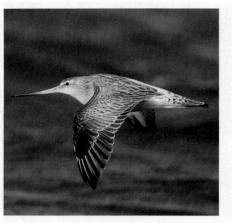

Like Sleeping on Air A female bar-tailed godwit flew over 10,000 miles, nonstop, from Alaska to Australia in a week. Were both sides of its brain awake the entire time?

the surface occasionally to breathe. Birds can also display unilateral sleep—one hemisphere sleeping while the other hemisphere watches for predators (Rattenborg, 2006). Unilateral sleep while gliding may also enable birds to fly long distances without stopping; for example, a bar-tailed godwit flew nonstop more than 10,000 miles, from Alaska to Australia, in a week (Gill et al., 2009). You can learn more about comparing patterns of sleep in different species in **A STEP FURTHER 10.2**, on the website.

HOW'S IT GOING ?

1. What are the different stages of sleep, and what measures define them?
2. What happens to our muscles during the sleep stage characterized by the most vivid dreams?
3. Contrast the mental activity present in REM sleep versus SWS.
4. Describe ways that certain species manage to sleep despite obstacles like living in water and nonstop flying.

The dark portions here indicate time asleep; the blank portions, time awake.

Weeks after birth

A stable pattern of sleep at night does not appear to be consolidated until about 16 weeks of age.

From N. Kleitman and T. Engelmann. 1953. *J. App. Physiol.* 6: 269

FIGURE 10.14 **The Trouble with Babies** This classic study may represent an extreme example of a baby slow to entrain to the day-night rhythm.

10.3 Our Sleep Patterns Change across the Life Span

THE ROAD AHEAD

The next section covers what we know about why we sleep, and how the brain switches from one stage to another. Studying this material should allow you to:

10.3.1 Describe the changes in sleep as we grow up and grow old.

10.3.2 Critically discuss the effects of partial versus total sleep deprivation.

10.3.3 Discuss various theories about the function of sleep.

10.3.4 Describe four brain systems that influence the sleep-waking cycle.

How much sleep and what kind of sleep we get changes across our lifetime. As infants, we sleep a lot; as we grow, we sleep less and less until we hit adolescence, when once again sleep seems precious. After that, we sleep less as we age, sometimes to our disappointment. These changes as we grow up and grow old suggest that the function(s) of sleep are more important during some stages of life than others.

Human infants sleep a lot, but a clear cycle of sleeping and waking takes several weeks (that feel like years) to settle in (**FIGURE 10.14**). A 24-hour rhythm is generally evident by 16 weeks of age. Infant sleep is characterized by shorter sleep cycles than those of adults, probably reflecting the relative immaturity of the brain, since sleep cycles in prematurely born infants are even shorter than in full-term newborns.

Infant mammals also show a large percentage of REM sleep. In humans, for example, half of sleep in the first 2 weeks of life is REM sleep. The prominence of REM sleep is even greater in premature infants. Unlike most adults, human infants can move directly from an awake state to REM sleep. The REM sleep of infants is quite active,

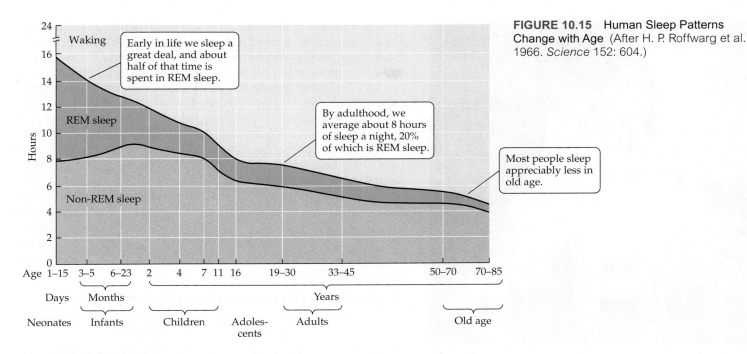

FIGURE 10.15 Human Sleep Patterns Change with Age (After H. P. Roffwarg et al. 1966. *Science* 152: 604.)

accompanied by muscle twitching, smiles, grimaces, and vocalizations. The preponderance of REM sleep early in life (**FIGURE 10.15**) suggests that this state provides stimulation that is essential to maturation of the nervous system. By contrast, killer whales and bottlenose dolphins appear to spend little or no time in REM sleep (or any other sleep stage) for the first month of life (Lyamin et al., 2005), presumably because they have to surface often to breathe. So, either REM sleep does not fill a crucial need in all mammalian infants, or dolphin and whale infants have evolved an alternative way to fill that need.

Most people sleep appreciably less as they age

The character of sleep changes in old age, though more slowly than in early development. **FIGURE 10.16** shows the sleep pattern typical of an elderly person. The total amount of sleep declines, while the number of awakenings increases (compare with Figure 10.12). Lack of sleep, or insomnia (which we discuss at the end of this chapter), is a common complaint of the elderly and is associated with a variety of physical and cognitive impairments (J. R. Cooke and Ancoli-Israel, 2011).

In humans and other mammals, the most dramatic decline is in stage 3 sleep; 60-year-old people spend only about half as much time in stage 3 as they did at age 20 (Mander et al., 2017). By 90 years of age, stage 3 sleep has disappeared. This decline

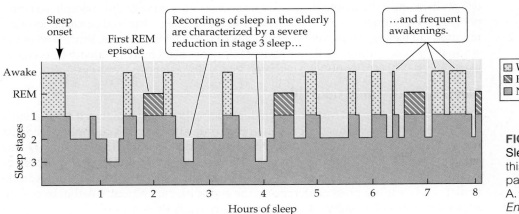

FIGURE 10.16 The Typical Pattern of Sleep in an Elderly Person Compare this recording with the young adult sleep pattern shown in Figure 10.12. (After A. Kales and J. D. Kales. 1974. *New England J. Med.* 290: 487.)

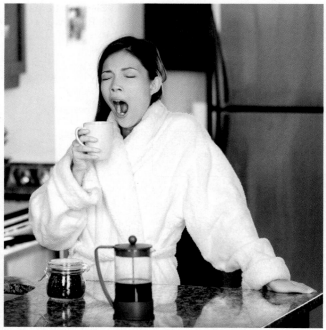

I Need Sleep! Doing without sleep has one clear effect: you feel sleepy.

in stage 3 sleep may be related to diminished cognitive functioning, since an especially marked reduction of stage 3 SWS characterizes the sleep of people who suffer from senile dementia. Growth hormone is secreted primarily during stage 3 SWS (see Table 10.1), so perhaps the loss of growth hormone due to disrupted sleep in the elderly leads to the cognitive deficits. Loss of SWS probably also impairs memory processes (discussed below) in older people and patients with dementia (Westerberg et al., 2012).

Most elderly people fall asleep easily enough, but then they may have a hard time staying asleep, which causes sleep "dissatisfaction." As in so many things, attitude may be important for how you experience sleep loss as you age. Objective measures of sleep suggest that elderly people who complain of poor sleep may actually sleep *more* than those who are satisfied with their sleep (McCrae et al., 2005). Perhaps if, as you grow older, you can regard waking up at 3:00 AM as a "bonus" (a little more time awake before you die), you will be more satisfied with the sleep you get.

Manipulating sleep reveals an underlying structure

Another persuasive clue that sleep is important is revealed when we go without it. First of all, our mental function is impaired. This is bad news for college students, who rarely get enough sleep, just when they're supposed to be learning how to make their way in the world. In addition, after sleep deprivation we tend to sleep more than we would have, as though catching up on something we need, as we'll see.

Most of us at one time or another have been willing or not-so-willing participants in informal **sleep deprivation** experiments. Thus, most of us are aware of the primary effect of partial or total sleep deprivation: it makes us sleepy. It has other effects as well. Early reports from sleep deprivation studies emphasized a similarity between schizophrenia and "bizarre" behavior provoked by sleep deprivation. But examination of people with schizophrenia does not fit this view. For example, these people can show sleep-waking cycles similar to those of typical adults, and sleep deprivation does not exacerbate their symptoms.

The behavioral effects of prolonged, total sleep deprivation vary appreciably and may depend on some general personality factors and on age. In studies employing prolonged total deprivation—205 hours (8.5 days!)—a few participants showed occasional episodes of hallucinations. But the most common behavior changes were increases in irritability, difficulty in concentrating, and episodes of disorientation.

You don't need to resort to total sleep deprivation to see effects. Moderate effects of sleep debt can accumulate with successive nights of little sleep. Voluntary experimental participants who got 6 or 4 hours of sleep per night for 2 weeks showed ever-mounting deficits in attention tasks and in speed of reaction, compared with those sleeping 8 hours per night (Van Dongen et al., 2003). Interestingly, the sleep-deprived participants often reported not feeling sleepy, yet they still exhibited behavioral deficits. By the end of the study, the people getting less than 8 hours of sleep per night had cognitive deficits equivalent to those of participants who had been totally sleep-deprived for 3 days!

Sleep recovery may take time

One of the most famous cases of sleep deprivation began as a high school student's science project. Researchers became involved only after Randy Gardner had started his deprivation schedule, which is why we have no data about his sleep before he decided to stay awake for, believe it or not, 11 days! As in other studies, Randy's performance on some tests was impaired, but he could still hold a conversation and was articulate and clear in a press conference at the end of his experiment. In other words, he showed no signs of insanity—he just acted really, really sleepy.

sleep deprivation The partial or total prevention of sleep.

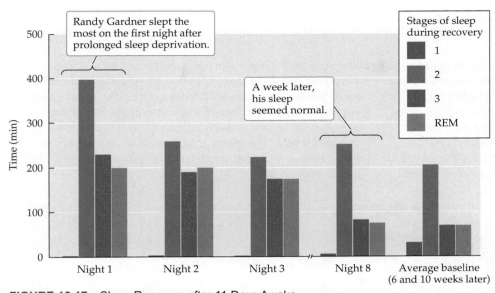

Randy Gardner slept the most on the first night after prolonged sleep deprivation.

A week later, his sleep seemed normal.

Stages of sleep during recovery
1
2
3
REM

FIGURE 10.17 Sleep Recovery after 11 Days Awake
(After G. Gulevich et al. 1966. *Arch. Gen. Psychiatry* 15: 29.)

sleep recovery The process of sleeping more than normally after a period of sleep deprivation, as though in compensation.

fatal familial insomnia An inherited disease that causes people in middle age to stop sleeping, which after a few months results in death.

Randy's **sleep recovery** after 11 days of sleep deprivation, depicted in **FIGURE 10.17**, shows the same pattern of sleep recovery as in controlled studies with shorter periods of deprivation. In the first night of sleep recovery, stage 3 sleep shows the greatest relative difference from normal. This increase in stage 3 sleep is usually at the expense of stage 2 sleep. However, the added stage 3 sleep during recovery never completely makes up for the deficit accumulated over the deprivation period. In fact, Randy had no more additional stage 3 sleep than do people deprived of sleep for half as long. REM sleep in recovery nights is more "intense" than normal, with a greater number of rapid eye movements per period of time. So you never recover all the sleep time you lost, but you may make up for the loss by having more intense sleep for a few nights. The sooner you get to sleep, the sooner you recover.

Finally, it is clear that prolonged, total sleep deprivation in mammals compromises the immune system and leads to death, as we'll see in Signs & Symptoms next.

Skipping Sleep for Science As a young man, Randy Gardner decided to see how long he could stay awake as a science fair project. The answer? Just over 11 days. Is that a record for the most demanding science fair project?

© San Diego History Center

SIGNS & SYMPTOMS

Total Sleep Deprivation Can Be Fatal

Sustained sleep deprivation in rats causes them to increase their metabolic rate, lose weight, and, within an average of 19 days, die (Everson et al., 1989). Allowing them to sleep prevents their death. After the fatal effect of sleep deprivation had been shown, researchers undertook studies in which they terminated the sleep deprivation before the fatal end point and looked for pathological changes in different organ systems. No single organ system seems affected in chronically sleep-deprived animals, but early in the deprivation they develop sores on their bodies. These sores mark the beginning of the end; shortly thereafter, blood tests reveal infections from a host of bacteria, which probably enter through the sores (Rechtschaffen and Bergmann, 2002).

These bacteria are not normally fatal, because the rat's immune system and body defenses keep the bacteria in check, but severely sleep-deprived rats fail to develop a fever in response to these infections. (Fever helps the body fight infection.) In fact, the sleep-deprived animals show a drop in body temperature, which probably speeds bacterial infections that in turn cause diffuse organ damage. The decline of these severely sleep-deprived rats is complicated, but it seems clear that getting sleep improves immune system function (Bryant et al., 2004). So perhaps Shakespeare's theory of the function of sleep, "Sleep that knits up the ravell'd sleave of care," isn't so far from the truth. Even fruit flies will die without sleep (P. J. Shaw et al., 2002).

(Continued)

Some unfortunate humans inherit a defect in the gene for the prion protein, which can transmit mad cow disease, and although they sleep normally at the beginning of life, in midlife they simply stop sleeping—with fatal effect. People with this disease, called **fatal familial insomnia**, die 7–24 months after the insomnia begins (K. Brown and Mastrianni, 2010). Autopsy reveals degeneration in the cerebral cortex (**FIGURE 10.18**) and thalamus, which may cause the insomnia. Like sleep-deprived rats,

sleep-deprived humans with this disorder don't have obvious damage to any single organ system, but they suffer from diffuse bacterial infections. Apparently, these patients die because they are chronically sleep-deprived, and these results, combined with research on rats, certainly support the idea that prolonged insomnia is fatal. The effects of sleep deprivation suggest that sleep plays an important function, or even several functions, that we'll consider next.

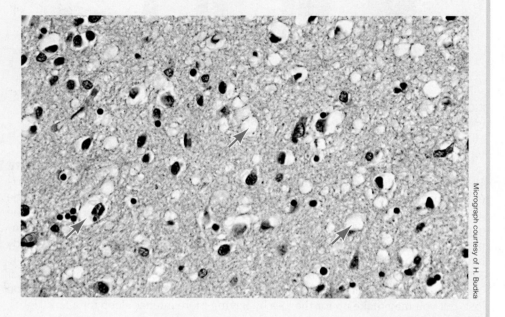

FIGURE 10.18 Fatal Sleeplessness Note the large holes (arrows) that have developed in this section of frontal cortex from a victim of fatal familial insomnia.

Micrograph courtesy of H. Budka

HOW'S IT GOING ❓

1. Describe how sleep changes as we grow up and grow old.
2. What happens when we are deprived of sleep?
3. Describe the outcome of Randy Gardner's famous self-study.

What are the biological functions of sleep?

Doesn't it seem like a big waste of time to spend one-third of our lifetime asleep? Most of us have fantasized about how great it would be if we could stay awake and chipper all the time, but we've seen that it's just not possible. What is so important about sleep that we can't seem to live without it? Let's consider the four functions that are most often ascribed to sleep:

1. Energy conservation
2. Niche adaptation
3. Body and brain restoration
4. Memory consolidation

CONSERVATION OF ENERGY We use up less energy when we sleep than when we're awake. For example, SWS is marked by reduced muscular tension, lowered heart rate, reduced blood pressure, reduced body temperature, and slower respiration. This diminished metabolic activity during sleep suggests that one role of sleep is to conserve energy. We can see the importance of this function by considering small animals. Small mammals and birds have very high metabolic rates (see Chapter 9). In general, the smaller the mammal, the higher its metabolic rate and the more time it spends asleep (Siegel, 2005). Larger mammals, like elephants, have low metabolic rates and sleep only a few hours per day (Gravett et al., 2017). That correlation supports the idea that sleep helps conserve energy. But energy savings from sleep seem modest at best (Lesku et al., 2009).

NICHE ADAPTATION   Almost all animals are either nocturnal or diurnal. This specialization for either nighttime or daytime activity is part of each species' **ecological niche**, that unique assortment of environmental opportunities and challenges to which each organism is adapted. Thanks to these adaptations, each species is better at gathering food either at night or in the daytime, and it is also better at avoiding predators either during the day or at night. If you're a nocturnal mammal, like a mouse, you are adept at sneaking around in the dark, using your acute senses of hearing and smell to navigate and find food. The rest of the time, during daylight, you should spend holed up somewhere safe to stay away from keen-eyed diurnal predators. Sleep debt and the unpleasant feelings of sleepiness have the effect of enforcing the circadian rhythm characteristic of your species. So, one important function of sleep, or of the results of sleep deprivation, is to force the individual to conform to the particular ecological niche for which it is well adapted (Meddis, 1975), and natural selection must have played an important role in its evolution.

PHYSICAL RESTORATION   If someone asked you why you wanted to go to sleep, you might answer that you "feel worn out." Indeed, one of the proposed functions of sleep is simply the rebuilding or restoration of materials used during waking, such as proteins (Pulak and Jensen, 2014). Maybe this is why most growth hormone release happens during slow wave sleep.

We've seen that prolonged and total sleep deprivation—either forced on rats or, in humans, as a result of inherited pathology—interferes with the immune system and leads to death. Even relatively mild deprivation, having sleep shortened or disrupted (e.g., by a nurse taking vital signs every hour), makes people more sensitive to pain the following day (Edwards et al., 2009). A study of over a million Americans found that those sleeping less than 6 hours per night were more likely to die over the next 6 years, although interestingly, people who slept *more than 8* hours per night were also at greater risk (Kripke et al., 2002). People who sleep less than 5 hours per night are more likely to develop diabetes (Gangwisch et al., 2007). Perhaps the most alarming link between sleep and health is the finding that people who work at night and sleep in the daytime are more likely to develop cancer (Erren et al., 2009). So the widespread belief that sleep helps the body ward off illness is well supported by research (S. Cohen et al., 2009; Imeri and Opp, 2009).

There's also evidence that sleep may help "clean out" the brain. Glia control the flow of cerebrospinal fluid through a network of microscopic channels throughout the brain, the glymphatic system we described in Chapter 1 (see Figure 1.33), collecting and disposing of toxins that build up. This flow is much faster during sleep than wakefulness (Xie et al., 2013), flushing out brain waste products as we snooze, including proteins—beta-amyloid and tau—that are implicated in Alzheimer's disease (Holth et al., 2019).

MEMORY CONSOLIDATION   A peculiar property of dreams is that, unless we describe them to someone or write them down soon after waking, we tend to forget them, as though the brain refuses to store anything that we experience during REM sleep. This seems like a good idea—why waste memory storage space on something

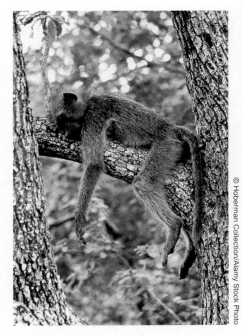

Finding Your Niche in Life   Species that can sleep in secure circumstances tend to sleep more than other species.

ecological niche   The unique assortment of environmental opportunities and challenges to which each organism is adapted.

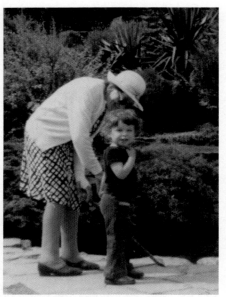

Courtesy of Ray Meddis

A Nonsleeper   When Ray Meddis brought this 70-year-old nurse into the lab for sleep recording, he confirmed that she slept only about an hour per night. Yet she was a healthy and energetic person. Here she's touring a garden with Meddis's son.

isolated brain   An experimental preparation in which an animal's brainstem has been separated from the spinal cord by a cut below the medulla.

isolated forebrain   An experimental preparation in which an animal's nervous system has been cut in the upper midbrain, dividing the forebrain from the brainstem.

basal forebrain   A ventral region in the forebrain that has been implicated in sleep.

tuberomammillary nucleus   A region of the basal hypothalamus, near the pituitary stalk, that plays a role in generating slow wave sleep.

general anesthetic   A drug that renders an individual unconscious.

that never happened? Similarly, and despite ads you might read in the backs of magazines, you cannot learn significant amounts of new material while you're sleeping (Druckman and Bjork, 1994). Putting a speaker under your pillow to recite material for a final exam will not help you, unless you stay awake to listen.

Sleep seems important for learning in another way, however. In 1924 an experiment suggested that sleep helps you learn or remember material or events experienced *before* you went to bed (Jenkins and Dallenbach, 1924). Some participants were trained in a verbal learning task at bedtime and tested 8 hours later on rising from sleep; other people were trained early in the day and tested 8 hours later (with no intervening sleep). The results showed better retention when a period of sleep intervened between a learning period and tests of recall. A surge of supporting evidence has shown that sleep helps with memory formation in many domains, not just verbal memory (Ellenbogen et al., 2007; Korman et al., 2007; Cherdieu et al., 2018; Navarro-Lobato and Genzel, 2018).

Despite early assumptions that REM sleep would play a bigger role in learning and memory, most research suggested that it is SWS that helps memory consolidation (Nishida and Walker, 2007). In fact, consolidation of a declarative memory task was even better if the person's cortical slow wave oscillations during SWS were boosted by electrically stimulating electrodes over the skull (Marshall et al., 2006). (Don't try this at home.) What's more, one man who had brainstem injuries that seemed to eliminate REM sleep could still learn, and he earned a law school degree (P. Lavie, 1996). So even if REM sleep *aids* learning, clearly it is not absolutely *necessary* for learning (Ackermann and Rasch, 2018).

Don't rule out a role for REM sleep in learning entirely, however, because synapses are being rearranged during that state (W. Li et al., 2017), and some memory consolidation seems dependent on REM (Boyce et al., 2016).

Some humans sleep remarkably little, yet function normally

One challenge to all the theories about the function of sleep is the existence of a few people who seem perfectly healthy, yet sleep hardly at all. These cases are more than just folktales. A Stanford University professor slept only 3–4 hours a night and lived to be 80 (Dement, 1974). Sleep researcher Ray Meddis (1977) found a cheerful 70-year-old retired nurse who said she had slept little since childhood. She was a busy person who easily filled up her 23 hours of daily wakefulness. During the night, she sat in bed reading or writing, and at about 2:00 AM she fell asleep for an hour or so, after which she readily awakened.

For her first two nights in Meddis's laboratory, she did not sleep at all, because it was all so interesting to her. On the third night, she slept a total of 99 minutes, and her sleep contained both SWS and REM sleep periods. In a later session, her sleep was recorded for 5 days. She didn't sleep the first night, but on subsequent nights she slept an average of 67 minutes. She never complained about not sleeping more, and she did not feel drowsy during either the day or the night. Meddis described several other people who slept only an hour or two per night. Some of these people reported having parents who slept little, so there may be a genetic tendency for little sleep. Whatever the function of sleep is, some people (and elephants) have a way of fulfilling it in just a few hours per night. Why aren't their immune systems compromised? We don't know, but perhaps their immune systems don't need much sleep either. Or perhaps the small amount of sleep they have almost every night is more efficient at doing whatever sleep does. The important point, though, is that no healthy person has ever been found who does not sleep at all.

HOW'S IT GOING ❓

1. Describe the four most prominent theories about the function of sleep and the evidence to support them.
2. What can we conclude about the function of sleep when we consider people who sleep very little?
3. What happens when we stop sleeping altogether?

RESEARCHERS AT WORK

The forebrain generates slow wave sleep

Some of the earliest studies of sleep indicated that a system in the forebrain promotes SWS. These are experiments in which an animal's brain is transected—literally cut into two parts: an upper part and a lower part. The entire brain can be isolated from the body by an incision between the medulla and the spinal cord. This preparation was first studied by the Belgian physiologist Frédéric Bremer (1892–1982), who called it the **isolated brain** (Bremer, 1938).

The EEGs of such animals showed signs of waking alternating with sleep (**FIGURE 10.19A**). During EEG-defined wakeful periods, the pupils were dilated and the eyes followed moving objects. During EEG-defined sleep, the pupils were small, as in normal sleep. REM sleep can also be detected in the isolated brain. These results demonstrated that wakefulness, SWS, and REM sleep are all mediated by *networks within the brain*.

When Bremer made the transection higher along the brainstem—in the midbrain—a very different result was seen. Bremer referred to such a preparation as an **isolated forebrain**, and he found that the EEG from the brain in front of the cut displayed constant SWS (**FIGURE 10.19B**), with no indications of wakefulness or REM sleep. This result demonstrates that the forebrain alone can generate SWS, without contributions from the lower brain regions.

The constant SWS seen in the cortex of the isolated forebrain appears to be generated by the **basal forebrain** in the ventral frontal lobe and anterior hypothalamus (**FIGURE 10.20A**). Electrical stimulation of the basal forebrain can induce SWS activity, while lesions there suppress sleep (McGinty and Sterman, 1968). Neurons in this region become active at sleep onset and release gamma-aminobutyric acid (GABA) (Gallopin et al., 2000) to stimulate $GABA_A$ receptors in the nearby **tuberomammillary nucleus** in the posterior hypothalamus. These same $GABA_A$ receptors are stimulated by **general anesthetics**—drugs such as barbiturates and anesthetic gases that render people unconscious during surgery. Thus, general anesthetics produce slow waves in the EEG that resemble those seen in SWS (Franks, 2008).

So the basal forebrain promotes SWS by releasing GABA into the nearby tuberomammillary nucleus, and if left alone, this system would keep the cortex asleep forever. But as we'll see next, the brainstem contains a system that arouses the forebrain from slumber.

FIGURE 10.19 Transecting the Brain at Different Levels

■ **Hypothesis**

The forebrain contains a neural system promoting SWS.

■ **Test**

Bremer transected the brain at one of two levels: between the spinal cord and medulla, or between the midbrain and the forebrain. If neural systems in the forebrain generate SWS, then the isolated forebrain should show SWS.

■ **Result**

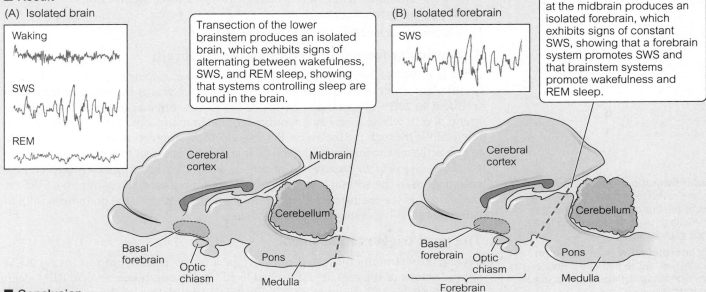

(A) Isolated brain

Waking

SWS

REM

Transection of the lower brainstem produces an isolated brain, which exhibits signs of alternating between wakefulness, SWS, and REM sleep, showing that systems controlling sleep are found in the brain.

Cerebral cortex

Midbrain

Cerebellum

Basal forebrain

Optic chiasm

Pons

Medulla

(B) Isolated forebrain

SWS

Transection of the brainstem at the midbrain produces an isolated forebrain, which exhibits signs of constant SWS, showing that a forebrain system promotes SWS and that brainstem systems promote wakefulness and REM sleep.

Cerebral cortex

Cerebellum

Basal forebrain

Optic chiasm

Pons

Medulla

Forebrain

■ **Conclusion**

The mechanism mediating SWS is in the forebrain and needs input from the brainstem to be roused from sleep.

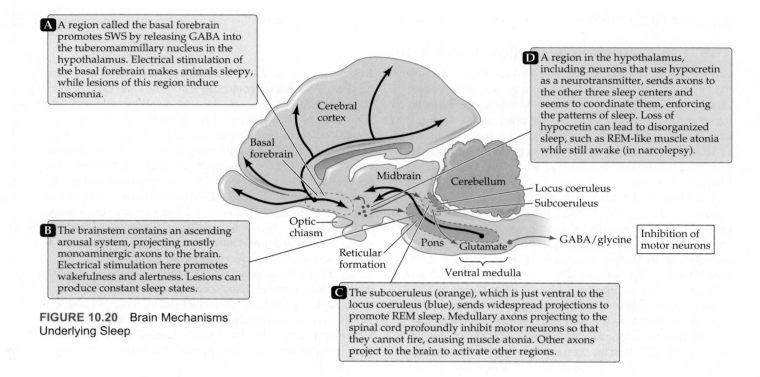

A A region called the basal forebrain promotes SWS by releasing GABA into the tuberomammillary nucleus in the hypothalamus. Electrical stimulation of the basal forebrain makes animals sleepy, while lesions of this region induce insomnia.

D A region in the hypothalamus, including neurons that use hypocretin as a neurotransmitter, sends axons to the other three sleep centers and seems to coordinate them, enforcing the patterns of sleep. Loss of hypocretin can lead to disorganized sleep, such as REM-like muscle atonia while still awake (in narcolepsy).

B The brainstem contains an ascending arousal system, projecting mostly monoaminergic axons to the brain. Electrical stimulation here promotes wakefulness and alertness. Lesions can produce constant sleep states.

C The subcoeruleus (orange), which is just ventral to the locus coeruleus (blue), sends widespread projections to promote REM sleep. Medullary axons projecting to the spinal cord profoundly inhibit motor neurons so that they cannot fire, causing muscle atonia. Other axons project to the brain to activate other regions.

FIGURE 10.20 Brain Mechanisms Underlying Sleep

View Activity 10.2:
Sleep Mechanisms

At least four interacting neural systems underlie sleep

At one time sleep was regarded as a passive state, as though most of the brain simply stopped working while we slept, leaving us unaware of events around us. We now know that sleep is an active state mediated by at least four interacting neural systems:

1. A *forebrain* system that generates SWS
2. A *brainstem* system that activates the sleeping forebrain into wakefulness
3. A *pontine* system that triggers REM sleep
4. A *hypothalamic* system that coordinates the other three brain regions to determine which state we're in

Let's examine each of these systems in some detail.

The reticular formation wakes up the forebrain

In the late 1940s, scientists found that they could wake sleeping animals by electrically stimulating an extensive region of the brainstem known as the **reticular formation** (**FIGURE 10.20B**) (Moruzzi and Magoun, 1949). The reticular formation is a diffuse group of cells whose axons and dendrites course in many directions, extending from the medulla through the thalamus. Because electrical stimulation anywhere along this region activates the forebrain, the reticular formation is sometimes called the *reticular activating system of the brainstem*. Conversely, lesions of these regions produced persistent sleep in the animals. So the basal forebrain region actively imposes SWS on the brain, and the brainstem reticular formation seems to push the brain from SWS to wakefulness. What system imposes REM sleep?

The pons triggers REM sleep

Several experiments indicated that a region of the pons is important for REM sleep. Lesions of the region just ventral to the **locus coeruleus** abolish REM sleep (**FIGURE 10.20C**) (B. E. Jones, 2020). Electrical stimulation of the same region, or

reticular formation Also called *reticular activating system*. An extensive region of the brainstem (extending from the medulla through the thalamus) that is involved in arousal.

locus coeruleus A small nucleus in the brainstem whose neurons produce norepinephrine and modulate large areas of the forebrain.

(A)

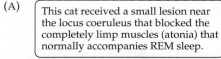

This cat received a small lesion near the locus coeruleus that blocked the completely limp muscles (atonia) that normally accompanies REM sleep.

(B)

The cat stands up wobbly, "looking" at something we cannot see. These behaviors indicate the cat is dreaming—seeing and interacting with objects that aren't really there.

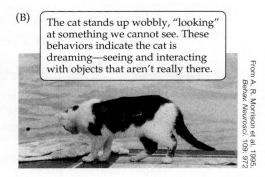

Following a bout of SWS, the cat in REM rises up as though about to pounce, but its eyes are nearly closed and nothing is there.

From A. R. Morrison et al. 1995. *Behav. Neurosci.* 109: 972

FIGURE 10.21   Acting Out a Dream

pharmacological stimulation of this region with cholinergic agonists, can induce or prolong REM sleep. Finally, some neurons in this region seem to be active only during REM sleep. So the pons has a REM sleep center near the locus coeruleus.

One important job of the pontine REM sleep center is to prevent motor neurons from firing. During REM sleep, the inhibitory transmitters GABA and glycine produce powerful inhibitory postsynaptic potentials (discussed in Chapter 3) in spinal motor neurons, preventing them from reaching threshold and producing an action potential (Kodama et al., 2003). Thus, the dreamer's muscles are not just relaxed, but flaccid. This loss of muscle tone during REM sleep can be abolished by small lesions that damage only a part of the REM center, suggesting that this subregion is what normally disables the motor system during REM.

Cats with such lesions seem to act out their dreams. They enter SWS as they normally would, but when they begin to display the EEG signs of REM sleep, instead of becoming completely limp as normal cats do, these cats stagger to their feet (A. R. Morrison, 2013). Are they awake or in REM sleep? They move their heads as though visually tracking moving objects (that aren't there), bat with their forepaws at nothing, and ignore objects that are present (**FIGURE 10.21**). In addition, the cats' *inner eyelids*, the translucent nictitating membranes, partially cover the eyes. Thus, the cats appear to be in REM sleep, but motor activity is not being inhibited by the brain. These results strongly suggest that animals dream too. What do cats dream of? If their actions while sleeping are any indication, they dream of stalking prey, perhaps a mouse or a ball of yarn.

So far, we've described three interacting brain systems controlling sleep: an SWS-promoting region in the forebrain, an arousing reticular formation in the brainstem, and a system in the pons that triggers REM sleep, including paralysis of the body during that state. There is a fourth important system, which seems to act as a "coordinating center" among these three centers, in the hypothalamus (**FIGURE 10.20D**). To understand how we learned about this fourth system, we need to consider sleep disorders because a rare but fascinating condition taught us about a specific neurotransmitter that is crucial in the control of sleep.

See Video 10.5:
Animal Sleep Activity

HOW'S IT GOING ❓

1. Describe the brain systems that control different stages of the sleep-waking cycle, discussing the experiments that revealed each.
2. What receptor systems do anesthetics act upon to render people unconscious?
3. What happens when brainstem systems to inhibit movement during REM sleep are damaged?

10.4 Sleep Disorders Can Be Serious, Even Life-Threatening

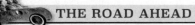

THE ROAD AHEAD

We close the chapter by considering disorders of sleep and wakefulness. Studying this material will enable you to:

10.4.1 Discuss narcolepsy and how the study of this disorder revealed a neural system controlling sleep.

10.4.2 Describe several different sleep disorders associated with particular sleep stages or partial arousals.

10.4.3 Distinguish between different types of insomnia, and offer advice for good sleep hygiene.

narcolepsy A disorder that involves frequent, intense episodes of sleep, which last from 5 to 30 minutes and can occur anytime during the usual waking hours.

For some people, the peace and comfort of regular, uninterrupted sleep is routinely disturbed by the inability to fall asleep, by prolonged sleep, or by unusual awakenings. Other people suffer from attacks where they cannot move, despite remaining conscious. Study of this disruptive disorder, first in dogs and then in people, revealed an important system for coordinating sleep states.

A hypothalamic sleep center was revealed by the study of narcolepsy

You might not consider getting lots of sleep an affliction, but some people are either drowsy all the time or suffer sudden attacks of sleep. At the extreme of such tendencies is **narcolepsy**, an unusual disorder in which the person is afflicted by frequent, intense attacks of sleep that last 5–30 minutes and can occur at any time during usual waking hours. These sleep attacks occur several times a day.

Most people display SWS for an hour or more before entering REM; individuals who have narcolepsy, however, tend to enter REM in the first few minutes of sleep. People with this disorder exhibit an otherwise normal sleep pattern at night, but they suffer abrupt, overwhelming sleepiness during the day. Some people with narcolepsy

See Video 10.6:
Narcoleptic Dogs

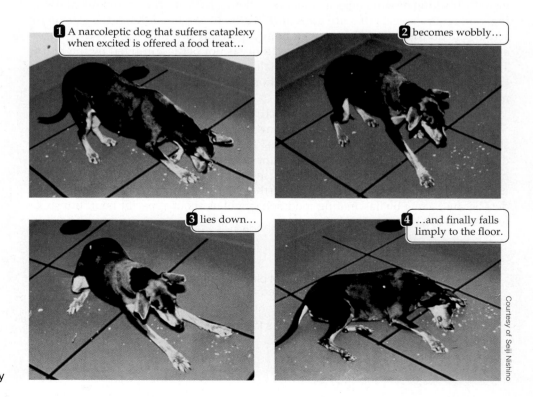

1 A narcoleptic dog that suffers cataplexy when excited is offered a food treat…

2 becomes wobbly…

3 lies down…

4 …and finally falls limply to the floor.

Courtesy of Seiji Nishino

FIGURE 10.22 Canine Narcolepsy

also show **cataplexy**, a sudden loss of muscle tone, leading to collapse of the body *without loss of consciousness*. Cataplexy can be triggered by sudden, intense emotional stimuli. Narcolepsy usually manifests itself between the ages of 15 and 25 years and continues throughout life. Remember Adrian from the start of this chapter? His narcolepsy was unusual in several ways: his only symptom was cataplexy, and that began unusually late in life, in his thirties. However, the trigger for Adrian's cataplexy, humor, is typical of others with narcolepsy; they become literally weak with laughter.

Several strains of dogs exhibit narcolepsy (Mignot, 2014), complete with sudden collapse, usually triggered by being excited, and very rapid sleep onset (**FIGURE 10.22**). Just like humans who have narcolepsy, these dogs often show REM signs immediately upon falling asleep. Abrupt collapse in these dogs is suppressed by the same drugs (discussed shortly) that are used to treat human cataplexy.

Finding the mutant gene responsible for narcoleptic dogs revealed a hypothalamic system that is responsible for narcolepsy in people too. This was the gene for a neuropeptide called **orexin** (also known as *hypocretin*; see Chapter 9) (Siegel et al., 2001). Mice with the *orexin* gene knocked out also display narcolepsy (M. Liu et al., 2017). Genetically normal rats can be made narcoleptic if injected with a toxin that destroys neurons possessing orexin receptors (Gerashchenko et al., 2001). The narcoleptic dogs start losing orexin neurons at about the age when symptoms of narcolepsy appear (John et al., 2004).

Similarly, humans with narcolepsy have lost about 90% of their orexin neurons (**FIGURE 10.23**) (Thannickal et al., 2000). This degeneration of orexin neurons seems to cause inappropriate activation of the cataplexy pathway that normally happens only during REM sleep. So, orexin normally keeps sleep at bay and prevents the transition from wakefulness directly into REM sleep.

The neurons that produce orexin are found almost exclusively in the hypothalamus. Where do these neurons send their axons to release the orexin? Not so coincidentally, the axons go to each of the three brain centers that we mentioned before: basal forebrain, reticular formation, and locus coeruleus (Sutcliffe and de Lecea, 2002). The orexin neurons also project axons to the hypothalamic tuberomammillary nucleus—the same structure that is inhibited by the basal forebrain to induce SWS. So, it looks as if the hypothalamus contains an orexin-based "switching station" (see Figure 10.20D) that switches the brain between states, from wakefulness to non-REM sleep to REM sleep (Saper et al., 2010). This system normally triggers paralysis only during REM, so loss of the system in narcolepsy leads to paralysis while awake (cataplexy).

The traditional treatment for narcolepsy was the use of amphetamines in the daytime. The drug GHB (gamma-hydroxybutyrate, trade name Xyrem, also called *sodium oxybate*) helps some narcoleptics (although there are concerns about potential abuse of this drug [Fuller and Hornfeldt, 2012]). A newer drug, modafinil (Provigil), is sometimes effective for preventing narcoleptic attacks and has been proposed as an "alertness drug"

cataplexy   Sudden loss of muscle tone, leading to collapse of the body without loss of consciousness. Cataplexy is sometimes a component of narcoleptic attacks.

orexin   Also called *hypocretin*. A neuropeptide produced in the hypothalamus that is involved in switching between sleep states, in narcolepsy, and in the control of appetite.

(A) Normal

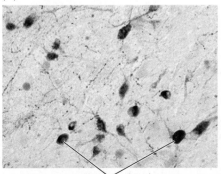

Immunocytochemistry reveals orexin-containing neurons in the lateral hypothalamus of a person who did not have narcolepsy.

(B) Narcoleptic

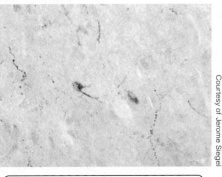

This same region of the brain from someone with narcolepsy has far fewer orexin neurons.

Courtesy of Jerome Siegel

FIGURE 10.23   Neural Degeneration in Humans with Narcolepsy

sleep paralysis A state, during the transition to or from sleep, in which the ability to move or talk is temporarily lost.

sleep enuresis Bed-wetting.

somnambulism Sleepwalking.

for people with attention deficit hyperactivity disorder. There is also debate about whether modafinil should be available to anyone who feels sleepy or needs to stay awake (Battleday and Brem, 2015), but at least one study found the drug no more effective than caffeine in this regard (Wesensten et al., 2002). Our friend Adrian, from the chapter opener, eventually found a combination of drugs that worked for him and continued a very successful career in the financial sector. Still, he finds he has to avoid trying to say or do anything amusing. "You just start to back away from the things that you know will almost without fail push you over the edge, which is a shame actually" (Leschziner, 2019, p. 131). Typical of people with narcolepsy, Adrian has low levels of orexin in CSF sampled through a spinal tap. Now that narcolepsy is known to be caused by a loss of orexin signaling, there is hope of developing synthetic drugs to stimulate orexin receptors, both for the relief of symptoms in narcolepsy and to combat sleepiness in people without narcolepsy.

Many people who do not suffer from narcolepsy nevertheless occasionally experience the cataplexy that accompanies narcolepsy (Denis, 2018). **Sleep paralysis** is the temporary inability to move or talk either just before dropping off to sleep or, more often, just after waking. In this state, people may experience sudden sensory hallucinations (Cheyne, 2002), including the belief that something is crushing their chest. Sleep paralysis never lasts more than a few minutes, so it's best to relax and avoid panic. One hypothesis is that sleep paralysis results when the pontine center (see Figure 10.20C) continues to impose paralysis for a short while after a person awakes from a REM episode.

Some minor dysfunctions are associated with non-REM sleep

Some dysfunctions associated with sleep are much more common in children than in adults. Two sleep disorders in children—night terrors (described earlier) and **sleep enuresis** (bed-wetting)—are associated with SWS. Most people grow out of these conditions without intervention, but pharmacological approaches can be used to reduce the amount of stage 3 sleep (as well as REM time) while increasing stage 2 sleep. For sleep enuresis, some doctors prescribe a nasal spray of the hormone vasopressin (see Chapter 9) before bedtime (Van Herzeele et al., 2017), which decreases urine production.

Somnambulism (sleepwalking) consists of getting out of bed, walking around the room, and appearing awake. Although more common in childhood, it sometimes persists into adulthood. These episodes last a few seconds to minutes, and the person

---

TABLE 10.2 Classification of Sleep Disorders with Some Examples

INSOMNIAS	PARASOMNIAS
Chronic insomnia (more than 3 months)	NREM-related parasomnias
Paradoxical insomnia (sleep state misperception)	Night terrors
Inadequate sleep hygiene	Sleepwalking (somnambulism)
Drug-related insomnia	REM-related parasomnias
Insomnia associated with psychiatric disorders	Nightmares
Short-term insomnia (less than 3 months)	Recurrent sleep paralysis
	REM behavior disorder (RBD)
SLEEP-RELATED BREATHING DISORDERS	Sleep enuresis (bed-wetting)
Obstructive sleep apnea	
Central sleep apnea	**SLEEP-RELATED MOVEMENT DISORDERS**
	Restless legs syndrome
CENTRAL DISORDERS OF HYPERSOMNOLENCE	Bruxism (teeth grinding)
Narcolepsy	Sleep-related myoclonus (sleep starts)
Hypersomnolence associated with psychiatric disorder	
Hypersomnolence due to medication or substance	**SLEEP-RELATED MEDICAL AND NEUROLOGICAL DISORDERS**
	Fatal familial insomnia
CIRCADIAN RHYTHM SLEEP-WAKE DISORDERS	Sleep epilepsy
Shift work disorder	Sleep headaches
Jet lag disorder	

Source: American Academy of Sleep Medicine, 2014. *International Classification of Sleep Disorders*, 3rd ed. American Academy of Sleep Medicine: Darien, IL.

usually does not remember the experience. Because such episodes occur during stage 3 SWS, they are more common in the first half of the night when that stage predominates. Likewise, episodes of "sexsomnia," when adults have sex but afterward have no memory of it (Muza et al., 2016), happen during non-REM sleep, early in the night. Narcolepsy and other sleep disorders (**TABLE 10.2**) have made sleep disorder clinics common in major medical centers.

Some people appear to be acting out their nightmares

While most sleepwalkers are not acting out a dream, there is a disorder where people appear to be acting out a dream. **REM behavior disorder** (**RBD**) is characterized by organized behavior—such as fighting an imaginary foe, eating a meal, or acting like a wild animal—by a person who appears to be asleep (St Louis and Boeve, 2017). Sometimes the person remembers a dream that fits well with his behavior (C. Brown, 2003), like the gentleman in the low-light video on our website (**FIGURE 10.24**). This disorder usually begins after the age of 50 and is more common in men than in women. Individuals with RBD are reminiscent of the cats with a lesion near the locus coeruleus, mentioned earlier, that were no longer paralyzed during REM and so acted out their dreams. In both cases, they no longer benefit from brainstem inhibition of motor neurons that would normally prevent them from moving. Unfortunately, the onset of RBD is often followed by symptoms of Parkinson's disease and dementia (Abbott and Videnovic, 2014), suggesting that the disorder marks the beginning of widespread neurodegeneration. The breakdown appears to begin in the brainstem region that imposes muscle atonia (see Figure 10.19) (Peever et al., 2014). RBD may be controlled by anti-anxiety drugs (benzodiazepines like Valium) taken at bedtime.

Insomniacs have trouble falling asleep or staying asleep

Almost all of us have trouble falling asleep on occasion, but many people persistently find it difficult to get as much sleep as they would like. Depending on the definition used for insomnia, its prevalence ranges from 10% to 40% of the adult population (Mai and Buysse, 2008). Insomnia is more commonly reported by older people, females, and users of drugs like tobacco, caffeine, and alcohol. It is not a trivial disorder; recall that adults who regularly sleep for short periods show a higher mortality rate than those who regularly sleep 7–8 hours each night (Kripke et al., 2002).

Insomnia seems to be the final common outcome for various conditions. Situational factors such as shift work, time zone changes, and changes in the daily routine (that hard motel bed) can lead to insomnia. Usually these conditions produce transient **sleep-onset insomnia**, a difficulty in falling asleep. Drugs, as well as neurological and psychiatric factors, seem to cause **sleep-maintenance insomnia**, a difficulty in remaining asleep. In this type of insomnia, sleep is punctuated by frequent nighttime arousals.

REM behavior disorder (RBD)
A sleep disorder in which a person physically acts out a dream.

sleep-onset insomnia   Difficulty in falling asleep.

sleep-maintenance insomnia
Difficulty in staying asleep.

See Video 10.7:
REM Behavior Disorder

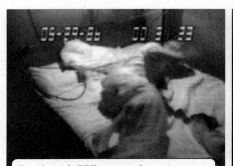

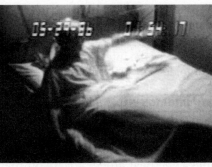

People with RBD seem to be acting out a dream, often of running away from or fighting an unseen foe.

FIGURE 10.24   Battling in Your Dreams

From M. W. Mahowald and C. H. Schenck, 2005. *Nature* 437: 1279

sleep state misperception
Commonly, the perception of not having been asleep when in fact the person has been. It typically occurs at the start of a sleep episode.

sleep apnea   A sleep disorder in which respiration slows or stops periodically, waking the sleeper. Excessive daytime sleepiness results from the frequent nocturnal awakening.

sudden infant death syndrome (SIDS)
Also called *crib death*. The sudden, unexpected death of an apparently healthy human infant who simply stops breathing, usually during sleep.

People with **sleep state misperception** (Lichstein, 2017; Rezaie et al., 2018) *report* that they didn't sleep even when the EEG showed signs of sleep and they failed to respond to stimuli. They are sleeping without knowing it. Sometimes these people, upon learning that they really are sleeping, are more satisfied with the sleep they get.

In some people, respiration becomes unreliable during sleep. Breathing may cease for a minute or so, or it may slow alarmingly; blood levels of oxygen drop markedly. This syndrome, called **sleep apnea**, arises either from the progressive relaxation of muscles of the chest, diaphragm, and throat cavity or from changes in the pacemaker respiratory neurons of the brainstem. In the former instance, relaxation of the throat obstructs the airway—a kind of self-choking. This mode of sleep apnea is common in very obese people, but it also occurs, often undiagnosed, in non-obese people. Sleep apnea is frequently accompanied by loud, interrupted snoring, so loud snorers should consult a physician about the possibility that they suffer from sleep apnea.

Investigators have speculated that **sudden infant death syndrome** (**SIDS**, or *crib death*) arises from sleep apnea as a result of immature systems that normally control respiration. Autopsies of SIDS victims reveal abnormalities in brainstem serotonin systems (Kinney, 2009); interfering with this system in mice renders them unable to regulate respiration effectively (Audero et al., 2008). Since the start of the Safe to Sleep campaign, which urges parents to place infants on their backs to sleep rather than on their stomachs, the incidence of SIDS is less than a third what it was before. Placing the baby face down may lead to suffocation if the baby cannot regulate breathing or arouse properly. Exposure to cigarette smoke also increases the risk of crib death.

Although many drugs affect sleep, there is no perfect sleeping pill

Throughout recorded history, humans have reached for substances to enhance sleep. Ancient Greeks used opium from the juice of the poppy, as well as products of the mandrake plant, to aid sleep. The preparation of barbituric acid in the mid-nineteenth century started the development of many drugs—barbiturates—that were widely used to combat insomnia.

Most modern sleeping pills—including benzodiazepines (see Chapter 4) like triazolam (Halcion) and nonbenzodiazepine sedatives, the "Z drugs" like zolpidem (Ambien) and eszopiclone (Lunesta)—bind to GABA receptors, inhibiting broad regions of the brain. But reliance on sleeping pills poses many problems (Carr, 2018). Viewed solely as a way to deal with sleep problems, current drugs fall far short of being a suitable remedy, for several reasons. First, even the newest class of sleeping pills produce little more sleep than placebos (Huedo-Medina et al., 2012). Second, continued use of sleeping pills causes them to lose effectiveness (Walker, 2017), and this declining ability to induce sleep often leads to increased self-prescribed dosages that can be dangerous. Another major drawback is that sleeping pills produce marked changes in the pattern of sleep, both while the drug is being used and for days afterward.

Use of sleeping pills may lead to a persistent "sleep drunkenness," coupled with drowsiness, that impairs waking activity, or to memory gaps about daily activity. Police have reported cases of "Ambien drivers," people who have taken a sleeping pill and then got up a few hours later to go for a spin, with sometimes disastrous results, while apparently asleep (Saul, 2006). In other cases, people taking such medicines eat snacks, shop over the internet, or even have sex, with no memory of these events the next day (Dolder and Nelson, 2008).

Everyone should practice good sleep hygiene

Certainly, the treatment for insomnia that has the fewest side effects, and that is very effective for most people, is not to use any drug, but to practice good sleep hygiene. One strategy is to develop a regular routine to exploit the body's circadian clock. The best advice for insomniacs is to use an alarm clock to wake up faithfully at the same time each day (weekends included, **FIGURE 10.25**) and then

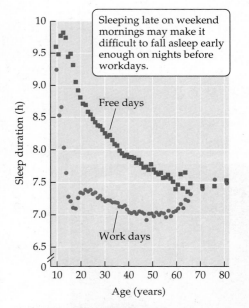

FIGURE 10.25 Sleeping In on the Weekend (After T. Roenneberg et al., 2012. *Curr. Biol.* 22: 939.)

simply go to bed once they feel sleepy. They should also avoid daytime naps and having caffeine at night. Going through a bedtime routine in a quiet, dark environment can also help to condition sleep onset. Melanopsin, the retinal photopigment that tells the SCN about light and dark, is especially sensitive to bluish light (Gooley et al., 2010), such as the light that comes from LCD screens. So avoiding the use of smartphones and laptops at bedtime (or at least dimming their light) can thus improve sleep (Bedrosian et al., 2013). These steps will let you get the sleep you need (**TABLE 10.3**), and sleeping pills will not (no matter what the millions of dollars in annual pharmaceutical advertising might say).

Unfortunately, many college students adopt schedules that virtually guarantee they won't get enough sleep. Waking up early on Monday and Wednesday to attend one class, sleeping a bit later on Tuesday and Thursday, and then sleeping a *lot* later on weekends disrupts your circadian sleep cycle, making it hard to fall asleep when you should on the nights before an early class. It's unpopular advice, but if you want enough sleep, get up at the same time *every* day, not just the days you have that early class, and go to bed about the same time each night. True, you'll miss out on some late-night activities with your friends, but you'll get to feel so self-righteous being awake and working while they are sleeping in. Plus you'll stay awake in lectures (we hope).

TABLE 10.3 Some Simple Tips to Promote Sleep Hygiene
Keep your internal clock set with a consistent sleep schedule (get up at the same time each day).
Seek sunlight in the daytime, avoid lights at night.
Turn your bedroom into a sleep-inducing environment.
Avoid caffeine, alcohol, and nicotine before bedtime.
Establish a soothing presleep routine.
Only go to sleep when you're truly tired.
If you're going to nap, do it early in the day.
Lighten up on evening meals.
Balance fluid intake to avoid night trips to the bathroom.
Avoid using computer screens before bedtime.
Don't exercise late in the day.

Source: Healthy Sleep, http://healthysleep.med.harvard.edu/healthy/getting/overcoming/tips

HOW'S IT GOING ❓

1. What is narcolepsy, and what brain system seems to be responsible for this disorder?
2. During what stage of sleep does sleepwalking tend to happen? During what time of night?
3. What are the different types of insomnia, and why are sleeping pills an imperfect long-term solution?
4. Describe REM behavior disorder.

Recommended Reading

Aserinsky, E., and Kleitman, N. (1955). Regularly occurring periods of eye motility, and concomitant phenomena, during sleep. *Science, 118,* 273–274.

Forger, D. B. (2017). *Biological Clocks, Rhythms, and Oscillations: The Theory of Biological Timekeeping.* Cambridge, MA: MIT Press.

Kryger, M. K., Roth, T., and Dement, W. C. (Eds.). (2016). *Principles and Practice of Sleep Medicine* (6th ed.). Philadelphia, PA: Saunders/Elsevier.

Leschziner, G. (2019). *The Nocturnal Brain: Nightmares, Neuroscience, and the Secret World of Sleep.* New York, NY: St. Martin's Press.

McNamara, P. (2019). *The Neuroscience of Sleep and Dreams.* Cambridge, UK: Cambridge University Press.

Walker, M. (2017). *Why We Sleep: Unlocking the Power of Sleep and Dreams.* New York, NY: Scribner.

You should be able to relate each summary to the adjacent illustration, including structures and processes. The online version of this **Visual Summary** includes links to figures, animations, and activities that will help you consolidate the material.

1 Animals show **circadian rhythms** of activity that can be **entrained** by light. These rhythms synchronize behavior to changes in the environment. In constant dim light, animals **free-run**, displaying a period of about 24 hours. Review **Figures 10.2** and **10.6**, **Animations 10.2** and **10.3**

2 Lesions of the **suprachiasmatic nucleus (SCN)** abolish activity rhythms in constant conditions. Transplanting the SCN from one animal into another results in a free-running rhythm of the donor, demonstrating that the SCN contains a clock that can drive circadian activity. Several proteins (including Clock and Cycle) interact, increasing and decreasing in a cyclic fashion that takes about 24 hours. This molecular clock, pooled from many SCN neurons, drives circadian rhythms. Review **Figures 10.3–10.10, Animation 10.4**

3 Almost all mammals show two sleep states: **rapid-eye-movement (REM) sleep** and **non-REM sleep**. Human non-REM sleep has three distinct stages—**stages 1, 2, 3**—defined by **electroencephalography (EEG)** criteria, including **sleep spindles** in stage 2 and large, slow **delta waves** in stage 3. Review **Figure 10.11, Table 10.1, Activity 10.1**

4 REM sleep is characterized by rapid, low-amplitude EEG waves (almost like an EEG while awake) but also by profound muscle relaxation because motor neurons are inhibited. People awakened from REM frequently report vivid dreams, while people awakened from SWS report ideas or thinking. Review **Table 10.1**

5 Sleep stages cycle through the night, with stage 3 SWS prominent early, while REM predominates later. Infants sleep a lot, with lots of REM, but as we grow up, we sleep less, with less REM. Elderly people sleep even less, and stage 3 sleep eventually disappears. Review **Figures 10.12–10.16**

6 Four proposed functions of sleep are energy conservation, **ecological niche** adaptation, body and brain restoration, and memory consolidation. **Sleep deprivation** leads to impairments in vigilance and reaction times. It also incurs sleep debt, although the lost SWS and REM may be partially restored in subsequent nights. Prolonged sleep deprivation compromises the immune system and leads to death. Review **Figure 10.18**

7 Four brain systems control sleep and waking. The **basal forebrain** promotes SWS, the brainstem **reticular formation** promotes arousal, a pontine system triggers REM sleep, and hypothalamic neurons releasing **orexin** regulate these three centers. Review **Figures 10.19–10.21, Activity 10.2, Video 10.5**

8 **Narcolepsy** is characterized by sudden, uncontrollable periods of sleep, which may be accompanied by **cataplexy**, paralysis while remaining conscious. Disruption of orexin signaling causes narcolepsy. Review **Figures 10.22** and **10.23, Video 10.6**

9 Sleep disorders fall into four categories: **sleep-onset** and **sleep-maintenance insomnia**; excessive drowsiness (e.g., narcolepsy); disruption of the sleep-waking schedule; and dysfunctions associated with sleep, sleep stages, or partial arousals (e.g., **somnambulism, RBD**). No pill guarantees a normal night's sleep. Review **Figure 10.24** and **10.25, Table 10.2, Video 10.7**

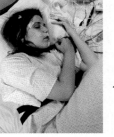

11 Emotions, Aggression, and Stress

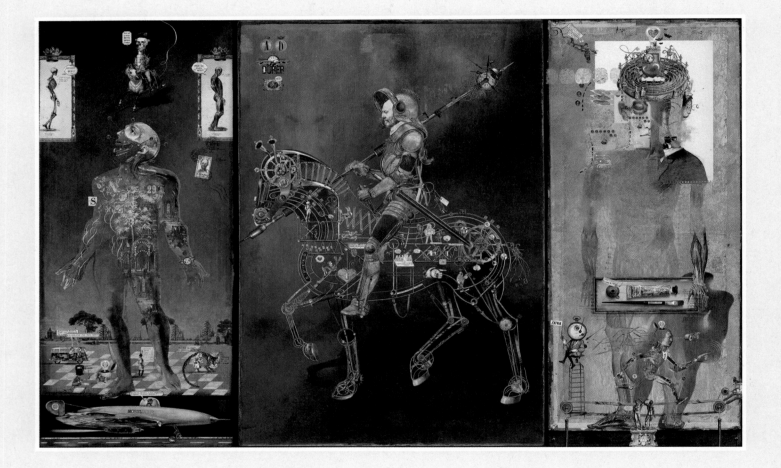

The Hazards of Fearlessness

"Fear has its use, but cowardice has none," wrote the Mahatma Gandhi. But wouldn't it be great to never feel fear at all? When we say that heroes are "fearless," what we really mean is that they manage to function effectively despite the fear they experience, not that they never feel afraid. However, there are people who literally do not experience fear. One such woman, known as S.M. in the scientific literature, lost her ability to feel fear in late childhood because of a genetic disorder so rare, fewer than 300 cases have been reported (Feinstein et al., 2011).

In Chapter 5 we saw how the absence of an unpleasant experience, pain, can be hazardous to your health. S.M. similarly shows us the survival value of fear. Not only is she unafraid of snakes or spiders, but she once walked right up to a knife-wielding robber and basically dared him to stab her. He was so disquieted by her strange response that he ran away! Another time she was nearly killed in an act of domestic violence. While her behavioral responses and self-report appear typical for other emotions, S.M. shows very little of the physiological response, organized by the sympathetic nervous system, that the rest of us experience in response to frightening situations. Similarly, S.M. produces almost no startle response to a sudden, loud noise (Aschwanden, 2013), and she seems not to notice expressions of fear in the faces of other people (L. F. Barrett, 2018).

S.M. is not deliberately reckless; she has learned to follow simple safety rules like looking both ways before crossing the street. But there are other consequences of S.M.'s fearlessness that you might not predict. When talking to someone, she tends to get much closer than other people do, sometimes just a foot away (D. P. Kennedy et al., 2009). When strangers talk to her in public, like the mugger she encountered, she tends to stroll right up to them. S.M. also fails to perceive risk in more mundane social situations, so she's an easy target for internet scams. Although she's very outgoing and might fondly address a waiter she's only met once before, she has few long-term friendships, perhaps because she speaks without caution. Maybe being fearless isn't all it's cracked up to be.

What happened to S.M. to make her this way, and is there really nothing she is afraid of?

Our chapter begins with a discussion of physiological and behavioral processes involved in varying emotional states, and then we turn to a more in-depth look at fear and aggression because both are important for survival and they are readily studied in animals. We'll then end the chapter by turning to one of the products of aggression—stress—and the impacts of stress on neural function.

See Video 11.1:
The Case of S.M.

emotion A subjective mental state that is usually accompanied by distinctive cognition, behaviors, and physiological changes.

sympathetic nervous system The part of the autonomic nervous system that acts as the fight-or-flight system, generally preparing the body for action.

parasympathetic nervous system The part of the autonomic nervous system that generally prepares the body to relax and recuperate.

View Animation 11.2: Brain Explorer

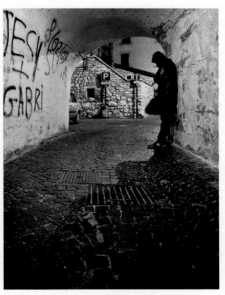

© istock.com/zodebala

Fear and Loathing Can Save You Strong emotions, like fear in unfamiliar and threatening circumstances, are evolved adaptations that swiftly activate behavioral and physiological responses appropriate to the situation.

11.1 Theories of Emotion Integrate Physiological and Behavioral Processes

THE ROAD AHEAD

We start by looking at theoretical accounts of the perception of emotions, and the display of emotion via facial expressions. After reading this section, you should be able to:

11.1.1 Describe and compare the dominant theories of the relationship between emotion and physiological changes.

11.1.2 Discuss the integration of autonomic responses with the perception of specific emotions.

11.1.3 Review the evidence for a core set of emotions as well as their role in guiding preprogrammed responses to environmental challenges.

11.1.4 Discuss the role of facial expressions of emotion, the ways in which cultural differences influence facial displays, and the neural pathways that control facial expressions.

11.1.5 Discuss the pros and cons of trying to measure emotional states using techniques like polygraphy.

Ranging from soaring joy to the depths of fear and loathing, our emotions are evolved programs that guide our responses to daily threats and opportunities. The topic of emotions is complicated by the fact that we apply the word emotion to several different things. Emotion is a private, subjective *feeling* that we may have without anyone else being aware of it. But the word *emotional* is also used to describe many *behaviors* that people show, such as fearful facial expressions, frantic arm movements, or angry shouting. Emotion may influence, and be influenced by, *cognitive* processes like memory and attention. Furthermore, during strong emotion we often experience *physiological* changes, such as a rapidly beating heart, shortness of breath, or excessive sweating. To encompass all four aspects of emotion, we will define **emotion** as a subjective mental state that is usually accompanied by distinctive cognition, behaviors, and physiological changes.

In many emotional states the heart races, the hands and face become warm, the palms sweat, and the stomach feels queasy. Common expressions capture this emotional-physical association: "my hair stood on end," "a sinking feeling in my stomach." These sensations are the result of activation of the autonomic nervous system—either the **sympathetic nervous system** (the "fight-or-flight" system that generally activates the body for action) or the **parasympathetic nervous system** (which generally prepares the body to relax and recuperate) (see Figure 1.9).

Several theories have tried to explain the close ties between the subjective feelings of emotions and the activity of the autonomic nervous system. Common sense suggests that the autonomic reactions are caused by the emotion—"I was so angry, my hands were shaking"—as though the anger produces the shaking (**FIGURE 11.1A**). Yet research indicates that the relationship between emotion and physiological arousal is more subtle.

Do emotions cause bodily changes, or vice versa?

William James (1842–1910) and Carl Lange (1834–1900) turned the commonsense notion on its head, suggesting that the emotions we experience are caused by the bodily changes. From this perspective, we experience fear because we perceive the activity that dangerous conditions trigger in our body (**FIGURE 11.1B**). Different emotions thus feel different because they are generated by different constellations of physiological responses.

The James-Lange theory inspired many attempts to link specific emotions to specific bodily responses. These attempts mostly failed because it turns out that there is no distinctive autonomic pattern for each emotion. Fear, surprise, and anger, for example, tend to be accompanied by sympathetic activation, while parasympathetic activation tends to accompany both joy and sadness.

In addition, the physiological reactions are rather slow, as physiologists Walter Cannon (1871–1945) and Philip Bard (1898–1977) pointed out (W. B. Cannon, 1929). According to the Cannon-Bard theory, it is the brain's job to decide which particular emotion is an appropriate response to the stimuli. According to this model, the cerebral cortex simultaneously decides on the appropriate emotional experience (fear, surprise, joy) and activates the autonomic nervous system to appropriately prepare the body, using either the parasympathetic system to help the body relax, or the sympathetic system to ready the body for action (**FIGURE 11.1C**).

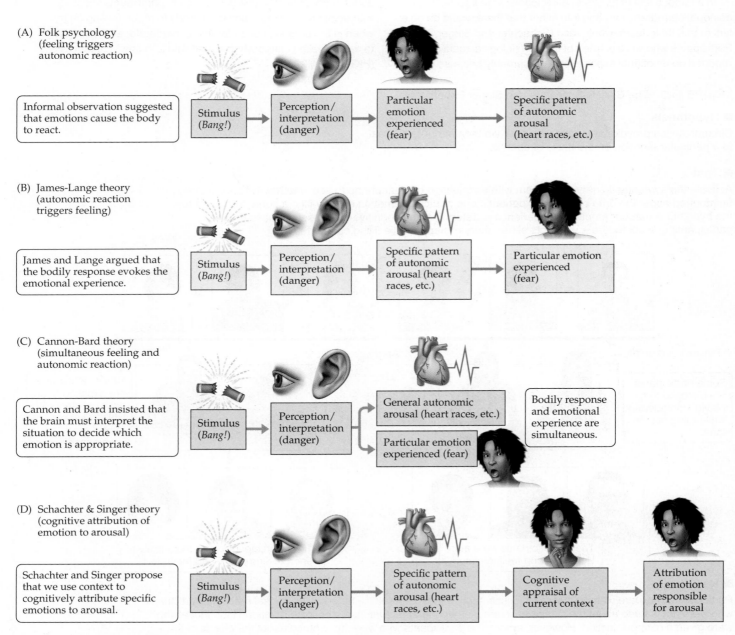

FIGURE 11.1 Different Views of the Chain of Events in Emotional Responses

RESEARCHERS AT WORK ||||||||||||||||||||||||||||||||||||||||||||||||||||||||||||||||||||||||||||||||||||||||||||||||||||||

Do we use context to attribute specific emotions to physiological arousal?

Like Cannon and Bard, Stanley Schachter and Jerome Singer (Schachter and Singer, 1962; Schachter, 1975) emphasized cognitive mechanisms in emotion. Under this model, however, emotional labels (e.g., anger, fear, joy) are attributed to relatively nonspecific feelings of physiological arousal (**FIGURE 11.1D**). The specific emotion we experience is thought to depend on cognitive systems that assess the context—our current social, physical, and psychological situation.

In a famous test of this idea, participants were injected with epinephrine (adrenaline) and told either that there would be no effect or that their hearts would race (Schachter and Singer, 1962). Participants who were warned of this physiological reaction reported no emotional experience—presumably because they

attributed the arousal to the injection rather than to an emotion—but some participants who were *not* forewarned experienced emotions when their bodies responded to the drug. Presumably, the participants who weren't forewarned misattributed their racing hearts to their current emotional context, rather than to the injection.

However, exactly *which* emotion was experienced could be affected by whether another person in the room (secretly an actor) acted angry or happy. The unsuspecting participants injected with epinephrine were much more likely to report feeling angry when in the presence of an "angry" confederate, and more likely to report feeling elated when paired with a "happy" confederate (**FIGURE 11.2A**).

FIGURE 11.2 The Classic Schachter and Singer Experiment

■ **Hypothesis**

Circumstances provoke autonomic arousal; we then attribute arousal to a particular emotion on the basis of context.

■ **Test**

Activate the sympathetic nervous system with an injection of epinephrine to see whether the participants, uninformed about the drug's effects, experience one particular emotion as they fill out some forms. To test the hypothesis that our emotional experience is determined by cognitive processes, expose the participants to a confederate who acts either angry or happy while filling out the forms.

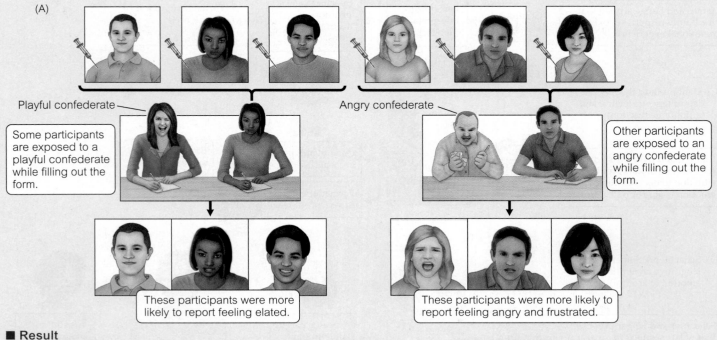

(A)

Playful confederate

Some participants are exposed to a playful confederate while filling out the form.

Angry confederate

Other participants are exposed to an angry confederate while filling out the form.

These participants were more likely to report feeling elated.

These participants were more likely to report feeling angry and frustrated.

■ **Result**

Participants who were warned that the injection might affect heart rate reported no emotional reaction. Participants who were not warned about the sympathetic arousal reported more intense emotional reactions than those who were given a control injection. However, among the participants who were not warned about the effects of the injection, *which* emotion they experienced (angry or happy) tended to match that of the confederate.

■ Conclusion

While autonomic responses can *intensify* our emotional experience, they cannot explain why we have different emotional experiences in different situations. Rather, our cognitive analysis of the environment affects which emotion we experience.

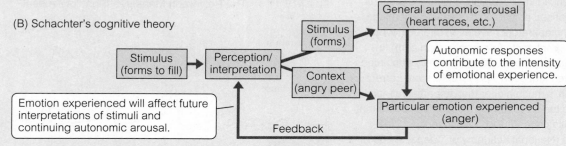

(B) Schachter's cognitive theory

These findings contradict the James-Lange prediction that feelings of anger or elation should each be associated with a unique profile of autonomic reactions. Schachter and Singer concluded that the participants experienced their epinephrine-induced physiological arousal as whichever emotion seemed appropriate, based on their cognitive assessment of the situation: "My heart's really pounding; I'm so angry!" or "My heart's really pounding; I'm so elated!" depending on the environment. Thus, they said, our emotional states are the results of interaction between two factors: physiological arousal, and cognitive interpretation of the concurrent context, including social cues like other people's emotional expressions. (This emphasis on the combination of physiological arousal and cognitive interpretation is why Schachter and Singer's model is also known as the *two-factor theory of emotion*). The cognitive theory also suggests that our emotional experience at one time may affect how we interpret later events (**FIGURE 11.2B**).

Another interesting outcome of the Schachter and Singer experiment is that the participants receiving epinephrine reported experiencing more *intense* emotions than other participants who were given saline. This result conforms with the James-Lange view that autonomic responses intensify emotion but are nonspecific (G. W. Hohmann, 1966). More recent evidence, however, has explored whether patterns of autonomic activity systematically differ between broad classes of positive and negative emotions—for example, happiness versus fear versus sadness versus anger—suggesting that the Schachter and Singer model may not provide a complete explanation of the relationship between arousal and emotion (B. H. Friedman, 2010; E. H. Siegel et al., 2018). Nevertheless, it is because the sympathetic system is activated to some degree by *any* threatening situation that so-called lie detectors are very poor at distinguishing liars from truthful people who are anxious, as we discuss next in Signs & Symptoms.

Lie Detector?

One of the most controversial attempts to apply biomedical science in legal settings is the so-called lie detector test. In this procedure, properly called a **polygraph** test (from the Greek *poly*, "many," and *graphein*, "to write"), multiple physiological measures are recorded in an attempt to detect lying during a carefully structured interview. The test is based on the assumption that people have emotional responses when lying because they fear detection and/or feel guilty about lying. Emotions are usually accompanied by bodily responses that are difficult to control, such as changes in respiratory rate, heart rate, blood pressure, and skin conductance (a measure of sweating). In

polygraph recordings like the one in **FIGURE 11.3**, each wiggly line, or *trace*, provides a measurement of one of these physiological variables. Taken together, the measurements are assumed to track the physiological arousal, over time, of the person being tested. When a person lies in response to a direct question (arrows), momentary changes in several of the measured variables may occur.

People who administer polygraph examinations for a living claim that polygraphs are accurate in 85–95% of tests, but the estimate from impartial research is an overall accuracy of about 65% (Nietzel, 2000; Gougler et al., 2011). Even if the higher figure

(Continued)

were correct, the fact that these tests are widely used would mean that thousands of truthful people could be branded as liars and fired, disciplined, or not hired. On the other hand, many criminals and spies have been able to pass the tests without detection (Wollan, 2015). For example, longtime CIA agent Aldrich Ames, who was sentenced in 1995 to life in prison for espionage, successfully passed polygraph tests after becoming a spy; former polygraph operators have even offered how-to guides to beating polygraph tests (www.polygraph.com). In the wake of the terrorist attacks of 2001, a federally appointed panel of scientists noted that even if polygraphs were correct 80% of the time (which is much higher than impartial research suggests), then giving the test to a group of 10,000 people that included 10 spies would condemn 1,600 innocent people— and let 2 spies go free (National Academy of Sciences, 2003)!

Some scientists believe that modern neuroscience may provide new methods of lie detection someday, perhaps using functional brain imaging technology such as PET or fMRI (Abe et al., 2007). However, attempts to use brain scanners as lie

detectors so far have yielded unreliable results (Rusconi and Mitchener-Nissen, 2013), and even if they are validated, such lie detectors will be more costly and less widely available than polygraphs.

FIGURE 11.3   The Polygraph Measures Signs of Arousal

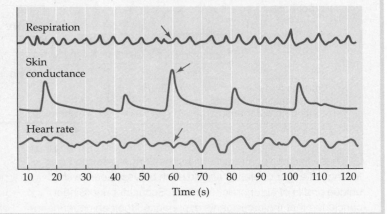

polygraph   Popularly but inaccurately referred to as a *lie detector*. A device that measures several bodily responses, such as heart rate and blood pressure.

Is there a core set of emotions?

Just as the colors of the spectrum combine into subtle hues, researchers think there may be a core set of basic emotions underlying the more varied and delicate nuances of our world of feelings. In his book *The Expression of the Emotions in Man and Animals* (1872), Charles Darwin noted that certain expressions of emotions appear to be universal among people of all regions of the world. Furthermore, Darwin asked whether nonhuman animals may show comparable expressions of some emotions, arguing that aspects of emotional expression may have originated in a common ancestor. He noted that nonhuman primates have the same facial muscles that humans have, and a century later, Redican (1982) noted distinct facial expressions in nonhuman primates that appeared to signal emotional states; for example, chimpanzees show a *play face*, which may be homologous to the human laugh (**FIGURE 11.4**). This connection may even extend beyond primates: for example, tickling and playing with rats can

(A)   (B)

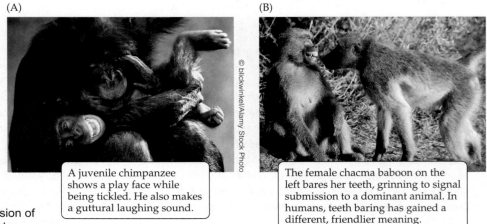

A juvenile chimpanzee shows a play face while being tickled. He also makes a guttural laughing sound.

The female chacma baboon on the left bares her teeth, grinning to signal submission to a dominant animal. In humans, teeth baring has gained a different, friendlier meaning.

FIGURE 11.4   Facial Expression of Emotions in Nonhuman Primates

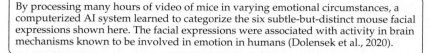

By processing many hours of video of mice in varying emotional circumstances, a computerized AI system learned to categorize the six subtle-but-distinct mouse facial expressions shown here. The facial expressions were associated with activity in brain mechanisms known to be involved in emotion in humans (Dolensek et al., 2020).

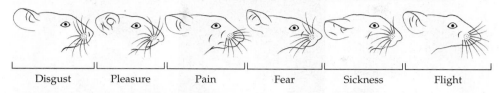

| Disgust | Pleasure | Pain | Fear | Sickness | Flight |

FIGURE 11.5 Facial Expressions in the Mouse (After N. Dolensek et al., 2020. *Science* 368: 89. Courtesy of Julia Kuhl.)

elicit ultrasonic vocalizations that resemble laughter, and playing may facilitate social contact and learning (Panksepp, 2007; Burgdorf et al., 2008). Amazingly, even mice make subtle but distinct emotion-related facial expressions, associated with activity in neural mechanisms of emotion (**FIGURE 11.5**) (Dolensek et al., 2020).

So, why did emotions and their expression evolve, and how do they help individuals survive and reproduce? Most of us have experienced the frightening nighttime perception of being stalked by a predator—real or imagined, human or nonhuman. Through natural selection, a program for dealing with this situation evolved: we call that program fear. The emotion of fear shifts our perception, attention, cognition, and action to focus on avoiding danger and seeking safety, while preparing us physiologically for fighting or fleeing. Other activities, such as seeking food, sleep, or mates, are suppressed. In the face of an imminent threat to survival, it is better to be afraid, thereby activating a recipe for action that was developed and tested over the ages, than to ad-lib something new.

Viewed in this way, emotions can be seen as evolved preprogramming that helps us deal quickly and effectively with a wide variety of situations. As another example, feelings of disgust for body fluids may help us avoid exposure to germs (Curtis et al., 2004), so it may be wise to recognize disgust in others. Our human tendency to make snap judgments about other people, based on their appearance and facial expressions, may be an unfortunate overgeneralization of mechanisms that evolved to help us recognize signs of threat or danger from others (Todorov et al., 2008).

One formulation (Plutchik, 2001) proposes there are eight basic emotions, grouped in four pairs of opposites—joy/sadness, affection/disgust, anger/fear, and expectation/surprise—with all other emotions arising from combinations of this basic array (**FIGURE 11.6**). But researchers do not yet agree about the number of basic emotions (six, seven, eight?). While there may be no way to determine once and for all the number of basic emotions, one clue comes from examining the number of different kinds of facial expressions that we produce and can recognize in others.

Facial expressions have complex functions in communication

How many different emotions can be detected in facial expressions? According to Paul Ekman and collaborators, there are distinctive expressions for anger, sadness, happiness, fear, disgust, surprise, contempt,

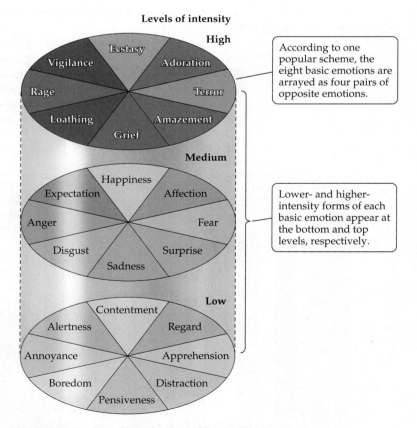

According to one popular scheme, the eight basic emotions are arrayed as four pairs of opposite emotions.

Lower- and higher-intensity forms of each basic emotion appear at the bottom and top levels, respectively.

FIGURE 11.6 One Classification of Basic Emotions (After R. Plutchik, 1994. *The psychology and biology of emotion.* HarperCollins. New York, NY.)

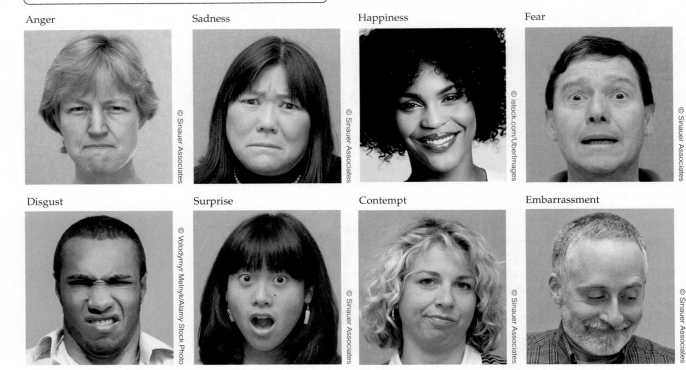

According to Paul Ekman and colleagues, the basic emotional facial expressions shown here are displayed in all cultures.

Anger   Sadness   Happiness   Fear

Disgust   Surprise   Contempt   Embarrassment

FIGURE 11.7   The Eight Universal Facial Expressions of Emotion

and embarrassment (**FIGURE 11.7**) (Keltner and Ekman, 2000). Facial expressions of these emotions are interpreted similarly across many cultures without explicit training. (In case you're keeping track, whereas Plutchik included affection and expectation in his eight basic emotions, Keltner and Ekman include, instead, facial expressions of contempt and embarrassment. The other six emotions—anger, sadness, happiness, fear, disgust, and surprise—are recognized in both schemes.)

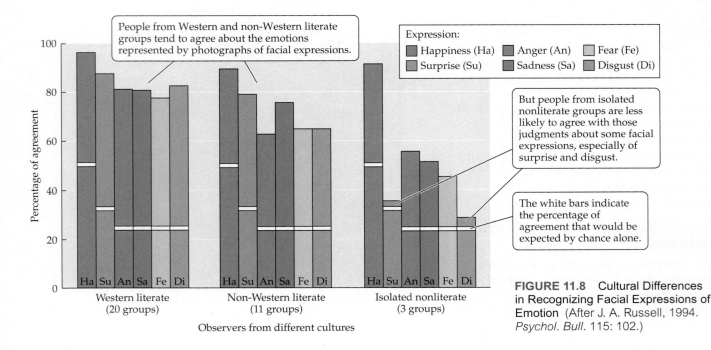

FIGURE 11.8   Cultural Differences in Recognizing Facial Expressions of Emotion (After J. A. Russell, 1994. *Psychol. Bull.* 115: 102.)

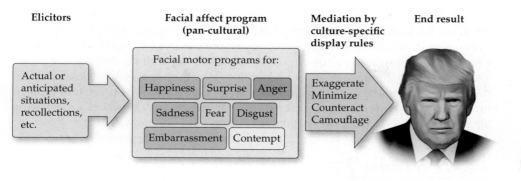

| Elicitors | Facial affect program (pan-cultural) | Mediation by culture-specific display rules | End result |

Facial motor programs for:

Happiness | Surprise | Anger

Sadness | Fear | Disgust

Embarrassment | Contempt

Actual or anticipated situations, recollections, etc.

Exaggerate
Minimize
Counteract
Camouflage

FIGURE 11.9 A Model for Emotional Facial Expressions across Cultures

Cross-cultural similarity is also noted in the production of expressions specific to particular emotions. For example, people in a nonliterate New Guinea society show emotional facial expressions like those of people in industrialized societies. However, facial expressions are not unfailingly universal. Although some degree of agreement is generally evident across cultures, researchers have repeatedly found isolated groups whose identifications of the emotions from facial expressions, such as those for surprise and disgust, did not fully agree with those of Westerners (**FIGURE 11.8**), suggesting that different cultures have adopted different ways to express some of the emotions (Crivelli et al., 2016).

These subtle cultural differences suggest that cultures prescribe rules for facial expression and that they control and enforce those rules by cultural conditioning. Everyone agrees that cultures affect the facial display of emotion; the remaining controversy is over the extent of that cultural influence (**FIGURE 11.9**).

Facial expressions are mediated by muscles, cranial nerves, and CNS pathways

The human face is a complicated object, a network of small muscles that are carefully controlled by the nervous system. We use subsets of those muscles to produce nuanced facial expressions, from grimace to grin, alongside less subtle facial behaviors, like eating and speaking. Facial muscles can be divided into two categories:

1. *Superficial facial muscles* mostly attach only between different points of facial skin (**FIGURE 11.10**), so when they contract, they change the shape of the mouth, eyes, or nose or maybe create a dimple.

2. *Deep facial muscles* attach to bone and produce larger-scale movements, like chewing.

These facial muscles are innervated by two cranial nerves: (1) the facial nerve (VII), which innervates the superficial muscles of facial expression; and (2) the motor branch of the trigeminal nerve (V), which innervates muscles that move the jaw (see Figure 1.7). The activity of the cranial nerves is governed by the face area of motor cortex: a disproportionately large brain region in humans (see Figure 5.10), probably reflecting the importance of emotional expression in our species.

An intriguing but controversial proposal—the *facial feedback hypothesis*—suggests that sensory feedback from our facial expressions can affect our mood, consistent with the James-Lange notion that sensations from our body inform us about our

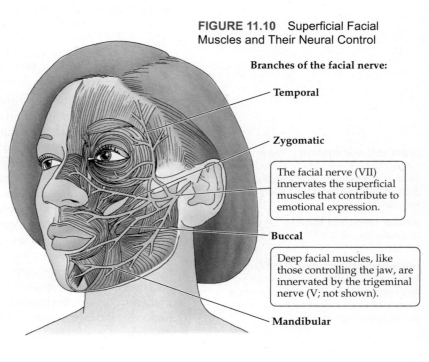

FIGURE 11.10 Superficial Facial Muscles and Their Neural Control

Branches of the facial nerve:

Temporal

Zygomatic

The facial nerve (VII) innervates the superficial muscles that contribute to emotional expression.

Buccal

Deep facial muscles, like those controlling the jaw, are innervated by the trigeminal nerve (V; not shown).

Mandibular

emotions. So, for example, people who have been simulating a smile (by holding a pencil between their teeth) reportedly experience more positive feelings than participants who have been simulating a frown (Davis et al., 2009). Important questions have arisen about the strength and reliability of this finding (Wagenmakers et al., 2016), but if further study confirms that forcing yourself to smile may actually help you feel happier, then the old song that tells us to "just put on a happy face" may be sound advice. Being forced to display false emotional expressions in stressful situations, however, may have negative consequences for well-being and job happiness (Hülsheger and Schewe, 2011).

HOW'S IT GOING ?

1. Compare and contrast the commonsense view of bodily responses to emotions with the James-Lange theory.
2. What two findings cast doubt on the James-Lange theory of emotions?
3. Describe the results of Schachter and Singer's experiment. What do these findings suggest about how autonomic reactions, emotional experience, and cognitive processing are related?
4. List some examples of particular facial expressions that are associated with particular emotions.
5. What is the evidence that emotions, and the facial expressions that accompany them, evolved by natural selection?
6. What evidence suggests that facial expressions of emotional state are inherited rather than taught by culture?

11.2 Do Distinct Brain Circuits Mediate Different Emotions?

THE ROAD AHEAD

Next we consider neural systems implicated in the experience and expression of emotions, and brain mechanisms involved in emotional learning. After studying this section, you should be able to:

11.2.1 Define and describe the phenomenon of brain self-stimulation.

11.2.2 Sketch and describe the major brain mechanisms involved in emotional behaviors, noting the behavioral manifestations of activity in the major pathways.

11.2.3 Describe the process of fear conditioning, the neural mechanisms responsible for fear reactions, and the role of this system in pathological states.

Studies that ask whether different emotions have their own distinct neural mechanisms have confirmed not only that some brain regions do specialize in emotions, but also that the same regions may be involved in multiple emotions. One way to study the neuroanatomy of emotion is to electrically stimulate brain sites in conscious animals and then observe the effects on behavior. Classic work in the 1950s produced an intriguing finding: rats will enthusiastically press a lever in order to give themselves brief electrical stimulation in a brain region called the *septum* (**FIGURE 11.11**) (Olds and Milner, 1954). This phenomenon, called **brain self-stimulation**, can also happen in humans. People receiving electrical stimulation in the septum feel a sense of pleasure or warmth, or sometimes sexual excitement (Heath, 1972).

Building on the discovery of self-stimulation, a rush of experimentation soon mapped brain sites that support self-stimulation responses. Almost all of these sites are subcortical and are especially concentrated in a large axon tract that ascends from the midbrain through the hypothalamus: the **medial forebrain bundle**. An important destination for the axons of the medial forebrain bundle is the **nucleus accumbens**, a major

brain self-stimulation The process in which animals will work to provide electrical stimulation to particular brain sites, presumably because the experience is very rewarding.

medial forebrain bundle A collection of axons traveling in the midline region of the forebrain.

nucleus accumbens A region of the forebrain that receives dopaminergic innervation from the ventral tegmental area, often associated with reward and pleasurable sensations.

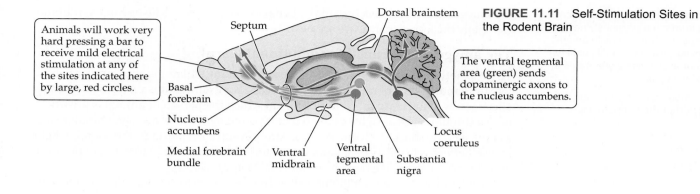

Animals will work very hard pressing a bar to receive mild electrical stimulation at any of the sites indicated here by large, red circles.

Dorsal brainstem

Septum

Basal forebrain

Nucleus accumbens

Medial forebrain bundle

Ventral midbrain

Ventral tegmental area

Substantia nigra

Locus coeruleus

The ventral tegmental area (green) sends dopaminergic axons to the nucleus accumbens.

FIGURE 11.11 Self-Stimulation Sites in the Rodent Brain

component of the brain's reward circuitry (see Figure 11.11 and Chapter 3). The release of dopamine into the nucleus accumbens appears to produce very pleasurable feelings.

One theory is that the electrical stimulation taps into dopaminergic circuits that are normally activated by behaviors that produce pleasurable feelings, such as feeding or sexual activity (White and Milner, 1992). As we discussed in Chapter 3, researchers have proposed that drugs of abuse are addictive because they activate these same neural circuits with an artificial intensity (E. L. Gardner, 2011).

Brain lesions also affect emotions

Early in the twentieth century, dogs in which the cortex had been removed were found to respond to routine handling with sudden intense **decorticate rage**—snarling, biting, and so on—sometimes referred to as *sham rage* because it seemed undirected. Clearly, then, emotional behaviors of this type must be organized at a subcortical level, with the cerebral cortex normally inhibiting rage responses. On the basis of studies such as these, combined with observations from brain autopsies of people with emotional disorders, James Papez (1937) proposed a subcortical circuit of emotion. Papez (whose name rhymes with "capes") noted associations between emotional changes and specific sites of brain damage. These interconnected regions, now known as the **limbic system** (MacLean, 1949), include the mammillary bodies of the hypothalamus, the anterior thalamus, the cingulate cortex, the hippocampus, the amygdala, and the fornix. The arrows in **FIGURE 11.12** schematically depict the interconnections of this circuit.

Early support for the limbic model of emotion came from studies of monkeys after removal of their temporal lobes (Klüver and Bucy, 1938). The animals' behavior changed dramatically following surgery; the highlight of this behavioral change was an extraordinary taming effect known as the **Klüver-Bucy syndrome**. Animals that had been wild and fearful of humans before surgery became tame and showed neither fear nor aggression afterward. They also showed strong oral tendencies, eating a variety of objects, including rocks! Frequent and often inappropriate sexual behavior was also observed. Because this type of behavior is also seen in monkeys in which *only* the left and right amygdalas have been destroyed—without damaging any adjacent tissue (Emery et al., 2001)—it appears that

decorticate rage Also called *sham rage*. Sudden intense rage characterized by actions (such as snarling and biting in dogs) that lack clear direction.

limbic system A loosely defined, widespread group of brain nuclei that innervate each other to form a network. These nuclei are implicated in emotions.

Klüver-Bucy syndrome A condition, brought about by bilateral amygdala damage, that is characterized by dramatic emotional changes including reduction in fear and anxiety.

FIGURE 11.12 The Limbic System: Medial Brain Regions Involved in Emotions

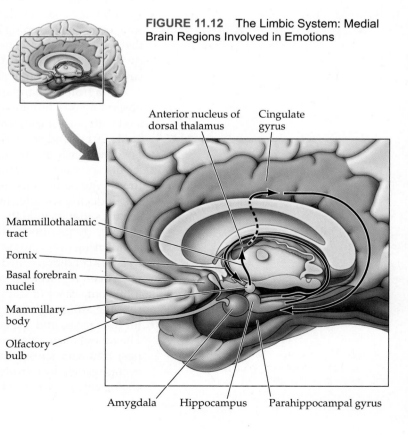

Anterior nucleus of dorsal thalamus

Cingulate gyrus

Mammillothalamic tract

Fornix

Basal forebrain nuclei

Mammillary body

Olfactory bulb

Amygdala

Hippocampus

Parahippocampal gyrus

fear conditioning A form of classical conditioning in which a previously neutral stimulus is repeatedly paired with an unpleasant stimulus, like foot shock, until the previously neutral stimulus alone elicits the responses seen in fear.

amygdala A group of nuclei in the medial anterior part of the temporal lobe.

the amygdala is a key structure in the behavioral changes in Klüver-Bucy syndrome, especially the loss of fear, as we see next.

The amygdala is crucial for emotional learning

There is nothing subtle about fear, and fear-provoking situations elicit similar behaviors from individuals of many different species. For example, it is very easy to reliably elicit fear by using classical conditioning, in which the person or animal is presented with a stimulus such as light or sound that is paired with a brief aversive stimulus such as mild electric shock (**FIGURE 11.13A**). After several such pairings, the sound or light by itself effectively elicits behaviors associated with fear, such as freezing in position, and autonomic signs like rapid heart rate and heavy breathing.

Studies of such **fear conditioning** allowed researchers to develop a map of the neural circuitry of emotional learning, which revealed the **amygdala** to be a key structure (**FIGURE 11.13B**). Located at the anterior medial portion of each temporal lobe, the amygdala is composed of about a dozen different nuclei, each with a distinctive set of connections. Lesioning just the central nucleus of the amygdala in rats prevents blood pressure increases and freezing behavior in response to a conditioned fear stimulus. Subsequent research has confirmed that the amygdala is crucial not only for aversive conditioning but also *appetitive learning*: conditioned positive emotional reactions to attractive stimuli, such as to sex-related stimuli, or other pleasurable signals. In both cases, the amygdala is thought to help form associations between emotional responses and specific memories of stimuli that are stored elsewhere in the brain (Paton et al., 2006; Janak and Tye, 2015).

On its way to the amygdala, sensory information about emotion-provoking stimuli reaches a fork in the road at the level of the thalamus (recall from Chapter 1 that the thalamus acts like a switchboard, directing sensory information to specific brain regions). A direct projection from the thalamus to the amygdala, nicknamed the "low road" for emotional responses in the original fear-conditioning studies (LeDoux, 1996), bypasses conscious processing and allows for immediate emotional reactions to stimuli (De Gelder et al., 2012; Celeghin et al., 2015). An alternate "high road" pathway routes the incoming information through sensory cortex, allowing for processing that, while slower, is conscious, fine-grained, and integrated with higher-level cognitive processes (**FIGURE 11.13C**). You can learn more details about the amygdala circuitry for fear and other emotions in **A STEP FURTHER 11.1**, on the website.

Data from rats and mice about the role of the amygdala in fear mesh well with observations of humans. For example, when people are shown visual stimuli associated with pain or fear, fear-specific activity is observed in amygdala neurons (S. Wang et al., 2014), and activation of the amygdala may be observed even if the person is not consciously aware of the stimuli (Pegna et al., 2005). Similarly, when people view facial expressions of fear, electrophysiological responses occur much more quickly in the amygdala than in visual cortex, reflecting the privileged low-road access of the fear-inducing stimulus (Méndez-Bértolo et al., 2016). People who have temporal lobe seizures that include the amygdala commonly report that intense fear accompanies seizures (Engel, 1992; Chong et al., 2016), and electrical stimulation of temporal lobe sites during brain surgery likewise may elicit feelings of fear (Nowacki et al., 2015). In a rare condition called *Capgras delusion*, people believe that their significant others have been replaced by impostors; although it is more typically a psychiatric symptom, some cases of Capgras delusion are thought to result from brain damage that robs the afflicted person of the privileged low-road connection between visual stimuli (like faces) and the emotions they would normally elicit (Ellis and Lewis, 2001). The neural mechanisms of fear conditioning are also thought to play a central role in post-traumatic stress disorder (PTSD; see Chapter 12), in which memories of horrible events repeatedly intrude into consciousness, reawakening all the autonomic and psychological symptoms of fear.

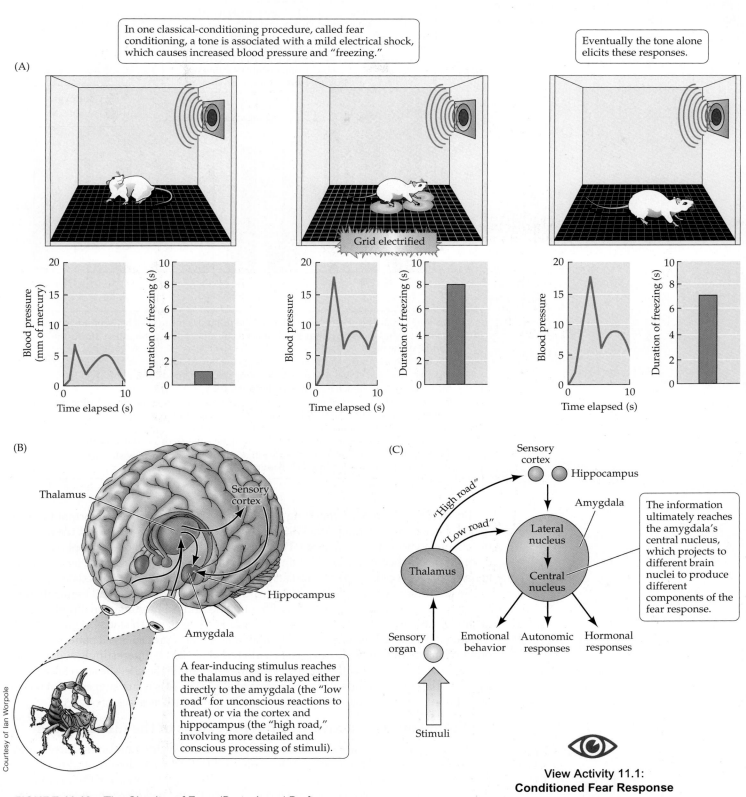

(A)

In one classical-conditioning procedure, called fear conditioning, a tone is associated with a mild electrical shock, which causes increased blood pressure and "freezing."

Eventually the tone alone elicits these responses.

Grid electrified

(B)

Thalamus

Sensory cortex

Hippocampus

Amygdala

Courtesy of Ian Worpole

A fear-inducing stimulus reaches the thalamus and is relayed either directly to the amygdala (the "low road" for unconscious reactions to threat) or via the cortex and hippocampus (the "high road," involving more detailed and conscious processing of stimuli).

(C)

Sensory cortex

Hippocampus

"High road"

"Low road"

Thalamus

Amygdala

Lateral nucleus

Central nucleus

The information ultimately reaches the amygdala's central nucleus, which projects to different brain nuclei to produce different components of the fear response.

Sensory organ

Stimuli

Emotional behavior

Autonomic responses

Hormonal responses

View Activity 11.1: Conditioned Fear Response

FIGURE 11.13   The Circuitry of Fear (Parts A and B after J. E. LeDoux, 1994. *Sci. Am.* 270: 50; C after J. E. LeDoux, 1996. *The emotional brain: The mysterious underpinnings of emotional life.* Simon & Schuster. London, England.)

FIGURE 11.14   The Woman Who Was Never Afraid
(After J. S. Feinstein et al., 2011. *Curr. Biol.* 21: 34.)

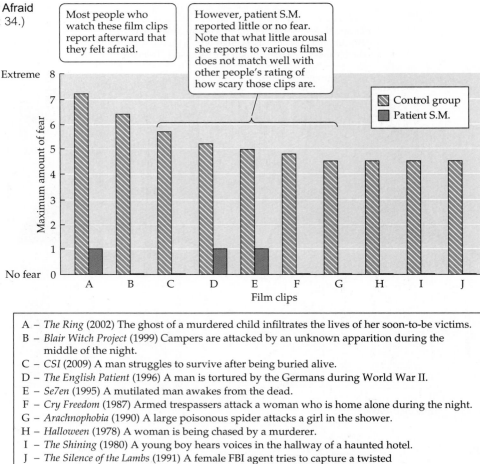

A – *The Ring* (2002) The ghost of a murdered child infiltrates the lives of her soon-to-be victims.
B – *Blair Witch Project* (1999) Campers are attacked by an unknown apparition during the middle of the night.
C – *CSI* (2009) A man struggles to survive after being buried alive.
D – *The English Patient* (1996) A man is tortured by the Germans during World War II.
E – *Se7en* (1995) A mutilated man awakes from the dead.
F – *Cry Freedom* (1987) Armed trespassers attack a woman who is home alone during the night.
G – *Arachnophobia* (1990) A large poisonous spider attacks a girl in the shower.
H – *Halloween* (1978) A woman is being chased by a murderer.
I – *The Shining* (1980) A young boy hears voices in the hallway of a haunted hotel.
J – *The Silence of the Lambs* (1991) A female FBI agent tries to capture a twisted serial killer who is hiding in a dark basement.

But perhaps the most compelling evidence that the amygdala is important for fear in our species comes from people like patient S.M., the woman we met at the start of the chapter, who is literally fearless. The fearlessness that she and other people with the disorder display seems almost certainly due to the loss of the amygdala. Her very rare genetic condition causes the accumulation of calcium deposits in the amygdala, starting in late childhood, which eventually destroys the nuclei in both cerebral hemispheres. When S.M. is shown movie clips that other people find frightening, she reports being unmoved (**FIGURE 11.14**). S.M. is also very poor at recognizing the facial expressions of fear in other people, but she recognizes other emotional expressions—a pattern seen in other people with damaged amygdalas (Adolphs et al., 2005). Interestingly, when S.M. was asked to breathe air with a high concentration of carbon dioxide, she soon felt a panicky fear, flailing her hands about (Feinstein et al., 2013). This result suggests that some other brain system mediates the fear of internal threats, such as a lack of oxygen.

Different emotions activate different regions of the human brain

Several forebrain areas are consistently implicated in varying emotions. Bartels and Zeki (2000) recruited volunteers who professed to be "truly, deeply, and madly in love." Each participant furnished four color photographs: one photo of their romantic partner, and three photos of friends who were of the same gender as the loved partner and who were similar in age and length of friendship. Functional-MRI brain scans were made while each participant was shown counterbalanced sequences of the four photographs. Brain activity elicited by viewing the loved person was compared with that elicited by viewing friends. Love, compared with friendship, involved increased

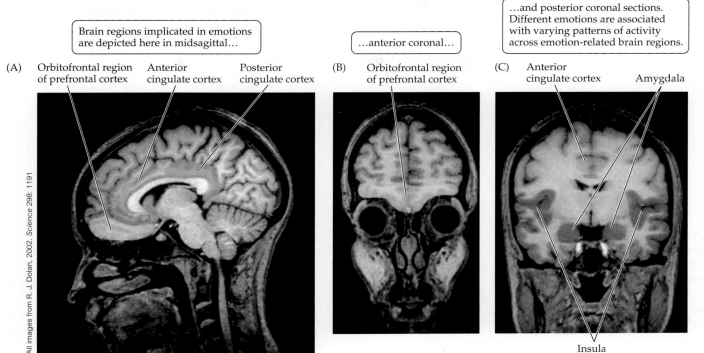

Brain regions implicated in emotions are depicted here in midsagittal...

...anterior coronal...

...and posterior coronal sections. Different emotions are associated with varying patterns of activity across emotion-related brain regions.

(A) Orbitofrontal region of prefrontal cortex   Anterior cingulate cortex   Posterior cingulate cortex

(B) Orbitofrontal region of prefrontal cortex

(C) Anterior cingulate cortex   Amygdala

Insula

All images from R. J. Dolan, 2002. *Science* 298: 1191

FIGURE 11.15   The Emotional Brain

activity in the insula and anterior cingulate cortex and reduced activity in the posterior cingulate and prefrontal cortices (**FIGURE 11.15**). Given its role in fear, you won't be surprised to learn that the amygdala also showed reduced activity when people were contemplating their romantic partners. Activity of the anterior insular cortex (see Figure 3.16) has been implicated in our conscious experience of these varied and nuanced emotional states; impairments in emotional awareness, termed *alexithymia*, are associated with dysfunction of the insula (Gu et al., 2013).

Another study compared brain activation during four different kinds of emotion, and again the insula, cingulate cortex, and prefrontal cortex were among the regions implicated. These studies indicate that there is no simple, one-to-one relation between a specific emotion and changed activity of a brain region. There is no "happy center" or "sad center." Instead, each emotion involves differential patterns of activation across a network of brain regions associated with emotion, as you can see in **A STEP FURTHER 11.2**, on the website. For example, activity of the cingulate cortex is altered in sadness, happiness, and anger, while the left somatosensory cortex is deactivated in both anger and fear. Although different emotions are associated with different patterns of activation, there is a good deal of overlap among patterns for different emotions (A. R. Damasio et al., 2000).

Let's focus next on the darker side of human emotional behavior—the forms and causes of aggression—before we turn our attention to stress and the toll these negative experiences take on our health.

HOW'S IT GOING ?

1. Describe brain self-stimulation and what this phenomenon suggests about emotional experience.
2. What is the limbic system, and what happens when portions of this system are damaged, such as in Klüver-Bucy syndrome?
3. Describe fear conditioning and the evidence that the amygdala plays a role in this process.
4. What evidence suggests that the amygdala mediates fear in humans?

11.3 Neural Circuitry, Hormones, and Synaptic Transmitters Mediate Violence and Aggression

THE ROAD AHEAD

Next we sharpen our focus on the neural and hormonal bases of violence and other aggressive behaviors. By the end of this section, you should be able to:

11.3.1 Define and distinguish between multiple forms of aggression.

11.3.2 Summarize research on the role of testosterone in aggression, contrasting between humans and nonhuman animals.

11.3.3 Identify the key neural systems implicated in aggression and the environmental stimuli that activate these systems.

11.3.4 Discuss the biopsychological origins of violent behavior in humans, and speculate about targets for reducing violent behavior.

aggression   Behavior that is intended to cause pain or harm to others.

intermale aggression   Aggression between males of the same species.

testosterone   A hormone, produced by male gonads, that controls a variety of bodily changes that become visible at puberty; one of a class of hormones called *androgens*.

Violence, assaults, and homicide exact a high price in modern society, and physical assault is not the only form of aggression. Verbal and symbolic aggression—name calling, horn honking, angry glares—also take their toll. We can define **aggression** as behavior that is intended to cause pain or harm (whether physical or emotional) to others, either individually or in groups. We will focus primarily on physical aggression between individuals, excluding the aggression of predators toward their prey, which is better viewed as feeding behavior (Glickman, 1977).

Intermale aggression (aggression between males of the same species) is observed in most vertebrates. The relevance to humans is reflected in the fact that males are 5 times as likely as females to be arrested on charges of murder in the United States. Whatever we may think about aggression, it seems clear that in many species aggressive behavior in males is adaptive for gaining access to food and mates. In the wild, groups of male chimpanzees sometimes band together to kill a rival male (Wilson et al., 2014), increasing the attackers' chances of mating in the future. In the USA in 2018, about 75% of people arrested for assault were male, and almost 90% of murder arrests involved male offenders (FBI, 2018). Aggressive behavior between boys, in contrast to that between girls, is evident early in life, in the form of vigorous and destructive play behavior (J. Archer, 2006). These and similar observations suggest that the hormone that prepares males for reproduction—testosterone—also plays a role in their aggressive behavior.

Androgens seem to increase aggression

At sexual maturity, as the testes begin secreting the steroid hormone **testosterone**, intermale aggression markedly increases in many species (Svare, 2013). In seasonally breeding animals as diverse as birds and primates, intermale aggression waxes and wanes in concert with seasonal changes in levels of testosterone (Bronsard and Bartolomei, 2013; Munley et al., 2018). Conversely, castrating males to remove the source of testosterone usually reduces aggressive behavior profoundly. Treating castrated males with testosterone restores fighting behavior (**FIGURE 11.16**).

The relationship between testosterone and aggression in humans is more complicated (for a review, see Geniole and Carré, 2018). Treating adult volunteers with extra testosterone does not increase their aggression (O'Connor et al., 2004). Similarly, young men going through puberty experience a sudden large increase in circulating testosterone, yet they do not show a correlated increase in aggressive behavior (J. Archer, 2006). Nevertheless, some human studies report that testosterone levels correlate with hostility, as measured by behavior rating scales, and are also associated with unprovoked versus defensive violence in both men and women (Denson et al., 2018).

At least two variables confound the correlations between testosterone and aggression. First is the observation that experience can affect testosterone levels. In mice and monkeys, the loser in aggressive encounters shows reduced androgen levels (Lloyd, 1971; I. S. Bernstein and Gordon, 1974), so measured levels of testosterone sometimes may be a *result*, rather than a *cause*, of behavior. In men, testosterone levels rise in

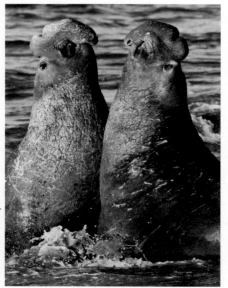

Nature, Red in Tooth and Flipper
Fighting male elephant seals draw blood. In most mammalian species, males must compete with one another, often in the form of physical aggression, for the chance to mate with females.

© David Osborn/Alamy

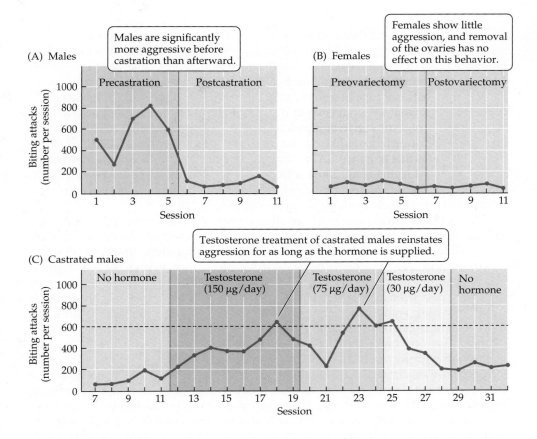

FIGURE 11.16 The Effects of Androgens on the Aggressive Behavior of Mice (After G. C. Wagner et al., 1980. *Aggress. Behav.* 6: 1.)

the winners and fall in the losers after competitions ranging from wrestling to chess (van Anders and Watson, 2006). Male sports fans even show a *vicarious* testosterone response to simply watching "their" team participate in sporting events (Van der Meij et al., 2012); in some studies the degree of the vicarious hormonal response relates to whether the team wins or loses (Bernhardt et al., 1998). During the 2008 U.S. presidential election, men who voted for John McCain experienced a sharp drop in circulating testosterone, compared with backers of Obama, who won (Stanton et al., 2009).

These observations suggest that a second confounding variable between testosterone and aggression is *dominance* (Mazur and Booth, 1998). According to this model, testosterone levels should be associated with behaviors that confer or protect the individual's social status (and thus reproductive fitness). This type of aggression is said to be *proactive*: part of an offense strategy to improve the individual's standing in comparison to others or achieve a desired social outcome. In contrast, *reactive* aggression encompasses the many forms of defensive behavior, ranging from freezing to preemptive attacks, that protect against external threats (Wrangham, 2018; LeDoux and Daw, 2018). Despite the lack of a close relationship between aggression and androgens, people have tried to modify the behavior of male criminals by manipulating sex hormones, through surgical castration or "chemical" castration with drugs that block androgen receptors or testosterone production. While lowered testosterone may reduce violence in some sex offenders (L. E. Weinberger et al., 2005), the main effect is a reduction in sexual motivation more than a direct effect on aggression. Many ethical issues raised by this approach to the rehabilitation of sex offenders, not to mention the intricacies of such intervention, have yet to be worked out.

Brain circuits mediate aggression

Aggressive behavior in various animals, including humans, is modulated by brain activity associated with several neurotransmitter systems, including dopamine, GABA, vasopressin, and especially serotonin (Numan, 2015; Rosell and Siever, 2015). For example, Higley et al. (1992) observed aggressive behavior in 28 monkeys from a large,

medial amygdala A portion of the amygdala that receives olfactory and pheromonal information.

ventromedial hypothalamus (VMH) A hypothalamic region involved in sexual behaviors, eating, and aggression.

maternal aggression Aggression of a mother defending her nest or offspring.

psychopath An individual incapable of experiencing remorse.

free-ranging colony, and they ranked the animals from least to most aggressive. When researchers gauged serotonin activity by measuring serotonin metabolites in the cerebrospinal fluid, they found evidence that the most aggressive monkeys had the lowest levels of serotonin being released in the brain. Similarly, genetically modified mice that lack a specific subtype of serotonin receptor are hyperaggressive (Bouwknecht et al., 2001)—just what we would expect if serotonin normally inhibits aggression. This inhibitory role of serotonin in aggression is probably evolutionarily ancient, since it is evident even in invertebrates like crayfish and locusts (Panksepp et al., 2003; Anstey et al., 2009). Drugs that enhance GABA transmission generally reduce aggressive behavior in humans (Lieving et al., 2008), although, paradoxically, these drugs—for example, benzodiazepine agonists and alcohol—occasionally *provoke* aggression in a minority of users (Albrecht et al., 2016; Guina and Merrill, 2018).

The **medial amygdala** analyzes olfactory and pheromonal information, allowing male rats and mice to distinguish between male rivals to be attacked and females to be courted. That information is relayed to the **ventromedial hypothalamus** (**VMH**), which serves as a trigger to activate aggressive behavior. In *optogenetic experiments*—the use of light to activate neurons in genetically modified mice—activation of VMH neurons can cause males that have been mating with females to suddenly attack them (H. Lee et al., 2014). Conversely, using optogenetic techniques to instead *inhibit* VMH activity reduces the likelihood of attack (Falkner et al., 2016). And a direct input to the VMH from the suprachiasmatic nucleus—the brain's circadian clock (see Chapter 10)—appears to regulate the daily variation in aggression seen in many species, including our own (Todd et al., 2018).

So far we've discussed aggression in males, but females are also aggressive at times, particularly when they are caring for their young. This **maternal aggression** is typically studied by introducing an intruder mouse, usually a male, into the cage of a mother nursing a litter. In such conditions, she may immediately attack the intruder. Maternal aggression, like male aggression, is controlled by neural circuits in the VMH, as well as other regions, including the preoptic area (POA), the premammillary nucleus (Motta et al., 2013), and a serotonergic projection originating from the midbrain (Holschbach et al., 2018).

The biopsychology of human violence is a controversial topic

Some forms of human violence are characterized by sudden, intense physical assaults. A long-standing controversy surrounds the idea that some forms of intense human violence are caused by temporal lobe disorders (Mark and Ervin, 1970). Aggression is sometimes a prominent symptom in people with temporal lobe seizures, and a significant percentage of people arrested for violent crimes have abnormal EEGs or other indicators of temporal lobe dysfunction (Cope et al., 2014).

Psychopathy is not a psychiatric disorder with formal diagnostic criteria in the *DSM-5*—instead it describes a cluster of personality traits that may be associated with antisocial behaviors. **Psychopaths** are often intelligent individuals with superficial charm who have poor self-control, a grandiose sense of self-worth, and little or no feelings of remorse (Hare et al., 1990). And while most people who score high on psychopathic tendencies lead normal, often highly successful lives, psychopaths have sometimes committed horribly violent acts without compunction. Compared with controls, psychopaths do not react as negatively to words about violence (N. S. Gray et al., 2003), and they show blunted responses to aversive cues associated with fear conditioning that typically cause strong reactions in other people (Glenn and Raine, 2014). Imaging studies suggest that psychopaths have reductions in both the size and activity of prefrontal cortex (**FIGURE 11.17**), which may impair their ability to control impulsive behavior (Yang et al., 2012; 2015).

Undoubtedly, human violence and aggression stem from many sources. Biological studies of aggression have been vigorously criticized by some politicians and social scientists. These critics argue that, as a result of emphasizing biological factors such as genetics or brain mechanisms, the preventable origins of human violence and aggression, such as poverty and child neglect, might be overlooked. But as we have seen throughout

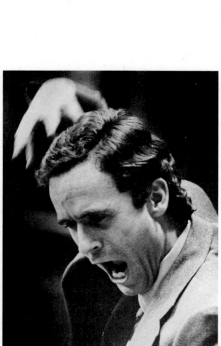

Psychopathic Impulsivity Serial killer Ted Bundy displayed many characteristics of a psychopath. He was superficially charming and, as shown here acting out in the courtroom when the judge was away, impulsive in nature. This scene also hints that, like other psychopaths, Bundy felt little or no remorse for his actions.

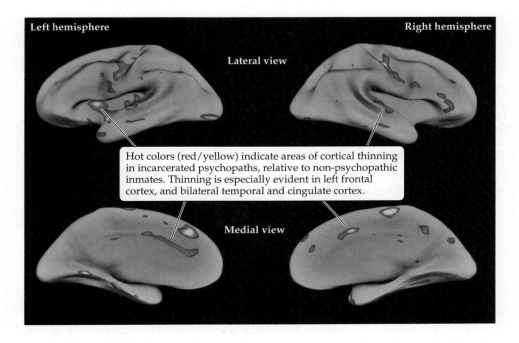

FIGURE 11.17 Brain Abnormalities in Psychopaths (After M. Ly et al., 2012. *Am. J. Psychiatry* 169: 743.)

the book, the brain is a malleable organ that is shaped by experience—and violent behavior must have its origins in the brain—so in principle it could be possible to reshape or at least moderate brain mechanisms of violence. The quality of life of some violent persons might be significantly improved if biological problems could be identified and addressed. For example, treatments that enhance serotonin activity in the brain might be a useful adjunct to psychotherapeutic intervention (George et al., 2011).

Next, let's look at one of the principal consequences of aggression and other aversive situations: stress.

HOW'S IT GOING ?

1. Why is intermale aggression common in so many species?
2. What is the relationship between androgens and aggression?
3. Which neurotransmitter has been most consistently implicated in aggression?

11.4 Stress Activates Many Bodily Responses

THE ROAD AHEAD

We conclude the chapter by looking at the ways in which reciprocal connections between the nervous system, the endocrine system, and the immune system allow them to regulate each other to preserve our health. By the end of this section, you should be able to:

11.4.1 Summarize the physiological correlates of stress, and contrast acute and chronic stress responses.

11.4.2 Discuss the ways in which people differ in their vulnerability and responses to stressful situations, and give examples of how early life experiences affect these individual differences.

11.4.3 Describe the communication between the nervous system and the immune system and how brain responses to stress can affect health.

11.4.4 Summarize the impact of chronic stress on health, as well as possible ways to mitigate these effects.

stress   Any circumstance that upsets homeostatic balance.

adrenal medulla   The inner core of the adrenal gland.

epinephrine   Also called *adrenaline*. A compound that acts both as a hormone (secreted by the adrenal medulla under the control of the sympathetic nervous system) and as a synaptic transmitter.

norepinephrine   Also called *noradrenaline*. A neurotransmitter produced and released by sympathetic postganglionic neurons to accelerate organ activity.

adrenal cortex   The steroid-secreting outer rind of the adrenal gland.

adrenal corticosteroid hormone A steroid hormone that is secreted by the adrenal cortex.

cortisol   A glucocorticoid stress hormone of the adrenal cortex.

We all experience stress, but what is it? Attempts to define this term have a certain vagueness. Hans Selye (1907–1982), whose work launched the modern field of stress research, broadly defined stress as "the rate of all the wear and tear caused by life" (Selye, 1956). Nowadays, researchers try to sharpen their focus by treating **stress** as a multidimensional concept that encompasses stressful stimuli, the stress-processing system (including cognitive assessment of the stimuli), and responses to stress. While many different parts of the body respond to stress, it's clear that the brain carefully monitors and controls those responses (McEwen et al., 2015).

The stress response progresses in stages

Selye called the initial response to stress the *alarm reaction*. As one part of the alarm reaction, the hypothalamus activates the sympathetic nervous system to ready the body for action; this is the fight-or-flight system we mentioned at the start of the chapter. The sympathetic system stimulates the core of the adrenal gland, which is called the **adrenal medulla**, to release the hormones **epinephrine** (also known as *adrenaline*) and **norepinephrine** (or *noradrenaline*). These hormones act on many parts of the body to boost heart rate, breathing, and other physiological processes that prepare the body for action. As another part of the alarm reaction, the hypothalamus stimulates the anterior pituitary to release a hormone that drives the outer layer of the adrenal gland, the **adrenal cortex**. Activation of this *hypothalamic-pituitary-adrenal axis* (*HPA axis*) results in the release of **adrenal corticosteroid hormones** such as **cortisol** (**FIGURE 11.18**). These hormones act more slowly than epinephrine, but they also ready the body for action, including releasing body stores of energy. Glucocorticoid receptors—the receptors that respond to cortisol—are found in many locations in the brain, where they are thought to mediate the formation of memories associated with stress and fear (De Quervain et al., 2017), as well as regulating the ongoing secretion of stress hormones via negative feedback (see Figure 8.11).

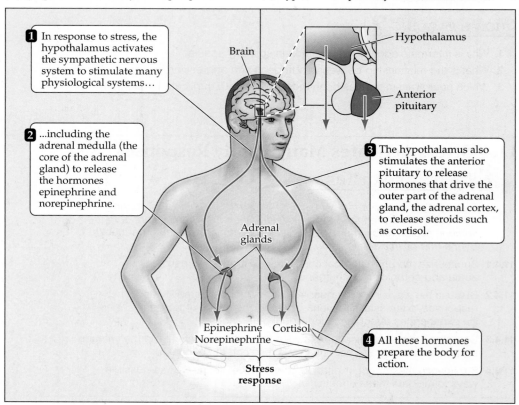

(A) Sympathetic nervous system: epinephrine   **(B) Hypothalamic-pituitary-adrenal axis: cortisol**

1 In response to stress, the hypothalamus activates the sympathetic nervous system to stimulate many physiological systems…

2 …including the adrenal medulla (the core of the adrenal gland) to release the hormones epinephrine and norepinephrine.

3 The hypothalamus also stimulates the anterior pituitary to release hormones that drive the outer part of the adrenal gland, the adrenal cortex, to release steroids such as cortisol.

4 All these hormones prepare the body for action.

Brain

Hypothalamus

Anterior pituitary

Adrenal glands

Epinephrine Norepinephrine   Cortisol

Stress response

FIGURE 11.18 Physiological Reactions to Stress

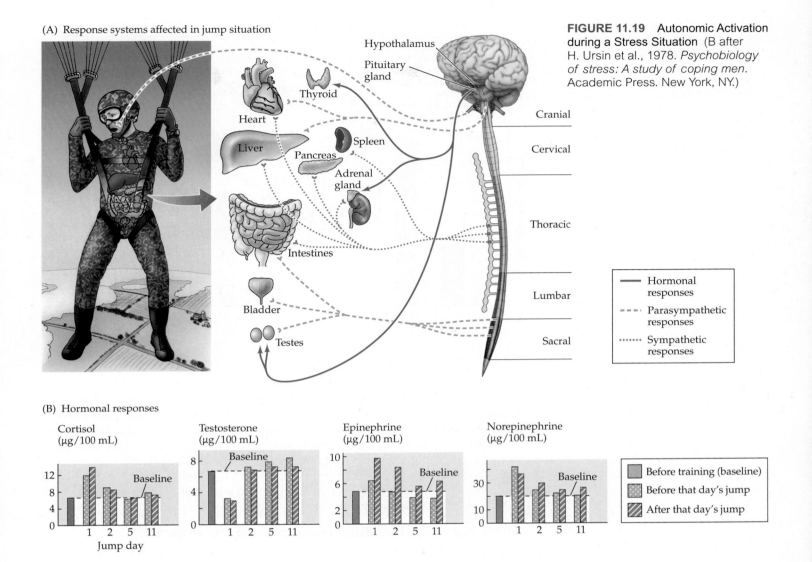

(A) Response systems affected in jump situation

FIGURE 11.19 Autonomic Activation during a Stress Situation (B after H. Ursin et al., 1978. *Psychobiology of stress: A study of coping men.* Academic Press. New York, NY.)

(B) Hormonal responses

In classic research, hormonal responses to stress were studied in a group of young recruits in the Norwegian military both before and during scary parachute training (Ursin et al., 1978). On each jump day, the anterior pituitary released enhanced levels of hormones, and both the sympathetic and parasympathetic systems were activated (**FIGURE 11.19A**). Initially, cortisol levels were elevated in the blood before each jump, but with more and more successful jumps over successive days, the pituitary-adrenal response soon declined. Epinephrine and norepinephrine were also elevated before the first jumps, but eventually they returned to normal before jumps. Testosterone showed the reverse pattern, falling far below control levels on the first day of training but returning to normal with subsequent jumps (**FIGURE 11.19B**). Once the soldiers mastered the jumps, they no longer showed increased hormonal responses, having adapted to the activity.

Less-dramatic real-life situations also evoke clear endocrine responses (Frankenhaeuser, 1978). For example, riding in a commuter train provokes the release of epinephrine; the longer the ride and the more crowded the train, the greater the hormonal response (**FIGURE 11.20A**). Factory work likewise leads to the release of epinephrine; the shorter the work cycle—that is, the more frequently the person has to repeat the same operations—the higher the levels of epinephrine. The stress of a PhD oral exam leads to a dramatic increase in both epinephrine and norepinephrine (**FIGURE 11.20B**), and medical students stressed by preparing for their licensing exams

FIGURE 11.20 Hormonal Changes in Humans in Response to Social Stresses (A after U. Lundberg, 1976. *J. Human Stress* 2: 26; B after M. Frankenhaeuser, 1978. *Nebr. Symp. Motiv.* 26: 123, edited by Richard A. Dienstbier by permission of the University of Nebraska Press. Copyright 1978 by the University of Nebraska Press.)

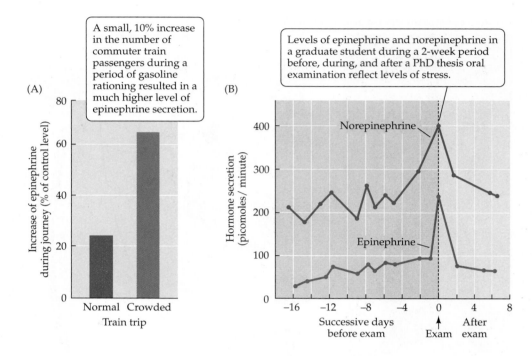

showed fMRI evidence of impairments in the brain mechanisms controlling attention; following the exam, their fMRI scans returned to normal (Liston et al., 2009). Sustained social stressors can also exact lasting medical costs: for example, young people with asthma who experience stress due to peer rejection or family conflict have a more responsive adrenal system, more severe respiratory symptoms, and impaired expression of anti-inflammatory genes (Murphy et al., 2015; Farrell et al., 2018). In general, childhood stress has an enduring impact on health in later life, including neural and cognitive development, emotional regulation, and measures of lifetime achievement (Cameron et al., 2017; see Chapter 4).

There are individual differences in the stress response

Why do individuals differ in their responses to stress (Infurna and Luthar, 2016)? One hypothesis focuses on early experience. Rat pups clearly find it stressful to have a human pick them up and handle them. Yet rats that have been briefly handled as pups are *less* susceptible to adult stress than are rats that have been left alone as pups (S. Levine et al., 1967). For example, the previously handled rats secrete lower adrenal steroid amounts in response to a wide variety of adult stressors. Researchers termed this effect *stress immunization* because a little stress early in life seemed to make the animals more resilient to later stress.

Follow-up research showed that there was more to the story. The pups did not benefit because they were stressed; they benefited because their *mothers comforted them after the stress*. When pups are returned to their mother after a separation, she spends considerable time licking and grooming them. And she will lick the pups much longer if they were handled by humans during the separation. Michael Meaney and colleagues suggest that this gentle tactile stimulation from Mom is crucial for the stress immunization effect. They found that, even among undisturbed litters, the offspring of mother rats that exhibited more licking and grooming behavior were more resilient in their responses to adult stress than other rats were (D. Liu et al., 1997). So the "immunizing" benefit of early stressful experience happens only if the pups are promptly comforted after each stressful event.

If the pups are deprived of their mother for long periods, receiving very little of her attention, then as adults they exhibit a greater stress response, have difficulty learning mazes, and show reduced neurogenesis in the hippocampus (Mirescu et al., 2004). Maternal deprivation exerts this negative effect on adult stress responses by causing long-lasting changes in the expression of adrenal steroid receptors in the brain. This change is termed **epigenetic regulation** because it represents a change in the expression of the gene, rather than a change in the encoding region of the gene (see Figure 4.14 and Figure 4.15).

Dramatic evidence for the same phenomenon has been seen in humans. For example, examination of the brains of suicide victims revealed the same epigenetic change in expression of the adrenal steroid receptor, but only in those victims who had a history of being abused or neglected as children (McGowan et al., 2009). The implication is that the early abuse epigenetically modified expression of the gene, making the person less able to handle stress and thus more likely to develop significant psychiatric disturbances—especially mood and anxiety disorders—that heighten the risk of suicide. Suicide victims who had no history of early neglect did not show the epigenetic change, so their suicidality may have been the result of mental health issues of different origin.

Stress and emotions affect our health

The field of **psychosomatic medicine** studies the distinctive psychological, behavioral, and social factors that influence individual susceptibility or resistance to diverse illnesses. The related field called **health psychology** (or *behavioral medicine*) emphasizes the role of social factors in the cause, progression, and consequences of health and illness (Ogden, 2012). For example, an active area of research is concerned with the association between heart disease and behavioral and social factors such as hostility, depression, loneliness, and stress at home and at work (Matthews, 2005; Rozanski, 2014).

The field of **psychoneuroimmunology** studies how the immune system—with its collection of cells that recognize and attack intruders—interacts with other organs, especially those of the hormonal systems and nervous system (Ader, 2001). Studies of both human and nonhuman subjects clearly show psychological and neurological influences on the immune system. For example, people with happy social lives are less likely to develop a cold when exposed to the virus (S. Cohen et al., 2006). People exposed to a cold virus have more severe symptoms if they are experiencing conflict with others. But individuals who feel they have more social support, and who receive more hugs from others, are protected from that effect of conflict (S. Cohen et al., 2015). Likewise, people who tend to feel positive emotions will also produce more antibodies in response to a flu vaccination (Rosenkranz et al., 2003), which should help them fight off sickness. These interactions go both ways: the brain influences responses of the immune system, and immune cells and their products affect brain activities, as **FIGURE 11.21** shows. You can learn details of how the immune system, endocrine system, and nervous system communicate with one another in **A STEP FURTHER 11.3**, on the website.

Periods of elevated stress—such as exam periods and pandemics!—frequently suppress the immune system. For students taking exams, individual perceptions of the stress of the academic program predict the degree of immune system suppression: those who perceive the program as stressful show the most suppression (Glaser and Kiecolt-Glaser, 2005). One experiment considered the effects of university examinations on wound healing in dental students (Marucha et al., 1998). Two small wounds were placed on the roof of the mouth of 11 dental students (sounds like revenge, doesn't it?). The first wound was timed during summer vacation; the second was inflicted 3 days before the first major examination of the term. Two independent daily measures showed that no student healed as rapidly during the exam period, when healing took 40% longer. One measure of immunological response declined 68% during the exam period. The experimenters concluded that even something as transient, predictable, and relatively benign as final exams (do students agree with this description?) can significantly impede wound healing.

epigenetic regulation   Changes in gene expression that are due to environmental effects rather than to changes in the nucleotide sequence of the gene.

psychosomatic medicine   A field of study that emphasizes the role of psychological factors in disease.

health psychology   Also called *behavioral medicine*. A field of study that focuses on psychological influences on health-related processes.

psychoneuroimmunology   The study of the immune system and its interaction with the nervous system and behavior.

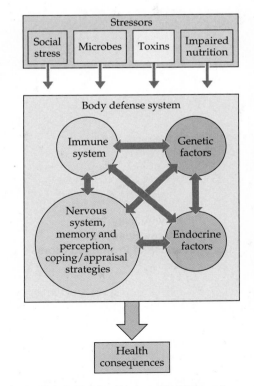

FIGURE 11.21   Factors That Interact during the Development and Progression of Disease

SIGNS & SYMPTOMS |||||||||||||||||||||||||||||||||||||||||||||||||||||||||||||||||||||||||||||||||||||||||||||||||||||||||||||

Long-Term Consequences of Childhood Bullying

There is growing recognition that children who are bullied, subjected to verbal or physical assault by other children, are at greater risk for mental and physical disorders when they grow up. A British study of children born in 1958 first gathered reports of whether they were being bullied at ages 7 and 11, then followed their health until they were age 50. After adjusting for IQ and other factors, the researchers found that those bullied as children were at increased risk for anxiety disorders and depression, as well as suicide (**FIGURE 11.22**) (Takizawa et al., 2014). Another study of both British and American children confirmed that those who were bullied were more likely to suffer these disorders. The authors were surprised to see that the effects of bullying were as strong as those of physical or sexual abuse (Lereya et al., 2015). Faced with such reports, schools are being encouraged to develop antibullying programs that teach children to recognize and report bullying and that train teachers to intervene rather than downplay bullying as a rite of passage or "normal" behavior. There is growing recognition many children today are subjected to another level of bullying—cyberbullying though social media (Hogan and Strasburger, 2020). Several

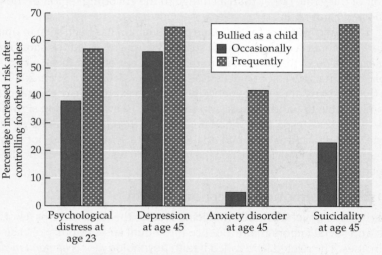

FIGURE 11.22   Being Bullied Is Bad for Your Health
(After R. Takizawa et al., 2014. *Am. J. Psychiatry* 171: 777.)

U.S. federal departments have collaborated to provide an online resource to increase understanding and combat bullying, including cyberbullying, at www.stopbullying.gov.

View Activity 11.2:
The Stress Response and
Consequences of Prolonged Stress

Why does chronic stress suppress the immune system?

Although brief stress doesn't impair immune function, and may even enhance it (Dhabhar, 2018), longer-lasting stress has a pronounced suppressive effect on the immune system. We discussed earlier how in response to stress, the brain causes adrenal steroid hormones such as cortisol to be released from the adrenal cortex. In chronic stress, these adrenal steroids directly suppress the immune system. But doesn't it seem like a bad idea to suppress immunity just when you are more likely to sustain an injury, and maybe an infection? Modern evolutionary theory offers some possible explanations for this seemingly maladaptive situation (for a very readable account, see Sapolsky, 2004).

To the extent that stress might be a sudden emergency, the temporary suppression of immune responses makes some sense because the stress response demands a rapid mobilization of energy. Slow and long-lasting immune responses consume energy that otherwise could be used for dealing with the emergency at hand. A zebra wounded by a lion must first escape and hide, and only then does infection of the wound pose a threat. So the stress of the encounter first suppresses the immune system, conserving resources until a safe haven is found. Later the animal can afford to mobilize the immune system to heal the wound. The adrenal steroids also suppress the swelling (inflammation) of injuries, especially of joints, to help the animal remain mobile long enough to find refuge (S. S. Cox et al., 2014). It is precisely this action that makes adrenal steroids like prednisone such useful medicines for treating inflammation.

In the wild, animals are under stress for only a short while; any animal stressed for a *prolonged* period dies. So natural selection has favored stress reactions as a drastic effort to deal with a short-term problem. What makes humans "special" is that, with our highly social lives and keen analytical minds, we are capable of experiencing stress for prolonged periods—months or even years. The bodily reactions to stress, which

TABLE 11.1 The Stress Response and Consequences of Prolonged Stress

Principal components of the stress response	Common pathological consequences of prolonged stress
Mobilization of energy at the cost of energy storage	Fatigue, muscle wasting, diabetes
Increased cardiovascular and cardiopulmonary tone	Hypertension (high blood pressure)
Suppression of digestion	Ulcers
Suppression of growth	Psychogenic dwarfism, bone decalcification
Suppression of reproduction	Suppression of ovulation, loss of libido
Suppression of immunity and of inflammatory response	Impaired disease resistance
Analgesia (painkilling)	Apathy
Neural responses, including altered cognition and sensory thresholds	Accelerated neural degeneration during aging

Source: R. M. Sapolsky, 2002, in J. B. Becker et al., (Eds.) *Behavioral endocrinology* (2nd. ed.). Cambridge, MA: MIT Press.

evolved to deal with short-term problems, become a handicap when extended too long (Sapolsky, 2004). **TABLE 11.1** lists a variety of stress responses that are beneficial in the short term but detrimental in the long term.

What we have described so far is a really depressing picture. If you are stressed for long periods of time, your health suffers, which brings another source of stress to your life. But don't give up hope. Even if there are some sources of stress you cannot avoid altogether, there are things you can do to reduce the impact of stress. *Relaxation training* involves focusing your attention on something calming while becoming more aware of your body, trying to relax muscles as much as you can (McGuigan and Lehrer, 2007). A program of therapy to deal with stress, partially inspired by various practices of meditation, is *mindfulness-based stress reduction (MBSR)*. MBSR pairs relaxation with efforts to focus attention on the present moment, including current sensations, thoughts, and bodily states, in an open, nonjudgmental way. MBSR is focused on results and does not require practitioners to adopt any particular religious or spiritual views. It has been shown to reduce activity in the amygdala (Goldin and Gross, 2010) and prevent relapses of anxiety disorders or depression (Hofmann et al., 2010).

See Video 11.3:
Stress

HOW'S IT GOING ?

1. What are the hormonal responses to stressful events, and how do those change as individuals adapt to those events?
2. What is stress immunization, and how is it mediated by epigenetic events?
3. Why do we suppress the immune system in times of stress, and how does that suppression impair health in brainy, social animals like us?
4. In what ways is a childhood history of being bullied evident in the psychological health of adults?

Recommended Reading

Adolphs, R., and Anderson, D. J. (2018). *The Neuroscience of Emotion: A New Synthesis*. Princeton, NJ: Princeton University Press.

Chen, A. (Ed.) (2019). *Stress Resilience: Molecular and Behavioral Aspects*. New York, NY: Academic Press.

Davis, K. L., and Panksepp, J. (2018). *The Emotional Foundations of Personality: A Neurobiological and Evolutionary Approach*. New York, NY: W. W. Norton.

Fernánadez-Dols, J.-M., and Russel, J. A. (Eds.) (2017). *The Science of Facial Expression*. New York, NY: Oxford University Press.

Fields, D. R. (2016). *Why We Snap: Understanding the Rage Circuits in Your Brain.* New York, NY: Dutton.

Gross, J. J. (2015). *Handbook of Emotion Regulation* (2nd ed.). New York, NY: Guilford Press.

Keltner, D., Oatley, K., and Jenkins, J. M. (2019). *Understanding Emotions* (4th ed.). New York, NY: Wiley.

LeDoux, J. (2015). *Anxious: Using the Brain to Understand and Treat Fear and Anxiety.* New York, NY: Viking.

Raine, A. (2013). *The Anatomy of Violence: The Biological Roots of Crime.* New York, NY: Pantheon.

Sapolsky, R. (2004). *Why Zebras Don't Get Ulcers* (3rd ed.). New York, NY: Holt.

11 • VISUAL SUMMARY

You should be able to relate each summary to the adjacent illustration, including structures and processes. The online version of this **Visual Summary** includes links to figures, animations, and activities that will help you consolidate the material.

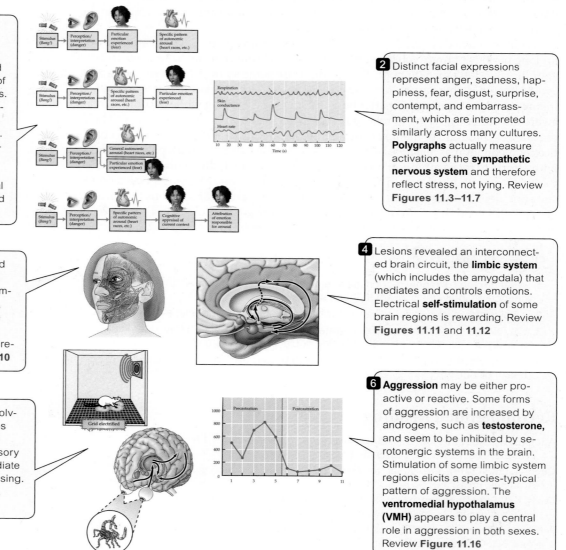

1 **Emotions** are a constellation of feelings, behaviors, and physiological reactions. The James-Lange theory considered emotions to be the perceptions of stimulus-induced bodily changes. The Cannon-Bard theory emphasized simultaneous emotional experience and bodily response. In Schachter and Singer's cognitive theory, we attribute visceral arousal to specific emotions by analyzing the physical and social context. Review **Figures 11.1** and **11.2**, **Animation 11.2**

2 Distinct facial expressions represent anger, sadness, happiness, fear, disgust, surprise, contempt, and embarrassment, which are interpreted similarly across many cultures. **Polygraphs** actually measure activation of the **sympathetic nervous system** and therefore reflect stress, not lying. Review **Figures 11.3–11.7**

3 Facial expressions are controlled by distinct sets of facial muscles controlled by the facial and trigeminal nerves. Emotions evolved as adaptations that trigger adaptive preprogrammed sequences of behavior, and they help in social relations. Review **Figures 11.8–11.10**

4 Lesions revealed an interconnected brain circuit, the **limbic system** (which includes the amygdala) that mediates and controls emotions. Electrical **self-stimulation** of some brain regions is rewarding. Review **Figures 11.11** and **11.12**

5 Fear is mediated by circuitry involving the **amygdala**, which receives information both through a rapid direct route and via cortical sensory regions, allowing for both immediate responses and cognitive processing. Review **Figures 11.13** and **11.14**, **Activity 11.1**

6 **Aggression** may be either proactive or reactive. Some forms of aggression are increased by androgens, such as **testosterone**, and seem to be inhibited by serotonergic systems in the brain. Stimulation of some limbic system regions elicits a species-typical pattern of aggression. The **ventromedial hypothalamus (VMH)** appears to play a central role in aggression in both sexes. Review **Figure 11.16**

7 **Stress** elevates levels of the hormones **cortisol**, from the **adrenal cortex**, and **epinephrine** and **norepinephrine**, from the **adrenal medulla**, while suppressing other hormones (testosterone). These responses to stress are adaptive in the short run, but in socially complex species that can experience stress for long periods, these hormonal responses decrease immune system competence, damaging our health. Review **Figures 11.18–11.20**, **Table 11.1**, **Activity 11.2**, **Video 11.3**

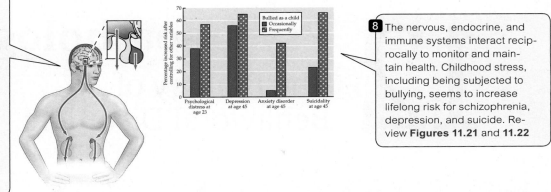

8 The nervous, endocrine, and immune systems interact reciprocally to monitor and maintain health. Childhood stress, including being subjected to bullying, seems to increase lifelong risk for schizophrenia, depression, and suicide. Review **Figures 11.21** and **11.22**

The Mind's Machine digital resources include additional videos, flashcards, and other study tools.

12 Psychopathology
The Biology of Behavioral Disorders

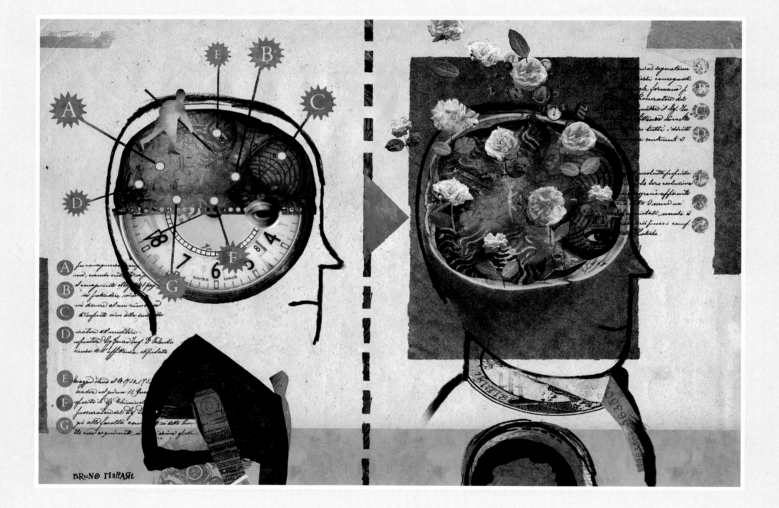

BRUNO MALLART

"My Lobotomy"

After Howard Dully's biological mother died unexpectedly when he was 4, his father married a woman named Lucille. For whatever reasons, Howard and Lucille did not get along. Howard was rebellious in the way that virtually all kids are—sassing back, breaking curfew, skipping out on church. But Howard was never violent with his stepmother (or anyone else). He sometimes got in trouble at school, for not paying attention in class or for smoking in the bathroom, but not for fighting or damaging school property. Howard's grades were erratic—an A on a test one day, an F on a test the next—but he was not flunking out.

Still, Lucille, frustrated with a headstrong boy in her house, took Howard to six different psychiatrists to find out "what was wrong with him." All concluded that his behavior was normal. But doctor number seven, the famous Walter Freeman, diagnosed the boy as schizophrenic. In 1960, Freeman gave 12-year-old Howard a lobotomy. First Freeman sedated the boy by giving him electro-shocks—jolts of electricity across the skull that induce a seizure and render the person unconscious. Then he lifted the boy's upper eyelids and used a hammer on an ice pick–like device to punch holes in Howard's skull above each eye. He then inserted a device to disconnect some of Howard's prefrontal cortex from the rest of his brain. Freeman was an old hand at the procedure, having lobotomized thousands of people, so the surgery took only 10 minutes. The total hospital charge was $200.

Family members report that Howard acted like a zombie for several days, so lethargic and disinterested in the events around him that, Freeman noted, they called Howard "lazy, stupid, dummy, and so on." One aunt said he acted like he was permanently tranquilized. And yet Lucille *still* wanted Howard out of her house. Soon Howard was institutionalized, and he would spend decades in various mental wards. Not until he was 50 did Howard find out what had happened to him as a child, a journey he movingly recounts in his memoir, *My Lobotomy* (Dully and Fleming, 2007).

Debilitating mental afflictions have plagued humans throughout history, plunging their victims into an abyss of disordered thought and emotional chaos. We have made great progress in understanding the causes of mental health issues like schizophrenia, depression, and anxiety disorders and have developed a wide variety of treatments that are at least partly effective, but the emotional and economic costs of these illnesses remain great. And they are widespread: psychopathology affects hundreds of millions of people throughout the world.

See Video 12.1: Lobotomy

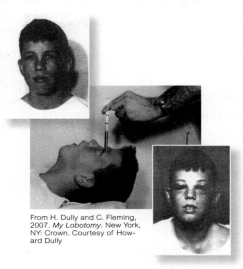

From H. Dully and C. Fleming, 2007. *My Lobotomy.* New York, NY: Crown. Courtesy of Howard Dully

Changed for Life   Twelve-year-old Howard Dully before, during, and after his transorbital lobotomy. The swelling around his eyes eventually went away, but Howard would spend the next four decades in various mental institutions.

View Animation 12.2: Brain Explorer

12.1 The Toll of Psychiatric Disorders Is Huge

THE ROAD AHEAD

We begin by considering schizophrenia, a severe disorder occurring in about 1% of the population, no matter where you go in the world. Learning this material should allow you to:

12.1.1 Know the most common symptoms of schizophrenia.

12.1.2 Understand the strong influence of both genes and the environment on the chances of developing schizophrenia.

12.1.3 Describe several of the structural brain differences of people with schizophrenia versus controls.

12.1.4 Discuss the several classes of antipsychotic drugs and their mechanisms of action.

The fifth edition of the American Psychiatric Association's *Diagnostic and Statistical Manual of Mental Disorders,* the *DSM-5,* provides a standardized system for diagnosing and classifying the major psychiatric illnesses according to current knowledge (American Psychiatric Association, 2013). Worldwide, between 15% and 50% of the population report psychiatric symptoms at some point in life, with North Americans positioned at the top end of this range (Kessler et al., 2007). About 19% of the adult population of the United States experiences psychiatric symptoms in the course of a year (SAMHSA, 2013), and of this number more than 4% (equating to almost 10 million people) are so ill that they are unable to carry out major life activities, like working or living independently. As shown in **FIGURE 12.1**, these rates are higher for females than for males, primarily because females are more likely to be depressed. (On the other hand, drug dependency and alcoholism, which are not reflected in Figure 12.1, are much more frequent in males.) Note also the high rates that are evident in 18- to 25-year-olds because certain psychiatric disorders—for example, schizophrenia—tend

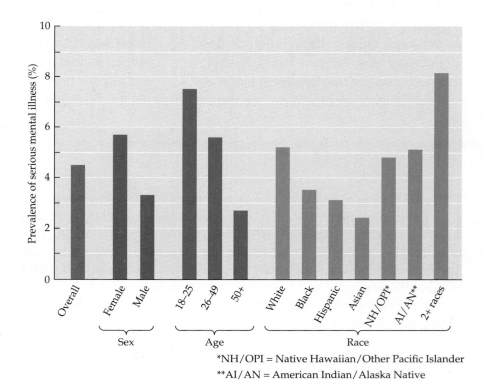

FIGURE 12.1   Prevalence of Serious Mental Illness among U.S. Adults in 2017   (After National Institute of Mental Health, 2018. *Past year prevalence of serious mental illness among U.S. adults (2017).* Bethesda, MD. Data courtesy of SAMHSA. Last updated February 2019. www.nimh.nih.gov/health/statistics/prevalence/serious-mental-illness-smi-among-us-adults.shtml)

*NH/OPI = Native Hawaiian/Other Pacific Islander

**AI/AN = American Indian/Alaska Native

to appear in adolescence and young adulthood. Clearly, mental disorders exact an enormous toll on our lives.

The seeds for a biological perspective in psychiatry were sown at the start of the twentieth century. At that time, almost a quarter of the patients in mental hospitals suffered from so-called paralytic dementia, featuring sudden onset of **delusions** (false beliefs strongly held in spite of contrary evidence), grandiosity (boastful self-importance), euphoria, poor judgment, impulsive behavior, disordered thought, and physiological signs like abnormal pupillary constriction (Argyll-Robertson, 1869). The disorder was originally believed to be caused by "weak character," but postmortem analyses of their brains revealed that their illness had a physiological cause: syphilis. With the advent of antibiotics to cure syphilis, paralytic dementia has virtually disappeared. This finding opened the door to biological explanations for other mental illnesses.

Schizophrenia is a major neurobiological challenge in psychiatry

Throughout the world and across the centuries, some people have been recognized as unusual because they hear voices that others don't, feel intensely frightened, sense persecution from unseen enemies, and generally act strangely (Bark, 2002; Heinrichs, 2003). For many, this disordered state—now known as **schizophrenia**—lasts a lifetime. For others, it appears and disappears unpredictably. Schizophrenia is also a public health problem because all too many people with schizophrenia become homeless.

The term *schizophrenia* (from the Greek *schizein*, "to split," and *phren*, "mind") was introduced early in the twentieth century to convey the idea that various functions of the mind—like memory, perception, and thinking—were split from each other (Bleuler, 1950, originally published in 1911). This poetic but vague description of schizophrenia was subsequently replaced with a more objective definition (K. Schneider, 1959) focusing on "first-rank symptoms," which include (1) auditory hallucinations, (2) highly personalized delusions, and (3) changes in affect (emotion). By the 1980s it became clear that many schizophrenia symptoms could be viewed as belonging to two general groups: positive and negative (McCutcheon et al., 2019). **Positive symptoms** are abnormal behavioral states that have been *gained*; examples include hallucinations, delusions, and excited motor behavior. **Negative symptoms** are abnormalities resulting from the *loss* of normal functions—for example, slow and impoverished thought and speech, emotional and social withdrawal, or blunted affect.

Researchers now recognize that schizophrenia is a complex syndrome in which individuals exhibit varying degrees of distinct but correlated categories of symptoms. The contemporary view of the symptoms of schizophrenia retains the distinction between positive symptoms (psychosis) and negative symptoms (emotional and motivational impairments) but recognizes an additional dimension: cognitive impairment (**TABLE 12.1**). The fact that the various categories of symptoms respond differently to drug treatments suggests that multiple neural mechanisms are involved in the disorder.

Schizophrenia has a heritable component

For many years, genetic studies of schizophrenia were controversial because some early researchers failed to understand that genes need not act in an all-or-none fashion. For any genotype there is often a large range of alternative outcomes determined by both developmental and environmental factors, as we'll see.

FAMILY STUDIES If schizophrenia can be inherited, relatives of people with schizophrenia should show a higher incidence (number of new cases during a period of time) than is found in the general population. In addition, the risk of schizophrenia among relatives should increase with the closeness of the relationship, because closer

delusion A false belief that is strongly held in spite of contrary evidence.

schizophrenia A severe psychopathological disorder characterized by negative symptoms such as emotional withdrawal and flat affect, by positive symptoms such as hallucinations and delusions, and by cognitive symptoms such as poor attention span.

positive symptom In psychiatry, an abnormal behavioral state. Examples include hallucinations, delusions, and excited motor behavior.

negative symptom In psychiatry, an abnormality that reflects insufficient functioning. Examples include emotional and social withdrawal, and blunted affect.

TABLE 12.1 Symptoms of Schizophrenia

Symptom dimension	Symptom category
POSITIVE SYMPTOMS Refers to symptoms that are present but should not be	**PSYCHOSIS** Hallucinations Delusions Disorganized thought and speech Bizarre behaviors
NEGATIVE SYMPTOMS Refers to characteristics of the individual that are absent but should be present	**EMOTIONAL DYSREGULATION** Lack of emotional expression Reduced facial expression (flat affect) Inability to experience pleasure in everyday activities (anhedonia) **IMPAIRED MOTIVATION** Reduced conversation (alogia) Diminished ability to begin or sustain activities Social withdrawal
COGNITIVE SYMPTOMS Refers to problems with processing and acting on external information	**NEUROCOGNITIVE IMPAIRMENT** Memory problems Poor attention span Difficulty making plans Reduced decision-making capacity Poor social cognition Abnormal movement patterns

concordance Sharing of a characteristic by both individuals of a pair of twins.

relatives share a greater number of genes. Indeed, parents and siblings of people with schizophrenia have a higher risk of developing schizophrenia than do individuals in the general population (**FIGURE 12.2**). However, the mode of inheritance of schizophrenia is not simple; that is, it does not involve a single recessive or dominant gene (Hyman, 2018). Rather, multiple genes play a role.

ADOPTION STUDIES It is easy to find fault with family studies. They confuse hereditary and environmental factors because members of a family share both. But what about children who are not raised with their biological parents? In fact, studies of adopted people confirm a strong genetic factor in schizophrenia. The biological parents of adoptees with schizophrenia are far more likely to have had this disorder than are the adopting parents (Foley et al., 2017).

TWIN STUDIES In twins, nature provides researchers with an excellent opportunity for a genetic experiment. In identical (or *monozygotic*) twins, who derive from a single fertilized egg and thus share the same set of genes, if one of the twins develops schizophrenia, the other twin has a roughly fifty-fifty chance of also developing the disorder. But in fraternal (or *dizygotic*) twin pairs, who come from two fertilized eggs and thus share about 50% of their genes, just like any pair of siblings, this **concordance** (sharing of a characteristic) drops to about 17% (see Figure 12.2) (Cardno and Gottesman, 2000). The higher concordance in the genetically identical twins is thus strong evidence of a genetic factor. Yet even with identical twins, the concordance rate for schizophrenia is only about 50%

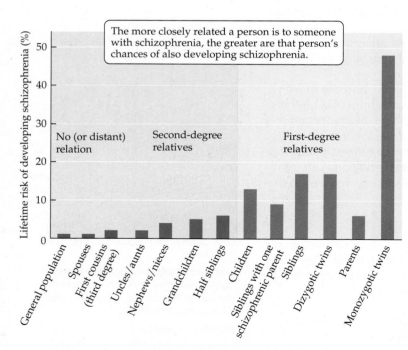

FIGURE 12.2 The Heritability of Schizophrenia (After I. I. Gottesman, 1991. *Schizophrenia genesis: The origins of madness.* Freeman. New York, NY.)

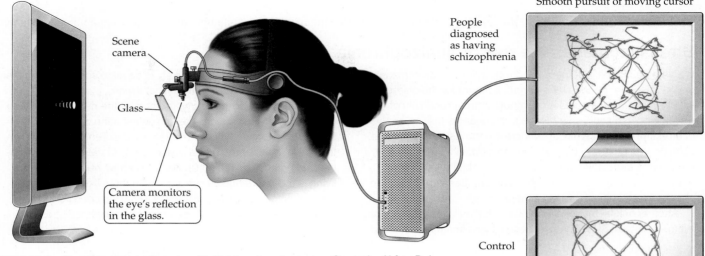

FIGURE 12.3   Eye Tracking in People with Schizophrenia versus Controls   (After P. J. Benson et al., 2012. *Biol. Psychiatry* 72: 716. Courtesy of Philip Benson.)

(some estimates are higher [Hilker et al., 2018], some lower [Joseph, 2013b]), so genes alone cannot fully explain whether a person will develop schizophrenia. Presumably, other factors, especially environmental influences, account for the 50% of identical twin pairs that are discordant (only one twin develops the disorder). Often, the twin who goes on to develop schizophrenia has an abnormal developmental history, such as lower birth weight, more physiological distress in early life, and behavior that seems more submissive, tearful, and sensitive than that of the unaffected twin (Torrey and Yolken, 2019). Subtle neurological signs, such as impaired motor coordination and difficulty with smooth movements of the eyes to follow a moving target (**FIGURE 12.3**), are also common (Avila et al., 2006). In short, the twin studies show that schizophrenia has both environmental and genetic origins.

INDIVIDUAL GENES   It has been difficult to identify any single gene that causes schizophrenia to develop or increases susceptibility (Hyman, 2018). In fact, genetic analyses suggest that over 100 genes influencing the likelihood of schizophrenia are scattered across many different human chromosomes (Birnbaum and Weinberger, 2017; Foley et al., 2017). Nonetheless, a few genes have been identified that appear to be abnormal in a small proportion of schizophrenia cases, including genes that are known to participate in synaptic plasticity (J. L. Kennedy et al., 2003; Mei and Xiong, 2008). In one large Scottish family, several members who had schizophrenia also carried a mutant, disabled version of a gene, which was therefore named *disrupted in schizophrenia 1* (*DISC1*). We'll discuss *DISC1* further a little later in the chapter.

An interesting *epigenetic* factor (see Chapter 13) in schizophrenia is paternal age: children fathered by older men have a greater risk of developing schizophrenia (de Kluiver et al., 2017). It is thought that, because they are the product of more cell divisions than the sperm of younger men, the sperm of older men have had more opportunity to accumulate mutations caused by errors in copying the chromosomes; these mutations may contribute to the development of schizophrenia in some cases.

Taken together, the studies make it clear that certain genes can indeed increase the risk of developing schizophrenia but that the environment also matters. As we'll see next, a big factor in whether a person will develop schizophrenia is stress.

RESEARCHERS AT WORK ||||||||||||||||||||||||||||||||||||||||||||||||||||||||||||||||||||||||||||||||||||||||||||||||||||||||||||||||||||||||||||||||

Stress increases the risk of schizophrenia

We've established that there is genetic influence on schizophrenia but also that genes alone cannot account for the disorder. What environmental factors contribute to the probability of developing schizophrenia? Research suggests that a variety of stressful events significantly increase the risk. For example, schizophrenia usually appears during a time in life that many people find stressful—the transition from childhood to adulthood, when people deal with physical, emotional, and lifestyle changes (e.g., going away to college).

Another risk factor seen in multiple studies is the stress of city living. As **FIGURE 12.4** shows, people living in a medium-sized city are about 1½ times more likely to develop schizophrenia than are people living in the country. What's more, the earlier in life a person begins living in the city, the greater the risk. People living in a *big* city are even more likely to develop the disorder (Pedersen and Mortensen, 2001). Conversely, children who move from the city to the country have a *reduced* risk of developing schizophrenia (Van Os et al., 2010). We don't know what it is about living in a city that makes schizophrenia more likely. Pollutants, greater exposure to minor diseases, crowded conditions, tense social interactions—all of these could be considered stressful.

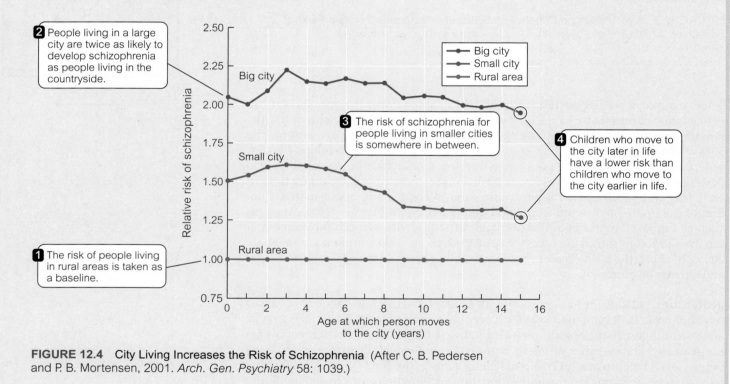

FIGURE 12.4 City Living Increases the Risk of Schizophrenia (After C. B. Pedersen and P. B. Mortensen, 2001. *Arch. Gen. Psychiatry* 58: 1039.)

An integrative model of schizophrenia emphasizes the interaction of factors

Prenatal stress, such as infection during pregnancy, increases the likelihood that the baby will develop schizophrenia later in life (P. H. Patterson, 2007; A. S. Brown, 2011). Likewise, if the mother and baby have incompatible blood types, or the mother becomes diabetic during pregnancy, or if there is a low birth weight for some reason, the baby is more likely to develop schizophrenia (S. King et al., 2010). Birth complications that deprive the baby of oxygen also increase the probability of schizophrenia (M. C. Clarke et al., 2011).

These findings suggest that relatively minor stress during development can make the difference in whether schizophrenia develops. It is fascinating, and frightening, to

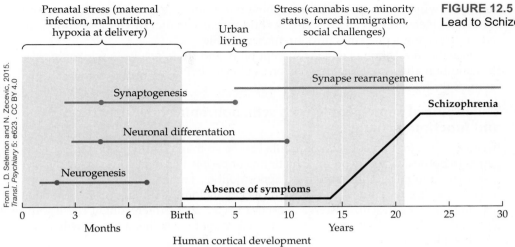

FIGURE 12.5 Developmental Periods When Stress Can Lead to Schizophrenia in Genetically Susceptible People

think that events in the womb or early childhood can affect the outcome 16 or 20 years later, when the schizophrenia appears.

Thus the evidence indicates that schizophrenia results from a complex interaction of genetic factors and stress. Each life stage has its own specific features that increase vulnerability to schizophrenia: infections before birth, complications at delivery, urban living in childhood and adulthood (Powell, 2010). From this perspective, the emergence of schizophrenia and related disorders depends on whether a genetically susceptible person is subjected to environmental stressors. These various stressors occur during critical phases of brain development (**FIGURE 12.5**), which may be affected by stress to lead to schizophrenia in genetically susceptible people. Alteration of brain development in people with schizophrenia is indicated by the acceleration of the normal thinning of cortical gray matter, a result of synapse rearrangement (**FIGURE 12.6**).

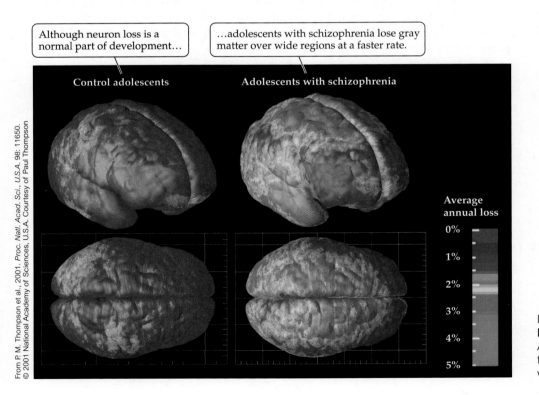

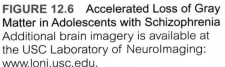

FIGURE 12.6 Accelerated Loss of Gray Matter in Adolescents with Schizophrenia Additional brain imagery is available at the USC Laboratory of NeuroImaging: www.loni.usc.edu.

Perhaps it will become possible to combine brain imaging, genetic screening, and behavioral measures, to identify at-risk children early in life, when interventions to reduce stress might prevent schizophrenia later in life.

Once the interaction of genetic susceptibility and stress results in schizophrenia, the condition affects not only the person's behavior but also the physical state of the brain, as we'll see next.

The brains of some people with schizophrenia show structural and functional changes

Because the symptoms of schizophrenia can be so marked and persistent, investigators hypothesized early on that the brains of people with this illness would show distinctive and measurable structural abnormalities. Later, CT and MRI scans confirmed this idea, revealing significant, consistent anatomical differences in the brains of many people with schizophrenia (Keshavan et al., 2020). Interestingly, these scans also confirm the idea that genes alone cannot account for whether a person will develop schizophrenia.

VENTRICULAR ABNORMALITIES   Most people with schizophrenia have enlarged cerebral ventricles, especially the lateral ventricles (Olabi et al., 2011) (**FIGURE 12.7**). What is the significance of enlarged ventricles? Because overall brain size does not seem to be affected in people with schizophrenia, or in a mouse model of schizophrenia, the enlarged ventricles must come at the expense of brain tissue. Therefore, interest has centered on possible changes in brain structures that run alongside the lateral ventricles, as discussed in **A STEP FURTHER 12.1**, on the website.

An important distinction is that twins with schizophrenia have decidedly enlarged lateral ventricles compared with their well counterparts, whose ventricles are of normal size (**FIGURE 12.8**). Among people with schizophrenia, those with larger ventricles benefit less from antipsychotic drugs (Garver et al., 2000).

Recall that a disabled version of the gene *DISC1* is associated with schizophrenia in one large family. The DISC1 protein normally regulates trafficking of molecules within neurons (Tomoda et al., 2017). When researchers inserted the schizophrenia-associated mutant version of *DISC1* into mice, they found that the mice developed enlarged lateral ventricles (**FIGURE 12.9**) that were reminiscent of the enlarged ventricles in people with schizophrenia (Pletnikov et al., 2008).

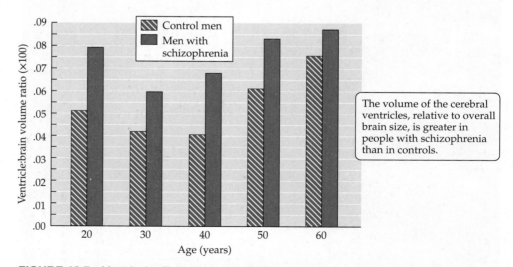

The volume of the cerebral ventricles, relative to overall brain size, is greater in people with schizophrenia than in controls.

FIGURE 12.7   Ventricular Enlargement in Schizophrenia
(After N. C. Andreasen et al., 1990. *Arch. Gen. Psychiatry* 47: 1008.)

FIGURE 12.8   Identical Genes, Different Fates

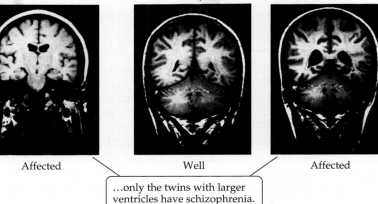

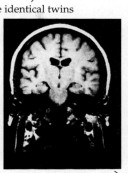

Although the two members of each set of identical twins shown here have the same genes…

35-year-old female identical twins

28-year-old male identical twins

Well   Affected   Well   Affected

…only the twins with larger ventricles have schizophrenia.

CORTICAL ABNORMALITIES   People with schizophrenia differ from controls in the structure and functional activity of the corpus callosum (Olabi et al., 2011). In addition to the accelerated cortical thinning (and reduction in subcortical volume) that we noted before (see Figure 12.6), people with schizophrenia tend to be impaired on neuropsychological tests that are sensitive to frontal cortical lesions. These findings raised the possibility that frontal cortex activity is abnormal in schizophrenia. Early observations using PET found that, compared with nonschizophrenic controls, people with schizophrenia had reduced metabolic activity in the frontal lobes relative to other regions of the brain (Buchsbaum et al., 1984). This observation led to the **hypofrontality hypothesis** that the frontal lobes are underactive in people with schizophrenia. Reviews of many studies over the past 35 years seem to support this idea (Minzenberg et al., 2009; Penadés et al., 2017).

In discordant identical twin pairs, where one twin is healthy and one has schizophrenia, reduced activity of the frontal cortex is evident only in the affected twin. Behavioral evidence indicates that hypofrontality is especially problematic during difficult cognitive tasks that depend on the frontal lobes for accurate

hypofrontality hypothesis   The idea that schizophrenia may reflect underactivation of the frontal lobes.

Transgenic mice expressing the *DISC1* mutation associated with schizophrenia in humans develop enlarged lateral ventricles (green) reminiscent of those in people with schizophrenia.

Control   Mutant

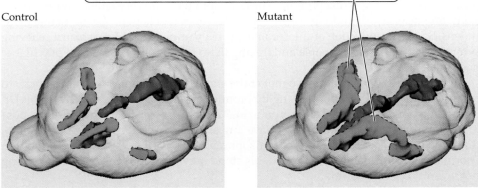

FIGURE 12.9   Enlarged Ventricles in a Mouse Model of Schizophrenia

lobotomy   The surgical separation of a portion of the frontal lobes from the rest of the brain, once used as a treatment for schizophrenia and many other ailments.

chlorpromazine   An early antipsychotic drug that revolutionized the treatment of schizophrenia.

dyskinesia   Difficulty or distortion in voluntary movement.

tardive dyskinesia   A disorder associated with first-generation antipsychotic use and characterized by involuntary movements, especially of the face and mouth.

supersensitivity psychosis   An exaggerated "rebound" psychosis that may emerge when doses of antipsychotic medication are reduced.

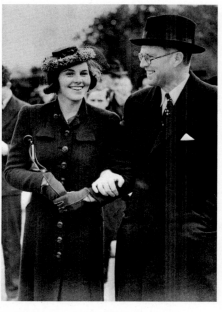

Another Victim of Lobotomy
Although it's unclear what psychological problems she had, if any, Rosemary Kennedy (1918–2005) was given a lobotomy at age 23, performed by Walter Freeman. A sister of President John F. Kennedy, Rosemary, shown here a few years before the surgery, was permanently incapacitated and spent the rest of her long life in an institution.

performance, such as the Wisconsin Card Sorting Task (see Figure 14.21). Unlike control participants, people with schizophrenia show little increase in their prefrontal activation during the task (D. R. Weinberger et al., 1994). In many cases, drugs that alleviate symptoms of schizophrenia, discussed next, also increase the activation of frontal cortex (Vogel et al., 2016).

The severity of schizophrenia led to desperate treatment attempts

In the 1930s, there were no effective treatments for schizophrenia. Because people with schizophrenia were often unable to take care of themselves, they were placed in caregiving institutions. In many cases, the health and welfare of patients in these (poorly funded) institutions were horribly neglected, leading to recurrent scandals. So perhaps it was in desperation that psychiatrists turned to **lobotomy**, the surgical separation of a portion of the frontal lobes from the rest of the brain, as a treatment for schizophrenia. Certainly there was little scientific evidence to think the surgery would be effective. But early practitioners reported nearly miraculous recoveries that, in retrospect, must be regarded as wishful thinking on the part of the physicians. The surgery may well have made the patients easier to handle, but they were rarely able to leave the mental institution. Used for almost any mental disorder, not just schizophrenia, lobotomies were performed on some 40,000 people in the United States alone (Kopell et al., 2005).

Antipsychotic medications revolutionized the treatment of schizophrenia

By the mid-twentieth century, more and more physicians were skeptical that lobotomy was effective for any disorder, and a drug discovered in the early 1950s—**chlorpromazine** (trade name Thorazine)—quickly replaced lobotomy as a treatment for schizophrenia. Although chlorpromazine was originally developed as an anesthetic (Charpentier et al., 1952; Ban, 2007), a lucky observation revealed that it could powerfully reduce the positive symptoms of schizophrenia. These symptoms—auditory hallucinations, delusions, and disordered thinking—were exactly the ones that kept people in mental institutions. So, the introduction of chlorpromazine truly revolutionized psychiatry, relieving symptoms for millions of people and freeing them from long-term beds in psychiatric hospitals.

Poor Howard Dully, whom we met at the start of the chapter, was very unlucky to run into a physician still performing lobotomies as late as the 1960s. Why didn't Dr. Freeman try giving Howard chlorpromazine? For one thing, the drug helps only positive symptoms, and Howard didn't have any of those. In fact, there's little reason to think the boy had *any* symptoms of schizophrenia (six psychiatrists had declared him "normal"). Unfortunately for Howard, his stepmother just happened upon the wrong physician at the wrong time.

Unfortunately, sometimes people taking antipsychotics develop undesirable side effects in movement, as we see in Signs & Symptoms, next.

SIGNS & SYMPTOMS ||||||||||||||||||||||||||||||||||||||||||||||||||||||||||||||||||||||||||||||||||||||||||||||||||||||||||||||||||||||||||||

Long-Term Effects of Antipsychotic Drugs

Few people would deny that antipsychotics are "miracle drugs." With drug treatment, many people who might otherwise have been in mental hospitals their whole lives can take care of themselves in nonhospital settings.

Unfortunately, antipsychotic drugs can have other, undesirable effects as well. Soon after beginning to take these drugs, some people develop maladaptive motor symptoms called **dyskinesia** (from the Greek *dys*, "bad," and *kinesis*, "motion"). Although many of these symptoms are transient and disappear when the dosage of drug is reduced, some drug-induced motor changes emerge only after prolonged drug treatment—after months, sometimes years—and are effectively permanent. This condition, called **tardive dyskinesia** (the Latin *tardus* means "slow"), is characterized by repetitive, involuntary movements, especially involving the face, mouth, lips, and tongue (**FIGURE 12.10**). Elaborate, uncontrollable movements of the tongue are particularly prominent, including incessant rolling movements, as well as sucking or smacking of the lips. Some people show twisting and sudden jerking movements of the arms or legs (Jain and Correll, 2018).

The underlying mechanism for tardive dyskinesia continues to be a puzzle. It may arise from the chronic blocking of dopamine receptors, which results in what is called *receptor supersensitivity*. Tardive dyskinesia frequently takes a long time to develop and tends to be irreversible. Long-term treatment with antipsychotic drugs can also have another undesirable effect. In some people, discontinuation of the drugs or a lowering of the dosage results in a sudden, marked increase in positive symptoms of schizophrenia, such as delusions or hallucinations. This **supersensitivity psychosis** (Yin et al., 2017) can often be reversed by the administration of increased dosages of dopamine receptor–blocking agents.

> Tardive dyskinesia may result in involuntary rolling of the tongue and smacking of the lips.

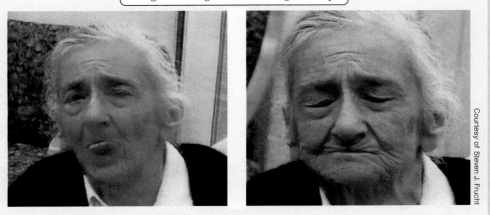

FIGURE 12.10   Tardive Dyskinesia The term describes a late onset of involuntary movements, often of the lower face. This woman with tardive dyskinesia has involuntary facial movements such as her tongue popping out (*left*) and intense grimacing (*right*).

Courtesy of Steven J. Frucht

THE DOPAMINE HYPOTHESIS   Chlorpromazine and other **antipsychotic** drugs (also known as *neuroleptics*) that came along a little later were eventually found to share a specific action: they block postsynaptic dopamine receptors, particularly dopamine D_2 receptors. Because antipsychotic drugs all blocked dopamine D_2 receptors to some extent, researchers proposed the **dopamine hypothesis**: that people with schizophrenia have an excess of either dopamine release or dopamine receptors. Interestingly, high doses of amphetamine cause an excess of dopamine to accumulate in synapses (see Chapter 4), resulting in a transient *amphetamine psychosis* that is strikingly similar to schizophrenia and is reversed by treatment with antischizophrenic medication. You might think that hallucinogenic drugs, like LSD, would similarly produce a schizophrenia-like state, but in fact there is little resemblance; for one thing, the effects of hallucinogens are primarily visual rather than auditory.

All of the various drugs that are now classified as **first-generation antipsychotics** (or *typical antipsychotics*) are D_2 receptor antagonists. In fact, the clinically effective dose of a first-generation antipsychotic can be predicted from its affinity for D_2

See Video 12.3:
Tardive Dyskinesia

antipsychotic   Also called *neuroleptic*. Any of a class of drugs that alleviate symptoms of schizophrenia, typically by blocking dopamine receptors.

dopamine hypothesis   The idea that schizophrenia results from either excessive levels of synaptic dopamine or excessive postsynaptic sensitivity to dopamine.

first-generation antipsychotic   Also called *typical antipsychotic*. An antischizophrenic drug that shows antagonist activity at dopamine D_2 receptors.

FIGURE 12.11 Traditional Antipsychotic Drugs Block Dopamine D$_2$ Receptors (After P. Seeman and T. Tallerico, 1998. *Mol. Psychiatry* 3: 123.)

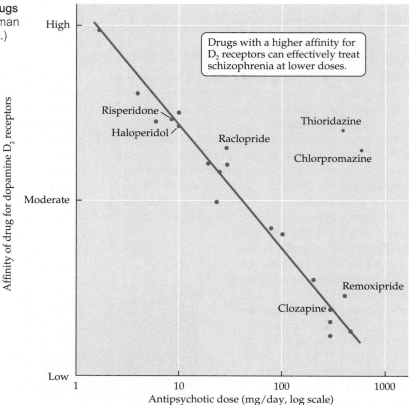

Drugs with a higher affinity for D$_2$ receptors can effectively treat schizophrenia at lower doses.

receptors (**FIGURE 12.11**), as the dopamine hypothesis would predict. For example, haloperidol, discovered a few years after chlorpromazine, has a greater affinity for D$_2$ receptors and quickly became the more widely used drug. Over the years, other clinical and experimental findings have bolstered the dopamine hypothesis; for example, treating people who have Parkinson's disease with L-dopa (the metabolic precursor of dopamine) may induce schizophrenia-like symptoms, presumably by boosting the synaptic availability of dopamine.

However, there are also several problems with the hypothesis. For example, there is no correspondence between the speed with which drugs block dopamine receptors (quite rapidly—within hours) and how long it takes for the symptoms to diminish (usually on the order of weeks). Thus, the relation of dopamine to schizophrenia is more complex than just hyperactive dopamine synapses. Furthermore, work with new types of antischizophrenic drugs, developed to reduce motor side effects we mentioned earlier, suggested that some symptoms of schizophrenia respond to modifications of other neurotransmitter systems. Called **second-generation antipsychotics** (or *atypical antipsychotics*), these drugs generally have only moderate affinity for the D$_2$ dopamine receptors that are the principal site of action of the first-generation antipsychotics. Instead, second-generation antipsychotics have their highest affinity for other transmitter receptors: **clozapine**, for example, blocks *serotonin* receptors (especially 5-HT$_{2A}$ receptors), as well as other receptor types.

Second-generation antipsychotics are just as effective as the older generation of drugs for relieving the symptoms of schizophrenia. So, if the problem is as simple as an overstimulation of dopamine receptors, why are the second-generation antipsychotics effective? For example, clozapine can *increase* dopamine release in frontal cortex (Bortolozzi et al., 2010)—hardly what we would expect if excess dopaminergic activity lies at the root of schizophrenia. In fact, it seems that supplementing antipsychotic treatments with L-dopa (thereby increasing dopaminergic activity) actually helps reduce symptoms of schizophrenia (Jaskiw and Popli, 2004).

second-generation antipsychotic Also called *atypical antipsychotic*. An antipsychotic drug that has primary actions other than or in addition to the dopamine D$_2$ receptor antagonism that characterizes the first-generation antipsychotics.

clozapine A second-generation antipsychotic that blocks 5HT$_{2A}$ receptors.

Until recently, almost all clinicians believed that second-generation antipsychotics were more effective than first-generation antipsychotics for treating schizophrenia, especially for relieving negative symptoms in addition to the positive symptoms relieved by first-generation antipsychotics. But several studies comparing the outcome for schizophrenic participants who had been given the two types of drugs found no difference (P. B. Jones et al., 2006; Crossley et al., 2010; Saha et al., 2016). Although the second-generation antipsychotics are less likely than first-generation antipsychotics to cause side effects in motor function (see Figure 12.10), they are more likely to cause weight gain (Sikich et al., 2008). So the overall outcome for quality of life appears equivalent for the two types of drugs (Heres et al., 2006).

Although antipsychotics were regarded as miracle drugs when they first became available, some are questioning whether their continued use is all that beneficial. Early studies typically ended 2 years after psychosis began, but later studies suggest a longer-lasting recovery without the drugs (**FIGURE 12.12**).

THE GLUTAMATE HYPOTHESIS   Another drug that, like chlorpromazine, was initially developed as an anesthetic has a much different relationship to schizophrenia. **Phencyclidine** (**PCP**) was soon found to be a potent **psychotomimetic**; that is, PCP produces phenomena strongly resembling both the positive and negative symptoms of schizophrenia. Users of PCP often experience auditory hallucinations, strange depersonalization, and disorientation, and they may become violent as a consequence of their drug-induced delusions. Prolonged psychotic states can develop with chronic use of PCP.

As illustrated in **FIGURE 12.13**, PCP acts as an NMDA receptor antagonist. PCP blocks the NMDA receptor's central calcium channel, thereby preventing the

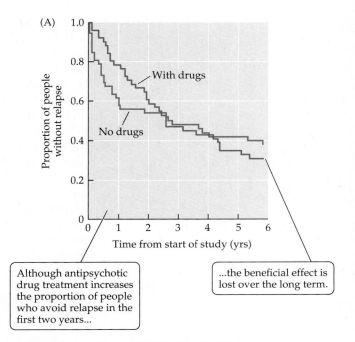

Although antipsychotic drug treatment increases the proportion of people who avoid relapse in the first two years...

...the beneficial effect is lost over the long term.

FIGURE 12.12   Long-term Outcomes with and without Antipsychotics (After L. Wunderink, 2019. *Ther Adv Psychopharmacol* 9: 1. CC BY-NC 4.0.)

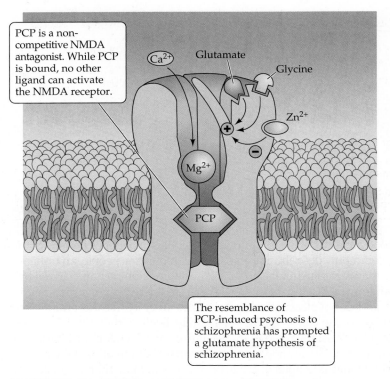

PCP is a noncompetitive NMDA antagonist. While PCP is bound, no other ligand can activate the NMDA receptor.

The resemblance of PCP-induced psychosis to schizophrenia has prompted a glutamate hypothesis of schizophrenia.

FIGURE 12.13   The Effects of PCP on the NMDA Receptor

phencyclidine (PCP)   Also called *angel dust*. An anesthetic agent that is also a psychedelic drug. PCP makes many people feel dissociated from themselves and their environment.

psychotomimetic   A drug that induces a state resembling schizophrenia.

endogenous ligand—glutamate—from having its usual effects. Treating monkeys with PCP for 2 weeks produces a schizophrenia-like syndrome, including poor performance on a test that is sensitive to prefrontal damage (Jentsch et al., 1997). Other antagonists of NMDA receptors, such as **ketamine**, have similar effects. These and other observations prompted researchers to propose a **glutamate hypothesis** of schizophrenia (Uno and Coyle, 2019), which suggests that schizophrenia results from an *under*activation of glutamate receptors, which might account for the reduced activity in frontal cortex (Marek et al., 2010)—the hypofrontality we described earlier. If this hypothesis is correct, you might ask whether compounds that increase glutamatergic activity would be effective antischizophrenic drugs. However, drugs that stimulate the ionotropic NMDA receptors tend to produce seizures, so NMDA receptor agonists are not an option. Instead, researchers are focusing on manipulations of the metabotropic glutamate receptors—mGluRs—of which there are at least eight different subtypes (Mueller et al., 2004). Although results from clinical trials with early candidate drugs have been disappointing (Stauffer et al., 2013), researchers hope that targeting the proper class of mGluRs with drugs that have novel modes of action may someday lead to a new generation of antipsychotics (Stansley and Conn, 2018).

HOW'S IT GOING ❓

1. Evaluate the evidence supporting the dopamine hypothesis of schizophrenia, and contrast it with the evidence casting doubt on this hypothesis.
2. What distinguishes first-generation antipsychotics from second-generation antipsychotics?
3. Which drugs can induce a psychosis resembling schizophrenia? What receptor(s) do these drugs act on?

12.2 Mood Disorders Are the Most Common Psychopathologies

THE ROAD AHEAD

Next we will discuss mood disorders, which include depression and bipolar disorder. Studying this material will enable you to:

12.2.1 Recognize the major symptoms of depression and the warning signs of suicide.

12.2.2 Understand the influence of genes on the risks for depression.

12.2.3 Describe the several treatments available for depression, and weigh the evidence for the effectiveness of antidepressant drugs.

12.2.4 Discuss the possible reasons that depression is more commonly reported among women than men.

12.2.5 Understand the symptoms of bipolar disorder, and describe the discovery that lithium can treat the condition.

Disturbances of mood are a fact of life for humans; most of us experience periods of unhappiness that we commonly describe as depression. But for some people, an unhappy mood state is more than a passing malaise. Clinically, **depression** is characterized by a combination of unhappy mood, loss of interests, reduced energy, changes in appetite and sleep patterns, and loss of pleasure in most things. Difficulty in concentration and restless agitation or torpor are common; the person may dwell on thoughts of death or even contemplate suicide. Pessimism seems to seep into every act (Solomon, 2001). Such depression can occur with no readily apparent stress, and without treatment the depression often lasts several months (Kupfer et al., 2012). Each year, more than 7% of American adults experience at least one episode of clinically significant depression (SAMHSA,

ketamine A dissociative anesthetic drug, similar to PCP, that acts as an NMDA receptor antagonist.

glutamate hypothesis The idea that schizophrenia may be caused, in part, by understimulation of glutamate receptors.

depression A psychiatric condition characterized by such symptoms as an unhappy mood; loss of interests, energy, and appetite; and difficulty concentrating.

2018). This condition is more common in people over 40 years of age, especially women, but depression can afflict people of any age, race, or ethnicity (CDC, 2010).

Along with other mental illnesses, depression can be lethal, as it may lead to suicide. Whether or not the person is depressed, many suicides appear to be impulsive acts, or are prompted by time-limited crises that would have eventually resolved themselves (Kleiman et al., 2017). For example, one classic study found that of the more than 500 people who were prevented from jumping off the Golden Gate Bridge in San Francisco, only 6% later went on to commit suicide (Seiden, 1978). Similarly, suicide rates went down by a third in Britain when that country switched from using coal gas, which contains lots of deadly carbon monoxide, to natural gas for heating. The suicide rate has remained at that reduced level in the 40+ years since (Thomas and Gunnell, 2010). Apparently those thousands of Britons who would have found it easy to follow a suicidal impulse by turning on the kitchen oven did not kill themselves when more planning was required. Thus, it is important for society to erect barriers, either literally (e.g., on bridges) or metaphorically, to make it difficult for people to kill themselves. Legal barriers, such as firearm legislation that mandates waiting periods, can likewise help reduce suicide rates in some regions (Anestis et al., 2019). Despite the myth that "people who want to kill themselves will succeed eventually," when suicide is averted the first time it is seriously considered or attempted, the person is unlikely to ever try it again. **TABLE 12.2** lists the warning signs that someone may be contemplating suicide. Despite public health initiatives to combat suicide in the United States, it has steadily risen this century (Carey, 2018).

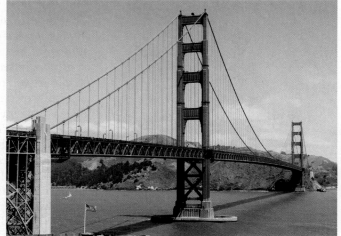

Wrong Impulse   The vast majority of people who were prevented from jumping off the Golden Gate Bridge never again attempted suicide. One of the few people to survive the jump has said "The very second I let go, I knew I had made a big mistake" (Hines 2013).

Inheritance is an important determinant of depression

Genetic studies of depressive disorders reveal strong hereditary contributions. The concordance rate for identical twins (about 40%) is substantially higher than for fraternal twins (about 20%) (K. E. Whitfield et al., 2008). The concordance rates for identical twins are similar whether the twins are reared apart or together. Although several early studies implicated specific chromosomes, subsequent research has failed to identify any particular gene (Risch et al., 2009). So, as is the case for schizophrenia, there is no single gene for depression. Rather, *many* genes contribute to making a person more or less susceptible, and environmental factors determine whether depression results.

TABLE 12.2 Warning Signs of Suicide[a]

Threatening to hurt or kill oneself or talking about wanting to hurt or kill oneself

Looking for ways to kill oneself by seeking access to firearms, pills, or other means

Talking or writing about death, dying, or suicide when these actions are out of the ordinary for the person

Feeling hopeless

Feeling rage or uncontrolled anger or seeking revenge

Acting reckless or engaging in risky activities—seemingly without thinking

Feeling trapped—like there's no way out

Increasing alcohol or drug use

Withdrawing from friends, family, and society

Feeling anxious, agitated, or unable to sleep, or sleeping all the time

Experiencing dramatic mood changes

Seeing no reason for living or having no sense of purpose in life

Source: https://www.nimh.nih.gov/health/topics/suicide-prevention/index.shtml

[a]Developed by the U.S. Department of Health and Human Services, these warning signs offer guidance about how to recognize someone at risk for suicide. If you or someone you know exhibits even a few of these signs, you can call the National Suicide Prevention Lifeline at 1-800-273-TALK (1-800-273-8255) at any time of day, any day of the year.

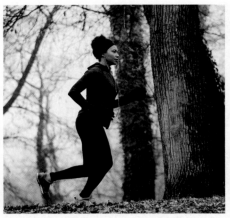

Breaking the Cycle   For many people, forcing themselves to engage in exercise, even as mild as walking, can improve their mood.

The brain changes with depression

Most reports of differences in the brains of depressed people focus on functional changes as detected by PET or fMRI. Depressed people show changes in activity in a number of brain regions, depending on whether the tasks being processed are principally cognitive or emotional in nature (S. M. Palmer et al., 2015). When depressed people are compared with control individuals, increased activation in the amygdala is especially evident during emotional processing, and increased activity in the frontal lobes is evident during more cognitively demanding tasks. Decreased activity is evident in the parietal and posterior temporal cortex and in the anterior cingulate cortex—systems that have been implicated in attention (see Chapter 14) (Davey et al., 2017). The increased activity in the amygdala—a structure involved in mediating fear (see Chapter 11)—persists even after the depression has lifted.

Descendants of people with severe depression also have a thinner cortex across large swaths of the right hemisphere than do control participants (B. S. Peterson et al., 2009), which might make them vulnerable to depression. There is also evidence that people who are depressed have difficulties regulating stress hormone release, as discussed in **A STEP FURTHER 12.2**, on the website.

Many studies report hippocampal volume is reduced in people with depression (Sexton et al., 2013), and there is reduced activation of the hippocampal region in depressed people during memory tasks (K. D. Young et al., 2012). But whether these changes in the hippocampus are present before the depression, and therefore may be a contributing cause of the disorder, or are a result of the depression remains unknown. In any case, there are effective treatments for depression, as we discuss next.

A wide variety of treatments are available for depression

Electroconvulsive shock therapy (**ECT**)—the intentional induction of a large-scale seizure (Payne and Prudic, 2009)—was originally a schizophrenia treatment, born of desperation during the 1930s. Although it proved to be of little help in schizophrenia, it soon became evident that ECT *could* rapidly reverse severe depression. The advent of antidepressant drugs has made ECT less common, but ECT remains an important tool for treating severe, drug-resistant depression (M. Fink and Taylor, 2007). A more modern technique for altering cortical electrical activity, called **repetitive transcranial magnetic stimulation** (**rTMS**) (see Chapter 1), is likewise being developed as a treatment for depression (D. R. Kim et al., 2009).

Today, the most common treatment for depression is the use of drugs that affect the monoamine transmitters: norepinephrine, dopamine, and serotonin. The first antidepressants were inhibitors of **monoamine oxidase** (**MAO**), the enzyme that normally inactivates monoamines in the synaptic cleft. This action of MAO inhibitors causes monoamine transmitters to accumulate to higher levels in synapses, so researchers proposed that depressed people do not get enough stimulation at monoamine synapses (this is sometimes called the *monoamine hypothesis of depression*). A second generation of antidepressants, called *tricyclics*, inhibits the reuptake of monoamines, which similarly boosts their synaptic activity. ECT may help depression by inducing the release of monoamines.

Among the monoamines, serotonin seems to play an especially important role in depression (Svenningsson et al., 2006). A major class of modern antidepressants, the **selective serotonin reuptake inhibitors** (**SSRIs**), such as Prozac (**TABLE 12.3**) (see Chapter 4), act to increase synaptic serotonin levels in the brain. In rats, SSRIs increase the birth of new neurons in the hippocampus (Sahay and Hen, 2007), which may mediate some of the mood effects of the drugs.

However, there are problems with the idea that reduced serotonin stimulation causes depression. We know that SSRI drugs increase synaptic serotonin within hours of administration. Yet it typically takes several weeks of SSRI treatment before people

electroconvulsive shock therapy (ECT)   A last-resort treatment for unmanageable depression, in which a strong electrical current is passed through the brain, causing a seizure.

repetitive transcranial magnetic stimulation (rTMS)   A noninvasive treatment in which repeated pulses of focused magnetic energy are used to stimulate the cortex through the scalp.

monoamine oxidase (MAO)   An enzyme that breaks down monoamine neurotransmitters, thereby inactivating them.

selective serotonin reuptake inhibitor (SSRI)   An antidepressant drug that blocks the reuptake of transmitter at serotonergic synapses.

TABLE 12.3 Drugs Used to Treat Depression

Symptom dimension	Symptom category	Examples[a]
Monoamine oxidase (MAO) inhibitors	Inhibit the enzyme monoamine oxidase, which breaks down serotonin, norepinephrine, and dopamine	Marplan, Nardil, Parnate
Tricyclics and heterocyclics	Inhibit the reuptake of norepinephrine, serotonin, and/or dopamine	Wellbutrin, Elavil, Aventyl, Ludiomil, Norpramin
Selective serotonin reuptake inhibitors (SSRIs)	Block the reuptake of serotonin, having little effect on norepinephrine or dopamine synapses	Prozac, Paxil, Zoloft
Second-generation antidepressants and investigational drugs	Norepinephrine and dopamine reuptake inhibitors (NDRIs), serotonin-norepinephrine reuptake inhibitors (SNRIs), noradrenergic and specific serotonergic antidepressants (NaSSAs), serotonin antagonist and reuptake inhibitors (SARIs), opioid receptor modulators, ketamine	Wellbutrin/Zyban (NDRI), Effexor (SNRI), Remeron (NaSSA), Oleptro (SARI), Buprenex (opioid receptor modulator)

[a]The names given are the more commonly used trade names rather than chemical names.

feel better. This paradox suggests that it is the brain's *response* to increased synaptic serotonin that relieves the symptoms, and that this response takes time. So even though boosting serotonin helps some people, their depression may originally have been caused by other factors in the brain.

A newer class of antidepressants is the serotonin-norepinephrine reuptake inhibitors (SNRIs) like Cymbalta (duloxetine) and Effexor (venlafaxine) (Hillhouse and Porter, 2015). Several other medications for depression are currently under study. For example, compounds being investigated as potential antidepressants include the glutamate receptor antagonist ketamine (see Chapter 3; Figure 12.13), a PCP-like drug that relieves depression almost instantly (E. E. Lee et al., 2015), in contrast to SSRIs and SNRIs, which typically must be taken for several weeks before they elevate mood.

Despite the popularity of SSRIs for treating depression, treatment with **cognitive behavioral therapy (CBT)**, a type of psychotherapy aimed at correcting negative thinking and improving interpersonal relationships, is about as effective as SSRI treatment (Butler et al., 2006). Furthermore, the rate of relapse is lower for CBT than for SSRI treatment (DeRubeis et al., 2008). Interestingly, CBT and SSRI treatment *together* are more effective in combating depression than either one is alone (Schramm et al., 2008). Typically, CBT helps the client to recognize self-defeating modes of thinking and encourages breaking out of a cycle of self-fulfilling depression (**FIGURE 12.14**) and has proven effective in avoiding suicide (Mewton and Andrews, 2016). Furthermore, while there is no doubt that current antidepressants do help many people who are depressed, evidence has accumulated that for a significant number of people, part of the benefit may actually be a placebo effect (Turner et al., 2008), as we discuss in Signs & Symptoms next.

cognitive behavioral therapy (CBT) Psychotherapy aimed at correcting negative thinking and consciously changing behaviors as a way of changing feelings.

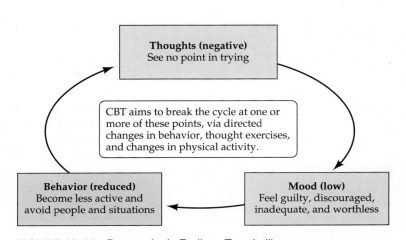

FIGURE 12.14 Depression's Endless Treadmill

SIGNS & SYMPTOMS ||||||||||||||||||||||||||||||||||||||||||||||||||||||||||||||||||||||||||||||||||||||||||||||||||||||||||||||||||||

Mixed Feelings about SSRIs

At their introduction, selective serotonin reuptake inhibitors (SSRIs) represented a major revolution in depression treatment. Heavily marketed to the public and to health professionals, SSRIs soon became one of the most widely prescribed medications, propelling an incredible 400% increase in antidepressant prescriptions by 2008. In fact, for 18- to 44-year-olds, antidepressants are prescribed more than any other drug; more than one in ten adult Americans is currently using antidepressant medication (Pratt et al., 2011). Needless to say, the development and sales of antidepressants have provided a huge windfall for the pharmaceuticals industry.

Now that SSRIs have been with us for more than 20 years, researchers have turned to retrospective analyses to reevaluate the efficacy of SSRIs. In part, these large-scale **meta-analyses** (analyses that combine the results of many previously published studies) have been prompted by the concern that for various reasons—public appetite, profit motives, the tendency of journals to publish only positive findings—studies that failed to find effects of SSRIs may historically have been underreported. The results of these meta-analyses have been mixed, but they at least give us cause to take a sober second look at SSRI usage.

As illustrated in **FIGURE 12.15**, systematic reviews of the clinical research seem to show that while modern antidepressant drugs are indeed effective, their effects are modest in size and evident in only the most severely depressed people (Fournier et al., 2010; Cipriani et al, 2018). Other large meta-analytic studies, also based on multiple clinical trials, find stronger

evidence of clear beneficial effects of SSRIs relative to placebos for people of all ages and with all levels of severity of depression (Gibbons et al., 2012). One possibility is that the relationship between symptom severity and SSRI efficacy is a statistical artifact of the methodology employed in order to combine studies in a meta-analysis. And while there are reservations about the efficacy of SSRIs for children or teenagers (Bower, 2006), millions of American children and teens have been given prescriptions for SSRIs despite a reported increased risk of suicide in these age groups (Olfson et al., 2006).

This controversy seems likely to rage on for a while. In the meantime, a prudent course of action is to deploy CBT as a first-rank treatment in moderate cases, supplemented with antidepressant medication in more severe or nonresponsive cases.

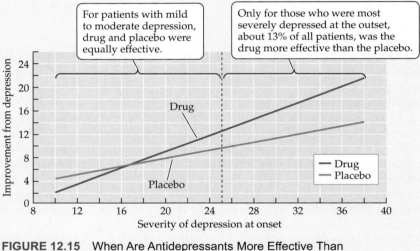

> For patients with mild to moderate depression, drug and placebo were equally effective.

> Only for those who were most severely depressed at the outset, about 13% of all patients, was the drug more effective than the placebo.

FIGURE 12.15   When Are Antidepressants More Effective Than Placebos? (After J. C. Fournier et al., 2010. *JAMA* 303: 47.)

An unusual treatment for depression involves a pacemaker that periodically applies mild electrical stimulation to the vagus nerve (cranial nerve X; see Chapter 1). This treatment is offered in cases where drugs or ECT have been ineffective, but it remains to be established whether vagal stimulation is a long-term solution (Grimm and Bajbouj, 2010; Blumberger et al., 2015). For extremely difficult cases of depression, researchers have turned again to psychosurgery—but nothing that resembles the ravages suffered by Howard Dully. In **deep brain stimulation** (**DBS**) surgery, delicate electrodes are surgically implanted in the cingulate cortex or other brain sites (Kringelbach et al., 2007). The effectiveness of DBS or vagal nerve stimulation for depression is difficult to evaluate, because most studies have no placebo control (R. Robinson, 2009). In the few placebo-controlled studies, where the participant was unaware of whether electrical stimulation was provided, the treatment appeared to be less effective than it seemed in initial, uncontrolled reports (Kisely et al., 2018; Widge et al., 2018), suggesting that the promising early results of DBS and vagal stimulation may have been due to placebo effects.

meta-analysis   A type of quantitative review of a field of research, in which the results of multiple previous studies are combined in order to identify overall patterns that are consistent across studies.

deep brain stimulation (DBS)
Mild electrical stimulation through an electrode that is surgically implanted deep in the brain.

Why do more females than males develop depression?

Studies all over the world show that more women than men experience major depression. In the United States, women are twice as likely as men to have major depression (Brody et al., 2018). Some researchers suggest that the apparent sex difference reflects different patterns of help-seeking behavior by males and females—that women are willing to use health facilities, while men see that as a sign of weakness. But sex differences in the incidence of depression also are evident in door-to-door surveys (J. S. Hyde and Mezulis, 2020), which would appear to rule out the simple explanation that women seek treatment more often than men do.

Some researchers have emphasized gender differences in endocrine physiology. The appearance of clinical depression often is related to events in the female reproductive cycle—for example, before menstruation, during use of contraceptive pills, following childbirth, and during menopause. Although there is little relation between circulating levels of individual hormones and measures of depression, the phenomenon of **postpartum depression**, a bout of depression immediately preceding and/or following childbirth, suggests that some combination of hormones can precipitate depression. About one out of every seven pregnant women will show symptoms of depression (Dietz et al., 2007). Because postpartum depression may affect the mother's relationship with her child, resulting in long-lasting negative effects on the child's behavior (Tronick and Reck, 2009), there is growing concern about this problem. However, there is also evidence that SSRIs taken by pregnant women may affect the later behavior of their children (Oberlander et al., 2010; Brandlistuen et al., 2015), and it is uncertain whether exposure to SSRIs via breast milk will have a long-term effect. Thus CBT offers the safest treatment for postpartum depression, and researchers continue to weigh the costs and benefits of supplementing that therapy with antidepressant medication (Grieb and Ragan, 2019).

Scientists are still searching for animal models of depression

Everyone agrees that an animal model of depression could be invaluable, as it might reveal underlying mechanisms or offer a convenient way to screen potential treatments (Nestler and Hyman, 2010). But it's not clear that any animal model has lived up to this promise so far. If depression were caused by the mutation of a particular gene, it might be possible to create a model by introducing that mutated gene in mice. But as we noted above, human depression is influenced by many genes, each having a modest effect alone. Plus, some of the most powerful symptoms of depression are internal—apathy and a feeling of hopelessness—and thus are difficult to assess in species we can't talk to.

Still, many of the signs of depression—such as decreased social contact, problems with eating, and changes in activity—are observable behaviors. So researchers have used these behaviors to evaluate animal models of depression. In one type of stress model—**learned helplessness**—an animal is exposed to a repetitive stressful stimulus, such as an electrical shock, that it cannot escape. Like depression, learned helplessness has been linked to a decrease in serotonin function (Maier and Seligman, 2016) and also to mechanisms that control the release of dopamine (B. Li et al., 2011), the main reward signal in the brain. Removing the olfactory bulb from rodents also creates a model of depression: the animals display irritability, preferences for alcohol, and elevated levels of corticosteroids—all of which are reversed by many antidepressants. A strain of rats created through selective breeding—the Flinders Sensitive Line—has been proposed as a model of depression because these animals show reduced overall activity, reduced body weight, learning difficulties, and exaggerated response to chronic stress (Overstreet and Wegener, 2013). These varied animal models may be useful in finding the essential mechanisms that cause and maintain depression in humans.

Sleep characteristics change in affective disorders

Difficulty falling asleep and inability to maintain sleep are common in depression. In addition, EEG sleep studies of people with depression show certain abnormalities that go beyond difficulty falling asleep. The sleep of people with major depressive disorders is marked by a striking reduction in stage 3, or slow wave, sleep (see Chapter 10) and a

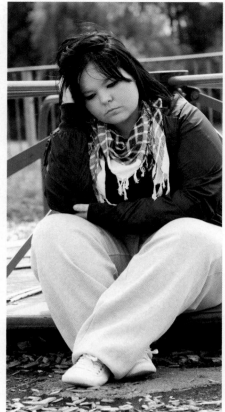

Depression For reasons that are not understood, women are more likely than men to develop depression.

postpartum depression A bout of depression that afflicts a woman either immediately before or after giving birth.

learned helplessness A learning paradigm in which individuals are subjected to inescapable, unpleasant conditions.

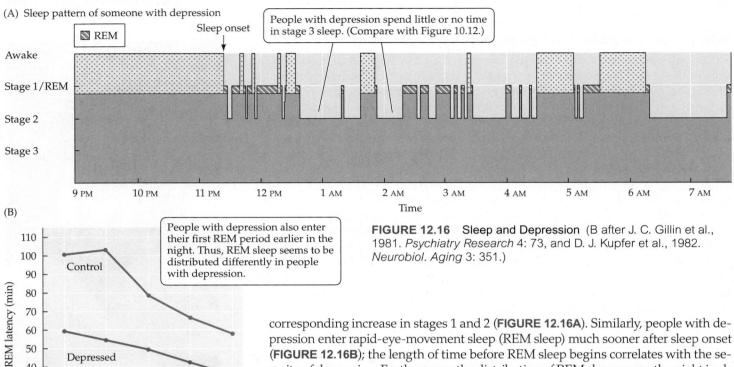

(A) Sleep pattern of someone with depression

People with depression spend little or no time in stage 3 sleep. (Compare with Figure 10.12.)

(B)

People with depression also enter their first REM period earlier in the night. Thus, REM sleep seems to be distributed differently in people with depression.

FIGURE 12.16 Sleep and Depression (B after J. C. Gillin et al., 1981. *Psychiatry Research* 4: 73, and D. J. Kupfer et al., 1982. *Neurobiol. Aging* 3: 351.)

corresponding increase in stages 1 and 2 (**FIGURE 12.16A**). Similarly, people with depression enter rapid-eye-movement sleep (REM sleep) much sooner after sleep onset (**FIGURE 12.16B**); the length of time before REM sleep begins correlates with the severity of depression. Furthermore, the distribution of REM sleep across the night is altered, with an increased amount of REM sleep occurring during the first half of sleep, as though REM sleep were displaced toward an earlier period in the night (Palagini et al., 2013).

As with these links between the daily rhythm of sleep and depression, seasonal rhythms have been implicated in a particular depressive condition known as *seasonal affective disorder* (*SAD*), which is described in **A STEP FURTHER 12.3**, on the website.

In bipolar disorder, mood cycles between extremes

Affecting about 2.6% of the U.S. population each year (Kessler et al., 2005), **bipolar disorder** is characterized by periods of depression alternating with periods of excessively expansive mood (or *mania*) that includes sustained overactivity, talkativeness, strange grandiosity, and increased energy. The rate at which the alternation occurs varies between individuals: some people exhibit *rapid-cycling* bipolar disorder, defined as consisting of four or more distinct cycles in one year (and some individuals have many more cycles than that; some may even show several cycles per *day*).

Men and women are equally affected by bipolar disorder, and the age of onset is usually much earlier than that of depression. Bipolar disorder is clearly heritable, with several different genes affecting the probability of the disorder (Smoller and Finn, 2003; Faraone et al., 2004).

The neural basis of bipolar disorder is not fully understood, but people with bipolar disorder exhibit enlarged ventricles on brain scans (Arnone et al., 2009), as is seen in schizophrenia (see Figure 12.8). The more manic episodes the person has experienced, the greater the ventricular enlargement, suggesting a worsening of brain loss over time (Moorhead et al., 2007).

The observed pattern of changes in the brain and behavior of people with bipolar disorder has led to a recognition that bipolar disorder has more in common with schizophrenia than with depression, so the older term *manic depression* has been largely abandoned. For example, the self-aggrandizing ideas and extreme talkativeness of people in the manic phase of bipolar disorder (e.g., "The president called me this morning to thank me for my efforts") may resemble the frank delusions seen in schizophrenia. In addition, families in which some individuals have been diagnosed with bipolar disorder are more likely than other families to have individuals with a diagnosis of schizophrenia

bipolar disorder A psychiatric disorder characterized by periods of depression that alternate with excessive, expansive moods.

(Lichtenstein et al., 2009; Van Os and Kapur, 2009). And although first-generation antipsychotics do not seem to help, the newer, second-generation antipsychotics seem to help dampen the manic phase in people with bipolar disorder. However, most people who have bipolar disorder benefit from taking the element **lithium** (Severus et al., 2018), a treatment discovered entirely by accident, as we discuss next.

lithium   A chemical element that often relieves the symptoms of bipolar disorder.

RESEARCHERS AT WORK ||||||||||||||||||||||||||||||||||||||||||||||||||||||||||||||||||||||||||||

The entirely accidental discovery of lithium therapy

The effect of lithium on bipolar disorder was discovered purely by accident when it was intended as an inert control in an experiment focusing on the urea in lithium urate (**FIGURE 12.17**), so the mechanism of action is not understood.

FIGURE 12.17   Surprisingly Calm Guinea Pigs   (After J. F. Cade, 1949. *Med. J. Aust.* 2: 349.)

■ **Question**

Do people with bipolar disorder have too much urea in circulation?

■ **Hypothesis**

Injecting urea into guinea pigs will make them manic.

■ **Test**

Cade (1949) found that he could dissolve higher concentrations of urea into solution if he used a urea-lithium combination, lithium urate, rather than urea alone. Other guinea pigs, the control group, got injections of lithium alone.

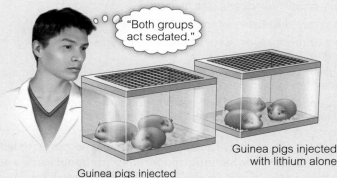

"Both groups act sedated."

Guinea pigs injected with lithium urate

Guinea pigs injected with lithium alone

■ **Results**

Instead of the lithium urate making the guinea pigs manic, it calmed them. But in another surprise, the control injections of lithium alone were just as effective for calming the animals (Howland, 2007). Intrigued, Cade took some lithium himself and, upon finding it harmless, tried giving it to people with bipolar disorder. Almost all of the treated people showed a remarkable recovery, and many who had been institutionalized for years could finally return home.

■ **Conclusion**

Lithium alone calms guinea pigs and relieves symptoms of bipolar disorder in humans. Note that this conclusion has nothing to do with the original question. This experiment demonstrates the importance of having a good control group. If Cade had not injected some guinea pigs with lithium alone, he might have wrongly concluded that urea has a calming effect.

Because lithium has a narrow range of safe doses (see Figure 3.6), care must be taken to avoid toxic side effects of an overdose. Nevertheless, well-managed lithium treatment produces marked relief for many people with bipolar disorder and even has been reported to increase the volume of gray matter in their brains (G. J. Moore et al., 2009).

anxiety disorder   Any of a class of psychological disorders that includes recurrent panic states and generalized persistent anxiety disorder.

The fact that the manic phases blocked by lithium are so exhilarating may be the reason that some people with bipolar disorder stop taking the medication. Unfortunately, doing so means that the depressive episodes return as well. As in depression, transcranial magnetic stimulation may provide a nonpharmacological treatment alternative in difficult cases of bipolar disorder (Michael and Erfurth, 2004). Furthermore, mounting evidence suggests that some forms of CBT for mild cases of bipolar disorder can be as effective as drug treatments (Salcedo et al., 2018) and perhaps can be beneficially combined with other forms of treatment.

HOW'S IT GOING ❓

1. What are the symptoms of depression, and how does depression differ from simple sadness?
2. What treatments for depression arose in the twentieth century, and which treatment is used most often today?
3. Summarize the evidence for and against the use of SSRIs in depression. Why is the use of SSRIs controversial?
4. What is bipolar disorder, and how does it compare with depression and with schizophrenia? How is it treated?

12.3 There Are Several Types of Anxiety Disorders

THE ROAD AHEAD

We conclude the chapter by considering anxiety disorders, among the most common of psychiatric conditions. The material will permit you to:

12.3.1 Describe the symptoms of several anxiety disorders.

12.3.2 Name the various medications used to treat anxiety disorders and their mechanisms of action.

12.3.3 Discuss the data indicating whether some people are initially more vulnerable to post-traumatic stress disorder (PTSD).

12.3.4 Describe the several treatments for obsessive-compulsive disorder (OCD), including controversial trials of brain surgery and stimulation.

All of us have at times felt apprehensive and fearful. But some people experience this state with an intensity that is overwhelming and includes irrational fears; a sense of terror; body sensations such as dizziness, difficulty breathing, trembling, and shaking; and a feeling of loss of control. Anxiety can be lethal: men with panic disorder are more likely than others to die from cardiovascular disease or suicide (De La Vega et al., 2018).

The *DSM-5* distinguishes several major types of **anxiety disorders**: *Phobic disorders* are intense, irrational fears that become centered on a specific object, activity, or situation that the person feels compelled to avoid. Another type of anxiety disorder is *panic disorder*, characterized by recurrent transient attacks of intense fearfulness. In *generalized anxiety disorder*, persistent, excessive anxiety and worry are experienced for months. There is a strong genetic contribution to each of these disorders (Shih et al., 2004; Oler et al., 2010) and distinctive underlying neurobiological predispositions to the development of anxiety disorders (Shackman et al., 2013).

Some people who experience recurrent panic attacks have temporal lobe abnormalities, especially in the left hemisphere (Vythilingam et al., 2000; Van Tol et al., 2010). Given the special role of the amygdala in mediating fear (see Chapter 11), changes may be particularly evident in the amygdala and associated circuitry within the temporal lobes (Rauch et al., 2003).

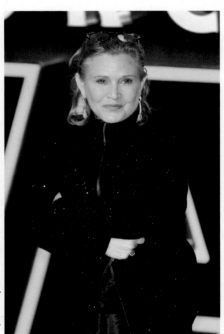

A Disturbance in the Force   Actress Carrie Fisher (1956–2016), who played Princess Leia/Leia Organa in five *Star Wars* movies, wrote about her struggles with bipolar disorder.

Drug treatments provide clues to the mechanisms of anxiety

Throughout history, people have consumed all sorts of substances in the hopes of controlling anxiety. The list includes alcohol, bromides, cannabis, opiates, and barbiturates. In the 1950s the tranquilizing drug meprobamate (Miltown) was introduced, and it became an instant best seller, ushering in the modern age of anxiety pharmacotherapy. Soon researchers discovered a new class of drugs called **benzodiazepines**, which quickly replaced Miltown as the favored drugs for treating anxiety. One type of benzodiazepine—diazepam (trade name Valium)—is one of the most prescribed drugs in history. Other commonly prescribed benzodiazepines include Xanax, Halcion, and Ativan. Such drugs that combat anxiety are termed **anxiolytics** ("anxiety-dissolving"), although they also may have anticonvulsant and sleep-inducing properties. The anxiolytic drugs are also discussed in Chapter 3.

Anxiolytic benzodiazepines interact with binding sites that are part of GABA receptors, especially the $GABA_A$ receptors, where they act as noncompetitive agonists. Recall from Chapter 3 that GABA is the most common inhibitory transmitter in the brain. When GABA is released from a presynaptic terminal and activates postsynaptic receptors, it hyperpolarizes the target neuron and therefore inhibits it from firing. Benzodiazepines alone have little effect on the $GABA_A$ receptor, but when benzodiazepines are present, GABA produces a markedly enhanced hyperpolarization. In other words, benzodiazepines boost GABA-mediated postsynaptic inhibition, reducing the excitability of postsynaptic neurons.

Interestingly, the brain probably makes its own anxiety-relieving substances that interact with the benzodiazepine-binding site on the GABA receptor; the neurosteroid allopregnanolone is a prime candidate for this function. Drugs developed to act at this site are effective anxiolytics in both rats and humans (Rupprecht et al., 2009). As you can see in **FIGURE 12.18**, benzodiazepine/ $GABA_A$ receptors are widely distributed throughout the brain, especially in the cerebral cortex and some subcortical areas, such as the hippocampus and the amygdala.

Although the benzodiazepines remain an important category of anxiolytics, especially for acute attacks, other anxiety-relieving drugs have been developed that lack the abuse potential of the benzodiazepines. A notable example is the drug buspirone (Buspar), an agonist at serotonin $5\text{-}HT_{1A}$ receptors that can provide relief from anxiety. This effect is consistent with functional-imaging research that reveals an abnormal density of $5\text{-}HT_{1A}$ receptors in the brains of people with anxiety disorders (Neumeister et al., 2004). SSRI antidepressants, such as paroxetine (Paxil) and fluoxetine (Prozac), which increase the stimulation of serotonin receptors, are also sometimes effective treatments for anxiety disorders.

In post-traumatic stress disorder, horrible memories won't go away

Some people experience especially awful moments in life that seem indelible, resulting in vivid impressions that persist the rest of their lives. The kind of event that seems particularly likely to produce subsequent stress disorders is intense and is usually associated with witnessing abusive violence and/or death. Examples include the sudden loss of a close friend, rape, torture, kidnapping, or profound social dislocation, such as in forced migration. In these cases, memories of horrible events intrude into consciousness and produce the same intense visceral arousal—the fear and trembling and general autonomic activation—that the original event caused. These traumatic memories are easily reawakened by stressful circumstances and even by harmless stimuli that somehow prompt recollection of the original event. An ever-watchful and fearful stance becomes the portrait of individuals afflicted with what is called **post-traumatic stress disorder** (PTSD), formerly called

> This PET scan of benzodiazepine receptors shows their wide distribution in the brain, especially the cortex. Highest concentrations are in red; lowest concentrations are in blue.

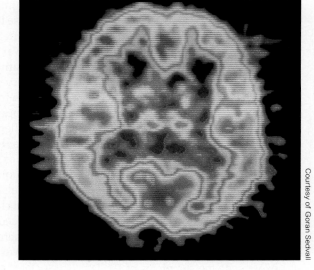

Courtesy of Goran Sedvall

FIGURE 12.18 The Distribution of Benzodiazepine Receptors in the Human Brain

benzodiazepine Any of a class of antianxiety drugs that are noncompetitive agonists of $GABA_A$ receptors in the central nervous system. One example is diazepam (Valium).

anxiolytic A substance that is used to reduce anxiety. Examples include alcohol, opiates, barbiturates, and the benzodiazepines.

post-traumatic stress disorder (PTSD) A disorder in which memories of an unpleasant episode repeatedly plague the person.

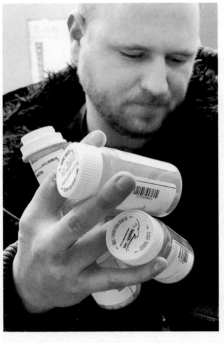

Delayed Reaction   Many combat veterans experience the symptoms of PTSD for years afterward.

fear conditioning   A form of classical conditioning in which fear comes to be associated with previously neutral stimuli.

combat fatigue, war neurosis, or *shell shock.* Although related in some ways to anxiety disorders, post-traumatic stress disorder is now recognized in the *DSM-5* as a separate entity.

Analysis of a random sample of Vietnam War veterans has indicated that 19% had PTSD at some point after service. This was the rate for *all* Vietnam veterans; when the researchers focused more specifically on veterans exposed to intense war zone stressors, more than 35% developed PTSD at some point, and most of them still had the symptoms of this disorder *decades* later (Dohrenwend et al., 2006). Gulf War veterans likewise have high rates of PTSD (Institute of Medicine, 2010).

Genetic factors affect vulnerability to PTSD, as indicated in twin studies of Vietnam War veterans who had seen combat, which showed that monozygotic twins were more similar than dizygotic twins. People who display combat-related PTSD show (1) memory changes such as amnesia for some war experiences, (2) flashbacks, and (3) deficits in short-term memory. These memory disturbances suggest involvement of the hippocampus (see Chapter 13), and indeed the volume of the right hippocampus is smaller in combat veterans with PTSD than in those without it, with no differences in other brain regions (Logue et al., 2018). It was once widely assumed that stressful episodes caused the hippocampus to shrink, but some veterans with PTSD had left their monozygotic twins at home, and it turns out that the nonstressed twins without PTSD also tended to have a smaller hippocampus (Gilbertson et al., 2002). So some inherited characteristic that's associated with having a small hippocampus, and perhaps a reduced rate of adult neurogenesis (J. S. Snyder et al., 2011; Kheirbek et al., 2012), may increase susceptibility to developing PTSD if the person is exposed to stress. In Gulf War veterans with more severe PTSD, marked hippocampal size difference is associated with markers of inflammatory processes (O'Donovan et al., 2015), which can strongly contribute to neural degeneration and decreased neurogenesis.

A comprehensive psychobiological model of the development of PTSD draws connections from PTSD's memory disturbances to the neural mechanisms of fear conditioning, behavioral sensitization, and extinction. Work in animals has revealed that **fear conditioning**—memory for a stimulus that the animal has learned to associate with a negative event—is very persistent and involves the amygdala and brainstem pathways that are part of a circuit of startle response behavior (see Chapter 11). The persistence of memory and fear in PTSD may depend on the failure of mechanisms to *forget*. There is also a hormonal link, because people with PTSD exhibit a paradoxical long-term *reduction* in cortisol (stress hormone) levels (Wichmann et al., 2017), perhaps due to persistent increases in *sensitivity* to cortisol. If, as a result, they feel the effect of stress hormones more strongly than other people do, that greater effect might repeatedly retrigger the fear response, making it harder for them to forget stressful events (**FIGURE 12.19**). In

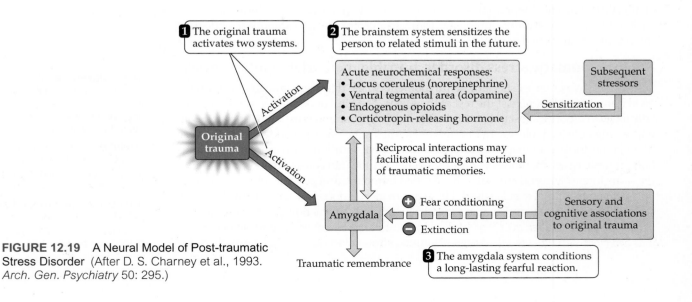

FIGURE 12.19   A Neural Model of Post-traumatic Stress Disorder   (After D. S. Charney et al., 1993. *Arch. Gen. Psychiatry* 50: 295.)

1 The original trauma activates two systems.

2 The brainstem system sensitizes the person to related stimuli in the future.

Acute neurochemical responses:
• Locus coeruleus (norepinephrine)
• Ventral tegmental area (dopamine)
• Endogenous opioids
• Corticotropin-releasing hormone

Subsequent stressors

Sensitization

Original trauma

Activation

Activation

Reciprocal interactions may facilitate encoding and retrieval of traumatic memories.

Amygdala

+ Fear conditioning

– Extinction

Sensory and cognitive associations to original trauma

Traumatic remembrance

3 The amygdala system conditions a long-lasting fearful reaction.

Chapter 13 we will discuss research-based methods that have been proposed to help people forget traumatic life events by having them recall the event while under the influence of a drug that dampens the stress response.

In obsessive-compulsive disorder, thoughts and acts keep repeating

Most of us aspire to be neat and clean, especially when we discover a thick layer of dust under the furniture or perhaps realize we've created yet another tottering pile of papers and bills. And of course, having certain small rituals in our lives—making coffee a certain way in the morning, wishing everyone good night before going to bed—can be a comfort amid the chaos of daily life. But when do orderliness and routine cross the line into pathology? People with **obsessive-compulsive disorder** (OCD) lead lives riddled with repetitive rituals and persistent thoughts that they feel powerless to control or stop, despite recognizing that the behaviors are abnormal. In people with OCD, routine acts that we all engage in, such as checking whether the door is locked when we leave our home, become *compulsions*, acts that are repeated over and over. Recurrent thoughts, or *obsessions*, such as fears of germs or other potential harms in the world, invade the consciousness. These symptoms progressively isolate a person from ordinary social engagement with the world. For many people with OCD, hours each day are consumed by compulsive acts such as repetitive hand washing. **TABLE 12.4** summarizes some of the symptoms of OCD.

Determining the number of people afflicted with OCD is difficult, especially because people with this disorder tend to hide their symptoms (Newth and Rachman, 2001). It is estimated that nearly 1% of adults in the United States will have "severe" OCD symptoms in any given year (Kessler et al., 2005). In many cases, the initial symptoms of this disorder appear in childhood; the peak age group for onset of OCD, however, is 25–44 years. People with OCD display increased metabolic rates in the orbitofrontal cortex, cingulate cortex, and caudate nuclei (Chamberlain et al., 2008).

Happily, OCD responds to treatment in most cases. OCD shows excellent response to cognitive behavioral therapy (Öst et al., 2016; Abramowitz et al., 2018) and also to

obsessive-compulsive disorder (OCD) An anxiety disorder in which the affected individual experiences recurrent unwanted thoughts and engages in repetitive behaviors without reason or the ability to stop.

TABLE 12.4 Symptoms of Obsessive-Compulsive Disorder

Symptoms (most to least common by type)

OBSESSIONS (THOUGHTS)
  Dirt, germs, or environmental toxins
  Something terrible happening (e.g., fire, death or illness of self or loved one)
  Symmetry, order, or exactness
  Religious obsessions
  Body wastes or secretions (urine, stool, saliva, etc.)
  Lucky or unlucky numbers
  Forbidden, aggressive, or perverse sexual thoughts, images, or impulses
  Fear of harming self or others
  Household items
  Intrusive nonsense sounds, words, or music

COMPULSIONS (ACTS)
  Performing excessive or ritualized hand washing, showering, bathing, tooth brushing,
    or grooming
  Repeating rituals (e.g., going in or out of a door, getting up from or sitting down on a chair)
  Checking (doors, locks, stove, appliances, emergency brake on car, paper route,
    homework, etc.)
  Engaging in miscellaneous rituals (such as writing, moving, speaking)
  Decontaminating
  Touching
  Counting
  Ordering or arranging
  Preventing harm to self or others
  Hoarding or collecting
  Cleaning household or inanimate objects

Source: After S. E. Swedo et al., 1989. *Arch. Gen. Psychiatry* 46: 335.

several drugs. What do effective OCD drugs—like fluoxetine (Prozac), fluvoxamine (Luvox), and clomipramine (Anafranil)—tend to have in common? They share the ability to inhibit the reuptake of serotonin at serotonergic synapses, thereby increasing the synaptic availability of serotonin. This observation suggests that the dysfunction of serotonergic neurotransmission plays a central role in OCD. Recall that we already discussed SSRIs like Prozac that inhibit the reuptake of serotonin when we discussed treatments for depression. How can the same drug help two disorders that seem so different? For one thing, depression often accompanies OCD, so the two disorders may be related. Furthermore, functional brain imaging suggests that the same SSRI drugs alter the activity of the orbitofrontal prefrontal cortex in people with OCD (Saxena et al., 2001) while affecting primarily ventrolateral prefrontal cortex in people with depression.

There is a heritable genetic component to OCD; as with schizophrenia and depression, several genes contribute to susceptibility to this disorder (Pauls et al., 2014), including genes related to serotonin signaling (Sinopoli et al., 2017). There is also evidence that OCD can be triggered by infections (Orlovska et al., 2017). Upon observing that numerous children exhibiting OCD symptoms had recently been treated for strep throat, Dale et al. (2005) found that many children with OCD are producing antibodies to brain proteins. Perhaps, in mounting an immune response to the streptococcal bacteria, these children also make antibodies that attack their own brains. The genetic link may be that some people are more likely than others to produce antibodies to the brain proteins.

In recent years, deep brain stimulation (DBS) has been tried for many psychiatric disorders that do not respond to medication, and OCD is no exception (Karas et al., 2019). But again there are few participants and many of the studies have no control condition (when no stimulation is provided to the electrode), so it is difficult to assess whether the DBS is effective (Naesström et al., 2016). Psychosurgery may be a treatment of last resort. Unlike lobotomies, these surgeries target much smaller regions. In one study, about one-third of severely disabled people with OCD who underwent cingulotomy (making lesions that interrupt pathways in the cingulate cortex) (**FIGURE 12.20**) benefited (Shah et al., 2008; Pepper et al., 2015). Even here it is difficult to rule out a placebo effect of the cingulotomy, as you cannot ethically ask some people to undergo sham neurosurgery, opening up their skull to then *not* make a lesion, to provide a control group. Frontal lobotomy, which causes much more extensive damage to the brain, is virtually never performed today. So we can be pretty confident that no one else will suffer the fate of Howard Dully, lobotomized for being a teenager.

Many researchers believe that OCD is part of a spectrum of related disorders (Olson, 2004), such as Tourette's, the topic of our final Signs & Symptoms for this chapter.

Tourette's syndrome   A disorder involving heightened sensitivity to sensory stimuli that may be accompanied by verbal or physical tics.

These MRIs show the brain of a person who underwent a cingulotomy—the disruption of cingulate cortex connections—in an attempt to treat OCD.

(A) Horizontal view

(B) Sagittal view

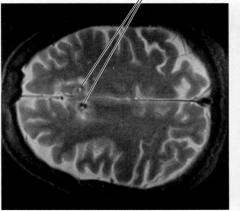
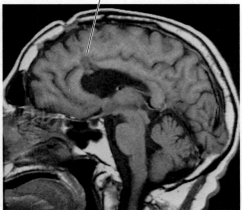

FIGURE 12.20   Neurosurgery to Treat Obsessive-Compulsive Disorder

From R. L. Martuza et al., 1990. *J. Neuropsychiatry Clin. Neurosci.* 2: 331, courtesy of Robert L. Martuza

SIGNS & SYMPTOMS |||||||||||||||||||||||||||||||||||||||||||||||||||||||||||||||||||||||||||||||||||||||||||||||||||||||||||||||||||||||||||||||||||||||||

Tics, Twitches, and Snorts: The Unusual Character of Tourette's Syndrome

The faces of people with Tourette's twitch in an insistent way, and every now and then, out of nowhere, they blurt out an odd sound. At times they fling their arms, kick their legs, or make violent shoulder movements. People with **Tourette's syndrome** are also supersensitive to tactile, auditory, and visual stimuli (J. H. Cox et al., 2018). Many people with Tourette's report that an urge to emit verbal or phonic tics builds up and that giving in to the urge brings relief. Although popular media often portray people with Tourette's as shouting out insults and profanities (a symptom called *coprolalia*), verbal tics of that sort are rare.

Tourette's syndrome begins early in life; the mean age of diagnosis is 6–7 years (Groth, 2018), and the syndrome is 3–4 times more common in males than in females. **FIGURE 12.21A** draws a portrait of the chronology of symptoms. Often people with Tourette's also exhibit attention deficit hyperactivity disorder (ADHD) or OCD (Eapen et al., 2016). Children with Tourette's display a thinning of primary somatosensory and motor cortex representing facial, oral, and laryngeal structures (Sowell et al., 2008), suggesting that the tics mediated by these regions may be underinhibited by cortex.

Family studies indicate that genetics plays an important role in this disorder. Among discordant monozygotic twin pairs, the twin with Tourette's has a greater density of dopamine D_2 receptors in the caudate nucleus of the basal ganglia than the unaffected twin has. This observation suggests that differences in the dopaminergic system (Mogwitz et al., 2013), especially in the basal ganglia (Maia and Conceição, 2018), may be important (D_2 receptor binding in an affected individual is illustrated in **FIGURE 12.21B**). The contemporary view is that Tourette's syndrome is mediated in a complex manner by many genes rather than just one (Hallett, 2015; Qi et al., 2017).

Treatment with haloperidol, a dopamine D_2 receptor antagonist that is better known as a first-generation antipsychotic drug (see Figure 12.11), significantly reduces tic frequency and is a primary treatment for Tourette's syndrome. Unfortunately, this treatment can have unpleasant side effects, as noted earlier, but some people with Tourette's also respond well to the second-generation antipsychotics, which may bring fewer side effects. Behavior modification techniques aimed at reducing the frequency of symptoms, especially tics, help some people learn how to replace their obvious tics with behaviors that are more subtle and socially acceptable (McGuire et al., 2015).

DBS, which we mentioned earlier, may also benefit people with Tourette's. In this case, battery-powered stimulating electrodes are aimed bilaterally at targets within the thalamus, in regions associated with the control of movement. Activation of the electrodes is reported to bring dramatic and almost immediate relief from symptoms (Porta et al., 2009; Baldermann et al., 2016).

FIGURE 12.21 Portrait of Tourette's Syndrome
(Part A after J. Jagger et al., 1982. *Schizophr. Bull.* 8: 267.)

(A) The chronology of Tourette's symptoms

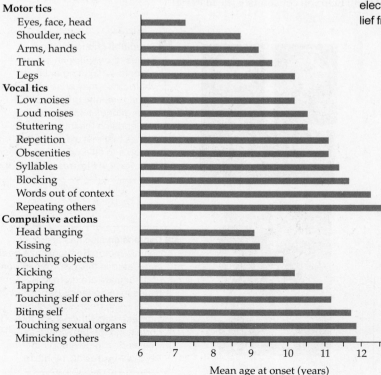

(B) D_2 receptor binding in Tourette's syndrome

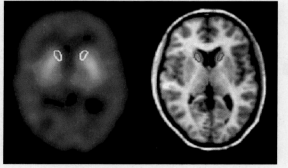

S. S. Wolf et al., 1996. *Science* 273: 1225. Courtesy of Steven Wolf

View Activity 12.1:
Concept Matching: Psychopathology

HOW'S IT GOING ❓

1. What are the main types of anxiety disorders?
2. What class of drugs is the most common anxiolytic, and what effect do these drugs have on transmitter systems?
3. Describe PTSD and the hypothesis that the disorder is a special case of fear conditioning.
4. What is OCD, and what treatments are available to combat it?

Recommended Reading

Beidel, D. C., and Frueh, B. C. (2018). *Adult Psychopathology and Diagnosis* (8th ed.). New York, NY: Wiley.

Charney, D. S., Nestler, E. J., Sklar, P., and Buxbaum, J. D. (Eds.). (2018). *Charney & Nestler's Neurobiology of Mental Illness* (5th ed.). New York, NY: Oxford University Press.

Huettel, S. A., Song, A. W., and McCarthy, G. (2014). *Functional Magnetic Resonance Imaging* (3rd ed.). Sunderland, MA: Oxford University Press/Sinauer.

Martino, D., and Leckman, J. F. (Eds.). (2013). *Tourette Syndrome.* Oxford, UK: Oxford University Press.

Meyer, J. S., and Quenzer, L. F. (2018). *Psychopharmacology: Drugs, the Brain, and Behavior* (3rd ed.). Sunderland, MA: Oxford University Press/Sinauer.

Solomon, A. (2001). *The Noonday Demon: An Atlas of Depression.* New York, NY: Scribner.

Steketee, G. (Ed.). (2011). *The Oxford Handbook of Obsessive Compulsive and Spectrum Disorders.* New York, NY: Oxford University Press.

12 • VISUAL SUMMARY

You should be able to relate each summary to the adjacent illustration, including structures and processes. The online version of this **Visual Summary** includes links to figures, animations, and activities that will help you consolidate the material.

1 Population studies find that psychiatric disorders are prevalent in modern society. Studies of families, twins, and adoptees demonstrate a strong role of genetic factors in **schizophrenia**. Rather than a single gene determining whether a person will develop schizophrenia, several genes contribute to the risk. Review **Figures 12.1** and **12.2**, **Table 12.1**, **Animation 12.2**

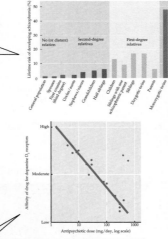

2 Structural changes in the brains of people with schizophrenia—including enlarged ventricles—may arise from early developmental problems. The emergence of schizophrenia depends on the interaction of genes that make a person vulnerable to environmental stressors. Review **Figures 12.3–12.9**

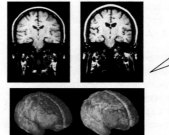

3 The frontal lobes are less active in people with schizophrenia than in people without it. Biochemical theories of schizophrenia emphasize the importance of the dopamine, glutamate, and serotonin receptors. **First-generation antipsychotics** block dopamine D_2 receptors, while **second-generation antipsychotics** block serotonin $5\text{-}HT_{2A}$ receptors in addition to acting on dopamine receptors. Review **Figures 12.11–12.13**, **Video 12.3**

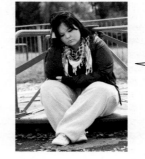

4 **Depression** also has a strong genetic factor. Serotonin has been implicated in this disorder. In general, females are more likely than males to experience depression. People with depression show increased activity in the frontal cortex and the amygdala, as well as disrupted sleep patterns. Review **Figures 12.14–12.16**

5 There is considerable evidence that suicide is often an impulsive act, so intervening in cases of people showing the warning signs of suicide can save lives. Review **Table 12.2**

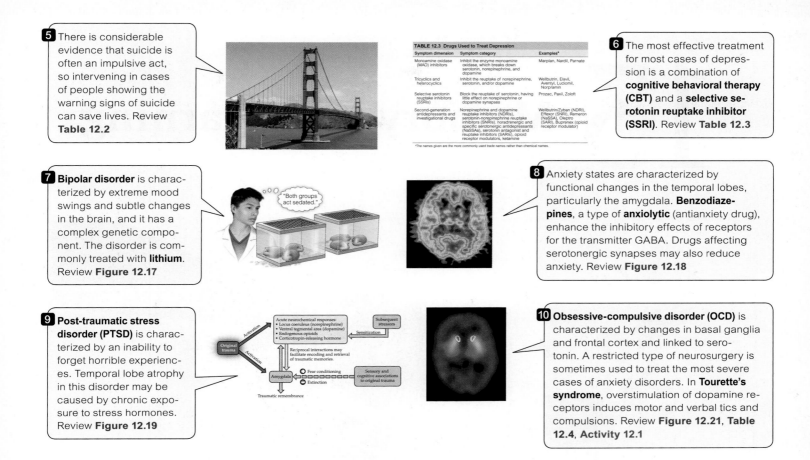

TABLE 12.3 Drugs Used to Treat Depression

Symptom dimension	Symptom category	Examples[a]
Monoamine oxidase (MAO) inhibitors	Inhibit the enzyme monoamine oxidase, which breaks down serotonin, norepinephrine, and dopamine	Marplan, Nardil, Parnate
Tricyclics and heterocyclics	Inhibit the reuptake of norepinephrine, serotonin, and/or dopamine	Wellbutrin, Elavil, Aventyl, Ludiomil, Norpramin
Selective serotonin reuptake inhibitors (SSRIs)	Block the reuptake of serotonin, having little effect on norepinephrine or dopamine synapses	Prozac, Paxil, Zoloft
Second-generation antidepressants and investigational drugs	Norepinephrine and dopamine reuptake inhibitors (NDRIs), serotonin-norepinephrine reuptake inhibitors (SNRIs), noradrenergic and specific serotonergic antidepressants (NaSSAs), serotonin antagonist and reuptake inhibitors (SARIs), opioid receptor modulators, ketamine	Wellbutrin/Zyban (NDRI), Effexor (SNRI), Remeron (NaSSA), Oleptro (SARI), Buprenex (opioid receptor modulator)

[a]The names given are the more commonly used trade names rather than chemical names.

6 The most effective treatment for most cases of depression is a combination of **cognitive behavioral therapy (CBT)** and a **selective serotonin reuptake inhibitor (SSRI)**. Review **Table 12.3**

7 **Bipolar disorder** is characterized by extreme mood swings and subtle changes in the brain, and it has a complex genetic component. The disorder is commonly treated with **lithium**. Review **Figure 12.17**

"Both groups act sedated."

8 Anxiety states are characterized by functional changes in the temporal lobes, particularly the amygdala. **Benzodiazepines**, a type of **anxiolytic** (antianxiety drug), enhance the inhibitory effects of receptors for the transmitter GABA. Drugs affecting serotonergic synapses may also reduce anxiety. Review **Figure 12.18**

9 **Post-traumatic stress disorder (PTSD)** is characterized by an inability to forget horrible experiences. Temporal lobe atrophy in this disorder may be caused by chronic exposure to stress hormones. Review **Figure 12.19**

10 **Obsessive-compulsive disorder (OCD)** is characterized by changes in basal ganglia and frontal cortex and linked to serotonin. A restricted type of neurosurgery is sometimes used to treat the most severe cases of anxiety disorders. In **Tourette's syndrome**, overstimulation of dopamine receptors induces motor and verbal tics and compulsions. Review **Figure 12.21**, **Table 12.4**, **Activity 12.1**

The Mind's Machine digital resources include additional videos, flashcards, and other study tools.

13 Memory and Learning

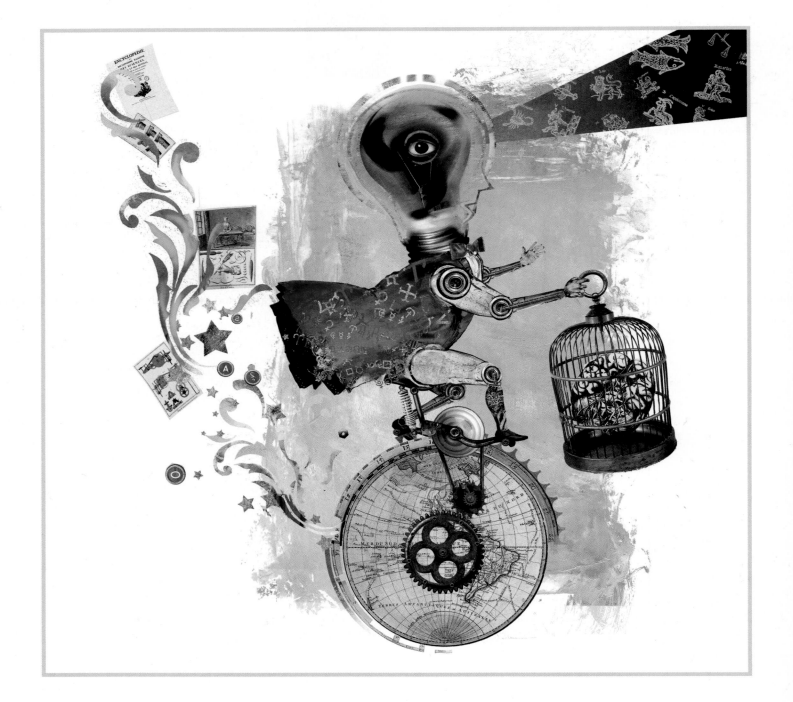

Trapped in the Eternal Now

Every day is alone in itself, whatever enjoyment I've had, and whatever sorrow I've had…. Right now, I'm wondering, have I done or said anything amiss? You see, at this moment everything looks clear to me, but what happened just before? That's what worries me. It's like waking from a dream. I just don't remember.

—Henry Molaison (B. Milner, 1970, p. 37)

Known as "Patient H.M." in a classic series of research articles, Henry Molaison was probably the most famous research participant in the history of neuroscience. Following a bicycle accident when Henry was an adolescent, he started to suffer seizures, and by his late twenties his epilepsy was out of control. Like the epilepsy patients we described at the end of Chapter 2, Henry decided to take the extreme measure of having a surgeon remove the brain sites where the seizures began. Because Henry's seizures began in both temporal lobes, a neurosurgeon removed most of his anterior temporal lobes in 1953.

Henry's surgery relieved his epilepsy, but at a terrible, unforeseen price: He couldn't seem to form new memories (Scoville and Milner, 1957). For more than 50 years after the surgery, until his death in 2008, Henry could retain any new fact only briefly; as soon as he was distracted, the newly acquired information vanished. He didn't know his age or the current date. For a while, he carried a note reminding himself that his father had died and his mother was in a retirement home. Henry knew that something was wrong with him, because he had no memories from the years since his surgery, or even memories from earlier the same day, as the quote above indicates.

Henry's inability to form new memories meant that he couldn't have a lasting relationship with anybody new. No matter what experiences he might share with someone he met, Henry would have to start the acquaintance anew the following day, because he would have no recollection of ever having met the person. In some ways, this dreadful loss of memory ended Henry's journey as a human being—he could no longer grow in his experience of historical events, his friendships, or even a sense of his own life story.

What happened to Henry, and what does his experience teach us about learning and memory?

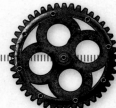

See Video 13.1: Memory

All the distinctively human aspects of our behavior are learned: the languages we speak, how we dress, the foods we eat and how we eat them, our skills, and the ways we reach our goals. So much of our own individuality depends on learning and memory. We begin this chapter with a discussion of memory because research in the twentieth century revealed that there are fundamentally different types of memory. Then we delve into what we know about how learning alters the structure of the brain, which differs for different types of memory.

View Animation 13.2:
Brain Explorer

learning   The process of acquiring new and relatively enduring information, behavior patterns, or abilities, characterized by modifications of behavior as a result of practice, study, or experience.

memory   1. The ability to learn and neurally encode information, consolidate the information for longer-term storage, and retrieve or reactivate the consolidated information at a later time. 2. The specific information that is stored in the brain.

amnesia   Severe impairment of memory.

retrograde amnesia   Difficulty in retrieving memories formed before the onset of amnesia.

Patient H.M.   The late Henry Molaison, a man who was unable to encode new declarative memories because of surgical removal of medial temporal lobe structures.

anterograde amnesia   Difficulty in forming new memories beginning with the onset of a disorder.

hippocampus   A medial temporal lobe structure that is important for learning and memory.

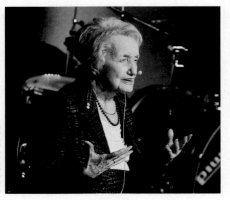

Eva Blue/CC BY 2.0

Brenda Milner   Earning her Ph.D. in 1952 a few years before working with Henry Molaison, Dr. Milner is still an active scholar, even after her 102nd birthday.

13.1 There Are Several Kinds of Learning and Memory

THE ROAD AHEAD

We begin our discussion about learning and memory by examining how they fail. Studying this material should allow you to:

13.1.1   Understand the two kinds of amnesia, one for memories before an event, and one for memories after an event.

13.1.2   Describe the two fundamentally different categories of memory.

13.1.3   Review the evidence that a particular circuit of three brain regions is crucial for forming certain types of memory.

13.1.4   Understand the two subtypes of declarative memories, the memories we can describe to other people.

The terms **learning**, the process of acquiring new information, and **memory**, the ability to store and retrieve that information, are so often paired that it sometimes seems as if one necessarily implies the other. We cannot be sure that learning has occurred unless a memory can be elicited later. Many kinds of brain damage, caused by disease or accident, impair both learning and memory. We'll start by looking at some brain damage cases that revealed different classes of learning and memory.

For Patient H.M., the present vanished into oblivion

Amnesia (Greek for "forgetfulness") is a severe impairment of memory, usually as a result of accident or disease. Loss of memories that formed prior to an event (such as surgery or trauma)—called **retrograde amnesia** (from the Latin *retro*, "backward," and *gradi*, "to go")—is not uncommon. After an accident that damages the brain, people often have retrograde amnesia regarding events that happened a few hours or days before the accident, or even a year before. Despite dramatic depictions you may see on TV, it is unlikely that longer-term (or "complete") retrograde memory loss has ever occurred.

   Patient H.M.—Henry Molaison, whom we met at the start of the chapter—suffered from a far more unusual symptom. In Henry's case, most old memories remained intact, but he had difficulty recollecting any events that took place *after* his surgery. What's more, he was unable to retain any new material for more than a brief period. The inability to form new memories after an event is called **anterograde amnesia** (the Latin *antero* means "forward").

   Over the very short term, Henry's memory was normal. If given a series of six or seven digits, he could immediately repeat the list without error. But when he was given a list of words to study and then tested on them after being distracted by another task, he could not repeat the list or even recall that there *was* a list. So Henry's case provided clear evidence that *short-term memory* differs from *long-term memory*—a distinction, long recognized by psychologists on behavioral grounds (W. James, 1890), that we will discuss in more depth later in this chapter.

   Henry's surgery removed the amygdala, most of the hippocampus, and surrounding cortex from both temporal lobes (**FIGURE 13.1**). The memory deficit seemed to be caused by loss of the *medial temporal lobe*, including the **hippocampus**, because people who had only the lateral temporal cortex removed had no memory impairment. Despite his obvious memory problems, Henry showed noticeable improvement over days of practice on a mirror-tracing task (**FIGURE 13.2A**) (B. Milner, 1965). Each day, when asked if he remembered the test, Henry said no, yet his performance was better than at the start of the first day (**FIGURE 13.2B**). So, was Henry's memory loss limited to tasks that relied on verbal processing? Not quite.

FIGURE 13.1 Brain Regions Crucial for Forming New Memories

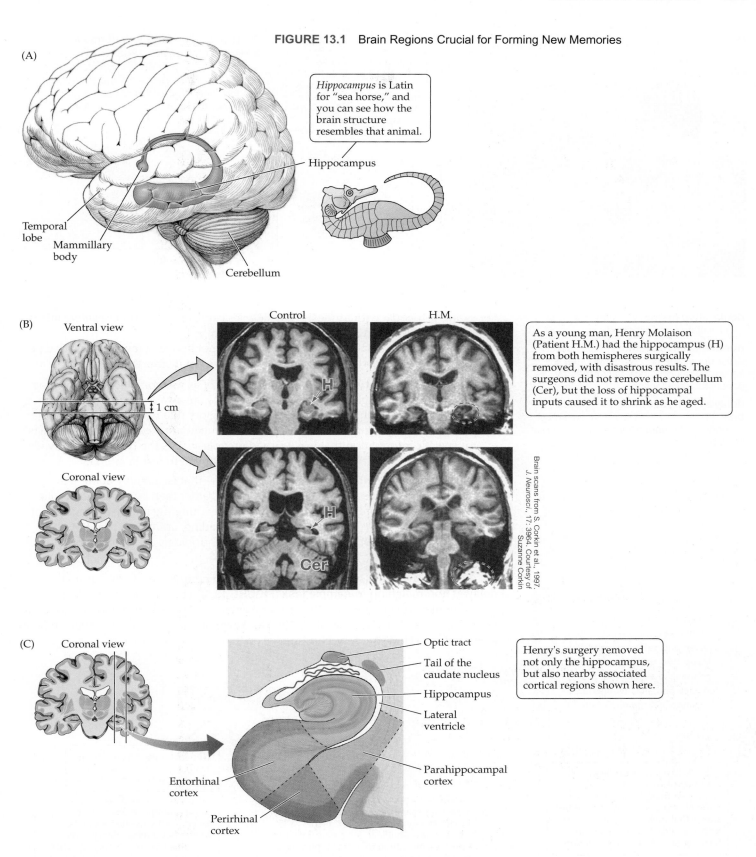

(A)

Hippocampus is Latin for "sea horse," and you can see how the brain structure resembles that animal.

Hippocampus

Temporal lobe

Mammillary body

Cerebellum

(B)

Ventral view

Coronal view

1 cm

Control   H.M.

H

H   Cer

As a young man, Henry Molaison (Patient H.M.) had the hippocampus (H) from both hemispheres surgically removed, with disastrous results. The surgeons did not remove the cerebellum (Cer), but the loss of hippocampal inputs caused it to shrink as he aged.

Brain scans from S. Corkin et al., 1997, *J. Neurosci.*, 17: 3964. Courtesy of Suzanne Corkin

(C)

Coronal view

Optic tract

Tail of the caudate nucleus

Hippocampus

Lateral ventricle

Parahippocampal cortex

Entorhinal cortex

Perirhinal cortex

Henry's surgery removed not only the hippocampus, but also nearby associated cortical regions shown here.

(A)

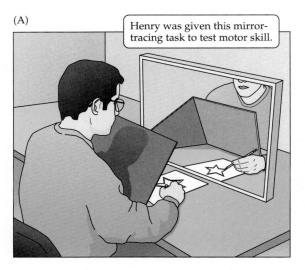

Henry was given this mirror-tracing task to test motor skill.

(B)

Although Henry never recognized the task, his performance progressively improved over successive days, demonstrating a type of long-term memory.

FIGURE 13.2 Henry's Performance on a Mirror-Tracing Task (After B. Milner, 1965 in P. M. Milner and S. E. Glickman [Eds.], *Cognitive processes and the brain; an enduring problem in psychology* [pp. 97–111]. Van Nostrand. USA.)

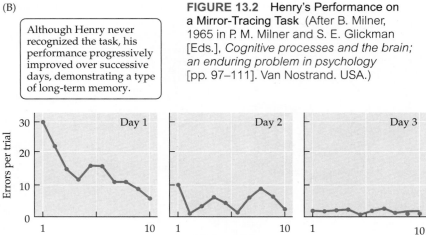

declarative memory A memory that can be stated or described.

nondeclarative memory Also called *procedural memory*. A memory that is shown by performance rather than by conscious recollection.

delayed non-matching-to-sample task A test in which the individual must respond to the unfamiliar stimulus in a pair of stimuli.

For example, people with amnesia like Henry's can learn the skill of *reading* mirror-reversed text (**FIGURE 13.3**), which is a verbal task.

The important distinction in Henry's deficit is not between motor and verbal performances, but rather between two general categories of memory:

1. **Declarative memory** is what we usually think of as memory: facts and information acquired through learning. It is memory we are aware of accessing, which we can *declare* to others. This is the type of memory that was so profoundly impaired by Henry's surgery. Tests of declarative memory take the form of requests for specific information that was learned previously. It is the type of memory we use to answer "what" questions—and thus is difficult to test in animals.

2. **Nondeclarative memory**, or *procedural memory*—that is, memory about perceptual or motor procedures—is shown by *performance* rather than by conscious recollection. Examples of procedural memory include learning the mirror-tracing task, at which Henry excelled, and the skill of mirror reading, or riding a bike (**FIGURE 13.4**). It is the type of memory we use for "how" problems and is often (but not always) nonverbal.

A clever way to measure declarative memory in monkeys and other animals is the **delayed non-matching-to-sample task** (**FIGURE 13.5**), a test of *object recognition* that requires monkeys to declare what they remember by identifying which of two objects was *not* seen previously (Winters et al., 2010). Monkeys with damage to the medial temporal lobe, similar to H.M., are severely impaired on this task, as we'll see next.

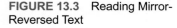

If you practice reading text that is mirror-reversed, you will become better and better at deciphering the text quickly. This is an example of learning a perceptual skill, and does not require an intact hippocampus.

Patients like Henry can learn to read mirror-reversed text quite well, even though they don't remember practicing it. This ability shows that their problem is not in learning verbal material, but in forming new declarative memories.

FIGURE 13.3 Reading Mirror-Reversed Text

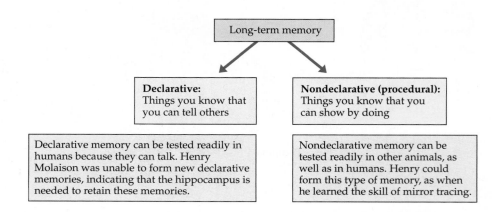

Long-term memory

Declarative: Things you know that you can tell others

Nondeclarative (procedural): Things you know that you can show by doing

Declarative memory can be tested readily in humans because they can talk. Henry Molaison was unable to form new declarative memories, indicating that the hippocampus is needed to retain these memories.

Nondeclarative memory can be tested readily in other animals, as well as in humans. Henry could form this type of memory, as when he learned the skill of mirror tracing.

FIGURE 13.4 Two Main Kinds of Memory: Declarative and Nondeclarative.

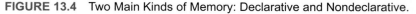

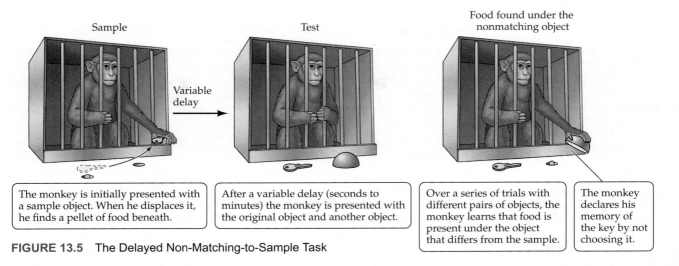

FIGURE 13.5 The Delayed Non-Matching-to-Sample Task

Sample

The monkey is initially presented with a sample object. When he displaces it, he finds a pellet of food beneath.

Test

After a variable delay (seconds to minutes) the monkey is presented with the original object and another object.

Food found under the nonmatching object

Over a series of trials with different pairs of objects, the monkey learns that food is present under the object that differs from the sample.

The monkey declares his memory of the key by not choosing it.

RESEARCHERS AT WORK

Which brain structures are important for declarative memory?

To determine which parts of the temporal lobe are crucial for declarative memory, researchers selectively removed specific parts of the medial temporal lobes of monkeys to confirm that the amygdala—one of the structures removed in Henry's surgery—is *not* crucial for performance on tests of declarative memory. However, removal of the adjacent hippocampus significantly impaired performance on these tests and, as shown in **FIGURE 13.6**, the deficit was even more pronounced when the hippocampal damage was paired with lesions of nearby cortical regions that communicate with the hippocampus: entorhinal, parahippocampal, and perirhinal cortices (Zola-Morgan et al., 1994). Humans similarly show larger impairments when both the hippocampus and medial temporal cortex are damaged (Squire and Wixted, 2011). So Henry's symptoms were probably caused by loss of the medial temporal lobe on both sides of the brain.

The experiments with monkeys, together with Henry's case, indicate that we need at least one intact medial temporal lobe (including the hippocampus) in order to make new declarative memories.

■ Hypothesis

Particular portions of the medial temporal lobe are required for the formation of new declarative memories.

■ Test

Selectively remove different portions of the temporal lobe from both sides of the brain, and test for declarative memories using the delayed non-matching-to-sample task (see Figure 13.5).

■ Result

(A) Ventral view of monkey brain showing areas of different medial temporal lesions

(B) Scores of groups with different lesions

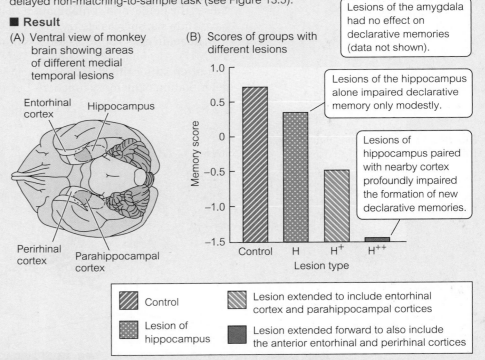

Lesions of the amygdala had no effect on declarative memories (data not shown).

Lesions of the hippocampus alone impaired declarative memory only modestly.

Lesions of hippocampus paired with nearby cortex profoundly impaired the formation of new declarative memories.

Control

Lesion of hippocampus

Lesion extended to include entorhinal cortex and parahippocampal cortices

Lesion extended forward to also include the anterior entorhinal and perirhinal cortices

■ Conclusion

The severe disruption of new declarative memories in Henry Molaison and patients like him is due to damage to both the hippocampus itself and to nearby cortex. But these regions aren't the only brain structures needed for new declarative memories, as we'll see next.

FIGURE 13.6 Memory Performance after Medial Temporal Lobe Lesions (Part A after L. R. Squire and S. Zola-Morgan, 1991. *Science* 253: 1380; B after S. Zola-Morgan et al., 1994. *Hippocampus* 4: 482.)

Damage to the medial diencephalon can also cause amnesia

Patient N.A.   A still-living man who is unable to encode new declarative memories, because of damage to the dorsomedial thalamus and the mammillary bodies.

dorsomedial thalamus   A limbic system structure that is connected to the hippocampus.

mammillary body   One of a pair of limbic system structures that are connected to the hippocampus.

Korsakoff's syndrome   A memory disorder, caused by thiamine deficiency, that is generally associated with chronic alcoholism.

confabulate   To fill in a gap in memory with a falsification. Confabulation is often seen in Korsakoff's syndrome.

In 1960, a young man known as **Patient N.A.** had a bizarre accident in which a miniature sword entered his nostril and injured his brain. Like Henry, N.A. has shown profound anterograde amnesia ever since his accident (Squire and Moore, 1979), and he can give little information about events since his accident, although his memory for earlier events is near normal (Kaushall et al., 1981). MRI study of N.A. (**FIGURE 13.7**) shows damage to several limbic system structures in the medial diencephalon that have connections to the hippocampus: the **dorsomedial thalamus** and the **mammillary bodies** (so called because they are shaped like a pair of breasts—see Figure 13.1A). Like Henry Molaison, N.A. shows normal short-term memory and can gain new nondeclarative/procedural memories, but he is impaired in forming declarative long-term memories. The similarity in symptoms suggests that the medial temporal lobe damaged in Henry's brain and these midline regions damaged in N.A. are parts of a larger memory system.

That idea is reinforced by studies of people with **Korsakoff's syndrome**, a degenerative disease in which damage is found in the mammillary bodies (**FIGURE 13.8**) and dorsomedial thalamus (Mair et al., 1979), but not in temporal lobe structures like the hippocampus. The mammillary bodies may serve as a processing system connecting the medial temporal lobes (which were removed from Henry Molaison) to the thalamus and, from there, to other cortical sites (Vann and Aggleton, 2004). People with Korsakoff's syndrome often fail to recognize or sense any familiarity with some items, even those presented repeatedly, yet frequently they deny that anything is wrong with them. They often **confabulate**—that is, fill a gap in memory with a falsification that they seem to accept as true. Damage to the frontal cortex, also found in people suffering from Korsakoff's syndrome, probably causes the denial and confabulation that differentiates them from other people who have amnesia, such as Henry.

The main cause of Korsakoff's syndrome is lack of the vitamin thiamine (Arts et al., 2017). Alcoholics who obtain most of their calories from alcohol and neglect their diet often suffer this deficiency. Treating them with thiamine can prevent further deterioration of memory functions but will not reverse the damage already done.

FIGURE 13.7   The Brain Damage in Patient N.A.

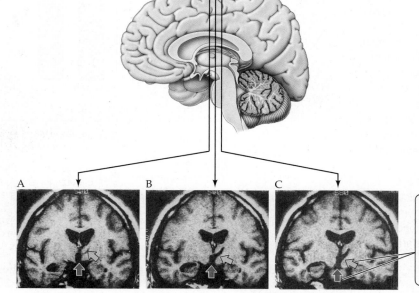

Anterior   Posterior

A   B   C

MRI scans show a prominent lesion of the dorsomedial thalamus on the left side of the brain (yellow arrows), as well as a lesion on the floor of the third ventricle where the mammillary bodies should be (red arrows).

Scans from L. R. Squire et al., 1989. *Exp. Neurol.* 105: 23

These studies make it clear that a brain circuit that includes the hippocampus, the mammillary bodies, and the dorsomedial thalamus is needed to *form* new declarative memories. But these case studies also clearly show that established declarative memories, formed before brain damage, are not *stored* in these structures for the long term. If they were, they would have been lost when the structures were damaged. So where are memories stored? We'll see next that a leading candidate is the cerebral cortex.

Brain damage can destroy autobiographical memories while sparing general memories

One striking case study suggests that at least some declarative memories are stored in the cortex, and it also illustrates an important distinction between two *subtypes* of declarative memory. Kent Cochrane, known to the world as **Patient K.C.**, suffered brain damage in a motorcycle accident at age 30. He could no longer retrieve any *personal memory* of his past, although his general knowledge remained good. He conversed easily and played a good game of chess but could not remember where he learned to play chess or who taught him the game. Detailed autobiographical declarative memory of this sort is known as **episodic memory**; you show episodic memory when you recall a specific *episode* in your life or relate an event to a particular time and place. In contrast, **semantic memory** is generalized declarative memory, such as knowing the meaning of a word without knowing where or when you learned that word (Tulving, 1972). If care was taken to space out the trials, Kent could acquire new semantic knowledge (Tulving et al., 1991). But even with this method, Kent could not acquire new *episodic* knowledge—he wouldn't remember where he had learned that new material.

Scans of Kent's brain revealed extensive damage to the left frontoparietal and the right parieto-occipital cerebral cortex, as well as severe shrinkage of both right and left hippocampus and nearby cortex (Rosenbaum et al., 2005). As with Henry, the bilateral hippocampal damage probably accounts for Kent's anterograde declarative amnesia. But that damage cannot account for Kent's selective loss of nearly all his autobiographical memory, because other people with damage restricted to the medial temporal lobe, like H.M., retain their autobiographical memories. Kent's inability to recall any autobiographical details of his life from many years before his accident may instead be a consequence of injuries to frontal and parietal cortex (Tulving, 1989). (Unlike dramatic portrayals of retrograde amnesia in fiction, Kent knew his name and recognized his family, although he couldn't remember any particular past events with those people.) **FIGURE 13.9** reviews our current view of the sequence of brain regions important for forming declarative memories.

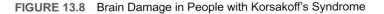

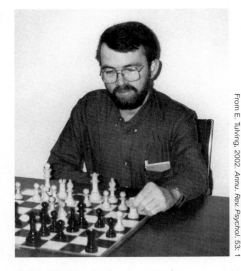

These oval-shaped mammillary bodies are darkened as a result of bleeding and cell death.

FIGURE 13.8 Brain Damage in People with Korsakoff's Syndrome

Patient K.C. The late Kent Cochrane, who sustained damage to the cortex that rendered him unable to form and retrieve episodic memories.

episodic memory Also called *autobiographical memory*. Memory of a particular incident or a particular time and place.

semantic memory Generalized declarative memory, such as knowing the meaning of a word.

Patient K.C. Brain damage from a severe motorcycle accident left Kent Cochrane (1951–2014) unable to retrieve episodic memories.

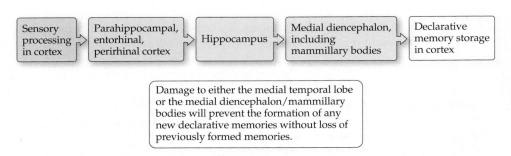

| Sensory processing in cortex | Parahippocampal, entorhinal, perirhinal cortex | Hippocampus | Medial diencephalon, including mammillary bodies | Declarative memory storage in cortex |

Damage to either the medial temporal lobe or the medial diencephalon/mammillary bodies will prevent the formation of any new declarative memories without loss of previously formed memories.

FIGURE 13.9 Current Model of Declarative Memory Formation

HOW'S IT GOING ?

1. What are the two main types of amnesia, and which deficit was more severe for Henry Molaison?
2. What are the two main types of memory, and which type was affected in Henry?
3. How did research with animals help pin down the brain regions required for forming new memories that we can declare to others?
4. Name the two brain regions, in addition to the medial temporal lobe, that are required to form new declarative memories.
5. What are the two main subtypes of declarative memory?

13.2 Different Forms of Nondeclarative Memory Involve Different Brain Regions

THE ROAD AHEAD

Now let's consider the different types of nondeclarative memory and the brain regions associated with each. Studying this material should allow you to:

13.2.1 List the different categories of nondeclarative memory.

13.2.2 Name the stages of memory formation and the vulnerability for losing information at each stage.

13.2.3 Describe a model of how we encode, consolidate, and retrieve memories.

13.2.4 Explain how retrieving a memory makes it vulnerable to distortion.

13.2.5 Describe the effects of emotional arousal for memory, and the prospects of a drug treatment to soften traumatic memories.

So far, we've seen that there are two different kinds of declarative memory: semantic and episodic. Likewise, there are several different types of nondeclarative memory, and we'll see that different brain regions are involved in these different forms.

Different types of nondeclarative memory serve varying functions

Skill learning is the process of learning how to perform a challenging task simply by doing it over and over. Improving at the mirror-tracing task performed by Henry Molaison (see Figure 13.2) or learning to read mirror-reversed text (see Figure 13.3) are examples of skill learning. So too is the acquisition of everyday skills like learning to ride a bike or to juggle (well, okay, maybe juggling isn't an "everyday" skill, but you get the idea). Henry demonstrated that the medial temporal lobe is not required to gain skills and retain them.

Imaging studies have investigated learning and memory for different kinds of skills, including *sensorimotor skills* (e.g., mirror tracing), *perceptual skills* (e.g., reading mirror-reversed text), and *cognitive skills* (tasks involving planning and problem solving, common in puzzles like the Tower of Hanoi problem. All three kinds of skill learning are impaired in people with damage to the **basal ganglia** (see Figure 1.14A). Damage to other brain regions, especially the motor cortex and cerebellum, also affects aspects of some skills. Neuroimaging studies confirm that the basal ganglia, cerebellum, and motor cortex are important for sensorimotor skill learning (Makino et al., 2016; Spampinato and Celnik, 2018).

Priming (or *repetition priming*) is a change in the way you process a stimulus, usually a word or a picture, because you've seen it, or something similar, previously. For example, if a person is shown the word *stamp* in a list and later is asked to complete the word stem *STA-*, then she is more likely to reply "stamp" than, say, "start." Priming does not require declarative memory of the stimulus—Henry Molaison and other

skill learning The process of learning to perform a challenging task simply by repeating it over and over.

basal ganglia A group of forebrain nuclei, including the caudate nucleus, globus pallidus, and putamen, found deep within the cerebral hemispheres. They are crucial for skill learning.

priming Also called *repetition priming*. The phenomenon by which exposure to a stimulus facilitates subsequent responses to the same or a similar stimulus.

FIGURE 13.10   Pavlovian (Classical) Conditioning

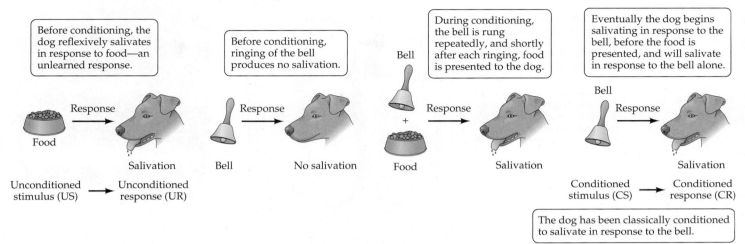

Before conditioning, the dog reflexively salivates in response to food—an unlearned response.

Before conditioning, ringing of the bell produces no salivation.

During conditioning, the bell is rung repeatedly, and shortly after each ringing, food is presented to the dog.

Eventually the dog begins salivating in response to the bell, before the food is presented, and will salivate in response to the bell alone.

Food   Response   Salivation

Unconditioned stimulus (US) → Unconditioned response (UR)

Bell   Response   No salivation

Bell + Food   Response   Salivation

Bell   Response   Salivation

Conditioned stimulus (CS) → Conditioned response (CR)

The dog has been classically conditioned to salivate in response to the bell.

people with amnesia have shown priming for words they don't remember having seen. In contrast with skill learning, priming is not impaired by damage to the basal ganglia. In functional-imaging studies, perceptual priming (priming based on the visual *form* of words) is related to reduced activity in bilateral occipitotemporal cortex (Schacter et al., 2007), while conceptual priming (priming based on word *meaning*) is associated with reduced activation of the left frontal cortex (Buckner and Koutstaal, 1998). So priming appears to be at least partly a function of the cortex.

Other types of nondeclarative memories include learning that involves relations between events—for example, between two or more stimuli, between a stimulus and a response, or between a response and its consequence—and is called **associative learning**. In the best-studied form, **classical conditioning**, an initially neutral stimulus comes to predict an event. In famous experiments, Ivan Pavlov (1849–1936) found that a dog would learn to salivate when presented with an auditory or visual stimulus if the stimulus came to predict the presentation of food. So, repeatedly ringing a bell before putting meat powder in a dog's mouth will eventually cause the dog to start salivating when it hears the bell alone. In this case the meat powder in the mouth is called the *unconditioned stimulus* (US), which already evokes an *unconditioned response* (UR; salivation in this example). The sound of the bell is called the *conditioned stimulus* (CS), and the learned response to the CS alone (salivation in response to the bell) is called the *conditioned response* (CR) (**FIGURE 13.10**). By the way, several sources on the web smugly declare that Pavlov never actually used a bell for a CS, but there's plenty of evidence that he did (R. K. Thomas, 1994; Tully, 2003). Some web "myths" are themselves myths!

Experimental evidence in lab animals shows that circuits in the **cerebellum** are crucial for simple eye-blink conditioning, in which a tone or other stimulus is associated with eye blinking in response to a puff of air. A PET study in humans confirmed this idea by showing a progressive increase in activity in the cerebellum during eye-blink conditioning (Logan and Grafton, 1995). People with hippocampal lesions can acquire the conditioned eye-blink response, but people with damage to the cerebellum on one side can acquire a conditioned eye-blink response *only on the side where the cerebellum is intact* (Papka et al., 1994).

In **instrumental conditioning** (also called *operant conditioning*), an association is formed between the animal's behavior and the consequence(s) of that behavior. An example of an apparatus designed to study instrumental conditioning is called the *Skinner box*, named for its originator, B. F. Skinner (**FIGURE 13.11**). In a common setup, the animal

associative learning   A type of learning in which an association is formed between two stimuli or between a stimulus and a response. It includes both classical and instrumental conditioning.

classical conditioning   Also called *Pavlovian conditioning*. A type of associative learning in which an originally neutral stimulus acquires the power to elicit a conditioned response when presented alone.

cerebellum   A structure located at the back of the brain, dorsal to the pons, that is involved in the central regulation of movement and in some forms of learning.

instrumental conditioning   Also called *operant conditioning*. A form of associative learning in which the likelihood that an act (instrumental response) will be performed depends on the consequences (reinforcing stimuli) that follow it.

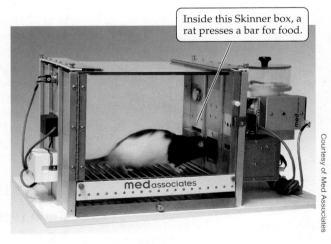

Inside this Skinner box, a rat presses a bar for food.

FIGURE 13.11   A Skinner Box

Courtesy of Med Associates

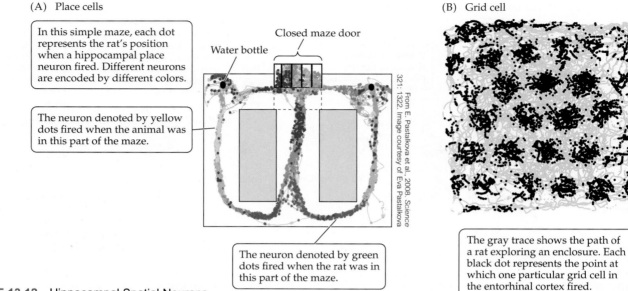

(A) Place cells

In this simple maze, each dot represents the rat's position when a hippocampal place neuron fired. Different neurons are encoded by different colors.

The neuron denoted by yellow dots fired when the animal was in this part of the maze.

Water bottle

Closed maze door

From E. Pastalkova et al., 2008. *Science* 321: 1322. Image courtesy of Eva Pastalkova

The neuron denoted by green dots fired when the rat was in this part of the maze.

(B) Grid cell

From E. I. Moser & M-B. Moser. 2013. *Neuron* 80: 765

The gray trace shows the path of a rat exploring an enclosure. Each black dot represents the point at which one particular grid cell in the entorhinal cortex fired.

FIGURE 13.12 Hippocampal Spatial Neurons

**View Activity 13.1:
Learning and Memory**

cognitive map A mental representation of the relative spatial organization of objects and information.

place cell A neuron in the hippocampus that selectively fires when the animal is in a particular location.

learns that performing a certain action (e.g., pressing a bar) is followed by a reward (such as a food pellet). Research in animals has not pinpointed the brain regions that are crucial for instrumental conditioning, perhaps because this type of learning taps so many different aspects of behavior.

Animal research confirms the various brain regions involved in different attributes of memory

The caricature of the white-coated scientist watching rats run in mazes, a staple of cartoonists to this day, has its origins in the intensive memory research of the early twentieth century. The early work indicated that rats and other animals don't just learn a series of turns but instead form a **cognitive map** (an understanding of the relative spatial organization of objects and information) in order to solve a maze (Tolman, 1949). Animals apparently learn at least some of these details of their spatial environment simply by moving through it (Tolman and Honzik, 1930).

We now know that, in parallel with its role in other types of declarative memory, the hippocampus is crucial for spatial learning. The rat hippocampus contains many neurons that selectively encode spatial location (O'Keefe and Burgess, 2005; Moser et al., 2017). These **place cells** become active when the animal is in—or moving toward—a particular location (**FIGURE 13.12A**). If the animal is moved to a new environment, place cell activity indicates that the hippocampus remaps to the new locations (Moita et al., 2004). Some rat hippocampal neurons act like "grid cells," likened to a latitude and longitude in a maze (**FIGURE 13.12B**), which have been recorded in people too (J. Jacobs et al., 2013). The Nobel Prize in Physiology or Medicine for 2014 was awarded to John O'Keefe, May-Britt Moser, and Edvard Moser for their work on understanding hippocampal cells.

Bird species that hide food in many locations have a larger hippocampus than other birds have (Croston et al., 2015), indicating that natural selection favors enlargement of the hippocampus to enhance spatial learning, as we discuss in **A STEP FURTHER 13.1**, on the website.

Brain regions involved in learning and memory: A summary

FIGURE 13.13 updates and summarizes the classification of long-term memory that we've been discussing. Several major conclusions should be apparent by now,

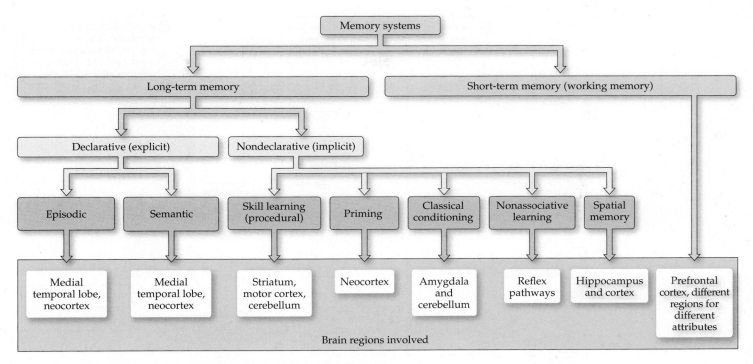

FIGURE 13.13   Subtypes of Declarative and Nondeclarative Memory
(After T. Bartsch and C. Butler. 2013. *Nat. Rev. Neurol.* 9: 86.)

especially (1) that many regions of the brain are involved in learning and memory; (2) that different forms of memory rely on at least partly different brain mechanisms, which may include several different regions of the brain; and (3) that the same brain structure can be a part of the circuitry for several different forms of learning. Next we'll discuss the stages by which memories, of any sort, can be preserved for a lifetime.

HOW'S IT GOING ?

1. Name three different types of nondeclarative memory, giving an example of each. What different parts of the brain have been implicated in each type?
2. What is a cognitive map?
3. What are hippocampal place cells, and why do they suggest a role for the hippocampus in spatial learning?

Successive processes capture, store, and retrieve information in the brain

The span of time over which a piece of information is retained in the brain varies. There are at least three different stages of memory. The briefest memories are called **sensory buffers** (for visual stimuli, they are sometimes called *iconic memories*); an example is the fleeting impression of a glimpsed scene that vanishes from memory seconds later. These brief memories are thought to be residual activity in sensory neurons.

Somewhat longer than sensory buffers are **short-term memories (STMs)**. If someone tells you a website name and you keep it in mind (perhaps through rehearsal) just until you type it into your browser, you are using STM. In the absence of rehearsal, STMs last only about 30 seconds (J. Brown, 1958; L. R. Peterson and Peterson, 1959). With rehearsal, you may be able to retain an STM until you turn to a new task a few minutes later, but when the STM is gone, it's gone for good. Eventually, some memories become really long-lasting—the address of your childhood

sensory buffer   A very brief type of memory that stores the sensory impression of a scene. In vision, it is sometimes called *iconic memory.*

short-term memory (STM)   A form of memory that usually lasts only seconds, or as long as rehearsal continues. Working memory can be considered a portion of STM where information can be manipulated.

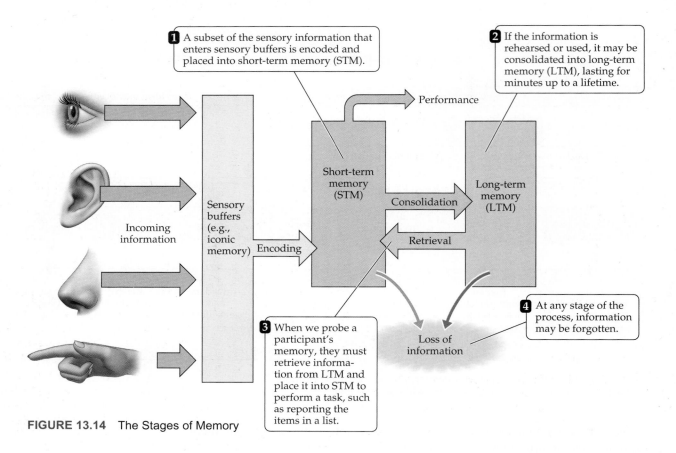

1 A subset of the sensory information that enters sensory buffers is encoded and placed into short-term memory (STM).

2 If the information is rehearsed or used, it may be consolidated into long-term memory (LTM), lasting for minutes up to a lifetime.

3 When we probe a participant's memory, they must retrieve information from LTM and place it into STM to perform a task, such as reporting the items in a list.

4 At any stage of the process, information may be forgotten.

FIGURE 13.14   The Stages of Memory

home, how to ride a bike, your first crush—and are called **long-term memories (LTMs)**. A related concept is *working memory*, which refers to the ability to actively manipulate information in your STM, perhaps retrieving information from LTM, to solve a problem or otherwise make use of the information (Aben et al., 2012). We will consider working memory to be a subset of STM where information can be analyzed and manipulated by some "executive" part of our mind.

As shown in **FIGURE 13.14**, the memory system consists of at least three processes: (1) **encoding** of raw information from sensory channels into STM, (2) **consolidation** of the volatile STM into more-durable LTM, and (3) eventual **retrieval** of the stored information from LTM for use in working memory. A problem at any stage can cause us to lose information. Although not depicted in the figure, this model suggests that the flow of information into and out of working memory is supervised by another part of the mind, an *executive function*, which we will discuss in more detail in Chapter 14.

Not all memories are created equal. We all know from firsthand experience that emotion can powerfully affect our memory for past events. For example, an emotionally arousing story is remembered significantly better than a closely matched but emotionally neutral story (Reisberg and Heuer, 1995). But if people are treated with propranolol (a beta-adrenergic antagonist, or beta-blocker, that blocks the effects of epinephrine), this emotional enhancement of memory vanishes. It's not that treated volunteers perceive the story as being any less emotional; in fact, they rate the emotional content of the stories just the same as untreated people do. Instead, the drug seems to directly interfere with the ability of adrenal stress hormones to act on the brain to enhance memory (Bolsoni and Zuardi, 2019), a topic we take up in Signs & Symptoms next.

long-term memory (LTM)   An enduring form of memory that lasts days, weeks, months, or years. LTM has a very large capacity.

encoding   The first process in the memory system, in which the information entering sensory channels is passed into short-term memory.

consolidation   The second process in the memory system, in which information in short-term memory is transferred to long-term memory.

retrieval   The third process of the memory system, in which a stored memory is used by an organism.

post-traumatic stress disorder (PTSD)   A disorder in which memories of an unpleasant episode repeatedly plague the victim.

Emotions and Memory

Almost everyone knows from personal experience that strong emotions can affect memory formation and retrieval. Examples of memories enhanced in this way might include a strong association between special music and a first kiss, or uncomfortably vivid recollection of the morning of September 11, 2001. A large-scale research effort in many labs has identified a suite of biochemical agents that participate in the emotional enhancement of memory.

Epinephrine (adrenaline), released from the adrenal glands during times of stress and strong emotion, appears to affect memory formation by influencing the amygdala, a brain region that is critical for fear conditioning (see Chapter 11). Electrical stimulation or lesions of the amygdala potently alter the memory-enhancing effects of epinephrine injections (Cahill and McGaugh, 1991), and tiny doses of epinephrine injected directly into the amygdala enhance memory formation in the same way that systemic injections do. This treatment appears to cause the release of norepinephrine within the amygdala, as do emotional experiences. Injecting propranolol, a blocker of beta-adrenergic receptors, into the amygdala blocks the memory-enhancing effects. In humans, the same drug can ease fears that have been conditioned in the lab (Kindt et al., 2009).

Can we develop pharmacological treatments to weaken or erase unwanted memories outside the lab? Some disorders would benefit greatly from such treatments. For example, people who have had life-threatening or other catastrophic experiences often develop **post-traumatic stress disorder** (**PTSD**) (see Chapter 12), characterized as "reliving experiences such as intrusive thoughts, nightmares, dissociative flashbacks to elements of the original traumatic event, and … preoccupation with that event" (Keane, 1998, p. 398). In PTSD, each recurrence of the strong emotions and memories of the traumatic event may reactivate memories that, when reconsolidated in the presence of stress signals like epinephrine, become even stronger. Therefore, one strategy to prevent PTSD formation could be to block the effects of epinephrine in the amygdala by treating victims with antiadrenergic drugs either shortly before a traumatic experience (e.g., in rescue workers) or as quickly as possible after it (in the case of victims of violence, for example) (Giustino et al., 2016). This treatment would not delete memories of the event but might diminish the traumatic aspects, and it might also be useful for weakening existing traumatic memories.

Perhaps one day it will be possible to selectively interfere with other neurotransmitters at work in the amygdala to provide more-specific and more-complete relief from traumatic memories. Whatever that treatment might be, it will probably have to be administered soon after the accident to effectively dull the painful memories.

Long-term memory has vast capacity but is subject to distortion

Henry Molaison's case and the research it inspired have already told us several ways in which STM and LTM differ from one another. While the medial temporal lobe is not needed to encode sensory information into STM, or to retrieve that information from STM (Henry could repeat back to you a list of words or numbers), it is crucial for moving information from STM into LTM. In terms of the model (see Figure 13.14), an intact hippocampus is required to *consolidate* declarative STMs into LTMs, indicating that the information is somehow transformed into a different format, one that may make it available for a lifetime.

How much information can be stored in LTM? There must be a limit, but no one has been able to come up with a way to measure it. In one classic experiment, people viewed long sequences of color photos of various scenes; several days later, they were shown pairs of images—in each case a new image plus one from the previous session—and asked to identify the images seen previously. Astonishingly, participants performed with a high degree of accuracy for series of up to 10,000 different stimuli (Standing, 1973)! For all practical purposes, there seems to be no upper bound to LTM capacity (Brady et al., 2014). Pigeons have a similarly impressive visual memory (Vaughan and Greene, 1984).

We take this capacity for granted and barely notice, for example, that knowledge of a language involves remembering at least 100,000 pieces of information. Most of us also store a huge assortment of information about faces, tunes, odors, skills, stories, and so on. The late Kim Peek (1951–2009) was a *savant* (from the French for "knowing"), a person with an unusually well-developed ability or skill. Born with several brain structural abnormalities, including an absence of the corpus callosum (Treffert and Christensen, 2005), Kim eventually memorized about 9,000 books, each taking

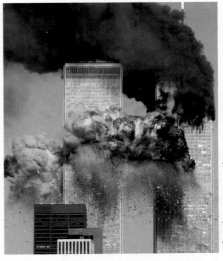

© Spencer Platt/Getty Images

Flashbulb Memories Many people have vivid, detailed memories of where they were when they learned of the September 11, 2001, terrorist attack on the World Trade Center towers in New York City.

memory trace Also called an *engram*. A persistent change in the brain that reflects the storage of memory.

reconsolidation The return of a memory trace to stable long-term storage after it has been temporarily made changeable during the process of recall.

about an hour. For example, he read the 656-page novel *The Hunt for Red October* in 75 minutes, and when asked, 4 months later, to name a minor character, not only did Kim know the name, but he cited the page number where the character appeared and quoted several passages on the page verbatim! Case studies of such individuals with exceptional memory indicate that without the usual process of pruning out unimportant memories, continual perfect recall can become uncontrollable, distracting, and exhausting (Luria, 1987; Parker et al., 2006).

Despite the vast capacity of LTM, forgetting is a normal aspect of memory, helping to filter out unimportant information and freeing up needed cognitive resources (Kuhl et al., 2007). Interestingly, research indicates that the **memory trace** (the record laid down in memory by a learning experience, also known as an *engram*) doesn't simply deteriorate from disuse and the passage of time; instead, memories tend to suffer interference from events before or after their formation.

For example, the process of retrieving information from LTM causes the memories to become temporarily unstable and susceptible to disruption or alteration before undergoing **reconsolidation** and returning to stable status (Nader and Hardt, 2009). Thus we can create false memories when we use leading questions to have people retrieve memories. Asking "Did you see the broken headlight?" rather than "Was the headlight broken?" can incorporate the false detail as the memory is reconsolidated (Loftus, 2003). This possibility of planting false memories clouds the issue of "recovered memories" of childhood sexual or physical abuse, because controversial therapeutic methods such as hypnosis or guided imagery (in which the person is encouraged to imagine hypothetical abuse scenarios) can inadvertently plant false memories.

On the other hand, you can use the power of reconsolidation when studying—as long as you're careful to check your facts. One of the best ways to improve learning is simply repeated retrieval (and thus, repeated reconsolidation) of the stored information with feedback to let you know what you got right or wrong (Karpicke and Roediger, 2008). In other words, test yourself repeatedly, as with the How's It Going? questions in this book. For your next exam, try making up some additional practice tests for yourself, or have a friend quiz you, instead of simply "cramming."

We still haven't talked about the nitty-gritty of memory in the brain—what exactly changes in the brain when we learn? That's our next topic.

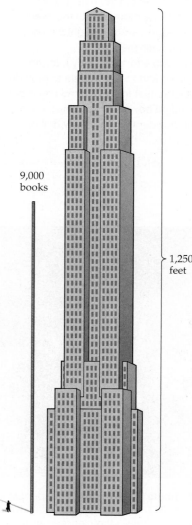

9,000 books

1,250 feet

Empire State Building

A Prodigious Memory Kim Peek (1951–2009) was a savant who memorized about 9,000 books.

HOW'S IT GOING ?

1. What are the stages of memory, and what do we call the processes by which information moves from one stage to the next?

2. What is the memory trace, and what are two explanations of why we sometimes cannot retrieve it?

3. Explain how reconsolidation makes us vulnerable to distorted memories.

13.3 Memory Storage Requires Physical Changes in the Brain

THE ROAD AHEAD

In this part of the chapter, we will look at some of the ways in which new learning involves changes in synapses. Reading this material should enable you to:

13.3.1 List the possible ways in which changes in neural function and structure could encode memories.

13.3.2 Review evidence that exposure to an enriched environment can affect brain structure and affect future behavior.

13.3.3 Describe how a circuit involving the cerebellum mediates certain types of conditioning.

In introducing the term *synapse*, Charles Sherrington (1897) speculated that synaptic alterations might be the basis of learning. Sherrington's notion anticipated what remains one of the most intensive efforts in all of neuroscience, since most theories of learning focus on **neuroplasticity** (or *neural plasticity*), changes in the structure and function of synapses.

Plastic changes at synapses can be physiological or structural

Synaptic changes that may store information can be measured physiologically. The changes can be presynaptic, postsynaptic, or both. They can include changes in the amount of neurotransmitter released and/or changes in the number or sensitivity of the postsynaptic receptors, resulting in larger (or smaller) postsynaptic potentials. Inhibiting inactivation of the transmitter (by altering reuptake or enzymatic degradation) can produce a similar effect (**FIGURE 13.15A**). Synaptic activity can also be influenced by inputs from other neurons, causing extra depolarization or hyperpolarization of the axon terminals and therefore changes in the amount of neurotransmitter released (**FIGURE 13.15B**).

neuroplasticity   Also called *neural plasticity*. The ability of the nervous system to change in response to experience or the environment.

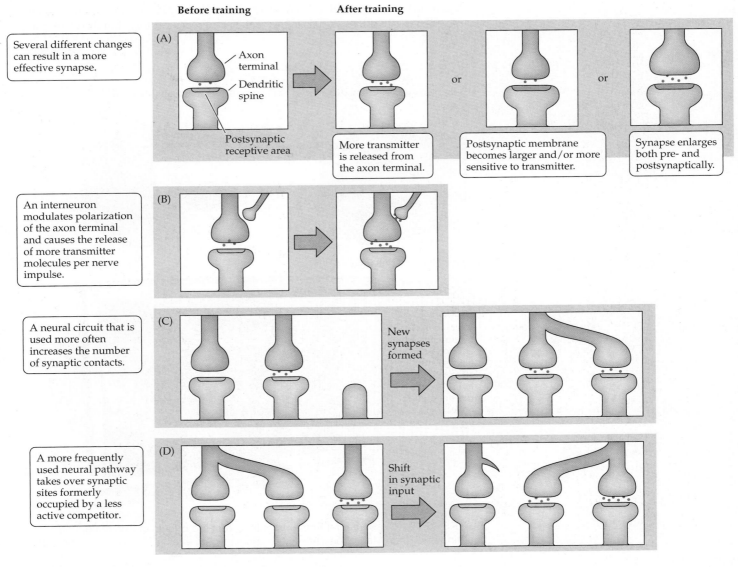

FIGURE 13.15   Synaptic Changes That May Store Memories

impoverished condition (IC)   Also called *isolated condition*. An environment for laboratory rodents in which each animal is housed singly in a small cage without complex stimuli.

standard condition (SC)   The usual environment for laboratory rodents, with a few animals in a cage and adequate food and water, but no complex stimulation.

Long-term memories may require changes in the nervous system so substantial that they can be directly observed (with the aid of a microscope, of course). After all, structural changes resulting from use are apparent in other parts of the body, as when exercise tones and shapes muscle. In a similar way, new synapses can form (or old synapses may die back) as a result of use (**FIGURE 13.15C**).

Training can also lead to the reorganization of synaptic connections. For example, it can cause a more active pathway to take over sites formerly occupied by a less active competitor (**FIGURE 13.15D**).

Varied experiences and learning cause the brain to change and grow

The remarkable plasticity of the brain is not all that difficult to demonstrate. Simply living in a complex environment, with its many opportunities for new learning, produces pronounced biochemical and anatomical changes in the brains of rats (Renner and Rosenzweig, 1987).

In standard studies of environmental enrichment, rats are randomly assigned to one of three housing conditions:

1. **Impoverished condition** (**IC**) Animals are housed individually in standard lab cages (**FIGURE 13.16A**).

2. **Standard condition** (**SC**) Animals are housed in small groups in standard lab cages (**FIGURE 13.16B**). This is the typical environment for laboratory animals.

(A) Impoverished condition (IC)   (B) Standard condition (SC)

(C) Enriched condition (EC)

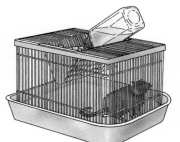

Interaction with an enriched environment has measurable effects on the brain, on stress reactions, and on learning.

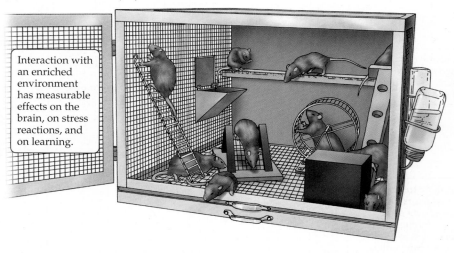

FIGURE 13.16 Experimental Environments to Test the Effects of Enrichment on Learning and Brain Measures (After M. R. Rosenzweig et al., 1972. *Sci. Am.* 226: 22.)

3. **Enriched condition (EC)** Animals are housed in large social groups in special cages containing various toys and other interesting features (**FIGURE 13.16C**). This condition provides enhanced opportunities for learning perceptual and motor skills, social learning, and so on.

In dozens of studies over several decades, a variety of changes in the brain were linked to environmental enrichment. For example, compared with IC animals:

- EC animals have a heavier, thicker cortex, especially in somatosensory and visual cortical areas (M. C. Diamond, 1967).

- EC animals show enhanced cholinergic activity throughout the cortex (Rosenzweig et al., 1961).

- EC animals have more dendritic branches on cortical neurons, and many more dendritic spines on those branches (**FIGURE 13.17**) (Greenough, 1976).

- EC animals have *larger* cortical synapses (M. C. Diamond et al., 1975), consistent with the storage of long-term memory in cortical areas through changes in synapses and circuits.

- EC animals have more neurons in the hippocampus because newly generated neurons (see Chapter 4) live longer (Kempermann et al., 1997).

- EC animals show enhanced recovery from brain damage (Will et al., 2004).

These cerebral effects of experience, which were surprising when first reported for rats in the early 1960s, are now seen to occur widely in the animal kingdom—from flies to philosophers (Mohammed, 2001; Chan et al., 2018). But how can we study the physiology of learning when the mammalian cortex has many billions of neurons, organized in vast networks, and upwards of a billion synapses per cubic centimeter (Merchán-Pérez et al., 2009)? Researchers made progress by studying simple learning circuits, in various species, uncovering basic cellular principles of memory formation that may generalize to neurons throughout the brain.

enriched condition (EC) Also called *complex environment*. An environment for laboratory rodents in which animals are group-housed with a wide variety of stimulus objects.

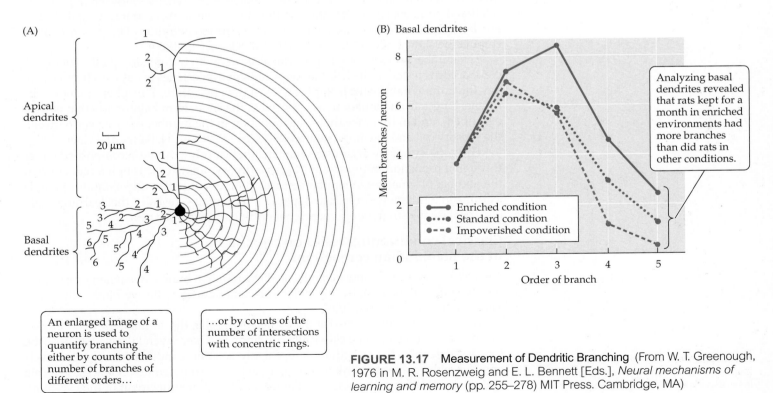

An enlarged image of a neuron is used to quantify branching either by counts of the number of branches of different orders…

…or by counts of the number of intersections with concentric rings.

FIGURE 13.17 Measurement of Dendritic Branching (From W. T. Greenough, 1976 in M. R. Rosenzweig and E. L. Bennett [Eds.], *Neural mechanisms of learning and memory* (pp. 255–278) MIT Press. Cambridge, MA)

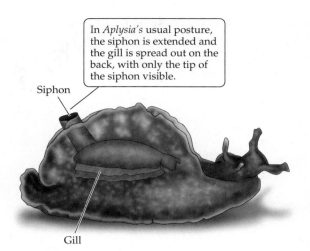

In *Aplysia*'s usual posture, the siphon is extended and the gill is spread out on the back, with only the tip of the siphon visible.

Siphon

Gill

FIGURE 13.18   The Sea Slug *Aplysia* (After E. R. Kandel, 1976. *Cellular basis of behavior.* Freeman. San Francisco.)

Invertebrate nervous systems show synaptic plasticity

As we've discussed, neuroplasticity and the ability to learn are ancient adaptations found throughout the animal kingdom. At the neuronal level, even species that are only remotely related likely share the same basic cellular processes for information storage. Indeed, one fruitful research strategy has been to focus on memory mechanisms in the very simple nervous systems of certain invertebrates. Invertebrate nervous systems have relatively few neurons (on the order of hundreds to tens of thousands). Because these neurons are arranged identically in different individuals, it is possible to construct detailed neural circuit diagrams for particular behaviors and study the same few identified neurons in multiple individuals.

Even in these "simple" organisms, the search for memory mechanisms began with the simplest types of learning. Earlier we discussed one of the most basic forms of learning—associative learning about two stimuli, such as the case of a dog learning to associate the sound of a bell with food. Even simpler than associative learning are the types of learning that involve only one stimulus, called *nonassociative learning*. Perhaps the simplest form of nonassociative learning is **habituation**—a decrease in response to a stimulus as it is repeated. To be true habituation, the decreased response cannot be due to failure of the sensory system to detect the stimulus or due to an inability of the motor system to respond. Sitting in a café, you may stop noticing the door chime when someone enters. Your ears still detect the chime, and your body is perfectly capable of looking up to see what happened, but you've habituated to the sound.

Scientists uncovered how the sea slug *Aplysia* learns to habituate to a stimulus (Kandel, 2009). If you squirt water at the slug's siphon—a tube through which it draws water—the animal protectively retracts its delicate gill (**FIGURE 13.18**). But with repeated stimulation the animal retracts the gill less and less, as it learns that the stimulation represents no danger to the gill. Eric Kandel and associates demonstrated that this short-term habituation is caused by changes in the synapse between the sensory cell that detects the squirt of water and the motor neuron that retracts the gill. As less and less transmitter is released at this synapse, the gill withdrawal in response to the stimulation slowly fades (**FIGURE 13.19A**) (M. Klein et al., 1980).

The number and size of synapses can also vary with training in *Aplysia*. For example, if a slug is tested in the habituation paradigm over a series of days, each successive day the animal habituates faster than it did the day before. This phenomenon represents long-term habituation (as opposed to the short-term habituation that we just described), and in this case there is a reduction in the number of synapses between the sensory cell and the motor neuron (**FIGURE 13.19B**) (C. H. Bailey and Chen, 1983).

Thus, a very simple organism taught us that learning can be accomplished either through a reduction in the strength of existing synapses or through a reduction in the number of synapses. A similar research program aimed at understanding simple learning in much more complicated species—mammals—revealed that learning could also increase the strength of synaptic connections, as we'll see next.

Classical conditioning relies on circuits in the mammalian cerebellum

Success at studying the more complicated mammalian brain came when researchers probed simple associative learning: classical conditioning of the eye-blink reflex (R. F. Thompson and Steinmetz, 2009).

When a puff of air is aimed at the cornea of a rabbit, the animal reflexively blinks. The eye-blink reflex can be classically conditioned. Over several trials, if an acoustic tone (CS) precedes the air puff (US) repeatedly, a simple conditioned response develops: the rabbit comes to blink (CR) when the tone is sounded (to review these terms and the basics of conditioning, see Figure 13.10). The neural circuit of the eye-blink reflex is also simple, involving cranial nerves and some interneurons that connect their

habituation   A form of nonassociative learning in which an organism becomes less responsive following repeated presentations of a stimulus.

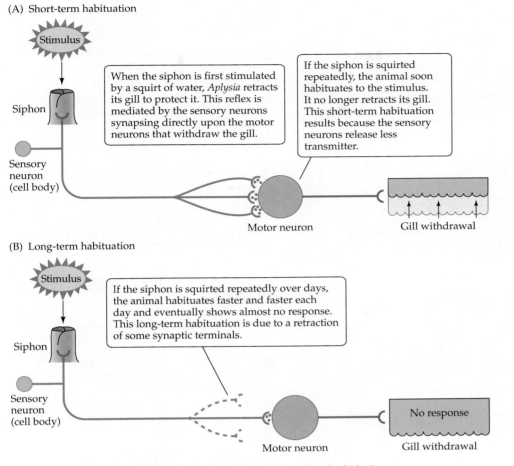

(A) Short-term habituation

Stimulus

Siphon

When the siphon is first stimulated by a squirt of water, *Aplysia* retracts its gill to protect it. This reflex is mediated by the sensory neurons synapsing directly upon the motor neurons that withdraw the gill.

If the siphon is squirted repeatedly, the animal soon habituates to the stimulus. It no longer retracts its gill. This short-term habituation results because the sensory neurons release less transmitter.

Sensory neuron (cell body)

Motor neuron

Gill withdrawal

(B) Long-term habituation

Stimulus

Siphon

If the siphon is squirted repeatedly over days, the animal habituates faster and faster each day and eventually shows almost no response. This long-term habituation is due to a retraction of some synaptic terminals.

Sensory neuron (cell body)

Motor neuron

No response

Gill withdrawal

FIGURE 13.19 Synaptic Plasticity Underlying Habituation in *Aplysia*

nuclei (**FIGURE 13.20A**). Sensory fibers from the eye's cornea run along cranial nerve V (the trigeminal nerve) to its nucleus in the brainstem. From there, some interneurons' axonal endings excite other cranial nerve motor nuclei (VI and VII), which in turn activate the muscles of the eyelids, causing the blink.

Early studies showed that destruction of the hippocampus and the rest of the medial temporal lobe has little effect on the conditioned eye-blink response in rabbits (Lockhart and Moore, 1975). Instead, researchers found that a *cerebellar* circuit is necessary for eye-blink conditioning (Poulos and Thompson, 2015).

The trigeminal (cranial nerve V) pathway that carries information about the corneal stimulation (the US) to the cranial motor nuclei also sends axons to the brainstem. These brainstem neurons, in turn, send axons called *climbing fibers* to synapse on cerebellar neurons. The same cerebellar cells also receive information about the auditory CS by a pathway through auditory centers (**FIGURE 13.20B**). So information about the US and CS converges in the cerebellum. After conditioning, the occurrence of the CS—the tone—has an enhanced effect on the cerebellar neurons, so they now trigger eye blink even in the absence of an air puff (**FIGURE 13.20C**). Imaging studies confirm that the cerebellum is important for conditioning of the eye-blink reflex and other simple conditioning in humans (Timmann et al., 2010). How does the training change the strength of those synapses, so that now the tone triggers a blink? At least some of these plastic changes in the cerebellar neurons rely on a special synaptic mechanism that has been best studied in the hippocampus (Mao and Evinger, 2001), so we'll turn our attention there to conclude the chapter.

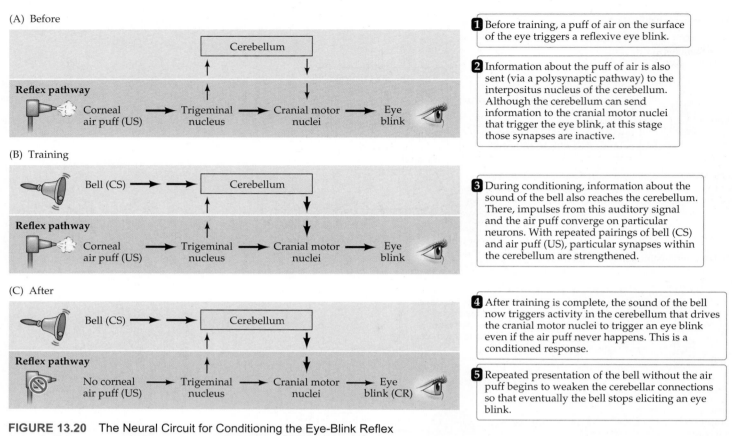

FIGURE 13.20 The Neural Circuit for Conditioning the Eye-Blink Reflex
(After R. F. Thompson and D. J. Krupa, 1994. *Annu. Rev. Neurosci.* 17: 519.)

HOW'S IT GOING ?

1. What are some of the ways that learning could alter synaptic structure or function?
2. Describe the effects of different environments on the brains of rats.
3. How does the circuitry in *Aplysia* change in the course of short-term and long-term habituation?
4. Which brain region is crucial for classical conditioning in mammals, and how does it play its role?

13.4 Synaptic Plasticity Can Be Measured in Simple Hippocampal Circuits

THE ROAD AHEAD

In the final part of the chapter, we will look at the biochemical signals that alter the strength of synapses that underlie memory. Reading this material should enable you to:

13.4.1 Explain the properties of a particular type of glutamate receptor that support long-term changes in synaptic strength.

13.4.2 Critically evaluate the possibility that such long-term changes in synaptic strength play a role in memory formation.

Modern ideas about synaptic plasticity have their origins in the theories of Donald Hebb, who proposed that when a presynaptic and a postsynaptic neuron were repeatedly activated together, the synaptic connection between them would become stronger and more stable (the phrase "Cells that fire together wire together" captures the basic idea). These **Hebbian synapses** could then act together to store memory traces (Hebb, 1949).

This idea was eventually confirmed in the 1970s when researchers discovered an impressive form of neuroplasticity in the hippocampus, which appeared to confirm Hebb's theories about synaptic changes (Bliss and Lømo, 1973; Schwartzkroin and Wester, 1975). In the classic experiments, electrodes are placed within the hippocampus, positioned so that the researchers can stimulate a group of *presynaptic* axons and record the electrical response of a group of *postsynaptic* neurons. Normal, low-level activation of the presynaptic cells produces stable and predictable excitatory postsynaptic potentials (EPSPs) (see Chapter 2), as expected. But when a brief high-frequency burst of electrical stimuli, called a **tetanus**, is applied to the presynaptic neurons, causing them to produce a high rate of action potentials that drive the postsynaptic cells to fire repeatedly, the response of the postsynaptic neurons changes. Now the postsynaptic cells produce much larger EPSPs; in other words, the synapses appear to have become stronger, more effective. This stable and long-lasting enhancement of synaptic transmission, termed **long-term potentiation** (**LTP**; *potentiation* means "strengthening"), is illustrated in **FIGURE 13.21**.

Hebbian synapse   A synapse that is strengthened when it successfully drives the postsynaptic cell.

tetanus   An intense volley of action potentials.

long-term potentiation (LTP)   A stable and enduring increase in the effectiveness of synapses following repeated strong stimulation.

FIGURE 13.21   Long-Term Potentiation Occurs in the Hippocampus

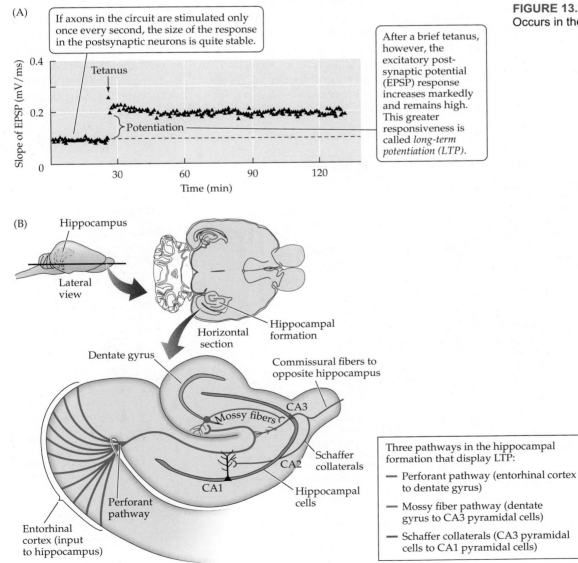

(A)

If axons in the circuit are stimulated only once every second, the size of the response in the postsynaptic neurons is quite stable.

After a brief tetanus, however, the excitatory post-synaptic potential (EPSP) response increases markedly and remains high. This greater responsiveness is called *long-term potentiation (LTP)*.

Tetanus

Potentiation

Slope of EPSP (mV/ms)

Time (min)

(B)

Hippocampus

Lateral view

Horizontal section

Hippocampal formation

Dentate gyrus

Commissural fibers to opposite hippocampus

Mossy fibers

CA3

Schaffer collaterals

CA2

CA1

Hippocampal cells

Perforant pathway

Entorhinal cortex (input to hippocampus)

Three pathways in the hippocampal formation that display LTP:

— Perforant pathway (entorhinal cortex to dentate gyrus)

— Mossy fiber pathway (dentate gyrus to CA3 pyramidal cells)

— Schaffer collaterals (CA3 pyramidal cells to CA1 pyramidal cells)

dentate gyrus   A strip of gray matter in the hippocampal formation.

glutamate   An amino acid transmitter; the most common excitatory transmitter.

NMDA receptor   A glutamate receptor that also binds the glutamate agonist NMDA (**N-m**ethyl-**D-a**spartate) and that is both ligand-gated and voltage-sensitive.

AMPA receptor   A fast-acting ionotropic glutamate receptor that also binds the glutamate agonist AMPA.

We now know that LTP can be generated in conscious and freely behaving animals, in anesthetized animals, and even in isolated slices of brain. LTP is also evident in a variety of invertebrate and vertebrate species. Once induced by a tetanus, LTP can last for weeks or more. So, at least superficially, LTP appears to have the hallmarks of a cellular mechanism of memory: a long-lasting change in synaptic strength. This hint at a cellular origin prompted research into the molecular and physiological mechanisms underlying LTP.

NMDA receptors and AMPA receptors collaborate in LTP

The region called the *hippocampal formation* consists of two interlocking C-shaped structures: the hippocampus itself and the **dentate gyrus**. At least three different pathways in the hippocampal formation display LTP, and it is seen in other brain regions too (Malenka and Bear, 2004). The most studied form of LTP occurs at synapses that use the excitatory neurotransmitter **glutamate**, and it is critically dependent on a glutamate receptor subtype called the **NMDA receptor** (after its selective ligand, **N-m**ethyl-**D-a**spartate). Treatment with drugs that selectively block NMDA receptors completely prevents new LTP in this region, but it does not affect synaptic changes that have already been established. As you might expect, these postsynaptic NMDA receptors—working in conjunction with other glutamate receptors called **AMPA receptors**—have some unique characteristics, which are responsible for LTP.

During normal, low-level activity, the release of glutamate at the synapse activates only the AMPA receptors. So the EPSP is mediated entirely by these AMPA receptors. The NMDA receptors cannot respond to the glutamate, because magnesium ions (Mg^{2+}) block the NMDA receptor's calcium ion (Ca^{2+}) channel (**FIGURE 13.22A**); thus, few Ca^{2+} ions can enter the neuron. The situation changes, however, if larger quantities of glutamate are released—say, in response to a barrage of action potentials caused by a tetanus. That stronger stimulation of the AMPA receptors depolarizes the

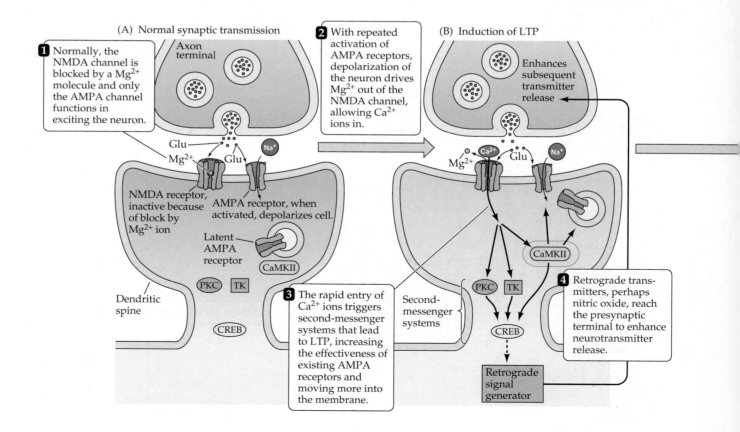

postsynaptic membrane so much that the Mg²⁺ plug is repulsed from the NMDA receptor's channel (**FIGURE 13.22B**). Now the NMDA receptors are also able to respond to glutamate, admitting large amounts of Ca²⁺ into the postsynaptic neuron. Thus, NMDA receptors are fully active only when "gated" by a combination of strong depolarization (via AMPA receptors) and the ligand (glutamate).

The large influx of Ca²⁺ at NMDA receptors activates a variety of intracellular enzymes that affect AMPA receptors in several important ways (**FIGURE 13.22C**) (Lisman et al., 2002; Kessels and Malinow, 2009). First, the enzymes cause existing nearby AMPA receptors to move to the active synapse (T. Takahashi et al., 2003), and they modify the AMPA receptors to increase their conductance of Na⁺ and K⁺ ions (Sanderson et al., 2008). In addition, more AMPA receptors are produced and inserted into the postsynaptic membrane. Thus, after the tetanus there are more AMPA receptors, and those receptors are more effective, so the synaptic response to glutamate is strengthened (see Figure 13.22B).

There are *presynaptic* changes in LTP too. When the postsynaptic cell is strongly stimulated and its NMDA receptors become active and admit Ca²⁺, an intracellular process causes the postsynaptic cell to release a **retrograde transmitter**—often a diffusible gas—that travels back across the synapse and alters the functioning of the presynaptic neuron (see Figure 13.22B). The retrograde transmitter induces the presynaptic terminal to release more glutamate than previously, thereby strengthening the synapse some more. So, LTP involves active changes on both sides of the synapse.

So far, we've talked about how activity can make existing Hebbian synapses stronger. However, evidence suggests that the same mechanisms can affect whether new synapses are formed and old synapses retracted. In these systems it appears that when several presynaptic neurons fire at the same time, they "gang up" on the postsynaptic cell, depolarizing it enough that the NMDA receptors are activated to strengthen those connections. Conversely, any presynaptic neurons that tend to fire *out* of synchrony

retrograde transmitter A neurotransmitter that is released by the postsynaptic neuron, diffuses back across the synapse, and alters the functioning of the presynaptic neuron.

View Animation 13.3: AMPA and NMDA Receptors

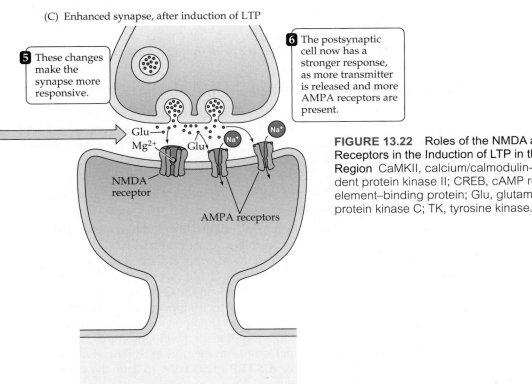

(C) Enhanced synapse, after induction of LTP

5 These changes make the synapse more responsive.

6 The postsynaptic cell now has a stronger response, as more transmitter is released and more AMPA receptors are present.

Glu
Mg²⁺ Glu
Na⁺ Na⁺

NMDA receptor

AMPA receptors

FIGURE 13.22 Roles of the NMDA and AMPA Receptors in the Induction of LTP in the CA1 Region CaMKII, calcium/calmodulin-dependent protein kinase II; CREB, cAMP responsive element–binding protein; Glu, glutamate; PKC, protein kinase C; TK, tyrosine kinase.

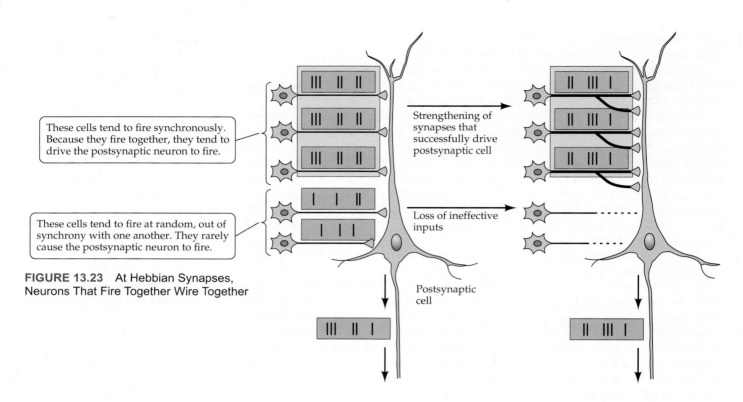

These cells tend to fire synchronously. Because they fire together, they tend to drive the postsynaptic neuron to fire.

These cells tend to fire at random, out of synchrony with one another. They rarely cause the postsynaptic neuron to fire.

Strengthening of synapses that successfully drive postsynaptic cell

Loss of ineffective inputs

Postsynaptic cell

FIGURE 13.23 At Hebbian Synapses, Neurons That Fire Together Wire Together

See Video 13.4:
Morris Water Maze

with the other inputs are not likely to depolarize the postsynaptic neurons enough to activate NMDA receptors. Eventually, the strengthened inputs seem to sprout new, additional connections, while the weakened synapses fade away (**FIGURE 13.23**).

Many scientists are excited about LTP because this momentary burst of neural activity, the tetanus, can change synaptic strength for a long time. It's easy to imagine how another momentary burst of neural activity, in this case triggered by a learning experience, could change synaptic strength, and that change in synaptic strength might be a memory trace. But is this just a case of an overactive imagination, or is LTP truly involved in learning?

Is LTP a mechanism of memory formation?

Even the simplest learning involves circuits of multiple neurons and many synapses, and more-complex declarative and procedural memory traces must involve vast networks of neurons, so we are unlikely to conclude that LTP is the *only* mechanism of learning. However, evidence from several research perspectives implicates LTP in at least some forms of memory:

1. *Correlational observations* The time course of LTP bears strong similarity to the time course of memory formation.

2. *Somatic intervention experiments* In general, pharmacological treatments that interfere with LTP also tend to impair learning. So, for example, NMDA receptor blockade interferes with performance in the Morris water maze (a test of spatial memory) and other types of memory tests (R. G. Morris et al., 1989). Knockout mice that lack functional NMDA receptors only in the CA1 region of the hippocampus appear normal in many respects, but their hippocampi are incapable of LTP and their declarative memory is impaired (Rampon et al., 2000). Conversely, mice engineered to *overexpress* NMDA receptors in the hippocampus have enhanced LTP and better-than-normal long-term memory (Y. P. Tang et al., 2001). (For the full story of these mice, see **A STEP FURTHER 13.2**, on the website.)

3. *Behavioral intervention experiments* In principle, the most convincing evidence for a link between LTP and learning would be "behavioral LTP": a demonstration that training an animal in a memory task induces LTP somewhere in the brain. Such research is difficult because of uncertainty about exactly where to put the recording electrodes in order to detect any induced LTP. Nevertheless, several examples of successful behavioral LTP have been reported (Whitlock et al., 2006).

Taken together, these findings support the idea that LTP is a kind of synaptic plasticity that underlies (or is very similar to) certain forms of learning and memory.

Thus it seems that the cause of Henry Molaison's tragic amnesia may have been the loss of medial temporal lobe structures like the hippocampus, which normally use LTP to consolidate short-term memories into long-term memories somewhere in the brain, probably the cortex. It's strange to think that microscopic changes in synapses in a particular brain region could be so crucial for living a full human life. Eventually Henry seemed to stop being shocked when he saw his reflection, and he learned he was no longer in his twenties. But it's not clear whether he understood, for long, that his parents had passed away. As a final act of generosity to a field of science that he helped launch, Henry arranged to donate his brain for further study after he died. Through webcasting technology, the dissection of Henry's brain was viewed live by thousands of people (see https://www.thebrainobservatory.org/project-hm), and a series of more than 2,000 brain sections are available.

To the end, although Henry could remember so little of his entire adult life, he was courteous and concerned about other people. Henry remembered the surgeon he had met several times before his operation: "He did medical research on people.... What he learned about me helped others too, and I'm glad about that" (Corkin, 2002, p. 158). Henry never knew how famous he was or how much his dreadful condition taught us about learning and memory; despite being deprived of one of the most important characteristics of a human being, he held fast to his humanity.

HOW'S IT GOING ❓

1. Describe how LTP is measured in the hippocampus.
2. What happens to AMPA receptors and NMDA receptors during LTP?
3. What evidence suggests that LTP may underlie some forms of learning and memory?

Recommended Reading

Baddeley, A. D., Eysenck, M., and Anderson, M. C. (2020). *Memory* (3rd ed.). London, UK: Routledge Press.

Clark, R. E., and Martin, S. J. (2018). *Behavioral Neuroscience of Learning and Memory*. Cham, Switzerland: Springer.

Gluck, M. A., Mercado, E., and Myers, C. E. (2020). *Learning and Memory: From Brain to Behavior* (4th ed.). New York, NY: Worth.

Rudy, J. W. (2021). *The Neurobiology of Learning and Memory* (3rd ed.). Sunderland, MA: Oxford University Press/Sinauer.

Slotnick, S. D. (2017). *Cognitive Neuroscience of Memory*. Cambridge, UK: Cambridge University Press.

You should be able to relate each summary to the adjacent illustration, including structures and processes. The online version of this **Visual Summary** includes links to figures, animations, and activities that will help you consolidate the material.

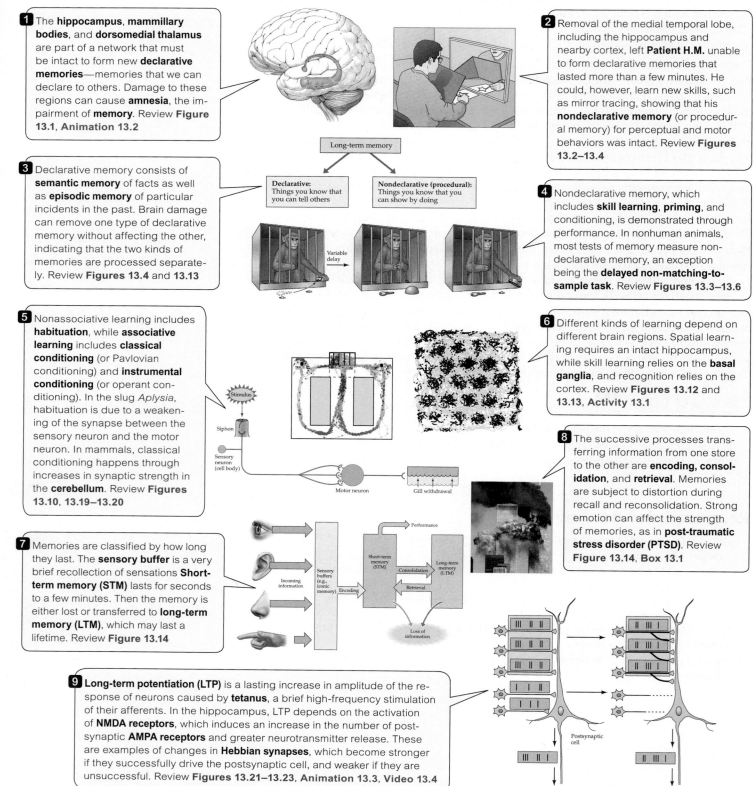

1 The **hippocampus, mammillary bodies**, and **dorsomedial thalamus** are part of a network that must be intact to form new **declarative memories**—memories that we can declare to others. Damage to these regions can cause **amnesia**, the impairment of **memory**. Review **Figure 13.1, Animation 13.2**

2 Removal of the medial temporal lobe, including the hippocampus and nearby cortex, left **Patient H.M.** unable to form declarative memories that lasted more than a few minutes. He could, however, learn new skills, such as mirror tracing, showing that his **nondeclarative memory** (or procedural memory) for perceptual and motor behaviors was intact. Review **Figures 13.2–13.4**

3 Declarative memory consists of **semantic memory** of facts as well as **episodic memory** of particular incidents in the past. Brain damage can remove one type of declarative memory without affecting the other, indicating that the two kinds of memories are processed separately. Review **Figures 13.4** and **13.13**

4 Nondeclarative memory, which includes **skill learning**, **priming**, and conditioning, is demonstrated through performance. In nonhuman animals, most tests of memory measure nondeclarative memory, an exception being the **delayed non-matching-to-sample task**. Review **Figures 13.3–13.6**

5 Nonassociative learning includes **habituation**, while **associative learning** includes **classical conditioning** (or Pavlovian conditioning) and **instrumental conditioning** (or operant conditioning). In the slug *Aplysia*, habituation is due to a weakening of the synapse between the sensory neuron and the motor neuron. In mammals, classical conditioning happens through increases in synaptic strength in the **cerebellum**. Review **Figures 13.10, 13.19–13.20**

6 Different kinds of learning depend on different brain regions. Spatial learning requires an intact hippocampus, while skill learning relies on the **basal ganglia**, and recognition relies on the cortex. Review **Figures 13.12** and **13.13, Activity 13.1**

7 Memories are classified by how long they last. The **sensory buffer** is a very brief recollection of sensations **Short-term memory (STM)** lasts for seconds to a few minutes. Then the memory is either lost or transferred to **long-term memory (LTM)**, which may last a lifetime. Review **Figure 13.14**

8 The successive processes transferring information from one store to the other are **encoding, consolidation**, and **retrieval**. Memories are subject to distortion during recall and reconsolidation. Strong emotion can affect the strength of memories, as in **post-traumatic stress disorder (PTSD)**. Review **Figure 13.14, Box 13.1**

9 **Long-term potentiation (LTP)** is a lasting increase in amplitude of the response of neurons caused by **tetanus**, a brief high-frequency stimulation of their afferents. In the hippocampus, LTP depends on the activation of **NMDA receptors**, which induces an increase in the number of postsynaptic **AMPA receptors** and greater neurotransmitter release. These are examples of changes in **Hebbian synapses**, which become stronger if they successfully drive the postsynaptic cell, and weaker if they are unsuccessful. Review **Figures 13.21–13.23, Animation 13.3, Video 13.4**

Long-term memory

Declarative:
Things you know that you can tell others

Nondeclarative (procedural):
Things you know that you can show by doing

Variable delay

Stimulus

Siphon

Sensory neuron (cell body)

Motor neuron

Gill withdrawal

Incoming information

Sensory buffers (e.g., iconic memory)

Encoding

Short-term memory (STM)

Consolidation

Retrieval

Long-term memory (LTM)

Performance

Loss of information

Postsynaptic cell

The Mind's Machine digital resources include additional videos, flashcards, and other study tools.

14 Attention and Higher Cognition

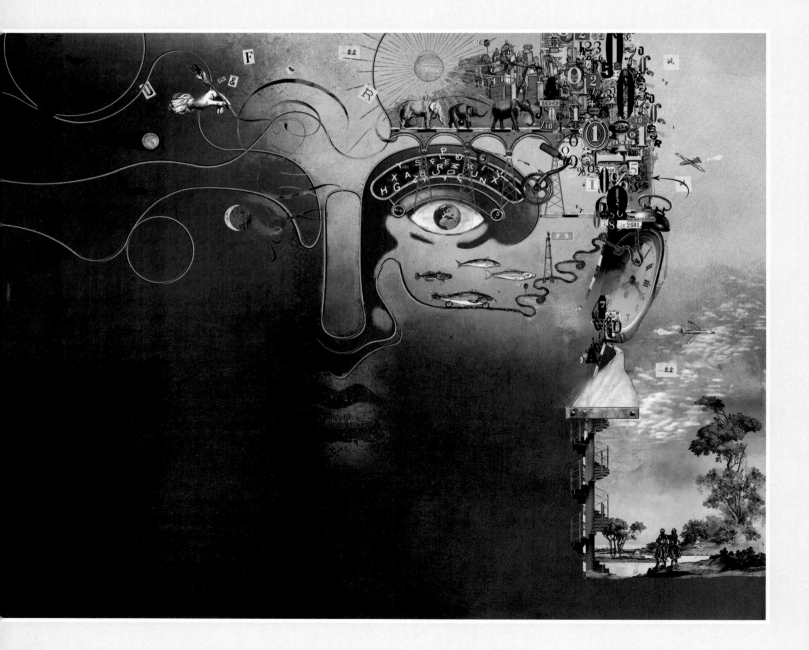

Attention to Details

Everyone agreed that Parminder and her family were bighearted—generous and friendly to a fault—but they were also "bad" hearted, in one sad sense. Many of Parminder's relatives had suffered early heart attacks and strokes, and now, in her 68th year, Parminder shared that unhappy fate. In February, and then again in September, blood clots that originated in Parminder's heart found their way into the complex of arteries in her brain, cutting off blood flow to the surrounding brain tissue. The two strokes that resulted were exceptional, however, because they were exact mirror images—they damaged identical regions of the left and right parietal lobes.

Parminder's unlikely lesions produced equally unlikely symptoms. A few weeks after her second stroke, Parminder had regained many of her intellectual powers—she could converse normally and remember things. Her visual fields were apparently normal too, but her visual *perception* was anything but normal. Parminder had lost the ability to perceive more than one thing at a time. For example, she could see her husband's face just fine, but she couldn't judge whether he had glasses on or not. It turned out that she could see the glasses *or* she could see the face, but she couldn't perceive them *both* at the same time. When shown a drawing of several overlapping items, she could perceive and name only one at a time. Furthermore, she couldn't understand where the objects she saw were located. It was as if Parminder was lost in space, able to pay attention to only one object or detail at a time, apparently alone in a world of its own. What could explain Parminder's symptoms?

What is attention? William James, the great American psychologist, wrote in 1890:

> *Everyone knows what attention is. It is the taking possession by the mind, in clear and vivid form, of one out of what seem several simultaneously possible objects or trains of thought. Focalization, concentration, of consciousness are of its essence. It implies withdrawal from some things in order to deal effectively with others, and is a condition which has a real opposite in the confused, dazed, scatterbrained state.*

Clearly, James understood that attention can be effortful, improves perception, and acts as a filter. This continual shifting of our focus from one interesting stimulus to the next lies at the heart of our innermost conscious experiences, our awareness of the world around us, and our place in it. So, we open this chapter by exploring the behavioral and neural dimensions of attention before turning to the more general question of our conscious experience of the world.

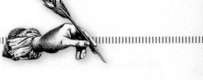

**See Video 14.1:
Attention and Perception**

14.1 Attention Focuses Cognitive Processing on Specific Objects

 THE ROAD AHEAD

The first part of this chapter concerns the consequences of attention processes: the ways attention filters the world and affects our processing of sensory information. At the conclusion of this section, you should be able to:

14.1.1 Provide a general definition of attention, and distinguish between overt and covert forms of attention, with examples.

14.1.2 Describe the limitations on our powers of attention, situations in which our attention may be overextended, and the behavioral manifestations of these limits on attention.

14.1.3 Speculate about the ways in which evolution may have shaped attention.

14.1.4 Distinguish between voluntary and reflexive attention, and describe general experimental designs for studying each.

14.1.5 Describe the use of focused attention to search the world for particular objects (using either a feature search or a conjunction search), and discuss the significance of the "binding problem."

Despite taking delight in pretending otherwise, the average 5-year-old knows exactly what it means when an exasperated parent shouts, "Pay attention!" We all share an intuitive understanding of the term *attention*, but it is tricky to formally define. In general, **attention** (or *selective attention*) is the process by which we select or focus on one or more specific stimuli—either external phenomena or internal thoughts—for enhanced processing and analysis. It is the *selective* quality of attention that distinguishes it from the related concept of **vigilance**, the global level of alertness of the individual. Most of the time we direct our eyes and our attention to the same target, a process known as **overt attention**. For example, as you read this sentence, it is both the center of your visual gaze and (we hope) the main item that your brain has selected for attention. But if we choose to, we can also shift the focus of our visual attention *covertly*, keeping our eyes fixed on one location while "secretly" scrutinizing something in peripheral vision (Helmholtz, 1962; original work published in 1894). Remember that teacher who, even when looking out the window, somehow knew instantly when someone read a text? That's an example of what is known as **covert attention** (**FIGURE 14.1**).

Selective attention isn't restricted to visual stimuli. Imagine yourself chatting with an old friend at a noisy party. Despite the background noise, you would probably find it relatively easy to focus on what your friend was saying, even if speaking quietly, because attention aids your sensory perception—paying close attention to a friend enhances your processing of their speech and helps filter out distracters. This phenomenon, known as the **cocktail party effect**,[1] nicely illustrates how attention acts to *focus* cognitive processing resources on a particular target. If your attention drifts to a different stimulus—for example, if you start eavesdropping on a more interesting conversation nearby—it becomes almost impossible to simultaneously follow what your friend is saying.

There are limits on attention

The powers of attention that help you to easily chat with a friend in a noisy room normally rely on cues in several different sensory modalities, such as where their speech sounds are coming from, the movements of their face while speaking, and what unique sounds their voice makes. But what if we restrict our attention to just one type of stimulus?

In **shadowing** experiments, participants must focus their attention on just one out of two or more simultaneous streams of stimuli. In a classic example of this technique,

---

View Animation 14.2: Brain Explorer

attention   Also called *selective attention.* A state or condition of selective awareness or perceptual receptivity, by which specific stimuli are selected for enhanced processing.

vigilance   The global, nonselective level of alertness of an individual.

overt attention   Attention in which the focus coincides with sensory orientation (e.g., you're attending to the same thing you're looking at).

covert attention   Attention in which the focus can be directed independently of sensory orientation (e.g., you're attending to one sensory stimulus while looking at another).

cocktail party effect   The selective enhancement of attention in order to filter out distracters, as you might do while listening to one person talking in the midst of a noisy party.

---

[1] The term *cocktail party effect* also sometimes describes what happens when a highly salient word (such as one's own name) captures attention in a noisy environment.

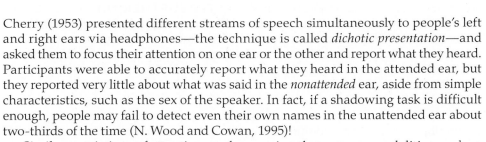

While holding our gaze steady on a central fixation point, we can independently center our visual attention on a different spatial location. This selective attention has sometimes been referred to as an *attentional spotlight*.

Visual fixation point

Location of covert spatial attention

FIGURE 14.1   Covert Attention

Cherry (1953) presented different streams of speech simultaneously to people's left and right ears via headphones—the technique is called *dichotic presentation*—and asked them to focus their attention on one ear or the other and report what they heard. Participants were able to accurately report what they heard in the attended ear, but they reported very little about what was said in the *nonattended* ear, aside from simple characteristics, such as the sex of the speaker. In fact, if a shadowing task is difficult enough, people may fail to detect even their own names in the unattended ear about two-thirds of the time (N. Wood and Cowan, 1995)!

Similar restrictions of attention can be seen in other sensory modalities, such as musical notes (Zendel and Alain, 2009) and visual stimuli. Participants closely attending to one complex visual event against a background of other moving stimuli—dancers weaving through a basketball game, for example—may show **inattentional blindness**: a surprising failure to perceive nonattended stimuli. And the unperceived stimuli can be things that you might think impossible to miss, like a gorilla strolling across the screen out of the blue (Simons and Chabris, 1999; Simons and Jensen, 2009). Even highly trained experts can have this problem. In one study 83% of radiologists screening CT scans for lung cancer didn't notice a seemingly obvious image of a gorilla inserted into one of the scans (Drew et al., 2013) (you can see an example on the website). Inattentional blindness even occurs when the nonattended stimulus could have life-or-death consequences for the observer; for example, a significant fraction of police officers and trainees will fail to notice a gun placed in plain view during a simulated traffic stop (Simons and Schlosser, 2017).

In general, **divided-attention tasks**—in which a person is asked to process two or more simultaneous stimuli—confirm that attention is a limited resource and that it's very difficult to attend to more than one thing at a time, particularly if the stimuli are spatially separated (Bonnel and Prinzmetal, 1998). So, our limited selective attention generally acts like an **attentional spotlight** (see Figure 14.1), shifting around the environment, highlighting stimuli for enhanced processing. It's an adaptation that we share with many other species because, like us, they are confronted with the problem of extracting important signals from a noisy background (Bee and Micheyl, 2008). Birds, for example, must isolate the vocalizations of specific individuals from a cacophony of calls and other noises

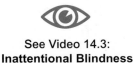

See Video 14.3:
Inattentional Blindness

shadowing   A task in which the participant is asked to focus attention on one ear or the other while different stimuli are being presented to the two ears, and to repeat aloud the material presented to the attended ear.

inattentional blindness   The failure to perceive nonattended stimuli that seem so obvious as to be impossible to miss.

divided-attention task   A task in which the participant is asked to focus attention on two or more stimuli simultaneously.

attentional spotlight   The steerable focus of our selective attention, used to select stimuli for enhanced processing.

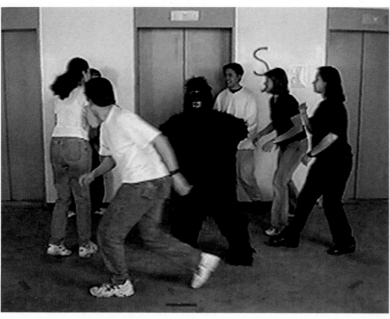

Gorillas in the Midst   Who could miss the gorilla in the video from which this still is taken? Most people do, if they are concentrating on some other task, such as counting the number of times people in white shirts touch a ball that is being passed around.

in the environment—an avian version of the cocktail party problem (Benney and Braaten, 2000). Having a single attentional spotlight helps us focus cognitive resources and behavioral responses toward the most important things in the environment at any given moment (the smell of smoke, the voice of a potential mate, a glimpse of a big spotted cat), while ignoring extraneous information.

In general, by acting as a filter, attention narrows our focus and directs our cognitive resources toward only the most important stimuli around us, thereby protecting the brain from being overwhelmed by the world. But the details of this **attentional bottleneck** have been elusive. Initial research gave evidence of an *early-selection model* of attention, in which unattended information is filtered out right away, at the level of the initial sensory input, as in the shadowing experiments we just described (Broadbent, 1958). But other researchers noted that important but unattended stimuli (such as your name) may undergo substantial unconscious processing, right up to the level of semantic meaning and awareness, before suddenly capturing attention (N. Wood and Cowan, 1995), thus illustrating a *late-selection model* of attention. Many contemporary models of attention now combine both early- and late-selection mechanisms (e.g., Wolfe, 1994), and debate continues over their relative importance (for a classic demonstration, see **A STEP FURTHER 14.1**, on the website).

A possible resolution to this debate involves the concept of **perceptual load**—the immediate processing demands presented by a stimulus. According to this view, when we focus on a very complex stimulus, the load on our perceptual processing resources is so great that there is nothing left over. We are thus unable to process competing unattended items, so those extra stimuli are excluded right from the outset: an early-selection process (N. Lavie et al., 2004; S. Murphy et al., 2017). But when we focus on stimuli that are easier to process, we may have enough perceptual resources left over to simultaneously process additional stimuli, all the way up to the level of semantic meaning and awareness. In this case the result is a late selection of stimuli to attend to (N. Lavie et al., 2009). In other words, if we view attention as a limited resource, then we only have enough of it to do one complex task at a time, or a few very simple ones. This research thus suggests that attention is continually rebalanced between early and late selection, depending on the difficulty of the task at hand. These more modern perspectives on attention are central to the development of computational models of attention in visual and auditory "scenes"; one hope is that mathematical descriptions of attentional processes will aid in the development of machine versions of vision and audition (Shic and Scassellati, 2007; Kaya and Elhilali, 2017).

Attention is deployed in several different ways

We've now seen that through an act of willpower we can direct our attention to specific stimuli without moving our eyes or otherwise reorienting. Early experiments on this phenomenon employed **sustained-attention tasks**, like the one depicted in Figure 14.1, where a single stimulus location must be held in the attentional spotlight for an extended period. Although these tasks are useful for studying basic phenomena, several key questions about attention require another approach. For example, how do we shift our attention around? How does attention enhance the processing of stimuli, and which brain regions are involved? To answer these questions, researchers devised clever tasks that employ *stimulus cuing* to control attention, which revealed two general categories of attention, as we'll discuss next.

The kind of attention that we have been discussing thus far in the chapter is what researchers call **voluntary attention** (or *endogenous attention*). As the name implies,

attentional bottleneck   A filter created by the limits intrinsic to our attentional processes, whose effect is that only the most important stimuli are selected for special processing.

perceptual load   The immediate processing demands presented by a stimulus.

sustained-attention task   A task in which a single stimulus source or location must be held in the attentional spotlight for a protracted period.

voluntary attention   Also called *endogenous attention*. The voluntary direction of attention toward specific aspects of the environment, in accordance with our interests and goals.

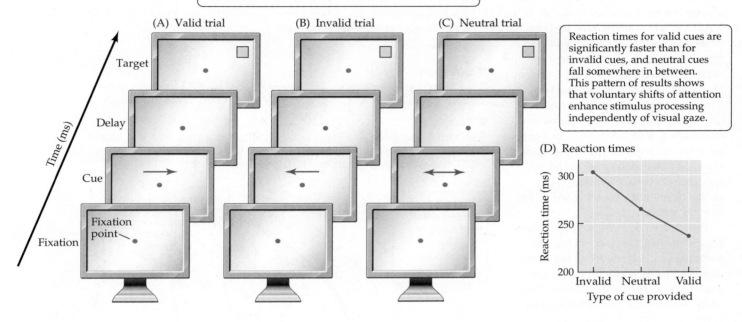

In three types of cuing trials, participants fixating on a central point are shown a symbol that gives an accurate clue to the location in which a subsequent stimulus item will briefly appear (A), a bogus cue that indicates an incorrect location (B), or a symbol that doesn't cue any particular location (C).

FIGURE 14.2 Measuring the Effects of Voluntary Shifts of Attention (After M. I. Posner, 1980. *Q. J. Exp. Psychol.* 32: 3.)

Reaction times for valid cues are significantly faster than for invalid cues, and neutral cues fall somewhere in between. This pattern of results shows that voluntary shifts of attention enhance stimulus processing independently of visual gaze.

(A) Valid trial   (B) Invalid trial   (C) Neutral trial

Target
Delay
Cue
Fixation
Fixation point
Time (ms)

(D) Reaction times

voluntary shifts of attention come from within; they are the conscious, *top-down* directing of our attention toward specific aspects of the environment, according to our interests and goals. **FIGURE 14.2** features the **symbolic cuing** task (or *spatial cuing* task), developed by Michael Posner and used extensively to study voluntary attention. Studies using cuing tasks have confirmed that consciously directing your attention to the correct location or stimulus improves processing speed and accuracy. Conversely, directing your attention to an *incorrect* location or stimulus impairs processing efficiency.

How much does it help to shift your attention to a location before a stimulus occurs there? Posner's (1980) symbolic cuing task allows us to quantify how voluntary attention benefits processing. In a symbolic cuing task, participants stare at a point in the center of a computer screen and must press a key as soon as a specific target (the stimulus) appears on the screen; this technique thus measures **reaction time**. The stimulus is preceded by a cue that briefly flashes on the screen, hinting where the stimulus will appear. Most of the time, as in **FIGURE 14.2A**, the participant is provided with a *valid cue*; for example, a right-ward arrow flashes on the screen moments before the stimulus appears on the right side of the screen. In a few trials, like the one in **FIGURE 14.2B**, the arrow points the wrong way and thus provides an *invalid cue*. And in "neutral" control trials (**FIGURE 14.2C**), the cue doesn't provide any hint at all. Both the cue and the stimulus are on the screen so briefly that participants don't have time to shift their gaze (and in any case, they have been told to stare at the fixation point).

Averaged over many trials, the reaction-time data (**FIGURE 14.2D**) clearly show that people swiftly learn to use cues to predict stimulus location, shifting their attention without shifting their gaze. Compared with neutral trials, processing is significantly faster for validly cued trials, and participants pay a price for misdirecting their attention on those few trials in which the cue is invalid, pointing to the wrong side of the display. Many variants of the symbolic cuing paradigm have been developed—varying the timing of the stimuli, altering their complexity, requiring a choice between different responses—all of which can affect reaction time, which we discuss next.

symbolic cuing   Also called *spatial cuing*. A technique for testing voluntary attention in which a visual stimulus is presented and participants are asked to respond as soon as the stimulus appears on a screen. Each trial is preceded by a meaningful symbol used as a cue to hint at where the stimulus will appear.

reaction time   The delay between the presentation of a stimulus and a participant's response to that stimulus, measured in milliseconds.

RESEARCHERS AT WORK ||||||||||||||||||||||||||||||||||||||||||||||||||||||||||||||||||||||||||||||||||||||||||||||||||||

Reaction times reflect brain processing, from input to output

Reaction-time measures are a mainstay of cognitive neuroscience research. In tests of *simple reaction time*, participants make a single response—for example, pressing a button—in response to an experimental stimulus (the appearance of a target, the solution to a problem, a tone, or whatever the experiment is testing). In tests of *choice reaction time*, the situation is slightly more complicated: a person is presented with alternatives and has to choose among them (e.g., correct versus incorrect, same versus different) by pressing one of two or more buttons.

Reaction times in an uncomplicated choice reaction time test, in which the participant indicates whether two stimuli are the same or different, average about 300–350 milliseconds (ms). The delay between stimulus and response varies depending on the amount of neural processing required between input and output. The neural systems involved in this sort of task, and the timing of events in the response circuit, are illustrated in **FIGURE 14.3**. Brain activity proceeds from the primary visual cortex (V1) through a ventral visual object identification pathway (see Chapter 7) to prefrontal cortex, and then through premotor and primary motor cortex, down to the spinal motor neurons and out to the finger muscles. In the sequence shown in the figure—proceeding from the presentation of visual stimuli to a discrimination response—notice that it takes about 110 ms for the sensory system to recognize the stimulus (somewhere in the inferior temporal lobe), about 35 ms more for that information to reach the prefrontal cortex, and then about 30 ms more to determine which button to push. After that, it takes another 75 ms or so for the movement to be executed (i.e., 75 ms of time elapses between the moment the signal from the prefrontal cortex arrives in premotor cortex and the moment the

finger pushes the button). It is fascinating to think that something like this sequence of neural events happens over and over

in more-complicated behaviors, such as recognizing a long-lost friend or composing an opera.

■ Question
Does the length of time required to respond to a stimulus increase with stimulus complexity?

■ Test
Compare the time taken to press a button after the appearance of a simple stimulus (such as a light turning on), versus time to react to more complex stimuli (for example, a green light but not an orange light).

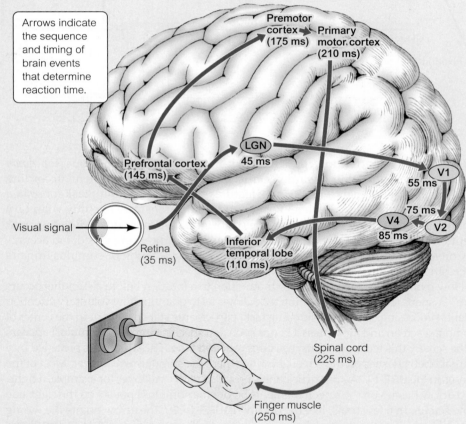

Arrows indicate the sequence and timing of brain events that determine reaction time.

Premotor cortex (175 ms) → Primary motor cortex (210 ms)

LGN 45 ms

Prefrontal cortex (145 ms)

V1 55 ms

75 ms

V4 85 ms V2

Visual signal →

Retina (35 ms)

Inferior temporal lobe (110 ms)

Spinal cord (225 ms)

Finger muscle (250 ms)

■ Result
The more complex the stimulus processing that is required, the longer the reaction time.

■ Conclusion
Complex stimuli require the participation of more brain pathways, slowing down reaction time proportionately.

FIGURE 14.3   A Reaction-Time Circuit in the Brain LGN, lateral geniculate nucleus; V1, primary visual cortex; V2 and V4, extrastriate visual areas. (Timings based on S. J. Thorpe and M. Fabre Thorpe, 2001. *Science* 291: 260.)

Some types of stimuli just grab our attention

There is a second way in which we pay attention to the world, involving more than just consciously steering our attentional spotlight around. Flashes, bangs, sudden movements—any striking or important change—can instantly snatch our attention away from whatever we're doing, unless we are very focused. Drop your glass in a restaurant, and every conversation stops, every head in the place swivels, seeking the source of the sound (you, embarrassingly). This sort of involuntary reorientation toward a sudden or important event is an example of **reflexive attention** (or *exogenous attention*). It is considered to be a *bottom-up* process, because attention is being seized by sensory inputs from lower levels of the nervous system, rather than being directed by voluntary, conscious *top-down* processes of the forebrain.

Researchers study reflexive attention using a different kind of cuing task, called **peripheral spatial cuing**. In this task, instead of a meaningful symbol like an arrow, the cue that is presented is a simple sensory stimulus, such as a flash of light, occurring *in the location to which attention is to be drawn*. Research with this type of simple cuing confirmed that valid reflexive cues enhance the processing of subsequent stimuli at the same location, but only when the target stimulus closely follows the cue. At longer intervals between the cue and target, starting at about 200 ms, a curious phenomenon is observed: detection of stimuli at the location where the valid cue occurred is actually *impaired* (Satel et al., 2019). It's as though attention has moved on from where the cue occurred and is reluctant to return to that location. This **inhibition of return** probably evolved because it prevented reflexive attention from settling on unimportant stimuli for more than an instant, an effective strategy in animals foraging for food or scanning the world for threats.

Normally, reflexive and voluntary attention work together to direct cognitive activities (**FIGURE 14.4**), probably relying on somewhat overlapping neural mechanisms. Anyone who has watched a squirrel at work has seen that twitchy interplay. When it comes to single-mindedly searching for tasty morsels (an example of voluntary attention), a squirrel has few rivals. But even slight noises and movements (cues that reflexively capture attention) cause the squirrel to stop and scan its surroundings—a sensible precaution if, like a squirrel, you are yourself a tasty morsel. So, it's no surprise that emotional cues—a sudden gasp from a companion, for example—can likewise reflexively capture attention and augment sensory processing (Carretié, 2014). And effective cues for reflexive attention may involve multiple sensory modalities: a sudden sound coming from a particular location, for example, can improve the *visual* processing of a stimulus that appears there (McDonald et al., 2000; Feng et al., 2017).

**View Animation 14.4:
From Input to Output**

reflexive attention   Also called *exogenous attention*. The involuntary reorienting of attention toward a specific stimulus source, cued by an unexpected object or event.

peripheral spatial cuing   A technique for testing reflexive attention in which a visual stimulus is preceded by a simple task-irrelevant sensory stimulus either in the location where the stimulus will appear or in an incorrect location.

inhibition of return   The phenomenon, observed in peripheral spatial cuing tasks when the interval between cue and target stimulus is 200 milliseconds or more, in which the detection of stimuli at the former location of the cue is increasingly impaired.

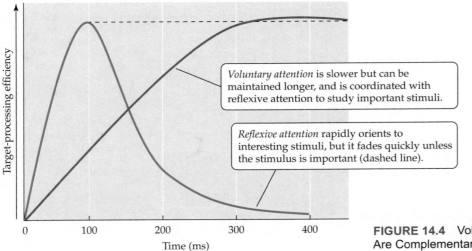

Voluntary attention is slower but can be maintained longer, and is coordinated with reflexive attention to study important stimuli.

Reflexive attention rapidly orients to interesting stimuli, but it fades quickly unless the stimulus is important (dashed line).

FIGURE 14.4 Voluntary and Reflexive Attention Are Complementary

Attention helps us to search for specific objects in a cluttered world

Another familiar way that we use attention is in *visual search*: systematically scanning the world to locate a specific object among many—your car in a parking lot, for example, or your friend's face in a crowd. If the sought-after item varies in just one key attribute, the task can be pretty easy—searching for your red car among a bunch of silver and black ones, for example. In a simple **feature search** like this (**FIGURE 14.5A**), the sought-after item "pops out" immediately, no matter how many distracters are present (Joseph et al., 1997). Effortful voluntary attention isn't needed.

More commonly, however, we must use a **conjunction search**—searching for an item on the basis of a *combination* of two or more features, such as size and color (**FIGURE 14.5B** and **C**). This can become very difficult when, for example, you must simultaneously consider the hair, nose, eyes, and smile of your friend's face in a crowd—and the bigger the crowd grows, the harder the task becomes (unless your friend waves, thereby reflexively grabbing your attention—phew!).

Experimental results (**FIGURE 14.5D**) confirm what you probably already know intuitively: conjunction searches can be relatively slow and laborious, involving a large cognitive effort. That's because your brain has to deal with what is known as the **binding problem** (A. M. Treisman, 1996), which is this: How do we know which

feature search A search for an item in which the target pops out right away, no matter how many distracters are present, because it possesses a unique attribute.

conjunction search A search for an item that is based on two or more features (e.g., size and color) that together distinguish the target from distracters that may share some of the same attributes.

binding problem The question of how the brain understands which individual attributes blend together into a single object, when these different features are processed by different regions in the brain.

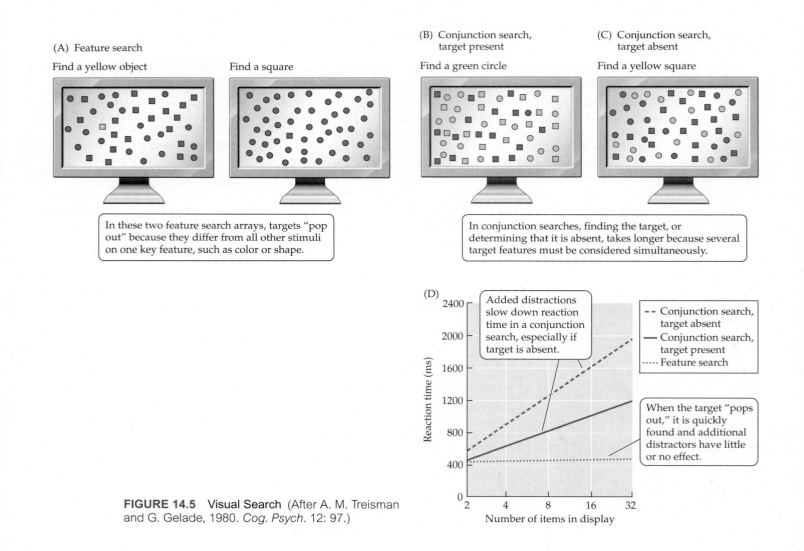

FIGURE 14.5 Visual Search (After A. M. Treisman and G. Gelade, 1980. *Cog. Psych.* 12: 97.)

different stimulus features—colors, shapes, sounds, etc., each processed by different regions of the brain—are bound together in a single object? And if those objects appear only infrequently—say, weapons in luggage or tumors in X-rays—they may go undetected with alarmingly high frequency, even by highly trained screeners (Wolfe et al., 2005). Our natural tendency is to let our attention wander between the various sources of stimuli in our environment.

To uncover finer details of attentional mechanisms, neuroscientists take two complementary perspectives on attention experimental strategies. First, we can look at *consequences of attention* in the brain, asking how neural systems are affected by selective attention to enhance the processing of stimuli. So, in these studies, the question is, What are the *targets* of attention? Second, we can try to uncover the *mechanisms of attention*, the brain regions that produce and control attention, shifting it between different stimuli in different sensory modalities. Here, the question is, What are the *sources* of attention? In selecting experimental techniques to address these different objectives, researchers must juggle the need for good **temporal resolution**—the ability to track changes in the brain that occur very quickly—with the need for excellent **spatial resolution**, the ability to observe the detailed structure of the brain. In general, electrophysiological approaches offer the speed (temporal resolution) necessary to distinguish the consequences of attention from the mechanisms that direct it, while brain-imaging techniques like fMRI offer the anatomical detail (spatial resolution) to figure out where these neural actions are taking place. This speed-versus-accuracy trade-off permeates the research that we discuss in the following section.

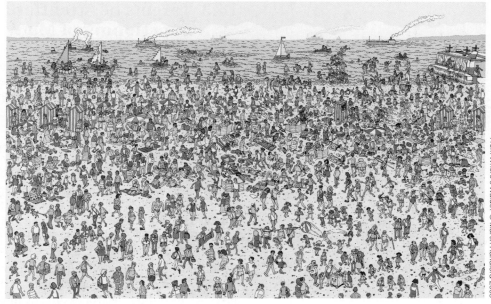

From *Where's Waldo?* © Martin Handford 2005

Where's Waldo?   Puzzles like the "Where's Waldo?" series are classic examples of conjunction searches: you can find Waldo only if you search for the right combination of striped sweater, hat, glasses, and slightly goofy expression. Imagine how much easier it would be to find Waldo if everyone else on the beach were wearing green! In that case, finding Waldo would be a feature search (the only person not wearing green) and he would "pop out" in the picture … but that wouldn't be any fun.

temporal resolution   The ability to track changes in the brain that occur very quickly.

spatial resolution   The ability to observe the detailed structure of the brain.

HOW'S IT GOING ❓

1. How do you define *attention*? Distinguish between overt and covert attention, giving examples of each. What is the attentional spotlight?

2. What is inattentional blindness, and under what circumstances might it occur?

3. How do early-selection effects of attention differ from late-selection effects? What single aspect of a stimulus may determine whether early or late selection occurs?

4. Summarize Posner's symbolic cuing task. What did this task reveal?

5. Compare and contrast voluntary attention and reflexive attention, and identify the principal ways in which they differ. What is inhibition of return, and does it relate to voluntary attention or to reflexive attention?

6. While conducting a visual search for something, we sometimes experience "pop-out." What is it? Is pop-out more closely associated with feature search or with conjunction search, and how do those differ?

7. Distinguish between temporal resolution and spatial resolution as they apply to brain-imaging techniques. How are they related?

14.2 Targets of Attention: Attention Alters the Functioning of Many Brain Regions

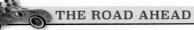

THE ROAD AHEAD

The next section turns to the impact of attention on brain processes. Once you have finished studying this section, you should be able to:

14.2.1 Describe how and why scientists use the electrical activity of the brain to study attention.

14.2.2 Name and describe the main components seen in event-related potentials (ERPs) as they relate to auditory versus visual attention, and particularly compare the auditory N1 effect and the visual P1 effect.

14.2.3 Describe the electrophysiological phenomena associated with visual search tasks.

14.2.4 Describe experimental evidence that selective attention to stimuli enhances neural activity in the brain regions processing the attended stimuli.

Recording electrical activity directly from the neurons of people's brains would be a way to obtain excellent temporal *and* excellent spatial resolution, but of course we can't just stick recording electrodes directly into the brains of healthy participants. Instead, we must find noninvasive ways to assess brain activity.

When many cortical neurons work together on a specific task, their activity becomes synchronized to some degree. You might think this would be easy to see in a standard EEG recording (i.e., an *electroencephalogram*, where the brain's electrical activity is recorded from the scalp, as we described in Chapter 3), but it isn't. Because of variation in the firing of the neurons, not to mention regional differences in the timing of brain activity, a real-time EEG recorded during an attention task looks surprisingly random. So instead, researchers record participants doing a task (**FIGURE 14.6A**) over and over again, and they *average* all the EEGs recorded during those repeated trials (**FIGURE 14.6B**). Over enough trials, the random variation averages out, and what's left is the overall electrical activity specifically associated with task performance (**FIGURE 14.6C**). This averaged activity, called the **event-related potential** (ERP) (Luck, 2005; Helfrich and Knight, 2019), tracks regional changes in brain activity much faster than brain-imaging techniques like fMRI do. For this reason, ERP has become the favorite tool of neuroscientists studying moment-to-moment consequences of attention in the brain.

Distinctive patterns of brain electrical activity mark shifts of attention

Consciously directing your attention to a particular auditory stimulus—for example, shadowing one ear, as we described earlier—has a predictable effect on the ERP. Between about 100 and 150 ms after the onset of a sound stimulus, two large waves are seen in the ERP from the auditory cortex: an initial positive-going wave called *P1*, immediately followed by a larger negative-going wave called *N1* (see Figure 14.6C). The N1 wave reflects an important aspect of auditory attention: it is much larger following a stimulus that is being attended to than it is for the very same stimulus presented at the same ear but *not* attended to (Hillyard et al., 1973). Because the only thing that changes between conditions is the participants' attention to the stimuli, this **auditory N1 effect** must be a result of selective attention somehow acting on neural mechanisms to enhance processing of that particular sound. Auditory attention may also affect much later ERP components, such as the wave called *P3* (or *auditory P300*) (see Figure 14.6C). Changes in late-occurring components like P3 are tricky to interpret, because they can be associated with multiple different cognitive operations, ranging from memory access to reactions to unexpected events (Wessel and Aron, 2017). Nevertheless, some researchers believe that P3 is

event-related potential (ERP) Also called *evoked potential*. Averaged EEG recordings measuring brain responses to repeated presentations of a stimulus. Components of the ERP tend to be reliable because the background noise of the cortex has been averaged out.

auditory N1 effect A negative deflection of the event-related potential, occurring about 100 milliseconds after stimulus presentation, that is enhanced for selectively attended auditory input compared with ignored input.

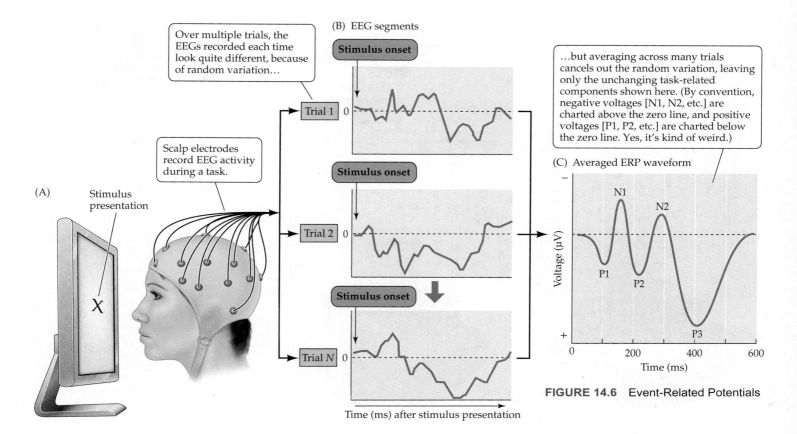

(B) EEG segments

Over multiple trials, the EEGs recorded each time look quite different, because of random variation…

Scalp electrodes record EEG activity during a task.

(A)

Stimulus presentation

Stimulus onset
Trial 1   0

Stimulus onset
Trial 2   0

Stimulus onset
Trial N   0

Time (ms) after stimulus presentation

…but averaging across many trials cancels out the random variation, leaving only the unchanging task-related components shown here. (By convention, negative voltages [N1, N2, etc.] are charted above the zero line, and positive voltages [P1, P2, etc.] are charted below the zero line. Yes, it's kind of weird.)

(C) Averaged ERP waveform

N1
N2
P1
P2
P3

Voltage (µV)

0   200   400   600
Time (ms)

FIGURE 14.6 Event-Related Potentials

especially sensitive to higher-order cognitive processing of the stimulus (Herrmann and Knight, 2001)—qualities like the underlying meaning of the stimulus, identity of the speaker, and so on—in which case the **P3 effect** provides an example of a late-selection effect of attention. Researchers are debating whether P3 therefore is (Dehaene and Changeux, 2011) or is not (Pitts et al., 2014) an electrophysiological marker of consciousness.

What about effects of attention on ERPs from *visual* stimuli? Because the neural systems involved in visual perception are different from those involved in audition, voluntary visual attention causes its own distinctive changes in the ERP. We can study these visual effects by collecting ERP data over occipital cortex—the primary visual area of the brain—while a participant performs a symbolic cuing task. **FIGURE 14.7** depicts this sort of experiment. On valid trials (remember, this is when the target appears as expected, in the location indicated by the cue, as in Figure 14.7A), electrodes over occipital cortex show a substantial enhancement of the ERP component P1, the positive wave that occurs about 70–100 ms after stimulus onset, often carrying over into an enhancement of the N1 component immediately afterward (**FIGURE 14.7C**). A similar effect on P1 is evident when attention is instead oriented *reflexively* to a flash or sound (Hopfinger and Mangun, 1998; McDonald et al., 2005), but only when the interval between the cue and the appearance of the target is brief. At longer intervals, the P1 effect may actually be *reduced* as an electrophysiological manifestation of the inhibition of return (McDonald et al., 1999) we discussed earlier. And for invalid trials (**FIGURE 14.7B**), where attention is being directed elsewhere, the **visual P1 effect** isn't evident at all, even though the visual stimulus is identical and in the same location as in the validly cued trials. Interestingly, the P1 effect is evident only in visual tasks involving manipulations of *spatial* attention (*where* is the target?)—not other features, like color, orientation, or more complex properties that would be characteristic of late-selection tasks.

P3 effect   A positive deflection of the event-related potential, occurring about 300 milliseconds after stimulus presentation, that is associated with higher-order auditory stimulus processing and late attentional selection.

visual P1 effect   A positive deflection of the event-related potential, occurring 70–100 milliseconds after stimulus presentation, that is enhanced for selectively attended visual input compared with ignored input.

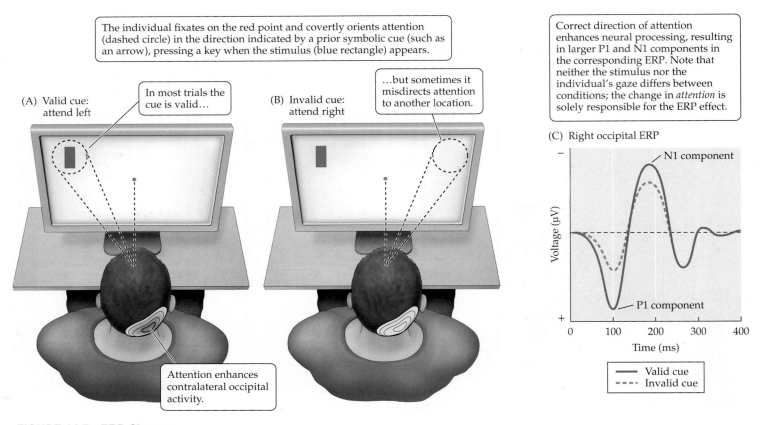

The individual fixates on the red point and covertly orients attention (dashed circle) in the direction indicated by a prior symbolic cue (such as an arrow), pressing a key when the stimulus (blue rectangle) appears.

(A) Valid cue: attend left

In most trials the cue is valid…

…but sometimes it misdirects attention to another location.

(B) Invalid cue: attend right

Attention enhances contralateral occipital activity.

Correct direction of attention enhances neural processing, resulting in larger P1 and N1 components in the corresponding ERP. Note that neither the stimulus nor the individual's gaze differs between conditions; the change in *attention* is solely responsible for the ERP effect.

(C) Right occipital ERP

N1 component

P1 component

Voltage (µV)

Time (ms)

— Valid cue
---- Invalid cue

FIGURE 14.7 ERP Changes in Voluntary Visual Attention

What happens to ERPs during visual search tasks, where we are directing attention so as to find a particular target in an array and ignore distracters? Under these conditions, a subcomponent of N2 (see Figure 14.6), called *N2pc,* is triggered at occipitotemporal sites contralateral to the visual target (Luck and Hillyard, 1994; Hickey et al., 2009).

The neural mechanisms of visual attention may be quite plastic. For example, extensive experience with action video games, which heavily rely on visual attention, is associated with neural changes (S. Tanaka et al., 2013; West et al., 2015) and corresponding enhancements of longer-latency ERP components (Mishra et al., 2011; Palaus et al., 2017). Possible trade-offs for all this gaming, however, may include impaired social and emotional function (no, we're not kidding: K. Bailey and West, 2013). And of course, some people could be drawn to gaming simply because they are already good at visuospatial processing (Boot et al., 2008).

Attention affects the activity of neurons

PET and fMRI operate too slowly to track the rapid changes in brain activity that occur in reaction-time tests. Instead, researchers have used "sustained-attention tasks" to confirm that attention enhances activity in brain regions that process key aspects of the target stimulus. In these experiments, participants are asked to pay close and lasting attention to one particular aspect of a complex stimulus—just the faces in a complex scene, or changes in the pattern of selected dots within an array, for example. Concurrent fMRI generally confirms that attention somehow acts directly on neurons, boosting the activity of those brain regions that process whichever stimulus characteristic has been targeted. So, in these particular examples, enhancement is seen in the cortical *fusiform face area* during attention to faces (O'Craven et al., 1999), or in the subcortical superior colliculus and lateral geniculate (important for spatial processing of visual stimuli) during attention to spatial arrays (Schneider and Kastner, 2009). In general, it seems that directed attention reduces variability and improves the signal-to-noise ratio in neural systems, perhaps by adjusting the influence of individual synapses (Briggs et al., 2013; Sprague et al., 2015).

In Chapter 7 we discussed the distinctive receptive fields of visual neurons and how stimuli falling within these fields can excite or inhibit the neurons, causing them to produce more or fewer action potentials. In an important early study, Moran and Desimone (1985) recorded the activity of individual neurons in visual cortex while attention was shifted *within each cell's receptive field*. Using a system of rewards, the researchers trained monkeys to covertly attend to one spatial location or another while recordings were made from single neurons in visual cortex. A display was presented that included the cell's most preferred stimulus, as well as an ineffective stimulus (one that, by itself, did not affect the cell's firing) a short distance away but still within the cell's receptive field. As long as attention was covertly directed at the preferred stimulus, the cell responded by producing many action potentials (**FIGURE 14.8**). But when the monkey's attention was shifted elsewhere within the cell's receptive field, even though the animal's gaze had not shifted, that same stimulus provoked far fewer action potentials from the neuron. Only the shift in attention could account for this sort of modulation of the cell's excitability. Subsequent work has confirmed that attention can also remold the receptive fields of neurons in a variety of ways (Womelsdorf et al., 2008; Speed et al., 2020).

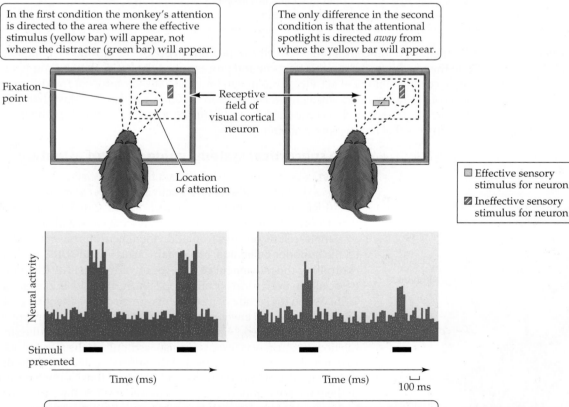

Here, a monkey has been trained to maintain central fixation while directing covert attention. Within the receptive field for the particular cortical neuron being recorded, the area being attended to is shown as a dashed circle.

In the first condition the monkey's attention is directed to the area where the effective stimulus (yellow bar) will appear, not where the distracter (green bar) will appear.

The only difference in the second condition is that the attentional spotlight is directed *away* from where the yellow bar will appear.

Fixation point

Receptive field of visual cortical neuron

Location of attention

□ Effective sensory stimulus for neuron

▨ Ineffective sensory stimulus for neuron

Neural activity

Stimuli presented

Time (ms)

Time (ms)

100 ms

The yellow bar is less effective at firing the cell in the second condition. Because (1) the stimuli are identical in both conditions, (2) the fixation point hasn't changed, and (3) the same cell is being recorded in both conditions, attentional mechanisms must have directly altered the individual neuron's responsiveness.

FIGURE 14.8 Effect of Selective Attention on the Activity of Single Visual Neurons (After J. Moran and R. Desimone, 1985. *Science* 229: 782.)

1. Define *EEG* and *ERP*, and explain how ERPs are measured. Why is the ERP a favored technique in cognitive neuroscience?

2. Match each of the following ERP phenomena—N1, P1, P3, N2pc—with one of these terms: *pop-out*, *early selection*, *auditory attention*, *late selection*, *visual attention*, *distractors*.

3. Describe an experimental procedure that can demonstrate the effects of selective attention on the activity of an individual neuron.

14.3 Sources of Attention: A Network of Brain Sites Creates and Directs Attention

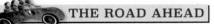 THE ROAD AHEAD

In the section that follows, we turn our attention to the anatomy of attention: the network of cortical and subcortical sites that govern voluntary and reflexive attention. After studying this material, you should be able to:

14.3.1 Discuss the functions of the principal subcortical sites—the superior colliculus and the pulvinar—that are associated with shifts of visual attention.

14.3.2 Summarize the dorsal frontoparietal network that is believed to govern voluntary attention, illustrating this action with examples of research.

14.3.3 Summarize the right temporoparietal network associated with reflexive shifts of attention, and again provide relevant research examples.

14.4.4 Describe some of the most striking forms of attentional disorders and some medical approaches to treat them.

View Activity 14.1:
Subcortical Sites Implicated in Visual Attention

superior colliculus A gray matter structure of the dorsal midbrain that processes visual information and is involved in direction of visual gaze and visual attention to intended stimuli.

Whether attention comes reflexively, from the bottom up, or is controlled voluntarily, from the top down, it strongly affects neural processing in the brain, thereby augmenting electrophysiological activity. That doesn't mean that the *sources* of the different forms of attention are identical, however, or even that they are similar—just that their *consequences* are somewhat comparable. So let's turn to some of the details of the brain mechanisms that are the *source* of attention.

Two subcortical systems guide shifts of attention

Subcortical structures can be difficult to study because, deep in the center of the brain and skull, their activity is harder to measure with EEG/ERP and other noninvasive techniques. Our knowledge of their roles in attention thus comes mostly from work with animals.

Single-cell recordings from individual neurons have implicated the **superior colliculus**, a midbrain structure (**FIGURE 14.9**), in controlling the movement of the eyes toward objects of attention, especially in overt forms of attention (Wurtz et al., 1982; Zhaoping, 2016). When the same eye movements are made but attention is directed elsewhere, a lower rate of firing by the collicular neurons is recorded. And in people with lesions in one superior colliculus, inhibition of return was *reduced* for visual stimuli on the affected side (Sapir et al., 1999). So it seems that the superior colliculus helps direct our gaze to attended objects, and it ensures that we don't return to them too soon after our gaze has moved on. The superior colliculus may also help direct the *covert* attentional spotlight: for example, monkeys in which the superior colliculus has been temporarily inactivated lose the ability to use selective attention cues (arrows, flashes, etc.) until the inactivation ends (Krauzlis et al., 2013).

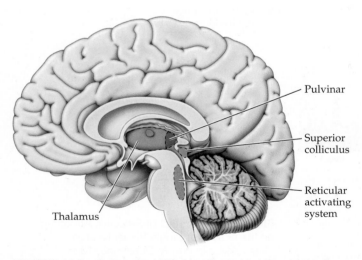

Pulvinar

Superior colliculus

Reticular activating system

Thalamus

FIGURE 14.9 Subcortical Sites Implicated in Visual Attention

The **pulvinar,** making up the posterior quarter of the human thalamus (see Figure 14.9), is heavily involved in visual processing, with widespread interconnections between lower visual pathways, the superior colliculus, and many cortical areas. The pulvinar is important for the orienting and shifting of attention. Monkeys whose pulvinars are inactivated with drugs, and humans with strokes affecting the pulvinar, may have great difficulty orienting *covert* attention toward visual targets (D. L. Robinson and Petersen, 1992; Kraft et al., 2015). The pulvinar is also needed to filter out and ignore distracting stimuli while we're engaged in covert attention tasks, and in general it coordinates activity in larger-scale cortical networks according to attentional demands (Saalman et al., 2012; Green et al., 2017). In humans, attention tasks with larger numbers of distracters induce greater activation of the pulvinar (M. S. Buchsbaum et al., 2006), indicating that this nucleus is also important for human attention.

Several cortical areas are crucial for generating and directing attention

The extensive connections between subcortical mechanisms of attention and the parietal lobes, along with observations from clinical cases that we will discuss shortly, point to a special role of the parietal lobes for attention control. Two integrated networks—dorsal frontoparietal and right temporoparietal—work together to continually select and shift between objects of interest, in coordination with subcortical mechanisms of attention.

A DORSAL FRONTOPARIETAL NETWORK FOR VOLUNTARY (TOP-DOWN) CONTROL OF ATTENTION   In monkeys, recordings from single cells show that a region called the **lateral intraparietal area**, or just **LIP**, is crucial for voluntary attention. LIP neurons increase their firing rate when attention—*not gaze*—is directed to particular locations, and it doesn't matter whether the voluntary attention is being directed toward visual or auditory targets (Bisley and Goldberg, 2003; Gottlieb, 2007). So it's the top-down steering of the attentional spotlight that is important to LIP neurons, not the sensory characteristics of the stimuli.

The human equivalent of this system is a region around the **intraparietal sulcus** (**IPS**) (**FIGURE 14.10**) that behaves much like the monkey LIP. For example, on tasks designed so that covert attention can be sustained long enough to make fMRI images, IPS activity is enhanced while participants are actively steering their attention (Corbetta and Shulman, 1998). And when researchers used transcranial magnetic stimulation (see Chapter 2) to temporarily inhibit the functioning of the IPS, the research participants found it difficult to voluntarily shift attention (Koch et al., 2005).

People with damage to a frontal lobe region called the **frontal eye field** (**FEF**) (see Figure 14.10) struggle to prevent their gaze from being drawn away toward peripheral distracters while they're performing a voluntary attention task (Paus et al., 1991). Neurons of the FEF appear to be crucial for ensuring that our gaze is directed among stimuli according to cognitive goals rather than eye-catching characteristics of the stimuli. In effect, the FEF ensures that cognitively controlled top-down attention gets priority. It's no surprise, then, that the FEF is closely connected to the superior colliculus, which, as we discussed earlier, is important for planned eye movements.

View Activity 14.2:
Cortical Regions Implicated in the Top-Level Control of Attention

pulvinar   In humans, the posterior portion of the thalamus. It is heavily involved in visual processing and direction of attention.

lateral intraparietal area (LIP)
A region in the monkey parietal lobe, homologous to the human intraparietal sulcus, that is especially involved in voluntary, top-down control of attention.

intraparietal sulcus (IPS)   A region in the human parietal lobe, homologous to the monkey lateral intraparietal area, that is especially involved in voluntary, top-down control of attention.

frontal eye field (FEF)   An area in the frontal lobe of the brain that contains neurons important for establishing gaze in accordance with cognitive goals (top-down processes) rather than with any characteristics of stimuli (bottom-up processes).

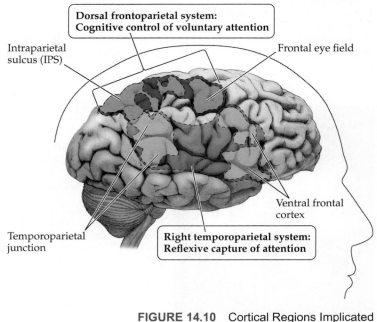

FIGURE 14.10   Cortical Regions Implicated in the Top-Level Control of Attention

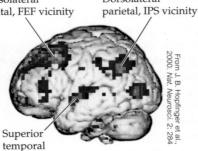

Dorsolateral
frontal, FEF vicinity

Dorsolateral
parietal, IPS vicinity

From J. B. Hopfinger et al.,
2000. *Nat. Neurosci. 2*: 284.

During conscious shifts of
covert attention, ER-fMRI
shows activation of the
frontal eye field and the
intraparietal sulcus (along
with some activation of
the temporal lobe).

Superior
temporal

FIGURE 14.11   The Frontoparietal Attention Network

A modified form of fMRI that links rapid behavioral events to changes in activity of selected brain regions (called, unsurprisingly, *event-related fMRI*, or *ER-fMRI*) reveals network activities during top-down attentional processing (Hopfinger et al., 2000, 2010). **FIGURE 14.11** shows patterns of activation while voluntary attention is shifting in response to a symbolic cue. Enhanced activity is evident in the vicinity of the frontal eye fields (dorsolateral frontal cortex) and, simultaneously, in the IPS. Electrophysiological studies of the timing of activity in the network indicate that the attentional control–related activity is first seen in the frontal and parietal components, followed by anticipatory activation of visual cortex (if the expected stimulus is visual) or auditory cortex (if the stimulus is a sound) (McDonald and Green, 2008; Green et al., 2011). Taken together, these studies support the view that a dorsal frontoparietal network provides top-down (voluntary) control of attention.

A RIGHT TEMPOROPARIETAL NETWORK FOR REFLEXIVE (BOTTOM-UP) SHIFTS OF ATTENTION   A second attention system, located at the border of the temporal and parietal lobes of the right hemisphere—and named, a little unimaginatively, the **temporoparietal junction** (**TPJ**) (see Figure 14.10)—is involved in reflexive steering of attention toward novel or unexpected stimuli (flashes, color changes, and so on). ER-fMRI studies (**FIGURE 14.12**) confirm that there's a spike in right-hemisphere TPJ activity if a relevant stimulus suddenly appears in an unexpected location (Corbetta and Shulman, 2002; Igelström and Graziano, 2017). Interestingly, the TPJ system receives direct input from the visual cortex, presumably providing direct access for information about visual stimuli. The TPJ also has strong connections with the ventral frontal cortex, a region that is involved in working memory (see Chapter 13). Because working memory tracks sensory inputs over short time frames, this system may specialize in analyzing *novelty* by comparing present stimuli with those of the recent past. Overall, the ventral TPJ system seems to act as an alerting signal, or "circuit breaker," overriding our current attentional priority if something new and unexpected happens.

Ultimately, the dorsal and ventral attention-control networks need to interact extensively and function as a single interactive system. According to one influential model (Corbetta and Shulman, 2002), the more dorsal stream of processing is responsible for *voluntary* attention, enhancing neural processing of stimuli and interacting with the pulvinar and superior colliculus to steer the attentional spotlight around. At the same time, the right-sided temporoparietal system scans the environment for novel salient stimuli (which then draw *reflexive* attention), rapidly reassigning attention as interesting stimuli pop up. This basic model seems to apply across sensory modalities, including both visual and auditory stimuli (Brunetti et al., 2008; Walther et al., 2010).

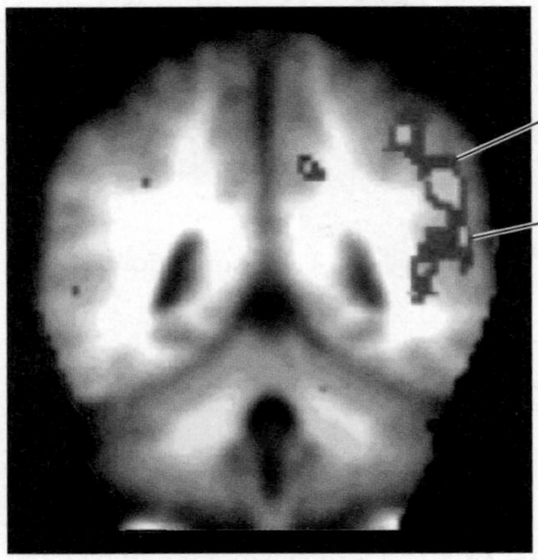

temporoparietal junction (TPJ)
The point in the brain where the temporal
and parietal lobes meet. It plays a role in
shifting attention to a new location after
target onset.

Brain disorders can cause specific impairments of attention

One way to learn about attention systems in the brain is to carefully analyze the behavioral consequences of damage to specific regions of the brain. Research on people with attentional disorders shows that damage of cortical or subcortical attention mechanisms can dramatically alter our ability to understand and interact with the environment.

Left   Right

From M. Corbetta et al., 2000. *Nat. Neurosci. 3*: 292

Intraparietal sulcus (IPS)

Temporoparietal junction (TPJ)

When attention is captured
by the sudden appearance
of stimuli (exogenous
attention), activity is
evident in this right-
hemisphere system.

FIGURE 14.12   The Right Temporoparietal System
for Reflexive Attention

RIGHT-HEMISPHERE LESIONS   We've discussed evidence that the right hemisphere normally plays a special role in attention (see Figure 14.12). Unfortunately, it is not uncommon for people to suffer strokes or other types of brain damage that particularly affect this part of the brain. The result—**hemispatial neglect**—is an extraordinary attention syndrome in which the person tends to completely disregard the left side of the world. People and objects to the left of the person's midline may be completely ignored, as if unseen, even though the person's vision is otherwise normal (Rafal, 1994). Someone with neglect may fail to dress the left side of their body, will not notice visitors if they approach from the left, and may fail to eat the food on the left side of their dinner plate. If touched lightly on both hands at the same moment, the person may notice only the right-hand touch—a symptom called *simultaneous extinction*. They may even deny ownership of their left arm or leg—"My sister must've left that arm in my bed; wasn't that an awful thing to do?!"—despite normal sensory function and otherwise intact intellectual capabilities.

It is as if the normally balanced competition for attention between the two sides has become skewed and now the input from the right side of the world overrules or extinguishes the input from the left. Lesions in people with hemispatial neglect (**FIGURE 14.13A**) neatly overlap the frontoparietal attention network that we discussed earlier (shown again in **FIGURE 14.13B**). This overlap suggests that hemispatial neglect is a disorder of attention itself, and not a problem with processing spatial relationships, as was once thought (Mesulam, 1985; Bartolomeo, 2007). With time, hemispatial neglect can significantly improve (although simultaneous extinction often persists), and targeted therapies may help. For example, researchers are experimenting with the use of special prism glasses to shift vision to the right during intense physical therapy, in order to recalibrate the visual attention system (Barrett et al., 2012; O'Shea et al., 2017).

BILATERAL LESIONS Parminder, whom we met at the beginning of the chapter, had *bilateral* lesions of the parietal lobe regions that are implicated in the attention network. While rare, biparietal damage can result in a dramatic disorder called **Balint's syndrome**, made up of three principal symptoms. First, people with Balint's syndrome have great difficulty steering their visual gaze appropriately (a symptom called *oculomotor apraxia*). Second, they are unable to accurately reach for objects using visual guidance (*optic ataxia*). And third—the most striking symptom—people with Balint's syndrome show a profound restriction of attention, to the point that only one object or feature can be consciously observed at any moment. This problem, called **simultagnosia**, can be likened to an extreme narrowing of the attentional spotlight, to the point that it can't encompass more than one object at a time. Hold up a comb or a pencil, and Parminder has no trouble identifying the object. But hold up both the comb *and* the pencil, and she can identify only one or the other. It's as though she is simply unable to consciously

Model | Patient's version

Diagnostic Test for Hemispatial Neglect
When asked to duplicate drawings of common symmetrical objects, people with hemispatial neglect ignore the left side of the model that they're copying. (After V. W. Mark. 2003. *Front. Biosci.* 8: e172.)

hemispatial neglect   Failure to pay any attention to objects presented to one side of the body.

Balint's syndrome   A disorder, caused by damage to both parietal lobes, that is characterized by difficulty in steering visual gaze (oculomotor apraxia), in accurately reaching for objects using visual guidance (optic ataxia), and in directing attention to more than one object or feature at a time (simultagnosia).

simultagnosia   A profound restriction of attention, often limited to a single item or feature.

(A) Critical areas damaged in hemispatial neglect

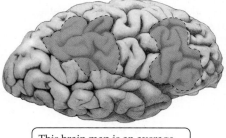

This brain map is an average of the lesions of several people with hemispatial neglect.

(B) Model of cortical attention control network

Intraparietal sulcus (IPS)   Frontal eye field   Ventral frontal cortex

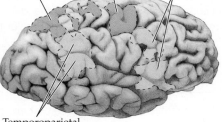

Temporoparietal junction

Note how the hemispatial-neglect lesions overlap with the proposed attentional networks discussed in the text and shown here.

FIGURE 14.13   Brain Damage in Hemispatial Neglect

experience more than one external feature at a time, despite having little or no loss of vision. Balint's syndrome thus illustrates the coordination of attention and awareness with mechanisms that orient us within our environment.

SIGNS & SYMPTOMS

Difficulty with Sustained Attention Can Sometimes Be Relieved with Stimulants

At least 5% of all children are diagnosed with **attention deficit hyperactivity disorder** (**ADHD**), characterized as difficulty with directing sustained attention to a task or activity, along with a higher degree of impulsivity than in other children of the same age. About three-fourths of those diagnosed are male. Estimating the prevalence of ADHD (**FIGURE 14.14**) is complicated and very controversial; for example, there is significant variation in ADHD diagnosis and medication between different (sometimes neighboring) states within the USA, raising questions about the reliability of current diagnostic practices (Fulton et al., 2009). Nevertheless, researchers have identified several neurological changes associated with this disorder. Affected children tend to have slightly reduced overall brain volumes (about 3–4% smaller than in unaffected children), with reductions especially evident in the cerebellum and the frontal lobes (Arnsten, 2006). As we discuss elsewhere in the chapter, frontal lobe function is important for myriad complex cognitive processes, including the inhibition of impulsive behavior, as we will discuss below. (But remember, correlational studies like these are mute with regard to causation; we don't know whether the brain differences cause, or are caused by, the behavior.)

In addition to structural changes, ADHD has been associated with abnormalities in connectivity between brain regions, such as within the default mode network, a neural system implicated in conscious reflection that we will discuss shortly (Cao et al., 2014). In fact, individual differences in the ability to sustain attention can be predicted with high accuracy from the strength of sets of brain connections (Rosenberg et al., 2016, 2017), even in the resting state, when the individual is not working on any particular task. Children with ADHD may have abnormal activity levels in some specific brain systems, such as the system that signals the rewarding aspects of activities (Furukawa et al., 2014). Based on a model of ADHD that implicates impairments in dopamine and norepinephrine neurotransmission, some researchers advocate treating these children with stimulant drugs like methylphenidate (Ritalin), which inhibits the synaptic reuptake of dopamine and norepinephrine, or with selective norepinephrine reuptake inhibitors

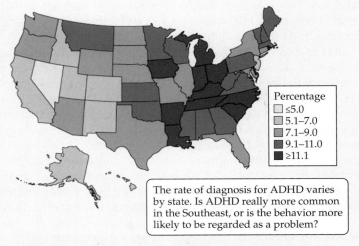

> The rate of diagnosis for ADHD varies by state. Is ADHD really more common in the Southeast, or is the behavior more likely to be regarded as a problem?

FIGURE 14.14   Prevalence of ADHD in the United States (After S. N. Visser et al., 2014. *J. Am. Acad. Child Adolesc. Psychiatry* 53: 34.)

Percentage
- ≤5.0
- 5.1–7.0
- 7.1–9.0
- 9.1–11.0
- ≥11.1

like atomexetine (Strattera) (Schwartz and Correll, 2014). Stimulant treatment often improves the focus and performance of children with ADHD within traditional school settings, but this treatment remains controversial because of the significant risk of side effects. Furthermore, stimulants improve focus in everybody, not just people with ADHD, which raises doubts about the orthodox view that impaired neurotransmission is the sole cause of ADHD (del Campo et al., 2013). An emerging alternative view is that what is diagnosed as ADHD may simply be an extreme on a continuum of normal behavior. Allowing kids diagnosed with ADHD to fidget and engage in more intense physical activity effectively reduces their symptoms and improves task performance (Hartanto et al., 2016; Den Heijer et al., 2017). You can read more about ADHD and another developmental disorder—autism spectrum disorder—in A Step Further 13.4, on the website.

---

attention deficit hyperactivity disorder (ADHD)   A syndrome characterized by distractibility, impulsiveness, and hyperactivity that, in children, interferes with school performance.

HOW'S IT GOING ?

1. Identify two subcortical structures that are implicated in the control of attention. What functions do they perform?
2. What is the general name for the cortical system responsible for conscious shifts of attention? What are its components, and what happens when those components are damaged?
3. Name the cortical system implicated in reflexive shifts of attention. Which specific regions are part of this system, and what happens if they are damaged?

14.4 Consciousness, Thought, and Decision Making Are Mysterious Products of the Brain

THE ROAD AHEAD

The final part of the chapter looks at the most enigmatic, top-level product of the brain—consciousness—and its relationships with attention, reflection, and the executive processes that direct thoughts and feelings. After reading this section, you should be able to:

14.4.1 Provide a reasonable definition of consciousness, and name the neural networks and structures that, when activated, may play a special role in coordinating conscious states.

14.4.2 Discuss the relationship between consciousness as experienced by healthy people and the diminished levels of consciousness experienced by people in comas and minimally conscious states.

14.4.3 Discuss the impediments to the scientific study of consciousness, distinguishing between the "easy" and "hard" problems of consciousness, and how free will relates to the study of consciousness.

14.4.4 Provide an overview of the organization and function of the frontal lobes, and especially prefrontal cortex, as they relate to high-level cognition and executive functions.

There can be no denying the close relationship between attention and consciousness; indeed, attention is the foundation on which consciousness is built. Whenever we are conscious, we're attending to *something*, be it internal or external. William James (1890) tried to capture the relationship between attention and consciousness when he wrote, "My experience is what I agree to attend to. Only those items which I notice shape my mind—without selective interest, experience is an utter chaos." We all experience consciousness, so we know what it is, but that experience is so personal, so subjective, that it's difficult to come up with an objective definition. Perhaps a reasonable attempt is to say that **consciousness** is the state of being *aware* that we are conscious and that we can perceive what's going on in our minds and all around us. However, "what's going on in our minds and all around us" covers an awful lot of ground. It includes our perception of time passing, our sense of being aware, our recollection of events that happened in the past, and our imaginings about what might happen in the future. Add to that our belief that we employ free will to direct our attention and make decisions, and we have a concept of immense scope.

Which brain regions are active when we are conscious?

Despite definitional complexities, consciousness is an active area of neuroscience research. So far, there are numerous competing theoretical models of consciousness, and a growing body of neuroscientific data. One approach is to look for patterns of synchronized activity in neural networks as people engage in conscious, inwardly focused thought. Using fMRI, researchers have identified a large circuit of brain regions—collectively called the **default mode network**, consisting of parts of the frontal, temporal, and parietal lobes—that seems to be selectively activated when we are at our most introspective and reflective, and relatively deactivated during behavior directed toward external goals (Raichle, 2015). In some ways you could think of it as a daydream network (and thereby also engage in metacognition: see Table 14.1). It has been proposed that dysfunction within the default mode network contributes to the symptoms of various cognitive problems, such as ADHD, autism spectrum disorder, schizophrenia, and dementia, in both adults and children (Whitfield-Gabrieli and Ford, 2012; Sato et al., 2015). Monkeys and lab rats have circuits that resemble the human default mode network on structural and functional grounds, raising the possibility that some nonhuman species may likewise engage in self-reflection or other introspective mental activity (Mantini et al., 2011; Sierakowiak et al., 2015). Some of the basic elements of human consciousness that researchers agree on are identified in **TABLE 14.1**, which also lists other species that may have comparable capacities and experiences.

consciousness   The state of awareness of one's own existence, thoughts, emotions, and experiences.

default mode network   A circuit of brain regions that is active during quiet introspective thought.

TABLE 14.1 Elements of Consciousness in Humans and Other Animals

Element	Definition	Other species
Theory of mind	Insight into the mental lives of others; understanding that other individuals act on their own unique beliefs, knowledge, and desires	Only chimpanzees, so far
Mirror recognition	Ability to recognize the self as depicted in a mirror	All great apes; dolphins; magpies; some elephants
Imitation	Ability to copy the actions of others; thought to be a stepping-stone to awareness and empathy	Many species, including cephalopods like the octopus
Empathy and emotion	Possession of complex emotions and the ability to imagine the feelings of other individuals	Most mammals, ranging from primates and dolphins, to hippos and rodents; most vertebrates able to experience pleasure (and other basic emotions)
Tool use	Ability to employ found objects to achieve intermediate and/or ultimate goals	Chimps and other primates; other mammals such as elephants, otters, and dolphins; birds such as crows and gulls
Language	Use of a system of arbitrary symbols, with specific meanings and strict grammar, to convey concrete or abstract information to any other individual that has learned the same language	Generally considered to be an exclusively human ability, with controversy over the extent to which the great apes can acquire language skills
Metacognition	"Thinking about thinking": the ability to consider the contents of one's own thoughts and cognitions	Nonhuman primates; dolphins

A practical alternative approach has been to study consciousness by focusing on people who lack it—people in comas or other states of reduced consciousness. Maps of brain activity in such people—or more precisely, maps of *deactivated* areas (Tsuchiya and Adolphs, 2007)—suggest that consciousness depends on a specific frontoparietal network (**FIGURE 14.15**) that includes much of the cortical attention network we've

These fMRI studies range from the temporary unconsciousness we all experience (sleep) to the profound and long-lasting unconsciousness of a persistent vegetative state. They share reduced activity of a frontoparietal network that includes dorsolateral prefrontal cortex (F), medial frontal cortex (MF), posterior parietal cortex (P), and posterior cingulate (Pr).

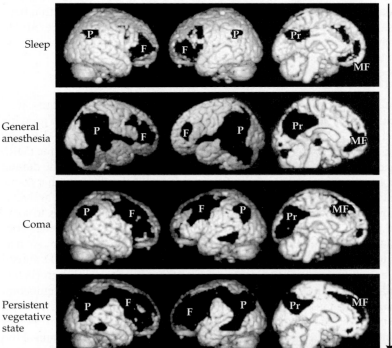

Sleep

General anesthesia

Deeper degrees of unconsciousness

Coma

Persistent vegetative state

FIGURE 14.15 The Unconscious Brain

From B. J. Baars et al., 2003. *Trends Neurosci.* 26: 671

been discussing, along with regions of medial frontal and cingulate cortices. Some researchers suspect that the *claustrum* (**FIGURE 14.16**)—a slender sheet of neurons buried within the white matter of the forebrain lateral to the basal ganglia—plays a critical role in generating the experience of being conscious (Crick and Koch, 2005; S. P. Brown et al., 2017), by virtue of its remarkable reciprocal connections with virtually every area of cortex, and especially prefrontal cortex. In one case, a woman with a stimulating electrode in the claustrum experienced a "switching off" of conscious awareness whenever a strong stimulation pulse was delivered through the electrode (Koubeissi et al., 2014); in another case, consciousness was interrupted by bilateral electrical stimulation in lateral frontal cortex (Quraishi et al., 2017), perhaps as a result of disrupting activity in complex networks associated with consciousness.

But is clinical unconsciousness really the inverse of consciousness? Perhaps it's not that simple. For one thing, some people in a *persistent vegetative state* (a very deep coma) can be instructed to use two different forms of mental imagery to create distinct "yes" and "no" patterns of activity on fMRI and then to use this mental activity to answer questions (**FIGURE 14.17**) (Monti et al., 2010; Fernández-Espejo and Owen, 2013).

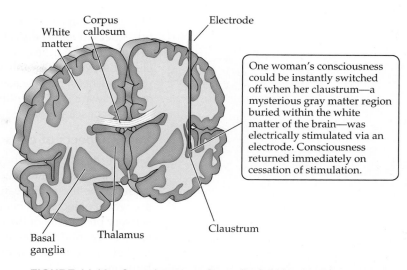

One woman's consciousness could be instantly switched off when her claustrum—a mysterious gray matter region buried within the white matter of the brain—was electrically stimulated via an electrode. Consciousness returned immediately on cessation of stimulation.

FIGURE 14.16   Consciousness Controller? (After M. Z. Koubeissi et al., 2014. *Epilepsy Behav.* 37: 32.)

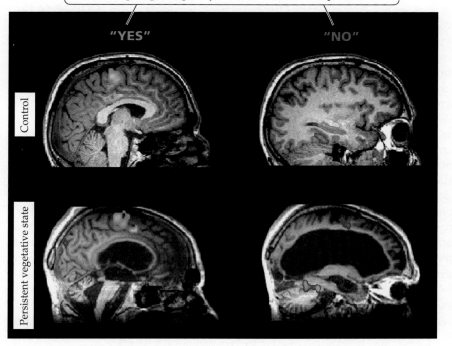

Functional MRI shows the brain activity of a healthy control participant asked to use two different mental images (playing tennis versus navigating) to signal "yes" or "no" answers to questions.

The strikingly similar brain activity of a person in a persistent vegetative state raises questions about the definition of unconsciousness. The person was able to correctly answer a variety of questions using this technique, despite being in a state of apparently deep unconsciousness due to profound brain damage (as evident in the grossly abnormal MRI scan) and lacking behavioral responses.

FIGURE 14.17   Communication in "Unconscious" People (After M. M. Monti et al., 2010. *NEJM* 362: 579.)

Most people in a vegetative state don't respond to questions and outside stimulation, but others in *minimally conscious states* may have considerable cognitive activity and awareness with little or no overt behavior (Gosseries et al., 2014). So, it's increasingly clear that we can't simply view a coma as an exact inverse of what we experience as consciousness. In any case, there seems to be more to consciousness than just being awake, aware, and attending. How can we identify and study the additional dimensions of consciousness?

Some aspects of consciousness are easier to study than others

Most of the activity of the central nervous system is unconscious. Scientists call unconscious brain functions **cognitively impenetrable**: they involve basic neural processing operations that cannot be experienced through introspection. For example, we see whole objects and hear whole words and can't really imagine what the primitive sensory precursors of those perceptions would feel like. Sweet food tastes sweet, and we can't mentally break it down any further. But those simpler mechanisms, operating below the surface of awareness, are the foundation that conscious experiences are built on.

In principle, then, we might someday develop technology that would let us directly reconstruct people's conscious experience—read their minds—by decoding the primitive neural activity and assembling identifiable patterns from it. This is sometimes called the **easy problem of consciousness**: understanding how particular patterns of neural activity create *specific* conscious experiences. Of course, it's almost a joke to call this problem "easy," but at least we can fairly say that, someday, the necessary technology and knowledge may be available to accomplish the task of eavesdropping on large networks of neurons, in real time.

Present-day technology offers a glimpse of that possible future. For example, if participants are repeatedly scanned while viewing several distinctive scenes, a computer can eventually learn to identify which of the scenes the participant is viewing on each trial, solely on the basis of the pattern of brain activation (**FIGURE 14.18A**) (Kay et al., 2008). Of course, this outcome relies on having the participants repeatedly view the same static images—hardly a normal state of consciousness. A much more complex problem is to reconstruct conscious experience from neural activity during a person's first exposure to a stimulus. So far, this has been accomplished for only relatively simple visual stimuli (**FIGURE 14.18B**) (Miyawaki et al., 2008) or brief video reconstructions (Nishimoto and Gallant, 2011). But it's a good start, and rapid progress seems likely as technological problems are solved.

Alas, there is also the **hard problem of consciousness**, and it may prove impossible to crack. How can we understand the brain processes that produce people's *subjective experiences* of their conscious perceptions? To use a simple example, everyone with normal vision will agree that a ripe tomato is "red." That's the label that children all learn to apply to the particular pattern of information, entering consciousness from the color-processing areas of visual cortex, that is provoked by looking at something like a tomato. But that doesn't mean that your friend's internal *personal* experience of "red" is the same as yours. These purely subjective experiences of perceptions are referred to as **qualia** (singular *quale*). Because they are subjective and impossible to communicate to others—how can your friend know if "redness" feels the same in your mind as it does in hers?—qualia may prove impossible to study (**FIGURE 14.18C**). At this point, anyway, we are unable to even conceive of a technology that would make it possible.

Our subjective experience of consciousness is closely tied up with the notion of **free will**: the belief that our conscious self is unconstrained in deciding our actions and decisions and that for any given moment, given exactly the same circumstances, we *could* have chosen to engage in a different behavior. After centuries of argument, there's still no agreement on whether we actually have free will, but most people behave as though there are always options, and in any event, there must be a neural substrate for the universal *feeling* of having free will. When participants *intend* to act (push a

**See Video 14.5:
Reconstructing Brain Activity**

cognitively impenetrable   Referring to basic neural processing operations that cannot be experienced through introspection—in other words, that are unconscious.

easy problem of consciousness   Understanding how particular patterns of neural activity create specific conscious experiences by reading brain activity directly from people's brains as they're having particular experiences.

hard problem of consciousness   Understanding the brain processes that produce people's subjective experiences of their conscious perceptions—that is, their qualia.

quale   A purely subjective experience of perception.

free will   The feeling that our conscious self is the author of our actions and decisions.

(A) Pattern identification

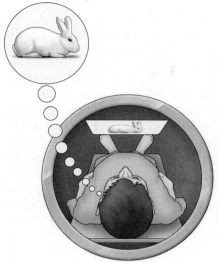

FIGURE 14.18 Easy and Hard Problems of Consciousness (Part A after K. N. Kay et al., 2008. *Nature* 452: 352; B after Y. Miyawaki et al., 2008. *Neuron* 60: 915.)

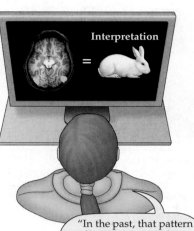

Interpretation

"In the past, that pattern of brain activity only appeared when he was looking at the rabbit."

For a person in a brain scanner, repeatedly viewing the same image causes the same pattern of brain activity to occur each time. Over enough trials, researchers can develop computer models that identify which of about 20 images the participant is looking at.

(B) Visual reconstruction

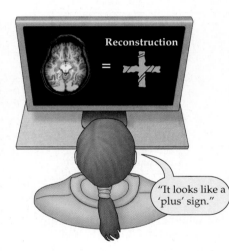

Reconstruction

"It looks like a 'plus' sign."

Scientists also know enough about how different parts of the brain are activated by light striking the retina that they can even predict what type of simple shapes a person is viewing.

(C) Subjective experience

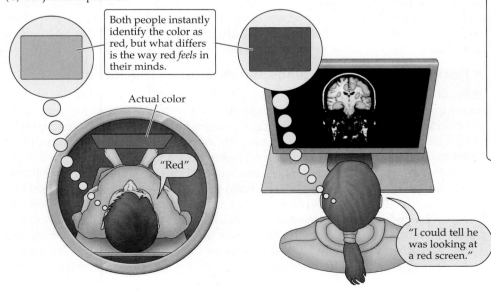

Both people instantly identify the color as red, but what differs is the way red *feels* in their minds.

Actual color

"Red"

"I could tell he was looking at a red screen."

The "hard" problem is to go beyond predicting what a person is seeing to knowing what that person's *subjective experience* is like. Here, the participant and the researcher would both immediately identify the color being viewed as "red" but, as suggested by their respective thought bubbles, the participant's personal, internal, *subjective* experience may be quite different from that of the researcher. It is difficult to see how we could ever be sure that we share any subjective experiences of consciousness.

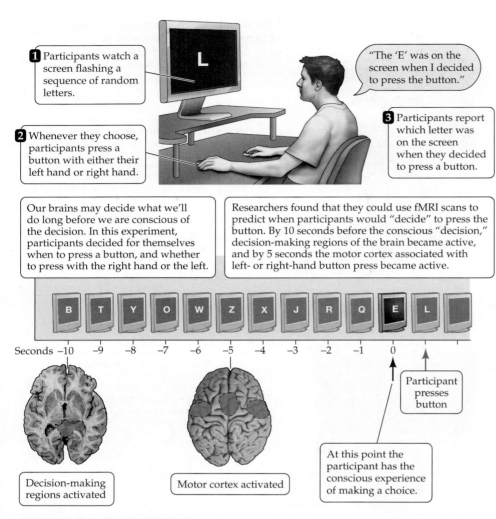

FIGURE 14.19 Reading the Future (After C. S. Soon et al., 2008. *Nat. Neurosci.* 11: 543.)

button, say), there is selective activation of the IPS (which we implicated earlier in top-down attention) and frontal regions including dorsal prefrontal cortex (Lau et al., 2004), suggesting that these regions are important for our feelings of control over our behavior. However, the conscious experience of intention may come relatively late in the process of deciding what to do. Early research (Libet, 1985), using EEG and a precise timer, found that an EEG component signaling movement preparation was evident 200 ms before participants consciously decided to move. Although controversy initially surrounded this work, later confirmatory research using fMRI (Soon et al., 2008; **FIGURE 14.19**) found, astonishingly, that brain activity associated with making a decision was evident in fMRI scans as much as 5–10 seconds *before* participants were consciously aware of making a choice!

These results are sometimes interpreted as meaning we have no free will, if our brain decides to push a button before our conscious self has decided. But remember, even if you are not aware that your brain has decided to push the left button, it was still *your brain* that made that decision, not someone else's brain. The conscious you may be a Johnny-come-lately in the decision-making process, but that doesn't tell us whether your brain was truly free to choose the left button rather than the right, or to take the blue pill or the red.

In any event, the earliest indications of the decision-making process are found in prefrontal cortex. Such involvement of prefrontal systems in most aspects of attention and consciousness, regardless of sensory modality or emotional tone, suggests that the prefrontal cortex is the main source of goal-driven behaviors (E. K. Miller and Cohen, 2001; Badre and Nee, 2018), as we discuss next.

A flexible frontal system plans and monitors our behavior

How do we translate our inner thoughts into behavior? Careful analysis of impairments in people with localized brain damage, along with functional imaging studies in healthy people, shows that a network of anterior forebrain sites dominated by the frontal lobes—but including several other cortical and subcortical sites—is crucial for **executive function**, the suite of high-level cognitive processes that control and organize lower-level cognitive functions in line with our thoughts and feelings (Alvarez and Emory, 2006; Yuan and Raz, 2014). Some scientists liken executive function to a "supervisory system" that analyzes important stimuli, weighs competing ideas and hypotheses, and governs the creation of suitable "plans" for future action by drawing on cognitive processes like working memory, attention, feedback utilization, and so on. Executive function involves at least three interrelated processes: (1) smooth *task switching* between different cognitive operations, (2) continual *updating* of the

executive function A neural and cognitive system that helps develop plans of action and organizes the activities of other high-level processing systems.

prefrontal cortex The most anterior region of the frontal lobe.

TABLE 14.2 Tests of Executive Functions

Test name	Procedure	Scoring	Functions sampled
Wisconsin Card Sorting Test (WCST) (Weigl, 1941; Heaton et al., 1993)	Sort cards into piles on the basis of the number, color, or shape of symbols on card face. Every 10 cards, discover and shift to a new sorting rule (see Figure 14.21).	Errors in sorting; perseveration in old sorting rule after rule change	Task switching and abstract reasoning
Controlled Oral Word Association Test (COWAT) (Benton and Hamsher, 1976)	Say as many words as possible that start with a specific letter (*F*, *A*, or *S*), in 60 seconds.	Total number of unique words uttered for all three starting letters	Verbal fluency, updating, working memory
Stroop Test of Color-Word Interference (Stroop, 1935; MacLeod, 1991)	Read aloud as quickly as possible color names that are printed in the congruent color (e.g., **BLUE**) or incongruent color (e.g., **BLUE**).	Time and total errors	Response inhibition

cognitive plan based on new information and the contents of working memory, and (3) timely *inhibition* of responses that would compromise the plan (A. Diamond, 2013). A closely related account proposes that the crucial function of the frontal network is *hierarchical cognitive control*: the ability to direct shorter-term actions while simultaneously keeping longer-term goals in mind (Koechlin et al., 2003; Badre and Nee, 2018). Accordingly, a person with executive dysfunction due to frontal lesions who is given a simple set of errands may be unable to complete them without numerous false starts, backtracking, and confusion (Shallice and Burgess, 1991; Rabinovici et al., 2019). Several of the most widely studied tests of executive functions are described in **TABLE 14.2**.

We have touched on some frontal lobe functions in earlier chapters—things like movement control, memory, language, psychopathology—but this mass of cortex also underlies other, more mysterious intellectual characteristics. Perhaps it reflects a bit of vanity about our species, but the large size of our frontal lobes— about one-third of the entire cortical surface (**FIGURE 14.20A**)—also led to the long-standing view that the frontal cortex is the seat of intelligence and abstract thinking. The remarkable story of Phineas Gage, one of the most famous case studies in the history of neurology, underscores the subtlety and complexity of behaviors governed by the frontal lobes. Like Gage, people with discrete prefrontal lesions express various unusual emotional, motor, and cognitive changes. Widespread frontal damage may be associated with a persistent strange apathy, broken by bouts of euphoria (an exalted sense of well-being). Ordinary social conventions are readily cast aside by impulsive behavior. Concern for the past or the future may be absent (Petrides and Milner, 1982; Duffy and Campbell, 1994). Forgetfulness is shown in many tasks requiring sustained attention. In fact, some people with frontal damage even forget their own warnings to "remember." However, standard IQ test performance often shows only slight changes after prefrontal injury or stroke.

On the basis of both structure and function, researchers distinguish between several major divisions of the human frontal lobes. The posterior portion of the frontal cortex includes motor and premotor regions (see Chapter 5). The anterior portion, usually referred to as **prefrontal cortex**, is immensely interconnected with the rest of the brain (Fuster, 1990; Mega and Cummings, 1994). It was prefrontal cortex that was surgically disrupted in frontal lobotomy—the notorious, now-discredited treatment for psychiatric disorders that we discussed in Chapter 12. Prefrontal cortex is further subdivided into *dorsolateral* and *orbitofrontal* regions (**FIGURE 14.20B**).

Dorsolateral prefrontal cortex is closely associated with executive control, as it is crucial for working memory (holding information in mind while using it to solve problems) and task switching. People with lesions that include the

The human prefrontal cortex can be subdivided into a dorsolateral region (blue) and an orbitofrontal region (green). Lesions in these different areas of prefrontal cortex have different effects on behavior.

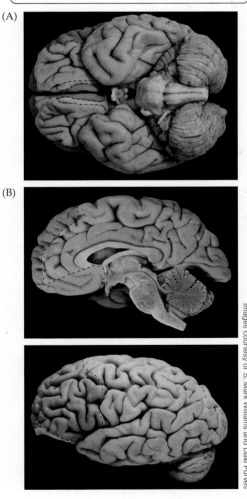

(A)

(B)

Images courtesy of S. Mark Williams and Dale Purves

FIGURE 14.20 The Prefrontal Cortex

Phineas Gage   Phineas P. Gage was a sober, polite, and capable member of a rail-laying crew, responsible for placing the charges used to blast rock from new rail beds. That's Gage on the left, holding a meter-long steel tamping rod. Perhaps the images on the right can help you guess why there appears to be something wrong with the left side of his face. In a horrific accident in 1848, a premature detonation blew that rod right through Gage's skull, on the trajectory shown in red, severely damaging both frontal lobes, especially in the orbitofrontal regions. Amazingly, Gage could speak shortly after the accident, and he walked up the stairs to a doctor's office, although no one expected him to live (Macmillan, 2000). In fact, Gage survived another 12 years, but he was definitely a changed man, so rude and aimless, and his powers of attention so badly impaired, "that his friends and acquaintances said that he was 'no longer Gage.'" The historical account of Gage's case, now a neuroscience classic, was eventually found to closely agree with the symptoms in modern cases of people with frontal lobe damage (H. Damasio et al., 1994; Wallis, 2007).

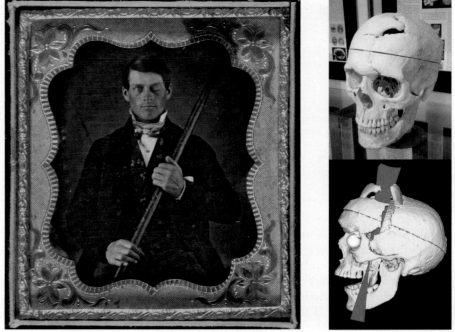

Left from the collection of Jack and Beverly Wilgus; *right after* J. D. Van Horn et al., 2012. *PLOS ONE* 7: e37454, courtesy of Warren Anatomical Museum, Harvard Medical School

dorsolateral prefrontal cortex may thus struggle with top-down conscious switching from one task to a new one, as in the Wisconsin Card Sorting Task (**FIGURE 14.21**), and tend to **perseverate** (continue beyond a reasonable degree) in any activity (B. Milner, 1963; Alvarez and Emory, 2006). Similarly, frontal lobe lesions may cause motor perseveration, repeating a simple movement over and over. However, the overall level of ordinary spontaneous motor activity is often quite diminished in people with frontal lesions. Along with movement of the head and eyes, facial expression of emotions may be greatly reduced. People with prefrontal lesions often have an inability to plan future acts and use foresight, as in the famous case of Phineas Gage. Their social skills may decline, especially the ability to inhibit inappropriate behaviors, and they may be unable to stay focused on any but short-term projects. They may agonize over even simple decisions. Some of the clinical features of damage to the subdivisions of prefrontal cortex are summarized in **TABLE 14.3**.

perseverate   Continue any activity beyond a reasonable degree.

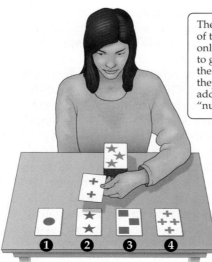

The participant starts sorting cards into piles on the basis of the number, color, or shape of the symbols, receiving only "correct" or "incorrect" feedback from the examiner to guide the sorting. The rule changes every 10 cards, so the participant must shift their sorting behavior until they discover the new rule. Here, the card should be added to pile 1 if the rule is "color," pile 2 if the rule is "number," or pile 4 if the rule is "shape."

FIGURE 14.21   The Wisconsin Card Sorting Task (WCST)

TABLE 14.3 Regional Prefrontal Syndromes

Prefrontal damage type	Syndrome type	Characteristics
Dorsolateral	Dysexecutive	Diminished judgment, planning, insight, and temporal organization; reduced cognitive focus; motor-programming deficits (possibly including aphasia and apraxia); diminished self-care
Orbitofrontal	Disinhibited	Stimulus-driven behavior; diminished social insight; distractibility; emotional lability
Mediofrontal	Apathetic	Diminished spontaneity; diminished verbal output; diminished motor behavior; urinary incontinence; lower-extremity weakness and sensory loss; diminished spontaneous prosody; increased response latency

A network that includes the orbitofrontal cortex appears to be crucial for goal-directed behaviors. For example, monkeys that must make decisions that could lead to rewards show increased orbitofrontal activation (Matsumoto et al., 2003); in general, orbitofrontal cortex seems to link pleasant experiences (e.g., eating a delicious meal) with reward signals generated elsewhere in the brain (Kringelbach, 2005). In fact, some researchers believe that orbitofrontal cortex is actually more important for anticipating outcomes than for learning (Schoenbaum et al., 2009), but either way the prospect of reward plays an important role. In humans performing tasks in which some stimuli have more reward value than others, the level of activation in prefrontal cortex correlates with how rewarding the stimulus is (Gottfried et al., 2003). This relationship seems to be a significant factor in gambling behavior and, more generally, is important for our decision-making processes, as we discuss next.

We make decisions using a frontal network that weighs risk and benefit

The waiter has brought over the dessert trolley, and it's decision time: do you go with the certain delight of the chocolate cake, or do you succumb to the glistening allure of the sticky toffee pudding? Or, do you allow yourself only a cup of black coffee, for the sake of your waistline? What happens in the brain when we make everyday decisions?

In the lab, researchers usually evaluate decision making by using monetary rewards (instead of desserts, darn it) because money is convenient: you can vary how much money is at stake, how great a reward is offered, and so on, to accurately gauge how we really make economic decisions. These studies show that most of us are very averse to loss and risk: we are more sensitive to losing a certain amount of money than we are to gaining that amount. In other words, losing $20 makes us feel a lot worse than gaining $20 makes us feel good. From a strictly logical point of view, the value of money, whether lost or gained, should be exactly the same. Our tendency to overemphasize loss is just one of several ways in which people fail to act rationally in the marketplace.

Neuroeconomics is the study of brain mechanisms at work during economic decision making, and our attention to environmental factors and evaluation of rewards has a tremendous impact on these decisions. In general, findings from human and animal research suggest that two main systems underlie decision processes (Kable and Glimcher, 2009). The first, consisting of the ventromedial prefrontal cortex (including the anterior cingulate cortex) plus the dopamine-based reward system of the brain (see Chapter 3), is a *valuation system*, a network that ranks choices on the basis of their perceived worth and potential reward. Impressively, using an optogenetic technique (see Chapter 2) to selectively activate neurons that express dopamine receptor D_2 in the nucleus accumbens—a central forebrain component of the brain's reward system—can instantaneously turn a risk-preferring rat into a risk-averse rat (Zalocusky et al., 2016)! Presumably, the activated cells cause the valuation system to devalue the reward relative to risk; a similar dopamine-dependent process appears to participate in human monetary decisions too (Ojala et al., 2018).

neuroeconomics The study of brain mechanisms at work during decision-making.

A costly decision is associated with activation of the amygdala and orbitofrontal cortex, signaling diminished reward and aversion to loss.

Amygdala   Orbitofrontal cortex

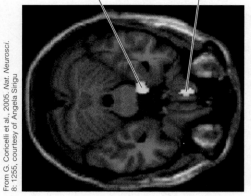

From G. Coricelli et al., 2005. *Nat. Neurosci.* 8: 1255, courtesy of Angela Sirigu

FIGURE 14.22   A Poor Choice

The second system involves dorsolateral prefrontal cortex, dorsal anterior cingulate cortex, and parietal regions (like the LIP or IPS discussed earlier in the chapter), and it is thought to be a *choice system*, sifting through the valuated alternatives and producing the conscious decision.

Neuroeconomics research is confirming that the prefrontal cortex normally inhibits impulsive decision making as a way to avoid loss (Tom et al., 2007; Muhlert and Lawrence, 2015). As people are faced with more and more uncertainty, the prefrontal cortex becomes more and more active (Hsu et al., 2005; Huettel et al., 2006), and the dorsal cingulate cortex may improve decisions by delaying action until full processing of a complex decision can be completed (Sheth et al., 2012; Heilbronner and Hayden, 2016). Likewise, when people have made wrong, costly decisions that they regret, activity increases in the amygdala and in the orbitofrontal aspect of the prefrontal cortex (**FIGURE 14.22**; Coricelli et al., 2005), probably reflecting the participant's perception of diminished reward and increasing aversion to loss.

We may never have a full understanding of the deepest secrets of consciousness, or an answer to the question of whether we *actually* make decisions based on the *free will* that our brain seems to perceive as an element of consciousness (Haggard, 2017). But that doesn't prevent us from marveling that our consciousness has become so self-aware that it can study itself to a high degree. Perhaps it's best to allow ourselves at least one or two mysteries, if only for the sake of art. Would life seem as rich if we could predict other people's behavior, or even our own, with perfect accuracy?

HOW'S IT GOING ❓

1. Define consciousness (or at least try!).
2. Discuss unconsciousness in states like deep coma. Is this unconsciousness the inverse of consciousness?
3. Contrast the easy and hard problems of consciousness, giving examples of each. What are qualia?
4. Name the main subdivisions of the prefrontal cortex. How do they differ in function?
5. What are some of the main symptoms of frontal lobe lesions?
6. What are the two main neural systems that are thought to operate in the process of decision making, as identified in neuroeconomics research?

Recommended Reading

Gazzaniga, M. S. (2018). *The Consciousness Instinct: Unraveling the Mystery of How the Brain Makes the Mind*. New York, NY: Farrar, Straus and Giroux.

Glimcher, P. W., and Fehr, E. (2013). *Neuroeconomics: Decision Making and the Brain* (2nd ed.). San Diego, CA: Academic Press.

Goldberg, E. (2017). *Executive Functions in Health and Disease*. New York, NY: Academic Press.

Koch, C. (2012). *Consciousness: Confessions of a Romantic Reductionist*. Cambridge, MA: MIT Press.

Laureys, S., and Tononi, G. (Eds.). (2015). *The Neurology of Consciousness: Cognitive Neuroscience and Neuropathology* (2nd ed.). New York, NY: Academic Press.

Mangun, G. R. (Ed.). (2012). *Neuroscience of Attention: Attentional Control and Selection*. Oxford, UK: Oxford University Press.

Nobre, K., and Kastner, S. (2018). *The Oxford Handbook of Attention*. Oxford, UK: Oxford University Press.

Owen, A. (2017). *Into the Gray Zone: A Neuroscientist Explores the Border between Life and Death*. New York, NY: Scribner.

Posner, M. I. (Ed.). (2012). *Cognitive Neuroscience of Attention* (2nd ed.). New York, NY: Guilford Press.

Stuss, D. T., and Knight, R. T. (2012). *Principles of Frontal Lobe Function* (2nd ed.). Oxford, UK: Oxford University Press.

You should be able to relate each summary to the adjacent illustration, including structures and processes.
The online version of this **Visual Summary** includes links to figures, animations, and activities that will help you consolidate the material.

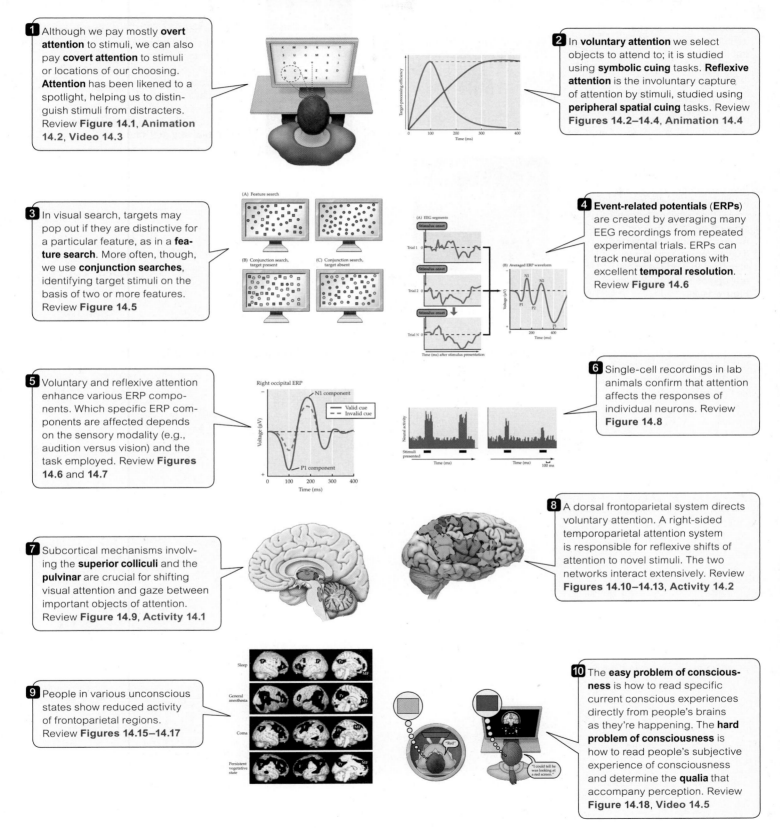

1 Although we pay mostly **overt attention** to stimuli, we can also pay **covert attention** to stimuli or locations of our choosing. **Attention** has been likened to a spotlight, helping us to distinguish stimuli from distracters. Review **Figure 14.1**, **Animation 14.2**, **Video 14.3**

2 In **voluntary attention** we select objects to attend to; it is studied using **symbolic cuing** tasks. **Reflexive attention** is the involuntary capture of attention by stimuli, studied using **peripheral spatial cuing** tasks. Review **Figures 14.2–14.4**, **Animation 14.4**

3 In visual search, targets may pop out if they are distinctive for a particular feature, as in a **feature search**. More often, though, we use **conjunction searches**, identifying target stimuli on the basis of two or more features. Review **Figure 14.5**

4 **Event-related potentials** (**ERPs**) are created by averaging many EEG recordings from repeated experimental trials. ERPs can track neural operations with excellent **temporal resolution**. Review **Figure 14.6**

5 Voluntary and reflexive attention enhance various ERP components. Which specific ERP components are affected depends on the sensory modality (e.g., audition versus vision) and the task employed. Review **Figures 14.6** and **14.7**

6 Single-cell recordings in lab animals confirm that attention affects the responses of individual neurons. Review **Figure 14.8**

7 Subcortical mechanisms involving the **superior colliculi** and the **pulvinar** are crucial for shifting visual attention and gaze between important objects of attention. Review **Figure 14.9**, **Activity 14.1**

8 A dorsal frontoparietal system directs voluntary attention. A right-sided temporoparietal attention system is responsible for reflexive shifts of attention to novel stimuli. The two networks interact extensively. Review **Figures 14.10–14.13**, **Activity 14.2**

9 People in various unconscious states show reduced activity of frontoparietal regions. Review **Figures 14.15–14.17**

10 The **easy problem of consciousness** is how to read specific current conscious experiences directly from people's brains as they're happening. The **hard problem of consciousness** is how to read people's subjective experience of consciousness and determine the **qualia** that accompany perception. Review **Figure 14.18**, **Video 14.5**

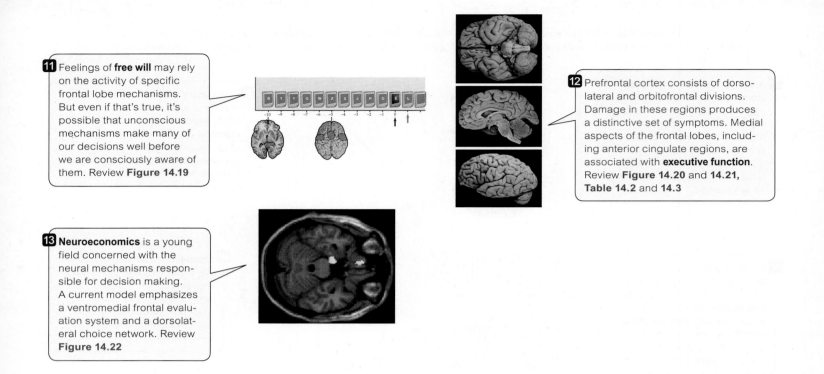

11 Feelings of **free will** may rely on the activity of specific frontal lobe mechanisms. But even if that's true, it's possible that unconscious mechanisms make many of our decisions well before we are consciously aware of them. Review **Figure 14.19**

12 Prefrontal cortex consists of dorso-lateral and orbitofrontal divisions. Damage in these regions produces a distinctive set of symptoms. Medial aspects of the frontal lobes, including anterior cingulate regions, are associated with **executive function**. Review **Figure 14.20** and **14.21, Table 14.2** and **14.3**

13 **Neuroeconomics** is a young field concerned with the neural mechanisms responsible for decision making. A current model emphasizes a ventromedial frontal evaluation system and a dorsolateral choice network. Review **Figure 14.22**

The Mind's Machine digital resources include additional videos, flashcards, and other study tools.

15 Language and Lateralization

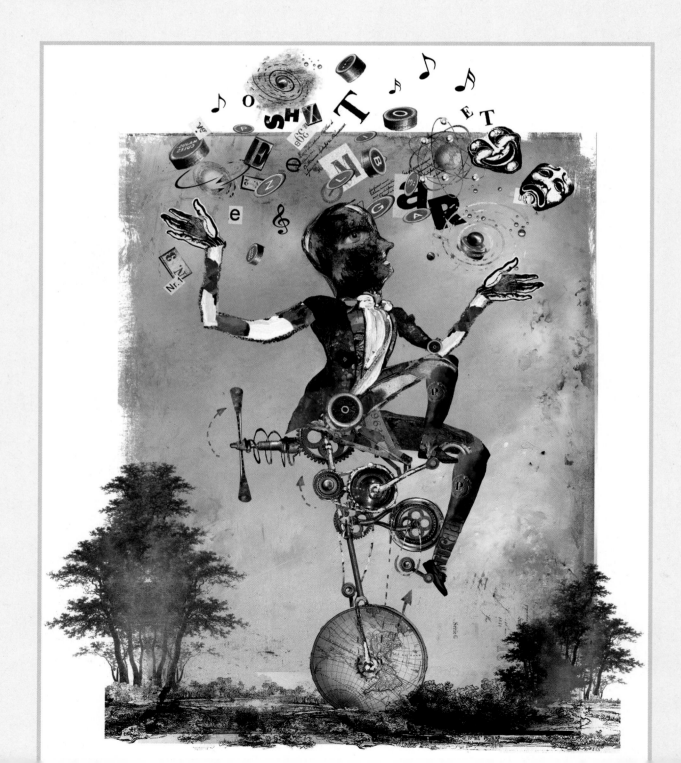

Silencing the Inner Me

We all have an inner voice: that mental narrator, sometimes annoying, whose dialogue wanders from calm abstraction ("What is love?") to urgent directives ("Pizza now!") to harsh self-criticism ("Way to go, fool!"). Some researchers, observing that the development of a child's sense of self is inextricably linked to the acquisition of language, have proposed that the inner voice is essential for the self-awareness that defines our consciousness. Nevertheless, sometimes we wish that Inner Me would just shut up for a while.

But what would life be like if our inner voice actually *were* silenced? This is just what happened to Tinna Geula Phillips. Suddenly one day, Tinna lost the ability to communicate in any of the six languages (yes, *six*) that she had mastered—a devastating neurological event. But even more profound was the immediate silencing of Tinna's inner voice. For several months, Tinna was unable to process thoughts in the way we take for granted. Tinna's internal silence had robbed her of a critical tool for organizing her activities, weighing her emotions, processing abstract concepts, and considering her memories. She would later describe the experience as a near-total loss of identity. What could have happened to cause Tinna to lose the ability to talk to anyone, even herself?

Faces, coloration, smells, sounds—many species use physical and behavioral signals to engage in **communication**, the transmission of information between individuals. But we humans may be alone in our use of **language**, the highly specialized form of communication in which arbitrary symbols or behaviors are assembled and reassembled in almost infinite variety and associated with a vast range of things, actions, and concepts. Because the speakers of a language all understand the same strict set of rules, or **grammar**, language allows us to assemble and share information on any topic, linking thinkers of the past with those of the future.

In almost everyone, verbal abilities are especially associated with the left hemisphere of the brain, while the right hemisphere plays a prominent role in *spatial cognition*, our ability to navigate and to understand the spatial relationships between objects. In this chapter we survey the neuroscience of this **cerebral lateralization**, with a special emphasis on the acquisition, use, and brain mechanisms of speech and language. Much of what we know about human brain organization comes from studies of people who have had strokes and other forms of brain injury, so we will also look at the ways in which the damaged brain can recover and adapt.

See Video 15.1:
Global Aphasia

15.1 The Left and Right Hemispheres of the Brain Are Different

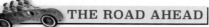 **THE ROAD AHEAD**

The first section of the chapter looks at the functional differences between the two hemispheres of the brain. After you've read through this material, you should be able to:

15.1.1 Describe techniques for studying the left and right hemispheres independently of each other.

15.1.2 Summarize the apparent cognitive specializations of each hemisphere as revealed by behavioral testing.

15.1.3 Discuss the relationship of handedness to cerebral lateralization.

**View Animation 15.2:
Brain Explorer**

communication Information transfer between two individuals.

language Communication in which arbitrary sounds or symbols are arranged according to a grammar in order to convey an almost limitless variety of concepts.

grammar All of the rules for usage of a particular language.

cerebral lateralization The division of labor between the two cerebral hemispheres such that each hemisphere is specialized for particular types of processing.

corpus callosum The main band of axons that connects the two cerebral hemispheres.

split-brain individual An individual whose corpus callosum has been severed, halting communication between the right and left hemispheres.

contralateral In anatomy, referring to a location on the opposite side of the body.

The discovery that some brain functions are lateralized should not be especially surprising; after all, other body organs also show considerable asymmetry between the right and left sides. But when we study the *behavior* of people, cerebral lateralization of function is masked by the rich neural connections between the hemispheres: they communicate with each other so quickly and thoroughly that they seem to act as one. So researchers have to devise clever experimental techniques for use with healthy participants and carefully analyze symptom patterns in people with neurological conditions, in order to understand the specific behavioral functions of each hemisphere.

Some rare and unfortunate people develop severe epilepsy that is very difficult to control with medication. Their frequent seizures start in one hemisphere and then spread to the other hemisphere through the **corpus callosum**—the huge white matter pathway consisting of hundreds of millions of axons that connect the two hemispheres. A surgical treatment of last resort—so invasive that it has been performed very infrequently (Gazzaniga, 2008)—is to cut the corpus callosum, preventing the spread of the seizure discharges from one hemisphere to the other. This operation, developed in the 1960s, significantly reduced the frequency and severity of seizures in affected people. It also changed their behavior in ways that presented a research opportunity: by analyzing the cognitive, perceptual, emotional, and motor behavior of these **split-brain individuals**, researchers were able to catalog the individual specializations of the newly isolated cerebral hemispheres.

In Nobel Prize–winning research, Roger Sperry and his collaborators applied techniques perfected in split-brain cats to study split-brain humans. The researchers realized that by exploiting the organization of the sensory systems, stimuli could be directed exclusively to one hemisphere or the other. For example, stimuli felt with the left hand, or seen only in the left visual field, are first processed in the sensory cortex of the **contralateral** (opposite side) hemisphere (in this case, the right hemisphere). Normally, information about the stimuli would be shared with the other hemisphere immediately, via the corpus callosum. But in split-brain individuals, the sensory information remains trapped within the receiving hemisphere, so the person's response to the stimuli reflects the processing specializations of that hemisphere in isolation.

In some studies of split-brain individuals, words were projected visually to either the left or the right hemisphere. The results were dramatic. Split-brain individuals could easily read and verbally report words projected to the left hemisphere (via the right visual field) but not words directed to the right hemisphere (**FIGURE 15.1**). Subsequent work (Zaidel, 1976) showed that the right hemisphere does have a limited amount of linguistic ability; for example, it can recognize simple words and the emotional content of verbal material. But in most people, vocabulary and grammar are the exclusive domain of the left hemisphere.

The capabilities of the "mute" right hemisphere had to be tested by nonverbal means. For example, a picture of a key might be projected to the left visual field and so reach only the right visual cortex. The participant would then be asked to touch

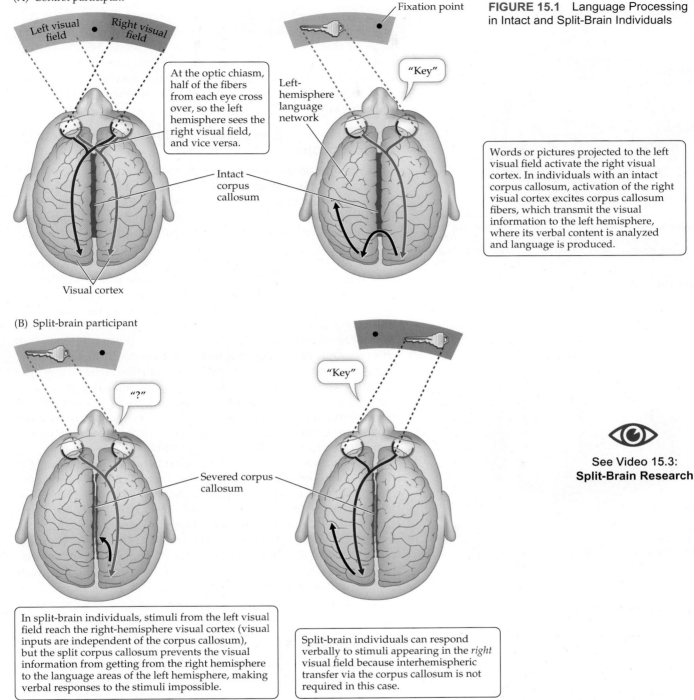

(A) Control participant

Left visual field   Right visual field

Fixation point

At the optic chiasm, half of the fibers from each eye cross over, so the left hemisphere sees the right visual field, and vice versa.

Left-hemisphere language network

"Key"

Intact corpus callosum

Visual cortex

Words or pictures projected to the left visual field activate the right visual cortex. In individuals with an intact corpus callosum, activation of the right visual cortex excites corpus callosum fibers, which transmit the visual information to the left hemisphere, where its verbal content is analyzed and language is produced.

FIGURE 15.1 Language Processing in Intact and Split-Brain Individuals

(B) Split-brain participant

"?"

"Key"

Severed corpus callosum

In split-brain individuals, stimuli from the left visual field reach the right-hemisphere visual cortex (visual inputs are independent of the corpus callosum), but the split corpus callosum prevents the visual information from getting from the right hemisphere to the language areas of the left hemisphere, making verbal responses to the stimuli impossible.

Split-brain individuals can respond verbally to stimuli appearing in the *right* visual field because interhemispheric transfer via the corpus callosum is not required in this case.

See Video 15.3:
Split-Brain Research

several different objects that they could not see and hold up the correct one. Such a task could be performed correctly by the left hand (controlled by the right hemisphere) but not by the right hand (controlled by the left hemisphere). So in this case, the left hemisphere literally does not know what the left hand is doing! In general, these and other studies with split-brain individuals provided evidence that, in most people, the right hemisphere is specialized for processing spatial information. Right-hemisphere mechanisms are also crucial for face perception, for processing emotional aspects of language, and for controlling attention (as we discussed in Chapter 14).

(A)

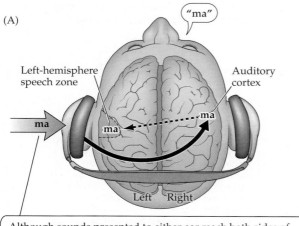

Left-hemisphere speech zone

Auditory cortex

"ma"

ma

ma   ma

Left   Right

Although sounds presented to either ear reach both sides of the brain, the auditory information is mostly processed by the contralateral hemisphere (see Chapter 6). So, verbal information presented to the left ear is first processed by the right auditory cortex and then transmitted to speech systems in the left hemisphere. Participant repeats the word.

(B)

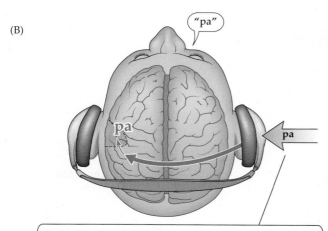

"pa"

pa

pa

Verbal information presented to the right ear is processed by the left auditory cortex and then passed directly to speech systems within the same hemisphere.

(C)

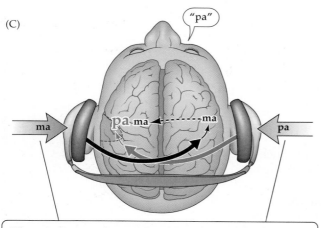

"pa"

ma   pa-ma   ma   pa

When conflicting information goes to both ears, the information to the right ear reaches the left hemisphere's speech system first. Subject repeats only the right-ear information.

Almost all types of behavior, from manual skills to intellectual activities, are performed better by the two hemispheres working together than by either hemisphere working alone. For this reason, and because better medical options have also been developed, the split-brain surgery has remained a very rare procedure, and the few modern forms of the operation generally cut only about a third of the corpus callosum.

The two hemispheres process information differently in most people

Most research on brain asymmetry in healthy people focuses on two sensory modalities: hearing and vision. That's because researchers have devised clever procedures for directing auditory or visual stimuli mostly to one hemisphere or the other and then inferring hemispheric specializations from the participants' behavior.

THE RIGHT-EAR ADVANTAGE Through earphones, we can present different sounds to the two ears at the same time—a technique called **dichotic presentation**. So, for example, a participant may hear a particular speech sound in one ear and, at the same time, a different vowel, consonant, or word in the other ear. The participant is asked to try to identify or recall both sounds. Although this procedure may seem designed to produce confusion, in general, right-handed people identify verbal stimuli delivered to the right ear more accurately than the stimuli simultaneously presented to the left ear. This result is described as a right-ear "advantage" for verbal information. In contrast, up to 50% of left-handed individuals may show a reduced or reversed pattern, with either no difference between the ears or a clear left-ear advantage.

As a consequence of the preferential connections between the right ear and the left hemisphere, the right-ear advantage for verbal stimuli confirms the idea that the left hemisphere is specialized for language (**FIGURE 15.2**). Although we can normally use either ear for processing speech sounds, speech presented to the right ear in dichotic presentation tests exerts stronger control over language mechanisms in the left hemisphere than does speech simultaneously presented to the left ear (Kimura, 1973). The competition between the left- and right-ear inputs is the key; presentation of speech stimuli to one ear at a time (*monaural* presentation) does not produce a right-ear advantage.

VISUAL PERCEPTION OF LINGUISTIC STIMULI Another way to study hemispheric specialization is to use a **tachistoscope test** to pit the two hemispheres against each other, using a device (called a *tachistoscope*, surprisingly; pronounced "ta-KISS-toe-scope") that very briefly presents visual stimuli to the left or right half of the visual field (see Figure 7.10 and Figure 15.1). If the stimulus exposure lasts less than 150 milliseconds or so, input is restricted to one hemisphere because there is not enough time for the eyes to shift their direction. In humans with intact brains, of course, further processing may involve the transmission of information through the corpus callosum to the other hemisphere.

FIGURE 15.2 The Right-Ear Advantage in Dichotic Presentation (After D. Kimura. 1973. *Sci. Am.* 228: 70.)

Most tachistoscopic studies confirm the general verbal-spatial division of labor between the hemispheres. Verbal stimuli (words and letters) presented to the right visual field (so the left hemisphere) are recognized more accurately than the same input presented to the left visual field (right hemisphere). Conversely, nonverbal visual stimuli (such as faces or geometric forms) presented to the left visual field (right hemisphere) are better recognized than the same stimuli presented to the other side. Simpler visual processing, such as the detection of light, hue, or simple patterns, is performed equivalently by the two hemispheres.

The left and right hemispheres differ in their auditory specializations

Anatomical studies of primary auditory cortex in the left and right hemispheres are consistent with the view that the two play different roles in auditory perception. In one early postmortem study of auditory cortex, the **planum temporale**—an auditory region on the superior surface of the temporal lobe—was found to be larger in the left hemisphere than in the right in most of the brains studied (Geschwind and Levitsky, 1968) (**FIGURE 15.3A**). In only 11% of adults was the right side larger. The planum temporale includes part of a posterior cortical region called *Wernicke's area*, which we'll see a little later is important for language, so it seems likely that the larger left planum temporale is related to that hemisphere's language specialization. Direct evidence of this relationship, however, remains somewhat elusive: in one MRI study, for example, asymmetry of the planum temporale did not correlate with direct measures of language lateralization (Dorsaint-Pierre et al., 2006).

As in adults, regions around the Sylvian fissure, including the planum temporale, are larger on the left than the right in the brains of infants and fetuses (Wada et al., 1975; Rajagopalan et al., 2011). The presence of this difference in our brains before we begin to speak therefore bolsters the view that we are born with a predisposition to acquire language in the left hemisphere. In fact, by just 12–14 weeks of gestation, a variety of genes show asymmetrical expression in the fetal human brain (Sun et al., 2005). The planum temporale likewise tends to be larger on the left than on the right in chimpanzees, but not in monkeys, indicating that this brain asymmetry evolved in an ancestral species before the hominids (including us) split off from the great apes (Gannon et al., 1998; Lyn et al., 2011). An anterior zone implicated in speech in humans (*Broca's area*, which we'll discuss shortly) is also larger on the left in chimps, bonobos, and gorillas, as it is in humans (Cantalupo and Hopkins, 2001). Furthermore, just as our left hemisphere is more activated than the right when we hear speech rather than other

dichotic presentation The simultaneous delivery of different stimuli to both the right and left ears at the same time.

tachistoscope test A test in which stimuli are very briefly presented to either the left or right visual half field.

planum temporale An auditory region of superior temporal cortex.

FIGURE 15.3 Structural Asymmetry of the Human Planum Temporale (After G. Schlaug et al. 1995. *Science* 267: 699.)

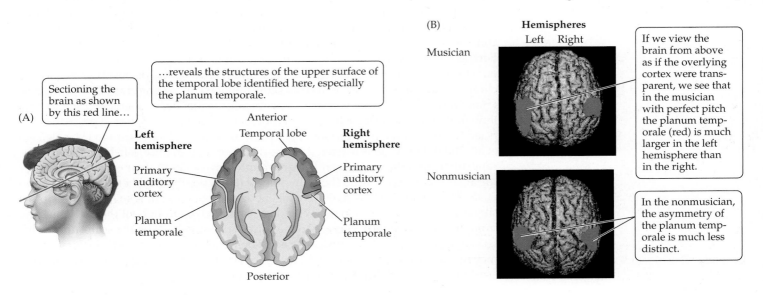

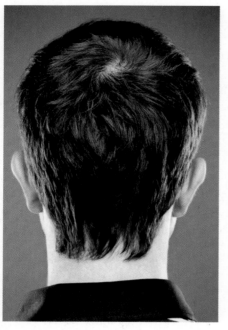

© istock.com/Marta Benavides

Whorls Apart   Because of the relationship between handedness and features such as the whorl of hair at the crown of the scalp—the whorl is clockwise in 93% of right-handers but randomly clockwise or counterclockwise in non-right-handers—it has been suggested that a single gene has a major (but not absolute) influence on asymmetries throughout the body (Klar, 2003; Corballis, 2014). Other aspects of development presumably account for the remaining variability in hand preference.

sounds, the left hemisphere of monkeys is more activated than the right when they hear monkey vocalizations rather than human speech (Poremba et al., 2004), and their perception of monkey vocalizations is far more impaired by left- than by right-hemisphere damage (Heffner and Heffner, 1984). These results and others indicate that primate brains are asymmetrically organized and contain a left-hemisphere specialization for communication (but not necessarily *language*) (Hopkins et al., 2015).

In contrast, the auditory areas of the *right* hemisphere play a major role in the perception of music. Musical perception is especially impaired after damage to the right hemisphere, and many aspects of music activate the right hemisphere more than the left (Zatorre et al., 1994; Nan and Friederici, 2013). In musicians, however, advanced skills and perfect pitch (the ability to accurately name a musical note just by listening to it) appear to strongly rely on *left*-hemisphere mechanisms (**FIGURE 15.3B**) and enhanced connectivity between the left and right planum temporale (Schlaug et al., 1995; Elmer et al., 2016), perhaps owing to its verbal aspects.

Despite these data, we cannot assign the perception of speech and pitch entirely to the left hemisphere and the perception of music entirely to the right hemisphere. We have seen that the right hemisphere can play a role in speech perception even in people in whom the left hemisphere is speech-dominant. In addition, the perception of emotional tone-of-voice aspects of language, termed **prosody**, is a *right*-hemisphere specialization. Furthermore, although damage to the right hemisphere can impair the perception of music, it does not abolish it. Damage to *both* sides of the brain can more completely impair or totally wipe out musical perception (Samson et al., 2002).

Thus, even though each hemisphere plays a greater role than the other in different kinds of auditory perception and other aspects of intellect, the two hemispheres appear to collaborate in most functions. The notions that the two hemispheres are so different that they need separate instruction and that some people are especially "right-brained" (supposedly more random, intuitive, and creative) or "left-brained" (supposedly logical, sequential, and analytical) lack any scientific foundation.

Handedness is associated with cerebral lateralization

Classic surveys of hand preferences, such as the incidence of left-handed writing in American college populations (Spiegler and Yeni-Komshian, 1983), indicated that 10–15% of the population is left-handed, although the estimated prevalence seems to vary somewhat through history and across geographic regions (Leask and Beaton, 2007). In a tiny minority of cases, early brain injuries may prompt a shift to left-handedness, but studies of achievement, ability, and cognitive function in school-age children find little evidence of any relationship between handedness and cognitive abilities (Faurie et al., 2006). Artifacts from prehistoric human societies suggest that a predominance of right-handedness is probably an ancient human characteristic, possibly in concert with hemispheric specializations for throwing and speech (Watson, 2001). Furthermore, a preference for one hand or the other seems to be a trait we share with our closest primate relatives: population-level hand preference is observed in gorillas, chimps, and bonobos (they're mostly right-handers) and orangutans (mostly lefties) (Hopkins et al., 2015). Some researchers even argue that hemispheric asymmetry and limb preferences reflect a left-right division of labor that, as a matter of processing efficiency, arose in the first vertebrates, hundreds of millions of years ago (MacNeilage et al., 2009). This view is bolstered by the discovery that in mice, left-hemisphere neurons differ from their right-hemisphere counterparts in both their expression of neurotransmitter receptors and their physiological functioning (Kohl et al., 2011; Shipton et al., 2014). Handedness may have a genetic component, but if so, it is not a simple single-gene effect. Genes that play a role in asymmetry throughout the body, ranging from the shape of internal organs to the pattern of hair whorls on the scalp, may be involved (Corballis, 2014). In any case, the evidence indicates that cerebral lateralization may be an ancient and ubiquitous adaptation. (For other examples of the evolution of asymmetry, see **A STEP FURTHER 15.1**, on the website.)

prosody   The perception of emotional tone-of-voice aspects of language.

RESEARCHERS AT WORK ||||||||||||||||||||||||||||||||||||||||||||||||||||||||||||||||||||||||||||||||||||||||||||||||||||||||||||||||

Reversibly shutting down one hemisphere reveals its specializations

Scientists estimate that 90–95% of humans have a left-hemisphere specialization for language. But how can we be certain which hemisphere is dominant for language (or other functions, such as spatial memory or music perception) in people who haven't had a stroke? In some cases, prior to brain surgery for example, it can be crucial to understand an individual's specific lateralization.

By injecting a short-acting anesthetic (amobarbital) into the carotid artery—first on one side (as shown in the figure) and then later, on the other—it is possible to simulate a massive stroke, shutting down each hemisphere for a few minutes (**FIGURE 15.4**) (Wada and Rasmussen, 1960; Sharan et al., 2011). This is just long enough to use behavioral measures to document the specializations of each hemisphere.

This **Wada test** confirms that most people have left-hemisphere specialization for language, regardless of handedness. The reverse pattern (right-hemisphere dominance for language) is uncommon, but when it occurs, it is more usually in left-handed people. Similar results can be obtained in healthy people by using transcranial magnetic stimulation (TMS) (Knecht et al., 2002) or fMRI.

FIGURE 15.4   A Simulated Stroke The Wada test uses anesthetic to shut down one hemisphere at a time.

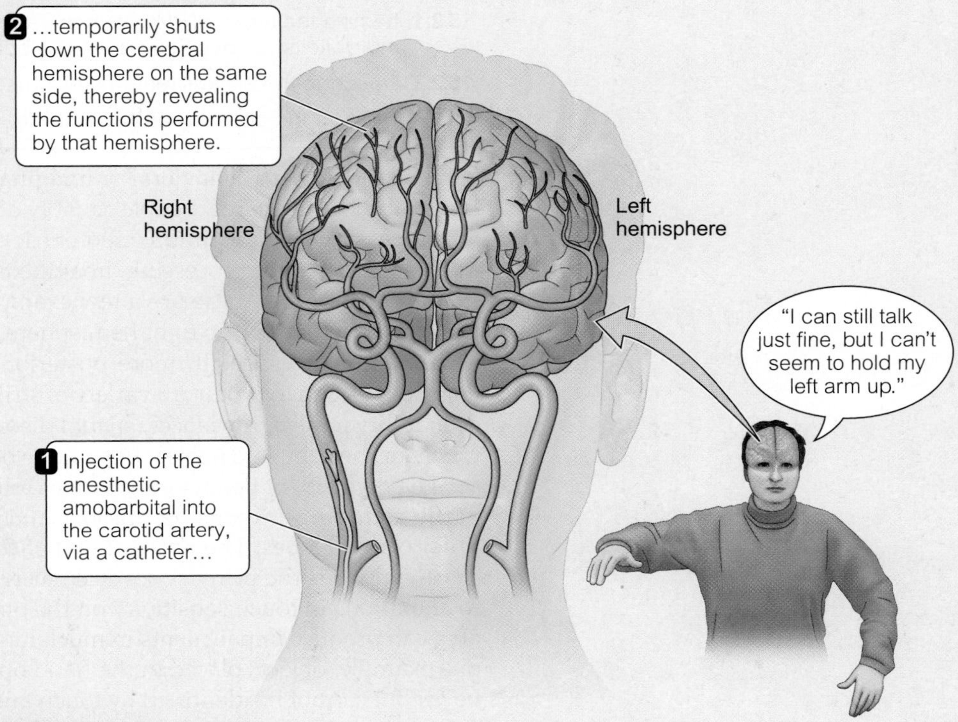

2 …temporarily shuts down the cerebral hemisphere on the same side, thereby revealing the functions performed by that hemisphere.

Right hemisphere

Left hemisphere

1 Injection of the anesthetic amobarbital into the carotid artery, via a catheter…

"I can still talk just fine, but I can't seem to hold my left arm up."

■ **Question**
Which hemisphere is specialized for language in an individual?

■ **Hypothesis**
That language is a left-hemisphere function in most people, irrespective of their handedness

■ **Test**
Silence one hemisphere by perfusing it with anaesthetic while the person performs cognitive tasks, including speech tests. Later, repeat with the other hemisphere.

In most people, shutting down the left hemisphere, but not the right hemisphere, interrupts language function

---

HOW'S IT GOING ❓

1. Summarize the cardinal differences between the left and right hemispheres of the human brain. How were these functional differences first identified?

2. Describe the dichotic presentation test and tachistoscope test. How do these tests reveal lateralization of function?

3. Discuss the representation of music in the human brain. What is the planum temporale, and how does its structure relate to musical experience?

4. Summarize the neural underpinnings of left-handedness. Do left-handers generally show reversed asymmetry, with language vested in the right hemisphere?

Wada test   A test in which a short-lasting anesthetic is delivered into one carotid artery to determine which cerebral hemisphere principally mediates language.

15.2 Right-Hemisphere Damage Impairs Specific Types of Cognition

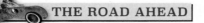 **THE ROAD AHEAD**

Our next section looks at some specific processing deficits that can result from right-hemisphere lesions. After studying this material you should be able to:

15.2.1 Itemize the types of deficits seen after right-hemisphere lesions, relating the deficits to specific anatomical locations within the hemisphere.

15.2.2 Describe the clinical features of prosopagnosia and related disorders.

15.2.3 Discuss the anatomy and specialized functions of the fusiform system.

When studied with behavioral or imaging techniques that highlight differences between the hemispheres, people reliably demonstrate a right-hemisphere advantage for processing spatial stimuli. Geometric shapes and their relations, direction sense and navigation, face processing, imagined three-dimensional rotation of objects held in the mind's eye—these are a few examples of the kinds of spatial processing that preferentially rely on the right hemisphere. It is therefore no surprise that right-hemisphere lesions—especially more-posterior lesions that involve the temporal and parietal lobes—tend to produce a variety of striking impairments of spatial cognition, such as inability to recognize faces, spatial disorientation, inability to recognize objects by touch, or the complete neglect of one side of the body that we discussed in Chapter 14.

The diversity of behavioral changes following injury to the parietal lobe is related partly to the large expanse of this lobe and its critical position, abutting all three of the other cortical lobes. The anterior end of the parietal region includes the postcentral gyrus, which is the primary cortical receiving area for somatic sensation. In addition to alterations in touch sensitivity on the opposite side of the body, brain injury in this area can produce impairments in much more complex forms of sensory processing. In one example, objects placed in the hand opposite the injured somatosensory area can be *felt* but cannot be identified by touch and active manipulation. This deficit is called **astereognosis** (from the Greek *a-*, "not"; *stereos*, "solid"; and *gnosis*, "knowledge").

More-extensive injuries in the parietal cortex, beyond the postcentral gyrus, affect interactions between or among sensory modalities, such as visual or tactile matching tasks, which require the participant to visually identify an object that is touched or to reach for an object that is identified visually.

In prosopagnosia, faces are unrecognizable

Suppose that one day you look in the mirror, and someone totally unfamiliar is looking back at you. As incredible as this scenario might seem, some individuals develop exactly this problem following damage to specific brain sites. In this rare syndrome, called **prosopagnosia** (from the Greek *prosop-*, "face"; *a-*, "not"; and *gnosis*, "knowledge") or *face blindness,* affected individuals fail to recognize not only their own faces but also the faces of relatives and friends. No amount of remedial training restores their ability to recognize anyone's face. In contrast, the ability to visually recognize *objects* may be retained, and the person may have no difficulty identifying people by their voices.

To people with prosopagnosia, faces simply lack meaning. No disorientation or confusion accompanies this condition, nor is there evidence of diminished intellectual abilities or significant visual impairment. Research with people whose right hemispheres have been impaired during strokes or shut down by Wada tests indicates that the right hemisphere is especially important for processing faces. For example, shutting down the right hemisphere with anesthetic during the Wada test can cause difficulty in recognizing faces, whereas anesthetizing the left hemisphere has less effect on facial recognition. This effect can be especially evident for recognizing one's own face (**FIGURE 15.5**).

astereognosis The inability to recognize objects by touching and feeling them.

prosopagnosia Also called *face blindness*. A condition characterized by the inability to recognize faces.

fusiform gyrus A region on the inferior surface of the cortex, at the junction of the temporal and occipital lobes, that has been associated with recognition of faces.

agnosia The inability to recognize objects, despite being able to describe them in terms of form and color. Agnosia may occur after localized brain damage.

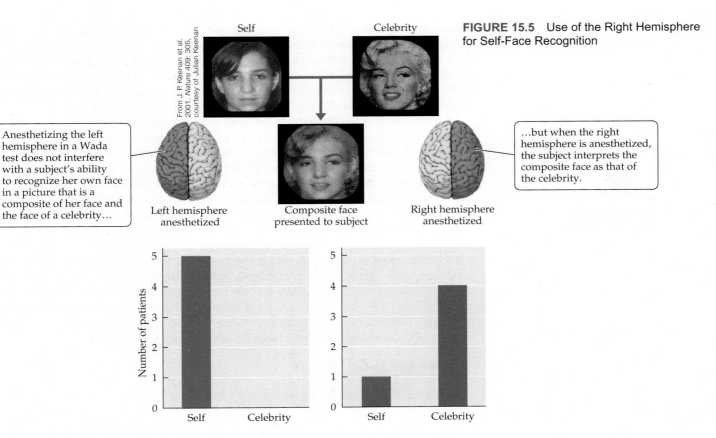

FIGURE 15.5 Use of the Right Hemisphere for Self-Face Recognition

Self   Celebrity

From J. P. Keenan et al. 2001. *Nature* 409: 305, courtesy of Julian Keenan

Anesthetizing the left hemisphere in a Wada test does not interfere with a subject's ability to recognize her own face in a picture that is a composite of her face and the face of a celebrity…

Left hemisphere anesthetized

Composite face presented to subject

Right hemisphere anesthetized

…but when the right hemisphere is anesthetized, the subject interprets the composite face as that of the celebrity.

Similarly, early work found that split-brain individuals do a better job of recognizing faces that are presented to the right hemisphere than to the left (Gazzaniga and Smylie, 1983). Still, data from split-brain individuals and functional-imaging studies make it clear that both hemispheres have *some* capacity for recognizing faces. Thus, although damage restricted to the right hemisphere can impair face processing, the most complete cases of prosopagnosia are caused by *bilateral* damage. The **fusiform gyrus**, a region of cortex on the inferior surface of the brain where the occipital and temporal cortices meet (**FIGURE 15.6**), is a central component of a network for face recognition (Rezlescu et al., 2014) and seems to play a special role in recognizing stimuli within specific categories (Weiner and Zilles, 2016; Grill-Spector et al., 2017). Individuals with prosopagnosia following brain damage almost always have damage here. Prosopagnosia may be accompanied by additional forms of **agnosia**, an inability to identify individual items—makes of cars, tools, bird species, sounds, and so on—in the absence of any specific sensory deficits or memory problems (Haque et al., 2018). Functional-MRI studies of healthy people show that, as with face recognition, the fusiform region is activated not

In this view from below the brain, the cerebellum has been removed to reveal the region of cortex that normally lies opposite to it.

The fusiform gyrus, at the juncture of the temporal and occipital lobes, is active during discrimination of objects within large categories, such as faces or birds or cars. Bilateral destruction of this region leads to prosopagnosia, the inability to recognize individual faces.

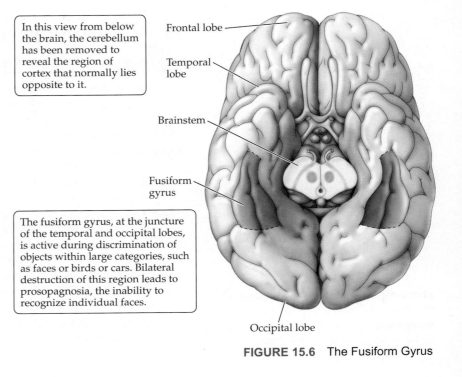

Frontal lobe

Temporal lobe

Brainstem

Fusiform gyrus

Occipital lobe

FIGURE 15.6 The Fusiform Gyrus

only when people are identifying faces, but also when identifying birds, or cars, or individual members of many other categories, especially if the participants have relevant expertise (birders, car enthusiasts, and so on) (McGugin et al., 2012; Ross et al., 2018). It remains to be seen exactly how many distinct categories are individually represented in the brain, and the extent to which brain regions other than the fusiform gyrus may participate (Connolly et al., 2012).

Until recently, it was believed that prosopagnosia occurred solely as a result of brain damage (*acquired prosopagnosia*), but a number of cases of *congenital prosopagnosia* (*congenital* means "present at birth") have now been identified. Unexpectedly, surveys reveal that about 2.5% of the general population is sufficiently impaired in processing faces to meet the criteria for congenital prosopagnosia (Kennerknecht et al., 2006; Duchaine et al., 2007). The congenital form of prosopagnosia appears to run in families, indicating a genetic aspect to the disorder (Grüter et al., 2008; De Luca et al., 2019). Congenital prosopagnosia is associated with reduced activation of the fusiform gyrus, in keeping with the anatomical findings in acquired prosopagnosia that we've already discussed. At the other end of the spectrum, some people are exceptionally good with faces. These "super-recognizers," who are about as good with faces as people with prosopagnosia are bad, are actively recruited by some police forces (Russell et al., 2009; Robertson et al., 2016), although efforts are underway to see if devices relying on artificial intelligence can do an even better job (Hill, 2020). (You can learn more, and test your own facial recognition ability, at www.testmybrain.org.)

**See Video 15.4:
Face Blindness**

HOW'S IT GOING ?

1. In general, what are the behavioral consequences of right-hemisphere damage in humans?

2. Define, compare, and contrast two of the most striking symptoms of right-hemisphere damage: astereognosis and prosopagnosia. Which areas of the brain appear to be involved in each?

3. Is prosopagnosia *always* associated with brain damage? What other behavioral abnormalities may co-occur with prosopagnosia?

15.3 Left-Hemisphere Damage Can Cause Aphasia

THE ROAD AHEAD

Brain damage restricted to the left hemisphere has predictable effects on behavior, especially language processes. After reading this section, you should be able to:

15.3.1 Distinguish among aphasia, apraxia, agraphia, and alexia.

15.3.2 Describe Broca's area and the behavioral consequences of lesions that include this area.

15.3.3 Define Wernicke's area and the behavioral consequences of lesions that include this area.

15.3.4 Describe global aphasia, its causes and prognosis, and its relationship to concepts of personal identity.

15.3.5 Contrast the motor theory of speech perception with the Wernicke-Geschwind model, and discuss research findings for and against each.

15.3.6 Summarize research using brain stimulation, functional brain imaging, and ERPs to map the brain's language network.

phoneme   A sound that is produced for language.

morpheme   The smallest grammatical unit of a language; a word or meaningful part of a word.

All human languages share certain basic features. Each language has basic speech sounds, or **phonemes**, that are assembled into simple units of meaning called **morphemes** (**FIGURE 15.7**). Morphemes are assembled into words: the word *unfathomable*, for example, consists of the morphemes *un-*, *fathom*, and *-able*, each of which adds meaning (termed *semantics* in linguistics). (Note that a morpheme is not the same thing as a *syllable*; there are two syllables but only one morpheme in *fathom*). In turn, the words are assembled into meaningful strings (which may be complete sentences or just phrases) according to the language's **syntax** (grammatical rules). Our speech is colored and clarified both by the context of the utterance, which is known as **pragmatics** in linguistics, and by the emotional tone and emphasis (called prosody) that we add to the things we say.

Physicians and scientists have known for centuries that brain damage can disrupt our use of the basic speech sounds and grammar that make up our language abilities, a disorder known as **aphasia** (Finger, 1994). Left-hemisphere damage in particular can impair language to varying degrees, depending on the location and extent of the injury. In cases of severe damage, people may lose the ability to produce any speech whatsoever. People with less severe damage may exhibit speech with **paraphasia**—insertion of incorrect sounds or words—along with labored, effortful speech production. Somewhere in the range of 25–50% of people who have a significant stroke (see Figure 1.17) will have aphasia as a primary symptom; for this reason, a sudden problem with language is considered to be one of the core warning signs of a stroke (see Figure 1.18), along with weakness or numbness on one side and dizziness, altered vision, or confusion. Such symptoms are reason to seek emergency treatment immediately. Most people with aphasia also show some impairment in writing, known as **agraphia**, and disturbances in reading, called **alexia**. Brain damage that produces aphasia also produces a distinctive motor impairment called **apraxia** (see Chapter 5), characterized by great difficulty in making precise *sequences* of movements, despite the absence of weakness or paralysis. In fact, as we discuss later, some theorists view aphasia as primarily a disorder of motor control. Research has distinguished several major categories of aphasia, differing from one another in the patterns of symptoms that occur (videos of people with aphasia can be seen on the website).

Damage to a left anterior speech zone causes nonfluent (or Broca's) aphasia

In the mid-1800s, French neurologist Paul Broca (1824–1880) examined a man who had lost the ability to utter more than the single syllable "tan" (**FIGURE 15.8**). Following postmortem analysis, Broca reported that this man, and other people with similar severe impairments of speech production, had sustained brain damage

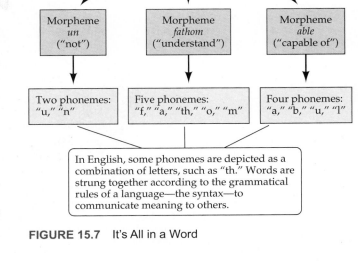

FIGURE 15.7   It's All in a Word

syntax   The grammatical rules for constructing phrases and sentences in a language.

pragmatics   In linguistics, the context in which a speech sound is uttered.

aphasia   An impairment in language understanding and/or production that is caused by brain injury.

paraphasia   A symptom of aphasia that is distinguished by the substitution of a word by a sound, an incorrect word, an unintended word, or a neologism (a meaningless word).

agraphia   The inability to write.

alexia   The inability to read.

apraxia   An impairment in the ability to carry out complex sequential movements, even though there is no muscle paralysis.

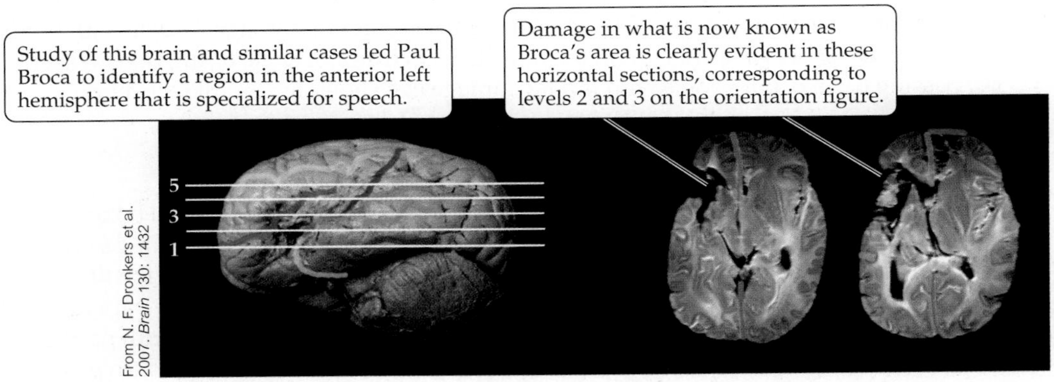

Study of this brain and similar cases led Paul Broca to identify a region in the anterior left hemisphere that is specialized for speech.

Damage in what is now known as Broca's area is clearly evident in these horizontal sections, corresponding to levels 2 and 3 on the orientation figure.

From N. F. Dronkers et al. 2007. *Brain* 130: 1432

5
3
1

FIGURE 15.8   The Brain of "Tan"   Photo and MRI image of the preserved brain of M. Leborgne, who could only utter the syllable "tan" after his brain injury.

FIGURE 15.9 Left-Hemisphere Speech and Language Areas in Humans

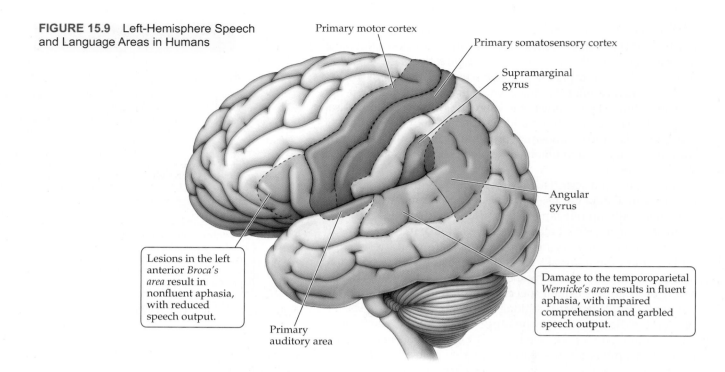

Primary motor cortex

Primary somatosensory cortex

Supramarginal gyrus

Angular gyrus

Lesions in the left anterior *Broca's area* result in nonfluent aphasia, with reduced speech output.

Damage to the temporoparietal *Wernicke's area* results in fluent aphasia, with impaired comprehension and garbled speech output.

Primary auditory area

View Activity 15.1: Speech and Language Areas

Broca's area   A region of the frontal lobe of the brain that is involved in the production of speech.

nonfluent aphasia   Also called *Broca's aphasia*. A language impairment characterized by difficulty with speech production but not with language comprehension. It is related to damage in Broca's area.

hemiplegia   Paralysis of one side of the body.

hemiparesis   Weakness of one side of the body.

Wernicke's area   A region of temporoparietal cortex in the brain that is involved in the perception and production of speech.

fluent aphasia   Also called *Wernicke's aphasia*. A language impairment characterized by fluent, meaningless speech and little language comprehension. It is related to damage in Wernicke's area.

that included a left inferior frontal region that now bears his name—**Broca's area** (**FIGURE 15.9**). Damage that includes Broca's area often produces a type of aphasia known as **nonfluent aphasia** (or *Broca's aphasia*). People with nonfluent aphasia have a lot of difficulty producing speech, talking only in a labored and hesitant manner. Reading and writing are also impaired. The ability to utter automatic speech, however, is often preserved. Such speech includes greetings ("Hello"); short, common expressions ("Oh my gosh!"); and swear words.

Compared with their difficulty with speech production, *comprehension* of language is relatively good in people with nonfluent aphasia. Because the primary and supplementary motor cortex is close to Broca's area (see Chapter 5), brain injuries that cause nonfluent aphasia often also cause **hemiplegia**—paralysis of one side of the body (usually the right side, which is controlled by the left hemisphere). Sometimes there is unilateral weakness, termed **hemiparesis**, rather than full paralysis.

The CT scans in **FIGURE 15.10A** and maps of lesion sites in **FIGURE 15.10B** are from several people with nonfluent aphasia. Seven years after a stroke, one such person still spoke slowly, using mainly nouns and very few verbs or function words (a selective loss of action words, called *averbia*, sometimes occurs in nonfluent aphasia), and spoke only with great effort. When asked to repeat the phrase "Go ahead and do it if possible," she could say only, "Go to do it," with a pause between each word. Her pattern is typical of people with extensive left anterior damage. People with brain lesions as extensive as hers tend to show little recovery of speech functions with the passing of time, but people with milder damage can show significant recovery.

Damage to a left posterior speech zone causes fluent (or Wernicke's) aphasia

Not long after Broca's groundbreaking discovery of the left anterior speech zone, German neurologist Carl Wernicke (pronounced "VER-nih-keh") (1848–1905) described a different form of aphasia, resulting from damage to a more posterior region of the left hemisphere, on the upper part of the temporal lobe near where it joins the parietal lobe, that is now known as **Wernicke's area** (see Figure 15.9). Unlike people with nonfluent aphasia, people who have this **fluent aphasia** (or *Wernicke's aphasia*) produce plenty of

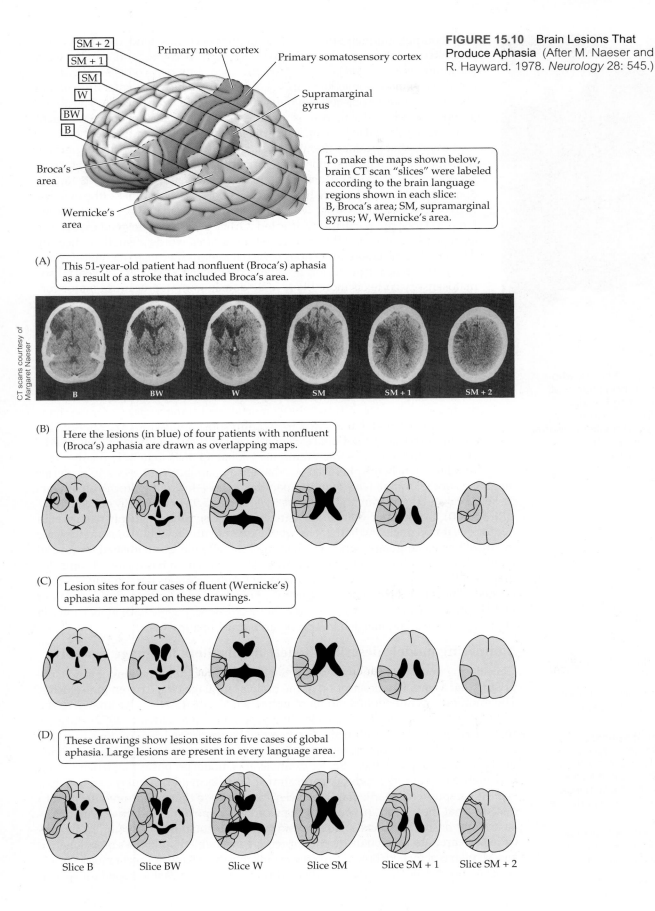

FIGURE 15.10 Brain Lesions That Produce Aphasia (After M. Naeser and R. Hayward. 1978. *Neurology* 28: 545.)

To make the maps shown below, brain CT scan "slices" were labeled according to the brain language regions shown in each slice: B, Broca's area; SM, supramarginal gyrus; W, Wernicke's area.

(A) This 51-year-old patient had nonfluent (Broca's) aphasia as a result of a stroke that included Broca's area.

CT scans courtesy of Margaret Naeser

(B) Here the lesions (in blue) of four patients with nonfluent (Broca's) aphasia are drawn as overlapping maps.

(C) Lesion sites for four cases of fluent (Wernicke's) aphasia are mapped on these drawings.

(D) These drawings show lesion sites for five cases of global aphasia. Large lesions are present in every language area.

Slice B   Slice BW   Slice W   Slice SM   Slice SM + 1   Slice SM + 2

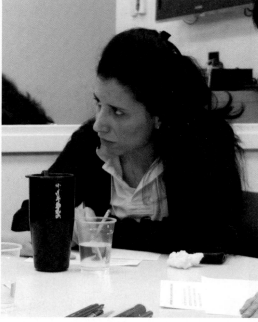

Speechless Tinna Geula Phillips, who sustained a stroke that robbed her of all language abilities, including her inner monologue, is profiled in a documentary entitled *Speechless*, by filmmaker Guillermo Florez (www.speechlessdoc.com).

verbal output, but their utterances, although speech-like, tend to contain many *paraphasias*, such as sound substitutions (e.g., "girl" becomes "curl") and/or word substitutions (e.g., *bread* becomes *cake*). Invented nonsense words—*neologisms*—are also common. Some fluent aphasias are marked by a particular difficulty in naming persons or objects—an impairment referred to as **anomia**. The ability to repeat words and sentences is impaired. For this reason, people with fluent aphasia are believed to have difficulty *comprehending* what they read or hear.

Lesions that produce fluent aphasia usually include the posterior parts of the superior left temporal lobe, extending into adjacent regions of parietal cortex. Examples of lesions causing fluent aphasia are shown in **FIGURE 15.10C**. Sometimes people who have had strokes experience *word deafness* (the inability to understand *spoken* words), which usually means that auditory regions of the temporal lobe are particularly affected. Other people may instead experience *word blindness* (the inability to understand *written* words), usually indicating damage that includes connections to visual regions. Because the typical lesion in fluent aphasia is posterior, involving Wernicke's area, the postcentral somatosensory cortex is more likely to be damaged than precentral motor cortex. As a result, people with fluent aphasia are somewhat more likely to have a right-sided numbness than the weakness common in nonfluent aphasia.

Widespread left-hemisphere damage can obliterate language capabilities

In some people, brain injury or disease results in total loss of the ability to understand or produce language. This syndrome, called **global aphasia**, was the diagnosis in the case of Tinna, the woman we met at the beginning of the chapter. People with global aphasia may retain some ability to make speech-like sounds, especially emotional exclamations. But they can utter very few words, and no semblance of syntax remains. Global aphasia generally results from very large left-hemisphere lesions that encompass both anterior and posterior language zones. Frontal, temporal, and parietal cortex—including Broca's area, Wernicke's area, and the supramarginal gyrus (see Figure 15.9)—are usually affected (**FIGURE 15.10D**). For nearly 2 years after Tinna had a massive left-hemisphere stroke, in her forties, it was unclear whether she would ever regain the ability to communicate in any of her six languages, and even her inner monologue was banished for several months, taking with it her personal identity. Although Tinna has regained some degree of both outward and inward language, her verbal abilities remain quite impoverished. This is in keeping with the generally poor prognosis for language recovery in global aphasia. And because of the extent of their lesions, people with global aphasia often experience additional debilitating neurological impairments.

Competing models describe the left-hemisphere language network

Considering how language is intertwined with so many other functions, it is not surprising that a complete description of the brain's language circuitry remains elusive. The traditional **connectionist model of aphasia** (**FIGURE 15.11**)—also known as the *Wernicke-Geschwind model* after its leading proponents (Geschwind, 1972)—argues that language deficits result from *disconnection* between the brain regions in a language network. Each of these regions is proposed to serve a particular feature of language analysis or production. So, for example, this model proposes that when a word or sentence is heard, the auditory cortex transmits information about the sounds to a speech reception mechanism in Wernicke's area, where the sounds are analyzed to decode what they mean. In order for the word to be spoken aloud, the connectionist account posits, Wernicke's area transmits this information, via a bundle of axons called the **arcuate fasciculus**, to the expressive mechanism in Broca's area, where a speech plan is activated. Broca's area then transmits this plan to adjacent motor cortex, which controls the muscles of the chest, throat, and mouth that are used for speech

anomia The inability to name persons or objects readily.

global aphasia The total loss of ability to understand language, or to speak, read, or write.

connectionist model of aphasia Also called the *Wernicke-Geschwind model*. A theory proposing that left-hemisphere language deficits result from disconnection between the brain regions in a language network, each of which serves a particular linguistic function.

arcuate fasciculus A fiber tract classically viewed as a connection between Wernicke's speech area and Broca's speech area.

(A) Speaking a *heard* word

1 Information about the sound is analyzed by primary auditory cortex and transmitted to Wernicke's area.

2 Wernicke's area analyzes the sound information to determine the word that was said.

3 Under the connectionist model this information is transmitted via the arcuate fasciculus. (Note, however, that anatomical research casts doubt on this projection.)

4 Broca's area forms a motor plan to repeat the word and sends that information to motor cortex.

5 Motor cortex implements the plan, manipulating the larynx and related structures to say the word.

Lesions of the arcuate fasciculus disrupt the transfer from Wernicke's area to Broca's area, so the patient has difficulty repeating spoken words (so-called conduction aphasia), but may retain comprehension of spoken language (because of intact Wernicke's area) and may still be able to speak spontaneously (because of intact Broca's area).

(B) Speaking a *written* word

1 Visual cortex analyzes the image and transmits the information about the image to the angular gyrus.

2 The angular gyrus decodes the image information to recognize the word and associate this visual form with the spoken form in Wernicke's area.

3 Information about the word is transmitted via the arcuate fasciculus to Broca's area.

4 Broca's area formulates a motor plan to say the appropriate word and transmits that plan to motor cortex for implementation.

5 Motor cortex implements the plan, manipulating the larynx and related structures to say the word.

A lesion of the angular gyrus disrupts the flow of information from visual cortex, so the person has difficulty saying words he has seen but not words he has heard.

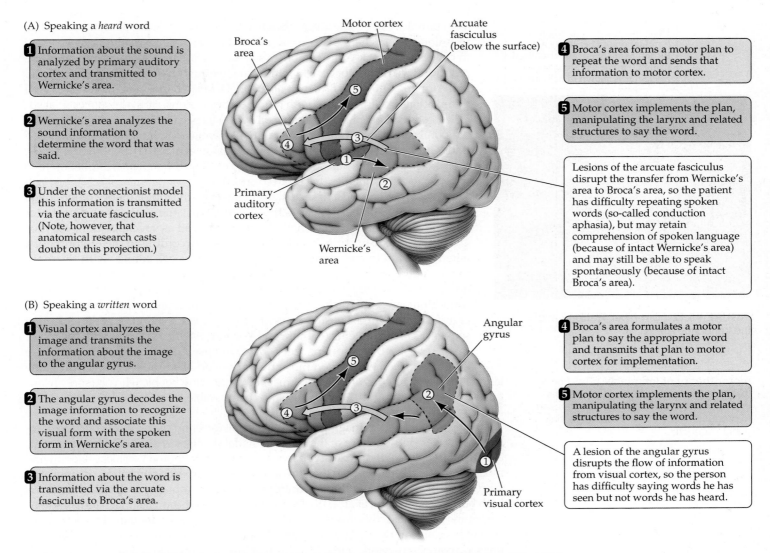

FIGURE 15.11 The Connectionist Model of Aphasia (After N. Geschwind. 1979. *Sci. Am.* 241: 180.)

production. The model therefore argues that people with lesions that selectively disrupt the arcuate fasciculus will especially struggle with *repetition* of words and phrases that they hear, despite good speech comprehension and production—a condition termed **conduction aphasia**.

Critics of the connectionist model argue that it oversimplifies the neural mechanisms of language, and furthermore, more modern fMRI data confirms that left-hemisphere language zones are not as rigidly modular as was previously believed (Blumstein and Amso, 2013). In addition, technological advances in the visualization of white matter pathways in the living brain have raised questions about the assumptions underlying the connectionist model.

In **diffusion tensor imaging** (**DTI**), MRI technology is used to specifically study white matter tracts—axon bundles—within the living brain. As we discussed in Chapter 1, MRI images are created from the radio-frequency energy that is emitted by relaxing protons within water molecules. In DTI, the unique behavior of water molecules that are constrained within axons (known as *fractional anisotropy*) is exploited to create images of axonal fiber pathways between areas, a procedure called **DTI tractography**, or *fiber tracking* (Assaf and Pasternak, 2008). Although the technology doesn't have the resolution to portray individual axons, the origin, orientation, course, and termination of

View Activity 15.2a and b: The Connectionist Model of Aphasia

conduction aphasia An impairment in the ability to repeat words and sentences.

diffusion tensor imaging (DTI) A modified form of MRI in which the diffusion of water in a confined space is exploited to produce images of axonal fiber tracts.

DTI tractography Also called *fiber tracking*. Visualization of the orientation and terminations of white matter tracts in the living brain via diffusion tensor imaging.

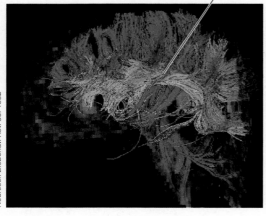

Here, the orientation, origin, and termination of fiber tracts within the left hemisphere are visualized using DTI. The left arcuate fasciculus is shown in light green.

From M. Vandermosten et al. 2012. *Neurosci. Biobehav. Rev.* 36: 1532

FIGURE 15.12 DTI Fiber Tracking and the Language Areas

motor theory of language The theory that speech is perceived using the same left-hemisphere mechanisms that are used to produce the complex movements that go into speech.

axon bundles can be effectively visualized, as shown in **FIGURE 15.12**. Using this technique, researchers have discovered that the arcuate fasciculus, long believed to connect Wernicke's area to Broca's area, instead appears to terminate in the precentral gyrus (motor cortex) in most people, just short of Broca's area (Bernal and Altman, 2010; E. C. Brown et al., 2014). Detailed brain-imaging research, and observations in clinical cases with purely cortical lesions, similarly suggest that so-called conduction aphasia is a consequence of a specific type of lesion of superior temporal cortex, rather than the disruption of white matter pathways as proposed under the connectionist model (B. R. Buchsbaum et al., 2011). So it remains to be seen exactly how the various mechanisms of the left hemisphere collaborate to give us the verbal abilities that seem so effortless.

An alternative model of speech mechanisms—the **motor theory of language** (Kimura, 1993; Lieberman, 2002)—suggests that the anterior and posterior left-hemisphere language zones originally evolved as specializations for programming and executing complex movements. According to the motor theory, when we listen to speech, we are analyzing the speech sounds with reference to the underlying movements of the throat and mouth that create them, and we do this analysis using the same neural systems that we would use to *make* those sounds ourselves. In this schema, simple phonemic units are programmed by an anterior system, and a posterior system strings speech sounds together into long sequences of movements (Kimura and Watson, 1989). Consistent with the motor theory of speech perception, deaf people who use American Sign Language—a language based entirely on movements instead of sounds—employ the same language-related regions of the left hemisphere as hearing people who use spoken language (Newman et al., 2015), and they show comparable aphasia-like symptoms after left-hemisphere damage (Corina et al., 2013).

In any event, detailed imaging studies show that the brain contains several speech-related areas well outside those of the classical model (E. Bates et al., 2003; Dronkers et al., 2004), implying greater complexity than was proposed under the Wernicke-Geschwind model. Further, recent evidence that low-level aspects of speech perception occur bilaterally (Cogan et al., 2014) and that semantic processing of natural speech relies heavily on both hemispheres (Huth et al., 2016; De Heer et al., 2017) shows that much remains to be determined about exactly what is, and what is not, the exclusive domain of the left-hemisphere language network. Whatever the details may be, it seems that the answer will involve a complex network of mechanisms that link perception to action.

HOW'S IT GOING ?

1. Distinguish among aphasia, agraphia, and alexia.
2. Identify the main types of aphasia, and summarize the distinctive symptoms of each. Which type of aphasia is most often associated with paralysis?
3. Provide a brief outline of the traditional "connectionist" model of aphasia. How does it get its name, and what shortcomings of the model have been identified by critics?
4. Briefly describe the motor theory of language. Can you think of ways that this theory may relate to the evolutionary origins of language?

Brain mapping helps us understand the organization of language in the brain

In healthy people with intact language capabilities, researchers can study the brain's language network by using two general experimental approaches. In some studies, researchers stimulate discrete regions of the cortex and measure associated changes in language function. Conversely, participants may be asked to engage in specific verbal behaviors while researchers measure associated changes in brain activity, using functional brain imaging. Together, these techniques have extended our understanding of the neural bases of language.

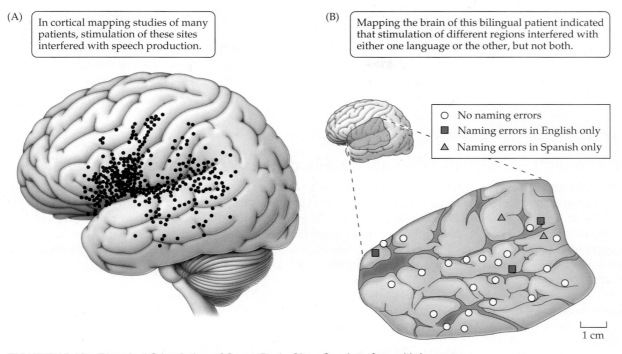

(A) In cortical mapping studies of many patients, stimulation of these sites interfered with speech production.

(B) Mapping the brain of this bilingual patient indicated that stimulation of different regions interfered with either one language or the other, but not both.

○ No naming errors
■ Naming errors in English only
△ Naming errors in Spanish only

1 cm

FIGURE 15.13 Electrical Stimulation of Some Brain Sites Can Interfere with Language (Part A after W. Penfield and L. Roberts. 1959. *Speech and brain-mechanisms.* Princeton University Press. Princeton, NJ; B after W. H. Calvin and G. Ojemann. 1994. *Conversations with Neil's brain: The neural nature of thought and language.* Addison-Wesley. Reading, MA.)

Early studies of the organization of language areas in the brain employed electrical stimulation mapping, in which a surgeon used a handheld electrode to electrically stimulate discrete regions of cortex while the effect on behavior was observed. Most of these studies collected data from people undergoing neurosurgery to remove a tumor or epileptic tissue (as in Wilder Penfield's experiments that we described in Chapter 1). Once the brain was exposed, small stimulating electrodes were touched to the surface, disrupting the normal functioning of neurons in the immediate vicinity. Because patients were given only local anesthesia, they were conscious and able to perform various cognitive tasks (the main aim of the procedure was to identify tissue that could be removed without impairing language). Data from numerous neurosurgical cases were superimposed to create a map of language-related zones of the left hemisphere (**FIGURE 15.13A**) (Penfield and Roberts, 1959). Stimulation anywhere within a large anterior zone often stopped speech outright. Other forms of language interference, such as misnaming or impaired repetition of words, occurred with stimulation throughout the anterior and posterior cortical speech zones.

Later cortical stimulation studies revealed anatomical compartmentalization of linguistic elements such as naming, verb generation, reading, speech production, and verbal memory (Calvin and Ojemann, 1994; Corina et al., 2005). An interesting example of the effects of cortical stimulation on naming is illustrated in **FIGURE 15.13B**, which shows the different places where stimulation caused naming errors in English and Spanish in a bilingual person. Note that this very fine-grained approach reveals different subregions that disrupt either English or Spanish function. People who are bilingual from an early age show completely overlapping organization of their two languages at the gross neuroanatomical level (Perani and Abutalebi, 2005), and evidence is mounting that early bilingualism has far-reaching beneficial effects on brain organization and resistance to cognitive decline in later life (Costa and Sebastián-Gallés, 2014; Perani et al., 2017).

Other studies employ a noninvasive cortical stimulation technology called *transcranial magnetic stimulation* to further probe the organization of language areas in healthy volunteers. As we discuss next, these studies have confirmed the general organization of the left-hemisphere language network and have revealed new details about the compartmentalization of functions within traditional speech areas.

RESEARCHERS AT WORK ||||||||||||||||||||||||||||||||||||||||||||||||||||||||||||||||||||||||||||||||||||||||

Noninvasive stimulation mapping reveals details of the brain's language areas

Transcranial magnetic stimulation (TMS; see Figure 1.20) allows researchers to stimulate small clusters of cortical neurons with good precision, from outside the scalp. By using MRI scans to select targets, TMS provides a noninvasive method for inducing a sort of temporary brain lesion, disrupting the activity of the selected brain region for up to an hour. Alternatively, TMS can be used along with PET or fMRI to precisely map regions of increased activity.

Using TMS mapping, researchers have generally replicated and extended the earlier findings regarding the cortical organization of language functions. For example, TMS mapping has revealed that speech production is associated with activation of not only face areas in motor cortex, but also hand areas, confirming the linkage and possible evolutionary relationship of hand gestures and speech (Meister et al., 2003; Onmyoji et al., 2015). Similarly, TMS mapping has been used to show that speech perception activates specific regions that TMS shows to be involved with speech production (S. K. Scott and Wise, 2004), providing support for the motor theory of language that we discussed earlier.

Impressively, the TMS temporary-lesion approach has revealed previously unknown functional subregions within Broca's area (**FIGURE 15.14**). In these studies, researchers found that anterior parts of Broca's area are involved in the semantic meaning of words, while a more posterior part of Broca's area is important for the patterning of speech sounds (Gough et al., 2005; Klaus and Hartwigsen, 2019). Other research has shown that the posterior speech zone

likewise contributes to both word meaning and sound-related aspects of language (Stoeckel et al., 2009; Sakreida et al., 2018). So the TMS procedure is providing new insights into the fine details of the cortical organization of language, especially in conjunction with traditional neuroimaging techniques (Devlin and Watkins, 2007; Lorca-Puls et al., 2017).

■ Question
How is Broca's area organized?

■ Hypothesis
Broca's area is made up of discrete subareas with differing linguistic functions.

■ Test
Guided by precise structural MRI scans, apply transcranial magnetic stimulation (TMS) to activate discrete regions within Broca's area.

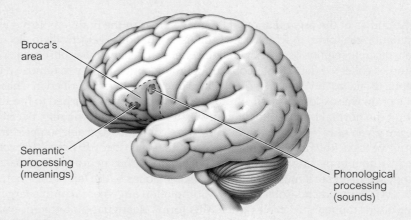

■ Result
Anterior regions of Broca's area appear to be important for semantic processing (word meanings), while more posterior regions within Broca's area specialize in phonological processing (sounds of words).

FIGURE 15.14   Subregions of Broca's Area Revealed by TMS (After P. M. Gough et al. 2005. *J. Neurosci.* 25: 8010.)

Functional neuroimaging technologies let us visualize activity in the brain's language zones during speech

Different aspects of language processing produce noticeably different patterns of brain activation, as shown in **FIGURE 15.15**. Passive *viewing* of words activates a posterior area within the left hemisphere (**FIGURE 15.15A**), but passive *hearing* of words shifts the focus of brain activation to the temporal lobes (**FIGURE 15.15B**). Repeating words orally activates the motor cortex of both sides, along with supplementary motor cortex and some of the cerebellum (**FIGURE 15.15C**). During word repetition or reading aloud, there is little activity in Broca's area. But when participants are required to generate an appropriate verb to go with a supplied noun, language-related regions in the left hemisphere, including Broca's area, suddenly become markedly activated (**FIGURE 15.15D**).

(A) Passively viewing words

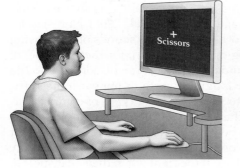

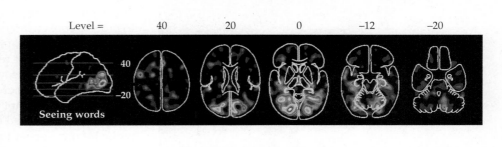

(B) Listening to words

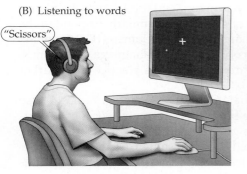

(C) Speaking words

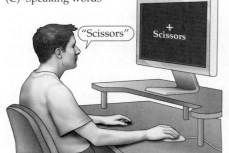

(D) Generating a verb associated with each noun shown

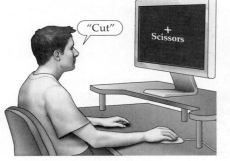

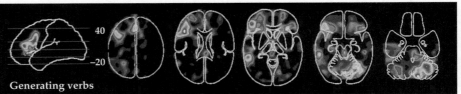

FIGURE 15.15 PET Scans of Brain Activation in Progressively More Complex Language Tasks (After M. I. Posner and M. E. Raichle. 1994. *Images of mind.* Scientific American Library. New York, NY.)

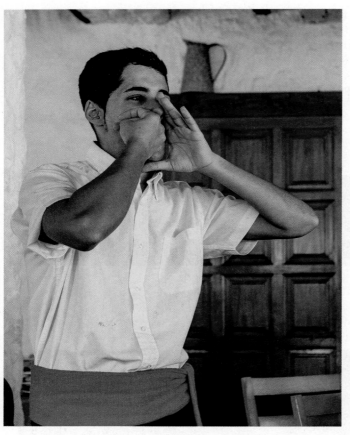

Whistle While You Work A *silbador* of the Canary Islands demonstrates *Silbo Gomero*, a whistled language used by shepherds to communicate over long distances.

Even languages that sound very, very different seem to activate much the same brain regions in native speakers. Silbo Gomero is a very unusual whistled surrogate language of the Canary Islands, used by shepherds (known as *silbadores*) to communicate over long distances. In Silbo, whistled notes serve as the phonemes and morphemes of a stripped-down form of Spanish (for an audio sample of Silbo, with translation, see **A STEP FURTHER 15.2**, on the website). Functional MRI showed that long-term *silbadores* process Silbo using the same left-hemisphere mechanisms that they (and everyone else) use to process spoken language (Carreiras et al., 2005). Non-*silbador* controls, in contrast, process the whistle sounds of Silbo using completely different regions of the brain; for these people, of course, the whistle sounds have no linguistic content. So the brain's left-hemisphere language systems appear to be sufficiently plastic to adapt to widely varying types of communication sounds, provided that they're heard early enough. In fact, while infants appear to be born with neural specializations for *speech* already in operation—they show more metabolic activity in the left hemisphere than in the right when they hear speech, even though they don't yet understand it (Dehaene-Lambertz et al., 2002)—those mechanisms don't similarly respond to the nonspeech sounds that make up Silbo Gomero (L. May et al., 2018). The incorporation of Silbo into the language system must therefore come about through extensive practice—the earlier the better.

Event-related potentials (ERPs; see Chapters 2 and 14) also provide hints about the brain's language network, by revealing the time base for language processing. For example, study participants can be asked to read a sentence in which there is a word that is grammatically correct but, because of its meaning, doesn't fit—such as "The man started the car engine and stepped on the pancake"—while brain electrical activity is recorded from scalp electrodes. About 400 milliseconds after the participant reads the word *pancake*, an enhancement of a distinctive ERP component called *N400* (*N* denotes "negative," and the number represents the response time in milliseconds; see Figure 14.6) is detectable (Kutas and Hillyard, 1984; Payne et al., 2015). Such N400 responses seem to be specific to word meanings and apparently originate from temporoparietal cortex (including Wernicke's area) (Kutas and Federmeier, 2011). In contrast, words that are inappropriate because of *grammar* rather than *meaning* tend to elicit a *positive* potential about 600 milliseconds after they are encountered (called a *P600 response*), indicating that detection of this level of error requires an extra 200 milliseconds of brain processing by other components of the language network (Osterhout, 1997; Mehravari et al., 2015). The degree to which meaning and grammar are processed independently in the brain, however, remains to be fully established and is an area of active investigation (Kuperberg, 2007; Brouwer et al., 2017).

HOW'S IT GOING ?

1. Summarize and discuss the organization of language systems in the human brain.

2. Discuss the patterns of brain activity that are observed in various verbal tasks, using functional-imaging technologies and ERPs. How well do these results align with traditional models of the organization of language areas in the brain?

3. What can we learn about general principles of language localization in the brain by studying unusual languages like Silbo Gomero?

15.4 Human Languages Share Basic Features

THE ROAD AHEAD

The next part of the chapter narrows its focus to our species' most distinctive characteristic: the everyday use of language, both in the form of speech and in the written word. After studying this material, you should be able to:

15.4.1 Provide a synopsis of the evolution and distribution of human languages.

15.4.2 Identify the principle linguistic components of speech.

15.4.3 Summarize the process of language development and the acquisition of grammar and reading skills.

15.4.4 Contrast human language with nonhuman animal communication.

15.4.5 Discuss in detail the forms of dyslexia and their possible neural underpinnings.

We've seen that all human languages share certain basic elements: phonemes, morphemes, and grammar. But how does each of us end up with the *right* set of sounds and rules—the ones we need for our particular native language?

The exact number of languages that we humans employ is unknown; our best guess is that there are 6,000–7,000 different languages, of which about 1,000 have been formally studied (Wuethrich, 2000). By applying the tools of evolutionary biology to linguistics, it is possible to track the cultural evolution of language, and this suggests a closer relation between languages than previously expected. In fact, the seven major language families found today in Europe and Asia appear to trace back to a single ancestral language in use about 15,000 years ago (**FIGURE 15.16**; Pagel et al., 2013). The subsequent explosion of new languages may have served cultural roles more than communicative ones; for example, the adoption of a new language would help a social group to identify its members and confound its rivals. But nowadays, in the increasingly globalized modern context, we seem to be inexorably sliding in the other direction as languages are lost or absorbed and we move toward a few common languages.

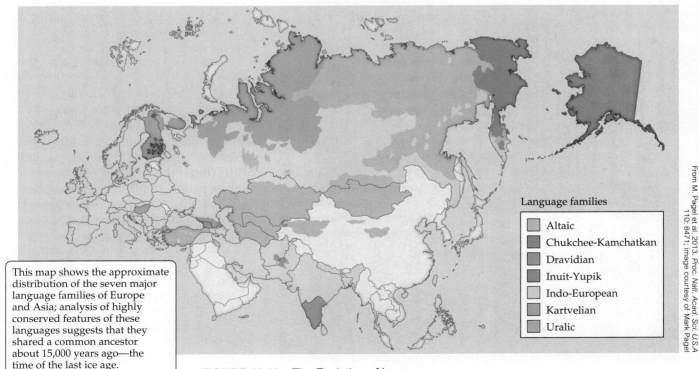

This map shows the approximate distribution of the seven major language families of Europe and Asia; analysis of highly conserved features of these languages suggests that they shared a common ancestor about 15,000 years ago—the time of the last ice age.

Language families

- Altaic
- Chukchee-Kamchatkan
- Dravidian
- Inuit-Yupik
- Indo-European
- Kartvelian
- Uralic

From M. Pagel et al. 2013. *Proc. Natl. Acad. Sci. U.S.A* 110: 8471; image courtesy of Mark Pagel

FIGURE 15.16 The Evolution of Languages

sensitive period   Also called *critical period*. The period during development in which an organism can be permanently altered by a particular experience or treatment.

stuttering   The tendency of otherwise healthy people to produce speech sounds only haltingly, tripping over certain syllables or being unable to start vocalizing certain words.

Williams syndrome   A disorder characterized by impairments of spatial cognition and IQ but superior linguistic abilities.

The King's Speech   England's King George VI—shown here during a wartime radio broadcast—stuttered severely. His struggle and eventual success in coping with speech difficulties, as portrayed in the film *The King's Speech*, shows that despite the possible genetic bases of the condition, effective therapy is possible.

© Hulton-Deutsch/Corbis Historical/Getty Images

Language has both unlearned and learned components

A child's brain is an incredible linguistic machine, rapidly acquiring the local language without need of formal instruction. Human babies start out babbling nearly all the known phonemes of all human languages, but they soon come to use only those phonemes that they hear in use around themselves. And each baby's developing language abilities are especially shaped by "parentese," the singsong speech of caregivers that helps babies to attach emotion and meaning to speech sounds (Falk, 2004). By 7 months of age, infants already have a sense of the grammar of the language used in their homes, and they react to exceptions (Marcus et al., 1999).

The human brain contains specialized mechanisms for language acquisition that show a clear-cut **sensitive period** (or *critical period*): a limited span of time during which exposure and practice with language must occur in order for language skills to develop normally. This sensitive period tapers down from the maximal sensitivity of early childhood to an eventual end of special sensitivity around puberty. Individuals who are exposed to language only late in the sensitive period or after it has ended show impaired language development; as many of us know from firsthand experience, learning a second language is much more difficult in adulthood, after the sensitive period is over (Curtiss, 1989; Norrman and Bylund, 2016). In fact, people who don't start to learn a second language until later in childhood or after puberty seem to use different brain networks for each language, compared with people who learn multiple languages simultaneously in early childhood (H. Liu and Cao, 2016; Cargnelutti et al., 2019), as we discussed earlier.

An important genetic aspect of language acquisition was discovered by studying an unusual family in England. Across at least three generations, about half of the members of the KE family have expressed a severe heritable language disorder. Affected family members take a long time to learn to speak and have difficulty with particular language tasks, such as learning verb tenses (Lai et al., 2001). Brain activation during language tasks is altered in these family members too (Liégeois et al., 2003).

By studying the KE family's pedigree, researchers soon identified a gene, called *FOXP2*, that must be important for the normal acquisition of human language, because affected members of the KE family all share a mutation in this gene (**FIGURE 15.17**). In fact, multiple variants of *FOXP2* tend to produce different abnormalities in language-associated areas of the brain (Pinel et al., 2012), probably because *FOXP2* is a transcription factor that can alter expression of a variety of other genes (Vernes et al., 2011). **Stuttering**—the tendency of otherwise healthy people to produce speech sounds only haltingly, tripping over certain syllables or being unable to start vocalizing certain words—is likewise at least partly heritable and associated with changes in other genes (C. Kang et al., 2010).

On the flip side of the coin, children born with **Williams syndrome**—caused by the deletion of 28 genes from chromosome 7—have various intellectual deficits but excellent verbal skills. No one knows exactly what developmental mechanism results in this

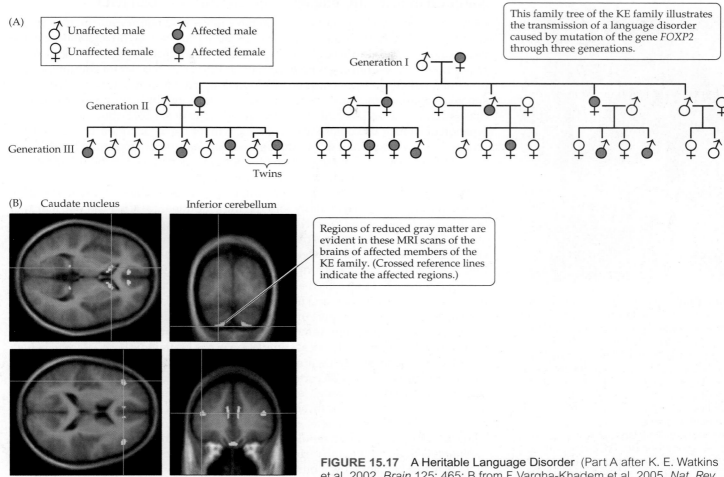

(A)

♂ Unaffected male	⚥ Affected male
♀ Unaffected female	⚥ Affected female

This family tree of the KE family illustrates the transmission of a language disorder caused by mutation of the gene *FOXP2* through three generations.

Generation I

Generation II

Generation III

Twins

(B)   Caudate nucleus   Inferior cerebellum

Regions of reduced gray matter are evident in these MRI scans of the brains of affected members of the KE family. (Crossed reference lines indicate the affected regions.)

Inferior frontal gyrus from two perspectives

FIGURE 15.17   A Heritable Language Disorder   (Part A after K. E. Watkins et al. 2002. *Brain* 125: 465; B from F. Vargha-Khadem et al. 2005. *Nat. Rev. Neurosci.* 6: 131, courtesy of Faraneh Vargha-Khadem.)

hyperverbal behavior (Paterson and Schultz, 2007), but possession of *extra* copies of the identified genes on chromosome 7—rather than deletions of these genes—produces a syndrome of very poor expressive language that is, in many ways, the converse of Williams syndrome (Somerville et al., 2005).

Taken together, the evidence confirms that basic mechanisms of language are heritable components of the human brain, and the product of a long evolutionary history. Speech mechanisms may have evolved from more-ancient systems controlling gestures of the face and hands (Corballis, 2020), in agreement with the motor theory of language that we discussed earlier. Even today there is a close relationship between speaking and gesturing with the hands (Gentilucci and Dalla Volta, 2008); in fact, most people find it difficult *not* to gesture when speaking. The use of language is one of the key adaptations of humans, so basic capabilities probably arose in an ancient ancestor of our species. For example, the Neandertals shared our version of *FOXP2* (Krause et al., 2007), so perhaps major differences in just a few genes like *FOXP2* and the stuttering genes are enough to explain why we write books and give speeches and chimps do not, despite our otherwise great genetic similarity (Fisher, 2017).

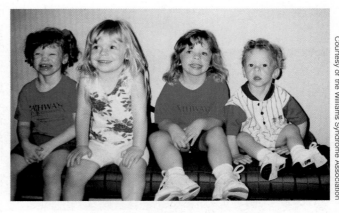

The Appearance of Williams Syndrome   Children with Williams syndrome often have a characteristic facial shape, caused by the loss of a copy of the elastin gene. The loss of copies of other nearby genes is thought to cause mild mental disability paired with verbal fluency.

Courtesy of the Williams Syndrome Association

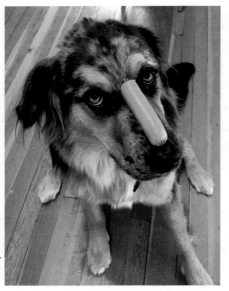

Good Dog!   Dog lovers know that their willing friends can learn to associate certain words with specific actions. Maisie here knows to "wait" until she hears "okay," at which time she will enjoy both a delicious sausage and a delighted human. Dogs can learn a small collection of words with sufficient practice (lots of practice, for some dogs), enabling communication between human and nonhuman, but instilling *language* is a different matter altogether. Because most animals appear to lack a capacity for grammar—the rule for assembling units of language into new combinations—it seems that language is a uniquely human skill.

Nonhuman primates engage in elaborate vocal behavior

Every day, you utter sentences that you have never said before, yet the meaning is clear to both you and your human listener because you share an understanding of the words and grammar involved. Animals generally are incapable of similar feats, instead requiring extensive training with each specific utterance in order for communication to occur at all. Speaking to your dog ("Good dog!") reportedly activates a left-hemisphere mechanism that processes meaning, as well as a right-hemisphere mechanism that assigns value and reward to those words (Andics et al., 2016), but each new combination of words that you use with your dog will have to be laboriously learned from scratch. In short, dogs and most other animals appear to lack grammar. For this reason, scientists have focused the search for nonhuman language capabilities mostly on our nearest relatives, the other primate species.

Apes and monkeys employ a wide range of vocal behaviors for communication between individuals, particularly for relaying emotional information like alarm or territoriality (Cheney and Seyfarth, 2018). The shrieking, purring, peeping, growling, and cackling sounds of squirrel monkeys, for example, can generally be related to specific social situations. Chimpanzees issue specific alarm calls to alert other members of their group to the presence of a viper (Crockford et al., 2012), and gibbons deploy a sizable repertoire of hooting calls that they recombine to communicate information about predators, social conditions, and mating opportunities (Clarke et al., 2015). But despite their apparent adaptive importance, most nonhuman primate vocalizations seem to have a somewhat "preprogrammed" quality, being repeatedly produced in much the same fashion and order. Electrical stimulation of the brain indicates that vocal behavior in monkeys and apes relies primarily on subcortical systems, especially sites in the limbic system, rather than on cortex. The vocalizations elicited by subcortical stimulation are associated with strongly emotional behaviors such as defense, attack, feeding, and sex (**FIGURE 15.18**). Vocalizations are more common if subcortical stimulation is provided to the left hemisphere, indicating a special role of the left hemisphere in the communicative behavior of monkeys and apes (Meguerditchian and Vauclair, 2006; Taglialatela et al., 2006), mirroring what we've seen for human speech. And some monkeys, like people, show a preference for using the right ear (which has preferential connections with the left hemisphere) to listen to vocalizations from conspecifics (Hopkins et al., 2015).

Nonhuman primates are unlikely to ever produce human speech, as their vocal tracts and vocal repertoires are suited to their own communication needs. But can these animals be taught other forms of communication, with features similar to those of human language? Can they learn to represent objects with symbols and to manipulate those symbols according to grammatical rules? Our closest primate relatives, the great apes (chimpanzees, gorillas, orangutans) reportedly use a variety of hand gestures for communication in the wild (Hobaiter and Byrne, 2014) and are quite capable of learning hundreds of hand gestures from American Sign Language (ASL). Classic research suggests that given enough training—it takes years—apes may learn to use ASL signs spontaneously, sometimes in novel sequences (R. A. Gardner and Gardner, 1969, 1984). Through extensive practice, apes can also be trained to communicate by assembling abstract symbols, such as colored plastic chips or computerized symbols, into new sentences (Premack, 1971; Rumbaugh, 1977).

Chimpanzees can learn to use arbitrary signs and/or symbols to communicate, but it is questionable whether this usage is equivalent to human language.

Chimpanzee Using Symbols   Some researchers argue that apes (chimpanzees, gorillas, and orangutans) are able to string arbitrary symbols together into meaningful, sentence-like statements. Others believe that while apes can learn subtle associations between symbols and meanings, their communicative behavior lacks the sense of grammar that is the hallmark of human language.

Some researchers contended that apes were thus able to acquire words (or equivalent symbols) and then string them together into novel, meaningful chains; that is, they seemed to employ a grammar to communicate ideas. Other researchers argued that these sequences were simply subtle forms of imitation (Terrace, 1979), perhaps unconsciously cued by the experimenter who provided the training. Observers who are native ASL users dispute the linguistic validity of the signs generated by apes; others, such as linguist Noam Chomsky, argue that teaching primates to emulate a quintessentially human behavior in which they do not naturally engage can tell us little about the behavior, other than the obvious conclusion that ape evolution did not favor the use of language. So although the debate remains unresolved, research on the linguistic abilities of nonhuman primates at least forced researchers to sharpen their criteria of what constitutes language. Researchers are now probing the extent to which the many components of "real" language are human adaptations that evolved independently of other cognitive capabilities, in order to solve specific problems in our evolutionary past (Pinker and Jackendoff, 2005; Corballis, 2020).

Many different species engage in vocal communication

Many nonprimate species use vocalizations—chirps, barks, meows, songs, and more—to communicate important information to members of their own or other species. Although these communication sounds do not constitute language, in that they lack the features of language that we've discussed, such sounds nevertheless broadcast crucial signals about readiness to mate, danger, territorial defense, emotional state, and so on. Whales sing and may perform songs that they've learned in distant oceans or from other species (Janik 2014); and some seal mothers and pups learn each other's vocalizations and remember them for years after separation (Insley, 2000; Pitcher et al., 2010). In fact, many species—from elephants to bats to birds to dolphins—are capable of vocal learning and use their vocalizations to help form social bonds and identify individuals (Tyack, 2003; Poole et al., 2005).

In the lab, measurement with special instruments reveals that rats and mice produce complex ultrasonic vocalizations that they use to communicate emotional information (Panksepp, 2005; Burgdorf et al., 2011). These ultrasonic vocalizations are associated with *FoxP2* gene expression (Shu et al., 2005; French and Fisher, 2014), providing an intriguing parallel to the situation in humans with *FOXP2* mutations that we discussed earlier.

Birds are particularly vocal animals. While many species of birds produce only simple vocalizations, species of songbirds—canaries, zebra finches, song sparrows, etc.—produce rich and melodious vocalizations that are crucial for their social behaviors and reproductive success. A select few, such as the grey parrot, can even learn to communicate using a significant vocabulary of human words (Pepperberg, 2008). Although birdsong has evolved quite independently of human speech, there are some interesting parallels between the two: for example, the songbird brain contains a specialized left-hemisphere system for vocal behavior (Moorman et al., 2012; Pfenning et al., 2014). What's more, juvenile birds must learn their songs from adult tutors during a distinct critical period in order for their own

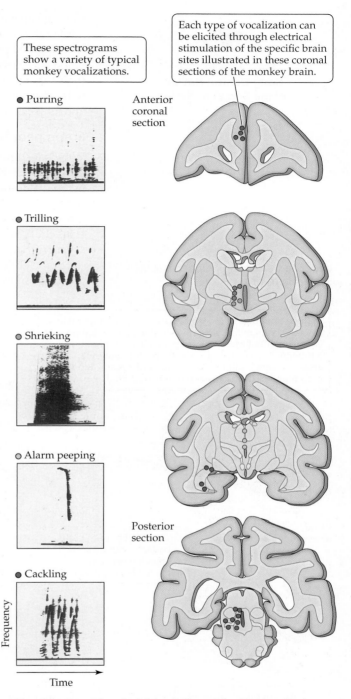

These spectrograms show a variety of typical monkey vocalizations.

Each type of vocalization can be elicited through electrical stimulation of the specific brain sites illustrated in these coronal sections of the monkey brain.

● Purring

● Trilling

● Shrieking

● Alarm peeping

● Cackling

Anterior coronal section

Posterior section

Frequency

Time

FIGURE 15.18 Electrical Stimulation of the Monkey Brain Elicits Vocalizations (After D. W. Ploog in A. Harrington. 1992. *So human a brain: Knowledge and values in the neurosciences*. Birkhauser. Boston, MA. Spectrograms courtesy of Uwe Jürgens.)

View Activity 15.3:
Song Control Nuclei
of the Songbird Brain

singing behavior to develop normally (Marler, 2004)—a requirement that also parallels human language. And yes, as with human speech, the *FoxP2* gene is implicated in the learning and production of birdsong (Bolhuis et al., 2010). When *FoxP2* expression is blocked in parts of the song control system, young males fail to properly learn and recite their tutor's song, producing errors that in some ways resemble those in the humans with abnormal *FOXP2* described earlier (Haesler et al., 2007). (For more on birdsong and its social roles, see **A STEP FURTHER 15.3**, on the website.)

Some people struggle throughout their lives to read

Why is it so much harder to learn to read and write than to speak? Compared with speech, the written word is a relatively new development for our species, so we haven't had enough time to evolve dedicated brain mechanisms for reading and writing of the sort we have for speech. Therefore, learning the written form of a language is a slow and laborious chore of childhood that is vulnerable to developmental disruptions that result in **dyslexia** (from the Greek *dys*, "bad," and *lexis*, "word"), a mild to severe difficulty with reading.

Some children just seem to take forever to learn to read, and not even extended practice can make their reading easy and accurate. Affecting about 5% of children—especially boys and left-handers—this *developmental dyslexia* is a problem unique to written language, not a general cognitive deficit. Indeed, children with dyslexia can have high IQs (B. Morris, 2002), and many have gone on to illustrious careers in varying fields. Instead, the problem seems to lie in connecting reading with the more ancient brain mechanisms for speech.

Developmental dyslexia has been associated with several types of neurological abnormalities (**FIGURE 15.19**). In both postmortem investigations and anatomical studies using MRI, the brains of dyslexic people have been found to have aberrant layering of the neurons of the cerebral cortex, along with excessive cortical folding and clusters of extra neurons in unexpected locations (Galaburda, 1994; Chang et al., 2005). Cortical abnormalities are especially evident in the frontal and temporal lobes, possibly because of defective migration of newborn neurons during fetal development (Galaburda et al., 2006). Studies using fMRI confirm that people with dyslexia show impaired neural activity in left posterior speech zones (Pugh et al., 2000; Shaywitz et al., 2003) while displaying a relative overactivation of anterior regions. Abnormality in the nearby temporoparietal region has been linked to the phonological (phoneme-processing) aspects of dyslexia (Hoeft et al., 2006). And it looks like some of these abnormalities have genetic bases; for example, disruption of genes involved in brain development

dyslexia   A reading disorder attributed to brain impairment.

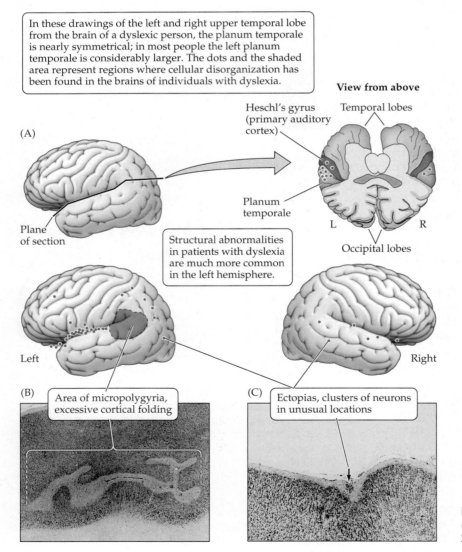

In these drawings of the left and right upper temporal lobe from the brain of a dyslexic person, the planum temporale is nearly symmetrical; in most people the left planum temporale is considerably larger. The dots and the shaded area represent regions where cellular disorganization has been found in the brains of individuals with dyslexia.

View from above

Heschl's gyrus (primary auditory cortex)

Temporal lobes

Planum temporale

L   R

Occipital lobes

(A)

Plane of section

Structural abnormalities in patients with dyslexia are much more common in the left hemisphere.

Left

Right

(B) Area of micropolygyria, excessive cortical folding

(C) Ectopias, clusters of neurons in unusual locations

FIGURE 15.19   Neural Disorganization in Dyslexia (After A. M. Galaburda et al. 1985. *Ann. Neurol.* 18: 222; micrographs courtesy of Albert Galaburda.)

and the migration of neurons into adult positions are associated with developmental dyslexia (Harold et al., 2006; Gabel et al., 2010).

Taken together, imaging and behavioral studies indicate that our brains rely on two different language systems during reading: one focused on the sounds of letters, the other on the meanings of whole words. Using fMRI, researchers found that people with dyslexia often have a disconnection between these systems, impairing the coordination of sounds with their meanings (Boets et al., 2013); it has been proposed that this disconnect is the result of hyperexcitability of reading-associated cortical networks (Hancock et al., 2017). Presumably, these systems are shaped by training: as with learning any highly skilled behavior, our brains mold themselves to accommodate our acquired expertise with written language, and lifelong avoidance of reading may be responsible for some of the sensory and word meaning problems that are evident in adults with dyslexia (Goswami, 2015). This could be why remedial training in people with dyslexia induces measurable changes in the left-hemisphere systems that are used for reading (Temple et al., 2003). And there are also positive findings: for example, evidence is accumulating that people with dyslexia actually outperform unaffected individuals in certain learning domains, such as aspects of spatial learning (Schneps et al., 2012). Findings like these may have important implications for developing new educational strategies in dyslexia. Perhaps, then, coupling education interventions with early genetic screening for dyslexia will help affected people completely overcome their trouble with words.

Brain damage may cause specific impairments in reading

Sometimes people who learned to read just fine as children suddenly become dyslexic in adulthood as a result of disease or injury, usually to the left hemisphere. This *acquired dyslexia* (sometimes called *alexia*) offers hints about how the brain processes written language. One type of acquired dyslexia, known as **deep dyslexia**, is characterized by semantic errors (i.e., errors related to the *meanings* of words); for example, the printed word *cow* is read as *horse*. People with deep dyslexia are also unable to read aloud words that are abstract as opposed to concrete, and they make frequent errors in which they seem to fail to see small differences in words. It's as though they grasp words whole, without noting the details of the letters, so they have a hard time sounding out nonsense words.

In another form of acquired dyslexia, **surface dyslexia**, the person makes different types of errors when reading. These people can read nonsense words without problems, indicating that they understand which letters make which sounds. But they find it difficult to recognize words in which the letter-to-sound rules are irregular. *The Tough Coughs as He Ploughs the Dough* by Dr. Seuss (1987), for example, would utterly confound them. In contrast to people with deep dyslexia, those with surface dyslexia have difficulties that are restricted to the details and sounds of letters. Interestingly, surface dyslexia doesn't occur in native speakers of languages that are perfectly phonetic (such as Italian, where every letter is pronounced). This finding indicates that what's lost in speakers of nonphonetic languages, like English, is purely a learned aspect of language. In contrast, deep dyslexia probably involves language mechanisms that are important for all languages.

Other kinds of brain damage can impair reading. For example, people with hemispatial neglect following right parietal lobe damage (discussed in Chapter 14) disregard the left half of the world, despite having otherwise normal vision. Such people thus also fail to notice the left halves of the words that they see, necessarily resulting in poor reading. In some severe cases of acquired dyslexia, the individuals exhibit *letter-by-letter reading*, a striking impairment in which they laboriously spell out each word to themselves (aloud or silently). In these cases, it seems that conscious attention to the spelling of each word is the only way by which words can be identified, so reading is dramatically slower.

deep dyslexia   Acquired dyslexia in which the person reads a word as another word that is semantically related.

surface dyslexia   Acquired dyslexia in which the person seems to attend only to the fine details of reading.

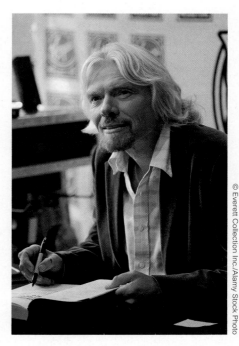

Overcoming Dyslexia   Many highly intelligent, highly successful people—like Virgin Group founder Sir Richard Branson, pictured here—have coped with dyslexia on their way to fame and fortune.

© Everett Collection Inc./Alamy Stock Photo

recovery of function The recovery of behavioral capacity following brain damage from stroke or injury.

HOW'S IT GOING ?

1. How many languages do humans use, and how have they spread over time?
2. Why do researchers think that a capacity for language is inborn in the human brain? Briefly describe some pertinent research findings that support this position, including genetic evidence.
3. What are the basic linguistic components of spoken language?
4. Discuss the process of language acquisition in infants. What is the significance of the term *sensitive period* in this regard?
5. Summarize some of the ways in which studies of nonhuman animals help us understand the neural mechanisms of language.
6. Why do researchers believe that it is so much harder to learn to read than to learn to speak?
7. What are the two principal types of acquired dyslexia? Summarize their respective features.

15.5 Recovery of Function after Brain Damage: Stabilization and Reorganization Are Crucial Stages

THE ROAD AHEAD

Because so much of the data on cerebral lateralization and language mechanisms has been drawn from studies of people with lateralized brain damage due to strokes and other types of brain injuries, the final section of the chapter turns to the processes by which the brain recovers at least some functions following damage. After reading this material, you should be able to:

15.5.1 Discuss the prevalence of various forms of brain damage and the reasons why so many people are living with the lasting effects of brain injury.

15.5.2 Describe the typical timeline for neurological recovery from a stroke or other brain damage, and identify factors that affect this process.

15.5.3 Discuss potential therapies that can aid the process of recovery.

15.5.4 Explore how it is that children can recover from brain injury much more completely than adults can.

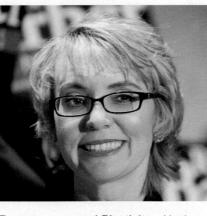

Perseverance and Plasticity Having survived a severe gunshot wound to the left cerebral hemisphere during an assassination attempt, former U.S. Representative Gabrielle Giffords has made striking progress in regaining her language and cognitive functions, thanks to intensive rehabilitation therapy and strategies for compensating for the damage.

Compared with the other organs of the body, it's all too easy to seriously damage the brain. A number of factors combine to make the brain so vulnerable: extreme complexity, delicate structure, metabolic neediness, limited capacity for regrowth, and an exposed location perched atop a thin and whippy neck. In the United States alone, according to the 2016 National Health Interview Survey (Blackwell and Villarroel, 2018), almost 7.5 million adults are survivors of stroke, and many more are living with the consequences of other disease processes, such as tumors and degenerative diseases. Traumatic brain injury (TBI) has many causes: motor vehicle accidents, injuries at work and in the home, and mishaps during recreational activities and sports (especially contact sports, as we'll see shortly). So, while prevention is always preferable to treatment, researchers are intensively studying **recovery of function**, with the aim of developing treatments that improve outcomes for people with brain damage.

In the months following a brain injury, people often show conspicuous improvements in neural function as the injury site stabilizes, unaffected tissue reorganizes, and compensation occurs. We now know that the nervous system has much more potential for plasticity and recovery than was previously believed. For example, damaged neurons can regrow their connections under some circumstances, through a process called *collateral sprouting*. (For more information on collateral sprouting,

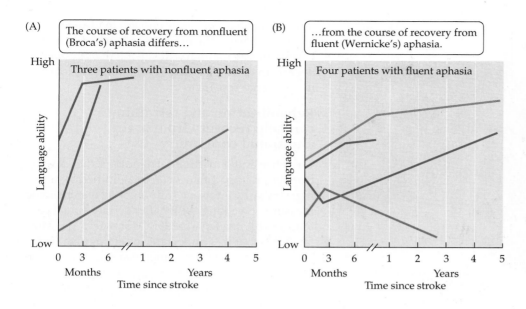

(A) The course of recovery from nonfluent (Broca's) aphasia differs...

Three patients with nonfluent aphasia

Language ability — High / Low

0 3 6 | 1 2 3 4 5
Months   Years
Time since stroke

(B) ...from the course of recovery from fluent (Wernicke's) aphasia.

Four patients with fluent aphasia

Language ability — High / Low

0 3 6 | 1 2 3 4 5
Months   Years
Time since stroke

FIGURE 15.20 Courses of Recovery for People with Aphasia (After A. Kertesz and P. McCabe. 1977. *Brain* 100: 1.)

see **A STEP FURTHER 15.4**, on the website.) And, as we've discussed in several places in this book, it has become evident that the adult brain is capable of producing new neurons; although this neurogenesis normally plays a minimal role in recovery from brain damage, perhaps we will learn how to bend these new neurons to our will and use them to replace damaged brain tissue.

One of the most exciting prospects for brain repair following stroke or injury or in many other neurological conditions is the use of **embryonic stem cells** (Casarosa et al., 2014; J. Takahashi, 2018). Derived from embryos, these cells have not yet differentiated into specific roles and therefore are able to develop, under the control of local chemical cues, into the types of cells needed. Controversy surrounds the use of human embryos as cell donors, so researchers are working to find ways of creating stem cells from other sources, such as skin, that can then be placed in the brain and helped to survive, migrate, and mature into functioning replacement neurons (Emborg et al., 2013; Morizane et al., 2017).

Several factors determine how thoroughly a person will recover from a brain injury. One of these is simply the passage of time. Immediate medical treatment at the onset of a stroke can greatly limit the extent of damage, reducing cell death and inflammation. (Mechanisms of brain damage, and the mitigation of brain injuries, are discussed in **A STEP FURTHER 15.5**, on the website.) However, it takes months for the extent of recovery to become evident. For people with aphasia following a stroke, most recovery occurs during the first 3 months following brain damage, but steady recovery continues for 1–1.5 years (**FIGURE 15.20**) (Kertesz et al., 1979), limited by the extent to which the left-hemisphere speech zones have been compromised. Recovery tends to be better when the brain injury is due to trauma, such as a blow to the head, rather than a stroke; this difference may be due to the generation of cell-damaging signaling chemicals in cells that have been starved of oxygen during a stroke. Older people and those with more-severe initial loss of language recover less completely (Nakagawa et al., 2019). And left-handed people show better recovery than those who are right-handed, perhaps because of reduced lateralization of function in some left-handers. Therapeutic approaches using alternate communication channels, such as singing, can help in some cases (Racette et al., 2006).

Recovery can be downright amazing in children, thanks to their greater neural plasticity: A child may show extensive language recovery even after losing the *entire* left hemisphere (Boshuisen et al., 2010; Lew, 2014) (**FIGURE 15.21**). Such observations show that undamaged brain regions *can* take over the functions of damaged regions,

embryonic stem cell A cell, derived from an embryo, that has the capacity to form any type of tissue.

In certain very rare cases of intractable childhood epilepsy, an entire hemisphere must be surgically removed to save the child's life (Griessenauer et al., 2015). The loss of the hemisphere produces severe symptoms such as complete paralysis of one side, speech loss, and visual impairments, but if the surgery occurs early enough the child may show almost complete recovery of function over a long period of time. Several years after a *hemispherectomy*—radical surgery to remove the left hemisphere—the 7-year-old pictured here had recovered normal language function (including bilingual capacity!) and near normal contralateral motor control.

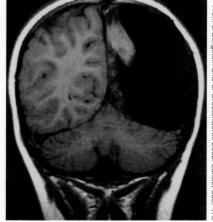

FIGURE 15. 21 The Amazing Resilience of a Child's Brain

From J. Borgstein and C. Grootendorst. 2002. *Lancet* 359: 473

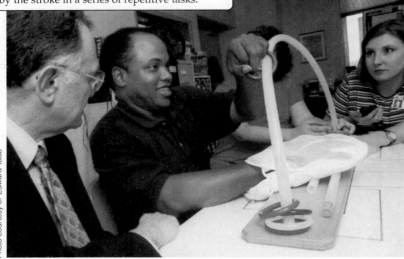

In this therapy, an unaffected limb is gently restrained (in this case in a white mitten) so that the patient must use the limb that was affected by the stroke in a series of repetitive tasks.

Photo courtesy of Edward Taub

FIGURE 15.22   Constraint-Induced Movement Therapy

if the damage occurs early enough in life. Unfortunately, as we age, the brain loses much of its ability to compensate for injury. Reversing this age-related decline in neuroplasticity is an important focus of neuroscience research.

Rehabilitation and retraining can help recovery from brain and spinal cord injury

Cognitive and/or perceptual handicaps that develop from brain impairments can be modified by training; similarly, intensive training may restore some measure of walking ability after certain spinal cord injuries (Barbeau et al., 1998; Morawietz and Moffat, 2013). But it is important to distinguish restoration of function from compensation. Practice can significantly reduce the impact of brain injury by fostering compensatory behavior (T. A. Jones, 2017). For example, vigorous eye movements can make up for the *scotomas* (blind spots) that commonly result from strokes or other injuries that affect the visual cortex. Indeed, people can develop a wide variety of behavioral strategies after a brain injury to enable successful performance on various tasks.

As with recovery of language functions after stroke, a growing body of evidence shows that people can substantially regain the use of limbs that have been paralyzed following brain injury, especially if they are *forced* to use the limbs repeatedly. **Constraint-induced movement therapy** (**CIMT**) persuades people to use a stroke-affected arm by simply tying the "good" arm to a splint for up to 90% of waking hours (Taub et al., 2002) in conjunction with daily rehabilitation therapy, including practice moving the affected limb repeatedly (**FIGURE 15.22**). People who receive this treatment reportedly regain up to 75% of normal use of the paralyzed arm after only 2 weeks of therapy. Although the underlying mechanisms are not well understood—they may involve a remapping of the motor cortex—it's clear that CIMT offers substantial benefits that persist over the long term (Liepert et al., 2000; Kwakkel et al., 2015).

Another surprising use of experience for rehabilitation involves a simple mirror. Altschuler et al. (1999) treated people who had reduced use of one arm after a stroke by placing them before a mirror with only their "good" arm visible. To these people, it looked as though they were seeing the entire body, but what they saw were mirror images of the good arm. The participants were told to make symmetrical fluid motions with both arms. In the mirror, the motions looked perfectly symmetrical (of course); surprisingly, even though their real arm movements weren't perfect, most of the participants soon learned to use the "weak" arm more extensively. It was as though the visible feedback, indicating that the weak arm was moving perfectly, overcame the brain's reluctance to use that arm. It is likely that the mirror neurons of the brain, discussed in Chapter 5, mediate some of the beneficial effects of this sort of rehearsal (Buccino et al., 2006).

Brain damage will remain a serious problem for the foreseeable future—one that will affect most of us in some way as our friends and relatives go through their lives. Perhaps the most important and encouraging message to convey to victims of stroke and other nervous system damage is that, with effort and perseverance, they can help their remarkably plastic brains to regain a significant amount of the lost behavioral capacity.

constraint-induced movement therapy (CIMT)   A therapy for recovery of movement after stroke or injury in which the person's unaffected limb is constrained while they are required to perform tasks with the affected limb.

SIGNS & SYMPTOMS |||||||||||||||||||||||||||||||||||||||||||||||||||||||||||||||||||||||||||||||||||||||||||||||||||||||||||||||||||||||||||||||||||||||||||||||||||||||

Contact Sports Can Be Costly

Jarring blows to the head are common in a number of sports—football, hockey, boxing, and wrestling, for example—sometimes resulting in **concussion** or *mild traumatic brain injury* (mTBI), with a range of possible symptoms including headache, mood disturbances, confusion, memory loss, and occasionally (but not usually) a brief loss of consciousness. Even one concussion, but especially a series of concussions or minor head impacts—even seemingly mild ones—puts a person at risk of permanent brain damage. Although uncomplicated concussions generally clear up with time, up to 25% of concussions may cause persistent cognitive symptoms (Ponsford, 2005), some of which may not become evident until later in the person's life (Thornton et al., 2008; Montenigro et al., 2016). In the USA alone, mTBIs result in more than 2.2 million hospital visits per year (CDC 2015); many more go unreported.

In an early large-scale CT study of 338 active boxers—athletes whose whole goal is to rain blows upon the head of an opponent—scans were abnormal in 7% (showing brain atrophy) and borderline in 12% (B. D. Jordan et al., 1992). The marked cognitive impairment that results from too many concussions, once called *dementia pugilistica* (the Latin *pugil* means "boxer") or *punch-drunk syndrome* (Erlanger et al., 1999), is known today as **chronic traumatic encephalopathy** (**CTE**). Evidence is mounting that

CTE is also alarmingly frequent in other athletes, especially American football players (Mez et al., 2017).

Researchers have not yet agreed on a definitive diagnostic marker for CTE in living people—typically, it can be diagnosed only in postmortem analysis (McKee et al., 2016)—but one possible approach uses a special type of PET scan to detect abnormal expression of the cytostructural protein tau in the brain (Barrio et al., 2015; see Figure 4.18). Neuropathological evidence indicates that, like Alzheimer's disease, CTE in athletes is a type of *tauopathy*, in which excess tau protein within neurons interferes with their functioning (McKee et al., 2009). The photos in **FIGURE 15.23** show the brain of a former boxer who, by his mid-thirties, was experiencing symptoms including memory loss, confusion, and a tendency to fall. As in other cases of CTE, an excessive amount of tau (brown in the photos) is evident in the brain, and it is found forming tangles within many neurons. CTE is a real and serious risk in contact sports, particularly where numerous blows to the head are sustained on a regular basis—which is why many researchers and physicians believe that the rules of some of these sports, especially where youths are participating, are in serious need of revision (*Nature*, 2017). And some sports, such as boxing, should perhaps retire from the ring altogether.

Unmagnified section of cortex

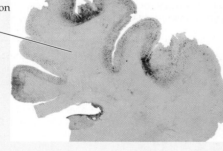

Cortical gray matter magnified x350

From McKee et al. 2009. *J. Neuropathol. Exp. Neurol.* 68: 709, courtesy of Ann McKee

FIGURE 15.23   Tau Protein in the Brain of a Boxer with CTE

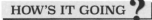
HOW'S IT GOING ❓

1. Just how prevalent is brain damage due to stroke, and to other diseases? Once the brain is damaged, is recovery more or less complete in a matter of hours, days, or months?

2. Discuss some of the factors that determine how thoroughly a person will recover from brain injury.

3. Is recovery better when brain damage is caused by trauma or when the damage is caused by stroke? What is believed to be responsible for the difference?

4. Discuss some of the types of therapy that appear to help maximize recovery following brain damage.

concussion   A form of closed head injury caused by a jarring blow to the head, resulting in damage to the tissue of the brain with short- or long-term consequences for cognitive function.

chronic traumatic encephalopathy (CTE)   A form of dementia that may develop following multiple concussions, such as in athletes engaged in contact sports.

Recommended Reading

Berwick, R. C., and Chomsky, N. (2015). *Why Only Us: Language and Evolution*. Cambridge, MA: MIT Press.

Bradbury, J. W., and Vehrencamp, S. L. (2011). *Principles of Animal Communication* (2nd ed.). Sunderland, MA: Oxford University Press/Sinauer.

Breedlove, S. M. (2017). *Foundations of Neural Development*. Sunderland, MA: Oxford University Press/Sinauer.

Fitch, W. T. (2010). *The Evolution of Language*. Cambridge, UK: Cambridge University Press.

Gazzaniga, M. S. (2016). *Tales from Both Sides of the Brain: A Life in Neuroscience*. New York, NY: Ecco.

Harrison, D. W. (2015). *Brain Asymmetry and Neural Systems: Foundations in Clinical Neuroscience and Neuropsychology*. New York, NY: Springer.

Honing, H., and Fitch, W. T. (2018). *The Origins of Musicality.* Cambridge, MA: MIT Press.

Koelsch, S. (2012). *Brain & Music.* New York, NY: Wiley-Blackwell.

Kolb, B., and Whishaw, I. Q. (2015). *Fundamentals of Human Neuropsychology* (7th ed.). New York, NY: Worth.

Meyer, J. (2015). *Whistled Languages: A Worldwide Enquiry on Human Whistled Speech.* New York, NY: Springer.

Purves, D., Cabeza, R., Huettel, S. A., LaBar, K. S., et al. (2012). *Principles of Cognitive Neuroscience* (2nd ed.). Sunderland, MA: Oxford University Press/Sinauer.

Tomasello, M. (2010). *Origins of Human Communication.* Cambridge, MA: Bradford Books/MIT Press.

15 • VISUAL SUMMARY

You should be able to relate each summary to the adjacent illustration, including structures and processes. Thwe online version of this **Visual Summary** includes links to figures, animations, and activities that will help you consolidate the material.

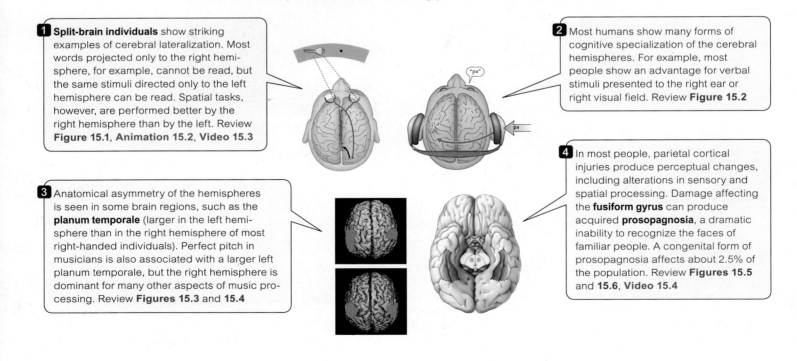

1 **Split-brain individuals** show striking examples of cerebral lateralization. Most words projected only to the right hemisphere, for example, cannot be read, but the same stimuli directed only to the left hemisphere can be read. Spatial tasks, however, are performed better by the right hemisphere than by the left. Review **Figure 15.1, Animation 15.2, Video 15.3**

2 Most humans show many forms of cognitive specialization of the cerebral hemispheres. For example, most people show an advantage for verbal stimuli presented to the right ear or right visual field. Review **Figure 15.2**

3 Anatomical asymmetry of the hemispheres is seen in some brain regions, such as the **planum temporale** (larger in the left hemisphere than in the right hemisphere of most right-handed individuals). Perfect pitch in musicians is also associated with a larger left planum temporale, but the right hemisphere is dominant for many other aspects of music processing. Review **Figures 15.3** and **15.4**

4 In most people, parietal cortical injuries produce perceptual changes, including alterations in sensory and spatial processing. Damage affecting the **fusiform gyrus** can produce acquired **prosopagnosia**, a dramatic inability to recognize the faces of familiar people. A congenital form of prosopagnosia affects about 2.5% of the population. Review **Figures 15.5** and **15.6, Video 15.4**

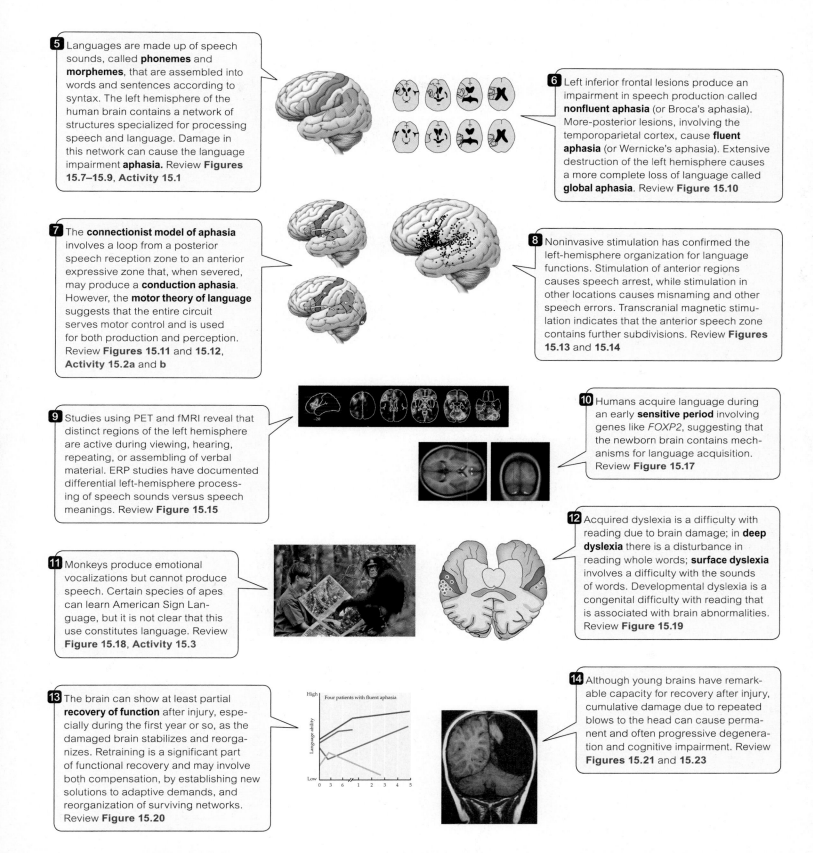

5 Languages are made up of speech sounds, called **phonemes** and **morphemes**, that are assembled into words and sentences according to syntax. The left hemisphere of the human brain contains a network of structures specialized for processing speech and language. Damage in this network can cause the language impairment **aphasia**. Review **Figures 15.7–15.9, Activity 15.1**

6 Left inferior frontal lesions produce an impairment in speech production called **nonfluent aphasia** (or Broca's aphasia). More-posterior lesions, involving the temporoparietal cortex, cause **fluent aphasia** (or Wernicke's aphasia). Extensive destruction of the left hemisphere causes a more complete loss of language called **global aphasia**. Review **Figure 15.10**

7 The **connectionist model of aphasia** involves a loop from a posterior speech reception zone to an anterior expressive zone that, when severed, may produce a **conduction aphasia**. However, the **motor theory of language** suggests that the entire circuit serves motor control and is used for both production and perception. Review **Figures 15.11** and **15.12, Activity 15.2a** and **b**

8 Noninvasive stimulation has confirmed the left-hemisphere organization for language functions. Stimulation of anterior regions causes speech arrest, while stimulation in other locations causes misnaming and other speech errors. Transcranial magnetic stimulation indicates that the anterior speech zone contains further subdivisions. Review **Figures 15.13** and **15.14**

9 Studies using PET and fMRI reveal that distinct regions of the left hemisphere are active during viewing, hearing, repeating, or assembling of verbal material. ERP studies have documented differential left-hemisphere processing of speech sounds versus speech meanings. Review **Figure 15.15**

10 Humans acquire language during an early **sensitive period** involving genes like *FOXP2*, suggesting that the newborn brain contains mechanisms for language acquisition. Review **Figure 15.17**

11 Monkeys produce emotional vocalizations but cannot produce speech. Certain species of apes can learn American Sign Language, but it is not clear that this use constitutes language. Review **Figure 15.18, Activity 15.3**

12 Acquired dyslexia is a difficulty with reading due to brain damage; in **deep dyslexia** there is a disturbance in reading whole words; **surface dyslexia** involves a difficulty with the sounds of words. Developmental dyslexia is a congenital difficulty with reading that is associated with brain abnormalities. Review **Figure 15.19**

13 The brain can show at least partial **recovery of function** after injury, especially during the first year or so, as the damaged brain stabilizes and reorganizes. Retraining is a significant part of functional recovery and may involve both compensation, by establishing new solutions to adaptive demands, and reorganization of surviving networks. Review **Figure 15.20**

14 Although young brains have remarkable capacity for recovery after injury, cumulative damage due to repeated blows to the head can cause permanent and often progressive degeneration and cognitive impairment. Review **Figures 15.21** and **15.23**

The Mind's Machine digital resources include additional videos, flashcards, and other study tools.

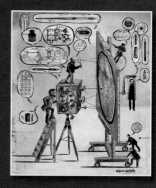

APPENDIX
A Primer on Concepts and Techniques in Molecular Biology

A.1 Genes Carry Information That Encodes Proteins

The most important thing about **genes** is that they are pieces of information, inherited from parents, that affect the development and function of our cells. Information carried by the genes is of a very specific sort: each gene carries the code for putting together a specific string of amino acids to form a particular **protein** molecule. This is all that genes do; they do not directly encode intelligence, or memories, or any other sort of complex behavior. The various proteins, each encoded by its own gene, make up the physical structure of the cell and most of its constituents, such as **enzymes**, which are proteins that enable chemical reactions in our cells. All these proteins make complex behavior possible, and in that context they are also the targets upon which the forces of evolution act.

Proteins are specific. For example, only cells that have liver-typical proteins will look like liver cells and be able to perform liver functions. Neurons, on the other hand, are cells that make neuron-typical proteins so that they can look and act like neurons. The genetic information for making these various proteins is crucial for an animal to live and for a nervous system to work properly.

One thing we hope this book will help you understand is that everyday experience can affect whether and when particular genetic recipes for making various proteins are used. To aid in that understanding, let's review how genetic information is stored and how proteins are made. Our discussion will be brief, but many online tutorials can provide you with more detailed information (see **A STEP FURTHER A.1**, on the website).

Genetic information is stored in molecules of DNA

The information for making all of our proteins could, in theory, be stored in any sort of format—on sheets of paper, a DVD, a smartphone—but organisms on this planet store their genetic information in a chemical called **deoxyribonucleic acid**, or **DNA**. Each molecule of DNA consists of a long strand of chemicals called **nucleotides** strung one after the other. DNA has only four nucleotides: guanine, cytosine, thymine, and adenine (abbreviated G, C, T, and A). The particular sequence of nucleotides (e.g., GCTTACC or TGGTCC or TGA) holds the information that will eventually make a protein. Because many millions of these nucleotides can be joined one after the other, a tremendous amount of information can be stored in very little space—on a single molecule of DNA.

A set of nucleotides that has been strung together can snuggle tightly against another string of nucleotides if it has the proper sequence: T nucleotides preferentially link with A nucleotides, and G nucleotides link with C nucleotides. Thus, T and A are said to be complementary nucleotides, and C and G are complementary nucleotides.

gene A length of DNA that encodes the information for constructing a particular protein.

protein A long string of amino acids. Proteins are the basic building material of organisms.

enzyme A complicated protein whose action increases the probability of a specific chemical reaction.

deoxyribonucleic acid (DNA) A nucleic acid that constitutes the chromosomes of cells and codes hereditary information.

nucleotide A portion of a DNA or RNA molecule that is composed of a single base and the adjoining sugar-phosphate unit of the strand.

FIGURE A.1 Duplication of DNA

Before cell division, all of the chromosomes in the cell must be duplicated, as illustrated here, so that each daughter cell has the full complement of genetic information.

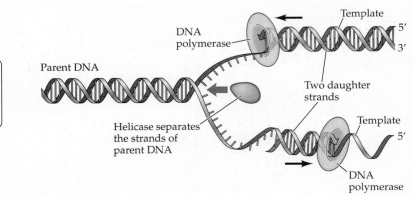

In fact, most of the time, our DNA consists not of a single strand of nucleotides, but of two complementary strands of nucleotides wrapped around one another.

The two strands of nucleotides are said to **hybridize** with (link to) one another, coiling slightly to form the famous double helix. The double-stranded DNA twists and coils further, becoming visible in microscopes as **chromosomes**, which resemble twisted lengths of yarn. Humans and the many other organisms known as **eukaryotes** store our chromosomes in a membranous sphere called a **cell nucleus** (plural nuclei). The ability of DNA to exist as two complementary strands of nucleotides is crucial for the duplication of the chromosomes (**FIGURE A.1**), but the details of that story will not concern us. Just remember that, with very few exceptions, every cell in your body has a faithful copy of all the DNA you received from your parents.

DNA is transcribed to produce messenger RNA

The information from DNA is used to assemble another molecule—**ribonucleic acid**, or **RNA**—that serves as a template for later steps in protein synthesis. Like DNA, RNA is made up of a long string of four types of nucleotides. For RNA, those nucleotides are G and C, which you'll recall are complementary to each other, plus A and U (uracil), which are also complementary to each other. Note that the T nucleotide is found only in DNA, and the U nucleotide is found only in RNA.

When a particular gene becomes active, the double strand of DNA unwinds enough so that one strand becomes free of the other and becomes available to special cellular machinery (including an enzyme called transcriptase) that begins **transcription**— the construction of a specific string of RNA nucleotides that are complementary to the exposed strand of DNA (**FIGURE A.2**). This length of RNA goes by several names: **messenger RNA (mRNA)**, transcript, or sometimes message. Each DNA nucleotide encodes a specific RNA nucleotide (an RNA G for every DNA C, an RNA C for every DNA G, an RNA U for every DNA A, and an RNA A for every DNA T). This transcript is made in the nucleus where the DNA resides; then the mRNA molecule moves to the cytoplasm, where protein molecules are assembled.

RNA molecules direct the formation of protein molecules

In the cytoplasm, special organelles called **ribosomes** attach themselves to a molecule of RNA, "read" the sequence of RNA nucleotides, and using that information, begin linking together amino acids to form a protein molecule. The structure and function of a protein molecule depend on which particular amino acids are put together and in what order. The decoding of an RNA transcript to manufacture a particular protein is called **translation** (see Figure A.2), as distinct from transcription, the construction of the mRNA molecule.

---

hybridization   The process by which one string of nucleotides becomes linked to a complementary series of nucleotides.

chromosome   A complex of condensed strands of DNA and associated protein molecules. Chromosomes are found in the nucleus of cells.

eukaryote   Any organism whose cells have the genetic material contained within a nuclear envelope.

cell nucleus   The spherical central structure of a cell that contains the chromosomes.

ribonucleic acid (RNA)   A nucleic acid that implements information found in DNA.

transcription   The process during which mRNA forms bases complementary to a strand of DNA. The resulting message (called a transcript) is then used to translate the DNA code into protein molecules.

messenger RNA (mRNA)   Also called transcript or message. A strand of RNA that carries the code of a section of a DNA strand to the cytoplasm.

ribosome   An organelle in the cell body where genetic information is translated to produce proteins.

translation   The process by which amino acids are linked together (directed by an mRNA molecule) to form protein molecules.

codon   A set of three nucleotides that encodes one particular amino acid.

peptide   A short string of amino acids. Longer strings of amino acids are called proteins.

Each trio of RNA nucleotides, or **codon**, encodes one of 20 or so different amino acids. Special molecules associated with the ribosome recognize the codon and bring a molecule of the appropriate amino acid so that the ribosome can fuse that amino acid to the previous one. If the resulting string of amino acids is short (say, 50 amino acids or less), it is called a **peptide**; if it is long, it is called a protein. Thus the ribosome assembles a very particular sequence of amino acids at the behest of a very particular sequence of RNA nucleotides, which were themselves encoded in the DNA inherited from our parents. In short, the biological secret of life is that DNA makes RNA, and RNA makes protein.

There are fascinating additions to this short story. Often the information from separate stretches of DNA is spliced together to make a single transcript; this so-called alternative splicing can create different transcripts from the same gene. Sometimes a protein is modified extensively after translation ends; special chemical processes can cleave long proteins to create one or several active peptides.

Keep in mind that each cell has the complete library of genetic information, collectively known as the **genome**, but makes only a fraction of all the proteins encoded in that DNA. In modern biology we say that each cell **expresses** only some genes; that is, the cell transcribes certain genes and makes the corresponding gene products (protein molecules). Thus, each cell must come to express all the genes needed to perform its function. Modern biologists refer to the expression of a particular subset of the genome as **cell differentiation**: the process by which different types of cells acquire their unique appearance and function. During development, individual cells appear to become more and more specialized, expressing progressively fewer genes. Many molecular biologists are striving to understand which cellular and molecular mechanisms "turn on" or "turn off" gene expression, in order to understand development and pathologies, such as cancer, or to provide crucial proteins to afflicted organs in a variety of diseases.

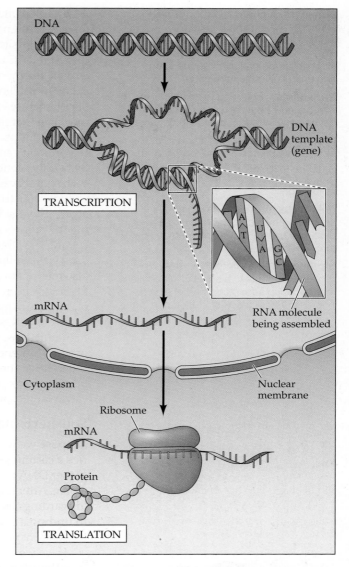

FIGURE A.2   DNA Makes RNA, and RNA Makes Protein

A.2 Molecular Biologists Have Craftily Enslaved Microorganisms and Enzymes

Many basic methods of molecular biology are not explicitly discussed in the text, so we will not describe them in detail here. However, you should understand what some of the terms mean, even if you don't know exactly how the methods are performed.

Molecular biologists have found ways to incorporate DNA from other species into the DNA of microorganisms such as bacteria and viruses. After the foreign DNA is incorporated, the microorganisms are allowed to reproduce rapidly, producing more and more copies of the (foreign) gene of interest. At this point the gene is said to be **cloned**, because researchers can make as many copies as they want. To ensure that the right gene is being cloned, the researcher generally clones many, many different genes—each into different bacteria—and then "screens" the bacteria rapidly to find the rare one that has incorporated the gene of interest.

When enough copies of the DNA have been made, the microorganisms are ground up and the DNA extracted. If sufficient DNA has been generated, chemical steps can then determine the exact sequence of nucleotides found in that stretch of DNA—a process known as **DNA sequencing**. Once the sequence of nucleotides has been determined, the sequence of complementary nucleotides in the messenger RNA for that

genome Also called genotype. All the genetic information that one specific individual has inherited.

expression For genes, the process by which a cell makes an mRNA transcript of a particular gene.

cell differentiation The developmental stage in which cells acquire distinctive characteristics, such as those of neurons, as the result of expressing particular genes.

clone Produce identical sequences of DNA or RNA, or a genetically identical organism.

DNA sequencing The process by which the order of nucleotides in a gene is identified.

polymerase chain reaction (PCR)
Also called gene amplification. A method for reproducing a particular RNA or DNA sequence manyfold, allowing amplification for sequencing or manipulating the sequence.

transgenic   Referring to an animal in which a new or altered gene has been deliberately introduced into the genome.

probe   In molecular biology, a manufactured sequence of DNA or RNA that is made to include a label (a colorful or radioactive molecule) that lets us track its location.

gel electrophoresis   A method of separating molecules of differing size or electrical charge by forcing them to flow through a gel.

blotting   Transferring DNA, RNA, or protein fragments to a sheet of nitrocellulose following separation via gel electrophoresis. The blotted substance can then be labeled.

**View Animation A.1:
Gel Electrophoresis**

gene can be inferred. The sequence of mRNA nucleotides tells the investigator the sequence of amino acids that will be made from that transcript, because biologists know which amino acid is encoded by each trio of DNA nucleotides. For example, scientists discovered the amino acid sequence of neurotransmitter receptors by this process.

The business of obtaining many copies of DNA has been boosted by a technique called the **polymerase chain reaction**, or **PCR**. This technique exploits a special type of polymerase enzyme that, like other such enzymes, induces the formation of a DNA molecule that is complementary to an existing single strand of DNA (see Figure A.1). Because this particular polymerase enzyme (called Taq polymerase) evolved in bacteria that inhabit geothermal hot springs, it can function in a broad range of temperatures. By heating double-stranded DNA, we can cause the two strands to separate, making each strand available to polymerase enzymes that, when the temperature has decreased enough, construct a new "mate" for each strand so that they are both double-stranded again. The first PCR yields only double the original number of DNA molecules; repeating the process results in 4 times as many molecules as at first. Repeatedly heating and cooling the DNA of interest in the presence of this heat-resistant polymerase enzyme soon yields millions of copies of the original DNA molecule, which is why this process is also referred to as gene amplification. In practice, PCR usually requires the investigator to provide primers—short nucleotide sequences synthesized to hybridize on either side of the gene of interest to amplify that particular gene more than others.

With PCR, sufficient quantities of DNA are produced for chemical analysis or other manipulations, such as introducing DNA into cells. For example, we might inject some of the DNA encoding a protein of interest into a fertilized mouse egg (a zygote) and then return the zygote to a pregnant mouse to grow. Occasionally the injected DNA becomes incorporated into the zygote's genome, resulting in a **transgenic** mouse that carries and expresses the foreign gene.

Southern blots identify particular genes

Suppose we want to know whether a particular individual or a particular species carries a certain gene. Because all cells contain a complete copy of the genome, we can gather DNA from just about any kind of cell population: blood, skin, or muscle, for example. After the cells are ground up, a chemical extraction procedure isolates the DNA (discarding the RNA and protein). Finding a particular gene in that DNA boils down to finding a particular sequence of DNA nucleotides. To do that, we can exploit the tendency of nucleic acids (DNA and RNA) to hybridize with one another.

If we were looking for the DNA sequence GCT, for example, we could manufacture the sequence CGA (there are machines to do that), which would then stick to (hybridize with) any DNA sequence of GCT. The manufactured sequence CGA is called a **probe** because it is made to include a label (a colorful or radioactive molecule) that lets us track its location. Of course, such a short length of nucleotides will be found in many genes. In order for a probe to recognize one particular gene, it has to be about 15 nucleotides long.

When we extract DNA from an individual, it's convenient to let enzymes cut up the very long stretches of DNA into more manageable pieces of 1,000–20,000 nucleotides each. A process called **gel electrophoresis** uses electrical current to separate these millions of pieces more or less by size (**FIGURE A.3**). Large pieces move slowly through a tube of gelatin-like material, and small pieces move rapidly. The tube of gel is then sliced and placed on top of a sheet of paper-like material called nitrocellulose. When fluid is allowed to flow through the gel and nitrocellulose, DNA molecules are pulled out of the gel and deposited on the waiting nitrocellulose. This process of making a "sandwich" of gel and nitrocellulose and using fluid to move molecules from the former to the latter is called **blotting** (see Figure A.3).

If the gene we're looking for is among those millions of DNA fragments sitting on the nitrocellulose, our labeled probe should recognize and hybridize with the sequence. The nitrocellulose sheet is soaked in a solution containing our labeled probe; we wait

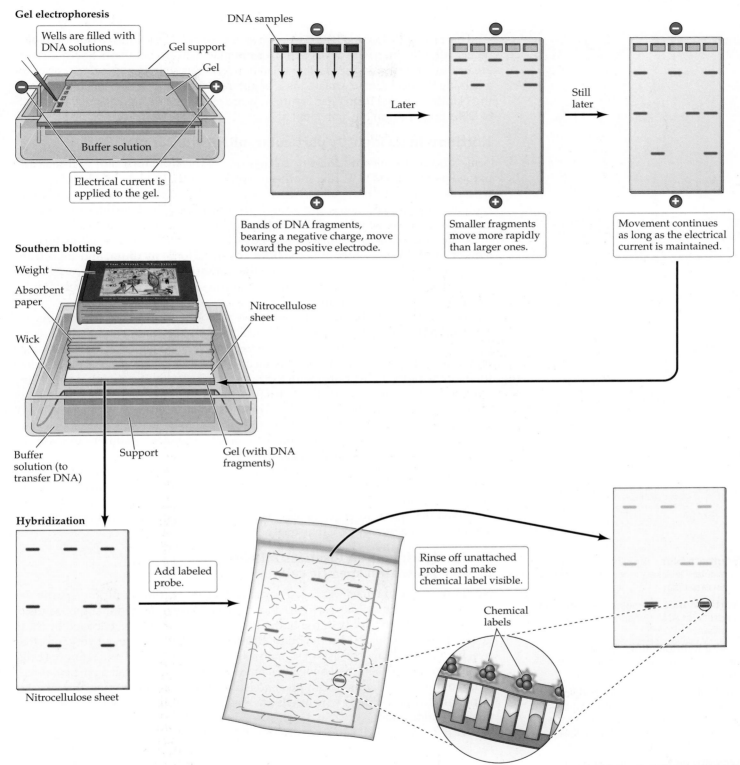

Gel electrophoresis

Wells are filled with DNA solutions.

Gel support

Gel

Buffer solution

Electrical current is applied to the gel.

DNA samples

Bands of DNA fragments, bearing a negative charge, move toward the positive electrode.

Later

Smaller fragments move more rapidly than larger ones.

Still later

Movement continues as long as the electrical current is maintained.

Southern blotting

Weight

Absorbent paper

Wick

Nitrocellulose sheet

Buffer solution (to transfer DNA)

Support

Gel (with DNA fragments)

Hybridization

Nitrocellulose sheet

Add labeled probe.

Rinse off unattached probe and make chemical label visible.

Chemical labels

FIGURE A.3 Gel Electrophoresis and Southern Blotting

for the probe to find and hybridize with the gene of interest (if it is present), and we rinse the sheet to remove probe molecules that did not find the gene. Then we visualize the probe, either by causing the label to show its color or, if radioactive, by letting the probe expose photographic film to identify the locations where the probe has accumulated. In either case, if the probe found the gene, a labeled band will be evident, corresponding to the size of DNA fragment that contained the gene (see Figure A.3).

This process of looking for a particular sequence of DNA is called a **Southern blot**, named after the man who developed the technique, Edward Southern. Southern blots are useful for determining whether related individuals share a particular gene or for assessing the evolutionary relatedness of different species. The developed blots, with their lanes of labeled bands (see Figure A.3), are often seen in popular-media accounts of DNA fingerprinting of individuals.

Northern blots identify particular mRNA transcripts

A method more relevant for our discussions is the **Northern blot** (whimsically named as the opposite of the Southern blot). A Northern blot can identify which tissues are making a particular RNA transcript. If liver cells are making a particular protein, for example, then some transcripts for the gene that encodes that protein should be present. So we can take the liver, grind it up, and use chemical processes to isolate most of the RNA (discarding the DNA and protein). The resulting mixture consists of RNA molecules of many different sizes: long, medium, and short transcripts. Gel electrophoresis will separate the transcripts by size, and we can blot the size-sorted mRNA molecules onto nitrocellulose sheets; the process is very similar to the Southern blot procedure.

To see whether the particular transcript we're looking for is among the mRNAs, we construct a labeled probe (of either DNA nucleotides or RNA nucleotides) that is complementary to the mRNA transcript of interest and long enough that it will hybridize only with that particular transcript. We incubate the nitrocellulose in the probe, allow time for the probe to hybridize with the targeted transcript (if present), rinse off any unused probe molecules, and then visualize the probe as before. If the transcript of interest is present, we should see a band on the film (see Figure A.3). The presence of several bands indicates that the probe has hybridized to more than one transcript and we may need to make a more specific probe or alter chemical conditions to make the probe less likely to bind similar transcripts.

Because different gene transcripts have different lengths, the transcript of interest should have reached a particular point in the electrophoresis gel: small transcripts should have moved far; large transcripts should have moved only a little. If our probe has found the right transcript, the single band of labeling should be at the point that is appropriate for a transcript of that length.

In situ hybridization localizes mRNA transcripts within specific cells

Northern blots can tell us whether a particular organ has transcripts for a particular gene product. For example, Northern blot analyses have indicated that thousands of genes are transcribed only in the brain. Presumably the proteins encoded by these genes are used exclusively in the brain. But such results alone are not very informative, because the brain consists of so many different kinds of glial and neuronal cells. We can refine Northern blot analyses somewhat, by dissecting out a particular part of the brain—say, the hippocampus—to isolate mRNAs. Sometimes, though, it is important to know exactly which cells are making the transcript. In that case we use **in situ hybridization**.

With in situ hybridization we use the same sort of labeled probe, constructed of nucleotides that are complementary to (and will therefore hybridize with) the targeted transcript, as in Northern blots. Instead of using the probe to find and hybridize with the transcript on a sheet of nitrocellulose, however, we use the probe to find the transcripts in situ (Latin for "in place")—that is, on a section of tissue. After rinsing off the probe molecules that didn't find a match, we visualize the probe in the tissue section. Any cells in the section that were transcribing the gene of interest will have transcripts in the cytoplasm that should have hybridized with our labeled probe. In situ hybridization therefore can tell us exactly which cells are expressing a particular gene (**FIGURE A.4** and Box 2.1).

Southern blot   A method of detecting a particular DNA sequence in the genome of an organism.

Northern blot   A method of detecting a particular RNA transcript in a tissue or organ.

in situ hybridization   A method for detecting particular RNA transcripts in tissue sections.

antibody   Also called immunoglobulin. A large protein that recognizes and permanently binds to particular shapes, normally as part of the immune system attack on foreign particles.

Western blot   A method of detecting a particular protein molecule in a tissue or organ.

immunocytochemistry (ICC)   A method for detecting a particular protein in tissues in which an antibody recognizes and binds to the protein and then chemical methods are used to leave a visible reaction product around each antibody.

Western blots identify particular proteins

Sometimes we wish to study a particular protein rather than its transcript. In such cases we can use antibodies. **Antibodies** are large, complicated molecules (proteins, in fact) that our immune system adds to the bloodstream to identify and fight invading microbes, thereby arresting and preventing disease. But if we inject a rabbit or mouse with a sample of a protein of interest, we can induce the animal to create antibodies that recognize and attach to that particular protein, just as if it were an invader.

Once these antibodies have been purified and chemically labeled, we can use them to search for the target protein. We grind up an organ, isolate the proteins (discarding the DNA and RNA), and separate them by means of gel electrophoresis. Then we blot these proteins out of the gel and onto nitrocellulose. Next we use the antibodies to tell us whether the targeted protein is among those made by that organ. If the antibodies identify only the protein we care about, there should be a single band of labeling (if there are two or more, then the antibodies may recognize more than one protein). Because proteins come in different sizes, the single band of label should be at the position corresponding to the size of the protein that we're studying. Such blots are called **Western blots**.

To review, Southern blots identify particular DNA pieces (genes), Northern blots identify particular RNA pieces (transcripts), and Western blots identify particular proteins (sometimes called products).

Antibodies can also tell us which cells possess a particular protein

If we need to know which particular cells within an organ such as the brain are making a particular protein, we can use the same sorts of antibodies that we use in Western blots, but in this case directed at that protein in tissue sections. We slice up the brain, expose the sections to the antibodies, allow time for them to find and attach to the protein, rinse off unattached antibodies, and use chemical treatments to visualize the antibodies. Cells that were making the protein will be labeled from the chemical treatments (see Figure 1.19C).

Because antibodies from the immune system are used to identify cells with the aid of chemical treatment, this method is called **immunocytochemistry**, or **ICC**. This technique can even tell us where, within the cell, the protein is found. Such information can provide important clues about the function of the protein. For example, if the protein is found in axon terminals, it may be a neurotransmitter.

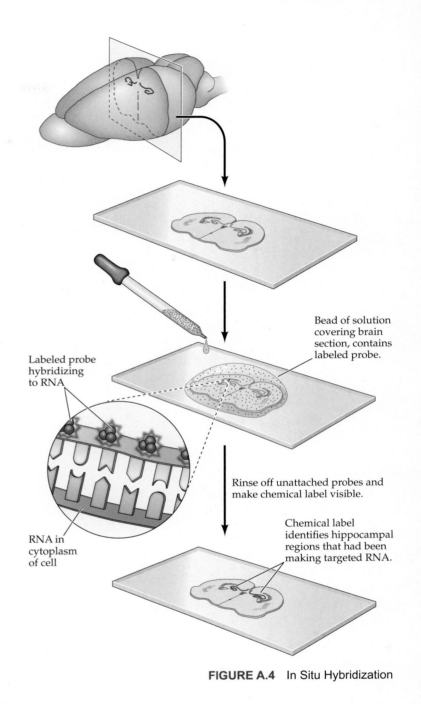

Bead of solution covering brain section, contains labeled probe.

Labeled probe hybridizing to RNA

RNA in cytoplasm of cell

Rinse off unattached probes and make chemical label visible.

Chemical label identifies hippocampal regions that had been making targeted RNA.

FIGURE A.4 In Situ Hybridization

Glossary

Numbers in brackets refer to the chapter(s) where the term is introduced.

5-alpha-reductase An enzyme that converts testosterone into dihydrotestosterone (DHT). [8]

5-HT See *serotonin*. [3]

17-beta-estradiol See *estradiol*. [8]

A

A delta (Aδ) fiber A moderately large, myelinated, and therefore fast-conducting axon that usually transmits pain information. Compare *C fiber*. [5]

absence attack See *simple partial seizure*.

absolute refractory phase A brief period of complete insensitivity to stimuli. Compare *relative refractory phase*. [2]

accommodation The process by which the ciliary muscles adjust the lens to bring nearby objects into focus. [7]

acetylcholine (ACh) A neurotransmitter that is produced and released by parasympathetic postganglionic neurons, by motor neurons, and by many neurons in the brain. See Table 3.1. [2, 3, 5]

acetylcholinesterase (AChE) An enzyme that inactivates the transmitter acetylcholine. [2, ASF 4.1]

ACh See *acetylcholine*. [2, 3, 5]

AChE See *acetylcholinesterase*. [2, ASF 4.1]

acid See *LSD*. [3]

act Complex behavior, as distinct from a simple movement. [5]

ACTH See *adrenocorticotropic hormone*. [ASF 8.4]

action potential Also called *spike*. A rapid reversal of the membrane potential that momentarily makes the inside of a neuron positive with respect to the outside. See Figures 2.6, 2.7. [2]

activational effect A temporary change in behavior resulting from the availability of a hormone to an adult animal. Compare *organizational effect*. [8]

acupuncture The insertion of needles at designated points on the skin to alleviate pain or neurological malfunction. [5]

adaptation 1. See *sensory adaptation*. [5] 2. In the context of evolution, a trait that increases the probability that an individual will leave offspring in subsequent generations.

ADH See *antidiuretic hormone*. [8, 9]

ADHD See *attention deficit hyperactivity disorder*. [ASF 13.4, 14]

adipose tissue Commonly called *fat tissue*. Tissue made up of fat cells. [9]

adrenal cortex The steroid-secreting outer rind of the adrenal gland. See Figure 8.1. Compare *adrenal medulla*. [11]

adrenal corticosteroid hormone A steroid hormone that is secreted by the adrenal cortex. [11]

adrenal medulla The inner core of the adrenal gland. The adrenal medulla secretes epinephrine and norepinephrine. See Figure 8.1. Compare *adrenal cortex*. [11]

adrenaline See *epinephrine*. [11]

adrenocorticotropic hormone (ACTH) A tropic hormone, secreted by the anterior pituitary gland, that controls the production and release of hormones of the adrenal cortex. [ASF 8.4]

adult neurogenesis The creation of new neurons in the brain of an adult. [Intro, 4]

afferent Refers to carrying action potentials toward the brain, or toward one region of interest. Compare *efferent*. [1]

affinity See *binding affinity*. [3]

afterpotential The positive or negative change in membrane potential that may follow an action potential. [2]

aggression Behavior that is intended to cause pain or harm to others. [11]

agnosia The inability to recognize objects, despite being able to describe them in terms of form and color. Agnosia may occur after localized brain damage. [15]

agonist A substance that mimics or boosts the actions of a transmitter or other signaling molecule. Compare *antagonist* (definition 1). [2, 3]

agraphia The inability to write. Compare *alexia*. [15]

AII See *angiotensin II*. [9]

AIS See *androgen insensitivity syndrome*. [8]

aldosterone A mineralocorticoid hormone, secreted by the adrenal cortex, that promotes the conservation of sodium by the kidneys. [9]

alexia The inability to read. See *dyslexia*. Compare *agraphia*. [15]

allele Any particular version of a gene.

allomone A chemical signal that is released outside the body by one species and affects the behavior of other species. See Figure 8.3. Compare *pheromone*. [8]

all-or-none property The condition that the size (amplitude) of the action potential is independent of the size of the stimulus. See Table 2.2. Compare *postsynaptic potential*. [2]

allostasis The varying behavioral and physiological adjustments that an individual makes in order to maintain optimal (rather than unchanging) functioning of a regulated system in the face of changing environmental stressors. [9]

alpha rhythm A brain potential of 8–12 Hz that occurs during relaxed wakefulness. See Figure 10.11. Compare *desynchronized EEG*. [10]

alpha-fetoprotein A protein found in the plasma of fetuses. In rodents, alpha-fetoprotein binds estrogens and prevents them from entering the brain. [ASF 8.7]

alpha-synuclein A protein that has been implicated in Parkinson's disease.

ALS See *amyotrophic lateral sclerosis*. [ASF 5.5]

Alzheimer's disease A form of dementia that may appear in middle age but is more frequent among the aged. [4]

amacrine cell A specialized retinal cell that contacts both bipolar cells and ganglion cells and is especially significant in inhibitory interactions within the retina. Compare *horizontal cell*. [7]

amblyopia Reduced visual acuity of one eye that is not caused by optical or retinal impairments. [4, 7, ASF 13.4]

AMH See *anti-müllerian hormone*. [8]

amine hormone Also called *monoamine hormone*. A hormone composed of a single amino acid that has been modified into a related molecule, such as melatonin or epinephrine. Compare *peptide hormone* and *steroid hormone*. [8]

amine neurotransmitter A neurotransmitter based on modifications of a single amino acid nucleus. Examples include acetylcholine, serotonin, and dopamine. See Table 3.1. Compare *amino acid neurotransmitter, gas neurotransmitter,* and *peptide neurotransmitter*. [3]

amino acid neurotransmitter A neurotransmitter that is itself an amino acid. Examples include GABA, glycine, and glutamate. See Table 3.1. Compare *amine neurotransmitter, gas neurotransmitter,* and *peptide neurotransmitter.* [3]

amnesia Severe impairment of memory. [13]

AMPA receptor A fast-acting ionotropic glutamate receptor that also binds the glutamate agonist AMPA. Compare *NMDA receptor.* [ASF 4.2, 13]

amphetamine A molecule that resembles the structure of the catecholamine transmitters and enhances their activity. [3]

ampulla (pl. ampullae) An enlarged region of each semicircular canal that contains the receptor cells (hair cells) of the vestibular system. See Figure 6.14. [6]

amusia A disorder characterized by the inability to discern or sing tunes accurately. [6]

amygdala A group of nuclei in the medial anterior part of the temporal lobe. See Figure 1.14. [11]

amyloid plaque Also called *senile plaque.* A small area of the brain that has abnormal cellular and chemical patterns. Amyloid plaques correlate with dementia. See Figure 4.17. [4]

amyloid precursor protein (APP) A protein that, when cleaved by several enzymes, produces beta-amyloid, which accumulates in Alzheimer's disease. [ASF 13.5]

amyotrophic lateral sclerosis (ALS) Also called *Lou Gehrig's disease.* A disease in which motor neurons and their target muscles waste away. [ASF 5.5]

analgesia Absence of or reduction in pain. [5]

analgesic Having painkilling properties. [3]

anandamide An endogenous substance that binds the cannabinoid receptor molecule. [3]

androgen Any of a class of hormones that includes testosterone and similar steroids. See Figure 8.13. [8]

androgen insensitivity syndrome (AIS) A syndrome caused by an androgen receptor gene mutation that renders tissues insensitive to androgenic hormones like testosterone. Affected XY individuals are phenotypic females, but they have internal testes and regressed internal genital structures. See Figure 8.27. [8]

angel dust See *phencyclidine.* [12]

angiotensin II (AII) A hormone produced in the blood by the action of renin and that may play a role in the control of thirst. [9]

angular gyrus A brain region in which strokes can lead to word blindness.

anion A negatively charged ion, such as a protein or a chloride ion. Compare *cation.* [2]

anomia The inability to name persons or objects readily. [15]

anorexia nervosa A syndrome in which individuals severely deprive themselves of food. [9]

anorexigenic neurons Neurons of the hypothalamic appetite system that inhibit feeding behavior. [9]

ANP See *atrial natriuretic peptide.* [9]

antagonist 1. A substance that blocks or attenuates the actions of a transmitter or other signaling molecule. Compare *agonist.* [2, 3] 2. A muscle that counteracts the effect of another muscle. Compare *synergist.* [5]

anterior Also called *rostral.* In anatomy, toward the head end of an organism. Compare *posterior.* [1]

anterior cerebral artery Either of two large arteries, arising from the carotid arteries, that provide blood to the anterior poles and medial surfaces of the cerebral hemispheres. Compare *middle cerebral artery* and *posterior cerebral artery.* [ASF 2.1]

anterior pituitary The front division of the pituitary gland. It secretes tropic hormones. See Figures 8.1, 8.12. Compare *posterior pituitary.* [8]

anterograde amnesia Difficulty in forming new memories beginning with the onset of a disorder. Compare *retrograde amnesia.* [12]

anterolateral system Also called *spinothalamic system.* A somatosensory system that carries most of the pain and temperature information from the body to the brain. See Figure 5.14. Compare *dorsal column system.* [5]

antibody Also called *immunoglobulin.* A large protein that recognizes and permanently binds to particular shapes, normally as part of the immune system attack on foreign particles. [ASF 11.4, App]

antidepressant A drug that relieves the symptoms of depression. Major categories include monoamine oxidase inhibitors, tricyclics, and selective serotonin reuptake inhibitors. [3]

antidiuretic hormone (ADH) See *vasopressin.* [8, 9]

anti-müllerian hormone (AMH) Also called *müllerian regression hormone.* A peptide hormone secreted by the fetal testes that inhibits müllerian duct development. [8]

antipsychotic Also called *neuroleptic.* Any of a class of drugs that alleviate symptoms of schizophrenia, typically by blocking dopamine receptors. [12]

anxiety disorder Any of a class of psychological disorders that includes recurrent panic states and generalized persistent anxiety disorder. [12]

anxiolytic A substance that is used to reduce anxiety. Examples include alcohol, opiates, barbiturates, and the benzodiazepines. [3, 12]

aphasia An impairment in language understanding and/or production that is caused by brain injury. [15]

apolipoprotein E (ApoE) A protein that may help break down beta-amyloid. Individuals carrying the *ApoE4* allele are more likely to develop Alzheimer's disease. [ASF 13.5]

apoptosis See *cell death.* [4]

APP See *amyloid precursor protein.* [ASF 13.5]

apraxia An impairment in the ability to carry out complex sequential movements, even though there is no muscle paralysis. [5, 15]

arachnoid The thin covering (one of the three meninges) of the brain that lies between the dura mater and the pia mater. See Figure 1.8. [1]

arcuate fasciculus A fiber tract classically viewed as a connection between Wernicke's speech area and Broca's speech area. See Figure 15.11. [15]

arcuate nucleus An arc-shaped hypothalamic nucleus implicated in appetite control. See Figure 9.16. [9]

area 17 See *primary visual cortex.* [7]

arginine vasopressin (AVP) See *vasopressin.* [8, 9]

aromatase An enzyme that converts many androgens into estrogens. [ASF 8.7]

aromatization The chemical reaction that converts testosterone to estradiol, and other androgens to other estrogens. [ASF 8.7]

aromatization hypothesis The hypothesis that testicular androgens enter the brain and are converted there into estrogens to masculinize the developing nervous system of some rodents. [ASF 8.7]

arousal The global, nonselective level of alertness of an individual.

Asperger's syndrome Also called *high-functioning autism.* A syndrome characterized by difficulties in social cognitive processing. It is usually accompanied by strong language skills. Compare *autism spectrum disorder.* [ASF 13.4]

associative learning A type of learning in which an association is formed between two stimuli or between a stimulus and a response. It includes both classical and instrumental conditioning. [13]

astereognosis The inability to recognize objects by touching and feeling them. [15]

astrocyte A star-shaped glial cell with numerous processes (extensions) that run in all directions. See Figure 1.5. [1]

ataxia A loss of movement coordination, often caused by disease of the cerebellum. [5]

atrial natriuretic peptide (ANP) A hormone, secreted by the heart, that normally reduces blood pressure, inhibits drinking, and promotes the excretion of water and salt at the kidneys. [9]

attention Also called *selective attention*. A state or condition of selective awareness or perceptual receptivity, by which specific stimuli are selected for enhanced processing. [14]

attention deficit hyperactivity disorder (ADHD) A syndrome characterized by distractibility, impulsiveness, and hyperactivity that, in children, interferes with school performance. [14, ASF 13.4]

attentional blink The reduced ability of subjects to detect a target stimulus if it follows another target stimulus by about 200–450 milliseconds.

attentional bottleneck A filter created by the limits intrinsic to our attentional processes, whose effect is that only the most important stimuli are selected for special processing. [14]

attentional spotlight The steerable focus of our selective attention, used to select stimuli for enhanced processing. [14]

atypical antipsychotic See *second-generation antipsychotic*. [3, 12]

auditory canal See *ear canal*. [6]

auditory N1 effect A negative deflection of the event-related potential, occurring about 100 milliseconds after stimulus presentation, that is enhanced for selectively attended auditory input compared with ignored input. Compare *visual P1 effect*. [14]

auditory P300 See *P3 effect*. [14]

aura In epilepsy, the unusual sensations or premonition that may precede the beginning of a seizure. [2]

autism spectrum disorder (ASD) A disorder, arising during childhood, that is characterized by social withdrawal and perseverative behavior. Compare *Asperger's syndrome*. [ASF 13.4]

autobiographical memory See *episodic memory*. [13]

autocrine Referring to a signal that is secreted by a cell into its environment and that feeds back to the same cell.

autoimmune disorder A disorder caused when the immune system mistakenly attacks a person's own body, thereby interfering with normal functioning. [ASF 5.5]

autonomic ganglion A collection of neuron bodies, belonging to the autonomic division of the peripheral nervous system, that is found in any of various locations and contributes to the innervation of major organs.

autonomic nervous system A part of the peripheral nervous system that provides the main neural connections to the internal organs. Its two divisions (sympathetic and parasympathetic) act in opposite fashion. See Figure 1.9. [1]

autoradiography A staining technique that shows the distribution of radioactive chemicals in tissues. See Box 8.1. [1, 8]

autoreceptor A receptor for a synaptic transmitter that is located in the presynaptic membrane and tells the axon terminal how much transmitter has been released. [3]

AVP See *arginine vasopressin*. [8, 9]

axo-axonic synapse A synapse at which a presynaptic axon terminal synapses onto the axon terminal of another neuron. Compare *axo-dendritic synapse*, *axo-somatic synapse*, and *dendro-dendritic synapse*. [2]

axo-dendritic synapse A synapse at which a presynaptic axon terminal synapses onto a dendrite of the postsynaptic neuron, either via a dendritic spine or directly onto the dendrite itself. Compare *axo-axonic synapse*, *axo-somatic synapse*, and *dendro-dendritic synapse*. [2]

axon Also called *nerve fiber*. A single extension from the neuron that carries action potentials from the cell body toward the axon terminals. Functionally, the axon is the conduction zone of the neuron. See Figures 1.1, 1.3. [1]

axon collateral A branch of an axon. [1]

axon hillock The cone-shaped area on the cell body from which the axon originates. See Figure 1.4. [1, 2]

axon terminal Also called *synaptic bouton*. The end of an axon or axon collateral, which forms a synapse onto a neuron or other target cell and thus serves as the output zone. See Figures 1.1, 1.3. [1]

axonal transport The transportation of materials from the neuronal cell body toward the axon terminals, and from the axon terminals back toward the cell body. [1]

axo-somatic synapse A synapse at which a presynaptic axon terminal synapses onto the cell body (soma) of the postsynaptic neuron. Compare *axo-axonic synapse*, *axo-dendritic synapse*, and *dendro-dendritic synapse*. [2]

B

B cell See *B lymphocyte*. [ASF 11.4]

B lymphocyte Also called *B cell*. An immune system cell, formed in the bone marrow (hence the *B*), that mediates humoral immunity. Compare *T lymphocyte*. [ASF 11.4]

Balint's syndrome A disorder, caused by damage to both parietal lobes, that is characterized by difficulty in steering visual gaze (oculomotor apraxia), in accurately reaching for objects using visual guidance (optic ataxia), and in directing attention to more than one object or feature at a time (simultagnosia). [14]

bar detector See *simple cortical cell*. [7]

barbiturate An early anxiolytic drug and sleep aid that has depressant activity in the nervous system. [3]

baroreceptor A pressure receptor in the heart or a major artery that detects a change in blood pressure. [9]

basal "Toward the base" or "toward the bottom" of a structure. [1]

basal forebrain A region, ventral to the basal ganglia, that is the major source of cholinergic projections in the brain and has been implicated in sleep. [3, 10]

basal ganglia A group of forebrain nuclei, including the caudate nucleus, globus pallidus, and putamen, found deep within the cerebral hemispheres. They are crucial for skill learning. See Figures 1.14, 5.29. [1, 5, 13]

basal metabolism The use of energy for processes such as heat production, maintenance of membrane potentials, and all the other basic life-sustaining functions of the body. [9]

basilar artery An artery, formed by the fusion of the vertebral arteries, that supplies blood to the brainstem and to the posterior cerebral arteries. [ASF 2.1]

basilar membrane A membrane in the cochlea that contains the principal structures involved in auditory transduction. See Figures 6.1, 6.2. [6]

behavioral intervention An approach to finding relations between body variables and behavioral variables that involves intervening in the behavior of an organism and looking for resultant changes in body structure or function. See Figure 1.24. Compare *somatic intervention*. [1]

behavioral medicine See *health psychology*. [11]

behavioral neuroscience Also called biological psychology, brain and behavior, and physiological psychology. The study of the biological bases of psychological processes and behavior. [Intro]

benzodiazepine Any of a class of anti-anxiety drugs that are noncompetitive agonists of GABAA receptors in the central nervous system. One example is diazepam (Valium). [3, 12]

beta activity See *desynchronized EEG*. [10]

beta-amyloid A protein that accumulates in amyloid plaques in Alzheimer's disease. [4]

beta-secretase An enzyme that cleaves amyloid precursor protein, forming beta-amyloid, present in plaques of people with Alzheimer's disease. See also *presenilin*. [ASF 13.5]

between-participants experiment An experiment in which an experimental group of individuals is compared with a control group of individuals that have been treated identically in every way except that they haven't received the experimental manipulation. Compare *within-participants experiment*. [1]

binaural Pertaining to two ears. Compare *monaural*.

binding affinity Also called simply *affinity*. The propensity of molecules of a drug (or other ligand) to bind to receptors. Drugs with high affinity for their receptors are effective even at low doses. [3]

binding problem The question of how the brain understands which individual attributes blend together into a single object, when these different features are processed by different regions in the brain. [14]

binge eating The rapid intake of large quantities of food, often poor in nutritional value and high in calories. [9]

binocular Referring to two-eyed processes. [7]

binocular deprivation Depriving both eyes of form vision, as by sealing the eyelids. Compare *monocular deprivation*. [4, ASF 13.4]

bioavailable Referring to a substance, usually a drug, that is present in the body in a form that is able to interact with physiological mechanisms. [3]

biological rhythm A regular fluctuation in any living process. [10]

biotransformation The process in which enzymes convert a drug into a metabolite that is itself active, possibly in ways that are substantially different from the actions of the original substance. [3]

bipolar cell An interneuron in the retina that receives information from rods and cones and passes the information

to retinal ganglion cells. See Figure 7.3. Compare *amacrine cell* and *horizontal cell*. [7]

bipolar disorder A psychiatric disorder characterized by periods of depression that alternate with excessive, expansive moods. [12]

bipolar neuron A neuron that has a single dendrite at one end and a single axon at the other end. See Figure 1.3. Compare *unipolar neuron* and *multipolar neuron*. [1]

blind spot The portion of the visual field from which light falls on the optic disc. [7]

blindsight The paradoxical phenomenon whereby, within a scotoma, a person cannot *consciously* perceive visual cues but may still be able to make some visual discrimination. [7]

blood-brain barrier The mechanisms that make the movement of substances from blood vessels into cells more difficult in the brain than in other body organs, thus affording the brain greater protection from exposure to some substances found in the blood. [1, 3]

blotting Transferring DNA, RNA, or protein fragments to nitrocellulose following separation via gel electrophoresis. The blotted substance can then be labeled. See Appendix Figure A.3. [App]

brain and behavior See *behavioral neuroscience*. [Intro]

brain self-stimulation The process in which animals will work to provide electrical stimulation to particular brain sites, presumably because the experience is very rewarding. [11]

brainstem The region of the brain that consists of the midbrain, the pons, and the medulla. [1]

brightness One of three basic dimensions of light perception, varying from dark to light. Compare *hue* and *saturation*. [7]

Broca's aphasia See *nonfluent aphasia*. [15]

Broca's area A region of the frontal lobe of the brain that is involved in the production of speech. See Figures 15.9, 15.10, 15.11. Compare *Wernicke's area*. [15]

brown fat Also called *brown adipose tissue*. A specialized type of fat tissue that generates heat through intense metabolism. [ASF 9.1]

bulimia Also called *bulimia nervosa*. A syndrome in which individuals periodically gorge themselves, usually with "junk food," and then either vomit or take laxatives to avoid weight gain. [9]

bungarotoxin A neurotoxin, isolated from the venom of the many-banded krait,

that selectively blocks acetylcholine receptors. [2]

C

C fiber A small, unmyelinated axon that conducts pain information slowly and adapts slowly. [5]

caffeine A compound found in coffee and other plants that exerts a stimulant action by blocking adenosine receptors. [3]

CAH See *congenital adrenal hyperplasia*. [8]

calcium ion (Ca²⁺) A calcium atom that carries a double positive charge. [2]

cannabidiol (CBD) One of the two major types of active compounds found in cannabis. The other is THC. [3]

cannabinoid receptor A receptor that responds to endogenous and/or exogenous cannabinoids. [3]

cannabis Also known as *marijuana*, although this name is considered pejorative. A psychoactive plant containing numerous active compounds in varying proportions. [3]

carotid artery Either of the two major arteries that ascend the left and right sides of the neck to the brain, supplying blood to the anterior and middle cerebral arteries. The branch that enters the brain is called the internal carotid artery. [ASF 2.1]

castration Removal of the gonads, usually the testes. [8]

CAT See *computerized axial tomography*. [1]

cataplexy Sudden loss of muscle tone, leading to collapse of the body without loss of consciousness. Cataplexy is sometimes a component of narcoleptic attacks. [10]

cation A positively charged ion, such as a potassium or sodium ion. Compare *anion*. [2]

cauda equina Literally, "horse's tail" (in Latin). The caudalmost spinal nerves, which extend beyond the spinal cord proper to exit the spinal column.

caudal See *posterior*. [1]

causality The relation of cause and effect, such that we can conclude that an experimental manipulation has specifically caused an observed result. [1]

CBT See *cognitive behavioral therapy*. [12]

CCK See *cholecystokinin*. [9]

cell body Also called *soma*. The region of a neuron that is defined by the presence of the cell nucleus. Functionally, the cell body is the integration zone of the neuron. See Figures 1.1, 1.3. [1]

cell death Also called *apoptosis*. The developmental process during which "surplus" cells die. See Figure 4.3. [4]

cell differentiation The developmental stage in which cells acquire distinctive characteristics, such as those of neurons, as a result of expressing particular genes. See Figure 4.3. [4, App]

cell membrane The lipid bilayer that encloses a cell. [2]

cell migration The movement of cells from site of origin to final location. See Figure 4.3. [4]

cell nucleus The spherical central structure of a cell that contains the chromosomes. [App]

cell-cell interaction The general process during development in which one cell affects the differentiation of other, usually neighboring, cells. [4]

central deafness A hearing impairment in which the auditory areas of the brain fail to process and interpret action potentials from sound stimuli in meaningful ways, usually as a consequence of damage in auditory brain areas. See Figure 6.10. Compare *conduction deafness* and *sensorineural deafness*. [6]

central modulation of sensory information The process in which higher brain centers, such as the cortex and thalamus, suppress some sources of sensory information and amplify others. [5]

central nervous system (CNS) The brain and the spinal cord. See Figures 1.6, 1.12. Compare *peripheral nervous system*. [1]

central sulcus A fissure that divides the frontal lobe from the parietal lobe. See Figure 1.11. [1]

cerebellum A structure located at the back of the brain, dorsal to the pons, that is involved in the central regulation of movement and in some forms of learning. See Figures 1.11, 1.12, 1.15, 5.29. [1, 5, 13]

cerebral arteries The three pairs of large arteries within the skull that supply blood to the cerebral cortex. [1]

cerebral cortex Also called simply *cortex*. The outer covering of the cerebral hemispheres, which consists largely of neuron bodies and their branches. See Figure 1.13. [1]

cerebral hemisphere One of the two halves—right or left—of the forebrain. See Figure 1.12. [1]

cerebral lateralization The division of labor between the two cerebral hemispheres such that each hemisphere is specialized for particular types of processing. [15]

cerebrocerebellum The lowermost part of the cerebellum, consisting especially of the lateral parts of each cerebellar hemisphere. It is implicated in planning complex movements. Compare *spinocerebellum* and *vestibulocerebellum*. [ASF 5.4]

cerebrospinal fluid (CSF) The fluid that fills the cerebral ventricles. See Figure 1.16. [1]

cervical Referring to the topmost eight segments of the spinal cord, in the neck region. See Figures 1.8, 1.9. Compare *thoracic, lumbar, sacral,* and *coccygeal*. [1]

c-fos An immediate early gene commonly used to identify activated neurons.

change blindness A failure to notice changes in comparisons of two alternating static visual scenes.

ChAT See choline acetyltransferase. [ASF 4.1]

chemical transmitter See *neurotransmitter*. [1, 2, 3]

chloride ion (Cl⁻) A chlorine atom that carries a negative charge. [2]

chlorpromazine An early antipsychotic drug that revolutionized the treatment of schizophrenia. [12]

cholecystokinin (CCK) A peptide hormone that is released by the gut after ingestion of food that is high in protein and/or fat. [9]

choline acetyltransferase (ChAT) An important enzyme in the synthesis of the neurotransmitter acetylcholine. [ASF 4.1]

cholinergic Referring to cells that use acetylcholine as their synaptic transmitter. [2, 3]

choroid plexus A specialized membrane lining the ventricles that produces cerebrospinal fluid by filtering blood. [1]

chromosome A complex of condensed strands of DNA and associated protein molecules. Chromosomes are found in the nucleus of cells. [App]

chronic traumatic encephalopathy (CTE) A form of dementia that may develop following multiple concussions, such as in athletes engaged in contact sports. It was formerly called *dementia pugilistica* or *punch-drunk syndrome*. [15]

ciliary muscle One of the muscles that control the shape of the lens inside the eye, focusing an image on the retina. See Figure 7.1. [7]

CIMT See constraint-induced movement therapy. [15]

cingulate cortex Also called *cingulum*. A region of medial cerebral cortex that lies dorsal to the corpus callosum. [5]

cingulate gyrus Also called *cingulate cortex* or *cingulum*. A strip of cortex, found in the frontal and parietal midline, that is part of the limbic system and is implicated in many cognitive functions. See Figures 1.14, 1.15. [1]

circadian rhythm A pattern of behavioral, biochemical, or physiological fluctuation that has a 24-hour period. [10]

circle of Willis A structure at the base of the brain that is formed by the joining of the carotid and basilar arteries. [ASF 2.1]

circumventricular organ Any of multiple distinct sites that lie in the wall of a cerebral ventricle and monitor the composition of the cerebrospinal fluid. See Figure 9.7. [9]

classical conditioning Also called *Pavlovian conditioning*. A type of associative learning in which an originally neutral stimulus acquires the power to elicit a conditioned response when presented alone. See Figure 13.10. Compare *instrumental conditioning*. [13]

clitoris The female phallus. Compare *penis*. [8]

cloacal exstrophy A rare medical condition in which individuals are born with an incompletely closed lower abdomen. [8]

clones Asexually produced organisms that are genetically identical. [4, App]

clozapine A second-generation antipsychotic that blocks 5-HT2A receptors. [12]

CNS See *central nervous system*. [1]

cocaine A drug of abuse, derived from the coca plant, that acts by enhancing catecholamine neurotransmission. [3]

coccygeal Referring to the lowest spinal vertebra (the coccyx, or "tailbone"). See Figures 1.8, 1.9. Compare *cervical, thoracic, lumbar,* and *sacral*. [1]

cochlea A snail-shaped structure in the inner ear canal that contains the primary receptor cells for hearing. See Figure 6.1. [6]

cochlear implant An implantable device that detects sounds and selectively stimulates nerves in different regions of the cochlea. [6]

cochlear nuclei Brainstem nuclei that receive input from auditory hair cells and send output to the superior olivary nuclei. See Figure 6.5. [6]

cocktail party effect The selective enhancement of attention in order to filter out distracters, as you might do while listening to one person talking in the midst of a noisy party. [14]

codon A set of three nucleotides that encodes one particular amino acid. A series of codons determines the structure of a peptide or protein. [App]

cognitive behavioral therapy (CBT) Psychotherapy aimed at correcting negative thinking and consciously changing behaviors as a way of changing feelings. [12]

cognitive map A mental representation of the relative spatial organization of objects and information. [13]

cognitively impenetrable Referring to basic neural processing operations that cannot be experienced through introspection—in other words, that are unconscious. [14]

coitus See *copulation*. [8]

collateral sprouting The formation of a new branch on an axon, usually in response to the uncovering of unoccupied postsynaptic sites. [ASF 15.4]

co-localization The synthesis and release of more than one type of neurotransmitter by a given presynaptic neuron. [3]

communication Information transfer between two individuals. [15]

complex cortical cell A cell in the visual cortex that responds best to a bar of a particular size and orientation anywhere within a particular area of the visual field and that needs movement to make it respond actively. Compare *simple cortical cell*. [7]

complex environment See *enriched condition*. [13]

complex partial seizure A type of seizure that doesn't involve the entire brain and therefore can cause a wide variety of symptoms. [2]

computerized axial tomography (CAT or CT scans) A noninvasive technique for examining brain structure through computer analysis of X-ray absorption at several positions around the head. See Figure 1.20. Compare *magnetic resonance imaging*. [1]

concordance Sharing of a characteristic by both individuals of a pair of twins. [12]

concussion A form of closed head injury caused by a jarring blow to the head, resulting in damage to the tissue of the brain with short- or long-term consequences for cognitive function. [15]

conduction aphasia An impairment in the ability to repeat words and sentences. [15]

conduction deafness A hearing impairment in which the ears fail to convert sound vibrations in air into waves of fluid in the cochlea. It is associated with defects of the external ear or middle ear. See Figure 6.10. Compare *central deafness* and *sensorineural deafness*. [6]

conduction velocity The speed at which an action potential is propagated along the length of an axon. [2]

conduction zone The part of a neuron—typically the axon—over which the action potential is actively propagated. See Figures 1.1, 1.3. Compare *input zone*, *integration zone*, and *output zone*. [1]

cone Any of several classes of photoreceptor cells in the retina that are re-sponsible for color vision. See Figure 7.3. Compare *rod*. [7]

confabulate To fill in a gap in memory with a falsification, often seen in Korsakoff's syndrome. [13]

congenital adrenal hyperplasia (CAH) Any of several genetic mutations that can cause a female fetus to be exposed to adrenal androgens, resulting in partial masculinization at birth. [8]

conjunction search A search for an item that is based on two or more features (e.g., size and color) that together distinguish the target from distracters that may share some of the same attributes. Compare *feature search*. [14]

connectionist model of aphasia Also called the *Wernicke-Geschwind model*. A theory proposing that left-hemisphere language deficits result from disconnection between the brain regions in a language network, each of which serves a particular linguistic function. Compare *motor theory of language*. [15]

consciousness The state of awareness of one's own existence, thoughts, emotions, and experiences. [Intro, 14]

conserved In the context of evolution, referring to a trait that is passed on from a common ancestor to two or more descendant species. [1]

consolidation The second process in the memory system, in which information in short-term memory is transferred to long-term memory. See Figure 13.14. Compare *encoding* and *retrieval*. [13]

constraint-induced movement therapy (CIMT) A therapy for recovery of movement after stroke or injury in which the person's unaffected limb is constrained while they are required to perform tasks with the affected limb. [15]

contralateral In anatomy, pertaining to a location on the opposite side of the body. Compare *ipsilateral*. [1, 15]

control group In research, a group of individuals that are identical to those in an experimental (or test) group in every way except that they do not receive the experimental treatment or manipulation. The experimental group is then compared with the control group to assess the effect of the treatment. [1]

convergence The phenomenon of neural connections in which many cells send signals to a single cell. [7, ASF 3.2]

Coolidge effect The propensity of an animal that appears sexually satisfied with a current partner to resume sexual activity when provided with a new partner. [8]

copulation Also called *coitus*. The transfer of sperm from a male to a female. [8]

cornea The transparent outer layer of the eye, whose curvature is fixed. The cornea bends light rays and is primarily responsible for forming the image on the retina. See Figure 7.1. [7]

coronal plane Also called *frontal plane* or *transverse plane*. The plane that divides the body or brain into front and back parts. Compare *horizontal plane* and *sagittal plane*. [1]

corpus callosum The main band of axons that connects the two cerebral hemispheres. See Figure 1.15. [1, 15]

corpus luteum (pl. corpora lutea) The structure that forms from the collapsed ovarian follicle after ovulation. The corpora lutea are a major source of progesterone. [8, ASF 8.4]

correlation The tendency of two measures to vary in concert, such that a change in one measure is matched by a change in the other. [1]

cortex (pl. cortices) The outer layer of a structure. See also *cerebral cortex*.

cortical column One of the vertical columns that constitute the basic organization of the cerebral cortex. [1]

cortical deafness A form of central deafness, caused by damage to both sides of the auditory cortex, that is characterized by difficulty in recognizing all complex sounds, whether verbal or nonverbal. [6]

corticospinal system See *pyramidal system*. [5]

cortisol A glucocorticoid stress hormone of the adrenal cortex. [11]

covert attention Attention in which the focus can be directed independently of sensory orientation (e.g., you're attending to one sensory stimulus while looking at another). Compare *overt attention*. [14]

cranial nerve A nerve that is connected directly to the brain. Compare *spinal nerve*. See Figure 1.7. [1]

crib death See *sudden infant death syndrome*. [10]

critical period See *sensitive period*. [4, 8, ASF 13.4, 15]

cross-tolerance A condition in which the development of tolerance for one drug causes an individual to develop tolerance for another drug. [3]

crystallization The final stage of birdsong formation, in which fully formed adult song is achieved. [ASF 15.3]

CSF See *cerebrospinal fluid*. [1

CT See *computerized axial tomography*. [1]

CTE See *chronic traumatic encephalopathy*. [15]

curare A neurotoxin that causes paralysis by blocking acetylcholine receptors in muscle. [2]

Cushing's syndrome A condition in which levels of adrenal glucocorticoids are abnormally high. [ASF 12.2]

cytokine A protein that has effects on other cells, as in the immune system. Examples include interleukins and interferons. [ASF 11.4]

cytoplasm See *intracellular fluid*. [2]

D

DA See *dopamine*. [3]

dB See *decibel*. [6]

DBS See *deep brain stimulation*. [12]

deafness Hearing loss so profound that speech perception is lost. [6]

decibel (dB) A measure of sound intensity, perceived as loudness. See Box 6.1. [6]

declarative memory A memory that can be stated or described. See Figure 13.4. Compare *nondeclarative memory*. [13]

decomposition of movement Difficulty of movement in which gestures are broken up into individual segments instead of being executed smoothly. It is a symptom of cerebellar lesions. [5]

decorticate rage Also called *sham rage*. Sudden intense rage characterized by actions (such as snarling and biting in dogs) that lack clear direction. [11]

deep brain stimulation (DBS) Mild electrical stimulation through an electrode that is surgically implanted deep in the brain. [12]

deep dyslexia Acquired dyslexia in which the person reads a word as another word that is semantically related. Compare *surface dyslexia*. [15]

default mode network A circuit of brain regions that is active during quiet introspective thought. [14]

degradation The chemical breakdown of a neurotransmitter into inactive metabolites. [2]

delayed non-matching-to-sample task A test in which the individual must respond to the unfamiliar stimulus in a pair of stimuli. See Figure 13.5. [13]

delta wave The slowest type of EEG wave, about 1 per second, characteristic of stage 3 sleep. See Figure 10.11. [10]

delta-9-tetrahydrocannabinol (THC) The major active ingredient in cannabis. [3]

delusion A false belief that is strongly held in spite of contrary evidence. [12]

dementia Drastic failure of cognitive ability, including memory failure and disorientation. [4]

dendrite An extension of the cell body that receives information from other neurons. Functionally, the dendrites are the input zone of the neuron. See Figures 1.1, 1.3. [1]

dendro-dendritic synapse A synapse at which a synaptic connection forms between the dendrites of two neurons. Compare *axo-axonic synapse*, *axo-dendritic synapse*, and *axo-somatic synapse*. [2]

dentate gyrus A strip of gray matter in the hippocampal formation. [13]

deoxyribonucleic acid (DNA) A nucleic acid that is present in the chromosomes of cells and codes hereditary information. Compare *ribonucleic acid*. [App]

dependent variable The factor that an experimenter measures to monitor a change in response to manipulation of an independent variable. [1]

depolarization A decrease in membrane potential (the interior of the neuron becomes less negative). See Figure 2.5. Compare *hyperpolarization*. [2]

depressant A drug that reduces the excitability of neurons. Compare *stimulant*. [3]

depression A psychiatric condition characterized by such symptoms as an unhappy mood; loss of interests, energy, and appetite; and difficulty concentrating. See also *bipolar disorder*. [12]

dermatome A strip of skin innervated by a particular spinal nerve. [5]

desynchronized EEG Also called *beta activity*. A pattern of EEG activity comprising a mix of many different high frequencies with low amplitude. Compare *alpha rhythm*. [10]

dexamethasone suppression test A test of pituitary-adrenal function in which the subject is given dexamethasone, a synthetic glucocorticoid hormone, which should cause a decline in the production of adrenal corticosteroids. [ASF 12.2]

DHT See *dihydrotestosterone*. [8]

diabetes mellitus A condition, characterized by excessive glucose in the blood and urine and by reduced glucose utilization by body cells, that is caused by the failure of insulin to induce glucose absorption. [9]

dichotic presentation The simultaneous delivery of different stimuli to the right and left ears at the same time. See Figure 15.2. [15]

diencephalon The posterior part of the fetal forebrain, which will become the thalamus and hypothalamus in adulthood. See Figure 1.12. Compare *telencephalon*. [1]

differentiation See *cell differentiation*. [4, App]

diffusion The spontaneous spread of solute molecules from an area of high concentration to an area of low concentration through a solvent until a uniform solute concentration is achieved. See Figure 2.3. Compare *osmosis*. [2, 9]

diffusion tensor imaging (DTI) A modified form of MRI in which the diffusion of water in a confined space is exploited to produce images of axonal fiber tracts. [1, 15]

digestion The process by which food is broken down to provide energy and nutrients. [ASF 9.3]

dihydrotestosterone (DHT) The 5-alpha-reduced metabolite of testosterone. DHT is a potent androgen that is principally responsible for the masculinization of the external genitalia in mammals. [8]

distal In anatomy, toward the periphery of an organism or toward the end of a limb. Compare *proximal*. [1]

divergence The phenomenon of neural connections in which one cell sends signals to many other cells. Compare *convergence*. [ASF 3.2]

divided-attention task A task in which the participant is asked to focus attention on two or more stimuli simultaneously. Compare *sustained-attention task*. [14]

DNA See *deoxyribonucleic acid*. [App]

DNA sequencing The process by which the order of nucleotides in a gene is identified. [App]

dopamine (DA) A monoamine transmitter found in the midbrain—especially the substantia nigra—and in the basal forebrain. See Figure 3.4, Table 3.1. [3]

dopamine hypothesis The idea that schizophrenia results from either excessive levels of synaptic dopamine or excessive postsynaptic sensitivity to dopamine. [12]

dopaminergic Referring to cells that use dopamine as their synaptic transmitter. [3]

dorsal In anatomy, toward the back of the body or the top of the brain. Compare *ventral*. [1]

dorsal column system A somatosensory system that delivers most touch stimuli to the brain via the dorsal columns of spinal white matter. See Figure 5.7. Compare *anterolateral system*. [5]

dorsomedial thalamus A limbic system structure that is connected to the hippocampus. [13]

dose-response curve (DRC) A formal graph of a drug's effects (on the y-axis) versus the dose given (on the x-axis). See Figure 3.6. [3]

down-regulation A compensatory decrease in receptor availability at the synapses of a neuron. Compare *up-regulation*. [3]

DRC See *dose-response curve*. [3]

drug tolerance Also called simply *tolerance*. A condition in which, with repeated exposure to a drug, an individual becomes less responsive to a constant dose. [3]

DTI See *diffusion tensor imaging*. [1, 15]

DTI tractography Also called *fiber tracking*. Visualization of the orientation and terminations of white matter tracts in the living brain via diffusion tensor imaging. [15]

dualism The notion, promoted by René Descartes, that the mind has an immaterial aspect that is distinct from the material body and brain. [Intro]

dura mater The outermost of the three meninges that surround the brain and spinal cord. See also *pia mater* and *arachnoid*. See Figure 1.8. [1]

dyskinesia Difficulty or distortion in voluntary movement. [12]

dyslexia Also called *alexia*. A reading disorder attributed to brain impairment. [15]

dysphoria Unpleasant feelings; the opposite of euphoria. [3]

dystrophin A protein that is needed for normal muscle function. Dystrophin is defective in some forms of muscular dystrophy. [ASF 5.5]

E

ear canal Also called *auditory canal*. The tube leading from the pinna to the tympanic membrane. [6]

eardrum See *tympanic membrane*. [6]

easy problem of consciousness Understanding how particular patterns of neural activity create specific conscious experiences by reading brain activity directly from people's brains as they're having particular experiences. Compare *hard problem of consciousness*. [14]

EC See *enriched condition*. [13]

ecological niche The unique assortment of environmental opportunities and challenges to which each organism is adapted. [10]

Ecstasy See *MDMA*. [3]

ECT See *electroconvulsive shock therapy*. [12]

ectoderm The outer cellular layer of the developing embryo, giving rise to the skin and the nervous system. [4]

ectotherm An animal whose body temperature is regulated by, and whose heat comes mainly from, the environment. Examples include snakes and bees. Compare *endotherm*. [9]

edge detector See *simple cortical cell*. [7]

EEG See *electroencephalogram* and *electroencephalography*. [2, 10]

efferent Carrying action potentials away from the brain, or away from one region of interest. Compare *afferent*. [1]

efficacy Also called *intrinsic activity*. The extent to which a drug activates a response when it binds to a receptor. Receptor antagonist drugs have low efficacy; receptor agonists have high efficacy. See Figure 3.6. [3]

egg See *ovum*. [8]

ejaculation The forceful expulsion of semen from the penis. [8]

electrical synapse Also called *gap junction*. The region between neurons where the presynaptic and postsynaptic membranes are so close that the action potential can jump to the postsynaptic membrane without first being translated into a chemical message. [ASF 3.1]

electroconvulsive shock therapy (ECT) A last-resort treatment for unmanageable depression, in which a strong electrical current is passed through the brain, causing a seizure. [12]

electroencephalogram (EEG) A recording of gross electrical activity of the brain via large electrodes placed on the scalp. See *electroencephalography*. [2]

electroencephalography (EEG) The recording of gross electrical activity of the brain via large electrodes placed on the scalp. See Figures 2.16, 10.11. [2, 10]

electromyography (EMG) The electrical recording of muscle activity. See Figure 5.17. [5]

electrostatic pressure The propensity of charged molecules or ions to move toward areas with the opposite charge. [2]

embryo The earliest stage in a developing animal. Humans are considered to be embryos until 8–10 weeks after conception. Compare *fetus*. [4]

embryonic stem cell A cell, derived from an embryo, that has the capacity to form any type of tissue. [15]

EMG See *electromyography*. [5]

emotion A subjective mental state that is usually accompanied by distinctive cognition, behaviors, and physiological changes. [11]

encoding The first process in the memory system, in which the information entering sensory channels is passed into short-term memory. See Figure 13.14. Compare *consolidation* and *retrieval*. [13]

endocannabinoid An endogenous ligand of cannabinoid receptors, thus an analog of cannabis that is produced by the brain. [3, 9]

endocrine Referring to glands that release chemicals to the interior of the body. These glands secrete the principal hormones used by the body. See Figure 8.3. [8]

endocrine gland A gland that secretes hormones into the bloodstream to act on distant targets. See Figure 8.1. [8]

endogenous Produced inside the body. Compare *exogenous*. [3]

endogenous opioid Any of a class of opium-like peptide transmitters that have been referred to as the body's own narcotics. The three kinds are enkephalins, endorphins, and dynorphins. See Table 3.1. [3]

endorphin One of three kinds of endogenous opioids. See Table 3.1. [5]

endotherm An animal whose body temperature is regulated chiefly by internal metabolic processes. Examples include mammals and birds. Compare *ectotherm*. [9]

enriched condition (EC) Also called *complex environment*. An environment for laboratory rodents in which animals are group-housed with a wide variety of stimulus objects. See Figure 13.16. Compare *impoverished condition* and *standard condition*. [13]

enterotype Each individual's personal composition of gut microbiota. [9]

entrainment The process of synchronizing a biological rhythm to an environmental stimulus. See Figure 10.2. [10]

enzyme A complicated protein that increases the probability of a specific chemical reaction. [App]

epigenetic regulation Changes in gene expression that are due to environmental effects rather than to changes in the nucleotide sequence of the gene. [11]

epigenetic transmission The passage from one individual to another of changes in the expression of targeted genes, without altering the sequence of nucleotides in the gene. [9]

epigenetics The study of factors that affect gene expression without making any changes in the nucleotide sequence of the genes themselves. [Intro, 4]

epilepsy A brain disorder marked by major, sudden changes in the electrophysiological state of the brain that are referred to as *seizures*. See Figure 2.17. [2]

epinephrine Also called *adrenaline*. A compound that acts both as a hormone (secreted by the adrenal medulla under the control of the sympathetic nervous system) and as a synaptic transmitter. See Tables 3.1, 8.1. [11]

episodic memory Also called *autobiographical memory*. Memory of a particular incident or a particular time and place. Compare *semantic memory*. [13]

EPSP See *excitatory postsynaptic potential*. [2]

equilibrium potential The point at which the movement of ions across the cell membrane is balanced, as the electrostatic pressure pulling ions in one direction is offset by the diffusion force pushing them in the opposite direction. [2]

ERP See *event-related potential*. [2, 14]

estradiol Formally called *17-beta-estradiol*. The primary type of estrogen secreted by the ovary. [8]

estrogen Any of a class of steroid hormones, including estradiol, produced by female gonads. See Figure 8.13. [8]

estrus The period during which female animals are sexually receptive. [8]

eukaryote Any organism whose cells have the genetic material contained within a nuclear envelope. [App]

event-related potential (ERP) Also called *evoked potential*. Averaged EEG recordings measuring brain responses to repeated presentations of a stimulus. Components of the ERP tend to be reliable because the background noise of the cortex has been averaged out. See Figures 2.16, 14.7. [2, 14]

evoked potential See *event-related potential*. [2, 14]

evolution by natural selection The Darwinian theory that evolution proceeds by differential success in reproduction.

evolutionary psychology A field of study devoted to asking how natural selection has shaped behavior in humans and other animals. [Intro]

excitatory postsynaptic potential (EPSP) A depolarizing potential in a neuron that is normally caused by synaptic excitation. EPSPs increase the probability that the postsynaptic neuron will fire an action potential. See Figure 2.15. Compare *inhibitory postsynaptic potential*. [2]

excitatory synapse A type of synapse that, when active, causes a local depolarization that increases the likelihood the neuron will fire an action potential. [3]

excitotoxicity The property by which neurons die when overstimulated, as with large amounts of glutamate. [ASF 15.5]

executive function A neural and cognitive system that helps develop plans of action and organizes the activities of other high-level processing systems. [14]

exogenous Arising from outside the body. Compare *endogenous*. [3]

expression See *gene expression*. [Intro, 4, App]

external ear The part of the ear that we readily see (the pinna) and the canal that leads to the eardrum. See Figure 6.1.

extracellular compartment The fluid of the body that exists outside the cells. See

Figure 9.6. Compare *intracellular compartment*. [9]

extracellular fluid Also called *interstitial fluid*. The fluid in the spaces between cells. Compare *intracellular fluid*. [2]

extraocular muscle One of the muscles attached to the eyeball that controls its position and movements. [7]

extrapyramidal system A motor system that includes the basal ganglia and some closely related brainstem structures. Axons of this system pass into the spinal cord outside the pyramids of the medulla. Compare *pyramidal system*. [5]

extrastriate cortex Visual cortex outside of the primary visual (striate) cortex. [7]

F

face blindness See *prosopagnosia*. [15]

FASD See *fetal alcohol spectrum disorder*. [3]

fat tissue See *adipose tissue*. [9]

fatal familial insomnia An inherited disease that causes people in middle age to stop sleeping, which after a few months results in death. [10]

fear conditioning A form of classical conditioning in which a previously neutral stimulus is repeatedly paired with an unpleasant stimulus, like foot shock, until the previously neutral stimulus alone elicits the responses seen in fear. [11, 12]

feature search A search for an item in which the target pops out right away, no matter how many distracters are present, because it possesses a unique attribute. Compare *conjunction search*. [14]

fecal transplantation A medical procedure in which gut microbiota, via fecal matter, are transplanted from a donor to a host. [9]

FEF See *frontal eye field*. [14]

fetal alcohol spectrum disorder (FASD) A family of developmental disorders that vary in severity, resulting from fetal exposure to alcohol consumed by the mother. Severe cases, associated with high levels of alcohol abuse by the mother, include intellectual disability and facial abnormalities. [3]

fetus A developing individual after the embryo stage. Humans are considered to be fetuses from 10 weeks after fertilization until birth. Compare *embryo*. [4]

fiber tracking See *DTI tractography*. [15]

final common pathway The motor neurons of the brain and spinal cord, so called because they receive and integrate all motor signals from the brain to direct movement. [5]

first-generation antipsychotic Also called *typical antipsychotic* or *neuroleptic*. An antischizophrenic drug that

shows antagonist activity at dopamine D2 receptors. [3, 12]

flavor The sense of taste combined with the sense of smell. Compare *taste*. [6]

fluent aphasia Also called *Wernicke's aphasia*. A language impairment characterized by fluent, meaningless speech and little language comprehension. It is related to damage in Wernicke's area. See Figure 15.10. Compare *nonfluent aphasia*. [15]

fMRI See *functional MRI*. [1]

follicle The structure of the ovary that contains an immature ovum (egg). [8, ASF 8.4]

follicle-stimulating hormone (FSH) A gonadotropin, named for its actions on ovarian follicles. See Figure 8.13. [8, ASF 8.4]

forebrain The frontal division of the neural tube, which in the mature vertebrate contains the cerebral hemispheres, the thalamus, and the hypothalamus. See Figure 1.12. Compare *hindbrain* and *midbrain*. [1, 4]

fornix A fiber tract that extends from the hippocampus to the mammillary body. See Figures 1.14, 1.15. [1]

Fourier analysis The mathematical decomposition of a complex pattern into a sum of sine waves. [ASF 7.2]

fourth ventricle The passageway within the pons that receives cerebrospinal fluid from the third ventricle and releases it to surround the brain and spinal cord. See Figure 1.16. Compare *lateral ventricle* and *third ventricle*. [1]

fovea The central portion of the retina, which is packed with the highest density of photoreceptors and is the center of our gaze. See Figure 7.1. [7]

fragile X syndrome A frequent cause of inherited intellectual disability produced by a fragile site on the X chromosome that seems prone to breaking because the DNA there is unstable. [4]

fraternal birth order effect A phenomenon in human populations, such that the more older biological brothers a boy has, the more likely it is he will grow up to be gay. [8]

free nerve ending An axon that terminates in the skin and has no specialized cell associated with it. Free nerve endings detect pain or itch, or changes in temperature. See Figure 5.3. [5]

free will The feeling that our conscious self is the author of our actions and decisions. [14]

free-running Referring to a rhythm of behavior shown by an animal deprived of external cues about time of day. See Figure 10.2. [10]

frequency The number of cycles per second in a sound wave, measured in hertz.

frontal eye field (FEF) An area in the frontal lobe of the brain that contains neurons important for establishing gaze in accordance with cognitive goals (top-down processes) rather than with any characteristics of stimuli (bottom-up processes). [14]

frontal lobe The most anterior portion of the cerebral cortex. See Figure 1.11. Compare *occipital lobe, parietal lobe*, and *temporal lobe*. [1]

frontal plane See *coronal plane*. [1]

FSH See *follicle-stimulating hormone*. [8, ASF 8.4]

functional MRI (fMRI) Magnetic resonance imaging that detects changes in blood flow and therefore identifies regions of the brain that are particularly active during a given task. See Figure 1.20. Compare *positron emission tomography*. [1]

functional tolerance The form of drug tolerance that arises when repeated exposure to the drug causes receptors to be up-regulated or down-regulated. Compare *metabolic tolerance*. [3]

fusiform gyrus A region on the inferior surface of the cortex, at the junction of the temporal and occipital lobes, that has been associated with recognition of faces. See Figure 15.6. [15]

G

G protein–coupled receptor (GPCR) A type of receptor that, when activated extracellularly, initiates a G protein signaling mechanism inside the cell. [3]

GABA See *gamma-aminobutyric acid*. [3]

gamete A sex cell (sperm or ovum) that contains only unpaired chromosomes and therefore has only half of the usual number of chromosomes. [8]

gamma-aminobutyric acid (GABA) A widely distributed amino acid transmitter, the main inhibitory transmitter in the mammalian nervous system. See Table 3.1. [3]

ganglion cell Any of a class of cells in the retina whose axons form the optic nerve. See Figure 7.15. Compare *amacrine cell, bipolar cell*, and *horizontal cell*. [7]

gap junction See *electrical synapse*. [ASF 3.1]

gas neurotransmitter A neurotransmitter that is a soluble gas. Examples include nitric oxide and carbon monoxide. Usually gas neurotransmitters act, in a retrograde fashion, on presynaptic neurons. See Table 3.1. Compare *amine neurotransmitter, amino acid neurotransmitter*, and *peptide neurotransmitter*. [3]

gel electrophoresis A method of separating molecules of differing size or electrical charge by forcing them to flow through a gel. See Appendix Figure A.3. [App]

gene A length of DNA that encodes the information for constructing a particular protein. [App]

gene amplification See *polymerase chain reaction*. [App]

gene expression The turning on or off of specific genes; the process by which a cell makes an mRNA transcript of a particular gene. [Intro, 4, App]

general anesthetic A drug that renders an individual unconscious. [10]

genital tubercle In the early fetus, a "bump" between the legs that can develop into either a clitoris or a penis. [8]

genome See *genotype*. [App]

genotype Also called *genome*. All the genetic information that one specific individual has inherited. Compare *phenotype*. [4, App]

GH See *growth hormone*. [8, ASF 8.4]

ghrelin A peptide gut hormone believed to act on the hypothalamic appetite system to increase hunger. See Figure 9.16. Compare PYY_{3-36}. [9]

glial cells Also called *glia*. Nonneuronal brain cells that provide structural, nutritional, and other types of support to the brain. See Figure 1.5. [1]

global aphasia The total loss of ability to understand language, or to speak, read, or write. See Figure 15.10. [15]

glomerulus (pl. glomeruli) A complex arbor of dendrites from a group of olfactory cells. [6]

GLP-1 See *glucagon-like peptide 1*. [9]

glucagon-like peptide 1 (GLP-1) A peptide gut hormone believed to act on the hypothalamic appetite system to suppress appetite. [9]

glucocorticoid Any of a class of steroid hormones, released by the adrenal cortex, that affect carbohydrate metabolism and inflammation.

glucodetector A specialized type of liver cell that detects and informs the nervous system about levels of circulating glucose. [9]

glucose An important sugar molecule used by the body and brain for energy. [9]

glutamate An amino acid transmitter, the most common excitatory transmitter. See Table 3.1. [3, 13]

glutamate hypothesis The idea that schizophrenia may be caused, in part, by understimulation of glutamate receptors. [12]

glycogen A complex carbohydrate made by the combining of glucose molecules for a short-term store of energy. [9]

glymphatic system A lymphatic system in the brain that participates in removal of wastes and the movement of nutrients and signaling compounds. [1]

GnRH See *gonadotropin-releasing hormone*. [8]

Golgi stain A tissue stain that completely fills a small proportion of neurons with a dark, silver-based precipitate. [1]

Golgi tendon organ A type of receptor found within tendons that sends impulses to the central nervous system when a muscle contracts. See Figure 5.21. Compare *muscle spindle*. [5]

gonad Any of the sexual organs (ovaries in females, testes in males) that produce gametes for reproduction. See Figure 8.1. [8]

gonadotropin An anterior pituitary tropic hormone that stimulates the cells of the gonads to produce sex steroids and gametes. See *luteinizing hormone* and *follicle-stimulating hormone*. [8, ASF 8.4]

gonadotropin-releasing hormone (GnRH) A hypothalamic hormone that controls the release of luteinizing hormone and follicle-stimulating hormone from the pituitary. See Figure 8.13. [8]

GPCR See *G protein–coupled receptor*. [3]

grammar All of the rules for usage of a particular language. [15]

grand mal seizure See *tonic-clonic seizure*. [2]

gray matter Areas of the brain that are dominated by cell bodies and are devoid of myelin. Gray matter mostly receives and processes information. See Figures 1.8, 1.10. Compare *white matter*. [1]

gross neuroanatomy Anatomical features of the nervous system that are apparent to the naked eye. [1]

growth hormone (GH) Also called *somatotropin* or *somatotropic hormone*. A tropic hormone, secreted by the anterior pituitary, that promotes the growth of cells and tissues. [8, ASF 8.4]

guevedoces Literally "eggs at 12" (in Spanish). A nickname for individuals who are raised as girls but at puberty change appearance and begin behaving as boys. [8]

gustatory system The sensory system that detects taste. See Figure 6.19. [6]

gut microbiota The microorganisms that normally inhabit the digestive system. [9]

gyrus (pl. gyri) A ridged or raised portion of a convoluted brain surface. Compare *sulcus*. [1]

H

habituation A form of nonassociative learning in which an organism becomes less responsive following repeated presentations of a stimulus. See Figure 13.19. [13]

hair cell One of the receptor cells for hearing in the cochlea, named for the stereocilia that protrude from the top of the cell and transduce vibrational energy in the cochlea into neural activity. See Figure 6.1. [6]

hallucinogen Also called *psychedelics* or *entheogens*. A drug that alters sensory perception and produces peculiar experiences. [3]

hard problem of consciousness Understanding the brain processes that produce people's subjective experiences of their conscious perceptions—that is, their qualia. Compare *easy problem of consciousness*. [14]

health psychology Also called *behavioral medicine*. A field of study that focuses on psychological influences on health-related processes. [11]

hearing loss Decreased sensitivity to sound, in varying degrees. [6]

Hebbian synapse A synapse that is strengthened when it successfully drives the postsynaptic cell. [4, 12, ASF 13.4]

hemiparesis Weakness of one side of the body. Compare *hemiplegia*. [15]

hemiplegia Paralysis of one side of the body. Compare *hemiparesis*. [15]

hemispatial neglect Failure to pay any attention to objects presented to one side of the body. [14]

hermaphrodite An individual possessing the reproductive organs of both sexes, either simultaneously or at different points in time. [ASF 8.6]

heroin Diacetylmorphine, an artificially modified, very potent form of morphine. [3]

hertz (Hz) Cycles per second, as of an auditory stimulus. Hertz is a measure of frequency. See Box 6.1. [6]

hindbrain The rear division of the brain, which in the mature vertebrate contains the cerebellum, pons, and medulla. See Figures 1.12, 4.1. Compare *forebrain* and *midbrain*. [1, 4]

hippocampus (pl. hippocampi) A medial temporal lobe structure that is important for spatial cognition, learning, and memory. See Figures 1.14, 13.1, 13.21. [1, 13]

histology The study of tissue structure. [1]

homeostasis The maintenance of a relatively constant internal physiological environment. [9]

horizontal cell A specialized retinal cell that contacts both photoreceptors and bipolar cells. Compare *amacrine cell* and *ganglion cell*. [7]

horizontal plane The plane that divides the body or brain into upper and lower parts. Compare *coronal plane* and *sagittal plane*. [1]

hormone A chemical, usually secreted by an endocrine gland, that is conveyed by the bloodstream and regulates target organs or tissues. See Table 8.1. [8]

hue One of three basic dimensions of light perception, varying through the spectrum from violet to red. Compare *brightness* and *saturation*. [7]

huntingtin A protein produced by a gene (called *HTT*) that, when containing too many trinucleotide repeats, results in Huntington's disease in a carrier. [ASF 5.5]

Huntington's disease A genetic disorder, with onset in middle age, in which the destruction of basal ganglia results in a syndrome of abrupt, involuntary writhing movements and changes in mental functioning. Compare *Parkinson's disease*. [5]

hybridization The process by which one string of nucleotides becomes linked to a complementary series of nucleotides. [App]

hydrocephalus A ballooning of the ventricles, at the expense of the surrounding brain, which may occur when the circulation of CSF is blocked. [1]

hyperpolarization An increase in membrane potential (the interior of the neuron becomes even more negative). See Figure 2.5. Compare *depolarization*. [2]

hypocretin See *orexin*. [9, 10]

hypofrontality hypothesis The idea that schizophrenia may reflect underactivation of the frontal lobes. [12]

hypothalamic-pituitary portal system An elaborate bed of blood vessels leading from the hypothalamus to the anterior pituitary. [8]

hypothalamus Part of the diencephalon, lying ventral to the thalamus. See Figures 1.12, 1.14, 1.15. [1]

hypovolemic thirst A desire to ingest fluids that is stimulated by a reduction in volume of the extracellular fluid. Compare *osmotic thirst*. [9]

Hz See *hertz*. [6]

I

IC See *impoverished condition*. [13]

ICC See *immunocytochemistry*. [8, App]

iconic memory See *sensory buffer*. [13]

IHC See *immunohistochemistry*. [1] See *inner hair cell*. [6]

IID See *interaural intensity difference*. [6]

immunocytochemistry (ICC) A method for detecting a particular protein in tissues in which an antibody recognizes and binds to the protein and then chemical methods are used to leave a visible reaction product around each antibody. See Box 8.1. [8, App]

immunoglobulin See *antibody*. [App, ASF 11.4]

immunohistochemistry (IHC) The use of antibodies to visualize the distribution of a particular protein in tissue. [1]

impoverished condition (IC) Also called *isolated condition*. An environment for laboratory rodents in which each animal is housed singly in a small cage without complex stimuli. See Figure 13.16. Compare *enriched condition* and *standard condition*. [13]

in situ hybridization A method for detecting particular RNA transcripts in tissue sections by providing a nucleotide probe that is complementary to, and will therefore hybridize with, the transcript of interest. See Box 8.1; Appendix Figure A.4. [1, 8, App]

inattentional blindness The failure to perceive nonattended stimuli that seem so obvious as to be impossible to miss. [14]

independent variable The factor that is manipulated by an experimenter. Compare *dependent variable*. [1]

indifferent gonads The undifferentiated gonads of the early mammalian fetus, which will eventually develop into either testes or ovaries. See Figure 8.23. [8]

inferior In anatomy, below. Compare *superior*. [1]

inferior colliculi (sing. colliculus) Paired gray matter structures of the dorsal midbrain that process auditory information. See Figure 1.15. Compare *superior colliculi*. [1, 6]

infradian Referring to a rhythmic biological event with a period longer than a day. Compare *ultradian*. [10]

infrasound Very-low-frequency sound, generally below the 20 Hz threshold for human hearing. Compare *ultrasound*. [6]

inhibition of return The phenomenon, observed in peripheral spatial cuing tasks when the interval between cue and target stimulus is 200 milliseconds or more, in which the detection of stimuli at the former location of the cue is increasingly impaired. [14]

inhibitory postsynaptic potential (IPSP) A hyperpolarizing potential in a neuron. IPSPs decrease the probability that the postsynaptic neuron will fire an action potential. See Figure 2.10. Compare *excitatory postsynaptic potential*. [2]

inhibitory synapse A type of synapse that, when active, causes a local hyperpolarization that decreases the likelihood the neuron will fire an action potential. [3]

inner ear The cochlea and vestibular apparatus. See Figure 6.1. [6]

inner hair cell (IHC) One of the two types of receptor cells for hearing in the cochlea. Compared with outer hair cells, IHCs are positioned closer to the central axis of the coiled cochlea. See Figure 6.1. [6]

innervate To provide neural input to. [1]

input zone The part of a neuron that receives information from other neurons or from specialized sensory structures. This zone usually corresponds to the cell's dendrites. See Figures 1.1, 1.3. Compare *conduction zone, integration zone,* and *output zone.* [1]

instrumental conditioning Also called *operant conditioning.* A form of associative learning in which the likelihood that an act (instrumental response) will be performed depends on the consequences (reinforcing stimuli) that follow it. Compare *classical conditioning.* [13]

insula A region of cortex lying below the surface, within the lateral sulcus, of the frontal, temporal, and parietal lobes. [3]

insulin A pancreatic hormone that lowers blood glucose, promotes energy storage, and facilitates glucose utilization by cells. Compare *glucagon.* [9]

integration zone The part of a neuron that initiates neural electrical activity. This zone usually corresponds to the neuron's cell body. See Figures 1.1, 1.3. Compare *conduction zone, input zone,* and *output zone.* [1]

intellectual disability A disability characterized by significant limitations in intellectual functioning and adaptive behavior. [4]

interaural intensity difference (IID) A perceived difference in loudness between the two ears, which the nervous system can use to localize a sound source. [6]

interaural temporal difference (ITD) A difference between the two ears in the time of arrival of a sound, which the nervous system can use to localize a sound source. [6]

intermale aggression Aggression between males of the same species. [11]

interneuron A neuron that is neither a sensory neuron nor a motor neuron. Interneurons receive input from and send output to other neurons. Compare *motor neuron* and *sensory neuron.* [1]

intersex Referring to an individual with atypical genital development and sexual differentiation, whose genitalia are generally intermediate in form between typical male and typical female genitalia. [8]

intracellular compartment The fluid of the body that is contained within cells. See Figure 9.6. Compare *extracellular compartment.* [9]

intracellular fluid Also called *cytoplasm.* The watery solution found within cells. Compare *extracellullar fluid.* [2]

intrafusal fiber Any of the small muscle fibers that lie within each muscle spindle. See Figure 5.21. [5]

intraparietal sulcus (IPS) A region in the human parietal lobe, homologous to the monkey lateral intraparietal area, that is especially involved in voluntary, top-down control of attention. [14]

intrinsic activity See *efficacy.* [3]

intromission Insertion of the penis into the vagina during copulation. [8]

ion An atom or molecule that has acquired an electrical charge by gaining or losing one or more electrons. [2]

ion channel A pore in the cell membrane that permits the passage of certain ions through the membrane when the channel is open. See Figure 2.2. [2]

ionotropic receptor Also called *ligand-gated ion channel.* A receptor protein containing an ion channel that opens when the receptor is bound by an agonist. See Figure 3.2. Compare *metabotropic receptor.* [3]

IPS See *intraparietal sulcus.* [3]

ipsilateral In anatomy, pertaining to a location on the same side of the body. Compare *contralateral.* [1]

IPSP See *inhibitory postsynaptic potential.* [2]

iris (pl. irides) The circular structure of the eye that provides an opening to form the pupil. See Figure 7.1. [7]

isolated brain An experimental preparation in which an animal's brainstem has been separated from the spinal cord by a cut below the medulla. [10]

isolated condition See *impoverished condition.* [13]

isolated forebrain An experimental preparation in which an animal's nervous system has been cut in the upper midbrain, dividing the forebrain from the brainstem. [10]

ITD See *interaural temporal difference.* [6]

K

K complex A sharp, negative EEG potential seen in stage 2 sleep. [10]

kcal See *kilocalorie.* [ASF 9.1]

ketamine A dissociative anesthetic drug, similar to PCP, that acts as an NMDA receptor antagonist. [12]

ketone An organic molecule, derived from the breakdown of fat, that can be used by cells as an energy source. [9]

khat Also spelled *qat.* An African shrub that, when chewed, acts as a stimulant. [3]

kilocalorie (kcal) A measure of energy commonly applied to food; formally defined as the quantity of heat required to raise the temperature of 1 kilogram of water by 1°C. [ASF 9.1]

Klüver-Bucy syndrome A condition, brought about by bilateral amygdala damage, that is characterized by dramatic emotional changes including reduction in fear and anxiety. [11]

knee-jerk reflex A variant of the stretch reflex in which stretching of the tendon beneath the knee leads to an upward kick of the leg. See Figure 2.15. [2]

knockout organism An individual in which a particular gene has been disabled by an experimenter. See Box 8.1. [8]

Korsakoff's syndrome A memory disorder, caused by thiamine deficiency, that is generally associated with chronic alcoholism. [13]

L

labeled lines The concept that each nerve input to the brain reports only a particular type of information. [5]

lamellated corpuscle See *Pacinian corpuscle.* [5]

language Communication in which arbitrary sounds or symbols are arranged according to a grammar in order to convey an almost limitless variety of concepts. [15]

lateral In anatomy, toward one side. Compare *medial.* [1]

lateral geniculate nucleus (LGN) The part of the thalamus that receives information from the optic tract and sends it to visual areas in the occipital cortex. [7]

lateral hypothalamus (LH) A hypothalamic region involved in the control of appetite and other functions. See Figure 9.13. [9]

lateral inhibition The phenomenon by which interconnected neurons inhibit their neighbors, producing contrast at the edges of regions. See Figure 7.15. [7]

lateral intraparietal area (LIP) A region in the monkey parietal lobe, homologous to the human intraparietal sulcus, that is especially involved in voluntary, top-down control of attention. [14]

lateral sulcus See *Sylvian fissure.* [1]

lateral tegmental area A brainstem region that provides some of the norepinephrine-containing projections of the brain. [3]

lateral ventricle A complex C-shaped lateral portion of the ventricular system within each hemisphere of the brain. See Figure 1.16. Compare *fourth ventricle* and *third ventricle*. [1]

l-dopa The immediate precursor of the transmitter dopamine. It is known to markedly reduce symptoms in patients with Parkinson's, decreasing tremors and increasing the speed of movements. [ASF 5.5]

learned helplessness A learning paradigm in which individuals are subjected to inescapable, unpleasant conditions. [12]

learning The process of acquiring new and relatively enduring information, behavior patterns, or abilities, characterized by modifications of behavior as a result of practice, study, or experience. [13]

lens A structure in the eye that helps focus an image on the retina. See Figure 7.1. [7]

leptin A peptide hormone released by fat cells. [9]

level of analysis The scope of an experimental approach. A scientist may try to understand behavior by monitoring molecules, neurons, brain regions, or social environments or using some combination of these levels of analysis. [1]

LGN See *lateral geniculate nucleus*. [7]

LH 1. See *lateral hypothalamus*. [9] 2. See *luteinizing hormone*. [8, ASF 8.4]

lie detector See *polygraph*. [11]

ligand A substance that binds to receptor molecules, such as a neurotransmitter or drug that binds to postsynaptic receptors. [2, 3]

ligand-gated ion channel See *ionotropic receptor*. [3]

limbic system A loosely defined, widespread group of brain nuclei that innervate each other to form a network. These nuclei are implicated in emotions. See Figure 1.14. [1, 11]

LIP See *lateral intraparietal area*. [14]

lipid A large molecule (frequently a fat) that consists of fatty acids and glycerol. Lipids are insoluble in water. [9]

lithium A chemical element that often relieves the symptoms of bipolar disorder. [12]

lobotomy The surgical separation of a portion of the frontal lobes from the rest of the brain, a former treatment, now discredited, for schizophrenia and many other ailments. [12]

local potential An electrical potential that is initiated by stimulation at a specific site, is a graded response that spreads passively across the cell membrane, and decreases in strength with time and distance. [2]

localization of function The concept that different brain regions specialize in specific behaviors. [Intro]

locus coeruleus A small nucleus in the brainstem whose neurons produce norepinephrine and modulate large areas of the forebrain. Compare *substantia nigra*. [3, 10]

long-term memory (LTM) An enduring form of memory that lasts days, weeks, months, or years. LTM has a very large capacity. Compare *sensory buffer* and *short-term memory*. See Figure 13.14. [13]

long-term potentiation (LTP) A stable and enduring increase in the effectiveness of synapses following repeated strong stimulation. See Figures 13.21, 13.22. [13]

lordosis A female receptive posture in four-legged animals in which the hindquarters are raised and the tail is turned to one side, facilitating intromission by the male. See Figures 8.16, 8.19. [8]

Lou Gehrig's disease See *amyotrophic lateral sclerosis*. [ASF 5.5]

LSD Also called *acid*. Lysergic acid diethylamide, a hallucinogenic drug. [3]

LTM See *long-term memory*. [13]

LTP See *long-term potentiation*. [13]

lumbar Referring to the five spinal segments in the upper part of the lower back. See Figures 1.8, 1.9. Compare *cervical*, *thoracic*, *sacral*, and *coccygeal*. [1]

luteinizing hormone (LH) A gonadotropin, named for its stimulatory effects on the ovarian corpora lutea. See Figure 8.13. [8, ASF 8.4]

M

M1 See *primary motor cortex*. [5]

magnetic resonance imaging (MRI) A noninvasive brain-imaging technology that uses magnetism and radio-frequency energy to create images of the gross structure of the living brain. See Figure 1.20. Compare *computerized axial tomography*. [1]

magnetoencephalography (MEG) A noninvasive brain-imaging technology that creates maps of brain activity during cognitive tasks by measuring tiny magnetic fields produced by active neurons. Compare *transcranial magnetic stimulation*. [1]

mammillary body One of a pair of limbic system structures that are connected to the hippocampus. See Figure 13.1. [13]

MAO See *monoamine oxidase*. [3, 12, ASF 4.1]

maternal aggression Aggression of a mother defending her nest or offspring. [11]

maternal behavior Behavior of adult females that has the goal of enhancing the well-being of their own offspring, often at some cost to the parents. [8]

MDMA Also called *Ecstasy* or *Molly*. 3,4-Methylenedioxymethamphetamine, a drug of abuse. [3]

medial In anatomy, toward the middle. Compare *lateral*. [1]

medial amygdala A portion of the amygdala that receives olfactory and pheromonal information. [8, 11]

medial forebrain bundle A collection of axons traveling in the midline region of the forebrain. [11]

medial geniculate nucleus Either of two nuclei—left and right—in the thalamus that receive input from the inferior colliculi and send output to the auditory cortex. See Figure 6.5. [6]

medial preoptic area (mPOA) A region of the anterior hypothalamus implicated in the control of many behaviors, including sexual behavior, gonadotropin secretion, and thermoregulation. [8]

median eminence A midline feature on the base of the brain that marks the point at which the pituitary stalk exits the hypothalamus to connect to the pituitary. The median eminence contains one end of the hypothalamic-pituitary portal system. See Figure 8.12. [8]

medulla The posterior part of the hindbrain, continuous with the spinal cord. See Figures 1.12, 1.15. [1]

MEG See *magnetoencephalography*. [1]

Meissner's corpuscle Also called *tactile corpuscle*. A skin receptor cell type that detects light touch, responding especially to changes in stimuli. See Figure 5.3. Compare *Merkel's disc*, *Pacinian corpuscle*, and *Ruffini corpuscle*. [5]

melanopsin A photopigment found in those retinal ganglion cells that project to the suprachiasmatic nucleus. See Figure 10.5. [10]

melatonin An amine hormone that is secreted by the pineal gland at night, thereby signaling day length to the brain. See Table 3.1. [ASF 8.1, 10]

memory 1. The ability to learn and neurally encode information, consolidate the information for longer-term storage, and retrieve or reactivate the consolidated information at a later time. 2. The specific information that is stored in the brain. [13]

memory trace Also called an *engram*. A persistent change in the brain that reflects the storage of memory. [13]

meninges The three protective membranes—dura mater, pia mater, and arachnoid—that surround the brain and spinal cord. See Figure 1.8. [1]

meningioma A noninvasive tumor of the meninges. [1]

meningitis An acute inflammation of the meninges, usually caused by a viral or bacterial infection. [1]

Merkel's disc A skin receptor cell type that detects light touch, responding especially to edges and isolated points on a surface. See Figure 5.3. Compare *Meissner's corpuscle, Pacinian corpuscle,* and *Ruffini corpuscle.* [5]

message See *messenger RNA.* [App]

messenger RNA (mRNA) Also called *transcript* or *message.* A strand of RNA that carries the code of a section of a DNA strand to the cytoplasm. [App]

meta-analysis A type of quantitative review of a field of research, in which the results of multiple previous studies are combined in order to identify overall patterns that are consistent across studies. [12]

metabolic tolerance The form of drug tolerance that arises when repeated exposure to the drug causes the metabolic machinery of the body to become more efficient at clearing the drug. Compare *functional tolerance.* [3]

metabolism The life-sustaining physiological processes wherein complex molecules are broken down into smaller molecules needed for cellular functions. [ASF 9.1]

metabotropic receptor A receptor protein that does not contain ion channels but may, when activated, use a second-messenger system to open nearby ion channels or to produce other cellular effects. See Figure 3.2. Compare *ionotropic receptor.* [3]

methylation A chemical modification of DNA that does not affect the nucleotide sequence of a gene but makes that gene less likely to be expressed. [4]

microbiome The collective term for a population of microorganisms that inhabit the body. [9]

microelectrode An especially small electrode used to record electrical potentials inside living cells. [2]

microglial cells Also called *microglia.* Extremely small motile glial cells that remove cellular debris from injured or dead cells. [1]

midbrain The middle division of the brain. See Figures 1.12, 4.1. Compare *forebrain* and *hindbrain.* [1, 4]

middle canal See *scala media.* See Figure 6.1. [6]

middle cerebral artery Either of two large arteries, arising from the carotid arteries, that provide blood to most of the forebrain. Compare *anterior cerebral artery* and *posterior cerebral artery.* [ASF 2.1]

middle ear The cavity between the tympanic membrane and the cochlea. See Figure 6.1. [6]

milk letdown reflex The reflexive release of milk by the mammary glands of a nursing female in response to stimuli associated with suckling. See Figure 8.9. [8]

millivolt (mV) A thousandth of a volt. [2]

mirror neuron A neuron that is active both when an individual makes a particular movement and when that individual sees another individual make the same movement. [5]

mitosis The process of division of somatic cells that involves duplication of DNA. [4]

monaural Pertaining to one ear. Compare *binaural.*

monoamine hormone See *amine hormone.* [8]

monoamine oxidase (MAO) An enzyme that breaks down monoamine neurotransmitters, thereby inactivating them. [3, ASF 4.1, 12]

monocular deprivation Depriving one eye of light. Compare *binocular deprivation.* [4, ASF 13.4]

monopolar neuron See *unipolar neuron.* [1]

morpheme The smallest grammatical unit of a language; a word or meaningful part of a word. [15]

morphine An opiate compound derived from the poppy flower. [3]

motion sickness The experience of nausea brought on by unnatural passive movement, as may occur in a car or boat. [6]

motivation The psychological process that induces or sustains a particular behavior. [9]

motoneuron See *motor neuron.* [1, 5]

motor nerve A nerve that transmits information from the central nervous system to the muscles and glands. Compare *sensory nerve.* [1]

motor neuron Also called *motoneuron.* A neuron that transmits neural messages to muscles (or glands). See Figure 5.20. Compare *interneuron* and *sensory neuron.* [1, 5]

motor plan Also called *motor program.* A plan for a series of muscular contractions, established in the nervous system prior to its execution. [5]

motor theory of language The theory that speech is perceived using the same left-hemisphere mechanisms that are used to produce the complex movements that go into speech. Compare *connectionist model of aphasia.* [15]

movement A single relocation of a body part, usually resulting from a brief muscle contraction. It is less complex than an act. [5]

mPOA See *medial preoptic area.* [8]

MRI See *magnetic resonance imaging.* [1]

mRNA See *messenger RNA.* [App]

müllerian duct A duct system in the embryo that will develop into female reproductive structures (oviducts, uterus, and upper vagina) in the absence of AMH. See Figure 8.23. Compare *wolffian duct.* [8]

müllerian regression hormone See *anti-müllerian hormone.* [8]

multiple sclerosis (MS) Literally "many scars." A disorder characterized by the widespread degeneration of myelin. [2, ASF 13.3]

multipolar neuron A neuron that has many dendrites and a single axon. See Figure 1.3. Compare *bipolar neuron* and *unipolar neuron.* [1]

multisensory See *polymodal.* [ASF 6.3]

muscle spindle A muscle receptor that lies parallel to a muscle and signals the central nervous system when the muscle is lengthened. See Figure 5.21. Compare *Golgi tendon organ.* [5]

muscular dystrophy A disease that leads to degeneration of and functional changes in muscles. [ASF 5.5]

musth An annual period of heightened aggressiveness and sexual activity in male elephants. [ASF 8.7]

mV See *millivolt.* [2]

myasthenia gravis A disorder characterized by a profound weakness of skeletal muscles. It is caused by a loss of acetylcholine receptors. [ASF 5.5]

myelin The fatty insulation around an axon, formed by glial cells. This myelin sheath boosts the speed at which action potentials are conducted. See Figures 1.5, 2.8. [1, 2]

myelination The process by which myelin sheaths develop around axons. See Figure 1.5. [ASF 13.3]

myopia Nearsightedness; the inability to focus the retinal image of objects that are far away. [7]

N

N1 effect See *auditory N1 effect.* [14]

naloxone A potent antagonist of opiates that is often administered to people who have taken drug overdoses. It blocks receptors for endogenous opioids. [5]

narcolepsy A disorder that involves frequent, intense episodes of sleep, which last from 5 to 30 minutes and can occur anytime during the usual waking hours. [10]

NE See *norepinephrine*. [3, 11]

negative feedback The process whereby a system monitors its own output and reduces its activity when a set point is reached. [8, 9]

negative symptom In psychiatry, an abnormality that reflects insufficient functioning. Examples include emotional and social withdrawal, and blunted affect. Compare *positive symptom*. [12]

neonatal Referring to newborns. [8]

nerve A collection of axons bundled together outside the central nervous system. See Figures 1.6, 1.7, 1.8. Compare *tract*. [1]

nerve cell See *neuron*. [Intro, 1]

nerve fiber See *axon*. [1]

neural chain A simple kind of neural circuit in which neurons are attached linearly, end-to-end. [ASF 3.2]

neural plasticity See *neuroplasticity*. [Intro, 1, 13]

neural tube An embryonic structure with subdivisions that correspond to the future forebrain, midbrain, and hindbrain. See Figure 4.1. [1, 4]

neuroeconomics The study of brain mechanisms at work during decision making. [Intro, 14]

neuroendocrine cell A neuron that releases hormones into local or general circulation. [8]

neurofibrillary tangle An abnormal whorl of neurofilaments within neurons that is seen in Alzheimer's disease. See Figure 4.17. [4]

neurogenesis The mitotic division of nonneuronal cells to produce neurons. See Figure 4.3. [4]

neuroleptic See *antipsychotic*. [12]

neuromuscular junction The region where the motor neuron terminal meets its target muscle fiber. It is the point where the nerve transmits its message to the muscle fiber. [5]

neuron Also called *nerve cell*. The basic unit of the nervous system, each composed of receptive extensions called *dendrites*, an integrating cell body, a conducting axon, and a transmitting axon terminal. See Figures 1.2, 1.3. [Intro, 1]

neuropathic pain Pain that persists long after the injury that started it has healed. [5]

neuropeptide See *peptide neurotransmitter*. [3]

neurophysiology The study of the life processes of neurons. [2]

neuroplasticity Also called neural plasticity. The ability of the nervous system to change in response to experience or the environment. [Intro, 1, 13]

neuroscience The scientific study of the nervous system. [Intro]

neurotransmitter receptor Also called simply *receptor*. A specialized protein that is embedded in the cell membrane, allowing it to selectively sense and react to molecules of a corresponding neurotransmitter or drug. [1, 2, 3]

neurotransmitter Also called *synaptic transmitter*, *chemical transmitter*, or simply *transmitter*. A signaling chemical, released by a presynaptic axon terminal, that diffuses across the synaptic cleft to alter the functioning of the postsynaptic neuron. It serves as the basis of communication between neurons. See Figure 2.12, Table 3.1. [1, 2, 3]

neurotrophic factor Also called simply *trophic factor*. A target-derived chemical that induces innervating neurons to survive. See Figure 4.6. [4]

nicotine A compound found in plants, including tobacco, that stimulates nicotinic acetylcholine receptors. [3]

night terror A sudden arousal from stage 3 sleep that is marked by intense fear and autonomic activation. Compare *nightmare*. [10]

nightmare A long, frightening dream that awakens the sleeper from REM sleep. Compare *night terror*. [10]

Nissl stain A tissue stain that fills all cell bodies because the dyes are attracted to RNA, which encircles the nucleus. [1]

NMDA receptor A glutamate receptor that also binds the glutamate agonist NMDA (N-methyl-d-aspartate) and that is both ligand-gated and voltage-sensitive. Compare *AMPA receptor*. [ASF 4.2, 13]

nociceptor A receptor that responds to stimuli that produce tissue damage or pose the threat of damage. [5]

node of Ranvier A gap between successive segments of the myelin sheath where the axon membrane is exposed. See Figures 1.5, 2.8. [1, 2]

nondeclarative memory Also called *procedural memory*. A memory that is shown by performance rather than by conscious recollection. See Figures 13.4, 13.13. Compare *declarative memory*. [13]

nonfluent aphasia Also called *Broca's aphasia*. A language impairment characterized by difficulty with speech production but not with language comprehension. It is related to damage in Broca's area. See Figure 15.10. Compare *fluent aphasia*. [15]

nonprimary motor cortex Frontal lobe regions adjacent to the primary motor cortex that contribute to motor control and modulate the activity of the primary motor cortex. See Figure 5.27. [5]

nonprimary sensory cortex Also called *secondary sensory cortex*. For a given sensory modality, the cortical regions receiving direct projections from primary sensory cortex for that modality. Compare *primary sensory cortex*. [5]

non-REM sleep Sleep, divided into stages 1–3, that is defined by the presence of distinctive EEG activity that differs from that seen in REM sleep. [10]

noradrenaline See *norepinephrine*. [3, 11]

noradrenergic Referring to cells using norepinephrine (noradrenaline) as a transmitter. [3]

norepinephrine (NE) Also called *noradrenaline*. A neurotransmitter active in both the brain and in the sympathetic nervous system. See Figure 3.4, Table 3.1. [3, 11]

Northern blot A method of detecting a particular RNA transcript in a tissue or organ by separating RNA from that source with gel electrophoresis, blotting the separated RNA molecules onto nitrocellulose, and then using a nucleotide probe to hybridize with, and highlight, the transcript of interest. Compare *Southern blot* and *Western blot*. [App]

NPY neuron A neuron in the hypothalamic appetite control system, that produces both neuropeptide Y and agouti-related peptide. Compare *POMC neuron*. [9]

NST See *nucleus of the solitary tract*. [9]

nucleotide A portion of a DNA or RNA molecule that is composed of a single base and the adjoining sugar-phosphate unit of the strand. [App]

nucleus (pl. nuclei) 1. A collection of neuronal cell bodies within the central nervous system (e.g., the caudate nucleus). [1] 2. See *cell nucleus*. [App]

nucleus accumbens A region of the forebrain that receives dopaminergic innervation from the ventral tegmental area, often associated with reward and pleasurable sensations. [3, 11]

nucleus of the solitary tract (NST) A complicated brainstem nucleus that receives visceral and taste information via several cranial nerves. See Figure 9.16. [9]

nutrients Chemicals required for the effective functioning, growth, and maintenance of the body. [9]

O

obsessive-compulsive disorder (OCD) An anxiety disorder in which the affected individual experiences recurrent unwanted thoughts and engages in repetitive behaviors without reason or the ability to stop. [12]

occipital cortex Also called *visual cortex*. The cortex of the occipital lobe of the brain, corresponding to the visual area of the cortex. See Figure 7.11. [7]

occipital lobe A large region of cortex that covers much of the posterior part of each cerebral hemisphere. See Figure 1.11. Compare *frontal lobe, parietal lobe,* and *temporal lobe*. [1]

OCD See *obsessive-compulsive disorder*. [12]

ocular dominance histogram A graph that portrays the strength of response of a brain neuron to stimuli presented to either the left eye or the right eye. [4, ASF 13.4]

odor The sensation of a smell. [6]

off-center bipolar cell A retinal bipolar cell that is inhibited by light in the center of its receptive field. See Figures 7.13, 7.14. Compare *on-center bipolar cell*. [7]

off-center ganglion cell A retinal ganglion cell that is activated when light is presented to the periphery, rather than the center, of the cell's receptive field. See Figures 7.13, 7.14. Compare *on-center ganglion cell*. [7]

off-center/on-surround Referring to a concentric receptive field in which stimulation of the center inhibits the cell of interest while stimulation of the surround excites it. See Figure 7.14. Compare *on-center/off-surround*. [7]

OHC See *outer hair cell*. [6]

olfaction The sensory system that detects smell; the act of smelling. [6]

olfactory bulb An anterior projection of the brain that terminates in the upper nasal passages and, through small openings in the skull, provides receptors for smell. See Figures 1.11, 1.15, 6.20. [1, 6]

olfactory epithelium A sheet of olfactory receptors and other cells that lines the dorsal portion of the nasal cavities and adjacent regions. See Figures 6.20, 6.21. [6]

oligodendrocyte A type of glial cell that ensheaths axons with myelin in the central nervous system. See Figure 1.5. Compare *Schwann cell*. [1]

on-center bipolar cell A retinal bipolar cell that is excited by light in the center of its receptive field. See Figures 7.13, 7.14. Compare *off-center bipolar cell*. [7]

on-center ganglion cell A retinal ganglion cell that is activated when light is presented to the center, rather than the periphery, of the cell's receptive field. See Figure 7.13. Compare *off-center ganglion cell*. [7]

on-center/off-surround Referring to a concentric receptive field in which stimulation of the center excites the cell of interest while stimulation of the surround inhibits it. See Figure 7.14. Compare *off-center/on-surround*. [7]

ontogeny The process by which individuals change over the course of their lifetimes. [Intro]

Onuf's nucleus The human homolog of the spinal nucleus of the bulbocavernosus (SNB) in rats. [8]

operant conditioning See *instrumental conditioning*. [13]

opioid peptide A type of endogenous peptide that mimics the effects of morphine in binding to opioid receptors and producing marked analgesia and reward. See Table 3.1. [3]

opioid receptor A receptor that responds to endogenous opioids and/or exogenous opiates. [3]

opium An extract of the opium poppy, *Papaver somniferum*. Drugs based on opium are potent painkillers. [3]

opponent-process hypothesis A hypothesis of color perception stating that different systems produce opposite responses to light of different wavelengths. [7]

optic ataxia Spatial disorientation in which the patient is unable to accurately reach for objects using visual guidance. [7]

optic chiasm The point at which parts of the two optic nerves cross the midline. See Figure 7.11. [7]

optic disc The region of the retina that is devoid of photoreceptors because ganglion cell axons and blood vessels exit the eyeball there. See Figure 7.7. [7]

optic nerve Cranial nerve II; the collection of ganglion cell axons that extends from the retina to the brain. See Figures 1.7, 7.11. [7]

optic radiation Axons from the lateral geniculate nucleus that terminate in the primary visual areas of the occipital cortex. See Figure 7.11. [7]

optic tract The axons of retinal ganglion cells after they have passed the optic chiasm. Most of these axons terminate in the lateral geniculate nucleus. See Figure 7.11. [7]

orexigenic neurons Neurons of the hypothalamic appetite system that promote feeding behavior. [9]

orexin Also called *hypocretin*. A neuropeptide produced in the hypothalamus that is involved in switching between sleep states, in narcolepsy, and in the control of appetite. [9, 10]

organ of Corti A structure in the inner ear that lies on the basilar membrane of the cochlea and contains the hair cells and terminations of the auditory nerve. See Figure 6.1. [6]

organizational effect A permanent alteration of the nervous system, and thus permanent change in behavior, resulting from the action of a steroid hormone on an animal early in its development. Compare *activational effect*. [8]

orgasm The climax of sexual behavior, marked by extremely pleasurable sensations. [8]

osmosensory neuron A specialized neuron that monitors the concentration of the extracellular fluid by measuring the movement of water into and out of the intracellular compartment. See Figures 9.6, 9.9. [9]

osmosis The passive movement of a solvent, usually water, through a semipermeable membrane until a uniform concentration of solute (often salt) is achieved on both sides of the membrane. See Figure 9.5. Compare *diffusion*. [9]

osmotic pressure The tendency of a solvent to move across a membrane in order to equalize the concentration of solute on both sides of the membrane. [9]

osmotic thirst A desire to ingest fluids that is stimulated by high concentration of solute (like salt) in the extracellular compartment. Compare *hypovolemic thirst*. [9]

ossicles Three small bones (incus, malleus, and stapes) that transmit vibration across the middle ear, from the tympanic membrane to the oval window. See Figure 6.1. [6]

otolith A small crystal on the in the gelatinous membrane overlying the hair cells of the saccule and utricle of the vestibular system.

outer hair cell (OHC) One of the two types of auditory receptor cells in the cochlea. Compared with inner hair cells, OHCs are positioned farther from the central axis of the coiled cochlea. See Figure 6.1. [6]

output zone The part of a neuron at which the cell sends information to another cell. This zone usually corresponds to the axon terminals. See Figures 1.1, 1.3. Compare *conduction zone, input zone,* and *integration zone*. [1]

oval window The location on the cochlea at which vibrations are transmitted from the ossicles to the interior of the cochlea. See Figure 6.1. [6]

ovaries The female gonads, which produce eggs (ova) for reproduction. See Figure 8.1. Compare *testes*. [8]

overt attention Attention in which the focus coincides with sensory orientation (e.g., you're attending to the same thing you're looking at). Compare *covert attention*. [14]

ovulation The production and release of an egg (ovum). [8]

ovulatory cycle The periodic occurrence of ovulation in females. See Figure 8.17. [8]

ovum (pl. ova) An egg, the female gamete. Compare *sperm*. [8]

oxytocin A peptide hormone, released from the posterior pituitary, that triggers milk letdown in the nursing female and is also associated with a variety of complex behaviors. See Figures 8.8, 8.9. [8]

P

P1 effect See *visual P1 effect*. [14]

P3 effect Also called *auditory P300*. A positive deflection of the event-related potential, occurring about 300 milliseconds after stimulus presentation, that is associated with higher-order auditory stimulus processing and late attentional selection. [14]

Pacinian corpuscle Also called *lamellated corpuscle*. A skin receptor cell type that detects vibration and pressure. See Figures 5.3, 5.4. Compare *Meissner's corpuscle*, *Merkel's disc*, and *Ruffini corpuscle*. [5]

pain The discomfort normally associated with tissue damage. [5]

pair-bond A durable and exclusive relationship between two individuals. [8]

papilla (pl. papillae) A small bump that projects from the surface of the tongue. Papillae contain most of the taste receptor cells. See Figures 6.15, 6.16. [6]

parabiotic Referring to a surgical preparation that joins two animals to share a single blood supply. [8]

paradoxical sleep See *rapid-eye-movement (REM) sleep*. [10]

paraphasia A symptom of aphasia that is distinguished by the substitution of a word by a sound, an incorrect word, an unintended word, or a neologism (a meaningless word). [15]

parasympathetic nervous system The part of the autonomic nervous system that generally prepares the body to relax and recuperate. See Figure 1.9. Compare *sympathetic nervous system*. [1, 11]

paraventricular nucleus (PVN) A nucleus of the hypothalamus involved in the release of peptide hormones and in the control of feeding and other behaviors. [9]

paresis Muscular weakness, often the result of damage to motor cortex. Compare *plegia*. [5]

parietal lobe The large region of cortex lying between the frontal and occipital lobes in each cerebral hemisphere. See Figure 1.11. Compare also *temporal lobe*. [1]

Parkinson's disease A degenerative neurological disorder, characterized by tremors at rest, muscular rigidity, and reduction in voluntary movement, caused by loss of the dopaminergic neurons of the substantia nigra. Compare *Huntington's disease*. [5]

partial agonist A drug that, when bound to a receptor, has only moderate effect, compared to other agonist ligands. The term *partial antagonist* is equivalent. [3]

Patient H.M. The late Henry Molaison, a man who was unable to encode new declarative memories because of surgical removal of medial temporal lobe structures. See Figure 13.1. [13]

Patient K.C. The late Kent Cochrane, who sustained damage to the cortex that rendered him unable to form and retrieve episodic memories. [13]

Patient N.A. A still-living man who is unable to encode new declarative memories, because of damage to the dorsomedial thalamus and the mammillary bodies. [13]

Pavlovian conditioning See *classical conditioning*. [13]

PCP See *phencyclidine*. [12]

PCR See polymerase chain reaction. [App]

penis The male phallus. Compare *clitoris*. [8]

peptide A short string of amino acids. Longer strings of amino acids are called *proteins*. [App]

peptide hormone Also called *protein hormone*. A hormone that consists of a string of amino acids. Compare *amine hormone*. [8]

peptide neurotransmitter Also called *neuropeptide*. A neurotransmitter consisting of a short chain of amino acids. See Table 3.1. Compare *amine neurotransmitter, amino acid neurotransmitter,* and *gas neurotransmitter*. [3]

perceptual load The immediate processing demands presented by a stimulus. [14]

periaqueductal gray A midbrain region involved in pain perception. [1, 3, 8]

period The interval of time between two similar points of successive cycles, such as sunset to sunset. [10]

peripheral nervous system The portion of the nervous system that includes all the nerves and neurons outside the brain and spinal cord. See Figures 1.6, 1.12. Compare *central nervous system*. [1]

peripheral spatial cuing A technique for testing reflexive attention in which a visual stimulus is preceded by a simple task-irrelevant sensory stimulus either in the location where the stimulus will appear or in an incorrect location. Compare *symbolic cuing*. [14]

perseverate Continue any activity beyond a reasonable degree. [ASF 13.4, 14]

PET See *positron emission tomography*. [1]

phagocyte An immune system cell that engulfs invading molecules or microbes. [ASF 11.4]

phallus The clitoris or penis. [8]

pharmacokinetics Collective name for all the factors that affect the movement of a drug into, through, and out of the body. [3]

phase shift A shift in the activity of a biological rhythm, typically provided by a synchronizing environmental stimulus, such as light. [10]

phasic receptor A receptor in which the frequency of action potentials drops rapidly as stimulation is maintained. Compare *tonic receptor*. [5]

phencyclidine (PCP) Also called *angel dust*. An anesthetic agent that is also a psychedelic drug. PCP makes many people feel dissociated from themselves and their environment. [12]

phenotype The sum of an individual's physical characteristics at one particular time. Compare *genotype*. [4]

phenylketonuria An inherited disorder in which the absence of an enzyme leads to a toxic buildup of phenylalanine metabolites, causing intellectual disability. [4]

pheromone A chemical signal that is released outside the body of an animal and affects other members of the same species. See Figure 8.3. Compare *allomone*. [6, 8]

phoneme A sound that is produced for language. [15]

photopic system A system in the retina that operates at high levels of light, shows sensitivity to color, and involves the cones. See Table 7.1. Compare *scotopic system*. [7]

photoreceptor adaptation The tendency of rods and cones to adjust their light sensitivity to match current levels of illumination. [7]

photoreceptor A neural cell in the retina that responds to light. [7]

phrenology The belief that bumps on the skull reflect enlargements of brain regions responsible for certain behavioral faculties. See Figure Intro.4. [Intro]

physiological psychology See *behavioral neuroscience*. [Intro]

pia mater The innermost of the three meninges that surround the brain and spinal cord. See Figure 1.8. Compare *dura mater* and *arachnoid*. [1]

pineal gland A secretory gland in the brain midline that is the main source of melatonin. See Figure 8.1. [ASF 8.1]

pinna (pl. pinnae) The external part of the ear. [6]

pituitary gland A small, complex endocrine gland located in a socket at the base of the skull. See Figures 1.15, 8.8, 8.12. [8]

pituitary stalk Also called *infundibulum*. A thin piece of tissue that connects the pituitary gland to the hypothalamus. [8]

place cell A neuron in the hippocampus that selectively fires when the animal is in a particular location. [13]

place coding theory Theory that the pitch of a sound is determined by the location of activated hair cells along the length of the basilar membrane. Compare *temporal coding theory*. [6]

placebo effect Relief of a symptom, such as pain, that results following a treatment that is known to be ineffective or inert. [5]

planum temporale An auditory region of superior temporal cortex. See Figure 15.3. [15]

plegia Paralysis; the loss of the ability to move. Compare *paresis*. [5]

poliovirus A virus that destroys motor neurons of the spinal cord and brainstem, causing permanent paralysis. [ASF 5.5]

polygraph Popularly but inaccurately referred to as a *lie detector*. A device that measures several bodily responses, such as heart rate and blood pressure. [11]

polymerase chain reaction (PCR) Also called *gene amplification*. A method for reproducing a particular RNA or DNA sequence manyfold, allowing amplification for sequencing or manipulating the sequence. [App]

polymodal Also called *multisensory*. Involving several sensory modalities. [ASF 6.3]

polymodal neuron A neuron upon which information from more than one sensory system converges. [5]

POMC neuron A neuron, involved in the hypothalamic appetite control system, that produces both pro-opiomelanocortin and cocaine- and amphetamine-regulated transcript. Compare *NPY neuron*. [9]

pons The portion of the brainstem that connects the midbrain to the medulla. See Figures 1.12, 1.15. [1]

positive symptom In psychiatry, an abnormal behavioral state. Examples include hallucinations, delusions, and excited motor behavior. Compare *negative symptom*. [12]

positron emission tomography (PET) A brain-imaging technology that tracks the metabolism of injected radioactive substances in the brain, in order to map brain activity. See Figure 1.20. Compare *functional MRI*. [1]

postcentral gyrus The strip of parietal cortex, just posterior to (behind) the central sulcus, that receives somatosensory information from the entire body. See Figure 1.11. Compare *precentral gyrus*. [1]

postcopulatory behavior The final stage in mating behavior. Species-specific postcopulatory behaviors include rolling (in the cat) and grooming (in the rat). [8]

posterior Also called *caudal*. In anatomy, toward the tail end of an organism. Compare *anterior*. [1]

posterior cerebral artery Either of two large arteries, arising from the basilar artery, that provide blood to posterior aspects of the cerebral hemispheres, cerebellum, and brainstem. Compare *anterior cerebral artery* and *middle cerebral artery*. [ASF 2.1]

posterior pituitary The rear division of the pituitary gland. See Figures 8.1, 8.8. Compare *anterior pituitary*. [8]

postpartum depression A bout of depression that afflicts a woman either immediately before or after giving birth. [12]

postsynaptic Referring to the region of a synapse that receives and responds to neurotransmitter. See Figure 1.4. Compare *presynaptic*. [1, 2, 3]

postsynaptic membrane The specialized membrane on the surface of a neuron that receives information by responding to neurotransmitter from a presynaptic neuron. See Figure 1.4. Compare *presynaptic membrane*. [1]

postsynaptic potential A local potential that is initiated by stimulation at a synapse, can vary in amplitude, and spreads passively across the cell membrane, decreasing in strength with time and distance. Compare *all-or-none property*. [2]

post-traumatic stress disorder (PTSD) A disorder in which memories of an unpleasant episode repeatedly plague the person. See Box 13.1. [12, 13]

potassium ion (K⁺) A potassium atom that carries a positive charge. [2]

pragmatics In linguistics, the context in which a speech sound is uttered. [15]

precentral gyrus The strip of frontal cortex, just in front of the central sulcus, that is crucial for motor control. See Figure 1.11. Compare *postcentral gyrus*. [1, 5]

prefrontal cortex The most anterior region of the frontal lobe. [14]

premotor cortex A region of nonprimary motor cortex just anterior to the primary motor cortex. See Figure 5.27. [5]

presenilin An enzyme that cleaves amyloid precursor protein, forming beta-amyloid, implicated in Alzheimer's disease. See also *beta-secretase*. [ASF 13.5]

presynaptic Referring to the "transmitting" side of a synapse. See Figure 1.4. Compare *postsynaptic*. [1, 2, 3]

presynaptic membrane The specialized membrane on the axon terminal of a neuron that transmits information by releasing neurotransmitter. See Figure 1.4. [1]

primary auditory cortex Also called *A1*. The cortical region, located on the superior surface of the temporal lobe, that processes complex sounds transmitted from lower auditory pathways. [6]

primary motor cortex (M1) The apparent executive region for the initiation of movement. It is primarily the precentral gyrus. Compare *nonprimary motor cortex*. [5]

primary sensory cortex For a given sensory modality, the region of cortex that receives most of the information about that modality via the thalamus (or, in the case of olfaction, directly from the secondary sensory neurons). See Figure 5.7. Compare *nonprimary sensory cortex*. [5]

primary somatosensory cortex Also called *somatosensory 1* or *S1*. Primarily the postcentral gyrus of the parietal lobe, where sensory inputs from the body surface are mapped. See Figure 5.7. [5]

primary visual cortex (V1) Also called *striate cortex* or *area 17*. The region of the occipital cortex where most visual information first arrives. See Figures 7.11, 7.12, 7.20. [7]

priming Also called *repetition priming*. The phenomenon by which exposure to a stimulus facilitates subsequent responses to the same or a similar stimulus. [13]

probe In molecular biology, a manufactured sequence of DNA that is made to include a label (a colorful or radioactive molecule) that lets us track its location. [App]

procedural memory See *nondeclarative memory*. [13]

proceptive Referring to a state in which a female advertises her readiness to mate through species-typical behaviors. [8]

progesterone The primary type of progestin secreted by the ovary. See Figure 8.13. [8]

progestin Any of a major class of steroid hormones that are produced by the ovary, including progesterone. See Figure 8.13. [8]

prolactin A protein hormone, produced by the anterior pituitary, that promotes mammary development for lactation in female mammals. [ASF 8.4]

proprioception Body sense; information about the position and movement of the body. [5]

prosody The perception of emotional tone-of-voice aspects of language. [15]

prosopagnosia Also called *face blindness*. A condition characterized by the inability to recognize faces. [15]

protein hormone See *peptide hormone*. [8]

protein A long string of amino acids. Proteins are the basic building material of organisms. Compare *peptide*. [App]

proximal In anatomy, near the trunk or center of an organism. Compare *distal*. [1]

psychoneuroimmunology The study of the immune system and its interaction with the nervous system and behavior. [11]

psychopath An individual who routinely engages in deception, violence, or other antisocial behavior and who has little capacity for empathy or remorse. [11]

psychosomatic medicine A field of study that emphasizes the role of psychological factors in disease. [11]

psychosurgery Any type of neurosurgery where the aim is to relieve the symptoms of severe psychiatric disorders.

psychotomimetic A drug that induces a state resembling schizophrenia. [12]

PTSD See *post-traumatic stress disorder*. [12, 13]

pulvinar In humans, the posterior portion of the thalamus. It is heavily involved in visual processing and direction of attention. [14]

pupil The opening, formed by the iris, that allows light to enter the eye. See Figures 7.1, 7.6. [7]

Purkinje cell A type of large neuron in the cerebellar cortex.

pyramidal cell A type of large neuron that has a roughly pyramid-shaped cell body and is found in the cerebral cortex. See Figure 1.13. [1]

pyramidal system Also called *corticospinal system*. The motor system that includes neurons within the cerebral cortex and their axons, which form the pyramidal tract. See Figure 5.24. Compare *extrapyramidal system*. [5]

PYY$_{3-36}$ A peptide gut hormone believed to act on the hypothalamic appetite system to suppress appetite. Compare *ghrelin*. [9]

Q

quale (pl. qualia) A purely subjective experience of perception. [14]

R

range fractionation The means by which sensory systems cover a wide range of intensity values, as each sensory receptor cell specializes in just one part of the overall range of intensities. [7]

raphe nuclei A string of nuclei in the midline of the midbrain and brainstem that contain most of the serotonergic neurons of the brain. [3]

rapid-eye-movement (REM) sleep Also called *paradoxical sleep*. A stage of sleep characterized by small-amplitude, fast EEG waves, no postural tension, and rapid eye movements. *REM* rhymes with "gem." See Figure 10.11. Compare *stage 3 sleep*. [10]

RBD See *REM behavior disorder*. [10]

reaction time The delay between the presentation of a stimulus and a participant's response to that stimulus, measured in milliseconds. [14]

receptive field The stimulus region and features that affect the activity of a cell in a sensory system. See Figures 5.5, 7.14, 7.17. [5, 7]

receptor See *neurotransmitter receptor*. [1, 2, 3]

receptor cell A specialized cell that responds to a particular energy or substance in the internal or external environment and converts this energy into a change in the electrical potential across its membrane. [5]

receptor potential Also called *generator potential*. A local change in the resting potential of a receptor cell in response to stimuli, which may initiate an action potential. [5]

receptor subtype Any type of receptor having functional characteristics that distinguish it from other types of receptors for the same neurotransmitter. For example, there are at least 15 different subtypes of serotonin receptors. [3]

reconsolidation The return of a memory trace to stable long-term storage after it has been temporarily made changeable during the process of recall. [13]

recovery of function The recovery of behavioral capacity following brain damage from stroke or injury. [15]

reductionism The scientific strategy of breaking a system down into increasingly smaller parts in order to understand it. [1]

reflex A simple, highly stereotyped, and unlearned response to a particular stimulus (e.g., an eye blink in response to a puff of air). See Figures 2.15, 5.23. [5]

reflexive attention Also called *exogenous attention*. The involuntary reorienting of attention toward a specific stimulus source, cued by an unexpected object or event. Compare *voluntary attention*. [14]

refraction The bending of light rays by a change in the density of a medium, such as the cornea and the lens of the eyes. [7]

refractory Temporarily unresponsive or inactivated. [2]

refractory phase 1. A period during and after an action potential in which the responsiveness of the axonal membrane is reduced. A brief period of complete insensitivity to stimuli (absolute refractory phase) is followed by a longer period of reduced sensitivity (relative refractory phase) during which only strong stimulation produces an action potential. 2. A period following copulation during which an individual does not recommence copulation. See Figure 8.22. [8]

relative refractory phase A period of reduced sensitivity during which only strong stimulation produces an action potential. Compare *absolute refractory phase*. [2]

releasing hormone Any of a class of hormones, produced in the hypothalamus, that traverse the hypothalamic-pituitary portal system to control the pituitary's release of tropic hormones. See Figure 8.12. [8]

REM behavior disorder (RBD) A sleep disorder in which a person physically acts out a dream. [10]

REM sleep See *rapid-eye-movement (REM) sleep*. [10]

repetition priming See *priming*. [13]

repetitive transcranial magnetic stimulation (rTMS) A noninvasive treatment in which repeated pulses of focused magnetic energy are used to stimulate the cortex through the scalp. [12]

resting potential The difference in electrical potential across the membrane of a neuron at rest. See Figures 2.1, 2.5. [2]

reticular formation Also called *reticular activating system*. An extensive region of the brainstem, extending from the medulla through the thalamus, that is involved in sleep and arousal. See Figure 10.20. [1, 10]

retina The receptive surface inside the eye that contains photoreceptors and other neurons. See Figures 7.1, 7.3. [7]

retinohypothalamic pathway The route by which specialized retinal ganglion cells send their axons to the suprachiasmatic nuclei. [10]

retrieval The third process of the memory system, in which a stored memory is used by an organism. See Figure 13.14. Compare *encoding* and *consolidation*. [13]

retrograde amnesia Difficulty in retrieving memories formed before the onset of amnesia. Compare *anterograde amnesia*. [13]

retrograde transmitter A neurotransmitter that is released by the postsynaptic neuron, diffuses back across the synapse, and alters the functioning of the presynaptic neuron. [3, 13]

reuptake The reabsorption of molecules of neurotransmitter by the neurons that released them, thereby ending the signaling activity of the transmitter molecules. [2, 3]

rhodopsin The photopigment in rods that responds to light. [7]

ribonucleic acid (RNA) A nucleic acid that implements information found in DNA. Compare *deoxyribonucleic acid*. [App]

ribosome An organelle in the cell body where genetic information is translated to produce proteins. See Appendix Figure A.2. [App]

RNA See *ribonucleic acid*. [App]

rod A photoreceptor cell in the retina that is most active at low levels of light. See Figure 7.3. Compare *cone*. [7]

rostral See *anterior*. [1]

Ruffini corpuscle A skin receptor cell type that detects stretching of the skin. See Figure 5.3. Compare *Meissner's corpuscle*, *Merkel's disc*, and *Pacinian corpuscle*. [5]

S

S1 See *primary somatosensory cortex*. [5]

sacral Referring to the five spinal segments in the lower part of the lower back. See Figures 1.8, 1.9. Compare *cervical*, *thoracic*, *lumbar*, and *coccygeal*. [1]

SAD See *seasonal affective disorder*. [ASF 12.3]

sagittal plane The plane that divides the body or brain into right and left portions. Compare *coronal plane* and *horizontal plane*. [1]

saltatory conduction The form of conduction that is characteristic of myelinated axons, in which the action potential jumps from one node of Ranvier to the next. [2]

saturation One of three basic dimensions of light perception, varying from rich to pale. Compare *brightness* and *hue*. [7]

SC See *standard condition*. [13]

scala media Also called *middle canal*. The central of the three spiraling canals inside the cochlea, situated between the vestibular canal and the tympanic canal. See Figure 6.1. [6]

scala tympani Also called *tympanic canal*. One of three principal canals running along the length of the cochlea. See Figure 6.1. Compare *scala media* and *scala vestibuli*. [6]

scala vestibuli Also called *vestibular canal*. One of three principal canals running along the length of the cochlea. See Figure 6.1. Compare *scala media* and *scala tympani*. [6]

schizophrenia A severe psychopathological disorder characterized by negative symptoms such as emotional withdrawal and flat affect, by positive symptoms such as hallucinations and delusions, and by cognitive symptoms such as poor attention span. [12]

Schwann cell A type of glial cell that forms myelin in the peripheral nervous system. Compare *oligodendrocyte*. [1]

SCN See *suprachiasmatic nucleus*. [10]

scotoma A region of blindness within the visual fields, caused by injury to the visual pathway or brain. [7]

scotopic system A system in the retina that operates at low levels of light and involves the rods. See Table 7.1. Compare *photopic system*. [7]

SDN-POA See *sexually dimorphic nucleus of the preoptic area*. [8]

seasonal affective disorder (SAD) A form of depression associated with the short days of winter. [ASF 12.3]

second messenger A slow-acting substance in a target cell that amplifies the effects of synaptic or hormonal activity and regulates activity within the target cell. [8]

secondary sensory cortex See *nonprimary sensory cortex*. [5]

second-generation antipsychotic Also called *atypical antipsychotic* and *atypical neuroleptic*. An antipsychotic drug that has primary actions other than or in addition to the dopamine D2 receptor antagonism that characterizes the first-generation antipsychotics. [3, 12]

seizure A wave of abnormally synchronous electrical activity in the brain. See Figure 2.17. [2]

selective attention See *attention*. [14]

selective permeability The property of a membrane that allows some substances to pass through, but not others. [2]

selective serotonin reuptake inhibitor (SSRI) A drug, used to treat depression and anxiety, that blocks the reuptake of transmitter at serotonergic synapses. [3, 12]

semantic memory Generalized declarative memory, such as knowing the meaning of a word. Compare *episodic memory*. [13]

semantics The meanings or interpretation of words and sentences in a language.

semen A mixture of fluid and sperm that is released during ejaculation. [8]

semicircular canal Any one of the three fluid-filled tubes in the inner ear that are part of the vestibular system. Each of the tubes, which are at right angles to each other, detects angular acceleration in a particular direction. See Figure 6.14. [6]

senile dementia A neurological disorder of the aged that is characterized by progressive psychological deterioration, including personality change and profound intellectual decline. It includes, but is not limited to, Alzheimer's disease.

senile plaque See *amyloid plaque*. [4]

sensitive period Also called *critical period*. The period during development in which an organism can be permanently altered by a particular experience or treatment. [4, 8, ASF 13.4, 15]

sensorineural deafness A hearing impairment most often caused by the permanent damage or destruction of hair cells or by interruption of the vestibulocochlear nerve that carries auditory information to the brain. See Figure 6.10. Compare *central deafness* and *conduction deafness*. [6]

sensory adaptation The progressive loss of receptor response as stimulation is maintained. See Figure 5.6. [5]

sensory buffer A very brief type of memory that stores the sensory impression of a scene. In vision, it is sometimes called *iconic memory*. See Figure 13.14. [13]

sensory nerve A nerve that conveys information from the body to the central nervous system. Compare *motor nerve*. [1]

sensory neuron A neuron that is directly affected by changes in the environment, such as light, odor, or touch. Compare *interneuron* and *motor neuron*. [1]

sensory transduction The process in which a receptor cell converts the energy in a stimulus into a change in the electrical potential across its membrane. [5]

serotonergic Referring to cells that use serotonin as their synaptic transmitter. [3]

serotonin (5-HT) A synaptic transmitter that is produced in the raphe nuclei and is active in structures throughout the cerebral hemispheres. See Figure 3.4, Table 3.1. [3]

serotonin-norepinephrine reuptake inhibitor (SNRI) Any of a class of drugs that promote the synaptic accumulation of serotonin and norepinephrine by blocking transmitter reuptake. [3]

set point The point of reference in a feedback system. An example is the temperature at which a thermostat is set. Compare *set zone*. [9]

set zone The optimal range of a variable that a negative feedback system tries to maintain. Compare *set point*. [9]

sexual attraction The first step in the mating behavior of many animals, in which animals emit stimuli that attract members of the opposite sex. [8]

sexual differentiation The process by which individuals develop either male-like or female-like bodies and behavior. See Figure 8.23. [8]

sexual dimorphism The condition in which males and females of the same species show pronounced sex differences in appearance. [8]

sexually dimorphic nucleus of the preoptic area (SDN-POA) A region of the preoptic area that is 5 to 6 times larger in volume in male than in female rats. See Figure 8.29. [8]

sexually receptive Referring to the state in which an individual (in mammals, typically the female) is willing to copulate. [8]

shadowing A task in which the participant is asked to focus attention on one ear or the other while different stimuli are being presented to the two ears, and to repeat aloud the material presented to the attended ear. [14]

sham rage See *decorticate rage*. [11]

shivering Rapid involuntary muscle contractions that generate heat in hypothermic animals. [ASF 9.1]

short-term memory (STM) A form of memory that usually lasts only seconds, or as long as rehearsal continues. Working memory can be considered a portion of STM where information can be manipulated. See Figure 13.14. Compare *sensory buffer* and *long-term memory*. [13]

SIDS See *sudden infant death syndrome*. [10]

simple cortical cell Also called *bar detector* or *edge detector*. A cell in the visual cortex that responds best to an edge or a bar that has a particular width, as well as a particular orientation and location in the visual field. Compare *complex cortical cell*. [7]

simple partial seizure Also called *petit mal seizure* or *absence attack*. A seizure that is characterized by a spike-and-wave EEG and often involves a loss of awareness and inability to recall events surrounding the seizure. [2]

simultagnosia A profound restriction of attention, often limited to a single item or feature. Simultagnosia is one of the three primary symptoms of Balint's syndrome. [14]

skill learning The process of learning to perform a challenging task simply by repeating it over and over. [13]

sleep apnea A sleep disorder in which respiration slows or stops periodically, waking the sleeper. Excessive daytime sleepiness results from the frequent nocturnal awakening. [10]

sleep cycle A period of slow-wave sleep followed by a period of REM sleep. In humans, a sleep cycle lasts 90–110 minutes.

sleep deprivation The partial or total prevention of sleep. [10]

sleep enuresis Bed-wetting. [10]

sleep paralysis A state, during the transition to or from sleep, in which the ability to move or talk is temporarily lost. [10]

sleep recovery The process of sleeping more than normally after a period of sleep deprivation, as though in compensation. [10]

sleep spindle A characteristic 12–14 Hz wave in the EEG of a person said to be in stage 2 sleep. See Figure 10.11. [10]

sleep state misperception Commonly, the perception of not having been asleep when in fact the person has been. It typically occurs at the start of a sleep episode. [10]

sleep-maintenance insomnia Difficulty in staying asleep. Compare *sleep-onset insomnia*. [10]

sleep-onset insomnia Difficulty in falling asleep. Compare *sleep-maintenance insomnia*. [10]

SMA See *supplementary motor area*. [5]

SNB See *spinal nucleus of the bulbocavernosus*. [8]

SNRI See *serotonin-norepinephrine reuptake inhibitor*. [3]

social neuroscience A field of study that uses the tools of neuroscience to discover both the biological bases of social behavior and the effects of social circumstances on brain activity. [Intro]

sodium ion (Na⁺) A sodium atom that carries a positive charge. [2]

sodium-potassium pump The energetically expensive mechanism that pushes sodium ions out of a cell, and potassium ions in. [2]

solute A solid compound that is dissolved in a liquid. Compare *solvent*. [2]

solvent The liquid (often water) in which a compound is dissolved. Compare *solute*. [2]

soma (pl. somata) See *cell body*. [1]

somatic intervention An approach to finding relations between body variables and behavioral variables that involves manipulating body structure or function and looking for resultant changes in behavior. See Figure 1.24. Compare *behavioral intervention*. [1]

somatic nerve See *spinal nerve*. [1]

somatic nervous system A part of the peripheral nervous system that supplies neural connections mostly to the skeletal muscles and sensory systems of the body. It consists of cranial nerves and spinal nerves. [1]

somatosensory 1 (S1) See *primary somatosensory cortex*. [5]

somatosensory system A set of specialized receptors and neural mechanisms responsible for body sensations such as touch and pain. [5]

somatotropic hormone Also called *somatotropin*. See *growth hormone*. [8]

somnambulism Sleepwalking. [10]

Southern blot A method of detecting a particular DNA sequence in the genome of an organism by separating DNA with gel electrophoresis, blotting the separated DNA molecules onto nitrocellulose, and then using a nucleotide probe to hybridize with, and highlight, the gene of interest. See Appendix Figure A.3. Compare *Northern blot* and *Western blot*. [App]

spasticity Markedly increased rigidity in response to forced movement of the limbs.

spatial resolution The ability to observe the detailed structure of the brain. Compare *temporal resolution*. [14]

spatial summation The summation of postsynaptic potentials that reach the axon hillock from different locations across the cell body. If this summation reaches threshold, an action potential is triggered. See Figure 2.11. Compare *temporal summation*. [2]

spatial-frequency model A model of visual perception that emphasizes the analysis of the different spatial frequencies present in various orientations and in various parts of a visual scene. [7, ASF 7.2]

spectral filtering The process by which the hills and valleys of the external ear alter the amplitude of some, but not all, frequencies in a sound. [6]

spectrally opponent cell Also called *color-opponent cell*. A visual system neuron that has opposite firing responses to different regions of the spectrum. See Figures 7.26, 7.27. [7]

sperm The gamete produced by males for the fertilization of eggs (ova). [8]

spike See *action potential*. [2]

spinal nerve Also called *somatic nerve*. A nerve that emerges from the spinal cord. There are 31 pairs of spinal nerves. See Figure 1.8. Compare *cranial nerve*. [1]

spinal nucleus of the bulbocavernosus (SNB) A group of motor neurons in the spinal cord of rats that innervate muscles controlling the penis. See Figure 8.31. Compare *Onuf's nucleus*. [8]

spinocerebellum The uppermost part of the cerebellum, consisting mostly of the vermis and the anterior lobe. It receives sensory information about the current spatial location of the parts of the body and anticipates subsequent movement. Compare *cerebrocerebellum* and *vestibulocerebellum*. [ASF 5.4]

spinothalamic system See *anterolateral system*. [5]

split-brain individual An individual whose corpus callosum has been severed, halting communication between the right and left hemispheres. [15]

SRY **gene** A gene on the Y chromosome that directs the developing gonads to become testes. The name *SRY* stands for sex-determining region on the Y chromosome. [8]

SSRI See *selective serotonin reuptake inhibitor*. [3, 12]

stage 1 sleep The initial stage of non-REM sleep, which is characterized by small-amplitude EEG waves of irregular frequency, slow heart rate, and reduced muscle tension. See Figure 10.11. [10]

stage 2 sleep A stage of sleep that is defined by bursts of EEG waves called *sleep spindles*. See Figure 10.11. [10]

stage 3 sleep Also called *slow wave sleep* (*SWS*). A stage of non-REM sleep that is defined by the presence of large-amplitude, slow delta waves. See Figure 10.11. [10]

standard condition (SC) The usual environment for laboratory rodents, with a few animals in a cage and adequate food and water, but no complex stimulation. See Figure 13.16. Compare *enriched condition* and *impoverished condition*. [13]

stem cell A cell that is undifferentiated and therefore can take on the fate of any cell that a donor organism can produce. [4]

stereocilium (pl. stereocilia) A tiny bristle that protrudes from a hair cell in the auditory or vestibular system. See Figure 6.1. [6]

steroid hormone Any of a class of hormones, each of which is composed of four interconnected rings of carbon atoms. Compare *amine hormone* and *peptide hormone*. [8]

stimulant A drug that enhances the excitability of neurons. Compare *depressant*. [3]

stimulus (pl. stimuli) A physical event that triggers a sensory response. [5]

stimulus cuing A technique for testing reaction time to sensory stimuli, in which a cue to where the stimulus will be presented is provided before the stimulus itself.

STM See *short-term memory*. [13]

stress Any circumstance that upsets homeostatic balance. [11]

stretch reflex The contraction of a muscle in response to stretch of that muscle. See Figure 5.23. [5]

striate cortex See *primary visual cortex*. [7]

striatum The caudate nucleus and putamen together.

stroke Damage to a region of brain tissue that results from the blockage or rupture of vessels that supply blood to that region. [1]

stuttering The tendency of otherwise healthy people to produce speech sounds only haltingly, tripping over certain syllables or being unable to start vocalizing certain words. [15]

substance P A peptide transmitter that is involved in pain transmission. [5]

substantia nigra A brainstem structure that innervates the basal ganglia and is a major source of dopaminergic projections. Compare *locus coeruleus*. [1, 3, 5]

sudden infant death syndrome (SIDS) Also called *crib death*. The sudden, unexpected death of an apparently healthy human infant who simply stops breathing, usually during sleep. [10]

sulcus (pl. sulci) A crevice or valley of a convoluted brain surface. Compare *gyrus*. [1]

superior In anatomy, above. Compare *inferior*. [1]

superior colliculus (pl. colliculi) A gray matter structure of the dorsal midbrain that processes visual information and is involved in direction of visual gaze and visual attention to intended stimuli. See Figures 1.15, 14.9. Compare *inferior colliculi*. [1, 14]

superior olivary nuclei Brainstem nuclei that receive input from both right and left cochlear nuclei and provide the first binaural analysis of auditory information. See Figure 6.5. [6]

supersensitivity psychosis An exaggerated "rebound" psychosis that may emerge when doses of antipsychotic medication are reduced, probably as a consequence of the up-regulation of receptors that occurred during drug treatment. [12]

supplementary motor area (SMA) A region of nonprimary motor cortex that receives input from the basal ganglia and modulates the activity of the primary motor cortex. See Figure 5.27. [5]

suprachiasmatic nucleus (SCN) A small region of the hypothalamus above the optic chiasm that is the location of a circadian clock. [10]

surface dyslexia Acquired dyslexia in which the person seems to attend only to the fine details of reading. Compare *deep dyslexia*. [15]

sustained-attention task A task in which a single stimulus source or location must be held in the attentional spotlight for a protracted period. Compare *divided-attention task*. [14]

SWS See *stage 3 sleep*. [10]

Sylvian fissure Also called *lateral sulcus*. A deep fissure that demarcates the temporal lobe. See Figure 1.11. [1]

symbolic cuing Also called *spatial cuing*. A technique for testing voluntary attention in which a visual stimulus is presented and participants are asked to respond as soon as the stimulus appears on a screen. Each trial is preceded by a meaningful symbol used as a cue to hint at where the stimulus will appear. Compare *peripheral spatial cuing*. [14]

sympathetic nervous system The part of the autonomic nervous system that acts as the fight-or-flight system, generally preparing the body for action. See Figure 1.9. Compare *parasympathetic nervous system*. [1, 11]

synapse The cellular location at which information is transmitted from a neuron to another cell. See Figure 1.4. [1, 3, 8]

synapse rearrangement Also called *synaptic remodeling*. The loss of some synapses and the development of others; a refinement of synaptic connections that is often seen in development. See Figure 4.3. [4]

synaptic bouton See *axon terminal*. [1]

synaptic cleft The space between the presynaptic and postsynaptic neurons at a synapse. This gap measures about 20–40 nanometers. See Figures 1.4, 2.12. [1, 2]

synaptic delay The brief delay between the arrival of an action potential at the axon terminal and the creation of a postsynaptic potential. [2]

synaptic remodeling See *synapse rearrangement*. [4]

synaptic transmitter See *neurotransmitter*. [1, 2, 3]

synaptic vesicle A small, spherical structure that contains molecules of neurotransmitter. See Figure 1.4. [1, 2]

synaptogenesis The establishment of synaptic connections as axons and dendrites grow. See Figure 4.3. [4]

synergist A muscle that acts together with another muscle. Compare *antagonist* (definition 2). [5]

synesthesia A condition in which stimuli in one modality evoke the involuntary experience of an additional sensation in another modality; for example, "tasting" shapes or "smelling" colors. [5]

syntax The grammatical rules for constructing phrases and sentences in a language. [15]

syrinx The vocal organ in birds. [ASF 15.3]

T

T cell See *T lymphocyte*. [ASF 11.4]

T lymphocyte Also called *T cell*. An immune system cell, formed in the thymus (hence the *T*), that attacks foreign microbes or tissue; "killer cell." Compare *B lymphocyte*. [ASF 11.4]

T1R A family of taste receptor proteins that, when particular members bind together, form taste receptors for sweet flavors and umami flavors. Compare *T2R*. [6]

T2R A family of bitter taste receptors. Compare *T1R*. [6]

TAAR See *trace amine–associated receptor*. [6]

tachistoscope test A test in which stimuli are very briefly presented to either the left or right visual half field. [15]

tactile Referring to touch.

tactile corpuscle See *Meissner's corpuscle*. [5]

tailbone See *coccygeal*. [1]

tardive dyskinesia A disorder associated with first-generation antipsychotic use and characterized by involuntary movements, especially of the face and mouth. [12]

taste Any of the five basic sensations detected by the tongue—sweet, salty, sour, bitter, and umami. Compare *flavor*. [6]

taste bud A cluster of 50–150 cells that detects tastes. Taste buds are found in papillae. See Figures 6.15, 6.16. [6]

tau A protein associated with neurofibrillary tangles in Alzheimer's and other neurodegenerative diseases.

tectorial membrane A gelatinous membrane located atop the organ of Corti. See Figure 6.1. [6]

tectum The dorsal portion of the midbrain, consisting of the inferior and superior colliculi. [1]

tegmentum The main body of the midbrain, containing the substantia nigra, periaqueductal gray, part of the reticular formation, and multiple fiber tracts. [1]

telencephalon The anterior part of the fetal forebrain, which will become the cerebral hemispheres in the adult brain. See Figure 1.12. Compare *diencephalon*. [1]

temporal coding theory Theory that the pitch of a sound is determined by the rate of firing of auditory neurons. Compare *place coding theory*. [6]

temporal lobe The large lateral region of cortex in each cerebral hemisphere. It is continuous with the parietal lobe posteriorly and separated from the frontal lobe by the Sylvian fissure. See Figure 1.11. Compare *occipital lobe*. [1]

temporal resolution The ability to track changes in the brain that occur very quickly. Compare *spatial resolution*. [14]

temporal summation The summation of postsynaptic potentials that reach the axon hillock at different times. The closer in time the potentials occur, the greater the summation. See Figure 2.11. Compare *spatial summation*. [2]

temporoparietal junction (TPJ) The point in the brain where the temporal and parietal lobes meet. It plays a role in shifting attention to a new location after target onset. [14]

TENS See *transcutaneous electrical nerve stimulation*. [5]

testes (sing. testis) The male gonads, which produce sperm and androgenic steroid hormones. See Figure 8.1. Compare *ovaries*. [8]

testosterone A hormone, produced by male gonads, that controls a variety of bodily changes that occur at puberty. It is one of a class of hormones called *androgens*. See Figure 8.13. [8, 11]

tetanus An intense volley of action potentials. [13]

tetrahydrocannabinol (THC) See *delta-9-tetrahydrocannabinol*. [3]

thalamus (pl. thalami) Paired structures to either side of the third ventricle, at the top of the brainstem, that direct the flow of sensory information to and from the cortex. See Figures 1.14, 1.15. [1, 5]

THC See *delta-9-tetrahydrocannabinol*. [3]

thermoregulation The active process of maintaining a relatively constant internal temperature through behavioral and physiological adjustments. [9]

third ventricle The midline ventricle that conducts cerebrospinal fluid from the lateral ventricles to the fourth ventricle. See Figure 1.16. Compare *fourth ventricle* and *lateral ventricle*. [1]

thoracic Referring to the 12 spinal segments below the cervical (neck) portion of the spinal cord, in the torso. See Figures 1.8, 1.9. Compare *cervical, lumbar, sacral,* and *coccygeal*. [1]

threshold The stimulus intensity that is just adequate to trigger an action potential in an axon. [2, 5]

thrombolytic A substance that is used to unblock blood vessels and restore circulation. [ASF 15.5]

thyroid-stimulating hormone (TSH) A tropic hormone, released by the anterior pituitary gland, that signals the thyroid gland to secrete its hormones. [ASF 8.4]

tinnitus A sensation of noises or ringing in the ears not caused by external sound. [6]

TMS See *transcranial magnetic stimulation*. [1]

tolerance See *drug tolerance*. [3]

tonic receptor A receptor in which the frequency of action potentials declines slowly or not at all as stimulation is maintained. Compare *phasic receptor*. [5]

tonic-clonic seizure Also called *grand mal seizure*. A type of generalized epileptic seizure in which neurons fire in high-frequency bursts, usually accompanied by involuntary rhythmic contractions of the body. [2]

tonotopic organization The organization of auditory neurons according to an orderly map of stimulus frequency, from low to high. [6]

topographic projection A mapping that preserves the point-to-point correspondence between neighboring parts of space. For example, a topographic projection extends from the retina to the cortex. [7]

Tourette's syndrome A disorder involving heightened sensitivity to sensory stimuli that may be accompanied by verbal or physical tics. [12]

TPJ See *temporoparietal junction*. [14]

trace amine–associated receptor (TAAR) Any one of a family of probable pheromone receptors produced by neurons in the main olfactory epithelium. [6]

tract A bundle of axons found within the central nervous system. Compare *nerve*. [1]

tract tracer A type of histological stain that is taken up by neurons and transported over the routes of their axons, allowing the sources and targets of axons to be visualized. [1]

transcranial magnetic stimulation (TMS) A noninvasive technique for examining brain function that applies strong magnetic fields to stimulate cortical neurons in order to identify discrete areas of the brain that are particularly active during specific behaviors. Compare *magnetoencephalography*. [1]

transcript See *messenger RNA*. [App]

transcription The process during which mRNA forms bases complementary to a strand of DNA. The resulting message (called a *transcript*) is then used to translate the DNA code into protein molecules. See Appendix Figure A.2. Compare *translation*. [App]

transcutaneous electrical nerve stimulation (TENS) The delivery of electrical pulses through electrodes attached to the skin, which excite nerves that supply the region to which pain is referred. [5]

transduction The conversion of one form of energy to another, such as from light to neuronal activity. [6, 7]

transgenic Referring to an animal in which a new or altered gene has been deliberately introduced into the genome. [App]

transient ischemic attack (TIA) A temporary blood restriction to part of the brain that causes stroke-like symptoms that quickly resolve, serving as a warning of elevated stroke risk. [1]

transient receptor potential type M3 (TRPM3) A receptor, found in some free nerve endings, that opens its channel in response to rising temperatures. [5]

translation The process by which amino acids are linked together (directed by an mRNA molecule) to form protein molecules. See Appendix Figure A.2. Compare *transcription*. [App]

transmitter See *neurotransmitter*. [1, 2, 3]

transporter A specialized membrane component that returns transmitter molecules to the presynaptic neuron for reuse. [2, 3]

transverse plane See *coronal plane*. [1]

trichromatic hypothesis A hypothesis of color perception stating that there are three different types of cones, each excited by a different region of the spectrum and each having a separate pathway to the brain. [7]

tricyclic antidepressant An antidepressant that acts by increasing the synaptic accumulation of serotonin and norepinephrine. [3]

trinucleotide repeat Repetition of the same three nucleotides within a gene, which can lead to dysfunction, as in Huntington's disease. [ASF 5.5]

trophic factor See *neurotrophic factor*. [4]

tropic hormone Any of a class of anterior pituitary hormones that affect the secretion of hormones by other endocrine glands. See Figure 8.12. [8]

TSH See *thyroid-stimulating hormone*. [ASF 8.4]

tuberomammillary nucleus A region of the basal hypothalamus, near the pituitary stalk, that plays a role in generating slow wave sleep. [10]

Turner's syndrome A condition, seen in individuals carrying a single X chromosome but no other sex chromosome, in which an apparent female has underdeveloped but recognizable ovaries. [8]

tympanic canal See *scala tympani*. [6]

tympanic membrane Also called *eardrum*. The taut membrane, at the inner end of the ear canal, that captures sound vibrations in air. See Figure 6.1. [6]

U

ultradian Referring to a rhythmic biological event with a period shorter than a day, usually from several minutes to several hours long. Compare *infradian*. [10]

ultrasound Very-high-frequency sound, generally beyond 20,000 Hz, which is the upper bound for a young adult human. Compare *infrasound*. [6]

umami One of the five basic tastes—the meaty, savory flavor. (The other four tastes are salty, sour, sweet, and bitter.) [6]

unipolar neuron Also called *monopolar neuron*. A neuron with a single branch that leaves the cell body and then extends in two directions; one end is the input zone, and the other end is the output zone. See Figure 1.3. Compare *bipolar neuron* and *multipolar neuron*. [1]

up-regulation A compensatory increase in receptor availability at the synapses of a neuron. Compare *down-regulation*. [3]

V

V1 See *primary visual cortex*. [7]

vagina The opening from the outside of the body to the cervix and uterus in females. [8]

vagus nerve Cranial nerve X, which transmits information between the brain and the viscera. The vagus both regulates visceral activity and transmits signals from the viscera to the brain. See Figures 1.7, 9.16. [9]

vasopressin Also called *arginine vasopressin (AVP)* or *antidiuretic hormone (ADH)*. A peptide hormone from the posterior pituitary that promotes water conservation and increases blood pressure. [8, 9]

ventral In anatomy, toward the belly or front of the body, or the bottom of the brain. Compare *dorsal*. [1]

ventral tegmental area (VTA) A portion of the midbrain that projects dopaminergic fibers to the nucleus accumbens. [3]

ventricular system A system of fluid-filled cavities inside the brain. See Figure 1.16. [1]

ventricular zone Also called *ependymal layer*. A region lining the cerebral ventricles from which new neurons and glial cells are born throughout life, via mitosis. See Figure 4.3. [4]

ventromedial hypothalamus (VMH) A hypothalamic region involved in sexual behaviors, eating, and aggression. See Figures 8.19, 9.12. [8, 9, 11]

vertex spike A sharp-wave EEG pattern that is seen during stage 1 sleep. See Figure 10.11. [10]

vestibular canal See *scala vestibuli*. See Figure 6.1. [6]

vestibular nuclei Brainstem nuclei that receive information from the vestibular organs through cranial nerve VIII (the vestibulocochlear nerve). [6]

vestibular system The sensory system that detects balance. It consists of several small inner-ear structures that adjoin the cochlea. [6]

vestibulocerebellum The middle portion of the cerebellum, sandwiched between the spinocerebellum and the cerebrocerebellum and consisting of the nodule and the flocculus. It helps the motor systems to maintain posture and appropriate orientation toward the external world. [ASF 5.4]

vestibulocochlear nerve Cranial nerve VIII, which runs from the cochlea to the brainstem auditory nuclei. See Figures 1.7, 6.1. [6]

vigilance The global, nonselective level of alertness of an individual. [14]

visual acuity Sharpness of vision. [7]

visual cortex See *occipital cortex*. [7]

visual field The whole area that you can see without moving your head or eyes. [7]

visual P1 effect A positive deflection of the event-related potential, occurring 70–100 milliseconds after stimulus presentation, that is enhanced for selectively attended visual input compared with ignored input. Compare *auditory N1 effect*. [14]

VMH See *ventromedial hypothalamus*. [8, 9, 11]

VNO See *vomeronasal organ*. [6, 8]

voltage-gated Na$^+$ channel A Na$^+$-selective channel that opens or closes in response to changes in the voltage of the local membrane potential. It mediates the action potential. Compare *ionotropic receptor*. [2]

voluntary attention Also called *endogenous attention*. The voluntary direction of attention toward specific aspects of the environment, in accordance with our interests and goals. Compare *reflexive attention*. [14]

vomeronasal organ (VNO) A collection of specialized receptor cells, near to but separate from the olfactory epithelium, that detect pheromones and send electrical signals to the accessory olfactory bulb in the brain. [6, 8]

VTA See *ventral tegmental area*. [3]

W

Wada test A test in which a short-lasting anesthetic is delivered into one carotid artery to determine the processing specializations of that hemisphere, such as language. [15]

wavelength The length between two peaks in a repeated stimulus such as a wave, light, or sound. See Figure 7.23. [7]

Wernicke's aphasia See *fluent aphasia*. [15]

Wernicke's area A region of temporoparietal cortex in the brain that is involved in the perception and production of speech. See Figure 15.9. Compare *Broca's area*. [15]

Wernicke-Geschwind model See *connectionist model of aphasia*. [15]

Western blot A method of detecting a particular protein molecule in a tissue or organ by separating proteins from that source with gel electrophoresis, blotting the separated proteins onto nitrocellulose, and then using an antibody that binds, and highlights, the protein of interest. Compare *Northern blot* and *Southern blot*. [App]

white matter A light-colored layer of tissue, consisting mostly of myelin-sheathed axons, that lies underneath the gray matter of the cortex. White matter mostly transmits information. See Figures 1.8, 1.10. Compare *gray matter*. [1]

Williams syndrome A disorder characterized by impairments of spatial cognition and IQ but superior linguistic abilities. [15]

withdrawal symptom An uncomfortable symptom that arises when a person stops taking a drug that they have used frequently, especially at high doses. [3]

within-participants experiment An experiment in which the same set of individuals is compared before and after an experimental manipulation. The experimental group thus serves as its own control group. Compare *between-participants experiment*. [1]

wolffian duct A duct system in the embryo that will develop into male reproductive structures (epididymis, vas deferens, and seminal vesicle) if androgens are present. See Figure 8.23. Compare *müllerian duct*. [8]

word deafness A form of central deafness that is characterized by the specific inability to hear words although other sounds can be detected. [6]

working memory See *short-term memory*. [13]

Z

zeitgeber Literally "time giver" (in German). The stimulus (usually the light-dark cycle) that entrains circadian rhythms. [10]

zygote The fertilized egg. [8]

References

A

Abbott, S. M., and Videnovic, A. (2014). Sleep disorders in atypical parkinsonism. *Movement Disorders Clinical Practice (Hoboken), 1*, 89–96.

Abe, N., Suzuki, M., Mori, E., Itoh, M., et al. (2007). Deceiving others: Distinct neural responses of the prefrontal cortex and amygdala in simple fabrication and deception with social interactions. *Journal of Cognitive Neuroscience, 19*, 287–295.

Aben, B., Stapert, S., and Blokland, A. (2012). About the distinction between working memory and short-term memory. *Frontiers in Psychology, 3*, 301.

Abramowitz, J. S., Blakey, S. M., Reuman, L., and Buchholz, J. L. (2018). New directions in the cognitive-behavioral treatment of OCD: Theory, research, and practice. *Behavior Therapy, 49*(3), 311–322.

Abtahi, S., Howell, E., Salvucci, J. T., Bastacky, J. M. R., et al. (2019). Exendin-4 antagonizes the metabolic action of acylated ghrelinergic signaling in the hypothalamic paraventricular nucleus. *General and Comparative Endocrinology, 270*, 75–81.

Ackermann, S., and Rasch, B. (2018). Differential effects of non-REM and REM sleep on memory consolidation? *Current Neurology and Neuroscience Reports, 14*(2), 430.

Ader, R. (2001). Psychoneuroimmunology. *Current Directions in Psychological Science, 10*(3), 94–98.

Adler, E., Hoon, M. A., Mueller, K. L., Chandrashekar, J., et al. (2000). A novel family of mammalian taste receptors. *Cell, 100*, 693–702.

Adolphs, R., Gosselin, F., Buchanan, T. W., Tranel, D., et al. (2005). A mechanism for impaired fear recognition after amygdala damage. *Nature, 433*, 68–72.

Agarwal, N., Pacher, P., Tegeder, I., Amay, F., et al. (2007). Cannabinoids mediate analgesia largely via peripheral type cannabinoid receptors in nociceptors. *Nature Neuroscience, 10*, 870–878.

Ajslev, T. A., Andersen, C. S., Gamborg, M., Sørensen, T. I., et al. (2011). Childhood overweight after establishment of the gut microbiota: The role of delivery mode, pre-pregnancy weight and early administration of antibiotics. *International Journal of Obesity (London), 35*(4), 522–529.

Albers, G. W., Marks, M. P., Kemp, S., Christensen, S., et al. (2018). Thrombectomy for stroke at 6 to 16 hours with selection by perfusion imaging. *New England Journal of Medicine.* PubMed PMID: 29364767.

Albrecht, B., Staiger, P. K., Hall, K., Kambouropoulos, N., et al. (2016). Motivational drive and alprazolam misuse: A recipe for aggression? *Psychiatry Research, 240*, 381–389.

Alhadeff, A. L., Mergler, B. D., Zimmer, D. J., Turner, C. A., et al. (2017). Endogenous glucagon-like peptide-1 receptor signaling in the nucleus tractus solitarius is required for food intake control. *Neuropsychopharmacology, 42*(7), 1471–1479.

Almanza-Sepulveda, M. L., Fleming, A. S., and Jonas, W. (2020). Mothering revisited: A role for cortisol? *Hormones and Behavior, 121*, 104679. https://doi.org/10.1016/j.yhbeh.2020.104679

Altschuler, E. L., Wisdom, S. B., Stone, L., Foster, C., et al. (1999). Rehabilitation of hemiparesis after stroke with a mirror. *Lancet, 353*, 2035–2036.

Alvarez, J. A., and Emory, E. (2006). Executive function and the frontal lobes: A meta-analytic review. *Neuropsychology Review, 16*, 17–42.

Alzheimer's Association. (2019). Alzheimer's disease facts and figures. *Alzheimer's & Dementia, 15*(3), 321–387. https://www.alz.org/alzheimers-dementia/facts-figures

American Psychiatric Association. (2013). *Diagnostic and statistical manual of mental disorders: DSM-5.* Washington, DC: American Psychiatric Association.

Amici, R., Bastianini, S., Berteotti, C., Cerri, M., et al. (2014). Sleep and bodily functions: The physiological interplay between body homeostasis and sleep homeostasis. *Archives Italiennes de Biologie, 152*, 66–78.

Amunts, K., Schlaug, G., Jaencke, L., Steinmetz, H., et al. (1997). Motor cortex and hand motor skills: Structural compliance in the human brain. *Human Brain Mapping, 5*, 206–215.

Anacker, C., Luna, V. M., Stevens, G. S., Millette, A., et al. (2018). Hippocampal neurogenesis confers stress resilience by inhibiting the ventral dentate gyrus. *Nature, 559*(7712), 98–102.

Anand, B. K., and Brobeck, J. R. (1951). Localization of a "feeding center" in the hypothalamus of the rat. *Proceedings of the Society for Experimental Biology and Medicine, 77*, 323–324.

Andersen, R. A., Andersen, K. N., Hwang, E. J., and Hauschild, M. (2014). Optic ataxia: From Balint's syndrome to the parietal reach region. *Neuron, 81*(5), 967–983.

Andics, A., Gábor, A., Gácsi, M., Faragó, T., et al. (2016). Neural mechanisms for lexical processing in dogs. *Science, 353*(6303), 1030–1032.

Anestis, M. D., Houtsma, C., Daruwala, S. E., and Butterworth, S. E. (2019). Firearm legislation and statewide suicide rates: The moderating role of household firearm ownership levels. *Behavioral Sciences & the Law, 37*(3), 270–280.

Anstey, M. L., Rogers, S. M., Ott, S. R., Burrows, M., et al. (2009). Serotonin mediates behavioral gregarization underlying swarm formation in desert locusts. *Science, 323*(5914), 627–630.

Apkarian, A. V., Sosa, Y., Sonty, S., Levy, R. M., et al. (2004). Chronic back pain is associated with decreased prefrontal and thalamic gray matter density. *Journal of Neuroscience, 24*, 10410–10415.

Archer, G. S., Friend, T. H., Piedrahita, J., Nevill, C. H., et al. (2003). Behavioral variation among cloned pigs. *Applied Animal Behaviour Science, 82*, 151–161.

Archer, J. (2006). Testosterone and human aggression: An evaluation of the challenge hypothesis. *Neuroscience and Biobehavioral Reviews, 30*, 319–345.

Argyll-Robertson, D. M. C. L. (1869). On an interesting series of eye symptoms in a case of spinal disease, with remarks on the action of belladonna on the iris. *Edinburgh Medical Journal, 14*, 696–708.

Arnone, D., Cavanagh, J., Gerber, D., Lawrie, S. M., et al. (2009). Magnetic resonance imaging studies in bipolar disorder and schizophrenia: Meta-analysis. *British Journal of Psychiatry, 195*, 194–201.

Arnsten, A. F. (2006). Fundamentals of attention-deficit/hyperactivity disorder: Circuits and pathways. *Journal of Clinical Psychiatry, 67*, 7–12.

Arts, N. J., Walvoort, S. J., and Kessels, R. P. (2017). Korsakoff's syndrome: A critical review. *Neuropsychiatric Disease and Treatment, 13*, 2875–2890.

Aschwanden, C. (2013, March 9). The curious lives of people who feel no fear. *New Scientist,* (2907), 36–39.

Aserinsky, E., and Kleitman, N. (1953). Regularly occurring periods of eye motility, and concomitant phenomena, during sleep. *Science, 118*, 273–274.

Assaf, Y., and Pasternak, O. (2008). Diffusion tensor imaging (DTI)-based white matter mapping in brain research: A review. *Journal of Molecular Neuroscience, 34*, 51–61.

Audero, E., Coppi, E., Mlinar, B., Rossetti, T., et al. (2008). Sporadic autonomic dysregulation and death associated with excessive serotonin autoinhibition. *Science, 321*, 130–133.

Augustine, V., Gokce, S. K., Lee, S., Wang, B., et al. (2018). Hierarchical neural architecture underlying thirst regulation. *Nature, 555*(7695), 204–209.

Aungst, J. L., Heyward, P. M., Puche, A. C., Karnup, S. V., et al. (2003). Centre-surround inhibition among olfactory bulb glomeruli. *Nature, 426*, 623–629.

Avila, M. T., Hong, L. E., Moates, A., Turano, K. A., et al. (2006). Role of anticipation in schizophrenia-related pursuit initiation deficits. *Journal of Neurophysiology, 95*, 593–601.

B

Baars, B. J., Ramsøy, T. Z., and Laureys, S. (2003). Brain, conscious experience and the observing self. *Trends in Neurosciences, 26*(12), 671–675.

Badre, D., and Nee, D. E. (2018). Frontal cortex and the hierarchical control of behavior. *Trends in Cognitive Sciences, 22*(2), 170–188.

Bagemihl, B. (1999). *Biological exuberance: Animal homosexuality and natural diversity.* New York, NY: St. Martin's Press.

Bagni, C., and Greenough, W. T. (2005). From mRNP trafficking to spine dysmorphogenesis: The roots of fragile X syndrome. *Nature Reviews Neuroscience, 6*, 376–387.

Bailey, C. H., and Chen, M. (1983). Morphological basis of long-term habituation and sensitization in *Aplysia. Science, 220*, 91–93.

Bailey, K., and West, R. (2013). The effects of an action video game on visual and affective information processing. *Brain Research, 1504*, 35–46.

Baillet, S. (2017). Magnetoencephalography for brain electrophysiology and imaging. *Nature Neuroscience, 20*(3), 327–339.

Baldermann, J. C., Schüller, T., Huys, D., Becker, I., et al. (2016). Deep brain stimulation for Tourette-syndrome: A systematic review and meta-analysis. *Brain Stimulation, 9*(2), 296–304.

Baldwin, M. W, Toda, Y., Nakagita, T., O'Connell, M. J., et al. (2014). Sensory biology: Evolution of sweet taste perception in hummingbirds by transformation of the ancestral umami receptor. *Science, 345*, 929–933.

Balthazart, J., and Ball, G. F. (2007). Topography in the preoptic region: Differential regulation of appetitive and consummatory male sexual behaviors. *Frontiers in Neuroendocrinology, 28*(4), 161–178.

Ban, T. A. (2007). Fifty years chlorpromazine: A historical perspective. *Neuropsychiatric Disease and Treatment, 3*(4), 495–500.

Barbeau, H., Norman, K., Fung, J., Visintin, M., et al. (1998). Does neurorehabilitation play a role in the recovery of walking in neurological populations? *Annals of the New York Academy of Sciences, 860*, 377–392.

Bark, N. (2002). Did schizophrenia change the course of English history? The mental illness of Henry VI. *Medical Hypotheses, 59*, 416–421.

Barnea, G., O'Donnell, S., Mancia, F., Sun, X., et al. (2004). Odorant receptors on axon termini in the brain. *Science, 304*, 1468.

Barnett, S. A. (1975). *The rat: A study in behavior.* Chicago, IL: University of Chicago Press.

Barrett, A. M., Goedert, K. M., and Basso, J. C. (2012). Prism adaptation for spatial neglect after stroke: Translational practice gaps. *Nature Reviews Neurology, 8*(10), 567–577.

Barrett, L. F. (2018). Seeing fear: It's all in the eyes? *Trends in Neurosciences, 41*(9), 559–563.

Barrio, J. R., Small, G. W., Wong, K. P., Huang, S. C., et al. (2015). In vivo characterization of chronic traumatic encephalopathy using [F-18]FDDNP PET brain imaging. *Proceedings of the National Academy of Sciences, USA, 112*(16), E2039–E2047.

Bartels, A., and Zeki, S. (2000). The neural basis of romantic love. *NeuroReport, 11*, 3829–3834.

Bartolomeo, P. (2007). Visual neglect. *Current Opinion in Neurology, 20*, 381–386.

Bartoshuk, L. M. (1993). Genetic and pathological taste variation: What can we learn from animal models and human disease? In D. Chadwick, J. Marsh, and J. Goode (Eds.), *The molecular basis of smell and taste transduction* (pp. 251–267). New York, NY: Wiley.

Basson, R. (2001). Human sex-response cycles. *Journal of Sex & Marital Therapy, 27*, 33–43.

Basson, R. (2008). Women's sexual function and dysfunction: Current uncertainties, future directions. *International Journal of Impotence Research, 20*, 466–478.

Bates, E., Wilson, S. M., Saygin, A. P., Dick, F., et al. (2003). Voxel-based lesion-symptom mapping. *Nature Neuroscience, 6*, 448–450.

Battleday, R. M., and Brem, A. K. (2015). Modafinil for cognitive neuroenhancement in healthy non-sleep-deprived subjects: A systematic review. *European Neuropsychopharmacology, 25*(11), 1865–1881.

Baumann, M. H., Walters, H. M., Niello, M., and Sitte, H. H. (2018). Neuropharmacology of synthetic cathinones. *Handbook of Experimental Pharmacology, 252*, 113–142.

Bautista, D. M., Siemens, J., Glazer, J. M., Tsuruda, P. R., et al. (2007). The menthol receptor TRPM8 is the principal detector of environmental cold. *Nature, 448*, 204–208.

Baynes, K. C., Dhillo, W. S., and Bloom, S. R. (2006). Regulation of food intake by gastrointestinal hormones. *Current Opinion in Gastroenterology, 22*, 626–631.

Bear, D. M., Lassance, J. M., Hoekstra, H. E., and Datta, S. R. (2016). The evolving neural and genetic architecture of vertebrate olfaction. *Current Biology, 26*(20), R1039–R1049.

Becker, J. B., McClellan, M. L., and Reed, B. G. (2017). Sex differences, gender and addiction. *Journal of Neuroscience Research, 95*(1–2), 136–147.

Bedrosian, T. A., Vaughn, C. A., Galan, A., Daye, G., et al. (2013). Nocturnal light exposure impairs affective responses in a wavelength-dependent manner. *Journal of Neuroscience, 33*, 13081–13087.

Bee, M. A., and Micheyl, C. (2008). The cocktail party problem: What is it? How can it be solved? And why should animal behaviorists study it? *Journal of Comparative Psychology, 122*, 235–251.

Beeli, G., Esslen, M., and Jäncke, L. (2005). When coloured sounds taste sweet. *Nature, 434*, 38.

Beggs, W. D., and Foreman, D. L. (1980). Sound localization and early binaural experience in the deaf. *British Journal of Audiology, 14*, 41–48.

Behrens, M., and Meyerhof, W. (2018). Vertebrate bitter taste receptors: Keys for survival in changing environments. *Journal of Agricultural and Food Chemistry, 66*(10), 2204–2213.

Behrens, M., and Meyerhof, W. (2019). A role for taste receptors in (neuro)endocrinology? *Journal of Neuroendocrinology, 31*, e12691.

Belelli, D., Brown, A. R., Mitchell, S. J., Gunn, B. G., et al. (2018). Endogenous neurosteroids influence synaptic $GABA_A$ receptors during postnatal development. *Journal of Neuroendocrinology, 30*(2).

Beliveau, V., Ganz, M., Feng, L., Ozenne, B., et al. (2017). A high-resolution in vivo atlas of the human brain's serotonin system. *Journal of Neuroscience, 37*(1), 120–128.

Bell, S., Daskalopoulou, M., Rapsomaniki, E., George, J., et al. (2017). Association between clinically recorded alcohol consumption and initial presentation of 12 cardiovascular diseases: Population based cohort study using linked health records. *BMJ*, 356, j909.

Belle, M. D. C., and Allen, C. N. (2018). The circadian clock: A tale of genetic-electrical interplay and synaptic integration. *Current Opinion in Physiology*, 5, 75–79.

Bennett, W. (1983). The nicotine fix. *Rhode Island Medical Journal*, 66, 455–458.

Benney, K. S., and Braaten, R. F. (2000). Auditory scene analysis in estrildid finches (*Taeniopygia guttata* and *Lonchura striata domestica*): A species advantage for detection of conspecific song. *Journal of Comparative Psychology*, 114, 174–182.

Benson, P. J., Beedie, S. A., Shephard, E., Giegling, I., et al. (2012). Simple viewing tests can detect eye movement abnormalities that distinguish schizophrenia cases from controls with exceptional accuracy. *Biological Psychiatry*, 72(9), 716–724.

Benton, A. L., and Hamsher, K. (1976). *Multilingual Aphasia Examination*. Iowa City: University of Iowa Press.

Berenbaum, S. A. (2001). Cognitive function in congenital adrenal hyperplasia. *Endocrinology and Metabolism Clinics of North America*, 30, 173–192.

Bernal, B., and Altman, N. (2010). The connectivity of the superior longitudinal fasciculus: A tractography DTI study. *Magnetic Resonance Imaging*, 28, 217–225.

Bernhardt, P. C., Dabbs, J. M., Jr., Fielden, J. A., and Lutter, C. D. (1998). Testosterone changes during vicarious experiences of winning and losing among fans at sporting events. *Physiology & Behavior*, 65(1), 59–62.

Bernstein, I. S., and Gordon, T. P. (1974). The function of aggression in primate societies. *American Scientist*, 62, 304–311.

Bernstein, L. E., Auer, E. T., Jr., Moore, J. K., Ponton, C. W., et al. (2002). Visual speech perception without primary auditory cortex activation. *NeuroReport*, 13, 311–315.

Bernstein, L., Burns, C., Sailer-Hammons, M., Kurtz, A., et al. (2017). Multiclinic observations on the simplified diet in PKU. *Journal of Nutrition and Metabolism*, 2017, 4083293.

Berthold, A. (1849). Transplantation der Hoden. *Archiv für Anatomie, Physiologie und Wissenschaftliche Medicin*, 16, 42–46.

Binder, J. R., Rao, S. M., Hammeke, T. A., Yetkin, F. Z., et al. (1994). Functional magnetic resonance imaging of human auditory cortex. *Annals of Neurology*, 35, 662–672.

Birnbaum, R., and Weinberger, D. R. (2017). Genetic insights into the neurodevelopmental origins of schizophrenia. *Nature Reviews Neuroscience*, 18(12), 727–740.

Bisley, J. W., and Goldberg, M. E. (2003). Neuronal activity in the lateral intraparietal area and spatial attention. *Science*, 299, 81–86.

Blackwell, D. L, Lucas, J. W, and Clarke, T. C. (2014). Summary health statistics for U.S. adults: National Health Interview Survey, 2012. *Vital and Health Statistics 10*(260), 1–161.

Blackwell, D. L., and Villarroel, M. A. (2018). Tables of Summary Health Statistics (for U.S. Adults: 2016 National Health Interview Survey), www.cdc.gov/nchs/nhis/SHS/tables.htm.

Blake, D. T., Heiser, M. A., Caywood, M., and Merzenich, M. M. (2006). Experience-dependent adult cortical plasticity requires cognitive association between sensation and reward. *Neuron*, 52, 371–381.

Blanchard, R., Cantor, J. M., Bogaert, A. F., Breedlove, S. M., et al. (2006). Interaction of fraternal birth order and handedness in the development of male homosexuality. *Hormones and Behavior*, 49, 405–414.

Bleuler, E. (1950). *Dementia praecox; or, The group of schizophrenias* (J. Zinkin, Trans.). New York, NY: International Universities Press.

Bliss, T. V. P., and Lømo, T. (1973). Long-lasting potentiation of synaptic transmission in the dentate area of the anaesthetized rabbit following stimulation of the perforant path. *Journal of Physiology (London)*, 232, 331–356.

Blum, I. D., Bell, B., and Wu, M. N. (2018). Time for bed: Genetic mechanisms mediating the circadian regulation of sleep. *Trends in Genetics*, 34(5), 379–388.

Blumberger, D. M., Hsu, J. H., and Daskalakis, Z. J. (2015). A review of brain stimulation treatments for late-life depression. *Current Treatment Options in Psychiatry*, 2(4), 413–421.

Blumstein, S. E., and Amso, D. (2013). Dynamic functional organization of language: Insights from functional neuroimaging. *Perspectives on Psychological Science*, 8(1), 44–48.

Boddhula, S. K., Boddhula, S., Gunasekaran, K., and Bischof, E. (2018). An unusual cause of thunderclap headache after eating the hottest pepper in the world—"The Carolina Reaper." *BMJ Case Reports*, pii: bcr-2017-224085.

Boets, B., Op de Beeck, H. P., Vandermosten, M., Scott, S. K., et al. (2013). Intact but less accessible phonetic representations in adults with dyslexia. *Science*, 342(6163), 1251–1254.

Bogaert, A. F. (2006). Biological versus nonbiological older brothers and men's sexual orientation. *Proceedings of the National Academy of Sciences, USA*, 103, 10771–10774.

Bogaert, A. F. (2007). Extreme right-handedness, older brothers, and sexual orientation in men. *Neuropsychology*, 21, 141–148.

Bogaert, A. F., Skorska, M. N., Wang, C., Gabrie, J., et al. (2018). Male homosexuality and maternal immune responsivity to the Y-linked protein NLGN4Y. *Proceedings of the National Academy of Sciences, USA*, 115(2), 302–306.

Bogenschutz, M. P., and Johnson, M. W. (2016). Classic hallucinogens in the treatment of addictions. *Progress in Neuro-Psychopharmacology and Biological Psychiatry*, 64, 250–258.

Boggs, D. L., Nguyen, J. D., Morgenson, D., Taffe, M. A., et al. (2018). Clinical and preclinical evidence for functional interactions of cannabidiol and Δ9-tetrahydrocannabinol. *Neuropsychopharmacology*, 43(1), 142–154.

Bogin, B. (1997). Evolutionary hypotheses for human childhood. *Yearbook of Physical Anthropology*, 40, 63–89.

Boldrini, M., Fulmore, C. A., Tartt, A. N., Simeon, L. R., et al. (2018). Human hippocampal neurogenesis persists throughout aging. *Cell Stem Cell*, 22(4), 589–599.

Bolhuis, J. J., Okanoya, K., and Scharff, C. (2010). Twitter evolution: Converging mechanisms in birdsong and human speech. *Nature Reviews Neuroscience*, 11, 747–759.

Bolsoni, L. M., and Zuardi, A. W. (2019). Pharmacological interventions during the process of reconsolidation of aversive memories: A systematic review. *Neurobiology of Stress*, 11, 100194. https://doi.org/10.1016/j.ynstr.2019.100194

Bonaz, B., Bazin, T., and Pellissier, S. (2018). The vagus nerve at the interface of the microbiota-gut-brain axis. *Frontiers in Neuroscience*, 12, 49. https://doi.org/10.3389/fnins.2018.00049

Bonnel, A. M., and Prinzmetal, W. (1998). Dividing attention between the color and the shape of objects. *Perception & Psychophysics*, 60, 113–124.

Boot, W. R., Kramer, A. F., Simons, D. J., Fabiani, M., et al. (2008). The effects of video game playing on attention, memory, and executive control. *Acta Psychologica (Amsterdam)*, 129, 387–398.

Borgstein, J., and Grootendorst, C. (2002). Clinical picture: Half a brain. *Lancet*, 359, 473.

Borota, D., Murray, E., Keceli, G., Chang, A., et al. (2014). Post-study caffeine administration enhances memory consolidation in humans. *Nature Neuroscience*, 17(2), 201–203.

Bortolozzi, A., Masana, M., Díaz-Mataix, L., Cortés, R., et al. (2010). Dopamine release induced by atypical antipsychotics in prefrontal cortex requires 5-HT(1A) receptors but not 5-HT(2A) receptors. *International Journal of Neuropsychopharmacology*, 13(10), 1299–1314.

Boshuisen, K., van Schooneveld, M. M., Leijten, F. S., de Kort, G. A., et al. (2010). Contralateral MRI abnormalities affect seizure and cognitive outcome after hemispherectomy. *Neurology, 75,* 1623–1630.

Bourque, C. W. (2008). Central mechanisms of osmosensation and systemic osmoregulation. *Nature Reviews Neuroscience, 9,* 519–531.

Bourque, J., Afzali, M. H., O'Leary-Barrett, M., and Conrod P. (2017). Cannabis use and psychotic-like experiences trajectories during early adolescence: The coevolution and potential mediators. *Journal of Child Psychology and Psychiatry, 58*(12), 1360–1369.

Bouwknecht, J. A., Hijzen, T. H., van der Gugten, J., Maes, R. A., et al. (2001). Absence of 5-HT(1B) receptors is associated with impaired impulse control in male 5-HT(1B) knockout mice. *Biological Psychiatry, 49,* 557–568.

Bower, B. (2003). Vision seekers. *Science News, 164,* 331–333.

Bower, B. (2006). Prescription for controversy: Medications for depressed kids spark scientific dispute. *Science News, 169,* 168–172.

Bowman, M. L. (1997). *Individual differences in posttraumatic response.* Mahway, NJ: Erlbaum.

Boyce, R., Glasgow, S. D., Williams, S., and Adamantidis, A. (2016). Causal evidence for the role of REM sleep theta rhythm in contextual memory consolidation. *Science, 352*(6287), 812–816.

Brady, T. F., Konkle, T., Alvarez, G. A., and Oliva, A. (2014). Visual long-term memory has a massive storage capacity for object details. *Proceedings of the National Academy of Sciences, USA, 105,* 14325–14329.

Brandlistuen, R. E., Ystrom, E., Eberhard-Gran, M., Nulman, I., et al. (2015). Behavioural effects of fetal antidepressant exposure in a Norwegian cohort of discordant siblings. *International Journal of Epidemiology, 44*(4), 1397–1407.

Brasser, S. M., Mozhui, K., and Smith, D. V. (2005). Differential covariation in taste responsiveness to bitter stimuli in rats. *Chemical Senses, 30,* 793–799.

Bray, G. A. (1969). Effect of caloric restriction on energy expenditure in obese patients. *Lancet, 2,* 397–398.

Breier, A., Malhotra, A. K., Pinals, D. A., Weisenfeld, N. I., et al. (1997). Association of ketamine-induced psychosis with focal activation of the prefrontal cortex in healthy volunteers. *American Journal of Psychiatry, 154*(6), 805–811.

Breitner, J. C., Wyse, B. W., Anthony, J. C., Welsh-Bohmer, K. A., et al. (1999). APOE-epsilon4 count predicts age when prevalence of AD increases, then declines: The Cache County Study. *Neurology, 53,* 321–331.

Bremer, F. (1938). L'activité électrique de l'écorce cérébrale. *Actualités Scientifiques et Industrielles, 658,* 3–46.

Brennan, S. C., Davies, T. S., Schepelmann, M., and Riccardi, D. (2014). Emerging roles of the extracellular calcium-sensing receptor in nutrient sensing: Control of taste modulation and intestinal hormone secretion. *British Journal of Nutrition, 111*(Suppl. 1), S16–22.

Bridges, R. S. (2015). Neuroendocrine regulation of maternal behavior. *Frontiers in Neuroendocrinology, 36,* 178–196. https://doi.org/10.1016/j.yfrne.2014.11.007

Briggs, F., Mangun, G. R., and Usrey, W. M. (2013). Attention enhances synaptic efficacy and the signal-to-noise ratio in neural circuits. *Nature, 499*(7459), 476–480.

Broadbent, D. A. (1958). *Perception and communication.* New York, NY: Pergamon Press.

Brody, D. J., Pratt, L. A., and Hughes, J. (2018). Prevalence of depression among adults aged 20 and over: United States, 2013–2016. *NCHS Data Brief, 303,* 1–8.

Bronsard, G., and Bartolomei, F. (2013). Rhythms, rhythmicity and aggression. *Journal of Physiology (Paris), 107*(4), 327–334.

Brooks, S. J., O'Daly, O. G., Uher, R., Schiöth, H. B., et al. (2012). Subliminal food images compromise superior working memory performance in women with restricting anorexia nervosa. *Consciousness and Cognition, 21*(2), 751–763.

Brouwer, H., Crocker, M. W., Venhuizen, N. J., and Hoeks, J. C. J. (2017). A neurocomputational model of the N400 and the P600 in language processing. *Cognitive Science, 41*(Suppl. 6), 1318–1352.

Brown, A. S. (2011). The environment and susceptibility to schizophrenia. *Progress in Neurobiology, 93,* 23–58.

Brown, C. (2003, February 2). The man who mistook his wife for a deer. *The New York Times,* Section 6, p. 32.

Brown, E. C., Jeong, J. W., Muzik, O., Rothermel, R., et al. (2014). Evaluating the arcuate fasciculus with combined diffusion-weighted MRI tractography and electrocorticography. *Human Brain Mapping, 35,* 2333–2347.

Brown, J. (1958). Some tests of the decay theory of immediate memory. *Quarterly Journal of Experimental Psychology, 10,* 12–21.

Brown, K., and Mastrianni, J. A. (2010). The prion diseases. *Journal of Geriatric Psychiatry and Neurology, 23*(4), 277–298.

Brown, S. P., Mathur, B. N., Olsen, S. R., Luppi, P. H., et al. (2017). New breakthroughs in understanding the role of functional interactions between the neocortex and the claustrum. *Journal of Neuroscience, 37*(45), 10877–10881.

Brownlee, S., and Schrof, J. M. (1997). The quality of mercy. Effective pain treatments already exist. Why aren't doctors using them? *U.S. News & World Report, 122,* 54–67.

Bruel-Jungerman, E., Rampon, C., and Laroche, S. (2007). Adult hippocampal neurogenesis, synaptic plasticity and memory: Facts and hypotheses. *Review in the Neurosciences, 18,* 93–114.

Brunetti, M., Della Penna, S., Ferretti, A., Del Gratta, C., et al. (2008). A frontoparietal network for spatial attention reorienting in the auditory domain: A human fMRI/MEG study of functional and temporal dynamics. *Cerebral Cortex, 18,* 1139–1147.

Bryant, P., Trinder, J., and Curtis, N. (2004). Sick and tired: Does sleep have a vital role in the immune system? *Nature Reviews Immunology, 4,* 457–467.

Buccino, G., Lui, F., Canessa, N., Patteri, I., et al. (2004). Neural circuits involved in the recognition of actions performed by nonconspecifics: An fMRI study. *Journal of Cognitive Neuroscience, 16,* 114–126.

Buccino, G., Solodkin, A., and Small, S. L. (2006). Functions of the mirror neuron system: Implications for neurorehabilitation. *Cognitive and Behavioral Neurology, 19,* 55–63.

Buchsbaum, B. R., Baldo, J., Okada, K., Berman, K. F., et al. (2011). Conduction aphasia, sensory-motor integration, and phonological short-term memory—An aggregate analysis of lesion and fMRI data. *Brain and Language, 119,* 119–128.

Buchsbaum, M. S., Buchsbaum, B. R., Chokron, S., Tang, C., et al. (2006). Thalamocortical circuits: fMRI assessment of the pulvinar and medial dorsal nucleus in normal volunteers. *Neuroscience Letters, 404,* 282–287.

Buchsbaum, M. S., Mirsky, A. F., DeLisi, L. E., Morihisa, J., et al. (1984). The Genain quadruplets: Electrophysiological, positron emission, and X-ray tomographic studies. *Psychiatry Research 13*(1), 95–108.

Buck, L., and Axel, R. (1991). A novel multigene family may encode odorant receptors: A molecular basis for odor recognition. *Cell, 65,* 175–187.

Buckner, R. L., and Koutstaal, W. (1998). Functional neuroimaging studies of encoding, priming, and explicit memory retrieval. *Proceedings of the National Academy of Sciences, USA, 95*(3), 891–898.

Burgdorf, J., Kroes, R. A., Moskal, J. R., Pfaus, J. G., et al. (2008). Ultrasonic vocalizations of rats (*Rattus norvegicus*) during mating, play, and aggression: Behavioral concomitants, relationship to reward, and self-administration of playback. *Journal of Comparative Psychology, 122,* 357–367.

Burgdorf, J., Panksepp, J., and Moskal, J. R. (2011). Frequency-modulated 50 kHz ultrasonic vocalizations: A tool for uncovering the molecular substrates of positive affect. *Neuroscience & Biobehavioral Reviews, 35,* 1831–1836.

Burgess, H. J., and Emens, J. S. (2018). Drugs used in circadian sleep-wake rhythm disturbances. *Sleep Medicine Clinics, 13*(2), 231–241.

Burmeister, M. A., Ayala, J. E., Smouse, H., Landivar-Rocha, A., et al. (2017). The hypothalamic glucagon-like peptide 1 receptor is sufficient but not necessary for the regulation of energy balance and glucose homeostasis in mice. *Diabetes, 66*(2), 372–384.

Bushdid, C., Magnasco, M. O., Vosshall, L. B., and Keller, A. (2014). Humans can discriminate more than 1 trillion olfactory stimuli. *Science, 343*(6177), 1370–1372.

Bushman, J. D., Ye, W., and Liman, E. R. (2015). A proton current associated with sour taste: Distribution and functional properties. *FASEB Journal, 29*, 3014–3026.

Buss, D. (2013). *Evolutionary psychology: The new science of the mind.* New York, NY: Psychology Press.

Butler, A. C., Chapman, J. E., Forman, E. M., and Beck, A. T. (2006). The empirical status of cognitive-behavioral therapy: A review of meta-analyses. *Clinical Psychology Review, 26*, 17–31.

Byne, W., Tobet, S., Mattiace, L. A., Lasco, M. S., et al. (2001). The interstitial nuclei of the human anterior hypothalamus: An investigation of variation with sex, sexual orientation, and HIV status. *Hormones and Behavior, 40*, 86–92.

C

Cade, J. F. (1949). Lithium salts in the treatment of psychotic excitement. *Medical Journal of Australia, 2*(10), 349–352.

Cahill, L. (2014). Equal ≠ the same: Sex differences in the human brain. *Cerebrum.* Apr 1, 5. eCollection 2014 (http://www.dana.org/Cerebrum/2014/Equal_%E2%89%A0_The_Same__Sex_Differences_in_the_Human_Brain/).

Cahill, L., and McGaugh, J. L. (1991). NMDA-induced lesions of the amygdaloid complex block the retention-enhancing effect of posttraining epinephrine. *Psychobiology, 19*, 206–210.

Calvert, G. A., Bullmore, E. T., Brammer, M. J., Campbell, R., et al. (1997). Activation of auditory cortex during silent lipreading. *Science, 276*, 593–596.

Calvin, W. H., and Ojemann, G. A. (1994). *Conversation's with Neil's brain: The neural nature of thought and language.* Reading, MA: Adison-Wesley.

Cameron, J. L., Eagleson, K. L., Fox, N. A., Hensch, T. K., et al. (2017). Social origins of developmental risk for mental and physical illness. *Journal of Neuroscience, 37*(45), 10783–10791.

Campbell, F. W., and Robson, J. G. (1968). Application of Fourier analysis to the visibility of gratings. *Journal of Physiology (London), 197*, 551–566.

Cannon, W. B. (1929). *Bodily changes in pain, hunger, fear and rage.* New York, NY: Appleton.

Cantalupo, C., and Hopkins, W. D. (2001). Asymmetric Broca's area in great apes. *Nature, 414*, 505.

Cantor, J. M., Blanchard, R., Paterson, A. D., and Bogaert, A. F. (2002). How many gay men owe their sexual orientation to fraternal birth order? *Archives of Sexual Behavior, 31*, 63–71.

Cao, M., Shu, N., Cao, Q., Wang, Y., et al. (2014). Imaging functional and structural brain connectomics in attention-deficit/hyperactivity disorder. *Molecular Neurobiology, 50*, 1111–1123.

Caramazza, A., Anzellotti, S., Strnad, L., and Lingnau, A. (2014). Embodied cognition and mirror neurons: A critical assessment. *Annual Review of Neuroscience, 37*, 1–15.

Cardenas, V. A., Studholme, C., Gazdzinski, S., Durazzo, T. C., et al. (2006). Deformation-based morphometry of brain changes in alcohol dependence and abstinence. *NeuroImage, 34*(3), 879–887.

Cardno, A. G., and Gottesman, I. I. (2000). Twin studies of schizophrenia: From bow-and-arrow concordances to Star Wars Mx and functional genomics. *American Journal of Medical Genetics, 97*, 12–17.

Carey, B. (2018, June 8). How suicide quietly morphed into a public health crisis. *The New York Times*, p. A21.

Cargnelutti, E., Tomasino, B., and Fabbro, F. (2019). Language brain representation in bilinguals with different age of appropriation and proficiency of the second language: A meta-analysis of functional imaging studies. *Frontiers in Human Neuroscience, 13*, 154.

Carhart-Harris, R. L., Bolstridge, M., Rucker, J., Day, C. M., et al. (2016). Psilocybin with psychological support for treatment-resistant depression: An open-label feasibility study. *Lancet Psychiatry, 3*(7), 619–627.

Carhart-Harris, R. L., Erritzoe, D., Williams, T., Stone, J. M., et al. (2012). Neural correlates of the psychedelic state as determined by fMRI studies with psilocybin. *Proceedings of the National Academy of Sciences, USA, 109*, 2138–2143.

Carlson, P. J., Diazgranados, N., Nugent, A. C., Ibrahim, L., et al. (2013). Neural correlates of rapid antidepressant response to ketamine in treatment-resistant unipolar depression: A preliminary positron emission tomography study. *Biological Psychiatry, 73*(12), 1213–1221.

Carr, G. V., and Lucki, I. (2011). The role of serotonin receptor subtypes in treating depression: A review of animal studies. *Psychopharmacology (Berlin), 213*(2–3), 265–287.

Carr, T. (2018). The problem with sleeping pills. *Consumer Reports* (https://www.consumerreports.org/drugs/the-problem-with-sleeping-pills/).

Carreiras, M., Lopez, J., Rivero, F., and Corina, D. (2005). Linguistic perception: Neural processing of a whistled language. *Nature, 433*, 31–32.

Carretié, L. (2014). Exogenous (automatic) attention to emotional stimuli: A review. *Cognitive, Affective, & Behavioral Neuroscience, 14*(4), 1228–1258.

Carter, C. S. (2017). The oxytocin-vasopressin pathway in the context of love and fear. *Frontiers in Endocrinology (Lausanne), 8*, 356.

Caruso, S., Mauro, D., Scalia, G., Palermo, C. I., et al. (2017). Oxytocin plasma levels in orgasmic and anorgasmic women. *Gynecological Endocrinology, 34*(1), 69–72. https://doi.org/10.1080/09513590.2017.1336219

Carvalho, L. S., Pessoa, D. M. A., Mountford, J. K., Davies, W. I. L., et al. (2017). The genetic and evolutionary drives behind primate color vision. *Frontiers in Ecology and Evolution*, 26 April 2017. |https://doi.org/10.3389/fevo.2017.00034

Casarosa, S., Bozzi, Y., and Conti, L. (2014). Neural stem cells: Ready for therapeutic applications? *Molecular and Cellular Therapies, 2*, 31.

Caterina, M. J., Leffler, A., Malmberg, A. B., Martin, W. J., et al. (2000). Impaired nociception and pain sensation in mice lacking the capsaicin receptor. *Science, 288*, 306–313.

CDC (Centers for Disease Control and Prevention). (2010). Current depression among adults—United States, 2006 and 2008. *Morbidity and Mortality Weekly Report, 59*, 1229–1235 (www.cdc.gov/mmwr/preview/mmwrhtml/mm5938a2.htm).

CDC (Centers for Disease Control and Prevention). (2015). *Report to Congress on traumatic brain injury in the United States: Epidemiology and rehabilitation.* Atlanta, GA: National Center for Injury Prevention and Control, Division of Unintentional Injury Prevention.

CDC (Centers for Disease Control and Prevention). (2016). Fetal alcohol spectrum disorders (FASDs), www.cdc.gov/ncbddd/fasd/alcohol-use.html.

Celeghin, A., de Gelder, B., and Tamietto, M. (2015). From affective blindsight to emotional consciousness. *Consciousness and Cognition, 36*, 414–425.

Chamberlain, S. R., Menzies, L., Hampshire, A., Suckling, J., et al. (2008). Orbitofrontal dysfunction in patients with obsessive-compulsive disorder and their unaffected relatives. *Science, 321*, 421–422.

Champagne, F., Diorio, J., Sharma, S., and Meaney, M. J. (2001). Naturally occurring variations in maternal behavior in the rat are associated with differences in estrogen-inducible central oxytocin receptors.

Proceedings of the National Academy of Sciences, USA, 98, 12736–12741.

Chan, M. Y., Na, J., Agres, P. F., Savalia, N. K., et al. (2018). Socioeconomic status moderates age-related differences in the brain's functional network organization and anatomy across the adult lifespan. *Proceedings of the National Academy of Sciences, USA, 115*(22), E5144–E5153.

Chandrashekar, J., Hoon, M. A., Ryba, N. J., and Zuker, C. S. (2006). The receptors and cells for mammalian taste. *Nature, 444*, 288–294.

Chandrashekar, J., Kuhn, C., Oka, Y., Yarmolinsky, D. A., et al. (2010). The cells and peripheral representation of sodium taste in mice. *Nature, 464*, 297–301.

Chandrashekar, J., Mueller, K. L., Hoon, M. A., Adler, E., et al. (2000). T2Rs function as bitter taste receptors. *Cell, 100*, 703–711.

Chandrashekar, J., Yarmolinsky, D., von Buchholtz, L., Oka, Y., et al. (2009). The taste of carbonation. *Science, 326*, 443–445.

Chang, B. S., Ly, J., Appignani, B., Bodell, A., et al. (2005). Reading impairment in the neuronal migration disorder of periventricular nodular heterotopia. *Neurology, 64*, 799–803.

Chapman, C. D., Dono, L. M., French, M. C., Weinberg, Z. Y., et al. (2012). Paraventricular nucleus anandamide signaling alters eating and substrate oxidation. *NeuroReport, 23*, 425–429.

Charney, D. S., Deutch, A. Y., Krystal, J. H., Southwick, S. M., et al. (1993). Psychobiologic mechanisms of posttraumatic stress disorder. *Archives of General Psychiatry, 50*, 295–305.

Charpentier, P., Gailliot, P., Jacob, R., Gaudechon, J., et al. (1952). Recherches sur les diméthylaminopropyl-N phénothiazines substituées. *Comptes rendus de l'Académie des Sciences (Paris), 235*, 59–60.

Chaudhari, N., Landin, A. M., and Roper, S. D. (2000). A metabotropic glutamate receptor variant functions as a taste receptor. *Nature Neuroscience, 3*, 113–119.

Chelikani, P. K., Haver, A. C., and Reidelberger, R. D. (2005). Intravenous infusion of peptide YY(3-36) potently inhibits food intake in rats. *Endocrinology, 146*, 879–888.

Cheney, D. L., and Seyfarth, R. M. (2018). Flexible usage and social function in primate vocalizations. *Proceedings of the National Academy of Sciences, USA, 115*(9), 1974–1979.

Cherdieu, M., Versace, R., Rey, A. E., Vallet, G. T., et al. (2018). Sleep on your memory traces: How sleep effects can be explained by Act-In, a functional memory model. *Sleep Medicine Reviews, 39*, 155–163.

Cherry, E. C. (1953). Some experiments on the recognition of speech, with one and with two ears. *Journal of the Acoustical Society of America, 25*, 975–979.

Cheyne, J. A. (2002). Situational factors affecting sleep paralysis and associated hallucinations: Position and timing effects. *Journal of Sleep Research, 11*, 169–177.

Chiaravalloti, A., Micarelli, A., Ricci, M., Pagani, M., et al. (2019). Evaluation of task-related brain activity: Is there a role for 18F FDG-PET imaging? *BioMed Research International, 4762404*. https://doi.org/10.1155/2019/4762404

Chiu, A. (2018, April 27). Female athletes with naturally high testosterone levels face hurdles under new IAAF rules. *Washington Post* (https://www.washingtonpost.com/news/morning-mix/wp/2018/04/27/female-athletes-with-naturally-high-testosterone-levels-face-hurdles-under-new-iaaf-rules/).

Cho, I., Yamanishi, S., Cox, L., Methé, B. A., et al. (2012). Antibiotics in early life alter the murine colonic microbiome and adiposity. *Nature, 488*(7413), 621–626.

Chong, D. J., and Dugan, P.; EPGP Investigators. (2016). Ictal fear: Associations with age, gender, and other experiential phenomena. *Epilepsy & Behavior, 62*, 153–158.

Choquet, D., and Triller, A. (2013). The dynamic synapse. *Neuron, 80*(3), 691–703.

Chung, W. S., Welsh, C. A., Barres, B. A., and Stevens, B. (2015). Do glia drive synaptic and cognitive impairment in disease? *Nature Neuroscience, 18*(11), 1539–1545.

Ciccocioppo, R., Martin-Fardon, R., and Weiss, F. (2004). Stimuli associated with a single cocaine experience elicit long-lasting cocaine-seeking. *Nature Neuroscience, 7*, 495–496.

Cipriani, A., Furukawa, T. A., Salanti, G., Chaimani, A., et al. (2018). Comparative efficacy and acceptability of 21 antidepressant drugs for the acute treatment of adults with major depressive disorder: A systematic review and network meta-analysis. *Lancet, 391*(10128), 1357–1366.

Clarke, E., Reichard, U. H., and Zuberbühler, K. (2015). Context-specific close-range "hoo" calls in wild gibbons (*Hylobates lar*). *BMC Evolutionary Biology, 15*, 56.

Clarke, M. C., Tanskanen, A., Huttunen, M., Leon, D. A., et al. (2011). Increased risk of schizophrenia from additive interaction between infant motor developmental delay and obstetric complications: Evidence from a population-based longitudinal study. *American Journal of Psychiatry, 168*, 1295–1302.

Cogan, G. B., Thesen, T., Carlson, C., Doyle, W., et al. (2014). Sensory-motor transformations for speech occur bilaterally. *Nature, 507*(7490), 94–98.

Coghill, R. C., McHaffie, J. G., and Yen, Y.-F. (2003). Neural correlates of interindividual differences in the subjective experience of pain. *Proceedings of the National Academy of Sciences, USA, 100*, 8538–8542.

Cohen, S., Alper, C. M., Doyle, W. H., Treanor, J. J., et al. (2006). Positive emotional style predicts resistance to illness after experimental exposure to rhinovirus or influenza A virus. *Psychosomatic Medicine, 68*, 809–815.

Cohen, S., Doyle, W. J., Alper, C. M., Janicki-Deverts, D., et al. (2009). Sleep habits and susceptibility to the common cold. *Archive of Internal Medicine, 169*, 62–67.

Cohen, S., Janicki-Deverts, D., Turner, R. B., and Doyle, W. J. (2015). Does hugging provide stress-buffering social support? A study of susceptibility to upper respiratory infection and illness. *Psychological Science, 26*(2), 135–147.

Cohen, S., Lichtenstein, E., Prochaska, J. O., Rossi, J. S., et al. (1989). Debunking myths about quitting: Evidence from 10 perspective studies of persons who attempt to quit smoking by themselves. *American Psychologist, 44*, 1355–1365.

Cole, J. (1995). *Pride and a daily marathon.* Cambridge, MA: MIT Press.

Cole, J. (2016). *Losing touch: A man without his body.* Oxford, UK: Oxford University Press.

Coleman, J. H., Lin, B., Louie, J. D., Peterson, J., et al. (2019). Spatial determination of neuronal diversification in the olfactory epithelium. *Journal of Neuroscience, 39*(5), 814–832.

Colman, R. J., Beasley, T. M., Kemnitz, J. W., Johnson, S. C., et al. (2014). Caloric restriction reduces age-related and all-cause mortality in rhesus monkeys. *Nature Communications, 5*, 3557.

Conel, J. L. (1939). *The postnatal development of the human cerebral cortex: Vol. 1. The cortex of the newborn.* Cambridge, MA: Harvard University Press.

Connolly, A. C., Guntupalli, J. S., Gors, J., et al. (2012). The representation of biological classes in the human brain. *Journal of Neuroscience, 32*(8), 2608–2618.

Cooke, B. M., Breedlove, S. M., and Jordan, C. L. (2003). Both estrogen receptors and androgen receptors contribute to testosterone-induced changes in the morphology of the medial amygdala and sexual arousal in male rats. *Hormones and Behavior, 43*, 336–346.

Cooke, J. R., and Ancoli-Israel, S. (2011). Normal and abnormal sleep in the elderly. *Handbook of Clinical Neurology, 98*, 653–665.

Cope, L. M., Ermer, E., Gaudet, L. M., Steele, V. R., et al. (2014). Abnormal brain structure in youth who commit homicide. *NeuroImage: Clinical, 4*, 800–807.

Corballis, M. C. (2014). Left brain, right brain: Facts and fantasies. *PLOS Biology, 12*(1), e1001767.

Corballis, M. C. (2020). Crossing the Rubicon: Behaviorism, language, and evolutionary continuity. *Frontiers in Psychology, 11*, 653.

Corbetta, M., Kincade, J. M., Ollinger, J. M., McAvoy, M. P., et al. (2000). Voluntary orienting is dissociated from target detection in human posterior parietal cortex. *Nature Neuroscience, 3*, 292–297.

Corbetta, M., and Shulman, G. L. (1998). Human cortical mechanisms of visual attention during orienting and search. *Philosophical Transactions of the Royal Society of London. Series B: Biological Sciences, 353*, 1353–1362.

Corbetta, M., and Shulman, G. L. (2002). Control of goal-directed and stimulus-driven attention in the brain. *Nature Reviews Neuroscience, 3*, 201–215.

Coricelli, G., Critchley, H. D., Joffily, M., O'Doherty, J. P., et al. (2005). Regret and its avoidance: A neuroimaging study of choice behavior. *Nature Neuroscience, 8*, 1255–1262.

Corina, D. P., Gibson, E. K., Martin, R., Poliakov, A., et al. (2005). Dissociation of action and object naming: Evidence from cortical stimulation mapping. *Human Brain Mapping, 24*(1), 1–10.

Corina, D. P., Lawyer, L. A., and Cates, D. (2013). Cross-linguistic differences in the neural representation of human language: Evidence from users of signed languages. *Frontiers in Psychology, 3*, 587.

Corkin, S. (2002). What's new with the amnesic patient H.M.? *Neuroscience, 3*, 153–159.

Corkin, S., Amaral., D. G., Gonzalez, R. G., Johnson, K. A., et al. (1997). H.M.'s medial temporal lobe lesion: Findings from magnetic resonance imaging. *Journal of Neuroscience, 17*, 3964–3979.

Correll, C. U., Rubio, J. M., Inczedy-Farkas, G., Birnbaum, M. L., et al. (2017). Efficacy of 42 pharmacologic cotreatment strategies added to antipsychotic monotherapy in schizophrenia: Systematic overview and quality appraisal of the meta-analytic evidence. *JAMA Psychiatry, 74*(7), 675–684.

Costa, A., and Sebastián-Gallés, N. (2014). How does the bilingual experience sculpt the brain? *Nature Reviews Neuroscience, 15*(5), 336–345.

Cox, J. H., Seri, S., and Cavanna, A. E. (2018). Sensory aspects of Tourette syndrome. *Neuroscience & Biobehavioral Reviews, 88*, 170–176.

Cox, J. J., Reimann, F., Nicholas, A. K., Thornton, G., et al. (2006). An *SCN9A* channelopathy causes congenital inability to experience pain. *Nature, 444*, 894–898.

Cox, L. M., and Blaser, M. J. (2015). Antibiotics in early life and obesity. *Nature Reviews Endocrinology, 11*(3), 182–190.

Cox, S. S., Speaker, K. J., Beninson, L. A., Craig, W. C., et al. (2014). Adrenergic and glucocorticoid modulation of the sterile inflammatory response. *Brain, Behavior, and Immunity, 36*, 183–192.

Cragg, B. G. (1975). The development of synapses in the visual system of the cat. *Journal of Comparative Neurology, 160*, 147–166.

Crews, F. T., Vetreno, R. P., Broadwater, M. A., and Robinson, D. L. (2016). Adolescent alcohol exposure persistently impacts adult neurobiology and behavior. *Pharmacological Reviews, 68*(4), 1074–1109.

Crick, F. C., and Koch, C. (2005). What is the function of the claustrum? *Philosophical Transactions of the Royal Society of London. Series B: Biological Sciences, 360*(1458), 1271–1279.

Crivelli, C., Russell, J. A., Jarillo, S., and Fernández-Dols, J. M. (2016). The fear gasping face as a threat display in a Melanesian society. *Proceedings of the National Academy of Sciences, USA, 113*(44), 12403–12407.

Crockford, C., Wittig, R. M., Mundry, R., and Zuberbühler, K. (2012). Wild chimpanzees inform ignorant group members of danger. *Current Biology, 22*, 142–146.

Crossley, N. A., Constante, M., McGuire, P., and Power, P. (2010). Efficacy of atypical v. typical antipsychotics in the treatment of early psychosis: Meta-analysis. *British Journal of Psychiatry, 196*(6), 434–439.

Croston, R., Branch, C. L., Kozlovsky, D. Y., Roth, T. C., II, et al. (2015). Potential mechanisms driving population variation in spatial memory and the hippocampus in food-caching chickadees. *Integrative and Comparative Biology, 55*(3), 354–371.

Crunelle, C. L., Kaag, A. M., van Wingen, G., van den Munkhof, H. E., et al. (2014). Reduced frontal brain volume in non-treatment-seeking cocaine-dependent individuals: Exploring the role of impulsivity, depression, and smoking. *Frontiers in Human Neuroscience, 8*, 7.

Cummings, D. E. (2006). Ghrelin and the short- and long-term regulation of appetite and body weight. *Physiology & Behavior, 89*, 71–84.

Curran, H. V., Freeman, T. P., Mokrysz, C., Lewis, D. A, et al. (2016). Keep off the grass? Cannabis, cognition and addiction. *Nature Reviews Neuroscience, 17*(5), 293–306.

Curtis, V., Aunger, R., and Rabie, T. (2004). Evidence that disgust evolved to protect from risk of disease. *Proceedings of the Royal Society of London. Series B: Biological Sciences, 271*(Suppl. 4), S131–S133.

Curtiss, S. (1989). The independence and task-specificity of language. In M. H. Bornstein and J. S. Bruner (Eds.), *Interaction in human development* (pp. 105–137). Hillsdale, NJ: Erlbaum.

Cussotto, S., Sandhu, K. V., Dinan, T. G., and Cryan, J. F. (2018, May 14). The neuroendocrinology of the microbiota-gut-brain axis: A behavioural perspective. *Frontiers in Neuroendocrinology*, pii: S0091-3022(18)30039-6.

D

Dale, R. C., Heyman, I., Giovannoni, G., and Church, A. W. (2005). Incidence of anti-brain antibodies in children with obsessive-compulsive disorder. *British Journal of Psychiatry, 187*, 314–319.

Damasio, A. R., Grabowski, T. J., Bechara, A., Damasio, H., et al. (2000). Subcortical and cortical brain activity during the feeling of self-generated emotions. *Nature Neuroscience, 3*, 1049–1056.

Damasio, H., Grabowski, T., Frank, R., Galaburda, A. M., et al. (1994). The return of Phineas Gage: Clues about the brain from the skull of a famous patient. *Science, 264*, 1102–1105.

Damassa, D. A., Smith, E. R., Tennent, B., and Davidson, J. M. (1977). The relationship between circulating testosterone levels and male sexual behavior in rats. *Hormones and Behavior, 8*, 275–286.

Daniels, D., and Marshall, A. (2012). Evaluating the potential for rostral diffusion in the cerebral ventricles using angiotensin II–induced drinking in rats. *Brain Research, 1486*, 62–67.

Darwin, C. (1872). The expression of the emotions in man and animals. London, UK: J. Murray.

Davey, C. G., Breakspear, M., Pujol, J., and Harrison, B. J. (2017). A brain model of disturbed self-appraisal in depression. *American Journal of Psychiatry, 174*(9), 895–903.

David, L. A., Maurice, C. F., Carmody, R. N., Gootenberg, D. B., et al. (2014). Diet rapidly and reproducibly alters the human gut microbiome. *Nature, 505*(7484), 559–563.

Davis, J. I., Senghas, A., and Ochsner, K. N. (2009). How does facial feedback modulate emotional experience? *Journal of Research in Personality, 43*, 822–829.

Davis, M. C., Horan, W. P., and Marder, S. R. (2014). Psychopharmacology of the negative symptoms: Current status and prospects for progress. *European Neuropsychopharmacology, 24*(5), 788–799.

Davis, N. (2018, April 10). Man eats world's hottest chilli pepper—and ends up in hospital. *Guardian*. ww.theguardian.com/science/2018/apr/09/competitive-eater-taken-to-hospital-after-eating-worlds-hottest-chilli-pepper.

De Boeck, P., and Jeon, M. (2018). Perceived crisis and reforms: Issues, explanations, and remedies. *Psychological Bulletin, 144*(7), 757–777.

De Gelder, B., Hortensius, R., and Tamietto, M. (2012). Attention and awareness each influence amygdala activity for dynamic bodily expressions: A short review. *Frontiers in Integrative Neuroscience, 6*, 54.

De Gelder, B., Tamietto, M., van Boxtel, G., Goebel, R., et al. (2008). Intact navigation skills after bilateral loss of striate cortex. *Current Biology, 18,* R1128–R1129.

De Groot, C. M., Janus, M. D., and Bornstein, R. A. (1995). Clinical predictors of psychopathology in children and adolescents with Tourette syndrome. *Journal of Psychiatric Research, 29,* 59–70.

De Groot, J. H., Semin, G. R., and Smeets, M. A. (2017). On the communicative function of body odors. *Perspectives on Psychological Science, 12*(2), 306–324.

De Heer, W. A., Huth, A. G., Griffiths, T. L., Gallant, J. L., et al. (2017). The hierarchical cortical organization of human speech processing. *Journal of Neuroscience, 37*(27), 6539–6557.

De Jong, M., Schoorl, M., and Hoek, H. W. (2018). Enhanced cognitive behavioural therapy for patients with eating disorders: A systematic review. *Current Opinion in Psychiatry, 31*(6), 436–444.

De Kloet, E. R., and Joëls, M. (2017). Brain mineralocorticoid receptor function in control of salt balance and stress-adaptation. *Physiology & Behavior, 178,* 13–20.

De Kluiver, H., Buizer-Voskamp, J. E., Dolan, C. V., and Boomsma, D. I. (2017). Paternal age and psychiatric disorders: A review. *American Journal of Medical Genetics Part B: Neuropsychiatric Genetics, 174*(3), 202–213.

De la Monte, S. M., and Kril, J. J. (2014). Human alcohol-related neuropathology. *Acta Neuropathologica, 127*(1), 71–90.

De La Vega, D., Giner, L., and Courtet, P. (2018). Suicidality in subjects with anxiety or obsessive-compulsive and related disorders: Recent advances. *Current Psychiatry Reports, 20*(4), 26. https://doi.org/10.1007/s11920-018-0885-z

De Luca, M., Pizzamiglio, M. R., Di Vita, A., Palermo, L., et al. (2019). First the nose, last the eyes in congenital prosopagnosia: Look like your father looks. *Neuropsychology, 33*(6), 855–861.

De Quervain, D., Schwabe, L., and Roozendaal, B. (2017). Stress, glucocorticoids and memory: Implications for treating fear-related disorders. *Nature Reviews Neuroscience, 18*(1), 7–19.

De Valois, R. L., and De Valois, K. K. (1988). *Spatial vision.* New York, NY: Oxford University Press.

De Valois, R. L., and De Valois, K. K. (1993). A multi-stage color model. *Vision Research, 33,* 1053–1065.

De Win, M. M., Jager, G., Booij, J., Reneman, L., et al. (2008). Sustained effects of ecstasy on the human brain: A prospective neuroimaging study in novel users. *Brain, 131*(Pt. 11), 2936–2945.

Dearborn, G. V. N. (1932). A case of congenital general pure analgesia. *Journal of Nervous and Mental Disease, 75,* 612–615.

Dehaene, S., and Changeux, J. P. (2011). Experimental and theoretical approaches to conscious processing. *Neuron, 70*(2), 200–227.

Dehaene-Lambertz, G., Dehaene, S., and Hertz-Pannier, L. (2002). Functional neuroimaging of speech perception in infants. *Science, 298,* 2013–2015.

Del Campo, N., Fryer, T. D., Hong, Y. T., Smith, R., et al. (2013). A positron emission tomography study of nigro-striatal dopaminergic mechanisms underlying attention: Implications for ADHD and its treatment. *Brain, 136*(11), 3252–3270.

Delgado, J. M. R. (1969). *Physical control of the mind: Toward a psychocivilized society.* New York, NY: Harper & Row.

Dement, W. C. (1974). *Some must watch while some must sleep.* San Francisco, CA: W.H. Freeman.

Dempsey-Jones, H., Wesselink, D. B., Friedman, J., and Makin, T. R. (2019). Organized toe maps in extreme foot users. *Cell Reports, 28*(11), 2748–2756.

Den Heijer, A. E., Groen, Y., Tucha, L., Fuermaier, A. B., et al. (2017). Sweat it out? The effects of physical exercise on cognition and behavior in children and adults with ADHD: A systematic literature review. *Journal of Neural Transmission (Vienna), 124*(Suppl. 1), 3–26.

Denis, D. (2018). Relationships between sleep paralysis and sleep quality: Current insights. *Nature and Science of Sleep, 10,* 355–367.

Denson, T. F., O'Dean, S. M., Blake, K. R., and Beames, J. R. (2018). Aggression in women: Behavior, brain and hormones. *Frontiers in Behavioral Neuroscience, 12,* 81.

Denton, D., Shade, R., Zamarippa, F., Egan, G., et al. (1999). Neuroimaging of genesis and satiation of thirst and an interoceptor-driven theory of origins of primary consciousness. *Proceedings of the National Academy of Sciences, USA, 96,* 5304–5309.

Depaepe, V., Suarez-Gonzalez, N., Dufour, A., Passante, L., et al. (2005). Ephrin signalling controls brain size by regulating apoptosis of neural progenitors. *Nature, 435,* 1244–1250.

DePaoli, A. M. (2014). 20 years of leptin: Leptin in common obesity and associated disorders of metabolism. *Journal of Endocrinology, 223*(1), T71–T81.

DeRubeis, R. J., Siegle, G. J., and Hollon, S. D. (2008). Cognitive therapy versus medication for depression: Treatment outcomes and neural mechanisms. *Nature, 9,* 788–796.

Devane, W. A., Dysarz, F. A., Johnson, M. R., Melvin, L. S., et al. (1988). Determination and characterization of a cannabinoid receptor in rat brain. *Molecular Pharmacology, 34,* 605–613.

Devane, W. A., Hanus, L., Breuer, A., Pertwee, R. G., et al. (1992). Isolation and structure of a brain constituent that binds the cannabinoid receptor. *Science, 258,* 1946–1949.

Devlin, J. T., and Watkins, K. E. (2007). Stimulating language: Insights from TMS. *Brain, 130*(Pt. 3), 610–622.

DeVoogd, T. J. (1994). Interactions between endocrinology and learning in the avian song system. *Annals of the New York Academy of Sciences, 743,* 19–41.

Dewan, A., Pacifico, R., Zhan, R., Rinberg, D., et al. (2013). Non-redundant coding of aversive odours in the main olfactory pathway. *Nature, 497*(7450), 486–489.

Dhabhar, F. S. (2018). The short-term stress response: Mother nature's mechanism for enhancing protection and performance under conditions of threat, challenge, and opportunity. *Frontiers in Neuroendocrinology, 49,* 175–192.

Di Marzo, V., and Matias, I. (2005). Endocannabinoid control of food intake and energy balance. *Nature Neuroscience, 8,* 585–589.

Diamond, A. (2013). Executive functions. *Annual Review of Psychology, 64,* 135–168.

Diamond, M. C. (1967). Extensive cortical depth measurements and neuron size increases in the cortex of environmentally enriched rats. *Journal of Comparative Neurology, 131,* 357–364.

Diamond, M. C., Lindner, B., Johnson, R., Bennett, E. L., et al. (1975). Differences in occipital cortical synapses from environmentally enriched, impoverished, and standard colony rats. *Journal of Neuroscience Research, 1,* 109–119.

Diana, M., Raij, T., Melis, M., Nummenmaa, A., et al. (2017). Rehabilitating the addicted brain with transcranial magnetic stimulation. *Nature Reviews Neuroscience, 18*(11), 685–693.

Dietz, P. M., Williams, S. B., Callaghan, W. M., Bachman, D. J., et al. (2007). Clinically identified maternal depression before, during, and after pregnancies ending in live births. *American Journal of Psychiatry, 164,* 1457–1459.

Dinh, H. T., Nishimaru, H., Matsumoto, J., Takamura, Y., et al. (2018). Superior neuronal detection of snakes and conspecific faces in the macaque medial prefrontal cortex. *Cerebral Cortex, 28*(6), 2131–2145.

Do, M. T. H., Kang, S. H., Zue, T., Zhong, H., et al. (2009). Photon capture and signalling by melanopsin retinal ganglion cells. *Nature, 457,* 281–287.

Dohanich, G. (2003). Ovarian steroids and cognitive function. *Current Directions in Psychological Science, 12,* 57–61.

Dohrenwend, B. P., Turner, J. B., Turse, N. A., Adams, B. G., et al. (2006). The psychological risks of Vietnam for U.S. veterans: A revisit with new data and methods. *Science, 313,* 979–982.

Dolan, R. J. (2002). Emotion, cognition, and behavior. *Science, 298*, 1191–1194.

Dolder, C. R., and Nelson, M. H. (2008). Hypnosedative-induced complex behaviours: Incidence, mechanisms and management. *CNS Drugs, 22*, 1021–1036.

Dolensek, N., Gehrlach, D. A., Klein, A. S., and Gogolla, N. (2020). Facial expressions of emotion states and their neural correlates in mice. *Science, 368*(6486), 89–94.

Dominguez, J., Riolo, J. V., Xu, Z., and Hull, E. M. (2001). Regulation by the medial amygdala of copulation and medial pre-optic dopamine release. *Journal of Neuroscience, 21*(1), 349–355.

Domjan, M., and Purdy, J. E. (1995). Animal research in psychology: More than meets the eye of the general psychology student. *American Psychologist, 50*, 496–503.

Donaldson, Z. R., and Young, L. J. (2008). Oxytocin, vasopressin, and the neurogenetics of sociality. *Science, 322*, 900–903.

Dorsaint-Pierre, R., Penhune, V. B., Watkins, K. E., Neelin, P., et al. (2006). Asymmetries of the planum temporale and Heschl's gyrus: Relationship to language lateralization. *Brain, 129*, 1164–1176.

Doyle, S., and Menaker, M. (2007). Circadian photoreception in vertebrates. *Cold Spring Harbor Symposia on Quantitative Biology, 72*, 499–508.

Dreger, A. (2018, April 27). Track's absurd new rules for women. *New York Times* (https://www.nytimes.com/2018/04/27/opinion/caster-semenya-intersex-athletes.html).

Drew, T., Võ, M. L., and Wolfe, J. M. (2013). The invisible gorilla strikes again: Sustained inattentional blindness in expert observers. *Psychological Science, 24*(9), 1848–1853.

Dronkers, N. F., Plaisant, O., Iba-Zizen, M. T., and Cabanis, E. A. (2007). Paul Broca's historic cases: High resolution MR imaging of the brains of Leborgne and Lelong. *Brain, 130* (5), 1432–1441.

Dronkers, N. F., Wilkins, D. P., Van Valin, R. D., Jr., Redfern, B. B., et al. (2004). Lesion analysis of the brain areas involved in language comprehension. *Cognition, 92*, 145–177.

Droutman, V., Read, S. J., and Bechara, A. (2015). Revisiting the role of the insula in addiction. *Trends in Cognitive Sciences, 19*(7), 414–420.

Druckman, D., and Bjork, R. A. (1994). *Learning, remembering, believing: Enhancing human performance*. Washington, DC: National Academies Press.

Duchaine, B., Germine, L., and Nakayama, K. (2007). Family resemblance: Ten family members with prosopagnosia and within-class object agnosia. *Cognitive Neuropsychology, 24*, 419–430.

Duchamp-Viret, P., Chaput, M. A., and Duchamp, A. (1999). Odor response properties of rat olfactory receptor neurons. *Science, 284*, 2171–2174.

Duffy, J. D., and Campbell, J. J. (1994). The regional prefrontal syndromes: A theoretical and clinical overview. *Journal of Neuropsychiatry and Clinical Neurosciences, 6*, 379–387.

Duffy, M. E., Twenge, J. M., and Joiner, T. E. (2019). Trends in mood and anxiety symptoms and suicide-related outcomes among U.S. undergraduates, 2007–2018: Evidence from two national surveys. *Journal of Adolescent Health, 65*(5), 590–598.

Dulac, C., and Torello, A. T. (2003). Molecular detection of pheromone signals in mammals, from genes to behaviour. *Nature Reviews Neuroscience, 4*, 551–562.

Dulak, J., Szade, K., Szade, A., Nowak, W., et al. (2015). Adult stem cells: Hopes and hypes of regenerative medicine. *Acta Biochimica Polonica, 62*(3), 329–337.

Dully, H., and Fleming, C. (2007). *My lobotomy*. New York, NY: Crown.

Durand-de Cuttoli, R., Mondoloni, S., Marti, F., Lemoine, D., et al. (2018). Manipulating midbrain dopamine neurons and reward-related behaviors with light-controllable nicotinic acetylcholine receptors. *eLife, 7*, e37487.

E

Eapen, V., Cavanna, A. E., and Robertson, M. M. (2016). Comorbidities, social impact, and quality of life in Tourette syndrome. *Frontiers in Psychiatry, 7*, 97.

Ebbinghaus, H. (1908). *Psychology: An elementary textbook*. Boston: Heath.

Edwards, R. R., Grace, E., Peterson, S., Klick, B., et al. (2009). Sleep continuity and architecture: Associations with pain-inhibitory processes in patients with temporomandibular joint disorder. *European Journal of Pain, 13*, 1043–1047.

Eklund, A., Nichols, T. E., and Knutsson, H. (2016). Cluster failure: Why fMRI inferences for spatial extent have inflated false-positive rates. *Proceedings of the National Academy of Sciences, USA, 113*(28), 7900–7905.

Ekström, P., and Meissl, H. (2003). Evolution of photosensory pineal organs in new light: The fate of neuroendocrine photoreceptors. *Philosophical Transactions of the Royal Society of London. Series B: Biological Sciences, 358*(1438), 1679–1700.

Ellenbogen, J. M., Hu, P. T., Payne, J. D., Titone, D., et al. (2007). Human relational memory requires time and sleep. *Proceedings of the National Academy of Sciences, USA, 104*, 7317–7318.

Ellis, H. D., and Lewis, M. B. (2001). Capgras delusion: A window on face recognition. *Trends in Cognitive Sciences, 5*(4), 149–156.

Elmer, S., Hänggi, J., and Jäncke, L. (2016). Interhemispheric transcallosal connectivity between the left and right planum temporale predicts musicianship, performance in temporal speech processing, and functional specialization. *Brain Structure and Function, 221*(1), 331–344.

Emborg, M. E., Liu, Y., Xi, J., Zhang, X., et al. (2013). Induced pluripotent stem cell–derived neural cells survive and mature in the nonhuman primate brain. *Cell Reports, 3*(3), 646–650.

Emery, N. J., Capitanio, J. P., Mason, W. A., Machado, C. J., et al. (2001). The effects of bilateral lesions of the amygdala on dyadic social interactions in rhesus monkeys (*Macaca mulatta*). *Behavioral Neuroscience, 115*, 515–544.

Engel, J., Jr. (1992). Recent advances in surgical treatment of temporal lobe epilepsy. *Acta Neurologica Scandinavica. Supplementum, 140*, 71–80.

English, P. J., Ghatei, M. A., Malik, I. A., Bloom, S. R., et al. (2002). Food fails to suppress ghrelin levels in obese humans. *Journal of Clinical Endocrinology and Metabolism, 87*, 2984–2987.

Erlanger, D. M., Kutner, K. C., Barth, J. T., and Barnes, R. (1999). Neuropsychology of sports-related head injury: Dementia pugilistica to post concussion syndrome. *Clinical Neuropsychologist, 13*, 193–209.

Eroglu, C., and Barres, B. A. (2010). Regulation of synaptic connectivity by glia. *Nature, 468*(7321), 223–231.

Erren, T. C., Morfeld, P., Stork, J., Knauth, P., et al. (2009). Shift work, chronodisruption and cancer?—The IARC 2007 challenge for research and prevention and 10 theses from the Cologne Colloquium 2008. *Scandinavian Journal of Work, Environment & Health, 35*, 74–79.

Evans, J. R., and Lawrenson, J. G. (2017). Antioxidant vitamin and mineral supplements for slowing the progression of age-related macular degeneration. *Cochrane Database of Systematic Reviews, 7*, CD000254.

Everson, C. A., Bergmann, B. M., and Rechtschaffen, A. (1989). Sleep deprivation in the rat: III. Total sleep deprivation. *Sleep, 12*, 13–21.

F

Falk, D. (2004). Prelinguistic evolution in early hominins: Whence motherese? *Behavioral and Brain Sciences, 27*, 491–503.

Falkner, A. L., Grosenick, L., Davidson, T. J., Deisseroth, K., et al. (2016). Hypothalamic control of male aggression-seeking behavior. *Nature Neuroscience, 19*(4), 596–604.

Faraone, S. V. (2018). The pharmacology of amphetamine and methylphenidate: Relevance to the neurobiology of attention-deficit/hyperactivity disorder and other psychiatric comorbidities. *Neuroscience & Biobehavioral Reviews, 87*, 255–270.

Faraone, S. V., Glatt, S. J., Su, J., and Tsuang, M. T. (2004). Three potential susceptibility loci shown by a genome-wide scan for regions influencing the age at onset of mania. *American Journal of Psychiatry, 161,* 625–630.

Farrell, A. K., Slatcher, R. B., Tobin, E. T., Imami, L., et al. (2018). Socioeconomic status, family negative emotional climate, and anti-inflammatory gene expression among youth with asthma. *Psychoneuroendocrinology, 91,* 62–67.

Farrell, M. J., Bowala, T. K., Gavrilescu, M., Phillips, P. A., et al. (2011). Cortical activation and lamina terminalis functional connectivity during thirst and drinking in humans. *American Journal of Physiology—Regulatory, Integrative and Comparative Physiology, 301,* R623–R631.

Faurie, C., Vianey-Liaud, N., and Raymond, M. (2006). Do left-handed children have advantages regarding school performance and leadership skills? *Laterality, 11*(1), 57–70. https://doi.org/10.1080/13576500500294620

Fay, R. R. (1988). *Hearing in vertebrates: A psychophysics databook.* Winnetka, IL: Hill-Fay Associates.

FBI. (2018). Crime in the United States, https://ucr.fbi.gov/crime-in-the-u.s/2018/crime-in-the-u.s.-2018. Tables 39 and 40.

Feduccia, A. A., Jerome, L., Yazar-Klosinski, B., Emerson, A., et al. (2019). Breakthrough for trauma treatment: Safety and efficacy of MDMA-assisted psychotherapy compared to paroxetine and sertraline. *Frontiers in Psychiatry, 10,* 650.

Feinstein, J. S., Adolphs, R., Damasio, A., and Tranel, D. (2011). The human amygdala and the induction and experience of fear. *Current Biology, 21,* 34–38.

Feinstein, J. S., Buzza, C., Hurelmann, R., Follmer, R. L., et al. (2013). Fear and panic in humans with bilateral amygdala damage. *Nature Neuroscience, 16,* 270–272.

Felleman, D. J., and Van Essen, D. C. (1991). Distributed hierarchical processing in the primate cerebral cortex. *Cerebral Cortex, 1,* 1–47.

Feng, W., Störmer, V. S., Martinez, A., McDonald, J. J., et al. (2017). Involuntary orienting of attention to a sound desynchronizes the occipital alpha rhythm and improves visual perception. *NeuroImage, 150,* 318–328.

Fernández-Espejo, D., and Owen, A. M. (2013). Detecting awareness after severe brain injury. *Nature Reviews Neuroscience, 14*(11), 801–809.

Ferri, S. L., Hildebrand, P. F., Way, S. E., and Flanagan-Cato, L. M. (2014). Estradiol regulates markers of synaptic plasticity in the hypothalamic ventromedial nucleus and amygdala of female rats. *Hormones and Behavior, 66*(2), 409–420.

Finch, C. E., and Kirkwood, T. B. L. (2000). *Chance, development, and aging.* New York, NY: Oxford University Press.

Finger, S. (1994). *Origins of neuroscience: A history of explorations into brain function.* New York, NY: Oxford University Press.

Fink, M., and Taylor, M. A. (2007). Electroconvulsive therapy: Evidence and challenges. *JAMA, 298,* 330–332.

Fisher, S. E. (2017). Evolution of language: Lessons from the genome. *Psychonomic Bulletin & Review, 24*(1), 34–40.

Flegal, K. M., Carroll, M. D., Ogden, C. L., and Johnson, C. L. (2002). Prevalence and trends in obesity among US adults, 1999–2000. *JAMA, 288*(14),1723–1727.

Fleming, A. S., Kraemer, G. W., Gonzalez, A., Lovic, V., et al. (2002). Mothering begets mothering: The transmission of behavior and its neurobiology across generations. *Pharmacology, Biochemistry, and Behavior, 73,* 61–75.

Foerster, O., and Penfield, W. (1930). The structural basis of traumatic epilepsy and results of radical operation. *Brain, 53,* 8–119.

Foley, C., Corvin, A., and Nakagome, S. (2017). Genetics of schizophrenia: Ready to translate? *Current Psychiatry Reports, 19*(9), 61.

Forger, N. G., and Breedlove, S. M. (1987). Seasonal variation in mammalian striated muscle mass and motoneuron morphology. *Journal of Neurobiology, 18,* 155–165.

Forger, N. G., Ruszkowski, E., Jacobs, A., and Wallen, K. (2018). Effects of sex and prenatal androgen manipulations on Onuf's nucleus of rhesus macaques. *Hormones and Behavior, 100,* 39–46.

Foster, G. D., Wyatt, H. R., Hill, J. O., McGuckin, B. G., et al. (2003). A randomized trial of a low-carbohydrate diet for obesity. *New England Journal of Medicine, 348,* 2082–2090.

Foster, R. G., Peirson, S. N., Wulff, K., Winnebeck, E., et al. (2013). Sleep and circadian rhythm disruption in social jetlag and mental illness. *Progress in Molecular Biology and Translational Science, 119,* 325–346.

Fothergill, E., Guo, J., Howard, L., Kerns, J. C., et al. (2016). Persistent metabolic adaptation 6 years after "The Biggest Loser" competition. *Obesity (Silver Spring), 24*(8), 1612–1619.

Fournier, J. C., DeRubeis, R. J., Hollon, S. D., Dimidjian, S., et al. (2010). Antidepressant drug effects and depression severity: A patient-level meta-analysis. *JAMA, 303,* 47–53.

Francis, D. D., Szegda, K., Campbell, G., Martin, W. D., et al. (2003). Epigenetic sources of behavioral differences in mice. *Nature Neuroscience, 6,* 445–446.

Frankenhaeuser, M. (1978). Psychoneuroendocrine approaches to the study of emotion as related to stress and coping. *Nebraska Symposium on Motivation, 26,* 123–162.

Franklin, T. R., Acton, P. D., Maldjian, J. A., Gray, J. D., et al. (2002). Decreased gray matter concentration in the insular, orbitofrontal, cingulate, and temporal cortices of cocaine patients. *Biological Psychiatry, 51,* 134–142.

Franks, N. P. (2008). General anaesthesia: From molecular targets to neuronal pathways of sleep and arousal. *Nature, 9,* 370–386.

Franssen, C. L., Bardi, M., Shea, E. A., Hampton, J. E., et al. (2011). Fatherhood alters behavioural and neural responsiveness in a spatial task. *Journal of Neuroendocrinology, 23,* 1177–1187.

Freeman, A. M., Petrilli, K., Lees, R., Hindocha, C., et al. (2019). How does cannabidiol (CBD) influence the acute effects of delta-9-tetrahydrocannabinol (THC) in humans? A systematic review. *Neuroscience & Biobehavioral Reviews, 107,* 696–712.

Freeman, T. P., Hindocha, C., Green, S. F., and Bloomfield, M. A. P. (2019). Medicinal use of cannabis based products and cannabinoids. *British Medical Journal, 365,* l1141.

Freiwald, W. A., Tsao, D. Y., and Livingstone, M. S. (2009). A face feature space in the macaque temporal lobe. *Nature Neuroscience, 12,* 1187–1196.

French, C. A., and Fisher, S. E. (2014). What can mice tell us about Foxp2 function? *Current Opinion in Neurology, 28,* 72–79.

Frey, S. H., Bogdanov, S., Smith, J. C., Watrous, S., et al. (2008). Chronically deafferented sensory cortex recovers a grossly typical organization after allogenic hand transplantation. *Current Biology, 18,* 1530–1534.

Fried, I., Wilson, C. L., MacDonald, K. A., and Behnke, E. J. (1998). Electric current stimulates laughter. *Nature, 391,* 650.

Friedman, B. H. (2010). Feelings and the body: The Jamesian perspective on autonomic specificity of emotion. *Biological Psychology, 84*(3), 383–393.

Fritz, J., Shamma, S., Elhilali, M., and Klein, D. (2003). Rapid task-related plasticity of spectrotemporal receptive fields in primary auditory cortex. *Nature Neuroscience, 6,* 1216–1223.

Fuller, D. E., and Hornfeldt, C. S. (2012). From club drug to orphan drug: Sodium oxybate (Xyrem) for the treatment of cataplexy. *Pharmacotherapy, 23*(9), 1205–1209.

Fulton, B. D., Scheffler, R. M., Hinshaw, S. P., Levine, P., et al. (2009). National variation of ADHD diagnostic prevalence and medication use: Health care providers and education policies. *Psychiatric Services, 60,* 1075–1083.

Fung, T. C., Olson, C. A., and Hsiao, E. Y. (2017). Interactions between the microbiota, immune and nervous systems in health and disease. *Nature Neuroscience, 20*(2), 145–155.

Furukawa, E., Bado, P., Tripp, G., Mattos, P., et al. (2014). Abnormal striatal BOLD responses to reward anticipation and reward delivery in ADHD. *PLOS ONE, 9*(2), e89129.

Fuster, J. M. (1990). Prefrontal cortex and the bridging of temporal gaps in the perception-action cycle. *Annals of the New York Academy of Sciences, 608*, 318–336.

G

Gabel, L. A., Gibson, C. J., Gruen, J. R., and LoTurco, J. J. (2010). Progress towards a cellular neurobiology of reading disability. *Neurobiology of Disease, 38*(2), 173–180.

Galaburda, A. M. (1994). Developmental dyslexia and animal studies: At the interface between cognition and neurology. *Cognition, 56*, 833–839.

Galaburda, A. M., LoTurco, J., Ramus, F., Fitch, R. H., et al. (2006). From genes to behavior in developmental dyslexia. *Nature Neuroscience, 9*, 1213–1217.

Galaburda, A. M., Sherman, G. F., Rosen, G. D., Aboitiz, F., et al. (1985). Developmental dyslexia: Four consecutive patients with cortical anomalies. *Annals of Neurology, 18*(2), 222–233. https://doi.org/10.1002/ana.410180210

Gallagher, M., Okonkwo, O. C., Resnick, S. M., Jagust, W. J., et al. (2019). What are the threats to successful brain and cognitive aging? *Neurobiology of Aging, 83*, 130–134.

Gallant, J. L., Braun, J., and Van Essen, D. C. (1993). Selectivity for polar, hyperbolic, and Cartesian gratings in macaque visual cortex. *Science, 259*, 100–103.

Gallese, V., and Sinigaglia, C. (2011). What is so special about embodied simulation? *Trends in Cognitive Sciences, 15*, 512–519.

Gallopin, T., Fort, P., Eggermann, E., Cauli, B., et al. (2000). Identification of sleep-promoting neurons in vitro. *Nature, 404*, 992–995.

Ganel, T., and Goodale, M. A. (2019). Still holding after all these years: An action-perception dissociation in patient DF. *Neuropsychologia, 128*, 249–254. https://doi.org/10.1016/j.neuropsychologia.2017.09.016

Gangwisch, J. E., Heymsfield, S. B., Boden-Albala, B., Buijs, R. M., et al. (2007). Sleep duration as a risk factor for diabetes incidence in a large U.S. sample. *Sleep, 30*, 1667–1673.

Gannon, P. J., Holloway, R. L., Broadfield, D. C., and Braun, A. R. (1998). Asymmetry of chimpanzee planum temporale: Human-like pattern of brain language area homolog. *Science, 279*, 220–222.

Gardner, E. L. (2011). Addiction and brain reward and antireward pathways. *Advances in Psychosomatic Medicine, 30*, 22–60.

Gardner, R. A., and Gardner, B. T. (1969). Teaching sign language to a chimpanzee. *Science, 165*, 664–672.

Gardner, R. A., and Gardner, B. T. (1984). A vocabulary test for chimpanzees (*Pan troglodytes*). *Journal of Comparative Psychology, 98*, 381–404.

Garfield, A. S., Li, C., Madara, J. C., Shah, B. P., et al. (2015). A neural basis for melanocortin-4 receptor-regulated appetite. *Nature Neuroscience, 18*(6), 863–871.

Garver, D. L., Holcomb, J. A., and Christensen, J. D. (2000). Heterogeneity of response to antipsychotics from multiple disorders in the schizophrenia spectrum. *Journal of Clinical Psychiatry, 61*, 964–972.

Gasser, P., Holstein, D., Michel, Y., Doblin, R., et al. (2014). Safety and efficacy of lysergic acid diethylamide-assisted psychotherapy for anxiety associated with life-threatening diseases. *Journal of Nervous and Mental Disease, 202*(7), 513–520.

Gassmann, M., and Bettler, B. (2012). Regulation of neuronal GABA$_B$ receptor functions by subunit composition. *Nature Reviews Neuroscience, 13*, 380–394.

Gates, N. J, and Sachdev, P. (2014). Is cognitive training an effective treatment for preclinical and early Alzheimer's disease? *Journal of Alzheimer's Disease, 42*, S551–S559.

Gazzaniga, M. S. (2008). *Human: The science behind what makes your brain unique.* New York, NY: Ecco.

Gazzaniga, M. S., and Smylie, C. S. (1983). Facial recognition and brain asymmetries: Clues to underlying mechanisms. *Annals of Neurology, 13*, 536–540.

Geers, A. E., Mitchell, C. M., Warner-Czyz, A., Wang, N. Y., et al. (2017). Early sign language exposure and cochlear implantation benefits. *Pediatrics, 140*(1), e20163489.

Gelber, R. P., Redline, S., Ross, G. W., Petrovitch, H., et al. (2015). Associations of brain lesions at autopsy with polysomnography features before death. *Neurology, 84*, 296–303.

Géléoc, G. S., and Holt, J. R. (2014). Sound strategies for hearing restoration. *Science, 344*(6184), 1241062.

Gelstein, S., Yeshurun, Y., Rozenkrantz, L., Shushan, S., et al. (2011). Human tears contain a chemosignal. *Science, 331*, 226–230.

Geniole, S. N., and Carré, J. M. (2018). Human social neuroendocrinology: Review of the rapid effects of testosterone. *Hormones and Behavior, 104*, 192–205.

Gentilucci, M., and Dalla Volta, R. (2008). Spoken language and arm gestures are controlled by the same motor control system. *Quarterly Journal of Experimental Psychology (Hove), 61*(6), 944–957. https://doi.org/10.1080/17470210701625683

George, D. T., Phillips, M. J., Lifshitz, M., Lionetti, T. A., et al. (2011). Fluoxetine

treatment of alcoholic perpetrators of domestic violence: A 12-week, double-blind, randomized, placebo-controlled intervention study. *Journal of Clinical Psychiatry, 72*(1), 60–65.

Georgiadis, J. R., Reinders, A. A., Paans, A. M., Renken, R., et al. (2009). Men versus women on sexual brain function: Prominent differences during tactile genital stimulation, but not during orgasm. *Human Brain Mapping, 10*, 3089–3101.

Georgopoulos, A. P., Kalaska, J. F., Caminiti, R., and Massey, J. T. (1982). On the relations between the direction of two-dimensional arm movements and cell discharge in primate motor cortex. *Journal of Neuroscience, 2*, 1527–1537.

Gerashchenko, D., Kohls, M. D., Greco, M. A., Waleh, N. S., et al. (2001). Hypocretin-2-saporin lesions of the lateral hypothalamus produce narcoleptic-like sleep behavior in the rat. *Neuroscience, 21*, 7273–7283.

Gerkin, R. C., and Castro, J. B. (2015). The number of olfactory stimuli that humans can discriminate is still unknown. *eLife, 4*, e08127.

Geschwind, N. (1972). Language and the brain. *Scientific American, 226*(4), 76–83.

Geschwind, N. (1979). Specializations of the human brain. *Scientific American, 241*(3), 180–199.

Geschwind, N., and Levitsky, W. (1968). Human brain: Left-right asymmetries in temporal speech region. *Science, 161*, 186–187.

Gibbons, R. D., Hur, K., Brown, C. H., Davis, J. M., et al. (2012). Benefits from antidepressants: Synthesis of 6-week patient-level outcomes from double-blind placebo-controlled randomized trials of fluoxetine and venlafaxine. *Archives of General Psychiatry, 69*, 572–579.

Gilbertson, M. W., Shenton, M. E., Ciszewski, A., Kasai, K., et al. (2002). Smaller hippocampal volume predicts pathologic vulnerability to psychological trauma. *Nature Neuroscience, 5*, 1242–1247.

Gill, R. E., Tibbitts, T. L., Douglas, D. C., Hanel, C. M., et al. (2009). Extreme endurance flights by landbirds crossing the Pacific Ocean: Ecological corridor rather than barrier? *Proceedings of the Royal Society of London. Series B: Biological Sciences, 276*, 447–457.

Gillin, J. C., Duncan, W. C., Murphy, D. L., Post, R. M., et al. (1981). Age-related changes in sleep in depressed and normal subjects. *Psychiatry Research, 4*, 73–78.

Giustino, T. F., Fitzgerald, P. J., and Maren, S. (2016). Revisiting propranolol and PTSD: Memory erasure or extinction enhancement? *Neurobiology of Learning and Memory, 130*, 26–33.

Glaser, R., and Kiecolt-Glaser, J. K. (2005). Stress-induced immune dysfunction:

Implications for health. *Nature Reviews Immunology, 5*(3), 243–251.

Glasser, M. F., Coalson, T. S., Robinson, E. C., Hacker, C. D., et al. (2016). A multi-modal parcellation of human cerebral cortex. *Nature, 536*(7615), 171–178.

Glenn, A. L., and Raine, A. (2014). Neurocriminology: Implications for the punishment, prediction and prevention of criminal behaviour. *Nature Reviews Neuroscience, 15*(1), 54–63.

Glickman, S. E. (1977). Comparative psychology. In P. Mussen and M. R. Rosenzweig (Eds.), *Psychology: An introduction* (2nd ed., pp. 625–703). Lexington, MA: Heath.

Gogtay, N., Giedd, J. N., Lusk, L., Hayashi, K. M., et al. (2004). Dynamic mapping of human cortical development during childhood through early adulthood. *Proceedings of the National Academy of Sciences, USA, 101*, 8174–8179.

Gold, B. P., Mas-Herrero, E., Zeighami, Y., Benovoy, M., et al. (2019). Musical reward prediction errors engage the nucleus accumbens and motivate learning. *Proceedings of the National Academy of Sciences, USA, 116*(8), 3310–3315.

Goldin, P. R., and Gross, J. J. (2010). Effects of mindfulness-based stress reduction (MBSR) on emotion regulation in social anxiety disorder. *Emotion, 10*, 83–91.

Goldstein, J. M., Seidman, L. J., Horton, N. J., Makris, N., et al. (2001). Normal sexual dimorphism of the adult human brain assessed by in vivo magnetic resonance imaging. *Cerebral Cortex, 11*, 490–497.

Golomb, J., de Leon, M. J., George, A. E., Kluger, A., et al. (1994). Hippocampal atrophy correlates with severe cognitive impairment in elderly patients with suspected normal pressure hydrocephalus. *Journal of Neurology, Neurosurgery and Psychiatry, 57*, 590–593.

Gonçalves, T. C., Londe, A. K., Albano, R. I., et al. (2014). Cannabidiol and endogenous opioid peptide-mediated mechanisms modulate antinociception induced by transcutaneous electrostimulation of the peripheral nervous system. *Journal of Neurological Sciences, 347*, 82–89.

Gooch, C. L., Pracht, E., and Borenstein, A. R. (2017). The burden of neurological disease in the United States: A summary report and call to action. *Annals of Neurology, 81*(4), 479–484.

Gooley, J. J., Rajaratnam, S. M., Brainard, G. C., Kronauer, R. E., et al. (2010). Spectral responses of the human circadian system depend on the irradiance and duration of exposure to light. *Science Translational Medicine, 2*, 31ra33.

Gorski, R. A. (2002). Hypothalamic imprinting by gonadal steroid hormones. *Advances in Experimental Medicine and Biology, 511*, 57–70.

Gorski, R. A., Gordon, J. H., Shryne, J. E., and Southam, A. M. (1978). Evidence for a morphological sex difference within the medial preoptic area of the rat brain. *Brain Research, 148*, 333–346.

Gorzalka, B. B., Mendelson, S. D., and Watson, N. V. (1990). Serotonin receptor subtypes and sexual behavior. *Annals of the New York Academy of Sciences, 600*, 435–444.

Gosseries, O., Di, H., Laureys, S., and Boly, M. (2014). Measuring consciousness in severely damaged brains. *Annual Review of Neuroscience, 37*, 457–478.

Goswami, U. (2015). Sensory theories of developmental dyslexia: Three challenges for research. *Nature Reviews Neuroscience, 16*(1), 43–54.

Gottesman, I. I. (1991). *Schizophrenia genesis: The origins of madness*. New York, NY: Freeman.

Gottfried, J. A., O'Doherty, J., and Dolan, R. J. (2003). Encoding predictive reward value in human amygdala and orbitofrontal cortex. *Science, 301*, 1104–1107.

Gottlieb, J. (2007). From thought to action: The parietal cortex as a bridge between perception, action, and cognition. *Neuron, 53*, 9–16.

Gough, P. M., Nobre, A. C., and Devlin, J. T. (2005). Dissociating linguistic processes in the left inferior frontal cortex with transcranial magnetic stimulation. *Journal of Neuroscience, 25*, 8010–8016.

Gougler, M., Nelson, R., Handler, M., Krapohl, D., et al. (2011). Meta-analytic survey of criterion accuracy of validated polygraph techniques. *Polygraph, 40*(4), 203–305.

Goutman, J. D., Elgoyhen, A. B., and Gómez-Casati, M. E. (2015). Cochlear hair cells: The sound-sensing machines. *FEBS Letters, 589*(22):3354–3361.

Gravett, N., Bhagwandin, A., Sutcliffe, R., Landen, K., et al. (2017). Inactivity/sleep in two wild free-roaming African elephant matriarchs: Does large body size make elephants the shortest mammalian sleepers? *PLOS ONE, 12*(3), e0171903.

Gray, J. D., Kogan, J. F., Marrocco, J., and McEwen, B. S. (2017). Genomic and epigenomic mechanisms of glucocorticoids in the brain. *Nature Reviews Endocrinology, 13*(11), 661–673.

Gray, N. S., MacCulloch, M. J., Smith, J., Morris, M., et al. (2003). Violence viewed by psychopathic murderers. *Nature, 423*, 497.

Graziano, M. (2006). The organization of behavioral repertoire in motor cortex. *Annual Review of Neuroscience, 29*, 105–134.

Graziano, M. S., and Aflalo, T. N. (2007). Mapping behavioral repertoire onto the cortex. *Neuron, 56*, 239–251.

Green, J. J., Boehler, C. N., Roberts, K. C., Chen, L. C., et al. (2017). Cortical and subcortical coordination of visual spatial attention revealed by simultaneous EEG-fMRI recording. *Journal of Neuroscience, 37*(33), 7803–7810.

Green, J. J., Doesburg, S. M., Ward, L. M., and McDonald, J. J. (2011). Electrical neuroimaging of voluntary audiospatial attention: Evidence for a supramodal attention control network. *Journal of Neuroscience, 31*(10), 3560–3564.

Greenough, W. T. (1976). Enduring brain effects of differential experience and training. In M. R. Rosenzweig and E. L. Bennett (Eds.), *Neural mechanisms of learning and memory* (pp. 255–278). Cambridge, MA: MIT Press.

Gregory, R. L., and Wallace, J. G. (1963). Recovery from early blindness: A case study. *Experimental Psychology Society Monograph, 2*, 1–44.

Grieb, Z. A., and Ragan, C. M. (2019). The effects of perinatal SSRI exposure on anxious behavior and neurobiology in rodent and human offspring. *European Neuropsychopharmacology, 29*(11), 1169–1184.

Grill-Spector, K., Weiner, K. S., Kay, K., and Gomez, J. (2017). The functional neuroanatomy of human face perception. *Annual Review of Vision Science, 3*, 167–196.

Grimm, S., and Bajbouj, M. (2010). Efficacy of vagus nerve stimulation in the treatment of depression. *Expert Review of Neurotherapeutics, 19*, 87–92.

Grob, C. S., Danforth, A. L., Chopra, G. S., Hagerty, M., et al. (2011). Pilot study of psilocybin treatment for anxiety in patients with advanced-stage cancer. *Archives of General Psychiatry, 68*(1), 71–78.

Gross, J. (2019). Magnetoencephalography in cognitive neuroscience: A primer. *Neuron, 104*(2), 189–204.

Groth, C. (2018). Tourette syndrome in a longitudinal perspective: Clinical course of tics and comorbidities, coexisting psychopathologies, phenotypes and predictors. *Danish Medical Journal, 65*(4), B5465.

Grover, G. J., Mellstrom, K., Ye, L., Malm, J., et al. (2003). Selective thyroid hormone receptor-β activation: A strategy for reduction of weight, cholesterol, and lipoprotein (a) with reduced cardiovascular liability. *Proceedings of the National Academy of Sciences, USA, 100*, 10067–10072.

Grumbach, M. M., and Auchus, R. J. (1999). Estrogen: Consequences and implications of human mutations in synthesis and action. *Journal of Clinical Endocrinology and Metabolism, 84*, 4677–4694.

Grunt, J. A., and Young, W. C. (1953). Consistency of sexual behavior patterns in individual male guinea pigs following castration and androgen therapy. *Journal of Comparative and Physiological Psychology, 46*, 138–144.

Grüter, T., Grüter, M., and Carbon, C. C. (2008). Neural and genetic foundations of face recognition and prosopagnosia. *Journal of Neuropsychology, 2,* 79–97.

Gu, X., Hof, P. R., Friston, K. J., and Fan, J. (2013). Anterior insular cortex and emotional awareness. *Journal of Comparative Neurology, 521*(15), 3371–3388.

Guarner, F., and Malagelada, J. R. (2003). Gut flora in health and disease. *Lancet, 361*(9356), 512–519.

Guina, J., and Merrill, B. (2018). Benzodiazepines I: Upping the care on downers: The evidence of risks, benefits and alternatives. *Journal of Clinical Medicine, 7*(2), E17. https://doi.org/10.3390/jcm7020017

Gulevich, G., Dement, W., and Johnson, L. (1966). Psychiatric and EEG observations on a case of prolonged (264 hours) wakefulness. *Archives of General Psychiatry, 15,* 29–35.

H

Haesler, S., Rochefort, C., Georgi, B., Licznerski, P., et al. (2007). Incomplete and inaccurate vocal imitation after knockdown of FoxP2 in songbird basal ganglia nucleus Area X. *PLOS Biology, 5,* e321.

Haggard, P. (2017). Sense of agency in the human brain. *Nature Reviews Neuroscience, 18*(4), 196–207.

Halford, J. C., Boyland, E. J., Blundell, J. E., Kirkham, T. C., et al. (2010). Pharmacological management of appetite expression in obesity. *Nature Reviews Endocrinology, 6*(5), 255–269.

Hall, K. D. (2018). The complicated relation between resting energy expenditure and maintenance of lost weight. *American Journal of Clinical Nutrition, 108*(4), 652–653.

Hallett, M. (2015). Tourette syndrome: Update. *Brain and Development, 37*(7), 651–655.

Halperin, A. (2018, January 29). Marijuana: Is it time to stop using a word with racist roots? *Guardian* (www.theguardian.com/society/2018/jan/29/marijuana-name-cannabis-racism).

Hamburger, V. (1975). Cell death in the development of the lateral motor column of the chick embryo. *Journal of Comparative Neurology, 160,* 535–546.

Hamson, D. K., Csupity, A. S., Ali, F. M., and Watson, N. V. (2009). Partner preference and mount latency are masculinized in androgen insensitive rats. *Physiology & Behavior, 98,* 25–30.

Hamson, D. K., and Watson, N. V. (2004). Regional brainstem expression of Fos associated with sexual behavior in male rats. *Brain Research, 1006,* 233–240.

Hancock, R., Pugh, K. R., and Hoeft, F. (2017). Neural noise hypothesis of developmental dyslexia. *Trends in Cognitive Sciences, 21*(6), 434–448.

Hanlon, C. A., Beveridge, T. J., and Porrino, L. J. (2013). Recovering from cocaine: Insights from clinical and preclinical investigations. *Neuroscience & Biobehavioral Reviews, 37*(9 Pt. A), 2037–2046.

Haque, S., Vaphiades, M. S., and Lueck, C. J. (2018). The visual agnosias and related disorders. *Journal of Neuro-Ophthalmology, 38*(3), 379–392.

Hare, R. D., Harpur, T. J., Hakstian, A. R., Forth, A. E., et al. (1990). The revised psychopathy checklist: Descriptive statistics, reliability, and factor structure. *Psychological Assessment, 2,* 338–341.

Harold, D., Paracchini, S., Scerri, T., Dennis, M., et al. (2006). Further evidence that the *KIAA0319* gene confers susceptibility to developmental dyslexia. *Molecular Psychiatry, 11,* 1085–1091, 1061.

Harrison, N. L., Skelly, M. J., Grosserode, E. K., Lowes, D. C., et al. (2017). Effects of acute alcohol on excitability in the CNS. *Neuropharmacology, 122,* 36–45.

Hartanto, T. A., Krafft, C. E., Iosif, A. M., and Schweitzer, J. B. (2016). A trial-by-trial analysis reveals more intense physical activity is associated with better cognitive control performance in attention-deficit/hyperactivity disorder. *Child Neuropsychology, 22*(5), 618–626.

Hartse, K. M. (2011). The phylogeny of sleep. *Handbook of Clinical Neurology, 98,* 97–109.

Haynes, K. F., Gemeno, C., Yeargan, K. V., Millar, J. G., et al. (2002). Aggressive chemical mimicry of moth pheromones by a bolas spider: How does this specialist predator attract more than one species of prey? *Chemoecology, 12,* 99–105.

He, D. Z., Lovas, S., Ai, Y., Li, Y., et al. (2014). Prestin at year 14: Progress and prospect. *Hearing Research, 311,* 25–35.

Heath, R. G. (1972). Pleasure and brain activity in man. *Journal of Nervous and Mental Diseases, 154,* 3–18.

Heaton, R. K., Chelune, G. J., Talley, J. L., Kay, G. G., et al. (1993). *Wisconsin Card Sorting Test manual: Revised and expanded.* Odessa, FL: Psychological Assessment Resources.

Hebb, D. O. (1949). *The organization of behavior.* New York, NY: Wiley.

Heffner, H. E., and Heffner, R. S. (1984). Temporal lobe lesions and perception of species-specific vocalizations by macaques. *Science, 226*(4670), 75–76.

Heidenreich, M., Lechner, S. G., Vardanyan, V., Wetzel, C., et al. (2011). KCNQ4 K(+) channels tune mechanoreceptors for normal touch sensation in mouse and man. *Nature Neuroscience, 15,* 138–145.

Heilbronner, S. R., and Hayden, B. Y. (2016). Dorsal anterior cingulate cortex: A bottom-up view. *Annual Review of Neuroscience, 39,* 149–170.

Heinrichs, R. W. (2003). Historical origins of schizophrenia: Two early madmen and

their illness. *Journal for the History of Behavioral Sciences, 39,* 349–363.

Helfrich, R. F., and Knight, R. T. (2019). Cognitive neurophysiology: Event-related potentials. *Handbook of Clinical Neurology, 160,* 543–558.

Helmholtz, H. von. (1962). *Treatise on physiological optics* (J. P. C. Southall, Trans.). New York, NY: Dover. (Original work published 1894.)

Henry, J. F., and Sherwin, B. B. (2012). Hormones and cognitive functioning during late pregnancy and postpartum: A longitudinal study. *Behavioral Neuroscience, 126,* 73–85.

Herbst, C. T., Stoeger, A. S., Frey, R., Lohscheller, J., et al. (2012). How low can you go? Physical production mechanism of elephant infrasonic vocalizations. *Science, 337*(6094), 595–599.

Herculano-Houzel, S. (2012). The remarkable, yet not extraordinary, human brain as a scaled-up primate brain and its associated cost. *Proceedings of the National Academy of Sciences, USA, 109*(Suppl. 1), 10661–10668.

Herculano-Houzel, S. (2014). The glia/neuron ratio: How it varies uniformly across brain structures and species and what that means for brain physiology and evolution. *Glia, 62*(9),1377–1391.

Herek, G. M., and McLemore, K. A. (2013). Sexual prejudice. *Annual Review of Psychology, 64,* 309–333.

Heres, S., Davis, J., Maino, K., Jetzinger, E., et al. (2006). Why olanzapine beats risperidone, risperidone beats quetiapine, and quetiapine beats olanzapine: An exploratory analysis of head-to-head comparison studies of second-generation antipsychotics. *American Journal of Psychiatry, 163,* 185–194.

Herrmann, C., and Knight, R. (2001). Mechanisms of human attention: Event-related potentials and oscillations. *Neuroscience and Biobehavioral Reviews, 25,* 465–476.

Hetherington, A. W., and Ranson, S. W. (1940). Hypothalamic lesions and adiposity in the rat. *Anatomical Record, 78,* 149–172.

Hickey, C., Di Lollo, V., and McDonald, J. J. (2009). Electrophysiological indices of target and distractor processing in visual search. *Journal of Cognitive Neuroscience, 21*(4), 760–775.

Hicks, M. J., De, B. P., Rosenberg, J. B., Davidson, J. T., et al. (2011). Cocaine analog coupled to disrupted adenovirus: A vaccine strategy to evoke high-titer immunity against addictive drugs. *Molecular Therapy, 19,* 612–619.

Hidaka, B. H. (2012). Depression as a disease of modernity: Explanations for increasing prevalence. *Journal of Affective Disorders, 140*(3), 205–214.

Higley, J. D., Mehlman, P. T., Taub, D. M., Higley, S. B., et al. (1992). Cerebrospinal fluid monoamine and adrenal correlates of aggression in free-ranging rhesus monkeys. *Archives of General Psychiatry, 49,* 436–441.

Hilker, R., Helenius, D., Fagerlund, B., Skytthe, A., et al. (2018). Heritability of schizophrenia and schizophrenia spectrum based on the nationwide Danish Twin Register. *Biological Psychiatry, 83*(6), 492–498.

Hill, K. (2020, January 19). The secretive company that might end privacy as we know it. *The New York Times* (https://www.nytimes.com/2020/01/18/technology/clearview-privacy-facial-recognition.html).

Hillhouse, T. M., and Porter, J. H. (2015). A brief history of the development of antidepressant drugs: From monoamines to glutamate. *Experimental and Clinical Psychopharmacology, 23*(1), 1–21.

Hillyard, S. A., Hink, R. F., Schwent, V. L., and Picton, T. W. (1973). Electrical signs of selective attention in the human brain. *Science, 182,* 177–180.

Hillyard, S. A., Störmer, V. S., Feng, W., Martinez, A., et al. (2016). Cross-modal orienting of visual attention. *Neuropsychologia, 83,* 170–178.

Hines, K. (2014) *Cracked, not broken.* Plymouth, UK: Rowman & Littlefield.

Hines, M. (2011). Prenatal endocrine influences on sexual orientation and on sexually differentiated childhood behavior. *Frontiers in Neuroendocrinology, 32*(2), 170–182. https://doi.org/10.1016/j.yfrne.2011.02.006

Hitt, E. (2007). Careers in neuroscience: From protons to poetry. *Science, 318,* 661–665.

Hobaiter, C., and Byrne, R. W. (2014). The meanings of chimpanzee gestures. *Current Biology, 24,* 1596–1600.

Hobson, J. A., and Friston, K. J. (2012). Waking and dreaming consciousness: Neurobiological and functional considerations. *Progress in Neurobiology, 98,* 82–98.

Hodgkin, A. L., and Katz, B. (1949). The effect of sodium ions on the electrical activity of the giant axon of the squid. *Journal of Physiology (London), 108,* 37–77.

Hoeft, F., Hernandez, A., McMillon, G., Taylor-Hill, H., et al. (2006). Neural basis of dyslexia: A comparison between dyslexic and nondyslexic children equated for reading ability. *Journal of Neuroscience, 26,* 10700–10708.

Hoekzema, E., Barba-Müller, E., Pozzobon, C., Picado, M., et al. (2017). Pregnancy leads to long-lasting changes in human brain structure. *Nature Neuroscience, 20*(2), 287–296.

Hofmann, S. G., Sawyer, A. T., Witt, A. A., and Oh, D. (2010). The effect of mindfulness-based therapy on anxiety and depression: A meta-analytic review. *Journal of Consulting and Clinical Psychology, 78,* 169–183.

Hogan, M., and Strasburger, V. (2020). Twenty questions (and answers) about media violence and cyberbullying. *Pediatric Clinics of North America, 67*(2), 275–291. https://doi.org/10.1016/j.pcl.2019.12.002

Hohmann, A. G., Suplita, R. L., Bolton, N. M., Neely, M. H., et al. (2005). An endocannabinoid mechanism for stress-induced analgesia. *Nature, 435,* 1108–1112.

Hohmann, G. W. (1966). Some effects of spinal cord lesions on experienced emotional feelings. *Psychophysiology, 3,* 143–156.

Hökfelt, T., Pernow, B., and Wahren, J. (2001). Substance P: A pioneer amongst neuropeptides. *Journal of Internal Medicine, 249*(1), 27–40.

Holschbach, M. A., Vitale, E. M., and Lonstein, J. S. (2018). Serotonin-specific lesions of the dorsal raphe disrupt maternal aggression and caregiving in postpartum rats. *Behavioural Brain Research, 348,* 53–64.

Holth, J. K., Fritschi, S. K., Wang, C., Pedersen, N. P., et al. (2019). The sleep-wake cycle regulates brain interstitial fluid tau in mice and CSF tau in humans. *Science, 363*(6429), 880–884.

Hopfinger, J. B., Buonocore, M. H., and Mangun, G. R. (2000). The neural mechanisms of top-down attentional control. *Nature Neuroscience, 3,* 284–291.

Hopfinger, J. B., Camblin, C. C., and Parks, E. L. (2010). Isolating the internal in endogenous attention. *Psychophysiology, 47*(4), 739–747.

Hopfinger, J., and Mangun, G. (1998). Reflexive attention modulates processing of visual stimuli in human extrastriate cortex. *Psychological Science, 6,* 441–447.

Hopkins, W. D., Misiura, M., Pope, S. M., and Latash, E. M. (2015). Behavioral and brain asymmetries in primates: A preliminary evaluation of two evolutionary hypotheses. *Annals of the New York Academy of Sciences, 1359,* 65–83.

Horn, H., Böhme, B., Dietrich, L., and Koch, M. (2018). Endocannabinoids in body weight control. *Pharmaceuticals (Basel), 11*(2), 55.

Horton, J. C., and Adams, D. L. (2005). The cortical column: A structure without a function. *Philosophical Transactions of the Royal Society of London. Series B: Biological Sciences, 360,* 837–862.

Howard-Jones, P. A. (2014). Neuroscience and education: Myths and messages. *Nature Reviews Neuroscience, 15*(12), 817–824.

Howland, R. H. (2007). Lithium: Underappreciated and underused? *Journal of Psychosocial Nursing and Mental Health Services, 45*(8), 13–17.

Hsu, M., Bhatt, M., Adolphs, R., Tranel, D., et al. (2005). Neural systems responding to degrees of uncertainty in human decision-making. *Science, 310,* 1680–1683.

Huang, A. L., Chen, X., Hoon, M. A., Chandrashekar, J., et al. (2006). The cells and logic for mammalian sour taste detection. *Nature, 442,* 934–938.

Huang, G., and Basaria, S. (2018). Do anabolic-androgenic steroids have performance-enhancing effects in female athletes? *Molecular and Cellular Endocrinology, 464,* 56–64.

Hubel, D. H., and Wiesel, T. N. (1959). Receptive fields of single neurones in the cat's striate cortex. *Journal of Physiology (London), 148,* 573–591.

Hubel, D. H., and Wiesel, T. N. (1962). Receptive fields, binocular interaction and functional architecture in the cat's visual cortex. *Journal of Physiology (London), 160,* 106–154.

Hubel, D. H., and Wiesel, T. N. (1965). Binocular interaction in striate cortex of kittens reared with artificial squint. *Journal of Neurophysiology, 28,* 1041–1059.

Huber, E., Webster, J. M., Brewer, A. A., MacLeod, D. I., et al. (2015). A lack of experience-dependent plasticity after more than a decade of recovered sight. *Psychological Science, 26*(4), 393–401.

Hudspeth, A. J. (2014). Integrating the active process of hair cells with cochlear function. *Nature Reviews Neuroscience, 15,* 600–614.

Hudspeth, A. J., Choe, Y., Mehta, A. D., and Martin, P. (2000). Putting ion channels to work: Mechanoelectrical transduction, adaptation, and amplification by hair cells. *Proceedings of the National Academy of Sciences, USA, 97,* 11765–11772.

Huedo-Medina, T. B., Kirsch, I., Middlemass, J., Klonizakis, M., et al. (2012). Effectiveness of non-benzodiazepine hypnotics in treatment of adult insomnia: Meta-analysis of data submitted to the Food and Drug Administration. *British Medical Journal, 345,* e8343.

Huettel, S. A., Stowe, C. J., Gordon, E. M., Warner, B. T., et al. (2006). Neural signatures of economic preferences for risk and ambiguity. *Neuron, 49,* 765–775.

Hughes, I. A., Houk, C., Ahmed, S. F., Lee, P. A., et al. (2006). Consensus statement on management of intersex disorders. *Journal of Pediatric Urology, 2*(3), 148–162.

Hughes, J., Smith, T. W., Kosterlitz, H. W., Fothergill, L. A., et al. (1975). Identification of two related pentapeptides from the brain with potent opiate agonist activity. *Nature, 258,* 577–580.

Hull, E. M., Muschamp, J. W., and Sato, S. (2004). Dopamine and serotonin: Influences on male sexual behavior. *Physiology & Behavior, 83*(2), 291–307. https://doi.org/10.1016/j.physbeh.2004.08.018

Hülsheger, U. R., and Schewe, A. F. (2011). On the costs and benefits of emotional labor: A meta-analysis of three decades of research. *Journal of Occupational Health Psychology, 16*(3), 361–389.

Human Rights Watch. (2017). *"I want to be like nature made me": Medically unnecessary surgeries on intersex children in the US.* New York, NY (https://www.hrw.org/sites/default/files/report_pdf/lgbtintersex0717_web_0.pdf).

Hurtado, M. D., Sergeyev, V. G., Acosta, A., Spegele, M., et al. (2013). Salivary peptide tyrosine-tyrosine 3-36 modulates ingestive behavior without inducing taste aversion. *Journal of Neuroscience, 33,* 18368–18380.

Hussain, S. J., and Cole, K. J. (2015). No enhancement of 24-hour visuomotor skill retention by post-practice caffeine administration. *PLOS ONE, 10*(6), e0129543.

Huston, N. J., Brenner, L. A., Taylor, Z. C., and Ritter, R. C. (2019). NPY2 receptor activation in the dorsal vagal complex increases food intake and attenuates CCK-induced satiation in male rats. *American Journal of Physiology—Regulatory, Integrative and Comparative Physiology, 316*(4), R406–R416.

Huth, A. G., de Heer, W. A., Griffiths, T. L., Theunissen, F. E., et al. (2016). Natural speech reveals the semantic maps that tile human cerebral cortex. *Nature, 532*(7600), 453–458.

Huttenlocher, P. R., and Dabholkar, A. S. (1997). Regional differences in synaptogenesis in human cerebral cortex. *Journal of Comparative Neurology, 387,* 167–178.

Hyde, J. S., and Mezulis, A. H. (2020). Gender differences in depression: Biological, affective, cognitive, and sociocultural factors. *Harvard Review of Psychiatry, 28*(1), 4–13.

Hyde, K. L., and Peretz I. (2004). Brains that are out of tune but in time. *Psychological Science, 15,* 356–360.

Hyde, K. L., Zatorre, R. J., Griffiths, T. D., Lerch, J. P., et al. (2006). Morphometry of the amusic brain: A two-site study. *Brain, 129,* 2562–2570.

Hyman, S. E. (2018). The daunting polygenicity of mental illness: Making a new map. *Philosophical Transactions of the Royal Society of London. Series B: Biological Sciences, 373*(1742), 20170031.

I

Ibrahim, C., Rubin-Kahana, D. S., Pushparaj, A., Musiol, M., et al. (2019). The insula: A brain stimulation target for the treatment of addiction. *Frontiers in Pharmacology, 10,* 720.

Igelström, K. M., and Graziano, M. S. A. (2017). The inferior parietal lobule and temporoparietal junction: A network perspective. *Neuropsychologia, 105,* 70–83.

Imai, T., Yamazaki, T., Kobayakawa, R., Kobayakawa, K., et al. (2009). Pre-target axon sorting establishes the neural map topography. *Science, 325,* 585–590.

Imeri, L., and Opp, M. R. (2009). How (and why) the immune system makes us sleep. *Nature Reviews Neuroscience, 10,* 199–210.

Imperato-McGinley, J. (2002). 5-alpha-reductase-2 deficiency and complete androgen insensitivity: Lessons from nature. *Advances in Experimental Medicine and Biology, 511,* 121–131; discussion 131–134.

Infurna, F. J., and Luthar, S. S. (2016). Resilience to major life stressors is not as common as thought. *Perspectives on Psychological Science, 11*(2), 175–194.

Insley, S. J. (2000). Long-term vocal recognition in the northern fur seal. *Nature, 406,* 404–405.

Institute of Medicine. (1990). *Broadening the base of treatment for alcohol problems.* Washington, DC: National Academies Press.

Institute of Medicine. (2010). *Gulf War and health: Vol. 8. Update of health effects of serving in the Gulf War.* Washington, DC: National Academies Press.

Intartaglia, B., White-Schwoch, T., Kraus, N., and Schön, D. (2017). Music training enhances the automatic neural processing of foreign speech sounds. *Scientific Reports, 7*(1), 12631.

Isles, A. R., Baum, M. J., Ma, D., Keverne, E. B., et al. (2001). Urinary odour preferences in mice. *Nature, 409,* 783–784.

J

Jackson, A. F., and Bolger, D. J. (2014). The neurophysiological bases of EEG and EEG measurement: A review for the rest of us. *Psychophysiology, 51*(11), 1061–1071.

Jacobs, G. H., Williams, G. A., Cahill, H., and Nathans, J. (2007). Emergence of novel color vision in mice engineered to express a human cone photopigment. *Science, 315,* 1723–1725.

Jacobs, J., Weidemann, C. T., Miller, J. F., Solway, A., et al. (2013). Direct recordings of grid-like neuronal activity in human spatial navigation. *Nature Neuroscience, 16*(9), 1188–1190.

Jain, R., and Correll, C. U. (2018). Tardive dyskinesia: Recognition, patient assessment, and differential diagnosis. *Journal of Clinical Psychiatry, Mar/Apr*(2), nu17034ah1c.

James, T. W., Culham, J., Humphery, G. K., Milner, A. D., et al. (2003). Ventral occipital lesions impair object recognition but not object-directed grasping: An fMRI study. *Brain, 126,* 2464–2475.

James, W. (1890). *Principles of psychology.* New York, NY: Holt.

Janak, P. H., and Tye, K. M. (2015). From circuits to behaviour in the amygdala. *Nature, 517*(7534), 284–292.

Janik, V. M. (2014). Cetacean vocal learning and communication. *Current Opinion in Neurobiology, 28,* 60–65. https://doi.org/10.1016/j.conb.2014.06.010

Jaskiw, G. E., and Popli, A. P. (2004). A meta-analysis of the response to chronic l-dopa in patients with schizophrenia: Therapeutic and heuristic implications. *Psychopharmacology (Berlin), 171,* 365–374.

Jasper, H., and Penfield, W. (1954). *Epilepsy and the functional anatomy of the human brain* (2nd ed.). New York, NY: Little, Brown.

Jenkins, J., and Dallenbach, K. (1924). Oblivescence during sleep and waking. *American Journal of Psychology, 35,* 605–612.

Jentsch, J. D., Redmond, D. E., Jr., Elsworth, J. D., Taylor, J. R., et al. (1997). Enduring cognitive deficits and cortical dopamine dysfunction in monkeys after long-term administration of phencyclidine. *Science, 277,* 953–955.

Jessen, N. A., Munk, A. S., Lundgaard, I., and Nedergaard, M. (2015). The glymphatic system: A beginner's guide. *Neurochemical Research, 40*(12), 2583–2599.

Johansson, R. S., and Flanagan, J. R. (2009). Coding and use of tactile signals from the fingertips in object manipulation tasks. *Nature Reviews Neuroscience, 10,* 345–358.

John, J., Wu, M. F., Maidment, N. T., Lam, H. A., et al. (2004). Developmental changes in CSF hypocretin-1 (orexin-A) levels in normal and genetically narcoleptic Doberman pinschers. *Journal of Physiology, 560*(Pt. 2), 587–592.

Jones, B. E. (2020). Arousal and sleep circuits. *Neuropsychopharmacology, 45*(1), 6–20.

Jones, H. J., Gage, S. H., Heron, J., Hickman, M., et al. (2018). Association of combined patterns of tobacco and cannabis use in adolescence with psychotic experiences. *JAMA Psychiatry.*

Jones, P. B., Barnes, T. R. E., Davies, L., Dunn, G., et al. (2006). Randomized controlled trial of the effect on Quality of Life of second- vs first-generation antipsychotic drugs in schizophrenia. *Archives of General Psychiatry, 39,* 1079–1087.

Jones, S. E., Lane, J. M., Wood, A. R., van Hees, V. T., et al. (2019). Genome-wide association analyses of chronotype in 697,828 individuals provides insights into circadian rhythms. *Nature Communications, 10*(1), 343.

Jones, T. A. (2017). Motor compensation and its effects on neural reorganization after stroke. *Nature Reviews Neuroscience, 18*(5), 267–280.

Jordan, B. D., Jahre, C., Hauser, W. A., Zimmerman, R. D., et al. (1992). CT of 338 active professional boxers. *Radiology, 185,* 509–512.

Jordan, G., Deeb, S. S., Bosten, J. M., and Mollon, J. D. (2010). The dimensionality of color vision in carriers of anomalous trichromacy. *Journal of Vision, 10*(8), 12.

Jordt, S.-E., Bautista, D. M., Chuang, H., McKemy, D. D., et al. (2004). Mustard oils and cannabinoids excite sensory nerve fibres through the TRP channel ANKTM1. *Nature, 427,* 260–265.

Joseph, J. (2013b). "Schizophrenia" and heredity: Why the emperor (still) has no genes. In J. Read and J. Dillon (Eds.), *Models of madness: Psychological, social and biological approaches to psychosis* (2nd ed., pp. 72–89). London, UK: Routledge.

Joseph, J. S., Chun, M. M., and Nakayama, K. (1997). Attentional requirements in a "preattentive" feature search task. *Nature, 387,* 805–807.

K

Kable, J. W., and Glimcher, P. W. (2009). The neurobiology of decision: Consensus and controversy. *Neuron, 63,* 733–745.

Kaiser, D. (2013). Infralow frequencies and ultradian rhythms. *Seminars in Pediatric Neurology, 20,* 242–245.

Kajimura, S., and Saito, M. (2014). A new era in brown adipose tissue biology: Molecular control of brown fat development and energy homeostasis. *Annual Review of Physiology, 76,* 225–249.

Kales, A., and Kales, J. (1970). Evaluation, diagnosis and treatment of clinical conditions related to sleep. *JAMA, 213,* 2229–2235.

Kales, A., and Kales, J. D. (1974). Sleep disorders. Recent findings in the diagnosis and treatment of disturbed sleep. *New England Journal of Medicine, 290,* 487–499.

Kalyani, H. H. N., Sullivan, K., Moyle, G., Brauer, S., et al. (2019). Effects of dance on gait, cognition, and dual-tasking in Parkinson's disease: A systematic review and meta-analysis. *Journal of Parkinson's Disease, 9*(2), 335–349.

Kandel, E. R. (1976). *Cellular basis of behavior.* San Francisco, CA: Freeman.

Kandel, E. R. (2009). The biology of memory: A forty-year perspective. *Journal of Neuroscience, 29,* 12748–12756.

Kandler, K., Clause, A., and Noh, J. (2009). Tonotopic reorganization of developing auditory brainstem circuits. *Nature Neuroscience, 12,* 711–716.

Kane, J. M., and Correll, C. U. (2010). Past and present progress in the pharmacologic treatment of schizophrenia. *Journal of Clinical Psychiatry, 71*(9), 1115–1124.

Kang, C., Riazuddin, S., Mundorff, J., Krasnewich, D., et al. (2010). Mutation in the lysosomal enzyme–targeting pathway and persistent stuttering. *New England Journal of Medicine, 362,* 677–685.

Karas, P. J., Lee, S., Jimenez-Shahed, J., Goodman, W. K., et al. (2019). Deep brain stimulation for obsessive compulsive disorder: Evolution of surgical stimulation target parallels changing model of dysfunctional brain circuits. *Frontiers in Neuroscience, 12,* 998.

Karch, S. B. (2006). *Drug abuse handbook* (2nd ed.). Boca Raton, FL: CRC Press.

Karlin, A. (2002). Emerging structure of the nicotinic acetylcholine receptors. *Nature Reviews Neuroscience, 3,* 102–114.

Karpicke, J. D., and Roediger, H. L., III. (2008). The critical importance of retrieval for learning. *Science, 319,* 966–968.

Karra, E., Chandarana, K., and Batterham, R. L. (2009). The role of peptide YY in appetite regulation and obesity. *Journal of Physiology, 587,* 19–25.

Kass, A. E., Kolko, R. P., and Wilfley, D. E. (2013). Psychological treatments for eating disorders. *Current Opinion in Psychiatry, 26,* 549–555.

Katsiki, N., Tziomalos, K., and Mikhailidis, D. P. (2014). Alcohol and the cardiovascular system: A double-edged sword. *Current Pharmaceutical Design, 20*(40), 6276–6288.

Katz, D. B., and Steinmetz, J. E. (2002). Psychological functions of the cerebellum. *Behavioral Cognitive Neuroscience Review, 1,* 229–241.

Katzenberg, D., Young, T., Finn, L., Lin, L., et al. (1998). A CLOCK polymorphism associated with human diurnal preference. *Sleep, 21,* 569–576.

Kauffmann, L., Ramanoël, S., Guyader, N., Chauvin, A., et al. (2015). Spatial frequency processing in scene-selective cortical regions. *NeuroImage, 112,* 86–95.

Kaushall, P. I., Zetin, M., and Squire, L. R. (1981). A psychosocial study of chronic, circumscribed amnesia. *Journal of Nervous and Mental Disease, 169,* 383–389.

Kay, K. N., Naselaris, T., Prenger, R. J., and Gallant, J. L. (2008). Identifying natural images from human brain activity. *Nature, 452,* 352–355.

Kaya, E. M., and Elhilali, M. (2017). Modelling auditory attention. *Philosophical Transactions of the Royal Society of London. Series B: Biological Sciences, 372*(1714), 1–10.

Kaye, W. H., Fudge, J. L., and Paulus, M. (2009). New insights into symptoms and neurocircuit function of anorexia nervosa. *Nature Reviews Neuroscience, 10,* 573–584.

Keane, T. M. (1998). Psychological and behavioral treatments of post-traumatic stress disorder. In P. E. Nathan and J. M. Gorman (Eds.), *A guide to treatments that work* (pp. 398–407). New York, NY: Oxford University Press.

Kee, N., Teixeira, C. M., Wang, A. H., and Frankland, P. W. (2007). Preferential incorporation of adult-generated granule cells into spatial memory networks in the dentate gyrus. *Nature Neuroscience, 10,* 355–362.

Keenan, J. P., Nelson, A., O'Connor, M., and Pascual-Leone, A. (2001). Self-recognition and the right hemisphere. *Nature, 409,* 305.

Keesey, R. E. (1980). A set-point analysis of the regulation of body weight. In A. J. Stunkard (Ed.), *Obesity* (pp. 144–165). Philadelphia, PA: Saunders.

Keesey, R. E., and Boyle, P. C. (1973). Effects of quinine adulteration upon body weight of LH-lesioned and intact male rats. *Journal of Comparative and Physiological Psychology, 84,* 38–46.

Keltner, D., and Ekman, P. (2000). Facial expression of emotion. In M. Lewis and J. M. Haviland-Jones (Eds.), *Handbook of emotions* (2nd ed., pp. 236–250). New York, NY: Guilford Press.

Kempermann, G., Kuhn, H. G., and Gage, F. H. (1997). More hippocampal neurons in adult mice living in an enriched environment. *Nature, 386,* 493–495.

Kennedy, D. P., Gläscher, J., Tyszka, J. M., and Adolphs, R. (2009). Personal space regulation by the human amygdala. *Nature Neuroscience, 12*(10), 1226–1227.

Kennedy, J. L., Farrer, L. A., Andreasen, N. C., Mayeux, R., et al. (2003). The genetics of adult-onset neuropsychiatric disease: Complexities and conundra? *Science, 302,* 822–826.

Kennerknecht, I., Grueter, T., Welling, B., Wentzek, S., et al. (2006). First report of prevalence of non-syndromic hereditary prosopagnosia (HPA). *American Journal of Medical Genetics Part A, 140,* 1617–1622.

Kerns, J. C., Guo, J., Fothergill, E., Howard, L., et al. (2017). Increased physical activity associated with less weight regain six years after "The Biggest Loser" competition. *Obesity (Silver Spring), 25*(11), 1838–1843.

Kertesz, A., Harlock, W., and Coates, R. (1979). Computer tomographic localization, lesion size, and prognosis in aphasia and nonverbal impairment. *Brain and Language, 8,* 34–50.

Kertesz, A., and McCabe, P. (1977). Recovery patterns and prognosis in aphasia. *Brain, 100*(Pt. 1), 1–18. https://doi.org/10.1093/brain/100.1.1

Keshavan, M. S., Collin, G., Guimond, S., Kelly, S., et al. (2020). Neuroimaging in schizophrenia. *Neuroimaging Clinics of North America, 30*(1), 73–83. https://doi.org/10.1016/j.nic.2019.09.007

Kessels, H. W., and Malinow, R. (2009). Synaptic AMPA receptor plasticity and behavior. *Neuron, 61,* 340–350.

Kessler, R. C., Angermeyer, M., Anthony, J. C., de Graaf, R., et al. (2007). Lifetime prevalence and age-of-onset distributions of mental disorders in the World Health Organization's World Mental Health Survey Initiative. *World Psychiatry, 6,* 168–176.

Kessler, R. C., Berglund, P., Demler, O., Jin, R., et al. (2005). Lifetime prevalence and age-of-onset distributions of *DSM-IV* disorders in the National Comorbidity Survey Replication. *Archives of General Psychiatry, 62,* 593–602.

Kheirbek, M. A., Klemenhagen, K. C., Sahay, A., and Hen, R. (2012). Neurogenesis and generalization: A new approach to stratify and treat anxiety disorders. *Nature Neuroscience, 15,* 1613–1620.

Kiang, N. Y. S. (1965). *Discharge patterns of single fibers in the cat's auditory nerve.* Cambridge, MA: MIT Press.

Kim, D. R., Pesiridou, A., and O'Reardon, J. P. (2009). Transcranial magnetic stimulation in the treatment of psychiatric disorders. *Current Psychiatry Reports, 11,* 447–452.

Kimura, D. (1973). The asymmetry of the human brain. *Scientific American, 228*(3), 70–78.

Kimura, D. (1993). *Neuromotor mechanisms in human communication.* Oxford, UK: Oxford University Press.

Kimura, D., and Watson, N. V. (1989). The relation between oral movement control and speech. *Brain and Language, 37,* 565–590.

Kindt, M., Soeter, M., and Vervliet, B. (2009). Beyond extinction: Erasing human fear responses and preventing the return of fear. *Nature Neuroscience, 12,* 256–258.

King, A. (2013). The nose knows: How to train a canine conservationist. *New Scientist, 219,* 40–43.

King, S., St-Hilaire, A., and Heidkamp, D. (2010). Prenatal factors in schizophrenia. *Current Directions in Psychological Science, 19,* 209–213.

Kinney, H. C. (2009). Brainstem mechanisms underlying the sudden infant death syndrome: Evidence from human pathologic studies. *Developmental Psychobiology, 51,* 223–233.

Kinsey, A. C., Pomeroy, W. B., and Martin, C. E. (1948). *Sexual behavior in the human male.* Philadelphia, PA: Saunders.

Kinsey, A. C., Pomeroy, W. B., Martin, C. E., and Gebhard, P. H. (1953). *Sexual behavior in the human female.* Philadelphia, PA: Saunders.

Kinsley, C. H., and Lambert, K. G. (2006). The maternal brain. *Scientific American, 294,* 72–79.

Kisely, S., Li, A., Warren, N., and Siskind, D. (2018). A systematic review and meta-analysis of deep brain stimulation for depression. *Depression and Anxiety, 35*(5), 468–480.

Klar, A. J. (2003). Human handedness and scalp hair-whorl direction develop from a common genetic mechanism. *Genetics, 165,* 269–276.

Klaus, J., and Hartwigsen, G. (2019). Dissociating semantic and phonological contributions of the left inferior frontal gyrus to language production. *Human Brain Mapping, 40*(11), 3279–3287.

Kleiman, E. M., Turner, B. J., Fedor, S., Beale, E. E., et al. (2017). Examination of real-time fluctuations in suicidal ideation and its risk factors: Results from two ecological momentary assessment studies. *Journal of Abnormal Psychology, 126*(6), 726–738.

Klein, M., Shapiro, K. M., and Kandel, E. R. (1980). Synaptic plasticity and the modulation of the Ca^{2+} current. *Journal of Experimental Biology, 89,* 117–157.

Kleitman, N., and Engelmann, T. (1953). Sleep characteristics of infants. *Journal of Applied Physiology, 6,* 269–282.

Kluger, M. J. (1978). The evolution and adaptive value of fever. *American Scientist, 66,* 38–43.

Klüver, H., and Bucy, P. C. (1938). An analysis of certain effects of bilateral temporal lobectomy in the rhesus monkey, with special reference to "psychic blindness." *Journal of Psychology, 5,* 33–54.

Knecht, S., Flöel, A., Dräger, B., Breitenstein, C., et al. (2002). Degree of language lateralization determines susceptibility to unilateral brain lesions. *Nature Neuroscience, 5,* 695–699.

Knibestol, M., and Valbo, A. B. (1970). Single unit analysis of mechanoreceptor activity from the human glabrous skin. *Acta Physiologica Scandinavica, 80,* 178–195.

Knudsen, L. B., Secher, A., Hecksher-Sørensen, J., and Pyke, C. (2016). Long-acting glucagon-like peptide-1 receptor agonists have direct access to and effects on pro-opiomelanocortin/cocaine- and amphetamine-stimulated transcript neurons in the mouse hypothalamus. *Journal of Diabetes Investigation, 7*(Suppl. 1), 56–63.

Koch, G., Oliveri, M., Torriero, S., and Caltagirone, C. (2005). Modulation of excitatory and inhibitory circuits for visual awareness in the human right parietal cortex. *Experimental Brain Research, 160,* 510–516.

Kodama, T., Lai, Y. Y., and Siegel, J. M. (2003). Changes in inhibitory amino acid release linked to pontine-induced atonia: An in vivo microdialysis study. *Journal of Neuroscience, 23,* 1548–1554.

Koechlin, E., Ody, C., and Kouneiher, F. (2003). The architecture of cognitive control in the human prefrontal cortex. *Science, 302*(5648), 1181–1185.

Koehler, K. R., Mikosz, A. M., Molosh, A. I., Patel, D., et al. (2013). Generation of inner ear sensory epithelia from pluripotent stem cells in 3D culture. *Nature, 500,* 217–221.

Kohl, M. M., Shipton, O. A., Deacon, R. M., Rawlins, J. N., et al. (2011). Hemisphere-specific optogenetic stimulation reveals left-right asymmetry of hippocampal plasticity. *Nature Neuroscience, 14,* 1413–1415.

Kokrashvili, Z., Mosinger, B., and Margolskee, R. F. (2009). T1r3 and alpha-gustducin in gut regulate secretion of glucagon-like peptide-1. *Annals of the New York Academy of Sciences, 1170,* 91–94.

Kondoh, K., Lu, Z., Ye, X., Olson, D. P., et al. (2016). A specific area of olfactory cortex involved in stress hormone responses to predator odours. *Nature, 532*(7597), 103–106.

Koob, G. F. (1995). Animal models of drug addiction. In F. E. Bloom and D. J. Kupfer (Eds.), *Psychopharmacology: The fourth generation of progress* (pp. 759–772). New York, NY: Raven Press.

Kopell, B. H., Machado, A. G., and Rezai, A. R. (2005). Not your father's lobotomy: Psychiatric surgery revisited. *Clinical Neurosurgery, 52,* 315–330.

Korman, M., Doyon, J., Doljansky, J., Carrier, J., et al. (2007). Daytime sleep condenses the time course of motor memory consolidation. *Nature Neuroscience, 10,* 1206–1213.

Korol, D. L., and Pisani, S. L. (2015). Estrogens and cognition: Friends or foes?: An evaluation of the opposing effects of estrogens on learning and memory. *Hormones and Behavior, 74,* 105–115.

Koubeissi, M. Z., Bartolomei, F., Beltagy, A., and Picard, F. (2014). Electrical stimulation of a small brain area reversibly disrupts consciousness. *Epilepsy & Behavior, 37,* 32–35.

Kraft, A., Irlbacher, K., Finke, K., Kaufmann, C., et al. (2015). Dissociable spatial and non-spatial attentional deficits after circumscribed thalamic stroke. *Cortex, 64,* 327–342.

Krashes, M. J., Lowell, B. B., and Garfield, A. S. (2016). Melanocortin-4 receptor-regulated energy homeostasis. *Nature Neuroscience, 19*(2), 206–219.

Krause, J., Lalueza-Fox, C., Orlando, L., Enard, W., et al. (2007). The derived *FOXP2* variant of modern humans was shared with Neandertals. *Current Biology, 17,* 1908–1912.

Krauzlis, R. J., Lovejoy, L. P., and Zénon, A. (2013). Superior colliculus and visual spatial attention. *Annual Review of Neuroscience, 36,* 165–182.

Kringelbach, M. L. (2005). The human orbitofrontal cortex: Linking reward to hedonic experience. *Nature Reviews Neuroscience, 6,* 691–702.

Kringelbach, M. L., Jenkinson, N., Owen, S. L. F., and Aziz, T. Z. (2007). Translational principles of deep brain stimulation. *Nature Reviews Neuroscience, 8,* 623–634.

Kripke, D. F., Garfinkel, L., Wingard, D. L., Klauber, M. R., et al. (2002). Mortality associated with sleep duration and insomnia. *Archives of General Psychiatry, 59*, 131–136.

Kuhl, B. A., Dudukovic, N. M., Kahn, I., and Wagner, A. D. (2007). Decreased demands on cognitive control reveal the neural processing benefits of forgetting. *Nature Neuroscience, 10*, 908–914.

Kulkarni, A., and Colburn, H. S. (1998). Role of spectral detail in sound-source localization. *Nature, 396*, 747–749.

Kuperberg, G. R. (2007). Neural mechanisms of language comprehension: Challenges to syntax. *Brain Research, 1146*, 23–49.

Kupfer, D. J., Frank, E., and Phillips, M. L. (2012). Major depressive disorder: New clinical, neurobiological, and treatment perspectives. *Lancet, 379*(9820), 1045–1055.

Kupfer, D. J., Reynolds, C. F., Ulrich, R. F., Shaw, D. H., et al. (1982). EEG sleep, depression, and aging. *Neurobiology of Aging, 3*, 351–360.

Kutas, M., and Federmeier, K. D. (2011). Thirty years and counting: Finding meaning in the N400 component of the event-related brain potential (ERP). *Annual Review of Psychology, 62*, 621–647.

Kutas, M., and Hillyard, S. A. (1984). Event-related potentials in cognitive science. In M. S. Gazzaniga (Ed.), *Handbook of cognitive neuroscience* (pp. 387–409). New York, NY: Plenum Press.

Kwakkel, G., Veerbeek, J. M., van Wegen, E. E., and Wolf, S. L. (2015). Constraint-induced movement therapy after stroke. *Lancet Neurology, 14*, 224–234.

Kyzar, E. J., Nichols, C. D., Gainetdinov, R. R., Nichols, D. E., et al. (2017). Psychedelic drugs in biomedicine. *Trends in Pharmacological Sciences, 38*(11), 992–1005.

L

Lagrèze, W. A., and Schaeffel, F. (2017). Preventing myopia. *Deutsches Arzteblatt International, 114*(35–36), 575–580.

Lai, C. S. L., Fisher, S. E., Hurst, J. A., Vargha-Khadem, F., et al. (2001). A forkhead-domain gene is mutated in a severe speech and language disorder. *Nature, 413*, 519–523.

Larroche, J.-C. (1977). *Developmental pathology of the neonate.* Amsterdam, Netherlands: Excerpta Medica.

Larsson, M., and Willander, J. (2009). Autobiographical odor memory. *Annals of the New York Academy of Sciences, 1170*, 318–323.

Lau, H. C., Rogers, R. D., Haggard, P., and Passingham, R. E. (2004). Attention to intention. *Science, 303*, 1208–1210.

Lavie, N., Hirst, A., de Fockert, J. W., and Viding, E. (2004). Load theory of selective attention and cognitive control. *Journal of Experimental Psychology: General, 133*, 339–354.

Lavie, N., Lin, Z., Zokaei, N., and Thoma, V. (2009). The role of perceptual load in object recognition. *Journal of Experimental Psychology: Human Perception and Performance, 35*, 1346–1358.

Lavie, P. (1996). *The enchanted world of sleep* (A. Berris, Trans.). New Haven, CT: Yale University Press.

Lavond, D. G., Kim, J. J., and Thompson, R. F. (1993). Mammalian brain substrates of aversive classical conditioning. *Annual Review of Psychology, 44*, 317–342.

Le Grand, R., Mondloch, C. J., Maurer, D., and Brent, H. P. (2001). Early visual experience and face processing. *Nature, 410*, 890.

Le Grange, D. (2005). The Maudsley family-based treatment for adolescent anorexia nervosa. *World Psychiatry, 4*, 142–146.

Leask, S. J., and Beaton, A. A. (2007). Handedness in Great Britain. *Laterality, 12*, 559–572.

LeDoux, J. E. (1994). Emotion, memory and the brain. *Scientific American, 270*(6), 50–57.

LeDoux, J. E. (1996). *The emotional brain: The mysterious underpinnings of emotional life.* London, UK: Simon & Schuster.

LeDoux, J., and Daw, N. D. (2018). Surviving threats: Neural circuit and computational implications of a new taxonomy of defensive behaviour. *Nature Reviews Neuroscience, 19*(5), 269–282.

Lee, E. E., Della Selva, M. P., Liu, A., and Himelhoch, S. (2015). Ketamine as a novel treatment for major depressive disorder and bipolar depression: A systematic review and quantitative meta-analysis. *General Hospital Psychiatry, 37*(2), 178–184.

Lee, H., Kim, D. W., Remedios, R., Anthony, T. E., et al. (2014). Scalable control of mounting and attack by Esr1+ neurons in the ventromedial hypothalamus. *Nature, 509*, 627–632.

Legras, R., Gaudric, A., and Woog, K. (2018). Distribution of cone density, spacing and arrangement in adult healthy retinas with adaptive optics flood illumination. *PLOS ONE, 13*(1), e0191141.

Leinders-Zufall, T., Lane, A. P., Puche, A. C., Ma, W., et al. (2000). Ultrasensitive pheromone detection by mammalian vomeronasal neurons. *Nature, 405*, 792–796.

Lepage, J. F., and Theoret, H. (2006). EEG evidence for the presence of an action observation-execution matching system in children. *European Journal of Neuroscience, 23*, 2505–2510.

Lereya, S. T., Copeland, W. E., Costello, E. J., and Wolke, D. (2015). Adult mental health consequences of peer bullying and maltreatment in childhood: Two cohorts in two countries. *Lancet Psychiatry, 2*, 524–531.

Leschziner, G. (2019). *The nocturnal brain: Nightmares, neuroscience, and the secret world of sleep.* New York, NY: St. Martin's Press.

Lesku, J. A., Roth, T. C., II, Rattenborg, N. C., Amlaner, C. J., et al. (2009). History and future of comparative analyses in sleep research. *Neuroscience and Biobehavioral Reviews, 33*, 1024–1036.

Leung, C. T., Coulombe, P. A., and Reed, R. R. (2007). Contribution of olfactory neural stem cells to tissue maintenance and regeneration. *Nature Neuroscience, 10*, 720–726.

LeVay, S. (1991). A difference in hypothalamic structure between heterosexual and homosexual men. *Science, 253*, 1034–1037.

Levine, J. D., Gordon, N. C., and Fields, H. L. (1978). The mechanism of placebo analgesia. *Lancet, 2*, 654–657.

Levine, S., Haltmeyer, G. C., and Karas, G. G. (1967). Physiological and behavioral effects of infantile stimulation. *Physiology & Behavior, 2*, 55–59.

Lew, S. M. (2014). Hemispherectomy in the treatment of seizures: A review. *Translational Pediatrics, 3*(3), 208–217.

Li, B., Piriz, J., Mirrione, M., Chung, C., et al. (2011). Synaptic potentiation onto habenula neurons in the learned helplessness model of depression. *Nature, 470*, 535–539.

Li, W., Ma, L., Yang, G., and Gan, W. B. (2017). REM sleep selectively prunes and maintains new synapses in development and learning. *Nature Neuroscience, 20*(3), 427–437.

Li, W., Wu, J., Yang, J., Sun, S., et al. (2015). Notch inhibition induces mitotically generated hair cells in mammalian cochleae via activating the Wnt pathway. *Proceedings of the National Academy of Sciences, USA, 112*(1), 166–171.

Li, X., Glaser, D., Li, W., Johnson, W. E., et al. (2009). Analyses of sweet receptor gene (*Tas1r2*) and preference for sweet stimuli in species of Carnivora. *Journal of Heredity, 100*(Suppl. 1), S90–S100.

Liberles, S. D. (2009). Trace amine-associated receptors are olfactory receptors in vertebrates. *Annals of the New York Academy of Science, 1170*, 168–172.

Liberles, S. D., and Buck, L. B. (2006). A second class of chemosensory receptors in the olfactory epithelium. *Nature, 442*, 645–650.

Libet, B. (1985). Unconscious cerebral initiative and the role of conscious will in voluntary action. *Behavioral and Brain Sciences, 8*, 529–566.

Lichstein, K. L. (2017). Insomnia identity. *Behaviour Research and Therapy, 97*, 230–241.

Lichtenstein, P., Yip, B. H., Björk, C., Pawitan, Y., et al. (2009). Common genetic determinants of schizophrenia and bipolar disorder in Swedish families: A population-based study. *Lancet, 373*, 234–239.

Lichtman, J. W., Livet, J., and Sanes, J. R. (2008). A technicolour approach to the connectome. *Nature Reviews Neuroscience, 9,* 417–422.

Lichtman, J. W., and Purves, D. (1980). The elimination of redundant preganglionic innervation to hamster sympathetic ganglion cells in early post-natal life. *Journal of Physiology (London), 301,* 213–228.

Liddelow, S. A., Guttenplan, K. A., Clarke, L. E., Bennett, F. C., et al. (2017). Neurotoxic reactive astrocytes are induced by activated microglia. *Nature, 541*(7638),481–487.

Lieberman, P. (2002). On the nature and evolution of the neural bases of human language. *American Journal of Physical Anthropology, 119*(S35), 36–62.

Liégeois, F., Baldeweg, T., Connelly, A., Gadian, D. G., et al. (2003). Language fMRI abnormalities associated with *FOXP2* gene mutation. *Nature Neuroscience, 6,* 1230–1237.

Liepert, J., Bauder, H., Wolfgang, H. R., Miltner, W. H., et al. (2000). Treatment-induced cortical reorganization after stroke in humans. *Stroke, 31,* 1210–1216.

Lieving, L. M., Cherek, D. R., Lane, S. D., Tcheremissine, O. V., et al. (2008). Effects of acute tiagabine administration on aggressive responses of adult male parolees. *Journal of psychopharmacology (Oxford), 22*(2), 144–152.

Lim, M. M., Wang, Z., Olazabal, D. E., Ren, X., et al. (2004). Enhanced partner preference in a promiscuous species by manipulating the expression of a single gene. *Nature, 429,* 754–757.

Lim, M. M., and Young, L. J. (2006). Neuropeptidergic regulation of affiliative behavior and social bonding in animals. *Hormones and Behavior, 50,* 506–557.

Lin, Y. C., Guo, Y. R., Miyagi, A., Levring, J., et al. (2019). Force-induced conformational changes in PIEZO1. *Nature, 573*(7773), 230–234.

Linde, K., Allais, G., Brinkhaus, B., Manheimer, E., et al. (2009). Acupuncture for tension-type headache. *Cochrane Database of Systematic Reviews, 1,* CD007587.

Lisman, J., Schulman, H., and Cline, H. (2002). The molecular basis of CAMKII function in synaptic and behavioural memory. *Nature Reviews Neuroscience, 3,* 175–190.

Liston, C., McEwen, B. S., & Casey, B. J. (2009). Psychosocial stress reversibly disrupts prefrontal processing and attentional control. *Proceedings of the National Academy of Sciences, USA, 106*(3), 912–917.

Liu, D., Diorio, J., Tannenbaum, B., Caldji, C., et al. (1997). Maternal care, hippocampal glucocorticoid receptors, and hypothalamic-pituitary-adrenal responses to stress. *Science, 277,* 1659–1662.

Liu, H., and Cao, F. (2016). L1 and L2 processing in the bilingual brain: A meta-analysis of neuroimaging studies. *Brain and Language, 159,* 60–73.

Liu, M., Blanco-Centurion, C., and Shiromani, P. J. (2017). Rewiring brain circuits to block cataplexy in murine models of narcolepsy. *Current Opinion in Neurobiology, 44,* 110–115.

Liu, Y., Gao, J.-H., Liu, H.-L., and Fox, P. T. (2000). The temporal response of the brain after eating revealed by functional MRI. *Nature, 405,* 1058–1062.

Liu, Y., Williamson, V., Setlow, B., Cottler, L. B., et al. (2018). The importance of considering polysubstance use: Lessons from cocaine research. *Drug and Alcohol Dependence, 192,* 16–28.

Lledo, P. M., and Valley, M. (2018). Adult olfactory bulb neurogenesis. *Cold Spring Harbor Perspectives in Biology, 8*(8), a018945.

Llewellyn, S., and Hobson, J. A. (2015). Not only ... but also: REM sleep creates and NREM Stage 2 instantiates landmark junctions in cortical memory networks. *Neurobiology of Learning and Memory, 122,* 69–87.

Lloyd, J. A. (1971). Weights of testes, thymi, and accessory reproductive glands in relation to rank in paired and grouped house mice (*Mus musculus*). *Proceedings of the Society for Experimental Biology and Medicine, 137,* 19–22.

Lo, J. C., Lee, S. M., Lee, X. K., Sasmita, K, et al. (2018). Sustained benefits of delaying school start time on adolescent sleep and well-being. *Sleep, 41*(6), zsy052.

Lockhart, M., and Moore, J. W. (1975). Classical differential and operant conditioning in rabbits (*Oryctolagus cuniculus*) with septal lesions. *Journal of Comparative and Physiological Psychology, 88,* 147–154.

Loconto, J., Papes, F., Chang, E., Stowers, L., et al. (2003). Functional expression of murine V2R pheromone receptors involves selective association with the M10 and M1 families of MHC class Ib molecules. *Cell, 112,* 607–618.

Loeb, G. E. (1990). Cochlear prosthetics. *Annual Review of Neuroscience, 13,* 357–371.

Loftus, E. F. (2003). Make-believe memories. *American Psychologist, 58,* 867–873.

Logan, C. G., and Grafton, S. T. (1995). Functional anatomy of human eyeblink conditioning determined with regional cerebral glucose metabolism and positron emission tomography. *Proceedings of the National Academy of Sciences, USA, 92,* 7500–7504.

Logue, M. W., van Rooij, S. J. H., Dennis, E. L., Davis, S. L., et al. (2018). Smaller hippocampal volume in posttraumatic stress disorder: A multisite ENIGMA-PGC study: Subcortical volumetry results from posttraumatic stress disorder consortia. *Biological Psychiatry, 83*(3), 244–253.

Lorca-Puls, D. L., Gajardo-Vidal, A., Seghier, M. L., Leff, A. P., et al. (2017). Using transcranial magnetic stimulation of the undamaged brain to identify lesion sites that predict language outcome after stroke. *Brain, 140*(6), 1729–1742.

Lotto, R. B., and Purves, D. (2000). An empirical explanation of color contrast. *Proceedings of the National Academy of Sciences, USA, 97,* 12834–12839.

Loui, P., Alsop, D., and Schlaug, G. (2009). Tone deafness: A new disconnection syndrome? *Journal of Neuroscience, 29,* 10215–10220.

Lübke, K. T., and Pause, B. M. (2015). Always follow your nose: The functional significance of social chemosignals in human reproduction and survival. *Hormones and Behavior, 68,* 134–144.

Luck, S. J. (2005). *An introduction to the event-related potential technique.* Cambridge, MA: MIT Press.

Luck, S. J., and Hillyard, S. A. (1994). Electrophysiological correlates of feature analysis during visual search. *Psychophysiology, 31,* 291–308.

Lundberg, U. (1976). Urban commuting: crowdedness and catecholamine excretion. *Journal of Human Stress, 2,* 26–32.

Luria, A. R. (1987). *The mind of a mnemonist.* Cambridge, MA: Harvard University Press.

Lush, I. E. (1989). The genetics of tasting in mice. VI. Saccharin, acesulfame, dulcin and sucrose. *Genetical Research, 53,* 95–99.

Ly, M., Motzkin, J. C., Philippi, C. L., Kirk, G. R., et al. (2012). Cortical thinning in psychopathy. *American Journal of Psychiatry, 169*(7), 743–739.

Lyamin, O. I., Manger, P. R., Ridgway, S. H., Mukhametov, L. M., et al. (2008). Cetacean sleep: An unusual form of mammalian sleep. *Neuroscience & Biobehavioral Reviews, 32*(8), 1451–1484.

Lyamin, O., Pryaslova, J., Lance, V., and Siegel, J. (2005). Continuous activity in cetaceans after birth: The exceptional wakefulness of newborn whales and dolphins has no ill-effect on their development. *Nature, 435,* 1177.

Lyn, H., Pierre, P., Bennett, A. J., Fears, S., et al. (2011). Planum temporale grey matter asymmetries in chimpanzees (*Pan troglodytes*), vervet (*Chlorocebus aethiops sabaeus*), rhesus (*Macaca mulatta*) and bonnet (*Macaca radiata*) monkeys. *Neuropsychologia, 49*(7), 2004–2012.

Lynch, G., Larson, J., Staubli, U., and Granger, R. (1991). Variants of synaptic potentiation and different types of memory operations in hippocampus and related structures. In L. R. Squire, N. M. Weinberger, G. Lynch, and J. L. McGaugh (Eds.), *Memory: Organization and locus of change* (pp. 330–363). New York, NY: Oxford University Press.

Lyons, J. I., Kerr, G. R., and Mueller, P. W. (2015). Fragile X syndrome: Scientific background and screening technologies. *Journal of Molecular Diagnostics.*

M

Macdonald, K., Germine, L., Anderson, A., Christodoulou, J., et al. (2017). Dispelling the myth: Training in education or neuroscience decreases but does not eliminate beliefs in neuromyths. *Frontiers in Psychology, 8,* 1314.

Mackey, S., Allgaier, N., Chaarani, B., Spechler, P., et al; ENIGMA Addiction Working Group. (2019). Mega-analysis of gray matter volume in substance dependence: General and substance-specific regional effects. *American Journal of Psychiatry, 176*(2), 119–128.

MacLean, P. D. (1949). Psychosomatic disease and the "visceral brain": Recent developments bearing on the Papez theory of emotion. *Psychosomatic Medicine, 11,* 338–353.

MacLeod, C. M. (1991). Half a century of research on the Stroop effect: An integrative review. *Psychological Bulletin, 109,* 163–203.

Macmillan, M. (2000). *An odd kind of fame: Stories of Phineas Gage.* Cambridge, MA: MIT Press.

MacNeilage, P. F., Rogers, L. J., and Vallortigara, G. (2009). Origins of the left & right brain. *Scientific American, 301*(1), 60–67.

MacNeilage, P. R., Banks, M. S., Berger, D. R., and Bülthoff, H. H. (2007). A Bayesian model of the disambiguation of gravitoinertial force by visual cues. *Experimental Brain Research, 179*(2), 263–290.

Maggioncalda, A. N., and Sapolsky, R. M. (2002). Disturbing behaviors of the orangutan. *Scientific American, 286*(6), 60–65.

Mahowald, M. W., and Schenck, C. H. (2005). Insights from studying human sleep disorders. *Nature, 437,* 1279–1285.

Mai, E., and Buysse, D. J. (2008). Insomnia: Prevalence, impact, pathogenesis, differential diagnosis, and evaluation. *Sleep Medicine Clinics, 3*(2), 167–174.

Maia, T. V., and Conceição, V. A. (2018, March 9). Dopaminergic disturbances in Tourette syndrome: An integrative account. *Biological Psychiatry,* pii: S0006-3223(18)31300-3.

Maier, S. F., and Seligman, M. E. (2016). Learned helplessness at fifty: Insights from neuroscience. *Psychological Review, 123*(4), 349–367.

Main, C. J. (2016). Pain assessment in context: A state of the science review of the McGill pain questionnaire 40 years on. *Pain, 157*(7), 1387–1399.

Mainland, J. D., Keller, A., Li, Y. R., Zhou, T., et al. (2014). The missense of smell: Functional variability in the human odorant receptor repertoire. *Nature Neuroscience, 17*(1), 114–120.

Mair, W. G. P., Warrington, E. K., and Wieskrantz, L. (1979). Memory disorder in Korsakoff's psychosis. *Brain, 102,* 749–783.

Makin, S. (2018). The amyloid hypothesis on trial. *Nature, 559*(7715), S4–S7.

Makino, H., Hwang, E. J., Hedrick, N. G., and Komiyama, T. (2016). Circuit mechanisms of sensorimotor learning. *Neuron, 92*(4), 705–721.

Malenka, R. C., and Bear, M. F. (2004). LTP and LTD: An embarrassment of riches. *Neuron, 44,* 5–21.

Malik, B., Elkaddi, N., Turkistani, J., Spielman, A. I., et al. (2019). Mammalian taste cells express functional olfactory receptors. *Chemical Senses, 44*(5), 289–301.

Malpas, C. B., Genc, S., Saling, M. M., Velakoulis, D., et al. (2016). MRI correlates of general intelligence in neurotypical adults. *Journal of Clinical Neuroscience, 24,* 128–134.

Mamluk, L., Edwards, H. B., Savović, J., Leach, V., et al. (2017). Low alcohol consumption and pregnancy and childhood outcomes: Time to change guidelines indicating apparently "safe" levels of alcohol during pregnancy? A systematic review and meta-analyses. *BMJ Open, 7*(7), e015410.

Mancuso, K., Hauswirth, W. W., Li, Q., Connor, T. B., et al. (2009). Gene therapy for red-green colour blindness in adult primates. *Nature, 461,* 784–788.

Mander, B. A., Winer, J. R., and Walker, M. P. (2017). Sleep and human aging. *Neuron, 94*(1), 19–36.

Manger, P. R., Fahringer, H. M., Pettigrew, J. D., and Siegel, J. M. (2002). The distribution and morphological characteristics of serotonergic cells in the brain of monotremes. *Brain, Behavior and Evolution, 60*(5), 315–332.

Mani, S. K., Fienberg, A. A., O'Callaghan, J. P., Snyder, G. L., et al. (2000). Requirement for DARPP-32 in progesterone-facilitated sexual receptivity in female rats and mice. *Science, 287,* 1053–1056.

Maniscalco, J. W., and Rinaman, L. (2018). Vagal interoceptive modulation of motivated behavior. *Physiology (Bethesda), 33*(2), 151–167.

Manoli, D. S., and Tollkuhn, J. (2018). Gene regulatory mechanisms underlying sex differences in brain development and psychiatric disease. *Annals of the New York Academy of Sciences, 1420*(1), 26–45.

Mantini, D., Gerits, A., Nelissen, K., Durand, J. B., et al. (2011). Default mode of brain function in monkeys. *Journal of Neuroscience, 31,* 12954–12962.

Mao, J. B., and Evinger, C. (2001). Long-term potentiation of the human blink reflex. *Journal of Neuroscience, 21,* RC151.

Marconi, A., Di Forti, M., Lewis, C. M., Murray, R. M., et al. (2016). Meta-analysis of the association between the level of cannabis use and risk of psychosis. *Schizophrenia Bulletin, 42*(5), 1262–1269.

Marcus, G. F., Vijayan, S., Bandi Rao, S., and Vishton, P. M. (1999). Rule learning by seven-month-old infants. *Science, 283,* 77–80.

Marek, G. J., Behl, B., Bespalov, A. Y., Gross, G., et al. (2010). Glutamatergic (*N*-methyl-D-aspartate receptor) hypofrontality in schizophrenia: Too little juice or a miswired brain? *Molecular Pharmacology, 77*(3), 317–326.

Mark, V. H., and Ervin, F. R. (1970). *Violence and the brain.* New York, NY: Harper & Row.

Marler, P. (2004). Bird calls: Their potential for behavioral neurobiology. *Annals of the New York Academy of Sciences, 1016,* 31–44.

Marshall, L., Helgadóttir, H., Mölle, M., and Born, J. (2006). Boosting slow oscillations during sleep potentiates memory. *Nature, 444,* 610–613.

Martin, C. K., Heilbronn, L., de Jonge, L., Delany, J. P., et al. (2007). Effect of calorie restriction on resting metabolic rate and spontaneous physical activity. *Obesity (Silver Spring), 15,* 2964–2973.

Martuza, R. L., Chiocca, E. A., Jenike, M. A., Giriunas, I. E., et al. (1990). Stereotactic radiofrequency thermal cingulotomy for obsessive compulsive disorder. *Journal of Neuropsychiatry and Clinical Neurosciences, 2,* 331–336.

Marucha, P. T., Kiecolt-Glaser, J. K., and Favagehi, M. (1998). Mucosal wound healing is impaired by examination stress. *Psychosomatic Medicine, 60,* 362–365.

Maruyama, Y., Pereira, E., Margolskee, R. F., Chaudhari, N., et al. (2006). Umami responses in mouse taste cells indicate more than one receptor. *Journal of Neuroscience, 26,* 2227–2234.

Marzullo, T. C. (2017). The missing manuscript of Dr. Jose Delgado's radio controlled bulls. *Journal of Undergraduate Neuroscience Education, 15*(2), R29–R35.

Masiulis, S., Desai, R., Uchański, T., Serna Martin, I., et al. (2019). GABA(A) receptor signalling mechanisms revealed by structural pharmacology. *Nature, 565*(7740), 454–459.

Masters, W. H., and Johnson, V. E. (1966). *Human sexual response.* Boston, MA: Little, Brown.

Masters, W. H., Johnson, V. E., and Kolodny, R. C. (1994). *Heterosexuality.* New York, NY: HarperCollins.

Mateo, J. M., and Johnston, R. E. (2000). Kin recognition and the "armpit effect": Evidence of self-referent phenotype matching. *Proceedings of the Royal Society of London. Series B: Biological Sciences, 267,* 695–700.

Matsumoto, K., Suzuki, W., and Tanaka, K. (2003). Neuronal correlates of goal-based motor selection in the prefrontal cortex. *Science, 301,* 229–232.

Mattes, R. D. (2011). Accumulating evidence supports a taste component for free fatty acids in humans. *Physiology & Behavior, 104*(4), 624–631.

Matthews, K. A. (2005). Psychological perspectives on the development of coronary heart disease. *American Psychologist, 60*(8), 783–796.

Mattson, M. P., and Arumugam, T. V. (2018). Hallmarks of brain aging: Adaptive and pathological modification by metabolic states. *Cell Metabolism, 27*(6), 1176–1199.

May, L., Gervain, J., Carreiras, M., and Werker, J. F. (2018). The specificity of the neural response to speech at birth. *Developmental Science, 21*(3), e12564.

Mazur, A., and Booth, A. (1998). Testosterone and dominance in men. *Behavioral and Brain Sciences, 21,* 353–363.

McBurney, D. H., Smith, D. V., and Shick, T. R. (1972). Gustatory cross adaptation: Sourness and bitterness. *Perception & Psychophysics, 11,* 2228–2232.

McCrae, C. S., Rowe, M. A., Tierney, C. G., Dautovich, N. D., et al. (2005). Sleep complaints, subjective and objective sleep patterns, health, psychological adjustment, and daytime functioning in community-dwelling older adults. *Journals of Gerontology. Series B, Psychological Sciences and Social Sciences, 60*(4), P182–P189.

McCutcheon, R. A., Reis Marques, T., and Howes, O. D. (2019). Schizophrenia: An overview. *JAMA Psychiatry, 7*(2), 201–210.

McDonald, J. J., and Green, J. J. (2008). Isolating event-related potential components associated with voluntary control of visuo-spatial attention. *Brain Research, 1227,* 96–109.

McDonald, J. J., Teder-Sälejärvi, W. A., Di Russo, F., and Hillyard, S. A. (2005). Neural basis of auditory-induced shifts in visual time-order perception. *Nature Neuroscience, 8*(9), 1197–1202.

McDonald, J. J., Teder-Sälejärvi, W. A., and Hillyard, S. A. (2000). Involuntary orienting to sound improves visual perception. *Nature, 407,* 906–908.

McDonald, J. J., Ward, L. M., and Kiehl, K. A. (1999). An event-related brain potential study of inhibition of return. *Perception & Psychophysics, 61*(7), 1411–1423.

McEwen, B. S. (2016). In pursuit of resilience: Stress, epigenetics, and brain plasticity. *Annals of the New York Academy of Sciences, 1373*(1), 56–64.

McEwen, B. S., Bowles, N. P., Gray, J. D., Hill, M. N., et al. (2015). Mechanisms of stress in the brain. *Nature Neuroscience, 18*(10), 1353–1363.

McEwen, B. S., and Wingfield, J. C. (2010). What is in a name? Integrating homeostasis, allostasis and stress. *Hormones and Behavior, 57,* 105–111.

McFadden, D. (2011). Sexual orientation and the auditory system. *Frontiers in Neuroendocrinology, 32*(2), 201–213.

McGann, J. P. (2017). Poor human olfaction is a 19th-century myth. *Science, 356*(6338), eaam7263.

McGinty, D. J., and Sterman, M. B. (1968). Sleep suppression after basal forebrain lesions in the cat. *Science, 160,* 1253–1255.

McGowan, P. O., Sasaki, A., D'Alessio, A. C., Dymov, S., et al. (2009). Epigenetic regulation of the glucocorticoid receptor in human brain associates with childhood abuse. *Nature Neuroscience, 12,* 342–348.

McGugin, R. W., Gatenby, J. C., Gore, J. C., and Gauthier, I. (2012). High-resolution imaging of expertise reveals reliable object selectivity in the fusiform face area related to perceptual performance. *Proceedings of the National Academy of Sciences, USA, 109*(42), 17063–17068.

McGuigan, F. J., and Lehrer, P. M. (2007). Progressive relaxation: Origins, principles and clinical application. In P. M. Lehrer, R. L. Woolfolk, and W. E. Sime (Eds.), *Principles and practices of stress management* (pp. 57–87). New York, NY: Guilford Press.

McGuire, J. F., Ricketts, E. J., Piacentini, J., Murphy, T. K., et al. (2015). Behavior therapy for tic disorders: An evidenced-based review and new directions for treatment research. *Current Developmental Disorders Reports, 2*(4), 309–317.

McKee, A. C., Cairns, N. J., Dickson, D. W., Folkerth, R. D., et al. (2016). The first NINDS/NIBIB consensus meeting to define neuropathological criteria for the diagnosis of chronic traumatic encephalopathy. *Acta Neuropathologica, 131*(1), 75–86.

McKee, A. C., Cantu, R. C., Nowinski, C. J., Hedley-Whyte, E. T., et al. (2009). Chronic traumatic encephalopathy in athletes: Progressive tauopathy after repetitive head injury. *Journal of Neuropathology and Experimental Neurology, 68,* 709–735.

McKim, W. A. (1991). *Drugs and behavior: An introduction to behavioral pharmacology* (2nd ed.). Englewood Cliffs, NJ: Prentice Hall.

McKinley, M. J., Denton, D. A., Ryan, P. J., Yao, S. T., et al. (2019). From sensory circumventricular organs to cerebral cortex: Neural pathways controlling thirst and hunger. *Journal of Neuroendocrinology, 31*(3), e12689.

McLaughlin, S. K., McKinnon, P. J., Spickofsky, N., Danho, W., et al. (1994). Molecular cloning of G proteins and phosphodiesterases from rat taste cells. *Physiology & Behavior, 56,* 1157–1164.

McLellan, T. M., Caldwell, J. A., and Lieberman, H. R. (2016). A review of caffeine's effects on cognitive, physical and occupational performance. *Neuroscience & Biobehavioral Reviews, 71,* 294–312.

McNamara, P., Johnson, P., McLaren, D., Harris, E., et al. (2010). REM and NREM sleep mentation. *International Review of Neurobiology, 92,* 69–86.

Meddis, R. (1975). On the function of sleep. *Animal Behavior, 23,* 676–691.

Meddis, R. (1977). *The sleep instinct.* London, UK: Routledge & Kegan Paul.

Mega, M. S., and Cummings, J. L. (1994). Frontal-subcortical circuits and neuropsychiatric disorders. *Journal of Neuropsychiatry and Clinical Neurosciences, 6,* 358–370.

Meguerditchian, A., and Vauclair, J. (2006). Baboons communicate with their right hand. *Behavioural Brain Research, 171,* 170–174.

Mehravari, A. S., Tanner, D., Wampler, E. K., Valentine, G. D., et al. (2015). Effects of grammaticality and morphological complexity on the P600 event-related potential component. *PLOS ONE, 10*(10), e0140850.

Mei, L., and Xiong, W.-C. (2008). Neuregulin 1 in neural development, synaptic plasticity and schizophrenia. *Nature Reviews Neuroscience, 9,* 437–452.

Meier, M. H., Caspi, A., Ambler, A., Harrington, H., et al. (2012). Persistent cannabis users show neuropsychological decline from childhood to midlife. *Proceedings of the National Academy of Sciences, USA, 109,* E2657–E2664.

Meister, I. G., Boroojerdi, B., Foltys, H., Sparing, R., et al. (2003). Motor cortex hand area and speech: Implications for the development of language. *Neuropsychologia, 41*(4), 401–406.

Meldrum, D. R., Burnett, A. L., Dorey, G., Esposito, K., et al. (2014). Erectile hydraulics: Maximizing inflow while minimizing outflow. *Journal of Sexual Medicine, 11*(5), 1208–1220.

Melzack, R., Coderre, T. J., Katz, J., and Vaccarino, A. L. (2001). Central neuroplasticity and pathological pain. *Annals of the New York Academy of Sciences, 933,* 157–174.

Melzack, R., and Wall, P. D. (1965). Pain mechanisms: A new history. *Science, 150,* 971–979.

Méndez-Bértolo, C., Moratti, S., Toledano, R., Lopez-Sosa, F., et al. (2016). A fast pathway for fear in human amygdala. *Nature Neuroscience, 19*(8), 1041–1049.

Menninger, W. C. (1948). Facts and statistics of significance for psychiatry. *Bulletin of the Menninger Clinic, 12,* 1–25.

Merchán-Pérez, A., Rodriguez, J. R., Alonso-Nanclares, L., Schertel, A., et al. (2009). Counting synapses using FIB/SEM microscopy: A true revolution for ultrastructural volume reconstruction. *Frontiers in Neuroanatomy, 3,* 18.

Meshberger, F. L. (1990). An interpretation of Michelangelo's *Creation of Adam* based on neuroanatomy. *JAMA, 264,* 1837–1841.

Mestre, H., Mori, Y., and Nedergaard, M. (2020). The brain's glymphatic system: Current controversies. *Trends in Neurosciences.*

Mesulam, M.-M. (1985). Attention, confusional states and neglect. In M.-M. Mesulam (Ed.), *Principles of behavioral neurology.* Philadelphia, PA: Davis.

Mewton, L., and Andrews, G. (2016). Cognitive behavioral therapy for suicidal behaviors: Improving patient outcomes. *Psychology Research and Behavior Management, 9,* 21–29.

Meyer-Bahlburg, H. F. L. (2011). Brain development and cognitive, psychosocial, and psychiatric functioning in classical 21-hydroxylase deficiency. *Endocrine Development, 20,* 88–95.

Mez, J., Daneshvar, D. H., Kiernan, P. T., Abdolmohammadi, B., et al. (2017). Clinicopathological evaluation of chronic traumatic encephalopathy in players of American football. *JAMA, 318*(4), 360–370.

Michael, N., and Erfurth, A. (2004). Treatment of bipolar mania with right prefrontal rapid transcranial magnetic stimulation. *Journal of Affective Disorders, 78,* 253–257.

Mignot, E. J. (2014). History of narcolepsy at Stanford University. *Immunological Research, 58*(2–3), 315–339.

Miller, E. K., and Cohen, J. D. (2001). An integrative theory of prefrontal cortex function. *Annual Review of Neuroscience, 24,* 167–202.

Miller, J. M., and Spelman, F. A. (1990). *Cochlear implants: Models of the electrically stimulated ear.* New York, NY: Springer-Verlag.

Miller, N. E., Sampliner, R. I., and Woodrow, P. (1957). Thirst-reducing effects of water by stomach fistula vs. water by mouth measured by both a consummatory and an instrumental response. *Journal of Comparative and Physiological Psychology, 50*(1), 1–5.

Milner, B. (1963). Effect of different brain lesions on card sorting. *Archives of Neurology, 9,* 90–100.

Milner, B. (1965). Memory disturbance after bilateral hippocampal lesions. In P. M. Milner and S. E. Glickman (Eds.), *Cognitive processes and the brain; an enduring problem in psychology* (pp. 97–111). Princeton, NJ: Van Nostrand.

Milner, B. (1970). Memory and the medial temporal regions of the brain. In D. H. Pribram and D. E. Broadbent (Eds.), *Biology of memory* (pp. 29–50). New York, NY: Academic Press.

Minzenberg, M. J., Laird, A. R., Thelen, S., Carter, C. S., et al. (2009). Meta-analysis of 41 functional neuroimaging studies of executive function in schizophrenia. *Archives of General Psychiatry, 66,* 811–822.

Mirescu, C., Peters, J. D., and Gould, E. (2004). Early life experience alters response of adult neurogenesis to stress. *Nature Neuroscience, 7,* 841–846.

Mishkin, M., and Ungerleider, L. (1982). Contribution of striate inputs to the visuospatial functions of parieto-preoccipital cortex in monkeys. *Behavioural Brain Research, 6,* 57–77.

Mishra, J., Zinni, M., Bavelier, D., and Hillyard, S. A. (2011). Neural basis of superior performance of action videogame players in an attention-demanding task. *Journal of Neuroscience, 31,* 992–998.

Mitidieri, E., Cirino, G., d'Emmanuele di Villa Bianca, R., and Sorrentino, R. (2020). Pharmacology and perspectives in erectile dysfunction in man. *Pharmacology & Therapeutics, 208,* 107493.

Miyawaki, Y., Uchida, H., Yamashita, O., Sato, M. A., et al. (2008). Visual image reconstruction from human brain activity using a combination of multiscale local image decoders. *Neuron, 60,* 915–929.

Mogwitz, S., Buse, J., Ehrlich, S., and Roessner, V. (2013). Clinical pharmacology of dopamine-modulating agents in Tourette's syndrome. *International Review of Neurobiology, 112,* 281–349.

Mohammed, A. (2001). *Enrichment and the brain. Plasticity in the adult brain: From genes to neurotherapy.* 22nd International Summer School of Brain Research, Amsterdam, Netherlands.

Mohrhardt, J., Nagel, M., Fleck, D., Ben-Shaul, Y., et al. (2018). Signal detection and coding in the accessory olfactory system. *Chemical Senses, 43*(9), 667–695.

Moita, M. A., Rosis, S., Zhou, Y., LeDoux, J. E., et al. (2004). Putting fear in its place: Remapping of hippocampal place cells during fear conditioning. *Journal of Neuroscience, 24,* 7015–7023.

Monfils, M. H., Plautz, E. J., and Kleim, J. A. (2005). In search of the motor engram: Motor map plasticity as a mechanism for encoding motor experience. *Neuroscientist, 11,* 471–483.

Monks, D. A., and Watson N. V. (2001). N-cadherin expression in motoneurons is directly regulated by androgens: A genetic mosaic analysis in rats. *Brain Research, 895,* 73–79.

Montenegro, P. H., Alosco, M. L., Martin, B., Daneshvar, D. H., et al. (2016). Cumulative head impact exposure predicts later-life depression, apathy, executive dysfunction, and cognitive impairment in former high school and college football players. *Journal of Neurotrauma, 34*(2), 328–340.

Monti, M. M., Vanhaudenhuyse, A., Coleman, M. R., Boly, M., et al. (2010). Willful modulation of brain activity in disorders of consciousness. *New England Journal of Medicine, 362,* 579–589.

Moore, C. L., Dou, H., and Juraska, J. M. (1992). Maternal stimulation affects the number of motor neurons in a sexually dimorphic nucleus of the lumbar spinal cord. *Brain Research, 572,* 52–56.

Moore, C., Gupta, R., Jordt, S. E., Chen, Y., et al. (2018). Regulation of pain and itch by TRP channels. *Neuroscience Bulletin, 34*(1), 120–142.

Moore, G. J., Cortese, B. M., Glitz, D. A., Zajac-Benitez, C., et al. (2009). A longitudinal study of the effects of lithium treatment on prefrontal and subgenual prefrontal gray matter volume in treatment-responsive bipolar disorder patients. *Journal of Clinical Psychiatry, 70*(5), 699–705.

Moore, R. Y. (2013). The suprachiasmatic nucleus and the circadian timing system. *Progress in Molecular Biology and Translational Science, 119,* 1–28.

Moore, R. Y., and Eichler, V. B. (1972). Loss of circadian adrenal corticosterone rhythm following suprachiasmatic lesions in the rat. *Brain Research, 42,* 201–206.

Moorhead, T. W., McKirdy, J., Sussmann, J. E., Hall, J., et al. (2007). Progressive gray matter loss in patients with bipolar disorder. *Biological Psychiatry, 62,* 894–900.

Moorman, S., Gobes, S. M., Kuijpers, M., Kerkhofs, A., et al. (2012). Human-like brain hemispheric dominance in birdsong learning. *Proceedings of the National Academy of Sciences, USA, 109*(31), 12782–12787.

Moran, J., and Desimone, R. (1985). Selective attention gates visual processing in the extrastriate cortex. *Science, 229,* 782–784.

Moratalla, R., Khairnar, A., Simola, N., Granado, N., et al. (2017). Amphetamine-related drugs neurotoxicity in humans and in experimental animals: Main mechanisms. *Progress in Neurobiology, 155,* 149–170.

Morawietz, C., and Moffat, F. (2013). Effects of locomotor training after incomplete spinal cord injury: A systematic review. *Archives of Physical Medicine and Rehabilitation, 94*(11), 2297–2308.

Mori, K., Nagao, H., and Yoshihara, Y. (1999). The olfactory bulb: Coding and processing of odor molecule information. *Science, 286,* 711–715.

Morizane, A., Kikuchi, T., Hayashi, T., Mizuma, H., et al. (2017). MHC matching improves engraftment of iPSC-derived neurons in non-human primates. *Nature Communications, 8*(1), 385.

Morris, B. (2002). Overcoming dyslexia. *Fortune, 145*(10), 1–7.

Morris, J. A., Jordan, C. L., and Breedlove, S. M. (2004). Sexual differentiation of the vertebrate nervous system. *Nature Neuroscience, 7*(10), 1034–1039.

Morris, R. G., Halliwell, R. F., and Bowery, N. (1989). Synaptic plasticity and learning. II: Do different kinds of plasticity underlie different kinds of learning? *Neuropsychologia, 27,* 41–59.

Morrison, A. R. (2013). Coming to grips with a "new" state of consciousness: The study of rapid-eye-movement sleep in the 1960s. *Journal of the History of the Neurosciences, 22*(4), 392–407.

Morrison, A. R., Sanford, L. D., Ball, W. A., Mann, G. L., et al. (1995). Stimulus-elicited behavior in rapid eye movement sleep without atonia. *Behavioral Neuroscience, 109,* 972–979.

Morrison, S. F. (2016). Central control of body temperature [version 1; peer review: 3 approved]. *F1000Research, 5*(F1000 Faculty Rev), 880. https://doi.org/10.12688/f1000research.7958.1

Moruzzi, G., and Magoun, H. W. (1949). Brain stem reticular formation and activation of the EEG. *Clinical Neurophysiology, 1,* 455–473.

Moser, E. I., Moser, M. B., and McNaughton, B. L. (2017). Spatial representation in the hippocampal formation: A history. *Nature Neuroscience, 20*(11), 1448–1464.

Mott, F. W. (1895). Experimental inquiry upon the afferent tracts of the central nervous system of the monkey. *Brain, 18,* 1–20.

Motta, S. C., Guimarães, C. C., Furigo, I. C., Sukikara, M. H., et al. (2013). Ventral premammillary nucleus as a critical sensory relay to the maternal aggression network. *Proceedings of the National Academy of Sciences, USA, 110,* 14438–14443.

Mountcastle, V. B. (1979). An organizing principle for cerebral function: The unit module and the distributed system. In F. O. Schmitt and F. G. Worden (Eds.), *The neurosciences: Fourth study program* (pp. 21–24). Cambridge, MA: MIT Press.

Mueller, H. T., Haroutunian, V., Davis, K. L., and Meador-Woodruff, J. H. (2004). Expression of the ionotropic glutamate receptor subunits and NMDA receptor-associated intracellular proteins in the substantia nigra in schizophrenia. *Brain Research. Molecular Brain Research, 121,* 60–69.

Muggli, E., Matthews, H., Penington, A., Claes, P., et al. (2017). Association between prenatal alcohol exposure and craniofacial shape of children at 12 months of age. *JAMA Pediatrics, 171*(8), 771–780.

Muhlert, N., and Lawrence, A. D. (2015). Brain structure correlates of emotion-based rash impulsivity. *NeuroImage, 115,* 138–146.

Mukhametov, L. M. (1984). Sleep in marine mammals. In A. Borbély and J. L. Valatx (Eds.), *Experimental Brain Research: Suppl. 8. Sleep mechanisms* (pp. 227–238). Berlin, Germany: Springer-Verlag.

Müller, M. J., Geisler, C., Heymsfield, S. B., and Bosy-Westphal, A. (2018). Recent advances in understanding body weight homeostasis in humans [version 1; peer review: 4 approved]. *F1000Research, 7*(F1000 Faculty Rev), 1025.

Munafo, J., Diedrick, M., and Stoffregen, T. A. (2017). The virtual reality head-mounted display Oculus Rift induces motion sickness and is sexist in its effects. *Experimental Brain Research, 235*(3), 889–901.

Munley, K. M., Rendon, N. M., and Demas, G. E. (2018). Neural androgen synthesis and aggression: Insights from a seasonally breeding rodent. *Frontiers in Endocrinology(Lausanne), 9,* 136.

Münte, T. F., Altenmüller, E., and Jäncke, L. (2002). The musician's brain as a model of neuroplasticity. *Nature Reviews Neuroscience, 3,* 473–478.

Murphy, M. L., Slavich, G. M., Chen, E., and Miller, G. E. (2015). Targeted rejection predicts decreased anti-inflammatory gene expression and increased symptom severity in youth with asthma. *Psychological Science, 26*(2), 111–121.

Murphy, S., Spence, C., and Dalton, P. (2017). Auditory perceptual load: A review. *Hearing Research, 352,* 40–48.

Murray, J., Burgess, S., Zuccolo, L., Hickman, M., et al. (2016). Moderate alcohol drinking in pregnancy increases risk for children's persistent conduct problems: Causal effects in a Mendelian randomisation study. *Journal of Child Psychology and Psychiatry, 57*(5), 575–584.

Muza, R., Lawrence, M., and Drakatos, P. (2016). The reality of sexsomnia. *Current Opinion in Pulmonary Medicine, 22*(6), 576–582.

N

Nader, K., and Hardt, O. (2009). A single standard for memory: The case for reconsolidation. *Nature Reviews Neuroscience, 10,* 224–234.

Naeser, M., and Hayward, R. (1978). Lesion localization in aphasia with cranial computed tomography and the Boston Diagnostic Aphasia Exam. *Neurology, 28,* 545–551.

Naesström, M., Blomstedt, P., and Bodlund, O. (2016). A systematic review of psychiatric indications for deep brain stimulation, with focus on major depressive and obsessive-compulsive disorder. *Nordic Journal of Psychiatry, 70*(7), 483–491.

Nakagawa, Y., Sano, Y., Funayama, M., and Kato, M. (2019). Prognostic factors for

long-term improvement from stroke-related aphasia with adequate linguistic rehabilitation. *Neurological Sciences, 40*(10), 2141–2146.

Nakazato, M., Murakami, N., Date, Y., Kojima, M., et al. (2001). A role for ghrelin in the central regulation of feeding. *Nature, 409,* 194–198.

Nan, Y., and Friederici, A. D. (2013). Differential roles of right temporal cortex and Broca's area in pitch processing: Evidence from music and Mandarin. *Human Brain Mapping, 34*(9), 2045–2054.

Naqvi, N. H., Rudrauf, D., Damasio, H., and Bechara, A. (2007). Damage to the insula disrupts addiction to cigarette smoking. *Science, 315,* 531–534.

Nation, E. F. (1973). William Osler on penis captivus and other urologic topics. *Urology, 2,* 468–470.

National Academy of Sciences. (2003). *The polygraph and lie detection.* Washington, DC: National Academies Press (www.nap.edu/openbook.php?isbn=0309084369).

National Institute of Mental Health, https://www.nimh.nih.gov/health/statistics.

National Institute of Mental Health. (2017). *Past year prevalence of serious mental illness among U.S. adults (2016).* (Data courtesy of SAMHSA. Last updated November 2017.) Bethesda, MD (www.nimh.nih.gov/health/statistics/prevalence/serious-mental-illness-smi-among-us-adults.shtml).

National Institute on Drug Abuse. (2016). Trends and Statistics, https://www.drugabuse.gov/related-topics/trends-statistics.

Nature. (2017). Head injuries in sport must be taken more seriously. *Nature, 548*(7668), 371.

Navarro-Lobato, I., and Genzel, L. (2018). The up and down of sleep: From molecules to electrophysiology. *Neurobiology of Learning and Memory,* pii: S1074-7427(18)30067-4.

Neff, W. D., and Casseday, J. H. (1977). Effects of unilateral ablation of auditory cortex on monaural cat's ability to localize sound. *Journal of Neurophysiology, 40,* 44–52.

Nelson, G., Chandrashekar, J., Hoon, M. A., Feng, L., et al. (2002). An amino-acid taste receptor. *Nature, 416,* 199–202.

Nelson, G., Hoon, M. A., Chandrashekar, J., Zhang, Y., et al. (2001). Mammalian sweet taste receptors. *Cell, 106,* 381–390.

Nestler, E. J., and Hyman, S. E. (2010). Animal models of neuropsychiatric disorders. *Nature Neuroscience, 13,* 1161–1169.

Neumeister, A., Bain, E., Nugent, A. C., Carson, R. E., et al. (2004). Reduced serotonin type 1A receptor binding in panic disorder. *Journal of Neuroscience, 24,* 589–591.

Newman, A. J., Supalla, T., Fernandez, N., Newport, E. L., et al. (2015). Neural systems supporting linguistic structure, linguistic experience, and symbolic communication in sign language and gesture. *Proceedings of the National Academy of Sciences, USA, 112*(37), 11684–11689. https://doi.org/10.1073/pnas.1510527112

Newth, S., and Rachman, S. (2001). The concealment of obsessions. *Behaviour Research and Therapy, 39*(4), 457–464.

Ng, M., Fleming, T., Robinson, M., Thomson, B., et al. (2014). Global, regional, and national prevalence of overweight and obesity in children and adults during 1980–2013: A systematic analysis for the Global Burden of Disease Study 2013. *Lancet, 384*, 766–781.

Ng, S. F., Lin, R. C., Laybutt, D. R., Barres, R., et al. (2010). Chronic high-fat diet in fathers programs β-cell dysfunction in female rat offspring. *Nature, 467*, 963–966.

Ngandu, T., Lehtisalo, J., Solomon, A., Levälahti, E., et al. (2015). A 2 year multidomain intervention of diet, exercise, cognitive training, and vascular risk monitoring versus control to prevent cognitive decline in at-risk elderly people (FINGER): A randomised controlled trial. *Lancet*, pii: S0140-6736(15)60461-5.

Nguyen, J. D., Bremer, P. T., Hwang, C. S., Vandewater, S. A., et al. (2017). Effective active vaccination against methamphetamine in female rats. *Drug and Alcohol Dependence, 175*, 179–186.

Niazi, R. K., Gjesing, A. P., Hollensted, M., Have, C. T., et al. (2018). Identification of novel LEPR mutations in Pakistani families with morbid childhood obesity. *BMC Medical Genetics, 19*(1), 199.

Nichols, M. J., and Newsome, W. T. (1999). The neurobiology of cognition. *Nature, 402*, C35–C38.

Nietzel, M. T. (2000). Police psychology. In A. E. Kazdin (Ed.), *Encyclopedia of psychology* (Vol. 6, pp. 224–226). Washington, DC: American Psychological Association.

Nishida, M., and Walker, M. P. (2007). Daytime naps, motor memory consolidation and regionally specific sleep spindles. *PLOS ONE, 2*, e341.

Nishimoto, S., and Gallant, J. L. (2011). A three-dimensional spatiotemporal receptive field model explains responses of area MT neurons to naturalistic movies. *Journal of Neuroscience, 31*, 14551–14564.

Norrman, G., and Bylund, E. (2016). The irreversibility of sensitive period effects in language development: Evidence from second language acquisition in international adoptees. *Developmental Science, 19*(3), 513–520.

Nowacki, A., Seidel, K., Schucht, P., Schindler, K., et al. (2015). Induction of fear by intraoperative stimulation during awake craniotomy: Case presentation and systematic review of the literature. *World Neurosurgery, 84*(2), 470–474.

Numan, M. (2015). Aggressive behavior. In M. Numan (Ed.), *Neurobiology of social behavior* (pp. 63–107). San Diego, CA: Academic Press.

Nutt, D. J., Lingford-Hughes, A., Erritzoe, D., and Stokes, P. R. (2015). The dopamine theory of addiction: 40 years of highs and lows. *Nature Reviews Neuroscience, 16*(5), 305–312.

O

O'Connell-Rodwell, C. E. (2007). Keeping an "ear" to the ground: Seismic communication in elephants. *Physiology (Bethesda), 22*, 287–294.

O'Connor, D. B., Archer, J., and Wu, F. C. (2004). Effects of testosterone on mood, aggression, and sexual behavior in young men: A double-blind, placebo-controlled, cross-over study. *Journal of Clinical Endocrinology & Metabolism, 89*, 2837–2845.

O'Connor, E. A., Evans, C. V., Burda, B. U., Walsh, E. S., et al. (2017). Screening for obesity and interventions for weight management in children and adolescents: A systematic evidence review for the U.S. Preventive Services Task Force. Evidence Synthesis No. 150. Rockville, MD: Agency for Healthcare Research and Quality (https://www.ncbi.nlm.nih.gov/books/NBK476325/pdf/Bookshelf_NBK476325.pdf).

O'Craven, K. M., Downing, P. E., and Kanwisher, N. (1999). fMRI evidence for objects as the units of attentional selection. *Nature, 401*, 584–587.

O'Donovan, A., Chao, L. L., Paulson, J., Samuelson, K. W., et al. (2015). Altered inflammatory activity associated with reduced hippocampal volume and more severe posttraumatic stress symptoms in Gulf War veterans. *Psychoneuroendocrinology, 51*, 557–566.

Oberlander, T. F., Papsdorf, M., Brain, U. M., Misri, S., et al. (2010). Prenatal effects of selective serotonin reuptake inhibitor antidepressants, serotonin transporter promoter genotype (SLC6A4), and maternal mood on child behavior at 3 years of age. *Archives of Pediatrics and Adolescent Medicine, 164*, 444–451.

O'Donnell, K. J., and Meaney, M. J. (2020). Epigenetics, development, and psychopathology. *Annual Review of Clinical Psychology, 16*, 327–350.

Ogden, J. (2012). *Health psychology*. New York, NY: Open University Press.

Ojala, K. E., Janssen, L. K., Hashemi, M. M., Timmer, M. H. M., et al. (2018). Dopaminergic drug effects on probability weighting during risky decision making. *eNeuro, 5*(2), ENEURO.0330-18.2018.

O'Keefe, J., and Burgess, N. (2005). Dual phase and rate coding in hippocampal place cells: Theoretical significance and relationship to entorhinal grid cells. *Hippocampus, 15*(7), 853–866.

O'Keefe, J. H., Bhatti, S. K., Bajwa, A., DiNicolantonio, J. J., et al. (2014). Alcohol and cardiovascular health: The dose makes the poison … or the remedy. *Mayo Clinic Proceedings, 89*(3), 382–393.

Olabi, B., Ellison-Wright, I., McIntosh, A. M., Wood, S. J., et al. (2011). Are there progressive brain changes in schizophrenia? A meta-analysis of structural magnetic resonance imaging studies. *Biological Psychiatry, 70*(1), 88–96.

Olds, J., and Milner, P. (1954). Positive reinforcement produced by electrical stimulation of septal area and other regions of rat brain. *Journal of Comparative and Physiological Psychology, 47*, 419–427.

Olender, T., Lancet, D., and Nebert, D. W. (2008). Update on the olfactory receptor (OR) gene superfamily. *Human Genomics, 3*(1), 87–97.

Oler, J. A., Fox, A. S., Shelton, S. E., Rogers, J., et al. (2010). Amygdalar and hippocampal substrates of anxious temperament differ in their heritability. *Nature, 466*, 864–868.

Olfson, M., Marcus, S. C., and Shaffer, D. (2006). Antidepressant drug therapy and suicide in severely depressed children and adults: A case-control study. *Archives of General Psychiatry, 63*, 865–872.

Olsen, R. W. (2018). GABA(A) receptor: Positive and negative allosteric modulators. *Neuropharmacology, 136*(Pt. A), 10–22.

Olson, S. (2004). Making sense of Tourette's. *Science, 305*, 1390–1392.

Oman, C. M. (2012). Are evolutionary hypotheses for motion sickness "just-so" stories? *Journal of Vestibular Research, 22*(2), 117–127.

Onmyoji, Y., Kubota, S., Hirano, M., Tanaka, M., et al. (2015). Excitability changes in the left primary motor cortex innervating the hand muscles induced during speech about hand or leg movements. *Neuroscience Letters, 594*, 46–50.

Opendak, M., and Gould, E. (2015). Adult neurogenesis: A substrate for experience-dependent change. *Trends in Cognitive Science, 19*, 151–161.

Oppenheim, K. (2006, February 3). Life full of danger for little girl who can't feel pain. *CNN* (http://www.cnn.com/2006/HEALTH/conditions/02/03/btsc.oppenheim).

Orlovska, S., Vestergaard, C. H., Bech, B. H., Nordentoft, M., et al. (2017). Association of streptococcal throat infection with mental disorders: Testing key aspects of the PANDAS hypothesis in a nationwide study. *JAMA Psychiatry, 74*(7), 740–746.

O'Shea, J., Revol, P., Cousijn, H., Near, J., et al. (2017). Induced sensorimotor cortex plasticity remediates chronic treatment-resistant visual neglect. *eLife, 6,* e26602.

Osorio, D., and Vorobyev, M. (2008). A review of the evolution of animal colour vision and visual communication signals. *Vision Research, 48,* 2042–2051.

Ossenkoppele, R., Jansen, W. J., Rabinovici, G. D., Knol, D. L., et al. (2015). Prevalence of amyloid PET positivity in dementia syndromes: A meta-analysis. *JAMA, 313,* 1939–1949.

Öst, L. G., Riise, E. N., Wergeland, G. J., Hansen, B., et al. (2016). Cognitive behavioral and pharmacological treatments of OCD in children: A systematic review and meta-analysis. *Journal of Anxiety Disorders, 43,* 58–69.

Osterhout, L. (1997). On the brain response to syntactic anomalies: Manipulations of word position and word class reveal individual differences. *Brain and Language, 59,* 494–522.

Ostrovsky, Y., Meyers, E., Ganesh, S., Mathur, U., et al. (2009). Visual parsing after recovery from blindness. *Psychological Science, 20,* 1484–1491.

O'Tuathaigh, C. M. P., Moran, P. M., Zhen, X. C., and Waddington, J. L. (2017). Translating advances in the molecular basis of schizophrenia into novel cognitive treatment strategies. *British Journal of Pharmacology, 174*(19), 3173–3190.

Overstreet, D. H., and Wegener, G. (2013). The Flinders Sensitive Line rat model of depression: 25 years and still producing. *Pharmacological Reviews, 65*(1), 143–155.

Overton, J. A., and Recanzone, G. H. (2016). Effects of aging on the response of single neurons to amplitude-modulated noise in primary auditory cortex of rhesus macaque. *Journal of Neurophysiology, 115*(6), 2911–2923.

P

Padawer, R. (2016, July 3). Too fast to be female. *New York Times Sunday Magazine* (https://www.nytimes.com/2016/07/03/magazine/the-humiliating-practice-of-sex-testing-female-athletes.html).

Pagel, J. F., and Helfter, P. (2003). Drug induced nightmares—An etiology based review. *Human Psychopharmacology, 18,* 59–67.

Pagel, M., Atkinson, Q. D., Calude, A. S., and Meade, A. (2013). Ultraconserved words point to deep language ancestry across Eurasia. *Proceedings of the National Academy of Sciences, USA, 110*(21), 8471–8476.

Palagini, L., Baglioni, C., Ciapparelli, A., Gemignani, A., et al. (2013). REM sleep dysregulation in depression: State of the art. *Sleep Medicine Reviews, 17*(5), 377–390.

Palaus, M., Marron, E. M., Viejo-Sobera, R., and Redolar-Ripoll, D. (2017). Neural basis of video gaming: A systematic review. *Frontiers in Human Neuroscience, 11,* 248.

Palmer, S. M, Crewther, S. G, Carey, L. M, and the START Project Team. (2015). A meta-analysis of changes in brain activity in clinical depression. *Frontiers in Human Neuroscience, 8,* 1045.

Panksepp, J. (2000). Emotions as natural kinds within the mammalian brain. In M. Lewis and J. M. Haviland-Jones (Eds.), *Handbook of emotions* (2nd ed., pp. 137–156). New York, NY: Guilford Press.

Panksepp, J. (2005). Beyond a joke: From animal laughter to human joy? *Science, 308,* 62–63.

Panksepp, J. (2007). Neuroevolutionary sources of laughter and social joy: Modeling primal human laughter in laboratory rats. *Behavioural Brain Research, 182,* 231–244.

Panksepp, J. B., Yue, Z., Drerup, C., and Huber, R. (2003). Amine neurochemistry and aggression in crayfish. *Microscopy Research and Technique, 60,* 360–368.

Pantev, C., Oostenveld, R., Engelien, A., Ross, B., et al. (1998). Increased auditory cortical representation in musicians. *Nature, 392,* 811–814.

Papez, J. W. (1937). A proposed mechanism of emotion. *Archives of Neurology and Psychiatry, 38,* 725–745.

Papka, M., Ivry, R., and Woodruff-Pak, D. S. (1994). Eyeblink classical conditioning and time production in patients with cerebellar damage. *Society of Neuroscience Abstracts, 20,* 360.

Paré, M., Behets, C., and Cornu, O. (2003). Paucity of presumptive Ruffini corpuscles in the index finger pad of humans. *Journal of Comparative Neurology, 456*(3), 260–266.

Park, K. M., Kim, S. E., and Lee, B. I. (2019). Antiepileptic drug therapy in patients with drug-resistant epilepsy. *Journal of Epilepsy Research, 9*(1), 14–26.

Parker, G., Cahill, L., and McGaugh, J. L. (2006). A case of unusual autobiographical remembering. *Neurocase, 12,* 35–49.

Parrott, A. C. (2013). Human psychobiology of MDMA or "Ecstasy": An overview of 25 years of empirical research. *Human Psychopharmacology, 28,* 289–307.

Parrott, A. C. (2014). The potential dangers of using MDMA for psychotherapy. *Journal of Psychoactive Drugs, 46*(1), 37–43.

Parton, A., Malhotra, P., and Husain, M. (2004). Hemispatial neglect. *Journal of Neurology, Neurosurgery and Psychiatry, 75,* 13–21.

Parton, L. E., Ye, C. P., Coppari, R., Enriori, P. J., et al. (2007). Glucose sensing by POMC neurons regulates glucose homeostasis and is impaired in obesity. *Nature, 449,* 228–232.

Pasquinelli, E. (2012). Neuromyths: Why do they exist and persist? *Mind, Brain, and Education, 6*(2), 89–96.

Pastalkova, E., Itskov, V., Amarasingham, A., and Buzsáki, G. (2008). Internally generated cell assembly sequences in the rat hippocampus. *Science, 321,* 1322–1327.

Paterson, S. J., Brown, J. H., Gsödl, M. K., Johnson, M. H., et al. (1999). Cognitive modularity and genetic disorders. *Science, 286,* 2355–2358.

Paterson, S. J., and Schultz, R. T. (2007). Neurodevelopmental and behavioral issues in Williams syndrome. *Current Psychiatry Reports, 9*(2), 165–171.

Paton, J. J., Belova, M. A., Morrison, S. E., and Salzman, C. D. (2006). The primate amygdala represents the positive and negative value of visual stimuli during learning. *Nature, 439*(7078), 865–870.

Patterson, P. H. (2007). Maternal effects on schizophrenia risk. *Science, 318,* 576–578.

Pauls, D. L., Abramovitch, A., Rauch, S. L., and Geller, D. A. (2014). Obsessive-compulsive disorder: An integrative genetic and neurobiological perspective. *Nature Reviews Neuroscience, 15*(6), 410–424.

Paus, T., Kalina, M., Patocková, L., Angerová, Y., et al. (1991). Medial vs lateral frontal lobe lesions and differential impairment of central-gaze fixation maintenance in man. *Brain, 114,* 2051–2067.

Paus, T., Keshavan, M., and Giedd, J. N. (2008). Why do many psychiatric disorders emerge during adolescence? *Nature Reviews Neuroscience, 9,* 947–956.

Payne, B. R., Lee, C. L., and Federmeier, K. D. (2015). Revisiting the incremental effects of context on word processing: Evidence from single-word event-related brain potentials. *Psychophysiology, 52*(11), 1456–1469.

Payne, N. A., and Prudic, J. (2009). Electroconvulsive therapy: Part I. A perspective on the evolution and current practice of ECT. *Journal of Psychiatric Practice, 15*(5), 346–368.

Pedersen, C. B., and Mortensen, P. B. (2001). Evidence of a dose-response relationship between urbanicity during upbringing and schizophrenia risk. *Archives of General Psychiatry, 58,* 1039–1046.

Pediatric Eye Disease Investigator Group. (2005). Randomized trial of treatment of amblyopia in children aged 7 to 17 years. *Archives of Ophthalmology, 13,* 437–447.

Pedreira, C., Mormann, F., Kraskov, A., Cerf, M., et al. (2010). Responses of human medial temporal lobe neurons are modulated by stimulus repetition. *Journal of Neurophysiology, 103,* 97–107.

Peever, J., Luppi, P. H., and Montplaisir, J. (2014). Breakdown in REM sleep circuitry underlies REM sleep behavior disorder. *Trends in Neurosciences, 37,* 279–288.

Pegna, A. J., Khateb, A., Lazeyras, F., and Seghier, M. L. (2005). Discriminating emotional faces without primary visual cortices involves the right amygdala. *Nature Neuroscience, 8,* 24–25.

Penadés, R., González-Rodríguez, A., Catalán, R., Segura, B., et al. (2017). Neuroimaging studies of cognitive remediation in schizophrenia: A systematic and critical review. *World Journal of Psychiatry, 7*(1), 34–43.

Penfield, W., and Rasmussen, T. (1950). *The cerebral cortex in man.* New York, NY: Macmillan.

Penfield, W., and Roberts, L. (1959). *Speech and brain-mechanisms.* Princeton, NJ: Princeton University Press.

Peplau, L. A. (2003). Human sexuality: How do men and women differ? *Current Directions in Psychological Science, 12,* 37–40.

Pepper, J., Hariz, M., and Zrinzo, L. (2015). Deep brain stimulation versus anterior capsulotomy for obsessive-compulsive disorder: A review of the literature. *Journal of Neurosurgery, 122,* 1028–1037.

Pepperberg, I. M. (2008). *Alex and me.* New York, NY: Harper.

Perani, D., and Abutalebi, J. (2005). The neural basis of first and second language processing. *Current Opinion in Neurobiology, 15,* 202–206.

Perani, D., Farsad, M., Ballarini, T., Lubian, F., et al. (2017). The impact of bilingualism on brain reserve and metabolic connectivity in Alzheimer's dementia. *Proceedings of the National Academy of Sciences, USA, 114*(7), 1690–1695.

Perea, G., Navarrete, M., and Araque, A. (2009). Tripartite synapses: Astrocytes process and control synaptic information. *Trends in Neurosciences, 32,* 421–431.

Pernía-Andrade, A. J., Kato, A., Witschi, R., Nyilas, R., et al. (2009). Spinal endocannabinoids and CB1 receptors mediate C-fiber–induced heterosynaptic pain sensitization. *Science, 325,* 760–764.

Peterson, B. S., Warner, V., Bansal, R., Zhu, H., et al. (2009). Cortical thinning in persons at increased familial risk for major depression. *Proceedings of the National Academy of Sciences, USA, 106,* 6273–6278.

Peterson, L. R., and Peterson, M. J. (1959). Short-term retention of individual verbal items. *Journal of Experimental Psychology, 58,* 193–198.

Petit, C., and Richardson, G. P. (2009). Linking genes underlying deafness to hair-bundle development and function. *Nature Neuroscience, 12,* 703–710.

Petrides, M., and Milner, B. (1982). Deficits on subject-ordered tasks after frontal- and temporal-lobe lesions in man. *Neuropsychologia, 20,* 249–262.

Petrone, A. B., Simpkins, J. W., and Barr, T. L. (2014). 17β-Estradiol and inflammation: Implications for ischemic stroke. *Aging and Disease, 5,* 340–345.

Petrovic, P., Kalso, E., Petersson, K. M., and Ingvar, M. (2002). Placebo and opioid analgesia imaging—A shared neuronal network. *Science, 295,* 1737–1740.

Pettit, H. O., and Justice, J. B., Jr. (1991). Effect of dose on cocaine self-administration behavior and dopamine levels in the nucleus accumbens. *Brain Research, 539,* 94–102.

Pfaff, D. W. (1980). Estrogens and brain function: Neural analysis of a hormone-controlled mammalian reproductive behavior. New York, NY: Springer-Verlag.

Pfaff, D. W., Gagnidze, K., and Hunter, R. G. (2018). Molecular endocrinology of female reproductive behavior. *Molecular and Cellular Endocrinology, 467,* 14–20.

Pfau, D., Jordan, C. L., and Breedlove, S. M. (2019). The de-scent of sexuality: Did loss of a pheromone signaling protein permit the evolution of same-sex sexual behavior in primates? *Archives of Sexual Behavior.*

Pfeffer, M., Wicht, H., von Gall, C., and Korf, H. W. (2015). Owls and larks in mice. *Frontiers in Neurology, 6,* 101.

Pfenning, A. R., Hara, E., Whitney, O., Rivas, M. V., et al. (2014). Convergent transcriptional specializations in the brains of humans and song-learning birds. *Science, 346*(6215), 1256846.

Phoenix, C. H., Goy, R. W., Gerall, A. A., and Young, W. C. (1959). Organizing action of prenatally administered testosterone propionate on the tissues mediating mating behavior in the female guinea pig. *Endocrinology, 65,* 369–382.

Pickens, R., and Thompson, T. (1968). Drug use by U.S. Army enlisted men in Vietnam: A followup on their return home. *Journal of Pharmacology and Experimental Therapeutics, 161,* 122–129.

Pin, J. P., and Bettler, B. (2016). Organization and functions of mGlu and GABA(B) receptor complexes. *Nature, 540*(7631), 60–68.

Pinel, P., Fauchereau, F., Moreno, A., Barbot, A., et al. (2012). Genetic variants of *FOXP2* and *KIAA0319/TTRAP/THEM2* locus are associated with altered brain activation in distinct language-related regions. *Journal of Neuroscience, 32,* 817–825.

Pinker, S., and Jackendoff, R. (2005). The faculty of language: What's special about it? *Cognition, 95*(2), 201–236.

Pirastu, N., Kooyman, M., Traglia, M., Robino, A., et al. (2016). A Genome-Wide Association Study in isolated populations reveals new genes associated to common food likings. *Reviews in Endocrine and Metabolic Disorders, 17*(2), 209–219.

Pitcher, B. J., Harcourt, R. G., and Charrier, I. (2010). The memory remains: Long-term vocal recognition in Australian sea lions. *Animal Cognition, 13*(5), 771–776.

Pitts, M. A., Padwal, J., Fennelly, D., Martínez, A., et al. (2014). Gamma band activity and the P3 reflect post-perceptual processes, not visual awareness. *NeuroImage, 101,* 337–350.

Pletnikov, M. V., Ayhan, Y., Nikolskaia, O., Xu, Y., et al. (2008). Inducible expression of mutant human *DISC1* in mice is associated with brain and behavioral abnormalities reminiscent of schizophrenia. *Molecular Psychiatry, 13,* 13–186.

Ploog, D. W. (1992). Neuroethological perspectives on the human brain: From the expression of emotions to intentional signing and speech. In A. Harrington (Ed.), *So human a brain: Knowledge and values in the neurosciences* (pp. 3–13). Boston, MA: Birkhauser.

Plutchik, R. (1994). *The psychology and biology of emotion.* New York, NY: HarperCollins.

Plutchik, R. (2001). The nature of emotions: Human emotions have deep evolutionary roots, a fact that may explain their complexity and provide tools for clinical practice. *American Scientist, 89*(4), 344–350.

Poldrack, R. A., Baker, C. I., Durnez, J., Gorgolewski, K. J., et al. (2017). Scanning the horizon: Towards transparent and reproducible neuroimaging research. *Nature Reviews Neuroscience, 18*(2), 115–126.

Ponsford, J. (2005). Rehabilitation interventions after mild head injury. *Current Opinion in Neurology, 18,* 692–697.

Poole, J. H., Tyack, P. L., Stoeger-Horwath, A. S., and Watwood, S. (2005). Animal behaviour: Elephants are capable of vocal learning. *Nature, 434,* 455–456.

Poremba, A., Malloy, M., Saunders, R. C., Carson, R. E., et al. (2004). Species-specific calls evoke asymmetric activity in the monkey's temporal poles. *Nature, 427,* 448–451.

Porta, M., Brambilla, A., Cavanna, A. E., Servello, D., et al. (2009). Thalamic deep brain stimulation for treatment-refractory Tourette syndrome: Two-year outcome. *Neurology, 73,* 1375–1380.

Posner, M. I. (1980). Orienting of attention. *Quarterly Journal of Experimental Psychology, 32,* 3–25.

Posner, M. I., and Raichle, M. E. (1994). *Images of mind.* New York, NY: Scientific American Library.

Poulet, J. F. A., and Petersen, C. C. H. (2008). Internal brain state regulates membrane potential synchrony in barrel cortex of behaving mice. *Nature, 454,* 881–885.

Poulos, A. M., and Thompson, R. F. (2015). Localization and characterization of an essential associative memory trace in the mammalian brain. *Brain Research, 1621,* 252–259.

Powell, S. B. (2010). Models of neurodevelopmental abnormalities in schizophrenia. *Current Topics in Behavioral Neurosciences, 4,* 435–481.

Pratt, L. A., Brody, D. J., and Gu, Q. (2011). *Antidepressant use in persons aged 12 and over: United States, 2005–2008* (NCHS

Data Brief, No. 76). Hyattsville, MD: National Center for Health Statistics.

Prehn, K., Jumpertz von Schwartzenberg, R., Mai, K., Zeitz, U., et al. (2017). Caloric restriction in older adults: Differential effects of weight loss and reduced weight on brain structure and function. *Cerebral Cortex, 27*(3), 1765–1778.

Premack, D. (1971). Language in a chimpanzee? *Science, 172,* 808–822.

Prendergast, B. J., Onishi, K. G., and Zucker, I. (2014). Female mice liberated for inclusion in neuroscience and biomedical research. *Neuroscience & Biobehavioral Reviews, 40,* 1–5.

Prentice, R. L. (2014). Postmenopausal hormone therapy and the risks of coronary heart disease, breast cancer, and stroke. *Seminars in Reproductive Medicine, 32,* 419–425.

Prudente, C. N., Stilla, R., Buetefisch, C. M., Singh, S., et al. (2015). Neural substrates for head movements in humans: A functional magnetic resonance imaging study. *Journal of Neuroscience, 35,* 9163–9172.

Pugh, K. R., Mencl, W. E., Shaywitz, B. A., Shaywitz, S. E., et al. (2000). The angular gyrus in developmental dyslexia: Task-specific differences in functional connectivity within posterior cortex. *Psychological Science, 11,* 51–56.

Pulak, L. M., and Jensen, L. (2014). Sleep in the intensive care unit: A review. *Journal of Intensive Care Medicine,* pii: 0885066614538749.

Purves, D., Augustine, G. J., Fitzpatrick, D., Katz, L., et al. (Eds.). (2001). *Neuroscience* (2nd ed.). Sunderland, MA: Oxford University Press/Sinauer.

Purves, D., Shimpi, A., and Lotto, R. B. (1999). An empirical explanation of the Cornsweet effect. *Journal of Neuroscience, 19,* 8542–4251.

Putman, C. T., Xu, X., Gillies, E., MacLean, I. M., et al. (2004). Effects of strength, endurance and combined training on myosin heavy chain content and fibre-type distribution in humans. *European Journal of Applied Physiology, 92,* 376–384.

Q

Qi, Y., Zheng, Y., Li, Z., and Xiong, L. (2017). Progress in genetic studies of Tourette's syndrome. *Brain Sciences, 7*(10), E134.

Quraishi, I. H., Benjamin, C. F., Spencer, D. D., Blumenfeld, H., et al. (2017). Impairment of consciousness induced by bilateral electrical stimulation of the frontal convexity. *Epilepsy & Behavior Case Reports, 8,* 117–122.

R

Rabinovici, G. D., Stephens, M. L., and Possin, K. L. (2015). Executive dysfunction. *Continuum: Lifelong Learning in Neurology, 21*(3: Behavioral Neurology and Neuropsychiatry), 646–659.

Racette, A., Bard, C., and Peretz, I. (2006). Making non-fluent aphasics speak: Sing along! *Brain, 129,* 2571–2584.

Racine, E., Bar-Ilan, O., and Illes, J. (2005). fMRI in the public eye. *Nature Reviews Neuroscience, 6,* 159–164.

Rafal, R. D. (1994). Neglect. *Current Opinion in Neurobiology, 4,* 231–236.

Rahman, Q. (2005). The neurodevelopment of human sexual orientation. *Neuroscience and Biobehavioral Reviews, 29,* 1057–1066.

Raichle, M. E. (2015). The brain's default mode network. *Annual Review of Neuroscience, 38,* 433–447.

Rajagopalan, V., Scott, J., Habas, P. A., Kim, J., et al. (2011). Local tissue growth patterns underlying normal fetal human brain gyrification quantified in utero. *Journal of Neuroscience, 31*(8), 2878–2887.

Rakic, P. (1979). In F. O. Schmitt and F. G. Worden (Eds.), *The neurosciences: Fourth study program.* Cambridge, MA: MIT Press.

Ralph, M. R., Foster, R. G., Davis, F. C., and Menaker, M. (1990). Transplanted suprachiasmatic nucleus determines circadian period. *Science, 247,* 975–978.

Ralph, M. R., and Menaker, M. (1988). A mutation of the circadian system in golden hamsters. *Science, 241,* 1225–1227.

Ramachandran, V. S., and Rogers-Ramachandran, D. (2000). Phantom limbs and neural plasticity. *Archives of Neurology, 57,* 317–320.

Rampon, C., Tang, Y. P., Goodhouse, J., Shimizu, E., et al. (2000). Enrichment induces structural changes and recovery from nonspatial memory deficits in CA1 *NMDAR1*-knockout mice. *Nature Neuroscience, 3,* 238–244.

Rasmussen, M. K., Mestre, H., and Nedergaard, M. (2018). The glymphatic pathway in neurological disorders. *Lancet Neurology, 17*(11), 1016–1024.

Rathelot, J. A., and Strick, P. L. (2006). Muscle representation in the macaque motor cortex: An anatomical perspective. *Proceedings of the National Academy of Sciences, USA, 103,* 8257–8262.

Rattenborg, N. C. (2006). Do birds sleep in flight? *Naturwissenschaften, 93,* 413–425.

Rauch, S. L., Shin, L. M., and Wright, C. I. (2003). Neuroimaging studies of amygdala function in anxiety disorders. *Annals of the New York Academy of Sciences, 985,* 389–410.

Rauschert, S., Melton, P. E., Burdge, G., Craig, J. M., et al. (2019). Maternal smoking during pregnancy induces persistent epigenetic changes into adolescence, independent of postnatal smoke exposure and is associated with cardiometabolic risk. *Frontiers in Genetics, 10,* 770.

Recanzone, G. (2018). The effects of aging on auditory cortical function. *Hearing Research, 366,* 99–105.

Rechtschaffen, A., and Bergmann, B. M. (2002). Sleep deprivation in the rat: An update of the 1989 paper. *Sleep, 25*(1), 18–24.

Rechtschaffen, A., and Kales, A. (1968). *A manual of standardized terminology, techniques and scoring system for sleep stages of human subjects.* Bethesda, MD: U.S. National Institute of Neurological Diseases and Blindness, Neurological Information Network.

Redican, W. K. (1982). An evolutionary perspective on human facial displays. In P. Ekman (Ed.), *Emotion in the human face* (2nd ed., pp. 212–280). Cambridge, UK: Cambridge University Press.

Reiner, W. G., and Gearhart, J. P. (2004). Discordant sexual identity in some genetic males with cloacal exstrophy assigned to female sex at birth. *New England Journal of Medicine, 350,* 333–341.

Reisberg, D., and Heuer, F. (1995). Emotion's multiple effects on memory. In J. L. McGaugh, N. M. Weinberger, and G. Lynch (Eds.), *Brain and memory: Modulation and mediation of neuroplasticity* (pp. 84–92). New York, NY: Oxford University Press.

Renner, M. J., and Rosenzweig, M. R. (1987). *Enriched and impoverished environments: Effects on brain and behavior.* New York, NY: Springer-Verlag.

Reppert, S. M., and Weaver, D. R. (2002). Coordination of circadian timing in mammals. *Nature, 418,* 935–941.

Rezaie, L., Fobian, A. D., McCall, W. V., and Khazaie, H. (2018). Paradoxical insomnia and subjective-objective sleep discrepancy: A review. *Sleep Medicine Reviews, 40,* 196–202.

Rezlescu, C., Barton, J. J., Pitcher, D., and Duchaine, B. (2014). Normal acquisition of expertise with greebles in two cases of acquired prosopagnosia. *Proceedings of the National Academy of Sciences USA, 111*(14), 5123–5128.

Richards, C., MacKenzie, N., Roberts, S., and Escorpizo, R. (2017). People with spinal cord injury in the United States. *American Journal of Physical Medicine & Rehabilitation, 96*(2 Suppl. 1), S124–S126.

Richter, C. (1967). Sleep and activity: Their relation to the 24-hour clock. *Proceedings of the Association for Research in Nervous and Mental Diseases, 45,* 8–27.

Risch, N., Herrell, R., Lehner, T., Liang, K. Y., et al. (2009). Interaction between the serotonin transporter gene (*5-HTTLPR*), stressful life events, and risk of depression: A meta-analysis. *JAMA, 301,* 2462–2471.

Ritchie, H., and Roser, M. (2019). Mental health. Our World in Data (https://ourworldindata.org/mental-health).

Rizzolatti, G., and Craighero, L. (2004). The mirror-neuron system. *Annual Review of Neuroscience, 27*, 169–192.

Roberto, M., and Varodayan, F. P. (2017). Synaptic targets: Chronic alcohol actions. *Neuropharmacology, 122*, 85–99.

Robertson, D. J., Noyes, E., Dowsett, A. J., Jenkins, R., et al. (2016). Face recognition by metropolitan police super-recognisers. *PLOS ONE, 11*(2), e0150036.

Robinson, D. L., and Petersen, S. E. (1992). The pulvinar and visual salience. *Trends in Neuroscience, 15*, 127–132.

Robinson, R. (2009). Intractable depression responds to deep brain stimulation. *Neurology Today, 9*, 7–10.

Roe, A. W., Chelazzi, L., Connor, C. E., Conway, B. R., et al. (2012). Toward a unified theory of visual area V4. *Neuron, 74*(1), 12–29.

Roebber, J. K., Roper, S. D., and Chaudhari, N. (2019). The role of the anion in salt (NaCl) detection by mouse taste buds. *Journal of Neuroscience, 39*(32), 6224–6232.

Roenneberg, T., Allebrandt, K. V., Merrow, M., and Vetter, C. (2012). Social jetlag and obesity. *Current Biology, 22*, 939–943.

Roenneberg, T., Kuehnle, T., Pramstaller, P. P., Ricken, J., et al. (2004). A marker for the end of adolescence. *Current Biology, 14*, R1038–R1039.

Roffwarg, H. P., Muzio, J. N., and Dement, W. C. (1966). Ontogenetic development of the human sleep-dream cycle. *Science, 152*, 604–619.

Roh, J. I., Lee, J., Park, S. U., Kang, Y. S., et al. (2018). CRISPR-Cas9-mediated generation of obese and diabetic mouse models. *Experimental Animals, 67*(2), 229–237.

Roland, P. E. (1993). *Brain activation.* New York, NY: Wiley-Liss.

Rose, K. A., Morgan, I. G., Smith, W., Burlutsky, G., et al. (2008). Myopia, lifestyle, and schooling in students of Chinese ethnicity in Singapore and Sydney. *Archives of Ophthalmology, 126*, 527–530.

Rosell, D. R., and Siever, L. J. (2015). The neurobiology of aggression and violence. *CNS Spectrums, 20*(3), 254–279.

Roselli, C. E., Larkin, K., Resko, J. A., Stellflug, J. N., et al. (2004). The volume of a sexually dimorphic nucleus in the ovine medial preoptic area/anterior hypothalamus varies with sexual partner preference. *Endocrinology, 145*, 475–477.

Roselli, C. E., and Stormshak, F. (2009). The neurobiology of sexual partner preferences in rams. *Hormones and Behavior, 55*, 611–620.

Rosenbaum, R. S., Köhler, S., Schacter, D. L., Moscovitch, M., et al. (2005). The case of K.C.: Contributions of a memory-impaired person to memory theory. *Neuropsychologia, 43*, 989–1021.

Rosenberg, M. D., Finn, E. S., Scheinost, D., Constable, R. T., et al. (2017).

Characterizing attention with predictive network models. *Trends in Cognitive Sciences, 21*(4), 290–302.

Rosenberg, M. D., Finn, E. S., Scheinost, D., Papademetris, X., et al. (2016). A neuromarker of sustained attention from whole-brain functional connectivity. *Nature Neuroscience, 19*(1), 165–171.

Rosenkranz, M. A., Jackson, D. C., Dalton, K. M., Dolski, I., et al. (2003). Affective style and in vivo immune response: Neurobehavioral mechanisms. *Proceedings of the National Academy of Sciences, USA, 100*, 11148–11152.

Rosenzweig, M. R., Bennett, E. L., and Diamond, M. C. (1972). Brain changes in response to experience. *Scientific American, 226*, 22–29.

Rosenzweig, M. R., Krech, D., and Bennett, E. L. (1961). Heredity, environment, brain biochemistry, and learning. In *Current trends in psychological theory* (pp. 87–110). Pittsburgh, PA: University of Pittsburgh Press.

Ross, D. A., Tamber-Rosenau, B. J., Palmeri, T. J., Zhang, J., et al. (2018). High-resolution functional magnetic resonance imaging reveals configural processing of cars in right anterior fusiform face area of car experts. *Journal of Cognitive Neuroscience, 30*(7), 973–984.

Rozanski, A. (2014). Behavioral cardiology: Current advances and future directions. *Journal of the American College of Cardiology, 64*(1), 100–110.

Rumbaugh, D. M. (1977). *Language learning by a chimpanzee: The LANA project.* New York, NY: Academic Press.

Rupprecht, R., Rammes, G., Eser, D., Baghai, T. C., et al. (2009). Translocator protein (18 kD) as target for anxiolytics without benzodiazepine-like side effects. *Science, 325*, 490–493.

Rusak, B., and Zucker, I. (1979). Neural regulation of circadian rhythms. *Physiological Reviews, 59*, 449–526.

Rusconi, E., and Mitchener-Nissen, T. (2013). Prospects of functional magnetic resonance imaging as lie detector. *Frontiers in Human Neuroscience, 7*, 594.

Russell, J. A. (1994). Is there universal recognition of emotion from facial expressions? A review of the cross-cultural studies. *Psychological Bulletin, 115*, 102–141.

Russell, R., Duchaine, B., and Nakayama, K. (2009). Super-recognizers: People with extraordinary face recognition ability. *Psychonomic Bulletin & Review, 16*(2), 252–257.

Russo, E. B., Jiang, H. E., Li, X., Sutton, A., et al. (2008). Phytochemical and genetic analyses of ancient cannabis from Central Asia. *Journal of Experimental Botany, 59*(15), 4171–4182.

Ruthazer, E. S., Akerman, C. J., and Cline, H. T. (2003). Control of axon branch

dynamics by correlated activity in vivo. *Science, 301*, 66–70.

S

Saalmann, Y. B., Pinsk, M. A., Wang, L., Li, X., et al. (2012). The pulvinar regulates information transmission between cortical areas based on attention demands. *Science, 337*(6095), 753–756.

Sack, R. L., and Lewy, A. J. (2001). Circadian rhythm sleep disorders: Lessons from the blind. *Sleep Medicine Reviews, 5*(3), 189–206.

Saha, K. B., Bo, L., Zhao, S., Xia, J., et al. (2016). Chlorpromazine versus atypical antipsychotic drugs for schizophrenia. *Cochrane Database of Systematic Reviews, 4*, CD010631.

Sahay, A., and Hen, R. (2007). Adult hippocampal neurogenesis in depression. *Nature Neuroscience, 10*, 1110–1114.

Sakmann, B. (2017). From single cells and single columns to cortical networks: Dendritic excitability, coincidence detection and synaptic transmission in brain slices and brains. *Experimental Physiology, 102*(5), 489–521.

Sakreida, K., Lange, I., Willmes, K., Heim, S., et al. (2018). High-resolution language mapping of Broca's region with transcranial magnetic stimulation. *Brain Structure and Function, 223*(3), 1297–1312.

Sakuma, Y. (2015). Estradiol-sensitive projection neurons in the female rat preoptic area. *Frontiers in Neuroscience, 9*, 67. https://doi.org/10.3389/fnins.2015.00067

Salazar, H., Llorente, I., Jara-Oseguera, A., García-Villegas, R., et al. (2008). A single N-terminal cysteine in TRPV1 determines activation by pungent compounds from onion and garlic. *Nature Neuroscience, 11*, 255–260.

Salcedo, S., Gold, A. K., Sheikh, S., Marcus, P. H., et al. (2018). Empirically supported psychosocial interventions for bipolar disorder: Current state of the research. *Journal of Affective Disorders, 201*, 203–214. https://doi.org/10.1016/j.jad.2016.05.018

Salimpoor, V. N., Zald, D. H., Zatorre, R. J., Dagher, A., et al. (2015). Predictions and the brain: How musical sounds become rewarding. *Trends in Cognitive Sciences, 19*(2), 86–91.

Samaha, F. F., Iqbal, N., Seshadri, P., Chicano, K. L., et al. (2003). A low-carbohydrate as compared with a low-fat diet in severe obesity. *New England Journal of Medicine, 348*, 2074–2081.

Samanta, D. (2019). Cannabidiol: A review of clinical efficacy and safety in epilepsy. *Pediatric Neurology, 96*, 24–29.

SAMHSA (Substance Abuse and Mental Health Services Administration). (2013). *Results from the 2012 National Survey on Drug Use and Health: Mental health findings* (NSDUH Series H-47, HHS Publication

No. [SMA] 13-4805). Rockville, MD: Substance Abuse and Mental Health Services Administration.

SAMHSA (Substance Abuse and Mental Health Services Administration). (2017). *Key Substance Use and Mental Health Indicators in the United States: Results from the 2016 National Survey on Drug Use and Health* (NSDUH Series H-52, HHS Publication No. [SMA] 17-5044). Rockville, MD: Substance Abuse and Mental Health Services Administration.

SAMHSA (Substance Abuse and Mental Health Services Administration). (2018). *Key Substance Use and Mental Health Indicators in the United States: Results from the 2017 National Survey on Drug Use and Health* (NSDUH Series H-53, HHS Publication No. [SMA] 18-5068). Rockville, MD: Substance Abuse and Mental Health Services Administration.

Samson, S., Zatorre, R. J., and Ramsay, J. O. (2002). Deficits of musical timbre perception after unilateral temporal-lobe lesion revealed with multidimensional scaling. *Brain, 125*(Pt. 3), 511–523.

Sánchez-Tena, M. Á., Alvarez-Peregrina, C., Valbuena-Iglesias, M. C., and Palomera, P. R. (2018). Optical illusions and spatial disorientation in aviation pilots. *Journal of Medical Systems, 42*(5), 79.

Sandberg, K., Umans, J. G.; Georgetown Consensus Conference Work Group. (2015). Recommendations concerning the new U.S. National Institutes of Health initiative to balance the sex of cells and animals in preclinical research. *FASEB Journal, 29*(5), 1646–1652.

Sanders, A. R., Beecham, G. W., Guo, S., Dawood, K., et al. (2017). Genome-wide association study of male sexual orientation. *Scientific Reports, 7*(1), 16950.

Sanderson, D. J., Good, M. A., Seeburg, P. H., Sprengel, R., et al. (2008). The role of the GluR-A (GluR1) AMPA receptor subunit in learning and memory. *Progress in Brain Research, 169*, 159–178.

Sansevero, G., Baroncelli, L., Scali, M., and Sale, A. (2019). Intranasal BDNF administration promotes visual function recovery in adult amblyopic rats. *Neuropharmacology, 145*(Pt. A), 114–122.

Saper, C. B., Fuller, P. M., Pedersen, N. P., Lu, J., et al. (2010). Sleep state switching. *Neuron, 68*, 1023–1042.

Sapir, A., Soroker, N., Berger, A., and Henik, A. (1999). Inhibition of return in spatial attention: Direct evidence for collicular generation. *Nature Neuroscience, 2*, 1053–1054.

Sapolsky, R. M. (1992). Neuroendocrinology of the stress-response. In J. B. Becker, S. M. Breedlove, and D. Crews (Eds.), *Behavioral endocrinology* (pp. 287–324). Cambridge, MA: MIT Press.

Sapolsky, R. M. (2004). *Why zebras don't get ulcers* (3rd ed.). New York, NY: Holt.

Satel, J., Wilson, N. R., and Klein, R. M. (2019). What neuroscientific studies tell us about inhibition of return. *Vision (Basel), 3*(4), 58.

Sato, J. R., Salum, G. A., Gadelha, A., Crossley, N., et al. (2015). Default mode network maturation and psychopathology in children and adolescents. *Journal of Child Psychology and Psychiatry*.

Saul, S. (2006, March 8). Some sleeping pill users range far beyond bed. *The New York Times*.

Saxena, S., Brody, A. L., Ho, M. L., Alborzian, S., et al. (2001). Cerebral metabolism in major depression and obsessive-compulsive disorder occurring separately and concurrently. *Biological Psychiatry, 50*, 159–170.

Scarmeas, N., Anastasiou, C. A., and Yannakoulia, M. (2018). Nutrition and prevention of cognitive impairment. *Lancet Neurology, 17*(11), 1006–1015.

SCENIHR (Scientific Committee on Emerging and Newly Identified Health Risks). (2008, September 23). *Potential health risks of exposure to noise from personal music players and mobile phones including a music playing function*. Brussels, Belgium: European Commission, Directorate General for Health & Consumers Protection (http://ec.europa.eu/health/ph_risk/committees/04_scenihr/docs/scenihr_o_018.pdf).

Schachter, S. (1975). Cognition and peripheralist-centralist controversies in motivation and emotion. In M. S. Gazzaniga and C. Blakemore (Eds.), *Handbook of psychobiology* (pp. 529–564). New York, NY: Academic Press.

Schachter, S., and Singer, J. (1962). Cognitive, social, and physiological determinants of emotional state. *Psychological Review, 69*, 379–399.

Schacter, D. L., Wig, G. S., and Stevens, W. D. (2007). Reductions in cortical activity during priming. *Current Opinion in Neurology, 17*(2), 17–16.

Schindler, E. A., Gottschalk, C. H., Weil, M. J., Shapiro, R. E., et al. (2015). Indoleamine hallucinogens in cluster headache: Results of the Clusterbusters Medication Use Survey. *Journal of Psychoactive Drugs, 47*(5), 372–381.

Schlaug, G., Jancke, L., Huang, Y., and Steinmetz, H. (1995). In vivo evidence of structural brain asymmetry in musicians. *Science, 267*, 699–701.

Schneider, K. (1959). *Clinical psychopathology*. New York, NY: Grune & Stratton.

Schneider, K. A., and Kastner, S. (2009). Effects of sustained spatial attention in the human lateral geniculate nucleus and superior colliculus. *Journal of Neuroscience, 29*(6), 1784–1795.

Schneider, P., Scherg, M., Dosch, H. G., Specht, H. J., et al. (2002). Morphology of Heschl's gyrus reflects enhanced activation in the auditory cortex of musicians. *Nature Neuroscience, 5*, 688–694.

Schneps, M. H., Brockmole, J. R., Sonnert, G., and Pomplun, M. (2012). History of reading struggles linked to enhanced learning in low spatial frequency scenes. *PLOS ONE, 7*, e35724.

Schoenbaum, G., Roesch, M. R., Stalnaker, T. A., and Takahashi, Y. K. (2009). A new perspective on the role of the orbitofrontal cortex in adaptive behaviour. *Nature Reviews Neuroscience, 10*, 885–892.

Schramm, E., Schneider, D., Zobel, I., van Calker, D., et al. (2008). Efficacy of Interpersonal Psychotherapy plus pharmacotherapy in chronically depressed inpatients. *Journal of Affective Disorders, 109*(1–2), 65–73.

Schulz, K. M., and Sisk, C. L. (2016). The organizing actions of adolescent gonadal steroid hormones on brain and behavioral development. *Neuroscience & Biobehavioral Reviews, 70*, 148–158.

Schummers, J., Yu, H., and Sur, M. (2008). Tuned responses of astrocytes and their influence on hemodynamic signals in the visual cortex. *Science, 320*, 1638–1643.

Schuster, C. R. (1970). Psychological approaches to opiate dependence and self-administration by laboratory animals. *Federation Proceedings, 29*, 1–5.

Schwartz, S., and Correll, C. U. (2014). Efficacy and safety of atomoxetine in children and adolescents with attention-deficit/hyperactivity disorder: Results from a comprehensive meta-analysis and metaregression. *Journal of the American Academy of Child and Adolescent Psychiatry, 53*, 174–187.

Schwartzkroin, P. A., and Wester, K. (1975). Long-lasting facilitation of a synaptic potential following tetanization in the in vitro hippocampal slice. *Brain Research, 89*, 107–119.

Sclafani, A., Springer, D., and Kluge, L. (1976). Effects of quinine adulterated diets on the food intake and body weight of obese and non-obese hypothalamic hyperphagic rats. *Physiology & Behavior, 16*(5), 631–640.

Scott, D. J., Stohler, C. S., Egnatuk, C. M., Wang, H., et al. (2008). Placebo and nocebo effects are defined by opposite opioid and dopaminergic responses. *Archives of General Psychiatry, 65*, 220–231.

Scott, S. K., and Wise, R. J. (2004). The functional neuroanatomy of prelexical processing in speech perception. *Cognition, 92*(1–2), 13–45.

Scoville, W. B., and Milner, B. (1957). Loss of recent memory after bilateral hippocampal lesions. *Journal of Neurology, Neurosurgery and Psychiatry, 20*, 11–21.

Seavey, C., Katz, P., and Zalk, S. R. (1975). Baby X: The effects of gender labels on adult responses to infants. *Sex Roles, 2*, 103–109.

Seeman, P., and Tallerico, T. (1998). Antipsychotic drugs which elicit little or no parkinsonism bind more loosely than dopamine to brain D2 receptors, yet occupy high levels of these receptors. *Molecular Psychiatry, 3*, 123–134.

Seiden, R. H. (1978). Where are they now? A follow-up study of suicide attempters from the Golden Gate Bridge. *Suicide and Life Threatening Behavior, 8*, 203–216.

Sekar, R., Wang, L., and Chow, B. K. (2017). Central control of feeding behavior by the secretin, pacap, and glucagon family of peptides. *Frontiers in Endocrinology (Lausanne), 8*, 18.

Selemon, L. D., and Zecevic, N. (2015). Schizophrenia: A tale of two critical periods for prefrontal cortical development. *Translational Psychiatry, 5*, e623.

Selkoe, D. J., and Hardy, J. (2016). The amyloid hypothesis of Alzheimer's disease at 25 years. *EMBO Molecular Medicine, 8*(6), 595–608.

Sellon, J. B., Ghaffari, R., and Freeman, D. M. (2019). The tectorial membrane: Mechanical properties and functions. *Cold Spring Harbor Perspectives in Medicine, 9*(10), a033514.

Selye, H. (1956). *The stress of life.* New York, NY: McGraw-Hill.

Sessa, B. (2017). MDMA and PTSD treatment: "PTSD: From novel pathophysiology to innovative therapeutics." *Neuroscience Letters, 649*, 176–180.

Seuss, Dr. (1987). *The tough coughs as he ploughs the dough: Early writings and cartoons by Dr. Seuss.* New York, NY: Morrow.

Severus, E., Bauer, M., and Geddes, J. (2018). Efficacy and effectiveness of lithium in the long-term treatment of bipolar disorders: An update 2018. *Pharmacopsychiatry, 51*(5), 173–176.

Sexton, C. E., Mackay, C. E., and Ebmeier, K. P. (2013). A systematic review and meta-analysis of magnetic resonance imaging studies in late-life depression. *American Journal of Geriatric Psychiatry, 21*, 184–195.

Shackman, A. J., Fox, A. S., Oler, J. A., Shelton, S. E., et al. (2013). Neural mechanisms underlying heterogeneity in the presentation of anxious temperament. *Proceedings of the National Academy of Sciences, USA, 110*, 6145–6150.

Shaffer, F., McCraty, R., and Zerr, C. L. (2014). A healthy heart is not a metronome: An integrative review of the heart's anatomy and heart rate variability. *Frontiers in Psychology, 5*, 1040.

Shah, D. B., Pesiridou, A., Baltuch, G. H., Malone, D. A., et al. (2008). Functional neurosurgery in the treatment of severe obsessive compulsive disorder and major depression: Overview of disease circuits and therapeutic targeting for the clinician. *Psychiatry (Edgmont), 5*(9), 24–33.

Shallice, T., and Burgess, P. W. (1991). Deficits in strategy application following frontal lobe damage in man. *Brain, 114*, 727–741.

Sharan, A., Ooi, Y. C., Langfitt, J., and Sperling, M. R. (2011). Intracarotid amobarbital procedure for epilepsy surgery. *Epilepsy & Behavior, 20*(2), 209–213.

Shaw, P., Greenstein, D., Lerch, J., Clasen, L., et al. (2006). Intellectual ability and cortical development in children and adolescents. *Nature, 440*, 676–679.

Shaw, P. J., Tononi, G., Greenspan, R. J., and Robinson, D. F. (2002). Stress response genes protect against lethal effects of sleep deprivation in *Drosophila. Nature, 417*, 287–291.

Shaywitz, S. E., Shaywitz, B. A, Fulbright, R. K., Skudlarski, P., et al. (2003). Neural systems for compensation and persistence: Young adult outcome of childhood reading disability. *Biological Psychiatry, 54*(1), 25–33.

Sheikh-Bahaei, N., Sajjadi, S. A., Manavaki, R., McLean, M., et al. (2018). Positron emission tomography-guided magnetic resonance spectroscopy in Alzheimer disease. *Annals of Neurology, 83*(4), 771–778.

Shein-Idelson, M., Ondracek, J. M., Liaw, H. P., Reiter, S., et al. (2016). Slow waves, sharp waves, ripples, and REM in sleeping dragons. *Science, 352*(6285), 590–595.

Sherrington, C. S. (1897). *A textbook of physiology. Part III. The central nervous system* (7th ed.), M. Foster (Ed.). London, UK: Macmillan.

Sherrington, C. S. (1898). Experiments in examination of the peripheral distribution of the fibres of the posterior roots of some spinal nerves. *Philosophical Transactions, 190*, 45–186.

Sherwin, B. B. (2002). Randomized clinical trials of combined estrogen-androgen preparations: Effects on sexual functioning. *Fertility and Sterility, 77*(Suppl. 4), 49–54.

Sherwin, B. B. (2009). Estrogen therapy: Is time of initiation critical for neuroprotection? *Nature Reviews Endocrinology, 5*, 620–627.

Sheth, S. A., Mian, M. K., Patel, S. R., Asaad, W. F., et al. (2012). Human dorsal anterior cingulate cortex neurons mediate ongoing behavioural adaptation. *Nature, 488*(7410), 218–221.

Shic, F., and Scassellati, B. (2007). A behavioral analysis of computational models of visual attention. *International Journal of Computer Vision, 73*(2), 159–177.

Shih, R. A., Belmonte, P. L., and Zandi, P. P. (2004). A review of the evidence from family, twin and adoption studies for a genetic contribution to adult psychiatric disorders. *International Review of Psychiatry, 16*, 260–283.

Shipton, O. A., El-Gaby, M., Apergis-Schoute, J., Deisseroth, K., et al. (2014). Left-right dissociation of hippocampal memory processes in mice. *Proceedings of the National Academy of Sciences, USA, 111*, 15238–15243.

Shu, W., Cho, J. Y., Jiang, Y., Zhang, M., et al. (2005). Altered ultrasonic vocalization in mice with a disruption in the *Foxp2* gene. *Proceedings of the National Academy of Sciences, USA, 102*, 9643–9648.

Siclari, F., Baird, B., Perogamvros, L., Bernardi, G., et al. (2017). The neural correlates of dreaming. *Nature Neuroscience, 20*(6), 872–878.

Siegel, E. H., Sands, M. K., Van den Noortgate, W., Condon, P., et al. (2018). Emotion fingerprints or emotion populations? A meta-analytic investigation of autonomic features of emotion categories. *Psychological Bulletin, 144*(4), 343–393.

Siegel, J. M. (2005). Clues to the function of mammalian sleep. *Nature, 437*, 1264–1271.

Siegel, J. M., Moore, R., Thannickal, T., and Nienhuis, R. (2001). A brief history of hypocretin/orexin and narcolepsy. *Neuropsychopharmacology, 25*(5 Suppl.), S14–20.

Sierakowiak, A., Monnot, C., Aski, S. N., Uppman, M., et al. (2015). Default mode network, motor network, dorsal and ventral basal ganglia networks in the rat brain: Comparison to human networks using resting state-fMRI. *PLOS ONE, 10*, e0120345.

Sikich, L, Frazier, J. A., McClellan, J., Findling, R. L., et al. (2008). Double-blind comparison of first- and second-generation antipsychotics in early-onset schizophrenia and schizo-affective disorder: Findings from the treatment of early-onset schizophrenia spectrum disorders (TEOSS) study. *American Journal of Psychiatry, 165*, 1420–1431.

Sikl, R., Simeccek, M., Porubanova-Norquist, M., Bezdicek, O., et al. (2013). Vision after 53 years of blindness. *i-Perception, 4*(8), 498–507.

Simons, D. J., and Chabris, C. F. (1999). Gorillas in our midst: Sustained inattentional blindness for dynamic events. *Perception, 28*, 1059–1074.

Simons, D. J., and Jensen, M. S. (2009). The effects of individual differences and task difficulty on inattentional blindness. *Psychonomic Bulletin & Review, 16*, 398–403.

Simons, D. J., and Schlosser, M. D. (2017). Inattentional blindness for a gun during a simulated police vehicle stop. *Cognitive Research: Principles and Implications, 2*(1), 37.

Singer, O., Marr, R. A., Rockenstein, E., Crews, L., et al. (2005). Targeting BACE1 with siRNAs ameliorates Alzheimer disease neuropathology in a transgenic model. *Nature Neuroscience, 8*, 1343–1349.

Singer, T., Seymour, B., O'Doherty, J., Kaube, H., et al. (2004). Empathy for pain involves the affective but not sensory components of pain. *Science, 303*, 1157–1162.

Sinopoli, V. M., Burton, C. L., Kronenberg, S., and Arnold, P. D. (2017). A review of the role of serotonin system genes in obsessive-compulsive disorder. *Neuroscience & Biobehavioral Reviews, 80*, 372–381.

Slee, S. J., and Young, E. D. (2014). Alignment of sound localization cues in the nucleus of the brachium of the inferior colliculus. *Journal of Neurophysiology, 111*, 2624–2633.

Smoller, J. W., and Finn, C. T. (2003). Family, twin, and adoption studies of bipolar disorder. *American Journal of Medical Genetics. Part C, Seminars in Medical Genetics, 123*, 48–58.

Snyder, J. S. (2019). Recalibrating the relevance of adult neurogenesis. *Trends in Neurosciences, 42*(3), 164–178.

Snyder, J. S., Soumier, A., Brewer, M., Pickel, J., et al. (2011). Adult hippocampal neurogenesis buffers stress responses and depressive behaviour. *Nature, 476*, 458–461.

Solomon, A. (2001). *The noonday demon: An atlas of depression.* New York, NY: Scribner.

Soltis, J., King, L. E., Douglas-Hamilton, I., Vollrath, F., et al. (2014). African elephant alarm calls distinguish between threats from humans and bees. *PLOS ONE, 9*, e89403.

Somerville, M. J., Mervis, C. B., Young, E. J., Seo, E. J., et al. (2005). Severe expressive-language delay related to duplication of the *Williams-Beuren* locus. *New England Journal of Medicine, 353*, 1694–1701.

Soon, C. S., Brass, M., Heinze, H. J., and Haynes, J. D. (2008). Unconscious determinants of free decisions in the human brain. *Nature Neuroscience, 11*, 543–545.

Sowell, E. R., Kan, E., Yoshii, J., Thompson, P. M., et al. (2008). Thinning of sensorimotor cortices in children with Tourette syndrome. *Nature Neuroscience, 11*, 637–639.

Spalding, K. L., Bergmann, O., Alkass, K., Bernard, S., et al. (2013). Dynamics of hippocampal neurogenesis in adult humans. *Cell, 153*(6), 1219–1227.

Spampinato, D., and Celnik, P. (2018). Deconstructing skill learning and its physiological mechanisms. *Cortex, 104*, 90–102.

Speakman, J. R., Levitsky, D. A., Allison, D. B., Bray, M. S., et al. (2011). Set points, settling points and some alternative models: Theoretical options to understand how genes and environments combine to regulate body adiposity. *Disease Models & Mechanisms, 4*(6), 733–745.

Speed, A., Del Rosario, J., Mikail, N., and Haider, B. (2020). Spatial attention

enhances network, cellular and subthreshold responses in mouse visual cortex. *Nature Communications, 11*(1), 505.

Spiegler, B. J., and Yeni-Komshian, G. H. (1983). Incidence of left-handed writing in a college population with reference to family patterns of hand preference. *Neuropsychologia, 21*, 651–659.

Spitzer, R. L. (2012). Spitzer reassesses his 2003 study of reparative therapy of homosexuality. *Archives of Sexual Behavior, 41*, 757.

Sprague, T. C., Saproo, S., and Serences, J. T. (2015). Visual attention mitigates information loss in small- and large-scale neural codes. *Trends in Cognitive Sciences, 19*(4), 215–226.

Squire, L. R., Amaral, D. G., Zola-Morgan, S., and Kritchevsky, M. P. G. (1989). Description of brain injury in the amnesic patient N.A. based on magnetic resonance imaging. *Experimental Neurology, 105*, 23–35.

Squire, L. R., and Moore, R. Y. (1979). Dorsal thalamic lesion in a noted case of chronic memory dysfunction. *Annals of Neurology, 6*, 503–506.

Squire, L. R., and Wixted, J. T. (2011). The cognitive neuroscience of human memory since H.M. *Annual Review of Neuroscience, 34*, 259–288.

Squire, L. R., and Zola-Morgan, S. (1991). The medial temporal lobe memor system. *Science, 253*, 1380–1386.

St Louis, E. K., and Boeve, B. F. (2017). REM sleep behavior disorder: Diagnosis, clinical implications, and future directions. *Mayo Clinic Proceedings, 92*(11), 1723–1736.

Standing, L. G. (1973). Learning 10,000 pictures. *Quarterly Journal of Experimental Psychology, 25*, 207–222.

Stansley, B. J., and Conn, P. J. (2018). The therapeutic potential of metabotropic glutamate receptor modulation for schizophrenia. *Current Opinion in Pharmacology, 38*, 31–36.

Stanton, S. J., Beehner, J. C., Saini, E. K., Kuhn, C. M., et al. (2009). Dominance, politics, and physiology: Voters' testosterone changes on the night of the 2008 United States presidential election. *PLOS ONE, 4*(10), e7543.

Stanton, S. J., Beehner, J. C., Saini, E. K., Kuhn, C. M., et al. (2009). Dominance, politics, and physiology: Voters' testosterone changes on the night of the 2008 United States presidential election. *PLOS ONE, 4*, e7543.

Staubli, U. V. (1995). Parallel properties of long-term potentiation and memory. In J. L. McGaugh, N. M. Weinberger, and G. Lynch (Eds.), *Brain and memory: Modulation and mediation of neuroplasticity* (pp. 303–318). New York, NY: Oxford University Press.

Staud, R., and Price, D. D. (2006). Mechanisms of acupuncture analgesia for clinical and experimental pain. *Expert Review of Neurotherapeutics, 6*(5), 661–667.

Stauffer, V. L., Millen, B. A., Andersen, S., Kinon, B. J., et al. (2013). Pomaglumetad methionil: No significant difference as an adjunctive treatment for patients with prominent negative symptoms of schizophrenia compared to placebo. *Schizophrenia Research, 150*, 434–441.

Stein, B. E., and Stanford, T. R. (2008). Multisensory integration: Current issues from the perspective of the single neuron. *Nature Reviews Neuroscience, 9*, 255–266.

Stephan, F. K., and Zucker, I. (1972). Circadian rhythms in drinking behavior and locomotor activity of rats are eliminated by hypothalamic lesions. *Proceedings of the National Academy of Sciences, USA, 69*, 1583–1586.

Stern, K., and McClintock, M. (1998). Regulation of ovulation by human pheromones. *Nature, 392*, 177–179.

Stoeckel, C., Gough, P. M., Watkins, K. E., and Devlin, J. T. (2009). Supramarginal gyrus involvement in visual word recognition. *Cortex, 45*, 1091–1096.

Stoeger, A. S., and Baotic, A. (2017). Male African elephants discriminate and prefer vocalizations of unfamiliar females. *Scientific Reports, 7*, 46414.

Stranahan, A. M., Khalil, D., and Gould, E. (2006). Social isolation delays the positive effects of running on adult neurogenesis. *Nature Neuroscience, 9*, 526–533.

Stroop, J. R. (1935). Studies of interference in serial verbal reactions. *Journal of Experimental Psychology, 18*, 643–662.

Suárez, L. E., Markello, R. D., Betzel, R. F., and Misic, B. (2020). Linking structure and function in macroscale brain networks. *Trends in Cognitive Sciences, 24*(4), 302–315.

Suez, J., and Elinav, E. (2017). The path towards microbiome-based metabolite treatment. *Nature Microbiology, 2*, 17075.

Suk, I., and Tamargo, R. J. (2010). Concealed neuroanatomy in Michelangelo's *Separation of Light from Darkness* in the Sistine Chapel. *Neurosurgery, 66*(5), 851–861.

Sumnall, H. R., and Cole, J. C. (2005). Self-reported depressive symptomatology in community samples of polysubstance misusers who report Ecstasy use: A meta-analysis. *Journal of Psychopharmacology, 19*, 84–92.

Sun, E. W. L., Martin, A. M., Young, R. L., and Keating, D. J. (2019). The regulation of peripheral metabolism by gut-derived hormones. *Frontiers in Endocrinology (Lausanne), 9*, 754.

Sun, T., Patoine, C., Abu-Khalil, A., Visvader, J., et al. (2005). Early asymmetry of gene transcription in embryonic human left and right cerebral cortex. *Science, 308,* 1794–1798.

Sunn, N., Egli, M., Burazin, T. C. D., Burns, P., et al. (2002). Circulating relaxin acts on subfornical organ neurons to stimulate water drinking in the rat. *Proceedings of the National Academy of Sciences, USA, 99,* 1701–1706.

Sunstein, C. R., and Nussbaum, M. C. (Eds.). (2004). *Animal rights: Current debates and new directions.* Oxford, UK: Oxford University Press.

Sutcliffe, J. G., and de Lecea, L. (2002). The hypocretins: Setting the arousal threshold. *Nature Reviews Neuroscience, 3,* 339–349.

Suzuki, S., Brown, C. M., and Wise, P. M. (2009). Neuroprotective effects of estrogens following ischemic stroke. *Frontiers in Neuroendocrinology, 30,* 201–211.

Svare, B. B. (2013). *Hormones and aggressive behavior.* New York, NY: Plenum.

Svenningsson, P., Chergui, K., Rachleff, I., Flajolet, M., et al. (2006). Alterations in 5-HT1B receptor function by p11 in depression-like states. *Science, 311,* 77–80.

Svoboda, K., and Li, N. (2018). Neural mechanisms of movement planning: Motor cortex and beyond. *Current Opinion in Neurobiology, 49,* 33–41.

Swedo, S. E., Rapoport, J. L., Leonard, H., Lenane, M., et al. (1989). Obsessive-compulsive disorder in children and adolescents: Clinical phenomenology of 70 consecutive cases. *Archives of General Psychiatry, 46,* 335–341.

Sylvia, K. E., and Demas, G. E. (2018). A gut feeling: Microbiome-brain-immune interactions modulate social and affective behaviors. *Hormones and Behavior, 99,* 41–49.

T

Taglialatela, J. P., Cantalupo, C., and Hopkins, W. D. (2006). Gesture handedness predicts asymmetry in the chimpanzee inferior frontal gyrus. *NeuroReport, 17,* 923–927.

Takahashi, J. (2018). Stem cells and regenerative medicine for neural repair. *Current Opinion in Biotechnology, 52,* 102–108.

Takahashi, T., Svoboda, K., and Malinow, R. (2003). Experience strengthening transmission by driving AMPA receptors into synapses. *Science, 299,* 1585–1588.

Takizawa, R., Maughan, B., and Arseneault, L. (2014). Adult health outcomes of childhood bullying victimization: Evidence from a five-decade longitudinal British birth cohort. *American Journal of Psychiatry, 171,* 777–784.

Tam, J., Duda, D. G., Perentes, J. Y., Quadri, R. S., et al. (2009). Blockade of VEGFR2 and not VEGFR1 can limit diet-induced fat tissue expansion: Role of local versus

bone marrow-derived endothelial cells. *PLOS ONE, 4,* e4974.

Tanaka, S., Hanako, I., Kazumi, K., Ryo, K., et al. (2013). Larger right posterior parietal volume in action video game experts: A behavioral and voxel-based morphometry (VBM) study. *PLOS ONE, 8,* e66998.

Tanda, G., Munzar, P., and Goldberg, S. R. (2000). Self-administration behavior is maintained by the psychoactive ingredient of marijuana in squirrel monkeys. *Nature Neuroscience, 3,* 1073–1074.

Tang, Y. P., Wang, H., Feng, R., Kyin, M., et al. (2001). Differential effects of enrichment on learning and memory function in NR2B transgenic mice. *Neuropharmacology, 41,* 779–790.

Tanji, J. (2001). Sequential organization of multiple movements: Involvement of cortical motor areas. *Annual Review of Neuroscience, 24,* 631–651.

Taub, E. (1976). Movement in nonhuman primates deprived of somatosensory feedback. *Exercise and Sport Sciences Reviews, 4,* 335–374.

Taub, E., Uswatte, G., and Elbert, T. (2002). New treatments in neurorehabilitation founded on basic research. *Nature Reviews Neuroscience, 3,* 228–235.

Teipel, S., Grothe, M. J., Zhou, J., Sepulcre, J., et al. (2016). Measuring cortical connectivity in Alzheimer's disease as a brain neural network pathology: Toward clinical applications. *Journal of the International Neuropsychological Society, 22*(2), 138–163.

Temple, E., Deutsch, G. K., Poldrack, R. A., Miller, S. L., et al. (2003). Neural deficits in children with dyslexia ameliorated by behavioral remediation: Evidence from functional MRI. *Proceedings of the National Academy of Sciences, USA, 100,* 2860–2865.

Terkel, J., and Rosenblatt, J. S. (1972). Humoral factors underlying maternal behavior at parturition: Cross transfusion between freely moving rats. *Journal of Comparative and Physiological Psychology, 80,* 365–371.

Terrace, H. S. (1979). *Nim.* New York, NY: Knopf.

Tetel, M. J., de Vries, G. J., Melcangi, R. C., Panzica, G., et al. (2018). Steroids, stress and the gut microbiome-brain axis. *Journal of Neuroendocrinology, 30*(2), e12548.

Thannickal, T. C., Moore, R. Y., Nienhuis, R., Ramanathan, L., et al. (2000). Reduced number of hypocretin neurons in human narcolepsy. *Neuron, 27,* 469–474.

Theunissen, F. E., and Elie, J. E. (2014). Neural processing of natural sounds. *Nature Reviews Neuroscience, 15*(6), 355–366.

Thomas, K., and Gunnell, D. (2010). Suicide in England and Wales 1861–2007: A time-trends analysis. *International Journal of Epidemiology, 39*(6), 1464–1475.

Thomas, M. A., Ryu, V., and Bartness, T. J. (2016). Central ghrelin increases food foraging/hoarding that is blocked by GHSR antagonism and attenuates hypothalamic paraventricular nucleus neuronal activation. *American Journal of Physiolog—Regulatory, Integrative and Comparative Physiology, 310*(3), R275–R285.

Thomas, R. K. (1994). Pavlov's dogs "dripped saliva at the sound of a bell." *Psycoloquy, 5*(80), Article 4.

Thompson, P. M., Vidal, C., Giedd, J. N., Gochman, P., et al. (2001). Mapping adolescent brain change reveals dynamic wave of accelerated gray matter loss in very early-onset schizophrenia. *Proceedings of the National Academy of Sciences, USA, 98,* 11650–11655.

Thompson, R. F. (1990). Neural mechanisms of classical conditioning in mammals. *Philosophical Transactions of the Royal Society of London. Series B: Biological Sciences, 329,* 161–170.

Thompson, R. F., and Krupa, D. J. (1994). Organization of memory traces in the mammalian brain. *Annual Review of Neuroscience, 17,* 519–549.

Thompson, R. F., and Steinmetz, J. E. (2009). The role of the cerebellum in classical conditioning of discrete behavioral responses. *Neuroscience, 162,* 732–755.

Thompson, T., and Schuster, C. R. (1964). Morphine self-administration, food reinforced and avoidance behaviour in rhesus monkeys. *Psychopharmacologia, 5,* 87–94.

Thornhill, R., and Palmer, C. T. (2000). *A natural history of rape.* Cambridge, MA: MIT Press.

Thornton, A. E., Cox, D. N., Whitfield, K., and Fouladi, R. T. (2008). Cumulative concussion exposure in rugby players: Neurocognitive and symptomatic outcomes. *Journal of Clinical and Experimental Neuropsychology, 30,* 398–409.

Thornton-Jones, Z. D., Kennett, G. A., Benwell, K. R., Revell, D. F., et al. (2006). The cannabinoid CB1 receptor inverse agonist, rimonabant, modifies body weight and adiponectin function in diet-induced obese rats as a consequence of reduced food intake. *Pharmacology, Biochemistry, and Behavior, 84,* 353–359.

Thorpe, S. J., and Fabre-Thorpe, M. (2001). Seeking categories in the brain. *Science, 291,* 260–263.

Timmann, D., Drepper, J., Frings, M., Maschke, M., et al. (2010). The human cerebellum contributes to motor, emotional and cognitive associative learning. A review. *Cortex, 46,* 845–857.

Todd, W. D., Fenselau, H., Wang, J. L., Zhang, R., et al. (2018). A hypothalamic circuit for the circadian control of aggression. *Nature Neuroscience, 21*(5), 717–724.

Todorov, A., Said, C. P., Engell, A. D., and Oosterhof, N. N. (2008). Understanding evaluation of faces on social dimensions. *Trends in Cognitive Science, 12,* 455–460.

Tolman, E. C. (1949). There is more than one kind of learning. *Psychological Review, 56,* 144–155.

Tolman, E. C., and Honzik, C. H. (1930). Introduction and removal of reward, and maze performance in rats. *University of California Publications in Psychology, 4,* 257–275.

Tom, S. M., Fox, C. R., Trepel, C., and Poldrack, R. A. (2007). The neural basis of loss aversion in decision-making under risk. *Science, 315,* 515–518.

Tomoda, T., Hikida, T., and Sakurai, T. (2017). Role of *DISC1* in neuronal trafficking and its implication in neuropsychiatric manifestation and neurotherapeutics. *Neurotherapeutics, 14*(3), 623–629.

Tootell, R. B. H., Hadjikhani, N. K., Vanduffel, W., Liu, A. K., et al. (1998). Functional analysis of primary visual cortex (V1) in humans. *Proceedings of the National Academy of Sciences, USA, 95,* 811–817.

Tootell, R. B., Silverman, M. S., Switkes, E., and De Valois, R. L. (1982). Deoxyglucose analysis of retinotopic organization in primate striate cortex. *Science, 218,* 902–904.

Tootell, R. B., Tsao, D., and Vanduffel, W. (2003). Neuroimaging weighs in: Humans meet macaques in "primate" visual cortex. *Journal of Neuroscience, 23,* 3981–3989.

Torrey, E. F., and Yolken, R. H. (2019). Schizophrenia as a pseudogenetic disease: A call for more gene-environmental studies. *Psychiatry Research, 278,* 146–150.

Trasande, L., Blustein, J., Liu, M., Corwin, E., et al. (2013). Infant antibiotic exposures and early-life body mass. *International Journal of Obesity (London), 37*(1), 16–23.

Treffert, D. A., and Christensen, D. D. (2005). Inside the mind of a savant. *Scientific American, 293*(6), 108–113.

Treisman, A. [M]. (1996). The binding problem. *Current Opinion in Neurobiology, 6,* 171–178.

Treisman, A. M., and Gelade, G. (1980). A feature-integration theory of attention. *Cognitive Psychology, 12,* 97–136.

Treisman, M. (1977). Motion sickness— Evolutionary hypotheses. *Science, 197,* 493–495.

Tremblay, S., Tuominen, L., Zayed, V., Pascual-Leone, A., et al. (2020). The study of noninvasive brain stimulation using molecular brain imaging: A systematic review. *Neuroimage.*

Tremlett, H., Bauer, K. C., Appel-Cresswell, S., Finlay, B. B., et al. (2017). The gut microbiome in human neurological disease: A review. *Annals of Neurology, 81*(3), 369–382.

Trimmer, C., Keller, A., Murphy, N. R., Snyder, L. L., et al. (2019). Genetic variation across the human olfactory receptor repertoire alters odor perception. *Proceedings of the National Academy of Sciences, USA, 116*(19), 9475–9480.

Tronick, R., and Reck, C. (2009). Infants of depressed mothers. *Harvard Review of Psychiatry, 17,* 147–156.

Tsai, L., and Barnea, G. (2014). A critical period defined by axon-targeting mechanisms in the murine olfactory bulb. *Science, 344*(6180), 197–200.

Tsuchiya, N., and Adolphs, R. (2007). Emotion and consciousness. *Trends in Cognitive Sciences, 11,* 158–167.

Tully, T. (2003). Reply: The myth of a myth. *Current Biology, 13*(11), r426.

Tulving, E. (1972). Episodic and semantic memory. In E. Tulving and W. Donaldson (Eds.), *Organization of memory* (pp. 381–403). New York, NY: Academic Press.

Tulving, E. (1989). Memory: Performance, knowledge, and experience. *European Journal of Cognitive Psychology, 1,* 3–26.

Tulving, E., Hayman, C. A., and Macdonald, C. A. (1991). Long-lasting perceptual priming and semantic learning in amnesia: A case experiment. *Journal of Experimental Psychology: Learning, Memory, and Cognition, 17,* 595–617.

Turel, O., He, Q., Brevers, D., and Bechara, A. (2018). Delay discounting mediates the association between posterior insular cortex volume and social media addiction symptoms. *Cognitive, Affective, & Behavioral Neuroscience, 18*(4), 694–704.

Turgeon, J. L., McDonnell, D. P, Martin, K. A, and Wise, P. M. (2004). Hormone therapy: Physiological complexity belies therapeutic simplicity. *Science, 304,* 1269–1273.

Turner, E. H., Matthews, A. M., Linardatos, E., Tell, R. A., et al. (2008). Selective publication of antidepressant trials and its influence on apparent efficacy. *New England Journal of Medicine, 358,* 252–260.

Tyack, P. L. (2003). Dolphins communicate about individual-specific social relationships. In F. de Waal and P. L. Tyack (Eds.), *Animal social complexity: Intelligence, culture, and individualized societies* (pp. 342–361). Cambridge, MA: Harvard University Press.

U

Umilta, M. A., Kohler, E., Galiese, V., Fogassi, L., et al. (2001). I know what you are doing: A neurophysiological study. *Neuron, 31,* 155–165.

Uno, Y., and Coyle, J. T. (2019). Glutamate hypothesis in schizophrenia. *Psychiatry and Clinical Neurosciences, 73*(5), 204–215.

Ursin, H., Baade, E., and Levine, S. (1978). *Psychobiology of stress: A study of coping men.* New York, NY: Academic Press.

V

Valenzuela, C. F., Morton, R. A., Diaz, M. R., and Topper, L. (2012). Does moderate drinking harm the fetal brain? Insights from animal models. *Trends in Neurosciences, 35*(5), 284–292.

Van Anders, S. M., and Watson, N. V. (2006). Social neuroendocrinology: Effects of social contexts and behaviors on sex steroids in humans. *Human Nature, 17,* 212–237.

Van der Meij, L., Almela, M., Hidalgo, V., Villada, C., et al. (2012). Testosterone and cortisol release among Spanish soccer fans watching the 2010 World Cup final. *PLOS ONE, 7*(4), e34814.

Van Dongen, H. P., Maislin, G., Mullington, J. M., and Dinges, D. F. (2003). The cumulative cost of additional wakefulness: Dose-response effects on neurobehavioral functions and sleep physiology from chronic sleep restriction and total sleep deprivation. *Sleep, 26,* 117–126.

Van Essen, D. C., and Glasser, M. F. (2018). Parcellating cerebral cortex: How invasive animal studies inform noninvasive mapmaking in humans. *Neuron, 99*(4), 640–663.

Van Essen, D. C., Lewis, J. W., Drury, H. A., Hadjikhani, N., et al. (2001). Mapping visual cortex in monkeys and humans using surface-based atlases. *Vision Research, 41*(10–11), 1359–5978.

Van Herzeele, C., Walle, J. V., Dhondt, K., and Juul, K. V. (2017). Recent advances in managing and understanding enuresis. *F1000Research, 6,* 1881.

Van Horn, J. D., Irimia, A., Torgerson, C. M., Chambers, M. C., et al. (2012). Mapping connectivity damage in the case of Phineas Gage. *PLOS ONE, 7*(5), e37454.

Van Os, J., and Kapur, S. (2009). Schizophrenia. *Lancet, 374,* 635–645.

Van Os, J., Kenis, G., and Rutten, B. P. (2010). The environment and schizophrenia. *Nature, 468,* 203–212.

Van Tol, M. J., van der Wee, N. J., van den Heuvel, O. A., Nielen, M. M., et al. (2010). Regional brain volume in depression and anxiety disorders. *Archives of General Psychiatry, 67,* 1002–1011.

Van Zoeren, J. G., and Stricker, E. M. (1977). Effects of preoptic, lateral hypothalamic, or dopamine-depleting lesions on behavioral thermoregulation in rats exposed to the cold. *Journal of Comparative and Physiological Psychology, 91,* 989–999.

Vance, C. G., Dailey, D. L., Rakel, B. A., and Sluka, K. A. (2014). Using TENS for pain control: The state of the evidence. *Pain Management, 4,* 197–209.

Vandermosten, M., Boets, B., Poelmans, H., Sunaert, S., et al. (2012). A tractography study in dyslexia: Neuroanatomic correlates of orthographic, phonological and speech processing. *Brain, 135*(Pt. 3), 935–948.

Vann, S. D., and Aggleton, J. P. (2004). The mammillary bodies: Two memory systems in one? *Nature Reviews Neuroscience, 5*, 35–44.

Vargha-Khadem, F., Gadian, D. G., Copp, A., and Mishkin, M. (2005). FOXP2 and the neuroanatomy of speech and language. *Nature Reviews Neuroscience, 6*(2), 131–138.

Vassar, R., Ngai, J., and Axel, R. (1993). Spatial segregation of odorant receptor expression in the mammalian olfactory epithelium. *Cell, 74*, 309–318.

Vaughan, W., and Greene, S. L. (1984). Pigeon visual memory capacity. *Journal of Experimental Psychology: Animal Behavior Processes, 10*, 256–271.

Vernes, S. C., Oliver, P. L., Spiteri, E., Lockstone, H. E., et al. (2011). Foxp2 regulates gene networks implicated in neurite outgrowth in the developing brain. *PLOS Genetics, 7*, e1002145.

Vincus, A. A., Ringwalt, C., Harris, M. S., and Shamblen, S. R. (2010). A short-term, quasi-experimental evaluation of D.A.R.E.'s revised elementary school curriculum. *Journal of Drug Education, 40*, 37–49.

Visser, S. N., Danielson, M. L., Bitsko, R. H., Holbrook, J. R., et al. (2014). Trends in the parent-report of health care provider–diagnosed and medicated attention-deficit/hyperactivity disorder: United States, 2003–2011. *Journal of the American Academy of Child and Adolescent Psychiatry, 53*(1), 34–46.e2.

Vitaterna, M. H., King, D. P., Chang, A. M., Kornhauser, J. M., et al. (1994). Mutagenesis and mapping of a mouse gene, Clock, essential for cicadian behavior. *Science, 29*, 719–725.

Vogel, T., Smieskova, R., Schmidt, A., Walter, A., et al. (2016). Increased superior frontal gyrus activation during working memory processing in psychosis: Significant relation to cumulative antipsychotic medication and to negative symptoms. *Schizophrenia Research, 175*(1–3), 20–26.

Vogt, B. A. (2005). Pain and emotion interactions in subregions of the cingulate gyrus. *Nature Reviews Neuroscience, 6*, 533–544.

Volkow, N., Benveniste, H., and McLellan, A. T. (2018). Use and misuse of opioids in chronic pain. *Annual Review of Medicine, 69*, 451–465.

Volkow, N. D., and Wise, R.A. (2005). How can drug addiction help us understand obesity? *Nature Neuroscience, 8*, 555–560.

Volkow, N. D., Wise, R. A., and Baler, R. (2017). The dopamine motive system: Implications for drug and food addiction. *Nature Reviews Neuroscience, 18*(12), 741–752.

Voskuhl, R., and Momtazee, C. (2017). Pregnancy: Effect on multiple sclerosis, treatment considerations, and breastfeeding. *Neurotherapeutics, 14*(4), 974–984.

Vriens, J, and Voets, T. (2018). Sensing the heat with *TRPM3. Pflügers Archiv, 470*(5):799–807.

Vrieze, A., Van Nood, E., Holleman, F., Salojärvi, J., et al. (2012). Transfer of intestinal microbiota from lean donors increases insulin sensitivity in individuals with metabolic syndrome. *Gastroenterology, 143*(4), 913–916.e7.

Vythilingam, M., Anderson, E. R., Goddard, A., Woods, S. W., et al. (2000). Temporal lobe volume in panic disorder—A quantitative magnetic resonance imaging study. *Psychiatry Research, 99*, 75–82.

W

Wada, J. A., Clarke, R., and Hamm, A. (1975). Cerebral hemispheric asymmetry in humans. Cortical speech zones in 100 adults and 100 infant brains. *Archives of Neurology, 32*, 239–246.

Wada, J. A., and Rasmussen, T. (1960). Intracarotid injection of sodium amytal for the lateralization of cerebral speech dominance: Experimental and clinical observations. *Journal of Neurosurgery, 17*, 266–282.

Wada, N., Hirako, S., Takenoya, F., Kageyama, H., et al. (2014). Leptin and its receptors. *Journal of Chemical Neuroanatomy, 61–62*, 191–199.

Wagenmakers, E.-J., Beek, T., Dijkhoff, L., Gronau, Q. F., et al. (2016). Registered Replication Report: Strack, Martin, & Stepper (1988). *Perspectives on Psychological Science, 11*, 917–928.

Wagner, G. C., Beuving, L. J., and Hutchinson, R. R. (1980). The effects of gonadal hormone manipulations on aggressive target-biting in mice. *Aggressive Behavior, 6*, 1–7.

Wahlstrom, K., Dretzke, B., Gordon, M., Peterson, K., et al. (2014). Examining the impact of later school start times on the health and academic performance of high school students: A multi-site study. Center for Applied Research and Educational Improvement. St. Paul, MN: University of Minnesota (https://conservancy.umn.edu/bitstream/handle/11299/162769/Impact%20of%20Later%20Start%20Time%20Final%20Report.pdf?sequence=1.pdf).

Waldrop, M. M. (2012). Brain in a box. *Nature 482*(7386), 456–458.

Walker, M. (2017). Why we sleep: Unlocking the power of sleep and dreams. New York, NY: Scribner.

Wallis, J. D. (2007). Orbitofrontal cortex and its contribution to decision-making. *Annual Review of Neuroscience, 30*, 31–56.

Walther, S., Goya-Maldonado, R., Stippich, C., Weisbrod, M., et al. (2010). A supramodal network for response inhibition. *NeuroReport, 21*, 191–195.

Wang, J., Ishikawa, M., Yang, Y., Otaka, M., et al. (2018). Cascades of homeostatic dysregulation promote incubation of cocaine craving. *Journal of Neuroscience, 38*(18), 4316–4328.

Wang, J., Wang, Y., Tong, M., Pan, H., et al. (2019). Medical cannabinoids for cancer cachexia: A systematic review and meta-analysis. *BioMed Research International, 2019*, Article 2864384.

Wang, S., Tudusciuc, O., Mamelak, A. N., Ross, I. B., et al. (2014). Neurons in the human amygdala selective for perceived emotion. *Proceedings of the National Academy of Sciences, USA, 111*(30), E3110-9.

Wang, Y. K., Zhu, W. W., Wu, M. H., Wu, Y. H., et al. (2018). Human clinical-grade parthenogenetic ESC-derived dopaminergic neurons recover locomotive defects of nonhuman primate models of Parkinson's disease. *Stem Cell Reports, 11*(1), 171–182. https://doi.org/10.1016/j.stemcr.2018.05.010

Watkins, K. E., Vargha-Khadem, F., Ashburner, J., Passingham, R. E., et al. (2002). MRI analysis of an inherited speech and language disorder: Structural brain abnormalities. *Brain, 125*(Pt. 3), 465–478.

Watson, N. V. (2001). Sex differences in throwing: Monkeys having a fling. *Trends in Cognitive Sciences, 5*, 98–99.

Watson, N. V., Freeman, L. M., and Breedlove, S. M. (2001). Neuronal size in the spinal nucleus of the bulbocavernosus: Direct modulation by androgen in rats with mosaic androgen insensitivity. *Journal of Neuroscience, 21*, 1062–1066.

Wee, R., Castrucci, A. M., Provencio, I., Gan, L., et al. (2002). Loss of photic entrainment and altered free-running circadian rhythms in math5-/- mice. *Journal of Neuroscience, 22*(23),10427–10433.

Weigl, E. (1941). On the psychology of so-called processes of abstraction. *Journal of Abnormal and Social Psychology, 36*, 3–33.

Weinberger, D. R., Aloia, M. S., Goldberg, T. E., and Berman, K. F. (1994). The frontal lobes and schizophrenia. *Journal of Neuropsychiatry and Clinical Neurosciences, 6*, 419–427.

Weinberger, L. E., Sreenivasan, S., Garrick, T., and Osran, H. (2005). The impact of surgical castration on sexual recidivism risk among sexually violent predatory offenders. *Journal of the American Academy of Psychiatry and the Law, 33*(1), 16–36.

Weinberger, N. M. (1998). Physiological memory in primary auditory cortex:

Characteristics and mechanisms. *Neurobiology of Learning and Memory, 70,* 226–251.

Weiner, K. S., and Zilles, K. (2016). The anatomical and functional specialization of the fusiform gyrus. *Neuropsychologia, 83,* 48–62.

Weiss, M. W., and Bidelman, G. M. (2015). Listening to the brainstem: Musicianship enhances intelligibility of subcortical representations for speech. *Journal of Neuroscience, 35*(4), 1687–1691.

Weissman, T. A., and Pan, Y. A. (2015). Brainbow: New resources and emerging biological applications for multicolor genetic labeling and analysis. *Genetics, 199*(2), 293–306.

Weitzman, E. D. (1981). Sleep and its disorders. *Annual Review of Neurosciences, 4,* 381–417.

Wesensten, N. J., Belenky, G., Kautz, M. A., Thorne, D. R., et al. (2002). Maintaining alertness and performance during sleep deprivation: Modafinil versus caffeine. *Psychopharmacology (Berlin), 159,* 238–247.

Wessel, J. R., and Aron, A. R. (2017). On the globality of motor suppression: Unexpected events and their influence on behavior and cognition. *Neuron, 93*(2), 259–280.

West, G. L., Drisdelle, B. L., Konishi, K., Jackson, J., et al. (2015). Habitual action video game playing is associated with caudate nucleus-dependent navigational strategies. *Proceedings of the Royal Society of London. Series B: Biological Sciences, 282*(1808), 20142952.

West, S. L., and O'Neal, K. K. (2004). Project D.A.R.E. outcome effectiveness revisited. *American Journal of Public Health, 94,* 1027–1029.

Westerberg, C. E., Mander, B. A., Florczak, S. M., Weintraub, S., et al. (2012). Concurrent impairments in sleep and memory in amnestic mild cognitive impairment. *Journal of the International Neuropsychological Society, 18,* 490–500.

Wever, R. A. (1979). Influence of physical workload on freerunning circadian rhythms of man. *Pflügers Archiv European Journal of Physiology, 381,* 119–126.

White, C. M. (2016). Mephedrone and 3,4-methylenedioxypyrovalerone (MDPV): Synthetic cathinones with serious health implications. *Journal of Clinical Pharmacology, 56*(11), 1319–1325.

White, N. M., and Milner, P. M. (1992). The psychobiology of reinforcers. *Annual Review of Psychology, 43,* 443–471.

Whitfield, K. E., Edwards, C. L., Brandon, D., and McDougald, C. (2008). Genetic and environmental influences on depressive symptoms by age and gender in African American twins. *Aging & Mental Health, 12*(2), 221–227.

Whitfield-Gabrieli, S., and Ford, J. M. (2012). Default mode network activity and connectivity in psychopathology. *Annual Review of Clinical Psychology, 8,* 49–76.

Whitlock, J. R., Heynen, A. J., Shuler, M. G., and Bear, M. F. (2006). Learning induces long-term potentiation in the hippocampus. *Science, 313,* 1093–1097.

Wichmann, S., Kirschbaum, C., Böhme, C., and Petrowski, K. (2017). Cortisol stress response in post-traumatic stress disorder, panic disorder, and major depressive disorder patients. *Psychoneuroendocrinology, 83,*135–141.

Widge, A. S., Malone, D. A., Jr., and Dougherty, D. D. (2018). Closing the loop on deep brain stimulation for treatment-resistant depression. *Frontiers in Neuroscience, 12,* 175.

Wiesel, T. N., and Hubel, D. H. (1965). Extent of recovery from the effects of visual deprivation in kittens. *Journal of Neurophysiology, 28,* 1060–1072.

Will, B., Galani, R., Kelche, C., and Rosenzweig, M. R. (2004). Recovery from brain injury in animals: Relative efficacy of environmental enrichment, physical exercise or formal training (1990–2002). *Progress in Neurobiology, 72,* 167–182.

Williams, J. H., Waiter, G. D., Gilchrist, A., Perrett, D. I., et al. (2006). Neural mechanisms of imitation and "mirror neuron" functioning in autistic spectrum disorder. *Neuropsychologia, 44,* 610–621.

Williams, N. R., and Schatzberg, A. F. (2016). NMDA antagonist treatment of depression. *Current Opinion in Neurology, 36,* 112–117.

Williams, T. J., Pepitone, M. E., Christensen, S. E., Cooke, B. M., et al. (2000). Finger-length ratios and sexual orientation. *Nature, 404,* 455–456.

Wilson, A. S., Koller, K. R., Ramaboli, M. C., Nesengani, L. T., et al. (2020). Diet and the human gut microbiome: An international review. *Digestive Diseases and Sciences, 65,* 723–740. https://doi.org/10.1007/s10620-020-06112-w

Wilson, M. L., Boesch, C., Fruth, B., Furuichi, T., et al. (2014). Lethal aggression in *Pan* is better explained by adaptive strategies than human impacts. *Nature, 513*(7518), 414–417.

Winters, B. D., Saksida, L. M., and Bussey, T. J. (2010). Implications of animal object memory research for human amnesia. *Neuropsychologia, 48*(8), 2251–2261.

Witte, A. V., Fobker, M., Gellner, R., Knecht, S., et al. (2009). Caloric restriction improves memory in elderly humans. *Proceedings of the National Academy of Sciences, USA, 106*(4), 1255–1260.

Wolf, M. E. (2016). Synaptic mechanisms underlying persistent cocaine craving. *Nature Reviews Neuroscience, 17*(6), 351–365.

Wolf, S. A., Boddeke, H. W., and Kettenmann, H. (2017). Microglia in physiology and disease. *Annual Review of Physiology, 79,* 619–643.

Wolf, S. S., Jones, D. W., Knable, M. B., Gorey, J. G., et al. (1996). Tourette syndrome: Prediction of phenotypic variation in monozygotic twins by caudate nucleus D2 receptor binding. *Science, 273,* 1225–1227.

Wolfe, J. M. (1994). Guided search 2.0: A revised model of visual search. *Psychonomic Bulletin & Review, 1,* 202–238.

Wolfe, J. M., Horowitz, T. S., and Kenner, N. M. (2005). Cognitive psychology: Rare items often missed in visual searches. *Nature, 435,* 439–440.

Wollan, M. (2015, April 10). How to beat a polygraph test. *New York Times Magazine,* p. MM25 (www.nytimes.com/2015/04/12/magazine/how-to-beat-a-polygraph-test.html).

Womelsdorf, T., Anton-Erxleben, K., and Treue, S. (2008). Receptive field shift and shrinkage in macaque middle temporal area through attentional gain modulation. *Journal of Neuroscience, 28,* 8934–8944.

Wood, N., and Cowan, N. (1995). The cocktail party phenomenon revisited: How frequent are attention shifts to one's name in an irrelevant auditory channel? *Journal of Experimental Psychology. Learning, Memory, and Cognition, 21,* 255–260.

Woolf, C. J., and Salter, M. W. (2000). Neuronal plasticity: Increasing the gain in pain. *Science, 288,* 1765–1769.

World Health Organization. (2001). *The world health report.* Geneva, Switzerland: World Health Organization.

Wrangham, R. W. (2018). Two types of aggression in human evolution. *Proceedings of the National Academy of Sciences, USA, 115*(2), 245–253.

Wren, A. M., Seal, L. J., Cohen, M. A., Brynes, A. E., et al. (2001). Ghrelin enhances appetite and increases food intake in humans. *Journal of Clinical Endocrinology and Metabolism, 86,* 5992–5995.

Wren, A. M., Small, C. J., Ward, H. L., Murphy, K. G., et al. (2000). The novel hypothalamic peptide ghrelin stimulates food intake and growth hormone secretion. *Endocrinology, 141,* 4325–4328.

Wu, Q., Qi, C., Long, J., Liao, Y., et al. (2018). Metabolites alterations in the medial prefrontal cortex of methamphetamine users in abstinence: A ^{1}H MRS study. *Frontiers in Psychiatry, 9,* 478.

Wuethrich, B. (2000). Learning the world's languages—before they vanish. *Science, 288,* 1156–1159.

Wunderink, L. (2019). Personalizing antipsychotic treatment: Evidence and thoughts on individualized tailoring of antipsychotic dosage in the treatment of psychotic disorders. *Therapeutic Advances in Psychopharmacology, 9,* 1–14.

Wurtz, R. H., Goldberg, M. E., and Robinson, D. L. (1982). Brain mechanisms of visual attention. *Scientific American, 246*(6), 124–135.

X

Xerri, C., Stern, J. M., and Merzenich, M. M. (1994). Alterations of the cortical representation of the rat ventrum induced by nursing behavior. *Journal of Neuroscience, 14,* 1710–1721.

Xie, L., Kang, H., Xu, Q., Chen, M. J., et al. (2013). Sleep drives metabolite clearance from the adult brain. *Science, 342,* 373–377.

Xu, J., Bartolome, C. L., Low, C. S., Yi, X., et al. (2018). Genetic identification of leptin neural circuits in energy and glucose homeostases. *Nature, 556*(7702), 505–509.

Y

Yamaguchi, Y., and Miura, M. (2015). Programmed cell death in neurodevelopment. *Developmental Cell, 32*(4), 478–490.

Yamazaki, S., Numano, R., Abe, M., Hida, A., et al. (2000). Resetting central and peripheral circadian oscillators in transgenic rats. *Science, 288,* 682–685.

Yang, T. T., Gallen, C. C., Ramachandran, V. S., Cobb, S., et al. (1994). Noninvasive detection of cerebral plasticity in adult human somatosensory cortex. *NeuroReport, 5,* 701–704.

Yang, Y., Choi, P. P., Smith, W. W., Xu, W., et al. (2017). Exendin-4 reduces food intake via the P13K/AKT pathway in the hypothalamus. *Scientific Reports, 7,* 6936.

Yang, Y., Narr, K. L., Baker, L. A., Joshi, S. H., et al. (2015). Frontal and striatal alterations associated with psychopathic traits in adolescents. *Psychiatry Research, 231*(3), 333–340.

Ycaza Herrera, A., and Mather, M. (2015). Actions and interactions of estradiol and glucocorticoids in cognition and the brain: Implications for aging women. *Neuroscience & Biobehavioral Reviews, 55,* 36–52.

Yin, J., Barr, A. M., Ramos-Miguel, A., and Procyshyn, R. M. (2017). Antipsychotic induced dopamine supersensitivity psychosis: A comprehensive review. *Current Neuropharmacology, 15*(1), 174–183.

Yoon, Y. J., Steele, C. R., and Puria, S. (2011). Feed-forward and feed-backward amplification model from cochlear cytoarchitecture: An interspecies comparison. *Biophysical Journal, 100*(1), 1–10.

Young, K. D., Erickson, K., Nugent, A. C., Fromm, S. J., et al. (2012). Functional anatomy of autobiographical memory recall deficits in depression. *Psychological Medicine, 42,* 345–357.

Yu, F., Han, W., Zhan, G., Li, S., et al. (2019). Abnormal gut microbiota composition contributes to the development of type 2 diabetes mellitus in db/db mice. *Aging (Albany, NY), 11*(22), 10454–10467.

Yu, Y. J., Atwal, J. K., Zhang, Y., Tong, R. K., et al. (2015). Therapeutic bispecific antibodies cross the blood-brain barrier in nonhuman primates. *Science Translational Medicine, 6,* 261ra154.

Yuan, J., Gong, H., Li, A., Li, X., et al. (2015). Visible rodent brain-wide networks at single-neuron resolution. *Frontiers in Neuroanatomy, 9,* 70.

Yuan, M., Cross, S. J., Loughlin, S. E., and Leslie, F. M. (2015). Nicotine and the adolescent brain. *Journal of Physiology, 593*(16), 3397–3412.

Yuan, P., and Raz, N. (2014). Prefrontal cortex and executive functions in healthy adults: A meta-analysis of structural neuroimaging studies. *Neuroscience & Biobehavioral Reviews, 42,* 180–192.

Z

Zabeau, L., Wauman, J., Dam, J., Van Lint, S., et al. (2019). A novel leptin receptor antagonist uncouples leptin's metabolic and immune functions. *Cellular and Molecular Life Sciences, 76*(6), 1201–1214.

Zahr, N. M., and Pfefferbaum, A. (2017). Alcohol's effects on the brain: Neuroimaging results in humans and animal models. *Alcohol Research, 38*(2), 183–206.

Zaidel, E. (1976). Auditory vocabulary of the right hemisphere following brain bisection or hemidecortication. *Cortex, 12,* 191–211.

Zalocusky, K. A., Ramakrishnan, C., Lerner, T. N., Davidson, T. J., et al. (2016). Nucleus accumbens D2R cells signal prior outcomes and control risky decision-making. *Nature, 531*(7596), 642–646.

Zatorre, R. J., Evans, A. C., and Meyer, E. (1994). Neural mechanisms underlying melodic perception and memory for pitch. *Journal of Neuroscience, 14,* 1908–1919.

Zawilska, J. B. (2014). Mephedrone and other cathinones. *Current Opinion in Psychiatry, 27*(4), 256–262.

Zehra, A., Burns, J., Liu, C. K., Manza, P., et al. (2018). Cannabis addiction and the brain: A review. *Journal of Neuroimmune Pharmacology, 13*(4), 438–452.

Zeki, S. (2015). Area V5: A microcosm of the visual brain. *Frontiers in Integrative Neuroscience, 9,* 21.

Zeman, A. (2002). *Consciousness: A user's guide.* New Haven, CT: Yale University Press.

Zendel, B. R., and Alain, C. (2009). Concurrent sound segregation is enhanced in musicians. *Journal of Cognitive Neuroscience, 21,* 1488–1498.

Zendel, B. R., Lagrois, M. É., Robitaille, N., and Peretz, I. (2015). Attending to pitch information inhibits processing of pitch information: The curious case of amusia. *Journal of Neuroscience, 35,* 3815–3824.

Zenner, H. P., Delb, W., Kröner-Herwig, B., Jäger, B., et al. (2017). A multidisciplinary systematic review of the treatment for chronic idiopathic tinnitus. *European Archives of Oto-Rhino-Laryngology, 274*(5), 2079–2091.

Zhang, C. L., Zou, Y., He, W., Gage, F. H., et al. (2008). A role for adult TLX-positive neural stem cells in learning and behaviour. *Nature, 451,* 1004–1007.

Zhang, F., Kurokawa, K., Lassoued, A., Crowell, J. A., et al. (2019). Cone photoreceptor classification in the living human eye from photostimulation-induced phase dynamics. *Proceedings of the National Academy of Sciences, USA, 116*(16), 7951–7956. https://doi.org/10.1073/pnas.1816360116

Zhang, T. Y., and Meaney, M. J. (2010). Epigenetics and the environmental regulation of the genome and its function. *Annual Review of Psychology, 61,* C1–C3.

Zhang, Y., Proenca, R., Maffei, M., Barone, M., et al. (1994). Positional cloning of the mouse *obese* gene and its human homologue. *Nature, 372,* 425–432.

Zhang, Z., Mocanu, V., Cai, C., Dang, J., et al. (2019). Impact of fecal microbiota transplantation on obesity and metabolic syndrome: A systematic review. *Nutrients, 11*(10), 2291.

Zhao, G. Q., Zhang, Y., Hoon, M. A., Chandrashekar, J., et al. (2003). The receptors for mammalian sweet and umami taste. *Cell, 115,* 255–266.

Zhao, Y., Tudorascu, D. L., Lopez, O. L., Cohen, A. D., et al. (2018). Amyloid β deposition and suspected non-Alzheimer pathophysiology and cognitive decline patterns for 12 years in oldest old participants without dementia. *JAMA Neurology, 75*(1), 88–96.

Zhaoping, L. (2016). From the optic tectum to the primary visual cortex: Migration through evolution of the saliency map for exogenous attentional guidance. *Current Opinion in Neurobiology, 40,* 94–102.

Zheng, J., Shen, W., He, D. Z., Long, K. B., et al. (2000). Prestin is the motor protein of cochlear outer hair cells. *Nature, 405,* 149–155.

Zieglgänsberger, W. (2019). Substance P and pain chronicity. *Cell and Tissue Research, 375*(1), 227–241.

Zihl, J., and Heywood, C. A. (2015). The contribution of LM to the neuroscience of movement vision. *Frontiers in Integrative Neuroscience, 9,* 6. https://doi.org/10.3389/fnint.2015.00006

Zimmer, C. (2004). *The soul made flesh: The discovery of the brain—and how it changed the world.* New York, NY: Basic Books.

Zimmerman, A., Bai, L., and Ginty, D. D. (2014). The gentle touch receptors of mammalian skin. *Science, 346*(6212), 950–954.

Zimmerman, C. A., Huey, E. L., Ahn, J. S., Beutler, L. R., et al. (2019). A gut-to-brain signal of fluid osmolarity controls thirst satiation. *Nature, 568*(7750), 98–102.

Zimmerman, C. A., Leib, D. E., and Knight, Z. A. (2017). Neural circuits underlying thirst and fluid homeostasis. *Nature Reviews Neuroscience, 18*(8), 459–469.

Zimmerman, C. A., Lin, Y. C., Leib, D. E., Guo, L., et al. (2016). Thirst neurons anticipate the homeostatic consequences of eating and drinking. *Nature, 537*(7622), 680–684.

Zocchi, D., Wennemuth, G., and Oka, Y. (2017). The cellular mechanism for water detection in the mammalian taste system. *Nature Neuroscience, 20*(7), 927–933.

Zola-Morgan, S., Squire, L. R., and Ramus, S. J. (1994). Severity of memory impairment in monkeys as a function of locus and extent of damage within the medial temporal lobe memory system. *Hippocampus, 4*, 483–495.

Zonooz, B., Arani, E., Körding, K. P., Aalbers, P. A. T. R., et al. (2019). Spectral weighting underlies perceived sound elevation. *Scientific Reports, 9*(1), 1642.

Zorumski, C. F., Izumi, Y., and Mennerick, S. (2016). Ketamine: NMDA receptors and beyond. *Journal of Neuroscience, 36*(44), 11158–11164.

Zou, M., Jie, Z., Cui, B., Wang, H., et al. (2020). Fecal microbiota transplantation results in bacterial strain displacement in patients with inflammatory bowel diseases. *FEBS Open Bio, 10*(1), 41–55.

Zucker, I. (1976). Light, behavior, and biologic rhythms. *Hospital Practice, 11*, 83–91.

Index

Somatic interventions, 47–48

Somatic nervous system, 26–28, 33

Somatogravic illusion, 196

Somatosensory cortex. *See* Primary somatosensory cortex

Somatosensory system
cortical maps and plasticity in processing, 153–154
defined, 148
determining the location of a stimulus, 148
information processing by the CNS, 150–152
pain perception, 154–160
receptive fields of sensory neurons, 148, *149*
See also Touch

Somatotropic hormone. *See* Growth hormone

Somatotropin. *See* Growth hormone

Somnambulism, 342–343

Songbirds, 491–492

Sound
hearing and, 178–190
properties of, 179
transduction of, 179, 180–184
See also Auditory system

Sound localization, 187–188, 189

Sound shadow, 187, *188*

Sour taste, 197, 198, 199

South American monkeys, 236

Southern, Edward, A–6

Southern blots, A–4, A–7

Spatial attention, 445

Spatial cognition, 469, 471

Spatial cuing, 439

Spatial learning, 416, *417*

Spatial processing, 474

Spatial resolution, 443

Spatial summation, 69

Spatial-frequency model of visual analysis, 227–228

Special K, 110, *111*
See also Ketamine

Spectral filtering, 188

Spectrally opponent cells, 236–237

Speech processing
primary auditory cortex, 185, 189
right-ear advantage, 470
See also Language behavior

Speechless (film), *480*

Sperm, 263

Sperry, Roger, 468

Spike, 60–61
See also Action potential

Spinal accessory nerve (cranial nerve XI), 26–27

Spinal block, *160*

Spinal cord
central nervous system and, 26
development, 32, *33*, 122, *123*
injuries to, *10*, 167–168
lordosis circuit, 266, *267*
mediation of genital reflexes, 266
motor neurons, 164
muscle reflexes, 166
neuromuscular system and movements, 162
neurotransmitter pathways, 90
pain pathways, *155*, 157
pyramidal and extrapyramidal systems, 166, 167
sexual dimorphism in mammals, 281–282
somatosensory projections, 150, *151*, *152*
spinal nerves, 27–28

Spinal cord reflexes, 55–56, 74–75
See also Reflexes

Spinal motor neurons, reaction-time circuit, 440

Spinal nerves, 27–28, *33*

Spinal nucleus of the bulbocavernosus (SNB), 281–282

Spinothalamic system, 157

Split-brain individuals, 468–470, 475

Spotted hyenas, 274

Squirrel monkeys, 490

SRY gene, 272

SSRIs. *See* Selective serotonin reuptake inhibitors

Stage 1 sleep, 326, *327*

Stage 2 sleep, 326, *327*

Stage 3 sleep (SWS sleep)
biological functions of, 334–335, 336
changes in the elderly, 331–332
definition and description of, 326, *327*
depression and, 395
dreaming and, 328, 329
in mammals, 329–330
release of growth hormone during, 327–328, 332, 335
sleep disorders associated with, 342–343
sleep recovery and, 333

Stage 4 sleep, 326

Standard condition (SC), 422

Stapedius, 180, *181*

Stapes, 180, *181*

Stem cells, 125–126

Stereocilia, *181*, 183

Steroid hormones
chemical structure, 249
defined, 249
examples of, *249*
gonadal sources and regulation of reproductive behavior, 258–260, 264, 271
interactions among, 260
mechanisms of action, 250
regulation of, *259*, 260
See also Androgens; Estrogens; Gonadal hormones

Stimulants
alcohol as, 107–108
amphetamine, 107
cocaine, 106–107
definition and description of, 105–106
nicotine, 106
treatment of ADHD, 452

Stimulation pain relief, 159, 160

Stimuli
defined, 144
determining the location of, 148
receptor cells, 144
sensory processing, 147–148 (*see also* Sensory processing)
sensory systems, *144*

Stimulus cuing, 438

STM. *See* Short-term memory

Stomach, ghrelin and appetite control, 306, 307, 308

Strain Black6 mice, *136*

Strattera, 452

Strep throat, 402

Streptomycin, 192

Stress
defined, 368
effect on health and the immune system, 371, 372–373
epigenetic effects of maternal care and, 3, 11–12, 136–137
individual differences in the stress response, 370–371
long-term consequences of childhood bullying, 372
pain relief and, 160
post-traumatic stress disorder, 399–401
schizophrenia, 382–384

stages of the stress response, 368–370
strategies to reduce, 373

Stress hormone
depression and, 392
post-traumatic stress disorder and, 399–401

Stress immunization, 370–371

Stress response
individual differences in, 370–371
stages in, 368–370

Stretch reflex, 165, 166

Striate cortex. *See* Primary visual cortex

Striate muscle, 163

Striatum, 91, *417*

Stroke
effects on attention, 435
effects on the motor system, 170
meningioma and, 43
prevalence, *10*
recovery of function, 494–495, 496
simulated to reveal cerebral hemisphere specializations, 473
See also Brain lesions

Stroop Test of Color-Word Interference, *459*

Stuttering, 488

Subarachnoid space, 38, *39*

Subcoeruleus, *338*

Subcutaneous injections, *97*

Subfornical organ, *298*, 299

Substance abuse
economic impact of, 116
as a global social problem, 112
medical interventions, 116
models of, 113–115
overdose deaths, *103*
prevalence, *10*, 113
substance use disorder, 112–113

Substance P, 92, 157

Substance use disorder, 112–113

Substantia nigra
basal ganglia and, 172
cannabinoid receptors, *104*, 105
defined, 36, 91, 173
mesostriatal pathway, *90*, 91
Parkinson's disease, 172–173

Subthalamic nucleus, 172

Subtractive analysis, 46

Sudden infant death syndrome (SIDS), 344